Atlas of UROLOGIC SURGERY

SECOND EDITION

FRANK HINMAN, JR., MD,
FACS, FAAP, FRCS ENG (HON)

Clinical Professor of Urology
Department of Urology
University of California
School of Medicine
San Francisco, California

Illustrated by

PAUL H. STEMPEN, MA, CMI

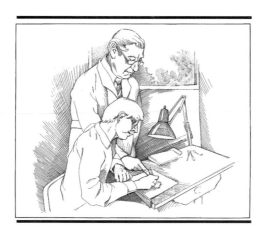

W.B. SAUNDERS COMPANY
A Division of Harcourt Brace & Company
Philadelphia   •   London   •   Toronto   •   Montreal   •   Sydney   •   Tokyo

W.B. SAUNDERS COMPANY
A Division of Harcourt Brace & Company

The Curtis Center
Independence Square West
Philadelphia, Pennsylvania 19106

Library of Congress Cataloging-in-Publication Data

Hinman, Frank
Atlas of urologic surgery / Frank Hinman, Jr.; illustrated by Paul H. Stempen.—
2nd ed.

p.   cm.

Includes bibliographical references and index.

ISBN 0–7216–6404–0

1. Genitourinary organs—Surgery—Atlases.   I. Title.
   [DNLM: 1. Urogenital System—surgery—atlases. WJ 17 H663a 1998]

RD571.H55 1998   617.4′6—dc21

DNLM/DLC   96–38015

Certain illustrations from this book have appeared previously in the *Atlas of Pediatric Urologic Surgery* and the *Atlas of UroSurgical Anatomy* by Frank Hinman, Jr., published by W.B. Saunders Company, 1994, and 1993.

ATLAS OF UROLOGIC SURGERY   ISBN 0-7216-6404-0

Printed in the United States of America.

Last digit is the print number: 9   8   7   6   5   4   3   2   1

To the well over 100 residents of the University of California and Children's Hospitals in San Francisco, who, by their inquiring minds and their manual help, have allowed me to develop my interests as a urologic surgeon.

To my teachers in Cincinnati: Mont Reid, my professor of surgery, and Rollo Hanlon, my counselor in residency

To my father, Frank Hinman, who advised, directed, and taught me the craft of urologic surgery.

Commentators

Paul Abrams, MD, FRCS
Consultant Urologist, Bristol Urological Institute, Bristol,
England
Colposuspension

Rolf Ackerman, MD
Professor of Urology, Department of Urology, Heinrich
Heine University, Dusseldorf, Germany
Repair of Pleural Tear

Rodney A. Appell, MD, FACS
Head, Section of Voiding Dysfunction and Female
Urology, The Cleveland Clinic Foundation, Cleveland,
OH
Insertion of Artificial Sphincter

Yoshio Aso, MD, PhD, FACS
Professor Emeritus, The University of Tokyo; Director,
Fujieda Municipal General Hospital, Fujieda, Japan
Gibson Incision

Thomas P. Ball, Jr., MD
Professor of Urology, University of Texas Health Science
Center at San Antonio, San Antonio, TX
Anterior Transverse (Chevron) Incision

Lynn H. W. Banowsky, MD, FACS
Clinical Professor of Urology, University of Texas Health
Science Center at San Antonio, San Antonio, TX
Living Donor Nephrectomy

John M. Barry, MD
Chairman, Division of Urology and Renal
Transplantation, Oregon Health Sciences University,
Portland, OR
Ureteroneocystostomy

Francis F. Bartone, MD, FACS, FAAP
Associate, Geisinger Clinic, Danville, PA
Suture Techniques

Laurence S. Baskin, MD
Assistant Professor of Urology and Pediatrics, University
of California, San Francisco, San Francisco, CA
Orchiopexy for the Nonpalpable Testis

Stuart B. Bauer, MD
Senior Associate in Surgery (Urology), The Children's
Hospital; Associate Professor of Surgery (Urology),
Harvard Medical School, Boston, MA
Circumcision

Mark F. Bellinger, MD
Professor, Department of Surgery, Division of Urology,
University of Pittsburgh; Chief, Pediatric Urologic
Surgery, Children's Hospital, Pittsburgh, PA
Ureteroneocystostomy

Abdelatif Benchekroun, MD
Professor of Urology, Head of Urology Department,
Avicenne Hospital, Rabat, Morocco
Ileal Hydraulic Valve Conduit

Mitchell C. Benson, MD, FACS
Professor of Urology, Columbia University College of
Physicians and Surgeons; Director, Urologic Oncology,
Columbia-Presbyterian Medical Center, New York, NY
Sigmoidocystoplasty

Ralph C. Benson, Jr., MD, FACS
Co-Director, The Center for Urological Treatment and
Research, Nashville, TN
Insertion of Inflatable Prosthesis

Jerry G. Blaivas, MD, FACS
Clinical Professor of Urology, Cornell University Medical
College, New York, NY
Urethrovaginal Fistula Repair

**John P. Blandy, CBE, DM, Mch, FRCS, FACS,
FRCSI (Hon)**
Emeritus Professor, The Royal London Hospital, London,
England
Operations for Priapism

David A. Bloom, MD
Professor of Urology, University of Michigan, Ann
Arbor, MI
Laparoscopic Orchiectomy

Guy A. Bogaert, MD
Pediatric Urologist, Heilkunde, Urologie Kinderurologie,
UZ Gasthuisberg, Leuven, Belgium
Laparoscopic Techniques for Impalpable Testes

William W. Bohnert, MD, AB, FACS
Section Chief—Urology, St. Joseph's Hospital and
Medical Center, Phoenix, AZ
Ureterolithotomy

William H. Boyce, MD, DSc, FACS
Professor of Surgery and Urology Emeritus, Bowman
Gray School of Medicine, Wake Forest University,
Winston-Salem, NC
Nephrolithotomy

Peter N. Bretan, Jr., MD
Associate Professor of Surgery and Urology, University of
California, San Francisco School of Medicine, San
Francisco, CA
Cadaver Donor Nephrectomy

v

Roberto Rocha Brito, MD
Urologist-in-Chief, Hospital Vera Cruz and Urological
Clinic, Campinas, SP, Brazil
Foley Muscle-Splitting Incision

Ronald B. Brown, FRCS, FRACS, FACS
Retired Head of Unit, Alfred Hospital, Melbourne,
Australia
Caliceal Diverticulectomy and Excision of Renal Cyst

Andrew W. Bruce, MD, FRCS, FRCS(C)
Emeritus Professor of Urology, University of Toronto,
Ontario, Canada
Repair of Incisional Hernia

Mark W. Burns, III, MD, FAAP, FACS
Clinical Associate Professor, University of Washington
School of Medicine, Seattle, WA
Gastrocystoplasty

Maurice Camey, MD
Professor of Urology (Retired), Faculty Paris Ouest,
Paris, France
Ileal Bladder Substitution

C. Eugene Carlton, Jr., MD, FACS
Professor of Urology, Baylor College of Medicine,
Houston, TX
Perineal Prostatectomy

Peter R. Carroll, MD
Professor of Urology and Chairman of the Department,
University of California, San Francisco, San Francisco,
CA
Nephroureterectomy

Culley C. Carson, III, MD, FACS
Professor and Chief of Urology, University of North
Carolina, Chapel Hill, NC
Simple Nephrectomy

Patrick C. Cartwright, MD, FACS, FAAP
Assistant Professor of Surgery and Pediatrics, University
of Utah, Primary Children's Medical Center, Salt Lake
City, UT
Autoaugmentation

Alexander S. Cass, MD, MBBS, FRCS, FACS
Staff Urologist, Hennepin County Medical Center,
Minneapolis, MN
Partial Penectomy

Paramjit S. Chandhoke, MD, PhD
Assistant Professor of Surgery (Urology) and Medicine
(Renal Diseases), University of Colorado Health Sciences
Center, Denver, CO
*Laparoscopic Modified Retroperitoneal Lymph Node
Dissection*

Warren H. Chapman, BS (Chem Eng), MD
Professor Emeritus of Urology, University of Washington,
Seattle, WA
Correction of Hydrocele

Bernard Churchill, MD, FRCS(C), FAAP
Professor of Surgery and Director, Clark Morrison
Children's Urological Center, University of California at
Los Angeles, Los Angeles, CA
Ureterocystoplasty

Philip B. Clark, MD, MChir, FRCS
The General Infirmary, Leeds, England
Perineal Urethrostomy

Ralph V. Clayman, MD, FACS
Professor of Urologic Surgery and Radiology, Washington
University School of Medicine, St. Louis, MO
Basic Laparoscopy

Lance J. Coetzee, MD, FCS(SA), MMed(Uro)
Uro-Oncology Fellow/Instructor in Urology, Duke
University Medical Center, Durham, NC
Modified Pelvic Lymph Node Dissection

Marc S. Cohen, MD, FACS
Associate Professor of Surgery/Urology, University of
Florida College of Medicine, Gainesville, FL
Renal Displacement and Autotransplantation

Joseph N. Corriere, Jr., MD
Professor of Surgery (Urology), University of Texas
Medical School at Houston, Houston, TX
Repair of Genital Injuries

E. David Crawford, MD
Professor and Chairman, Division of Urology, University
of Colorado Health Sciences Center, Denver, CO
Total Penectomy

William J. Cromie, MD, MBA, FACS, FAAP
Professor of Surgery and Pediatrics, University of
Chicago, Chicago, IL
Surgery for the Horseshoe Kidney

Jean B. deKernion, MD
Professor of Surgery/Urology; Chief, Division of Urology,
University of California, Los Angeles Medical Center, Los
Angeles, CA
Pelvic Lymphadenectomy

**Charles J. Devine, Jr., MD, FAAP, FASPRS
(Hon), DSc (Hon)**
Professor Emeritus, Eastern Virginia Medical School,
Norfolk, VA
*Basic Instructions for Hypospadias Repair; Perimeatal-
Based Tube Repair (Mustardé)*

Roger R. Dmochowski, MD, FACS
Assistant Professor of Urology, University of Tennessee,
Memphis, TN
Cystostomy

John P. Donohue, MD, FACS
Distinguished Professor Emeritus, Indiana University
Medical Center, Indianapolis, IN
Retroperitoneal Lymph Node Dissection

Michael J. Droller, MD
Professor and Chairman, Department of Urology, The Mount Sinai School of Medicine, New York, NY
Psoas Hitch Procedure

John W. Duckett, Jr., MD (deceased)
Professor of Urology in Surgery, University of Pennsylvania School of Medicine; Director, Pediatric Urology, Children's Hospital of Philadelphia, Philadelphia, PA
Onlay Preputial Island Flap

Mitchell Edson, MD, FACS
Clinical Professor of Surgery, Uniformed Services University of the Health Sciences, Bethesda, MD
Repair of Renal Injuries

Jack S. Elder, MD, FACS, FAAP
Professor of Urology and Pediatrics, Case Western Reserve University School of Medicine; Director of Pediatric Urology, Rainbow Babies and Children's Hospital, Cleveland, OH
Excision of Utricular Cyst

Roger C. L. Feneley, MD, MA, MChir, FRCS
Consultant Urologist, Southmead Hospital, Bristol, England
Laparoscopic Colposuspension; Closure of Female Vesical Neck

Robert C. Flanigan, MD, FACS
Professor and Chairman, Department of Urology, Loyola University Medical Center, Maywood, IL
Seminal Vesiculectomy

Stuart M. Flechner, MD, FACS
Section of Renal Transplantation, Department of Urology, The Cleveland Clinic Foundation, Cleveland, OH
Renal Transplant Recipient

Eric W. Fonkalsrud, MD, FACS
Professor and Chief of Pediatric Surgery, University of California, Los Angeles, School of Medicine, Los Angeles, CA
Inguinal Hernia Repair

René Frontera, MD
Assistant Professor of Urology, Wayne State University, Detroit, MI
Strictures of the Penile Urethra

William L. Furlow, MD, FACS
Emeritus Professor of Urology, Mayo Medical School, Mayo Clinic, Rochester, MN
Insertion of Inflatable Prosthesis

John P. Gearhart, MD, FAAP, FACS
Director of Pediatric Urology, Johns Hopkins Hospital, Baltimore, MD
Vaginal Reconstruction; Urethrovaginal Fistula Repair

Louis G. Gecelter, MB, Bch, FRCS, FACS
Senior Lecturer, Witwatersrand Medical School, Johannesburg, South Africa
Closure of Rectourethral Fistula; Excision of Urachus

Mohamed A. Ghoneim, MD
Professor of Urology; Director, Urology and Nephrology Center, Mansoura, Egypt
Ureterosigmoidostomy

James F. Glenn, BA, MD, FRCS Eng (Hon)
Professor of Surgery, University of Kentucky College of Medicine, Lexington, KY
Closure of Vesicosigmoid Fistula; Preparation and Approaches for Adrenal Excision

Marc Goldstein, MD, FACS
Professor of Urology, Cornell University Medical College; Director, Center for Male Reproductive Medicine and Microsurgery, The Department of Urology, The New York Hospital–Cornell Medical Center, New York, NY
Simple Orchiectomy

Ricardo Gonzalez, MD, FAAP
Chief of Pediatric Urology, Children's Hospital of Michigan, Detroit, MI
Operations for Ureteral Duplication

Sam D. Graham, MD
Professor of Surgery (Urology), Emory University School of Medicine, Atlanta, GA
Closure of Rectourethral Fistula

Peter A. Harbison, MB, BS, FRCS, FRACS
Senior Visiting Urologist (Retired), Queen Elizabeth Hospital, North Adelaide, Queensland, South Australia
Subcostal Incision

W. Hardy Hendren, III, MD, FACS, FRCS(I) Hon
Chief of Surgery, Children's Hospital; Robert E. Gross Professor of Surgery, Harvard Medical School; Visiting Surgeon, Massachusetts General Hospital, Boston, MA
Ureteroneocystostomy with Tailoring

Terry W. Hensle, MD
Professor of Urology; Director of Pediatric Urology, Columbia University College of Physicians and Surgeons, New York, NY
Vascular Access; Pyeloureteroplasty

Norman B. Hodgson, MD
Clinical Professor of Urology, Medical College of Wisconsin, Milwaukee, WI
Double-Faced Transverse Island Flap

John P. Hopewell, MB, BS, FRCS
Honorary Consulting Surgeon, Royal Free Hospital Department of Surgery, London, England
Midline Transperitoneal Incision

Stuart S. Howards, MD, FACS
Professor of Urology, University of Virginia, Charlottesville, VA
Vasovasostomy and Vasoepididymostomy

Günter Janetschek, MD
Professor of Urology, Department of Urology, University
of Innsbruck, Innsbruck, Austria
Laparoscopic Nephrectomy

Gerald H. Jordan, MD, FACS
Professor of Urology, Eastern Virginia Medical School,
Norfolk, VA
*Plastic Surgical Techniques; Procedures for Peyronie's
Disease; Strictures of the Fossa Navicularis*

Klaus-Peter Jünemann, MD
Associate Professor of Urology, Department of Urology,
Klinikum Mannheim of the University of Heidelberg,
Mannheim, Germany
Sigmoid Conduit

George W. Kaplan, MD, MS, FAAP, FACS
Clinical Professor of Urology and Pediatrics, Chief of
Pediatric Urology, University of California, San Diego,
San Diego, CA
Ventral Tube Repair

Louis R. Kavoussi, MD
Associate Professor in Urologic Surgery, Johns Hopkins
University, Baltimore, MD
Laparoscopic Ileal Conduit

**Keith W. Kaye, MB, BCh, BSc (Hon), FCS(SA),
FRCS(Edin), FRACS**
Chair of Urology, Director of Urological Research
Centre, University of Western Australia, Nedlands,
Western Australia
Laparoscopic Varicocele Ligation

Panayotis P. Kelalis, MD
Professor of Urology, Mayo Medical School, Rochester
MN; Mayo Clinic, Jacksonville, FL
Ileal Conduit

**Nils G. Kock, MD, MD (Hon), FRCS Eng (Hon),
FACS (Hon), PhD**
Professor of Surgery (Emeritus), Department of Surgery,
University of Göteborg, Göteborg, Sweden
Ileal Reservoir

Barry A. Kogan, MD
Professor and Chief, Division of Urology, The Albany
Medical College, Albany, NY
Meatoplasty and Glanuloplasty (MAGPI)

Warren W. Koontz, Jr., MD, FACS
Professor Emeritus (Urology), Medical College of
Virginia; Executive Director, Virginia Board of Medicine,
Richmond, VA
Subcapsular Nephrectomy

Ken Koshiba, MD, FACS
Professor and Chairman, Department of Urology,
Kitasato University School of Medicine; President,
Kitasato Institute Medical Center Hospital, Sagamihara,
Japan
Ureterolithotomy

R. Lawrence Kroovand, MD, FAAP
Professor of Surgery (Pediatric Urology) and Pediatrics;
Head, Section on Pediatric, Adolescent, and
Reconstructive Urology, Wake Forest University,
Winston-Salem, NC
Basic Instructions for Hypospadias Repair

Kenneth A. Kropp, MD, FACS
Professor of Urology, Medical College of Ohio,
Toledo, OH
Intravesical Urethral Lengthening

William H. Lakey, BSc, MD, FRCS(C)
Emeritus Professor of Surgery (Urology), University of
Alberta, Edmonton, Alberta, Canada
Nephrostomy and Ureterostomy

Gary E. Leach, MD
Associate Clinical Professor of Urology, University of
California, Los Angeles; Director, Tower Urology
Institute for Incontinence, Los Angeles, CA
Vesicovaginal Fistula Repair

Guy W. Leadbetter, Jr., MD, AB
Professor of Surgery and Chief of Urology (Emeritus),
University of Vermont Medical School, Medical Center
Hospital of Vermont, Burlington, VT
Trigonal Tubularization

Joe Y. Lee, MD
Staff Urologist, Hennepin County Medical Center,
Minneapolis, MN
Partial Penectomy

Laurence A. Levine, MD
Associate Professor of Urology, Rush Medical College,
Rush-Presbyterian-St Luke's Medical Center, Chicago, IL
Construction of Penis

John A. Libertino, MD, FACS
Chairman of Urology and Chief of Surgery, Lahey-
Hitchcock Clinic Medical Center, Burlington, MA
*Ileal Ureteral Replacement; Lateral Approach to the
Adrenal Gland*

R. Wyndham Lloyd-Davies, MB, MS, FRCS
Consulting Urologist, St. Thomas's Hospital, London,
England
Midline Lower Abdominal Extraperitoneal Incision

Jorge L. Lockhart, MD
Professor of Surgery, University of South Florida, College
of Medicine, Tampa, FL
Ileocecal Reservoir

Tom F. Lue, MD, FACS
Professor of Urology, University of California, San
Francisco, San Francisco, CA
Penile Arterial Revascularization

**John S. P. Lumley, MS, FRCS, FGA, FMAA
(Hon), PPICS**
Professor of Vascular Surgery, St. Bartholomew's
Hospital, London, England
Microsurgical Techniques

J. Warwick F. Macky, OBE, MB, MS, FRCS(Eng), FRACS
Consultant Urologist, Auckland Hospital, Auckland, New Zealand
Paramedian Incision

Michael Marberger, MD
Professor and Chairman, Department of Urology, University of Vienna, Vienna, Austria
Extracorporeal Renal Surgery

Victor F. Marshall, MD, ScD
Emeritus Professor of Urology at Cornell University Medical College, New York, NY, and University of Virginia, Charlottesville, VA
Cystourethropexy

Donald C. Martin, MD
Professor of Surgery/Urology (Emeritus), University of California, Irvine, Irvine, CA
Vascular Access

Etienne Mazeman, MD
Professor and Chairman of Department of Urology, University of Lille, Lille, France
Female Urethral Diverticulectomy

Jack W. McAninch, MS, MD, FACS
Professor of Urology, University of California, San Francisco; Chief of Urology, San Francisco General Hospital, San Francisco, CA
General Considerations for Urethral Strictures; Strictures of the Bulbar Urethra

R. Dale McClure, MD, FRCS(C)
Director of Microsurgery and Infertility, Virginia Mason Medical Center; Clinical Associate Professor of Urology, University of Washington, Seattle, WA
Testis Biopsy

David L. McCullough, MD, FACS
Professor and Chairman of Department of Urology, William H. Boyce Professor of Urology, Bowman Gray School of Medicine of Wake Forest University, Winston-Salem, NC
Urethrectomy

T. E. D. McDermott, LRCP, FRCSI
Consultant Urologist, Meath Hospital, St. James' Hospital and National Rehabilitation Centre, Dublin, Ireland
Transcostal Incision

W. Scott McDougal, MD, FACS
Professor of Surgery, Harvard Medical School; Chief of Urology, Massachusetts General Hospital, Boston, MA
Pelvic Exenteration

Edward J. McGuire, MD
Professor and Director, Division of Urology, University of Texas Medical School, Houston, TX
Pubovaginal Sling

Warren R. McKay, MD
Associate Clinical Professor, Department of Anesthesia and Co-Director of Anesthesia, Moffitt-Long Hospital, University of California, San Francisco, San Francisco, CA
Methods of Nerve Block

Winston K. Mebust, MD
Valk Professor and Chairman, Section of Urology, University of Kansas Medical Center, Kansas City, KS
Excision of Urethral Caruncle and Urethral Prolapse

Mani Menon, MD
Professor and Chairman, University of Massachusetts Medical Center, Worcester, MA
Dorsal Lumbotomy

Hrair-George J. Mesrobian, MD, FAAP, FACS
Associate Professor, Department of Urology, Medical College of Wisconsin; Chief, Division of Pediatric Urology, MACC Fund Research Center, Milwaukee, WI
Cutaneous Ureterostomy and Pyelostomy

Euan J. G. Milroy, FRCS
Consultant Urologist, St. Peter's Hospitals and Institute of Urology at the Middlesex Hospital, London, England
Ureteral Stricture Repair and Ureterolysis

David T. Mininberg, MD, FAAP, FACS
Associate Professor of Clinical Urology and Director, Pediatric Urology, The New York Hospital, Cornell University Medical College, New York, NY
Inguinal Orchiopexy

Michael E. Mitchell, MD
Professor of Pediatric Urology, Children's Hospital and Medical Center, Seattle, WA
Gastric Bladder Replacement

Paul Mitrofanoff, MD
Professor of Pediatric Surgery, Hospital Charles Nicolle, Centre Hospitalier Universitaire, Rouen, France
Appendicovesicostomy

John J. Mulcahy, MD, MS, PhD, FACS
Professor of Urology, Indiana University Medical Center, Indianapolis, IN
Insertion of Flexible Prosthesis

Anthony Richard Mundy, MS, FRCS, MRCP
Professor of Urology, The Institute of Urology, London, England
Ileocystoplasty

George R. Nagamatsu, BSEE, MD, FACS
Research Professor and Past-Chairman, Department of Urology, New York Medical College, New York, NY
Dorsal Flap Incision

Harris M. Nagler, MD
Professor of Urology, The Albert Einstein College of Medicine of Yeshiva University; Chairman, Department of Urology, Beth Israel Medical Center, New York, NY
Spermatocelectomy; Epididymectomy

Perinchery Narayan, MD, FACS
Professor and Chairman of Urology, Division of Urology,
University of Florida, College of Medicine, Gainesville, FL
Ilioinguinal Lymphadenectomy

Johannes H. Naude, MD, ChB, FCS(SA)Urol
Professor of Urology, University of Cape Town and
Groote Schuur Hospital, Cape Town, South Africa
Vesicostomy

Andrew C. Novick, MD
Chairman, Department of Urology, The Cleveland Clinic
Foundation, Cleveland, OH
Partial Nephrectomy; Vena Caval Thrombectomy

Helen E. O'Connell, MD, MBBS, FRACS(Urol)
Clinical Fellow, University of Texas Medical School,
Division of Urology, Houston, TX
Pubovaginal Sling

**J. Dermot O'Flynn, MCh, FRCSI, FRCS(Ed),
FRC Paul S(Glas) (Hon), FRES(Eng) (Hon)**
Urological Department, Meath Hospital, Dublin, Ireland
Bladder Flap Repair

Carl A. Olsson, MD
John K. Lattimer Professor and Chairman, Department
of Urology, Columbia University College of Physicians
and Surgeons, New York, NY
Ileocecal Reservoir

Michael G. Packer, MD, FAAP
Assistant Clinical Professor of Surgery/Urology,
University of California, San Diego, San Diego, CA
Microvascular Orchiopexy

Vito Pansadoro, MD
Urologist, Department of Urology, San Camillo Hospital,
Rome, Italy
Pyelolithotomy

Thomas S. Parrott, III, MD
Late Clinical Associate Professor of Surgery (Urology),
Emory University School of Medicine, Atlanta, GA
Heminephrectomy

David F. Paulson, MD, FACS
Professor and Chief, Division of Urology, Duke
University Medical Center, Durham, NC
Modified Pelvic Lymph Node Dissection

Michele Pavone-Macaluso, MD
Professor and Chairman, Department of Urology,
University of Palermo, Palermo, Italy
Anterior Subcostal Incision

Carlos A. Pellegrini, MD, FACS
Professor and Chairman, Department of Surgery,
University of Washington, Seattle, WA
Appendectomy

Alan D. Perlmutter, MD, FACS
Professor Emeritus, Department of Urology, Wayne State
University School of Medicine, Detroit, MI
Pediatric Extended Anterior Incision

Craig A. Peters, MD
Assistant Professor of Surgery (Urology), Harvard
Medical School and Children's Hospital, Boston, MA
Reduction of Testis Torsion

Paul C. Peters, MD, FACS
Ashbel Smith Professor Emeritus of Urology, The
University of Texas Southwestern Medical Center,
Dallas, TX
Sigmoid Conduit

Silas Pettersson, MD, PhD
Head of the Department of Urology, Sahlgrenska
University Hospital; Professor of Urology, Faculty of
Medicine, Department of Urology, Institute for Surgical
Sciences, Göteborg University, Göteborg, Sweden
Renal Artery Reconstruction

J. Edson Pontes, MD
Professor and Chairman, Department of Urology, Wayne
State University School of Medicine, Detroit, MI
Strictures of the Penile Urethra

Julio E. Pow-Sang, MD
Instituto National de Infermedades Neoplasicas, Urology
Department, Lima, Peru
Ileocecocystoplasty

Joseph C. Presti, Jr., MD, FACS
Assistant Professor of Urology, University of California,
San Francisco, San Francisco, CA
Radical Orchiectomy

John P. Pryor, MS, FRCS
Senior Lecturer, Institute of Urology; Senior Surgeon, St.
Peter's Hospitals, London, England
Penile Curvature

Ronald Rabinowitz, MD, FAAP, FACS
Professor of Urologic Surgery and Professor of
Pediatrics, University of Rochester School of Medicine,
Rochester, NY
Tubed Preputial Island Flap

Schlomo Raz, MD
Professor of Surgery/Urology, Center for Health
Sciences, University of California, Los Angeles, Los
Angeles, CA
Vaginal Needle Suspension

Pratap K. Reddy, MD
Professor of Urology, University of Minnesota; Chief of
Urology, VA Medical Center, Minneapolis, MN
Colonic Bladder Substitution

John F. Redman, MD
Professor and Chairman, Department of Urology,
University of Arkansas College of Medicine,
Little Rock, AR
Transverse Lower Abdominal Incision

Martin I. Resnick, MD, FACS
Lester Persky Professor and Chairman, Department of
Urology, Case Western Reserve University, Cleveland,
OH
Total Perineal Prostatectomy

Alan B. Retik, MD, FACS
Professor of Surgery (Urology), Harvard Medical School,
Boston, MA
Basic Instructions for Hypospadias Repair

Jerome P. Richie, MD, FACS
Elliott Carr Cutler Professor of Surgery, Harvard Medical
School; Chairman, Harvard Program in Urology
(Longwood Area); Chief of Urology, Brigham and
Women's Hospital, Boston, MA
Thoracoabdominal Incision

Richard C. Rink, MD, FACS, FAAP
Associate Professor of Urology, Chief of Pediatric
Urology, James Whitcomb Riley Hospital for Children,
Indiana University School of Medicine, Indianapolis, IN
Gastric Reservoir

Randall G. Rowland, MD, PhD
Professor of Urology, Indiana University School of
Medicine, Indianapolis, IN
Ileocecal Reservoir

Thomas R. Russell, MD, FACS
Clinical Professor of Surgery, University of California,
San Francisco; Chairman, Department of Surgery,
California-Pacific Medical Center, San Francisco, CA
Closure of Bowel Lacerations

Peter N. Schlegel, MD, FACS
Associate Professor of Urology, The New York
Hospital–Cornell Medical Center; Staff Scientist, The
Population Council Center for Biomedical Research,
New York, NY
Preperitoneal Inguinal Herniorrhaphy

Joseph D. Schmidt, MD, FACS
Professor and Head, Division of Urology, University of
California, San Diego, San Diego, CA
Radical Cystectomy

Richard A. Schmidt, MD
Professor of Surgery (Urology) and Director of
Neurourology, University of Colorado Health Sciences
Center, Denver, CO
*Sacral Laminectomy and Dorsal Rhizotomy for
Placement of Pacemaker*

Stanwood S. Schmidt, MD
Research Associate in Urology, University of California,
San Francisco, San Francisco, CA
Vasoligation

Theodore R. Schrock, MD, FACS
Professor of Surgery, University of California, San
Francisco, San Francisco, CA
Loop Ileostomy and Colostomy

William W. Schuessler, MD
Private Practice, San Antonio, TX
Laparoscopic Colposuspension

Claude C. Schulman, MD, PhD
Professor of Urology, University Clinics of Brussels,
Erasme Hospital, Brussels, Belgium
Repair of Ureterocele

Ahmed Shafik, MD, PhD
Professor and Chairman, Department of Surgery and
Experimental Research. Faculty of Medicine, Cairo
University, Cairo, Egypt
Free Tube Graft and Partial Island Flap

George F. Sheldon, MD, FACS
Professor and Chairman, Department of Surgery,
University of North Carolina School of Medicine, Chapel
Hill, NC
Splenorrhaphy and Splenectomy

Joseph A. Smith, Jr., MD
William L. Bray Professor and Chairman, Department of
Urologic Surgery, Vanderbilt University, Nashville, TN
Bowel Stapling Techniques

Joseph C. Smith, MA, MS, FRCS
Consultant Urological Surgeon, Churchill Hospital,
Oxford, England
Ureteroureterostomy and Transureteroureterostomy

M. J. Vernon Smith, MD, PhD
Professor of Urology, Medical College of Virginia,
Richmond, VA
Repair of Ureterovaginal Fistula

Howard M. Snyder, III, MD
Associate Director of Pediatric Urology, Children's
Hospital of Philadelphia; Professor of Surgery in Urology,
University of Pennsylvania School of Medicine,
Philadelphia, PA
Inguinal Orchiopexy

Mark S. Soloway, MD, FACS
Chairman, Department of Urology, University of Miami,
Miami, FL
Partial Cystectomy

Gary D. Steinberg, MD
Assistant Professor of Surgery, Section of Urology,
University of Chicago, Chicago, IL
Excision of Vesical Diverticulum

Mitchell S. Steiner, MD
Associate Professor of Urology and Pharmacology and
Director of Urologic Oncology and Urological Research,
University of Tennessee, Memphis, TN
*Laparoscopic and Minilaparotomy Pelvic Lymph Node
Dissection*

F. Douglas Stephens, AO, DSO, MB, MS, FRACS
Emeritus Professor, Urology and Surgery, Northwestern
University; Honorary Senior Research Fellow, Royal

Children's Hospital Research Foundation, Melbourne, Victoria, Australia
Orchiopexy with Vascular Division

Marshall L. Stoller, MD
Associate Professor of Urology, University of California, San Francisco, San Francisco, CA
Ureteral Stents

Lynn Stothers, MD
Assistant Professor of Urology, University of British Columbia, Vancouver, British Columbia, Canada
Vaginal Needle Suspension

Ralph A. Straffon, MD, FACS
Vice-Chairman, Board of Governors, and Chief of Staff, The Cleveland Clinic Foundation, Cleveland, OH
Repair of Vascular Injuries

Ray E. Stutzman, MD, FACS
Associate Professor, Urology, Johns Hopkins University School of Medicine, Baltimore, MD
Suprapubic Prostatectomy

Emil A. Tanagho, MD
Professor of Urology, University of California, San Francisco, San Francisco, CA
Vesical Neck Tubularization

Joachim W. Thüroff, MD
Professor of Urology, Witten/Herdecke University, Klinikum Barmen, Wuppertal-Barmen, Germany
Ileocecal Bladder Substitution

Donald D. Trunkey, MD, FACS
Chairman, Department of Surgery, Oregon Health Sciences University, Portland, OR
Suture Techniques; Gastrostomy

Paul J. Turek, MD
Assistant Professor-in-Residence, Department of Urology; Assistant Chief of Urology, Veterans Affairs Hospital, University of California, San Francisco, San Francisco, CA
Varicocele Ligation

Richard Turner-Warwick, CBE, DMDSe, FRCP, FRCS, FRCOG, FACS, FRACS (Hon), FACS (Hon)
Emeritus Surgeon, The Middlesex Hospital; Senior Lecturer, London University, Institute of Urology, London, England
Mobilization of the Omentum; Suprapubic V-Incision

E. Darracott Vaughan, Jr., MD
Chairman, Department of Urology and James J. Colt Professor of Urology, The New York Hospital–Cornell Medical Center, New York, NY
Posterior Approach to the Adrenal Gland

Jeffrey Wacksman, MD
Associate Professor of Clinical Surgery, University of Cincinnati Medical Center; Associate Director, Division of Pediatric Urology, Children's Hospital Medical Center, Cincinnati, OH
Meatotomy

George D. Webster, MB, FRCS
Professor of Urologic Surgery, Duke University Medical Center, Durham, NC
Bulbomembranous Urethral Strictures

Robert M. Weiss, MD, FAAP, FACS
Professor and Chief, Section of Urology, Yale University School of Medicine, New Haven, CT
Calicoureterostomy

Eric Wespes, MD, PhD
Professor of Urology, University Clinic of Brussels, Brussels, Belgium
Correction of Penile Venous Leakage

Hugh N. Whitfield, MA, MChir, FRCS
Senior Lecturer, Institute of Urology and Nephrology, London, England
Open Renal Biopsy

Howard N. Winfield, MD, FACS, FRCS(C)
Associate Professor of Urology, University of Iowa College of Medicine, Iowa City, IA
Laparoscopic and Minilaparotomy Pelvic Lymph Node Dissection

Ross O'Neil Witherow, MB, BS, MS, FRCS, FEBU
Consultant Urologist and Clinical Senior Lecturer, St. Mary's Hospital, London, England
Retropubic Prostatectomy

John R. Woodard, MD, FACS, FAAP
Clinical Professor of Surgery (Urology), Emory University School of Medicine, Atlanta, GA
Two-Stage Orchiopexy

Ernst J. Zingg, MD
Professor of Urology (Emeritus), Department of Urology, Inselspital, University of Berne, Berne, Switzerland
Radical Nephrectomy

Leonard M. Zinman, MD, FACS
Associate Clinical Professor, Harvard Medical School, Boston; Attending Urological Surgeon, Lahey Clinic Medical Center, Burlington, MA
Cecocystoplasty and Antireflux Cecocystoplasty

Foreword

When, in 1989, the Royal College of Surgeons of England presented its Honorary Fellowship to Frank Hinman, Jr.—a rare honor indeed for a urologic surgeon—the late Dr. Harry Spence of Dallas, who was then widely regarded as the current "Father of Urology," wrote, specially for inclusion in the citation, "His pre-eminence in all facets of urology, including its surgical writings and organizational activities, plus versatility in his many interests, entitle Frank Hinman, Jr. to be known as 'a Man for all Seasons.'"

For more than 80 years "The Hinmans of San Francisco"—father and son—have together created an era of outstanding contribution and devotion to urology that has virtually spanned the duration of its history. Frank Hinman, Sr. was appointed Founder Chairman of the Department of Urology at the University of California in 1916 and his book, *The Principles and Practice of Urology,* was a pioneer urologic text. Like Frank, Jr., he was an insatiable clinical investigator. It is recorded that, as a junior physician, Frank found his father working in an attic laboratory on a fine summer day; when Frank asked him why he was not out playing golf, or some such, his father's response was, "A man is entitled to some fun, isn't he?"

One of the hallmarks of the pinnacle of success in the urologic world—in the sense of peer review, approbation, and appreciation—is election to the presidency of the American Association of Genitourinary Surgeons. Frank, Sr. was president of this august body in 1937, and Frank, Jr. was its president in 1981.

Frank, Jr. qualified in 1937 and his personal catalog of appointments, contributions, and honors has spanned an extraordinarily active 60 years—and still there is no sign of its waning. His career was punctuated by military service in the Pacific as a surgeon on the much-hit aircraft carrier Intrepid. In 1962, like his father, he became Chief of Urology at San Francisco General Hospital. In the course of time he was elected President of the Society of Pediatric Urologists, a Regent of the American College of Surgeons, and, eventually, Vice President of the American College of Surgeons. He was awarded the Barringer Medal of the GU Surgeons, the Guiteras Medal of the American Urological Association, and in 1991, the St. Paul's Medal of the British Association of Urological Surgeons.

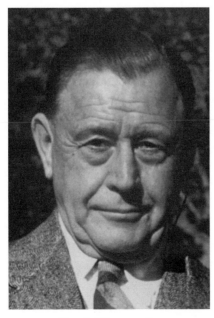

Frank Hinman, Sr.

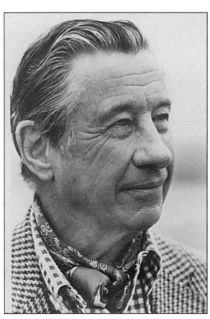

Frank Hinman, Jr.

The demand for a second edition of the *Atlas of Urologic Surgery* with updating of its excellent instructional details of more than 200 operations, together with comments on each by national or international authorities, every one a personal friend, is a fine tribute in itself. But such things do not just happen, they have to be made to happen. The accomplishment of this reflects not only Frank's immense surgical experience in both adult and pediatric urology and his personal innovative contributions, but also his outstanding talent as a teacher and his immense enthusiasm—always tempered, wise, and enduring.

The creation of such an atlas is naturally dependent upon a particularly skilled and devoted medical artist, and Frank certainly regards himself as most fortunate in his association with Paul Stempen. However, the special key is his own ability as an artist that has enabled him to select and sketch the illustrations that best demonstrate the critical stages of every operation he describes—a formidable accomplishment indeed.

But what of the man? Outstandingly kind and a friend of all who know him, an accomplished skier, an ardent duck hunter, a fine carpenter, a talented artist of "one-man show" caliber, and national yacht racing champion in the Triton Class on three occasions. In 1948, he met and married Marion Modesta Eaves, herself a fine sailor, a skier, a duck hunter, a gardener, and subsequently a civic organizer—equal in caliber to Frank and a constant companion.

Frank is clearly the modern equivalent of the ever-youthful Peter Pan and just as surely our current "Father of Urology." We are all immensely grateful to him for his latest offspring—*Atlas of Urologic Surgery*—its gestation and his prolonged labor will be greatly appreciated worldwide.

RICHARD TURNER-WARWICK

Preface to the Second Edition

In the eight years since the first edition of the *Atlas of Urologic Surgery* was published, two companion volumes, one on urosurgical anatomy and one on pediatric urologic surgery, have been published that may be used to supplement this surgical atlas. The original *Atlas* was translated into Spanish, German, Italian, and Chinese.

The basic premise for this *Atlas* has not changed. It is to give you, the urologic surgeon, a practical book that instructs, guides, reminds, and warns.

New procedures, improvements in standard techniques, and entirely new methodologies have made a second edition necessary. For example, when the first edition was being prepared in the mid-1980s, laparoscopic methods were still experimental. Now these new techniques are being applied generally. As a consequence, much of the text has been either rewritten or revised. Many of the illustrations have been modified or redrawn, and over 200 new illustrations have been added, bringing the number of figures to over 1800. To provide a more anatomic approach, we have placed illustrations of the relevant structures before the description of the operation.

As a result, we think the contents of the *Atlas* have changed for the better. I have gone over each of the standard operations to amplify and modernize it and have asked a different Commentator to review the steps of the operation and give another point of view. New technical developments that are just now coming into general use have been inserted in the operative instructions. Because urologic surgery has progressed, many new operations have been added, described in detail, and given focus by a knowledgeable Commentator.

You will find that you will use this edition of the *Atlas,* as the first one, in several ways. When confronted with a new operation or one performed infrequently, you can review it and orient it in your mind step-by-step the night before. In this way, the operation not only will flow smoothly without wasted time but also will be improved by the addition of important fine points and the avoidance of pitfalls. We expect in the near future to have the book on a CD ROM so that the relevant page can be displayed over the operating table for the education of assistants and students, if not for the surgeon. Even for a familiar operation, the *Atlas* can provide the opportunity to branch out and discover a better way to do it. However the book is used, Paul and I trust it will improve the practice of urologic surgery.

FRANK HINMAN, JR.

Preface to the First Edition

Soon after completing residency training, I began to record with sketches and brief notations the techniques I was learning and teaching to the residents, as we worked in the operating rooms of the University of California (UC) and the old San Francisco General Hospitals. At that time, I intended to put together a "how-to" atlas, modeled after that of my fourth year surgery teachers, Cutler and Zollinger. Soon I became busy with other academic pursuits. It wasn't until later when my private practice was cut back that time was found.

Today, as more urologists do fewer operations, a ready source of technical review before some operations is needed. Many procedures that have been routine will now be only occasionally performed. Changes in methods of reimbursement for care of patients may make fewer cases available for resident teaching. Remarkable advances, such as the lithotriptor, have already greatly reduced the frequency of several open operations; more are liable to be done rarely, except in remote areas. Still, they must be done well.

This atlas is written primarily for review by the trained urologist. I trust residents and registrars as well as the operating room staff will also make good use of it.

There are many excellent texts on urologic surgery. However, most are multi-authored; thus, the quality of the chapters varies greatly. Space is given to matters such as descriptions of diseases, "work-ups," and indications for operations, at the expense of the precise description of technique that this atlas provides.

The fortunate confluence of a long-considered format, enough time, an enthusiastic publisher, and the availability of the most promising graduate of our UC medical illustration program, who is also accomplished in the fine arts, made possible this single-authored atlas of urologic operations.

The method of constructing this atlas was complex but logical. First, I made a list of the important operations that should be described, a list that became longer as the work progressed. I reviewed my sketches and postoperative notes made over the last 35 years. Current and classic publications were then consulted to be sure that each important step of every operation was covered. References are not cited in the text, but all are included in the reference section and listed separately for each operation. By combining this previously published information with my notes, made at urologic meetings, and conceptions from my own experiences, I was able to compose written protocols. In these, I described the operation step by step, just as I would tell you how to do it at the operating table, "Cut here, suture there." I hope the user won't take offense at this approach. A deliberate attempt was made to use the simplest words possible to make each segment of the text easy to follow for all readers, including those surgeons who do not speak English as their native language. Each of the steps of the operation was numbered. For each, I either made a rough sketch, as painting is my avocation, or pasted an appropriately revised photocopy alongside my surgical instructions.

Illustrator Paul Stempen reviewed each protocol before witnessing the selected operation so that he could appreciate which steps were important. He photographed each procedure, using a Nikon single-lens reflex camera with a 35-105 mm zoom lens and Ektachrome 160 film with ambient light. For supplementation, he worked from still frames of movies made by accomplished urologic surgeons and from cadaver dissections in our laboratory. At the drawing board, Mr. Stempen made a series of realistic, yet still generally applicable, pencil drawings of the operation from the viewpoint of the surgeon to coincide with the steps described in the protocol. Every attempt was made to have each drawing an original one. At 4 o'clock in the afternoon I joined him in our workroom and checked his sketches against the protocol. We reviewed the day's work for accuracy and clarity. It was similar to teaching a new resident, yet at the same time I learned from him by being forced to clarify my concepts. As in the operating room, we learned together.

Early samples of operations were prepared, taken to the W.B. Saunders Company in Philadelphia, and reviewed with the staff.

The protocol text was processed into an IBM-XT computer by Miss Mary Jane Still and then edited by Miss Aileen Andrus. As the work proceeded, a great many notes on new ideas were obtained at meetings and from current journals. These and previously overlooked points were filed to be added to the protocols in due course.

Photocopies of the drawings and text were sent to almost 200 friends and colleagues whom I knew to have contributed, usually to a particular operation. These authorities included not only urologists, but also general, plastic, vascular, pediatric, and gynecologic surgeons. I asked each of them to use a red pencil liberally on both text and drawings to eliminate inaccuracies and ambiguities. I also asked them to write a personal *Commentary* to follow the text. When these were returned to me, the text and drawings were revised appropriately. Mr. Stempen then redrew the corrected pencil drawings in the clear pen-and-ink technique required for publication.

The team at Saunders composed the pages from the text and drawings, for continuity and readability. The effort was very successful, as you can see. In this atlas you will find precautions on the preparation of the patient and on the surgical procedure itself and assistance with the management of problems in the immediate postoperative period. Long-term follow-up and management of late complications are left to other sources. A list of instruments specific to the procedure is included for the use of the operating room staff as well as the surgeon.

You will not find the history of operations or much discussion of the diseases requiring surgery. The diagnostic steps and assessments and the indications and contraindications are only briefly touched upon; this information can be found in the bibliography, where articles and texts cover these aspects thoroughly. *Advice:* It is safer to read the appropriate references before attempting an unfamiliar procedure. Finally, an atlas can't teach judgment, yet this is the most important ingredient of a successful operation.

The illustrations depict a right-handed surgeon but can be adapted by any surgeon who is left-handed or ambidextrous. Warnings have been inserted wherever there seemed a possibility for going astray.

There are other ways of performing many of the operations. However, after some 5600 operations, I have taken the prerogative of telling others how I would do it. In these instances, I have the support of published surgical descriptions of hundreds of surgeons, for whom credit is given in the reference section, along with the backing of my collaborators who reviewed the individual protocols and sketches.

These open operations are as close to "standard" as they can be described. (Endoscopic procedures are not included.) Some operations that appeared to me to be no longer useful are omitted, but some older operations based on useful principles are included. As John Duckett has pointed out, it is important to know about historical techniques when you have to operate on a patient who was subjected to such a procedure in the past. Newer operations that have yet to prove themselves are in-

cluded; some will be out of date by the time of publication, others may be discredited, to be deleted in a future edition. Certain incisions and approaches appear more than once but with different drawings in order to make a particular operation clear without the need to refer repeatedly to other procedures. The space devoted to several operations is not proportional to the frequency of their performance.

Although I believe all descriptions and directions in the atlas have been "kitchen tested" and are correct, it does not mean that one can read the book and then perform the operation. Thorough training in urologic surgery is a prerequisite before trying any operation, including those described here. Even then, experience with similar operations or performing these operations under supervision is necessary if the patient is not to be at risk of harm. Complicated or difficult operations that occur infrequently in general urologic practice, such as neonatal procedures, repair of severe hypospadias or complicated urethral strictures, and radical excisions for cancer, might best be referred to a subspecialist who has performed enough of these types of operations to have gained special expertise.

You may use this atlas in several ways. Usually, review the appropriate protocol just before doing an infrequently performed operation, thus obtaining a refresher course. You can use the atlas to discover if there is a better way to do a routine operation, expanding your surgical horizon. I hope that each procedure will contain at least a few suggestions or precautions that you have not yet encountered and so provide solutions to immediate problems, before they become insoluble.

FRANK HINMAN, JR.

Acknowledgments

The author and the illustrator appreciate the generous cooperation of the members of the Department of Urology and the support of our past chairman, Emil A. Tanagho, and of the editorial and secretarial staffs who have provided a fine environment for the preparation of this atlas. The organizational assistance of the staff at W.B. Saunders has made for an attractive, readable volume.

The authenticity of each set of verbal and visual instructions derives from the collaboration of nearly 200 of our national and international colleagues. These experts have reviewed the text and the figures and not only have made valuable suggestions for additions and changes but also have written the practical Commentaries that bring the details of the procedures into focus.

Introduction

When Frank Hinman, Jr. invited me to write an introduction to the second edition of his *Atlas of Urologic Surgery,* I was pleased and flattered. One glance at the condition of the cover and pages of the library copy of the *Atlas* confirmed that this specialized book had been subjected to heavy use, and with good reason. The critical anatomic and technical aspects of operative procedures are detailed with remarkable clarity. The line drawings reflect the unusual combined expertise in surgery and artistic presentation of the author. His regular interaction with his collaborating artist, Paul Stempen, undoubtedly helped to target and illustrate the important technical considerations of the procedures selected for presentation. Accuracy and clarity were enhanced by the process of utilizing almost 200 colleagues with special expertise for critical review and comments before finalizing the content of the *Atlas*. Maintaining single author responsibility for the manuscript, however, has undoubtedly maximized communication and minimized duplication and contradiction.

That book, resulting from this combination of experience and effort by a very talented surgeon, presents an accurate, easily understood recipe for operations in urology that were in use when it was published. In the foreword to the first edition of the *Atlas,* Willard Goodwin predicted that this "is the kind of book that every urologic resident will want to review just before trying a given operation for the first time and that every urologic surgeon will want to review before beginning an infrequently done procedure." In my opinion, time has proven this assessment accurate. However, in the past few years, an expanding array of alternative procedures, especially those employing minimally invasive or alternative tissue or pathology destructive approaches, have been developed and are utilized to accomplish our surgical goals. As a result, the original *Atlas* had gaps that needed to be filled. Fortunately, Frank, Jr. has undertaken this task with a new edition.

To those who know Frank, the effort he made in producing the first edition of the *Atlas of Urologic Surgery* and the results achieved are expected. He was blessed and possibly burdened by being the son of a famous urologist who made many contributions to Urology. His urologic text *Principles and Practice of Urology,* published in 1935 by W.B. Saunders, was a gold mine of information and practical insights that were very helpful to many of us during and after our residency. Frank and his father seem to share many characteristics. He has persistently demonstrated a very inquisitive attitude and commitment to excellence and hard work. Frank, Jr. has established his own identity and niche. I recently watched with admiration as one urologist after another came forward to thank him for various types of help he had given them. Although Frank and I are of the same generation, he was always sufficiently far ahead of my development as a urologist to have his big foot firmly imprinted into what was new ground to me. I gradually recognized that his talents were not limited to the diverse abilities he displayed in urology but were complemented by a host of others, such as sailing and art. He has clearly added luster to the Hinman name.

Frank accepted the challenge to produce a needed revision of the *Atlas of Urologic Surgery* at a time in life when most choose not to take on additional chores. I think we are fortunate that he did. The newly developed operative approaches needed to be added to the *Atlas* and presented side by side with the established ones. As alternatives to open surgery take an increasingly prominent place in the treatment of urologic problems, the classic surgical approaches and procedures will be utilized less often overall. Furthermore, the proportion of complex problems in which they will be employed will very probably increase. If this scenario is correct, the importance of this *Atlas* in refreshing and preserving the accumulated open surgical experience for the urologists to come is likely to increase. I still utilize Frank Hinman, Sr.'s book to look up specific information and I find it detailed and referenced often enough to continue the practice. In my opinion, the *Atlas of Urologic Surgery* has the same permanency as an invaluable reference source. This book expands the debt of gratitude urology, urologists, and their patients owe the Hinman clan for their many contributions.

JOHN T. GRAYHACK

Abbreviations, Sutures

CCG   Chromic catgut

NAS   Nonabsorbable suture

PCG   Plain catgut

PDS   Polydioxanone suture

SAS   Synthetic absorbable suture

Contents

SECTION

1

Surgical Basics

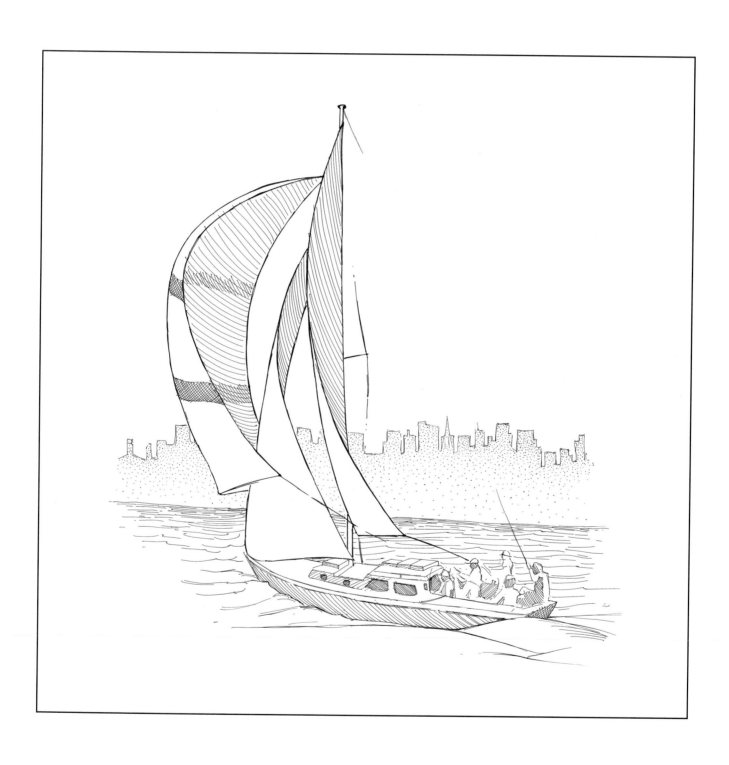

Strategy and Tactics

Racing a yacht is a lot like performing a surgical operation. For yacht racing, the winning skipper develops a strategy before going out to race: What is the game plan? Competition may disrupt the plan; how can competitors be thwarted? What will the winds be, so that the most efficient sails can be set? How much will the boat be set by the tides and in what direction? What will be the shortest course around the buoys? Are the skipper and crew well trained and practiced, and do they have a winning attitude? Is the boat well equipped and able to go fast? Once on the course, how can the strategy be adapted to the conditions, using the tactics developed for going fast: starting with the gun in clear air; obtaining boat speed; covering the moves of the adversaries; applying the rules to gain advantages and keep out of trouble; staying out of shoals and calms; and, most important, finishing the winner?

For operations, too, the surgeon must have a strategy in order to win: What is the game plan and what are the steps to achieve it? Does the surgeon understand the problem to be treated and know the structure and function of the body? "If you know how it works, you can fix it." Tactics at the operating table are as important as strategy. Has the surgeon learned the manual and mental skills required to execute the successive steps of the operation, acquired the basic surgical rules, and learned the maneuvers needed to get to the finish?

In this book, the surgeon can first understand the overall scheme of the operations. Then, by following step by step the detailed instructions that are illustrated and described in this atlas, the operation can be steered to a rapid and successful finish.

It is axiomatic that no exploratory operations are done in urology. The reason is that instrumental and imaging techniques define the problem before the operation starts and make the approach, exposure, and procedure straightforward.

For surgery, strategy comes first. Select the optimal operation, plan the steps of the procedure before starting, have the operating room well equipped and well staffed, and assemble a capable and experienced crew who can work as a team. Then use tactics. Apply surgical techniques that are appropriate to the overall strategy to the different conditions that are encountered. Start with good exposure; fend off difficult planes and vascular traps; and avoid becoming becalmed by making ineffective movements or running into obstructions off the course. And persist with a winning attitude even when you seem to be coming in last because the race isn't over until the finish line is reached in the recovery room. Tactics, of course, have to be learned at the operating table; only general precepts can be given in this book.

This atlas describes the steps of an operation, asks some questions, and provides some warnings. Use one of the good urology textbooks to review the pathophysiology of the disease and the necessary diagnostic steps. If possible, read the description of the operation written by its originator, and obtain details and alternatives from other authors in the selected bibliographic list given for each type of operation.

EQUANIMITY

Surgery is very intense work. You get keyed up and can't understand why everyone else at the table isn't equally attentive. Don't lose your temper. You are the captain, but the crew has to work along with you.

Tension causes a lot of water to evaporate during an operation. It's surprising how thirsty you are when you finish. Of course, antidiuresis may allow you to finish a long operation without leaving the table.

SUMMARY

Surgery is much more than dissecting. Know the anatomy and function involved before starting the operation. Review the operation in your mind the night before, and picture each step ahead of time. Know the details of your patient's abnormalities, and review the findings before you go to the operating room. Attention to detail before, during, and after the operation makes good results possible. Be compulsive about detail.

Act logically for each move. Control yourself, and don't fall apart under stress. Become adept at manipulating instruments and tissues. Don't hesitate, and don't waste motion. Have a good team, with enough trained hands, and be the leader of your crew. Be sure all the needed pieces of equipment are available, and know that you have available consultants and back-up facilities. Use delicate surgical technique, irrigate debris, obtain good hemostasis, close dead spaces, and provide adequate drainage. Be gentle but not indecisive. Tie sutures only to approximate the tissues. Dissect and follow the natural tissue planes. Work from the known to the unknown. Fulgurate or ligate only those vessels involved and do it accurately. Avoid blind dissection with either instruments or fingers. Keep tissues moist and covered. Ensure adequate exposure and proper lighting. A sufficiently large incision, good help, and retraction are basic. Finally, your responsibility to the patient continues through recovery and convalescence.

Preoperative Evaluation

The patient is best served if you—rather than a member of the house staff—take the history and perform the physical examination. In children this is essential to establish rapport. For the patient who is well, few tests are needed before most operations other than complete blood tests and urinalysis, and these may be done within a month of the procedure. For *collection of urine* specimens, midstream samples are needed. To obtain a specimen from an indwelling catheter, clamp the tubing, wipe the wall with an alcohol sponge, and aspirate a sample with a syringe and fine needle. Avoid disconnecting the sterile pathway.

EVALUATION OF RISKS

First, assess the *operative risk*. It influences the preparation, procedure, and outcome. Use a checklist for *risk factors* (Table 1) to help determine the degree of risk. Place the patient in one of four categories in the Physical Status Scale proposed by the American Society of Anesthesiologists: Class 1, a normal, healthy individual; Class 2, a patient with mild systemic disease; Class 3, a patient with severe systemic disease that is not incapacitating; and Class 4, a patient with an incapacitating systemic disease that is a constant threat to life. Consider age, morbid obesity, and nutritional status in the evaluation.

Cardiac status is particularly important. The chance of death in the first 48 hours after operation averages about 0.3 percent, principally from cardiac dysfunction. Ten percent of that risk is during induction of anesthesia, 35 percent during the operation, and the rest in the following 2 days. Demand for oxygen may be excessive from tachycardia, hypertension, increased peripheral resistance, fever, or fluid overload. Or oxygen delivery may be inadequate from hypotension, pulmonary disease, hypoxia, anemia, hypovolemia, or dysrhythmia. Because cardiac functional status determines how well the patient withstands the operation, it must be carefully evaluated preoperatively by history and physical examination. Postoperative risk is related to evidence of heart failure, rhythm disturbances, the type of surgical procedure, age greater than 70 years, significant aortic stenosis, and the appearance of a patient in generally poor condition. Delay operation for 6 months after a myocardial infarction. Also in the postoperative period, realize that infarction not infrequently occurs within the first 7 days, and in half of the patients it takes place without chest pain. This necessitates postoperative serial screening of high-risk patients with electrocardiograms (ECGs) and enzyme determinations.

It is advisable to have patients stop taking aspirin 1 to 2 weeks before operation, especially if bleeding may be a problem. For major operations on older patients, consider digitalization, giving digoxin, 0.5 mg, in the morning of the day before operation; 0.25 mg that afternoon; and 0.125 mg that evening. It is well to hydrate the patient overnight with lactated Ringer's solution.

Evaluate *pulmonary function* by measuring maximum mid-expiratory flow rate, related to the ability to cough and thus avoid pneumonia. If the patient retains carbon dioxide, ventilatory support will be needed postoperatively. Perform spirometry with and without bronchodilators to test the reversibility of bronchospasm with these agents preoperatively. Have the patient stop smoking at least 2 weeks before surgery.

Assess *nutrition*. Patients having a weight loss greater than 10 percent are at increased risk for complications, as are those who have a serum albumin level of less than 3.2 g/dl, a transferrin level greater than 220 mg/dl, or skin test anergy. These chronically ill patients coming to operation require restoration of their nutritional deficit to avoid poor wound healing, immunologic deficiencies (total lymphocyte count should be above 1500), and organ malfunction. Hyperalimentation alone can reduce morbidity and mortality significantly. Treat the patient for at least 1 or 2 weeks before operation with tube feedings to bring the child or elderly patient into positive nitrogen balance. Give supplemental vitamins, particularly vitamin C.

For the *chronically ill patient*, often with marginal renal function, obtain consultations to look for immunologic or hematologic abnormalities secondary to the disease or to the treatment for it. Correct electrolyte imbalances, especially hyperkalemia (greater than 7 mmol/L) or uncompensated metabolic acidosis (capillary blood pH less than 7.30), with oral solutions if possible because intravenous administration is harder to control. Correct any defects in coagulation. Restore blood volume with donor-designated blood. Look for defects in coagulation, detected by platelet count, bleeding time, prothrombin time, and partial thromboplastin time. Restore blood volume and give packed cells to obtain a level of hemoglobin of 13 or 14 g/dl, even though 10 g/dl has been considered a safe lower level for anesthesia. Be sure that the protein level is at least 5 g/dl.

Patients with reduced renal function should be admitted to the hospital to allow evaluation. There the intake and output may be monitored and abnormalities in serum electrolytes corrected.

EVALUATION BY THE ANESTHESIOLOGIST

Discuss the projected procedure with the anesthesiologist, and give any information about the patient's status that was gained from your history and physical examination. In particular, discuss details about drugs that may cause intraoperative hypotension and provide data from previous operations, such as hyperpyrexia, drug reactions, and bleeding problems. Do not hesitate to cancel an elective operation if the anesthesiologist believes that the patient has an upper respiratory infection. Be certain to have the patient arrive with an empty stomach, having taken nothing by mouth in the previous 2 hours.

PROCEDURE REVIEW

The night before the operation, go over the steps of the operation in your mind. Be sure to review the operation from an atlas or journal article, especially if it is a procedure done infrequently. More important than reading through the steps in a book, however, is visualizing the procedure step by step in your mind's eye. This allows the actual operation to progress easily and with greater accuracy.

Table 1. Checklist of Risk Factors (Gapta)

	Low Risk	Moderate Risk	High Risk
Anemia	11 to 12 g/dl	8 to 10 g/dl	<8 g/dl
Creatinine >2 mg/dl	Reversible	—	Irreversible
Cerebrovascular accidents	>6 mo	3 to 6 mo	<6 mo
Diabetes	Mild	Moderate	Uncontrolled
Hypertension	150/90 mm Hg	200/120 mm Hg	280/150 mm Hg
Heart block	Incomplete	—	Pacemaker
Myocardial infarction	>6 mo	3 to 6 mo	<3 mo
Dyspnea from airway obstruction	Unusual exertion	Moderate exertion	At rest

Preparation for Surgery

PREOPERATIVE PREPARATION

Manage *hypertension* preoperatively to stabilize the blood pressure so that it does not swing during anesthetic induction and intubation. Try to achieve normal blood pressure, or at least reduce the diastolic blood pressure below 100 mm Hg. Consider hydrating the patient overnight with lactated Ringer's solution.

If *blood loss* is anticipated, arrange for the patient to store blood prior to the operation to reduce the risk of viral acquisition. Autologous donations are suitable for cystectomy, pelvic and retroperitoneal lymph node dissection, nephrectomy and nephroureterectomy, radical penectomy, open and transurethral prostatectomy, and urethroplasty. Reinfusion of recovered blood may be indicated if the loss is large.

Hypokalemia, seen in older patients preoperatively, is usually due to depletion of total body potassium. For blood levels above 3 mEq/L, oral supplementation is sufficient, but replacement is slow and may delay the operation. For lower levels, intravenous potassium administration may be resorted to, but the rate should not exceed 10 mEq/hr. Rescheduling the procedure may be the wiser course.

OUTPATIENT SURGERY

Operations in a "come-and-go" setting are becoming the standard, one reason being economic. Procedures such as inguinal, penile, and scrotal surgery and many endoscopic procedures may be done as same-day surgery with the expectation of few postoperative hospitalizations and very few complications, either surgical or anesthetic. Such operations are clearly better in pediatric urology because they are well tolerated by children and they keep children and parents together.

Prior to the day of surgery, arrange for the adult patient or the child and parents to be interviewed by the anesthesiologist and, if feasible, examined by a member of the house staff.

Admit the patient to the same-day surgery unit at least 1 hour before the operation. If the procedure is to be done with local anesthesia, provide sedoanalgesia (page 8) at this time. After stopping by the same-day surgery waiting room to reassure the patient's family, go to the operating room before the patient is put to sleep (thereby providing more reassurance). After the operation and the necessary stay in the recovery room, the patient can be transferred to a less supervised room to recover fully before discharge. A subsequent telephone call to the patient or family from the unit nurse allows immediate detection of any problems.

INSTRUMENTS

With the help of the operating room nurse or technician, make out a card for each operation you commonly do, listing the position of the patient, the instruments you need, and the sutures to have ready. In this atlas, lists of instruments are provided with the descriptions of many operations, and the composition of the basic specialty sets is listed in the back of the book under "Instruments" (page 1081). Make your own instrument cards by photocopying the appropriate list, revising it to suit your own technique, and then having it typed on a card to be filed in the operating room. Have the appropriate card out on the counter in the operating room while the patient is being anesthetized. Check the cards and keep them up to date. In some cases, go over the card with the scrub nurse at the instrument table to be sure everything is at hand.

A "GU cart" is a necessity. Obtain a roll-around cart with five or six drawers of the type that mechanics use to hold tools. Paint it a color that prevents it from being mistaken for an emergency cart. Outfit it with catheters, sounds, stents, and special instruments and have it parked in your operating room during the operation. Suggested contents are found in the "Instruments" section (page 1081). A separate cart for sutures is also useful, especially for procedures on infants and children which require special sutures and needles.

1 Two useful tools that can be made are the Rumel tourniquet (**A**) and a pair of 12-inch intrarenal retractors (**B**).

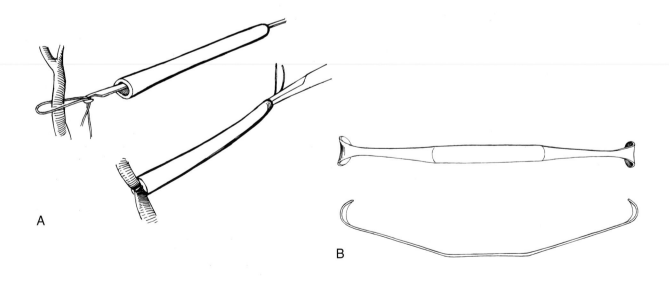

A

B

Table 1. Preparation of Coagulum

1. Cryoprecipitate from Blood Bank, 2 bags of 15 ml each. (Call ahead to thaw for 30 minutes.)
2. $CaCl_2$ 10%; 1 amp.
3. Methylene blue.
4. 18-gauge angiocatheter; cut off extra length, add stopcock.
5. 35-ml syringe.
6. IV extension tubing without stopcock. Attach to angiocatheter.
7. 60-ml syringe for irrigation.
8. 8 F infant feeding tube.
9. 200-ml bowl.
10. Saline irrigation solution.

Draw cryoprecipitate into the 60-ml syringe, add 6 ml $CaCl_2$ tinted with methylene blue, and mix in a bowl. Draw the mixture into a 35-ml syringe and instill it into the pelvis through an angiocatheter. After removal of the clot, flush the ureter with saline via the 8 F infant feeding tube.

For coagulum pyelolithotomy, assemble the requisites before the operation (Table 1).

Proper retractors are necessary. Perineal prostatectomy, for example, requires a special set of posterior and lateral retractors, as well as prostatic tractors with blades that open to elevate the gland. Ring retractors are needed for pediatric procedures and for work on the urethra. A Balfour retractor with malleable blades is useful for adults, but a self-retaining retractor, with universal joints and detachable disposable blades, fastened to the table top, such as the Omni-Tract, is better for major cases.

PREOPERATIVE CHECKLIST

To avoid missing important orders, refer to a preoperative checklist (Table 2).

PREPARATION OF THE OPERATIVE SITE

Shaving increases bacterial colonization and should be done as near to the time of operation as feasible. A razor with a recessed blade causes the least damage. Shave only those areas where the hair would get in the way; use scissors for the rest. Follow this with a brief mechanical wash to expose bacteria so that they can be reached by topical antiseptic agents. An iodophor, such as povidone-iodine (Betadine), in which iodine is complexed with a surfactant compound, releases iodine slowly to act on contaminants. Wash the area for 5 to 10 minutes with such a solution, then paint it with concentrated iodophor. Avoid spreading these solutions on the delicate skin of the genitalia.

Table 2. Preoperative Checklist

Assess Operative Risk
  Nutrition (serum albumin <3 g/dl)
  Immune competence (total lymphocyte count <1000/µl; allergies)
  Drug therapy (aspirin, corticosteroids, immunosuppressives, antibiotics, chemotherapy)
  Pulmonary dysfunction (chest radiograph, blood gas values, pulmonary function test; preoperative pulmonary preparation)
  Wound healing (protein and vitamin C deficiency; dehydration with hypovolemia, anemia, irradiation)
  Obesity
Prepare the Patient
  Informed consent and permit
  Banked blood
  Skin preparation
  Bowel preparation
  Preanesthetic medication
  Blood transfusion
  Hydration
  Medications
  Antibiotics

If you can, have the circulating nurse do the preparation while you scrub. Make the skin preparation brief, especially in children, using warmed solutions and avoiding agents that evaporate on the skin or that run under the body.

For children, it is advisable to focus an infrared lamp during the interval between placement on the table and application of the drapes. For long operations, warm the intravenous fluids to body temperature. Apply a small grounding plate to minimize heat loss.

Contamination. Bacteria colonize the shedding superficial cells of the skin and the hair follicles. Contamination from the surgeon and staff comes less from the hands than from hairs falling from the head into the wound or from fallen pubic hairs redistributed from the floor. Appropriate coverings for the head, neck, and perineum reduce contamination of the operative field and the adjacent floor. Remember to shower your head after a haircut, and develop the habit of cleaning under the nails each morning with soap and a fingernail of the other hand. We probably scrub our hands too long—5 minutes should be enough, if the subungual spaces are mechanically cleaned. There is no need to run the water continuously during the scrub; this not only wastes water but also makes conversation with your assistant difficult. Rinse and wipe the powder from your gloves, or better, wear powderless gloves (Hunt et al, 1994).

Epilation

To remove hairs from areas of skin that will be incorporated into the urethra, obtain a 12-volt DC generator. Wear a three-power loupe, and insert a fine straight milliner's needle into the follicle alongside the hair. Touch it with the tip of the active electrode while applying very gentle traction on the hair with forceps. Withdraw the hair together with the needle after a few moments of coagulation.

Draping

Adhesive drapes are barriers to bacteria and also form a thermal barrier. Cover the areas adjacent to the site of the incision with sterile dry towels and keep them in place with small clips. Try to keep the towels dry. Nonabsorbent, plastic stick-on drapes may reduce contamination but foster bacterial proliferation under them unless they are porous to vapor. Fold the covering drape upon itself to form a lateral pocket to hold instruments.

AVOIDANCE OF POSTOPERATIVE COMPLICATIONS PREOPERATIVELY

Nutrition

Before operation, have the patient in optimal nutritional state if possible, resorting to tube feeding and even parenteral nutrition if necessary.

For major operations such as total cystectomy in a debilitated patient, punch a 14 F Silastic self-retaining catheter into the stomach, or perform a gastrostomy. Anchor the tube to the abdominal wall with a purse-string suture, and do not remove the tube before the tract has matured. A feeding jejunostomy may be warranted in some cases. With the help of a clinical nutritionist, select an enteral formula based on the patient's digestive and absorptive capacity, specific nutrient needs, tolerance, allergies, and age. Use isotonic feedings initially, do not increase the volume and the concentration at the same time, use intermittent (bolus) feeding only in patients with a gastrostomy, and use only continuous feedings to the small bowel through the jejunostomy. When the patient becomes intolerant, fall back to the previous tolerated volume and concentration and progress more slowly. When to start oral alimentation is always a problem.

BOWEL PREPARATION

Balanced Lavage Method

Weigh the patient and check serum electrolyte values. Order a clear liquid diet. At noon or 4 PM the day before surgery, give 240 ml of a balanced bowel preparation solution (GoLYTELY) every 10 minutes for 4 hours for a total of 6 L. If nausea is a problem, give prochlorperazine maleate 10 mg IM. Alternatively, start an IV infusion of metoclopramide at noon, the purpose of which is to tighten the esophagogastric junction and stimulate peristalsis, thereby providing an antiemetic effect. (This is in contrast to prochlorperazine maleate, which acts centrally to achieve an antiemetic effect but peripherally retards the activity of the entire bowel.) Recheck the patient's weight and serum electrolyte values. Give neomycin (1 g orally) at 1 PM, 2 PM, and 11 PM, and give metronidazole (500 mg IV) 1 hour before starting the operation. Erythromycin base (1 g orally) given at 1 PM, 2 PM, and 11 PM may be substituted for the metronidazole. If metronidazole is used preoperatively, give two more doses at 8-hour intervals after the procedure. Stop oral intake 4 hours before the operation.

Children with a neurogenic bladder have impaired bowel motility and require 3 days of liquid diet and enemas, in addition to the balanced bowel preparation solution, given through a nasogastric tube.

For the *oral mannitol method,* start a clear liquid diet 3 to 4 days preoperatively. On the day before operation, have the patient take 100 g of mannitol diluted in 1 L of water. Replace the resulting fluid loss with IV fluids of lactated Ringer's solution or 5 percent dextrose in normal saline at 100 to 125 ml/hr.

VASCULAR ACCESS

The anesthetist obtains vascular access by percutaneous methods in 90 percent of cases using local or topical anesthetic. Femoral vein catheterization carries risk of infection. Percutaneous subclavian vein puncture done by an interventional radiologist does not require general anesthesia but does carry a slight risk of pneumothorax or arterial puncture. Techniques for vascular access are described on page 90.

PREOPERATIVE MEDICATION

On the patient's initial visit, make a judgment about the need for premedication. Give the narcotic 45 to 60 minutes before the patient is called; atropine may be combined with the narcotic in the same syringe. It is essential that oxygen, suction equipment, and drugs and equipment for airway support and resuscitation be available. For monitoring, the pulse oximeter is ideal. Now that most operations are done without admission to the hospital, avoid a needle stick by having the anesthetist give the atropine IV at the time of induction.

Which narcotic agent is best has not been determined. Morphine is an effective tranquilizer but may promote nausea and vomiting. Pentazocine may be a good substitute. In children, because needles hurt and rectal drugs are not dependable, drugs may be administered orally.

Commonly administered drugs are listed in Table 3.

Table 3. Dosages for Preoperative Medication

Morphine	0.1–0.2 mg/kg
Meperidine	1.0–1.5 mg/kg
Pentobarbital	2–3 mg/kg IM or orally, 5 mg/kg rectally
Pentazocine	1 mg/kg
Diazepam	0.4 mg/kg
Chlorpromazine	0.5 mg/kg
Atropine	0.03 mg/kg (max. 0.6 mg/kg)

Data from Luck SR: Preoperative evaluation and preparation. In Roffensperger JG (ed): Swenson's Pediatric Surgery, 5th ed. Norwalk, CT, Appleton & Lange, 1990, p 7.

PERIOPERATIVE INFECTION

A few precepts are generally accepted:

1. Favor outpatient operations to reduce the chance for cross-infection.
2. Clear infections if present preoperatively.
3. Have the patient bathe immediately before operation. A hexachlorophene shower is advisable before a genital operation. Prior to vaginal procedures, douches with an iodophor preparation are indicated the night before.
4. Prepare the bowel thoroughly.
5. Provide antibacterial prophylaxis for patients undergoing major surgery.

Perioperative Antibiotics

For *clean* cases, prophylactic antibiotics are probably not necessary; the incidence of infection is too low. If used in the absence of bacteriuria or tissue infection, antibacterial agents in sufficient concentrations need to be present in the body only during the actual operation, when the wound could become contaminated, and during the immediate postoperative period to prevent any introduced bacteria from becoming established. The exception is during insertion of prosthetic devices. A dose of a broad-spectrum antibiotic, given IM 1 hour preoperatively and repeated two times at 8-hour intervals, is adequate in most cases. If an indwelling catheter has been in place, add ampicillin IV to cover any enterococcus species that may be present. Trimethoprim-sulfamethoxazole may be given for several days following removal of a catheter.

Antibacterial presence in *clean/contaminated* cases is needed at most only at the time of operation and for the subsequent 3 or 4 hours. In *contaminated* cases, antibiotics assume a therapeutic rather than a prophylactic role and are selected by the type of bacteria expected. For abdominal contamination, clindamycin plus gentamicin is effective.

Specific Prophylactic Situations. For placement of a *balloon catheter* or for a cystoscopic examination, give a cephalosporine (cephalexin) 25 mg/kg IV. With *ventriculoperitoneal shunt,* give vancomycin IV immediately before surgery and for 2 days following for non–urinary tract–related operations; add gentamicin if the urinary tract is involved. For *operations involving bowel,* prepare the bowel as described and 30 minutes before the operation give a second-generation antibiotic, cefoxitin, repeat it intraoperatively, and continue for 3 to 5 days, or give cefotetan as a single dose.

Patients who have *valvular heart disease* and are thus susceptible to bacterial endocarditis should receive antibiotic prophylaxis. Give ampicillin, 2.0 g, and gentamicin, 1.5 mg/kg IM or IV, 30 minutes before the procedure; after 6 hours, give oral amoxicillin, 1.5 g, or repeat the initial parenteral medications. If the patient is allergic to penicillin, substitute vancomycin, 1.0 g given over 60 minutes.

Table 4 lists appropriate drugs for several conditions.

Table 4. Preoperative Antibiotics

	Regimen
Clean Procedures	
Scrotal	None
Pelvic without instrumentation	None
Prosthetic	Prophylaxis
Clean/Contaminated Procedures	
Renal, ureteral, vesical	None
High-risk patient	Prophylaxis
Contaminated Procedures	
Enteroplasty	Prophylaxis
Urethral instrumentation	Prophylaxis
Reoperation	Prophylaxis
Dirty Procedures	
After trauma and emergencies (unprepared bowel)	Prophylaxis, then continue

PROCEDURE REVIEW

Going over the steps of the operation in your mind the night before guarantees a more precise and quicker procedure. Review the operation from a book chapter or an article in a journal. More importantly, on the morning of surgery, you must visualize the details of the procedure in your mind's eye, moving from step to step. This is necessary to make the actual operation flow much more easily and accurately.

OPERATING ROOM SURVEY

Arrive in the operating room before the patient is put to sleep. This not only provides reassurance to the patient but also allows you, the surgeon, to supervise each step of anesthetization and preparation, for which you are ultimately responsible. Learn the names of the scrub and circulating nurses; things will then run a lot more smoothly. If necessary, teach the anesthetist how to adjust the top of that particular operating table before the operation. Put the radiographs and scans on the view boxes; don't operate without them. Check the radiographs. Be certain that you are operating on the patient's diseased side. The radiographs may also help determine the site of the incision and may help in checking the findings during the operation, especially in stone removal cases. After the operation, always go to the recovery room to evaluate the patient and the orders; do this even when you have a resident.

PROTECTION DURING SURGERY

Set the room temperature: 70° to 72° F for adults, 72° to 74° F for children, and 74° to 76° F for infants.

The appropriate position for the patient is shown in this atlas for each operation, but the details for protection of the patient vary. Be thorough in placing foam rubber padding over all bony prominences to avoid damage to adjacent nerve trunks, especially the ulnar and peroneal nerves. When the patient is in the lateral position, place a pad in the axilla to protect the brachial plexus. The lithotomy position is especially likely to cause nerve injury. Avoid positions that put a strain on muscles, ligaments, and joints. For minor procedures in children, use a restraining wrap (papoose board).

Anesthesia

PREPARATION FOR ANESTHESIA

Arrive in the operating room in time to brief the anesthetist and operating team on the procedure. Reassure the patient, and avoid noisy talk. The patient may be given a choice between mask and needle, but the surgeon should stand by for reassurance and restraint. The surgeon must also be ready to help if difficulty is encountered in placing an airway or giving drugs to control laryngospasm. Consider placement of a nasogastric tube to avoid vomiting and consequent aspiration postoperatively.

Follow *body temperature during induction* with a rectal or esophageal probe.

FLUID AND ELECTROLYTE REPLACEMENT

Fluid losses increase during surgery because of drapes and heat from the lights. The anesthetist provides sufficient fluid to replace insensible losses and third-space losses incurred at the operative site, giving lactated Ringer's solution in 5 percent dextrose in water at a rate of 10 ml/kg/hr. You can assist the anesthetist in monitoring blood loss and can advocate replacing it with whole blood or packed cells after you believe 10 percent of the blood volume has been lost. The state of hydration can be monitored by changes in the blood pressure, although for difficult cases a central venous pressure line is needed. The urinary output, serum electrolytes, blood glucose, and hematocrit should also be monitored.

Watch for *hypoglycemia*, evidenced by a blood sugar level below 45 mg/dl. Supply 10 percent dextrose at 3 to 4 ml/hr, but do not allow the blood sugar level to get above approximately 130 mg/dl for fear of intraventricular bleeding and of dehydration-hyponatremia from the resulting diuresis.

SEDATION FOR SAME-DAY SURGERY

Sedoanalgesia is suitable for adults undergoing surgery on a come-and-go basis under local anesthesia. Give midazolam, 100 μg/kg for healthy individuals 20 to 30 minutes before the procedure, along with a diclofenac suppository, 100 mg, and an intramuscular antibiotic. For American Society of Anesthesiologists Class 4 patients, reduce the dose of midazolam to 35 μg/kg (Briggs et al, 1995). If needed, add midazolam in 0.5-mg increments. Give nasal oxygen, monitored by a pulse oximeter. Reverse the effects of midazolam with flumazenil if necessary.

LOCAL ANESTHESIA

Anesthesia with lidocaine hydrochloride is achieved in 5 minutes and lasts from 1.5 to 2.5 hours. As a regional block and as a subcutaneous anesthesia in adults, do not use more than 30 ml of a 1 percent solution, without epinephrine, through a 27-gauge needle. For *ilioinguinal and penile block* and for *caudal block*, use bupivacaine (Marcaine), 0.5 to 1.0 ml/kg of a 0.25 percent solution. Suggested maximum doses (with and without epinephrine) are as follows: procaine (Novocain) 14 to 18 mg/kg, lidocaine (Xylocaine) 7 to 9 mg/kg, and bupivacaine 2 to 3 mg/kg. The addition of epinephrine 1:200,000 decreases local blood flow and the rate of absorption of the agent, with a resulting prolongation of anesthesia and a 25 percent reduction in blood levels. However, epinephrine can produce systemic side effects and potentiates infection. Great care must be used when injecting bupivacaine; entry into the venous system may cause irreversible cardiomyopathy with asystole, a sequela that is not dose related.

Treat a toxic reaction to a local anesthetic by starting oxygen administration, then give barbiturates or benzodiazepines IV (e.g., diazepam 5 to 10 mg as the initial dose). Make provisions for positive-pressure ventilation (mask or endotracheal tube) whenever large doses of local anesthetics are used. Short, beveled needles are less likely to injure nerves and provide more precise localization of the agent. When walking a needle off bone, place the bevel toward the edge of the bone.

GENERAL ANESTHESIA
Monitoring

Careful monitoring of body temperature, ECG, blood pressure, and blood loss is essential. Central venous pressure monitoring may be added. For major cases, monitoring must be provided for (1) heart rate, (2) ECG, (3) blood pressure (Doppler meter), (4) central venous pressure (CVP, indwelling lines), (5) filling pressure, (6) pulse oximeter, and (7) P_{O_2}.

Body temperature must be maintained, especially in infants. Temperature is followed via a rectal (or esophageal) thermoprobe. *Malignant hyperthermia* is a serious complication and may be suggested by change in blood gases and by tachypnea or paralysis, dark blood in the wound, and cardiac arrhythmias. It must be treated immediately (Table 1). Because it is not known which agent precipitated the hyperthermia, stop all anesthetic agents and rapidly terminate the procedure. Hyperventilate the patient with 100 percent oxygen at a rate three to five times normal to rid the body of excess CO_2, and give sodium bicarbonate for the acidosis and hyperkalemia. Start diuretics and insert a catheter to monitor the urine color and volume. Give dantrolene, 1 to 10 mg/kg intravenously at a rate of 1 mg/kg/min, and repeat the dose in 15 minutes if the response is not adequate. Place the patient in an ice pack. Consider cardiopulmonary bypass with heat exchange. Give hypertonic glucose solution for hypoglycemia.

Monitoring of the *cardiovascular system* is achieved by observing vital signs and blood pressure, ECG, and oxygen saturation. An arm cuff is usually satisfactory for following the blood pressure. For difficult cases, direct arterial cannulation not only is more precise but also allows blood sampling. Alternatively, a Doppler ultrasound flowmeter also provides direct measurements. It may be necessary also to monitor end-expiratory CO_2. A precordial stethoscope allows the heart and breath sounds to be followed.

Monitoring blood loss is discussed on page 11.

Table 1. Checklist for Malignant Hyperthermia

Action	Dosage, Instructions
Remove triggering agent	
Hyperventilate with 100% O_2	O_2 requirement 3–5× normal
Sodium bicarbonate	
Dantrolene	1–10 mg/kg at 1 mg/kg/min
Ice pack	
Diuretics	
Insert urethral catheter	Monitor urine color, pH, volume
Monitor for elevated serum K	Give insulin in 50% glucose
Monitor for decreased serum K	Replace K

Operative Management

POSITION OF THE PATIENT

The position of the patient is illustrated before each representative operation, accompanied by instructions for obtaining that position. Padding at all points of contact is essential, and the position should not put stress on joints or on the respiratory system.

ASSISTANCE

An assistant capable of taking over should you become ill should always be with you when you perform major surgery. The assistant should be familiar with the operation. The best assistants anticipate you. As Joseph Kaufman says, "Don't assist me, help me." In a teaching setting, quiz the assistant as the operation proceeds. What is this tissue? And that structure? In this way you will do some teaching, and the next time you will get more help and better understanding.

The main function of an assistant is to provide exposure. This is accomplished not only by retraction (which is really the job of a self-retaining retractor or a second assistant) but by anticipating the next move and grasping the appropriate tissue layer at the right time and place. A good first assistant can essentially do the operation this way; the surgeon merely follows the lead. We know this from "assisting" first-year residents. And like the crew in a yacht race, the assistant should be encouraging and optimistic. Surgeons, like skippers, need all the support they can get.

The second assistant, who stands sideways and out of the way at the surgeon's side, provides exposure with retractors and stick sponges. He or she also removes the loose ends of sutures from the field. It's only fair to let this assistant tie some knots, do the appendectomy, or help close the wound.

Much can be learned by watching Richard Turner-Warwick operate. He is such a master at arranging his retractors and stay sutures that an assistant quickly and lamentably becomes an observer. Maximal utilization of self-retaining retractors and stay sutures needs to be cultivated. The various ring retractors now available allow the use of all combinations of blades, hooks, and stay sutures to maintain exposure during each step of the operation.

Those of us who instruct developing urologic surgeons must remember that we need to foster learning on several levels. Our demonstrations and examples at the operating table, along with suggesting readings from texts and atlases, plus lectures and video tapes, provide for *receptive learning*. More important is integrated learning gained by *guided inquiry*, by having the trainees explain the problems and options. Inexperienced urologists then learn on their own by *autonomous learning*, a process that continues throughout their careers.

Robert Gross was a great teacher. He had a sign in his operating room that said, "If an operation is difficult you are not doing it properly." According to Gross's student, Hardy Hendren, "Silence meant approval; a soft groan of exasperation signaled that the resident needed to figure out quickly what he was doing incorrectly and what should be done differently to meet his approval. A soft tapping of the foot was as effective as a spoken word, and meant 'get on with it'" (Hendren, 1989).

PROTECTION OF THE SURGICAL TEAM FROM VIRAL INFECTION

Human Immunodeficiency Virus

Whether every patient should be tested preoperative for human immunodeficiency virus (HIV) reaction is not clear. The assumptions must be made, however, that every surgical patient would test positively and that it is the surgeon's responsibility to operate upon all patients, regardless of their HIV status. Thus, extreme care must be exercised by all of the team exposed to blood or secretions.

Surgeons, anesthetists, and scrub personnel should wear protective glasses during invasive procedures and should wear protective boots or impervious shoe coverings routinely. Double gloves should also be used routinely. The risk to surgeons who operate with open skin lesions is unknown, but covering any small cuts or abrasions on your hands with sterile Tegaderm seals them in case of glove puncture.

When wearing gloves that have been contaminated, be careful not to handle objects in the operating room that may not receive routine cleaning. If the gloves of unscrubbed personnel become contaminated with blood or other body fluids, they should be changed as soon as possible. Similarly, if a gown becomes contaminated with blood, it should be changed as soon as possible. Remove all garments, such as gowns, gloves, and shoe covers, before leaving the operating room.

Exposed skin surfaces should be washed with detergent immediately after contamination with blood or body fluids. Hands should be washed immediately after gloves are removed at the end of a procedure.

Extreme caution should be exercised with needles and sharp instruments. Meticulous technique is required both in the immediate operative field and in the entire operating room to minimize accidental HIV exposure. Instead of having the nurse pass a sharp instrument directly, have the nurse set it on a neutral area from which you can pick it up. Extreme care should also be taken during operative procedures to avoid needle sticks. Needles should not be recapped, bent, or broken. After use, needles and disposable sharp instruments should be immediately placed in puncture-resistant containers for disposal.

Although needles are the greater hazard, a scalpel in the hand of the surgeon or the assistant can puncture through two layers of glove. Some surgeons may want to have a whetstone on the instrument table so that the tip of the blade can be dulled before the operation begins. The point of a scalpel is seldom needed because the cut is made with its belly.

Personnel entering the operative field in the middle of a procedure should put on their own gowns and gloves to prevent contamination of the inside of the garments with the patient's blood or bodily fluids, which may be on the scrub nurse's gloves.

Hepatitis B Virus

The overall risk of hepatitis B virus (HBV) infection is greater than that for HIV infection because, even though the frequency and type of exposure are similar, the prevalence of infective patients is somewhat greater and the risk of infection associated with each exposure is much higher. The reasons for the increased risk after exposure are that the titer of the HBV virus is much higher and infectivity is maintained on environmental surfaces much longer. Fortunately, most HBV infections are not manifested clinically and are self-limited. However, between 5 and 10 percent of those infected develop chronic infection (carriers), accompanied by an increase in the risk of cirrhosis and hepatocellular carcinoma.

Even though the risk for infection is greater with HBV than HIV, the surgeon can be vaccinated against HBV if he or she has not acquired natural immunity from previous exposure. Postexposure prophylaxis is provided by hepatitis B immune globulin (Rhodes, 1995).

POSITION OF THE SURGEON

Decide beforehand on which side of the table to stand. In this atlas, position is shown for right-handed surgeons. The exposure and procedure are also illustrated from that point of view.

Start with the table at a height that allows your elbows to be flexed at right angles, with your hands resting on the surface of the patient. Avoid putting your head down; your eyes (or corrective glasses) have a reading distance of greater than 30 cm. If you need more magnification, wear a loupe. Blocking the wound with your head makes it difficult for the light to penetrate and for your assistants to help you. And it looks amateurish. A shorter assistant should wear elevator sandals or stand on a lift.

For operations involving the perineum, you can sit on an adjustable stool. This is easier for you and allows your assistants to get a better view and be more helpful. Babies are exceptions; because they have short legs, the surgeon and assistants can work best while standing. Sitting is necessary for long, delicate operations, such as vasovasostomy. If you do choose to stand, make sure that no wires or tubing is underfoot and that the arm board is angled toward the head of the table to allow you free movement. Too much angulation, however, may injure the patient's brachial plexus.

SURGICAL TECHNIQUE

Good surgical technique is essential to get through complicated procedures. It is recognized by the absence of wasted motion and wasted time. The mind, eye, and hand all work together smoothly. Some surgeons tend to be fast but rough—a combination that saves time but unduly injures tissues and may even lead to disaster. So that you will not be hurried by the following surgeon and team, when you schedule a case add 25 percent to what you think your actual operating time will be.

Continuously think ahead to the next step. Don't wait until you need another kind of instrument or suture; ask for it ahead of time so that the scrub nurse will have it ready. Good surgeons keep moving. At the same time they watch every detail and are not afraid to stop during the procedure to consider alternatives.

Dissection

The tissue, the organ, and what needs to be done determine how each instrument is applied. For a node dissection, a sweeping motion with closed scissors may do the job. For a pyeloplasty, careful dissection is done by supporting the tissues with stay sutures, occasionally applying fine smooth forceps and incising with Lahey scissors. Sometimes a little hand traction or dissection with the finger helps, but blind finger dissection does not. Don't cut where you can't see. As John Donohue says, operating at the apex of one's exposure is dangerous. Obtain pointers by assisting good surgeons or by watching films of their techniques.

Don't depend on antibacterial agents to avoid infection. Rather, handle the tissues gently because healthy cells can resist infection. Plastic surgeon Bengt Johanson once told me that the

problem is not infection; it is "hematoma and tissue damage." The tools of careful surgeons are stay sutures and skin hooks. They use needle or bipolar electrodes for point fulguration, fine ligatures and sutures, and moist gauze. Fine forceps are useful, but remember that all forceps cause some injury to tissue. Vascular forceps with a longitudinal groove are excellent for deep tissues; Wangensteen or Russian forceps are useful for areolar tissue; and Adson forceps are best for skin. If forceps grasping your skin cause you pain, they will also damage tissue.

Visibility

The intensity of the light in the wound determines visual acuity. At least two light sources are required, with one shining over the surgeon's right shoulder. Focused beams should reach the bottom of the wound without interference from heads. For deep wounds, a head lamp or a fiber light on the sucker may help. In any case, don't put your head close to the wound.

The ability to see also increases with magnification. You should own a pair of binocular loupes permanently attached to plain or prescription glasses, which are ready to be flipped down when a closer view is needed. Be sure that the glasses fit well behind the ears; otherwise they may fall into the wound. Alternatively, keep less expensive industrial-type loupes on plastic headbands in the operating room, to be slipped on when needed.

Incision

Cut with a single stroke through the skin and subcutaneous tissue, using a good-sized scalpel. Multiple small cuts injure the vulnerable subcutaneous tissue and promote infection. Do not use the cutting current in the subcutaneous tissue; it damages a wider path than does the knife. Select a very sharp knife for the same reason. Let the scalpel float down through the fat until it meets the fascia. You do not need to discard the skin knife unless it is dull; it has been shown that it does not pick up significant bacteria from the skin.

The electrosurgical unit is useful for incising muscle, but not skin or subcutaneous tissue. Switch to the undamped cutting current and deliver it through the smallest available electrode. A needle electrode is often the best. Use an electrosurgical blade that is activated by a foot pedal rather than one with a button on the handle; the pedal leaves the hand free to grasp the handle in the most effective position. A laser knife decreases blood loss but greatly increases tissue damage; however, it may be found useful for massive excisions.

1 Realize that the surgical electrode is similar to a ray gun. It does not cut or coagulate through contact but rather through the arc that emanates from its tip. Avoid burrowing under the muscle before dividing it; burrowing only opens more tissue planes. Rather, progressively cut through the muscle with the cutting current, using long strokes and taking care not to go deeply in any one area. The muscle retracts so that the edge is exposed for hemostasis with the coagulating current. The next layer is uncovered for division. It is therefore not necessary to clamp, cut, and ligate muscles, a process that causes more necrosis than does electrosurgery.

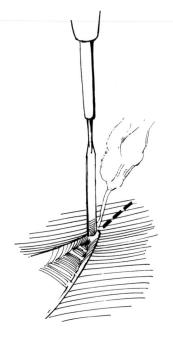

Hemostasis

Use pinpoint coagulation with damped current to control vessels less than 2 mm in diameter; this is quicker and produces less local destruction than suture ligation. Special bipolar coagulating forceps operated by the first assistant produce minimal damage to delicate tissues and can speed up the operation. An insulated knife or scissors connected to monopolar current may also reduce operating time. In any case, don't wave the electrode back and forth but be precise and touch only the bleeding vessel. For small bleeders in retractile muscle, insert the electrode first and then apply the current. For larger vessels, do not try to fulgurate them, but clamp first and then divide and ligate. These methods damage less tissue than when the vessel is cut and then roughly clamped and fulgurated. Electrocoagulation, similar to electroincision, increases the chance of infection three-fold; therefore, avoid its use in the skin and subcutaneous tissue.

Packing the Abdominal Contents

To expose the retroperitoneum and pelvis, follow this sequence: Hold the intestines in position with the left hand. Take an open laparotomy pad in the right hand and insinuate it under the palm of the left hand, tucking the pad under the viscera. (Always remember to place a ring or a large clamp on any sponge or pad introduced into the wound.) Pack the right gutter first, then the left, and finally the intervening small bowel with a third laparotomy pad. Place a moist rolled towel across the pads above the bifurcation of the aorta. Then place a Deaver retractor on the towel for higher exposure. Keep the wound edges and especially the surface of the bowel covered with moist laparotomy pads throughout the operation to reduce wound infection in dehydrated tissue.

Fixation of Organs and Tissues

Before closing a wound, restore all structures to a position as close to normal as possible. Pull the omentum down and spread it out over the intestines to separate them from the incision. In the flank, tack Gerota's fascia and the perirenal fat back together with 3-0 PCG sutures to isolate the repair site in the pelvis or ureter from the body wall. If the kidney has been dissected from its bed, it should be repositioned with a *nephropexy stitch* by inserting a mattress suture in the lower pole of the kidney at the appropriate place (insert pieces of fat under the sutures to prevent cutting into the parenchyma), and placing the stitch into the psoas muscle. After construction of intestinal segments, be sure to close the proximal edge of the mesentery against the retroperitoneal surface to prevent an internal hernia in the "trap."

Contamination and Infection

Before closure, wash the fat and tissue debris from the wound with sterile water by repeatedly filling and aspirating the wound bed. This significantly reduces the size of any inoculum. Washing allows primary closure in contaminated wounds because an inoculum must contain at least 10^6 bacteria to cause infection, no matter what the species. If contamination is especially feared, use a solution of bacitracin, 500,000 units, and neomycin, 0.5 gm in 1000 ml of saline, as extraperitoneal (not intraperitoneal) irrigation. Erythematous, infected wounds or those grossly contaminated should be left open, covered with gauze, and then closed secondarily 3 or more days after the operation.

BLOOD LOSS AND TRANSFUSION

Because 7 percent of body weight is blood, a man weighing 70 kg has a circulating blood volume of about 5000 ml. A loss at operation of up to 15 percent of this volume does not affect blood pressure, pulse pressure, respiration rate, or the capillary blanch test. Unless other fluid losses are occurring, you can count on transcapillary refill and other compensatory mechanisms to restore blood volume.

A volume loss between 15 and 30 percent, however, representing 800 to 1500 ml of blood in an adult (this is Class II hemorrhage on the scale of trauma surgeons), causes tachycardia, tachypnea, and most significantly, a decrease in pulse pressure. Realize that the systolic pressure may be fairly well sustained, but a rise in diastolic pressure is ominous. The capillary blanch test becomes positive, and the urinary output falls moderately to between 20 and 30 ml/hr. These patients require transfusions.

A loss of more than 30 percent (2000 ml) produces a measurable drop in systolic blood pressure (Class III hemorrhage).

Initially replace blood loss with lactated Ringer's solution, giving a bolus of 1 to 2 L in an adult and 20 ml/kg in a child. Observe the response. If the signs are not reversed or are only transiently improved and if urinary output remains low, give packed red blood cells, if they are already matched, and establish a central venous pressure (CVP) line. Replace crystalloids in a ratio of three volumes for each volume of blood lost. In a real emergency, use type-specific or type O blood. Matched whole blood is best, of course, if it can be obtained. Transfusion requirements are listed in Table 1.

Coagulopathy becomes a problem after 10 units of blood have been replaced, mainly because of hemodilution. Should abnormal bleeding appear after replacement, obtain a "clotting screen" and give a platelet pack. If clotting factors are found to be significantly deficient, give at least 300 ml of fresh frozen plasma. Hypothermia exacerbates clotting abnormalities; therefore, warm all fluids and gases, provide warm blankets, and irrigate the abdominal cavity with warm saline.

Fluid overload may occur even though the CVP has not reached normal levels. Instead of depending upon the CVP, watch for return of adequate perfusion by observing urinary output, skin color, and return of pulse rate and blood pressure readings toward normal. However, if overload does occur, avoid diuretics because they render measurement of urine output useless as a guide and may precipitate hypovolemia.

If severe blood loss is expected, consider autotransfusion if a machine is available. Controlled sodium nitroprusside–induced hypotension can be used in younger patients.

Table 1. Effects of Blood Loss (70-kg Male)

Estimated loss	750–1500 ml (<15%)	1500–2000 ml (15–30%)
Pulse	>100	>120
Respiration	20–30/min	30–40/min
Blood pressure	Normal	Decreased
Pulse pressure	Decreased	Decreased
Capillary blanch test	+	+
Urine output	20–30 ml/hr	5–15 ml/hr
Fluid replacement	Crystalloid	Crystalloid and blood

Adapted from ACS Committee on Trauma: Advanced Trauma Life Support Student Manual. Chicago: American College of Surgeons, 1993, p 86.

DRAINS

Drainage tubes produce harmful effects, but these are usually outweighed by their benefits in urologic patients. Drains do render the tissue more susceptible to bacterial invasion and provide the route for bacterial entry from the skin and external environment, but they also facilitate the exit of potentially contaminated urine, serum, and blood, as well as collections of pus. The most common purpose for a drain is prophylaxis, that is, preventing the accumulation of potentially infected blood, serum, or urine. Any surgical wound is susceptible to infection, and hematomas increase the risk. The indications for drainage are still controversial, and neither drains nor antibiotics are substitutes for an atraumatic surgical technique. Make a decision about drainage at the end of the operation based on the operation and the patient's condition. For example, after a retroperitoneal operation, a drain allows trapped air and blood to escape; it may be removed the next day. When the urinary tract has been opened, a drain placed extraperitoneally is especially important to provide an escape route for urinary leakage; remove it 2 or 3 days after you are sure drainage has stopped.

Currently, two types of drains are in use: passive drains, such as the Penrose, and the more costly, active-suction drains, such as the closed (Jackson-Pratt or Hemovac) or open (sump) drain. Passive drainage depends upon intra-abdominal or wound pressure; active drainage, upon suction. Passive drainage is adequate for most urologic wounds, as it permits escape of air and any accumulated blood; if the urinary passages have been opened, it prevents formation of urinomas. Active, closed-suction drainage is valuable in more superficial operations, such as inguinal node dissection and, with miniaturization, in certain cases of hypospadias, to obliterate the space beneath the skin flaps. It may also be useful after major pelvic operations to detect postoperative bleeding.

Take care to keep the end of the drain away from contact with the site of repair or an anastomosis. One way is to suture the Penrose drain to a structure adjacent to the repair so that it is not displaced during closure. Use a plain catgut (PCG) stitch. A more secure way is to stitch the drain in place with a removable suture.

2 **Long Suture Technique** (see also page 917). First place a 3-0 SAS through one end of the Penrose drain and tie it. Then pass the suture through the adjacent fat or muscle so that the end of the drain lies within 2 or 3 cm of the repair site (**A**). Now stitch the suture through the side of the drain at a place that will be outside the body after the wound is closed, take up the slack, and tie it to itself. In all cases, transfix it with a safety pin (**B**). To remove the drain, cut the suture flush with the skin. The remaining suture follows the drain as it is withdrawn (**C**).

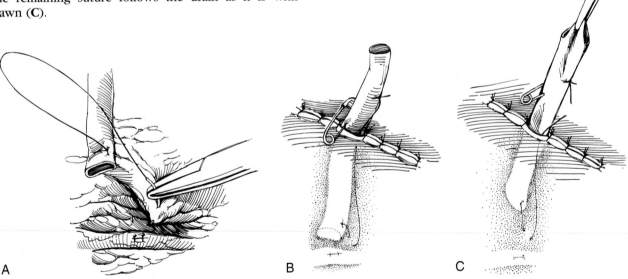

A   B   C

Generally a drain causes less harm if brought out through a separate stab wound. Only with poor hemostasis, urinary leakage, or gross contamination is it safer to have it exit through the wound itself.

CATHETERS AND TUBES

Catheters are inserted before an operation to empty the bladder and get it out of the way, to fill the bladder preparatory to its incision, to instill antibacterial or antineoplastic agents, or to allow identification of the urethra and vesical neck. For these purposes, a 22 F or 24 F balloon catheter is usually satisfactory. One made of silicone is preferable, even if it is to remain only a few days.

Intraoperatively, the catheter may be replaced with one of a smaller size (16 F), always made of silicone so that it is better tolerated by the urethral wall, as it is to be left indwelling. If clots are anticipated, use a larger catheter. In complicated cases such as radical perineal prostatectomy, the catheter should be stitched to the glans and taped to the penis and abdomen or leg, because its inadvertent removal could lead to serious complications.

Taping the Urethral Catheter in Place

3 If tape is to support catheters or tubing, it must be waterproof and applied over tincture of benzoin. Once applied, check it each day at evening rounds. Tubes don't just "fall out," despite frequent reports on rounds to that effect. A straight urethral catheter, if taped as described and monitored daily, remains indwelling in the male for 5 to 6 days.

Cut 0.5-inch tape into six 8-inch and two 2-inch lengths, then cut 1-inch tape into two 4-inch lengths. Coat the penis and its base as well as the catheter with tincture of benzoin and let it dry. Apply four long strips to the four quadrants of the penis and catheter. Allow the lateral and dorsal strips to extend up over the base of the penis onto the pubis. Wrap the two narrow short strips around the catheter to hold the long tapes. Place the two remaining long narrow strips around 90 percent of the penis, allowing room for erectile expansion. Place the last 1-inch pieces to hold the long strips onto the base of the penis.

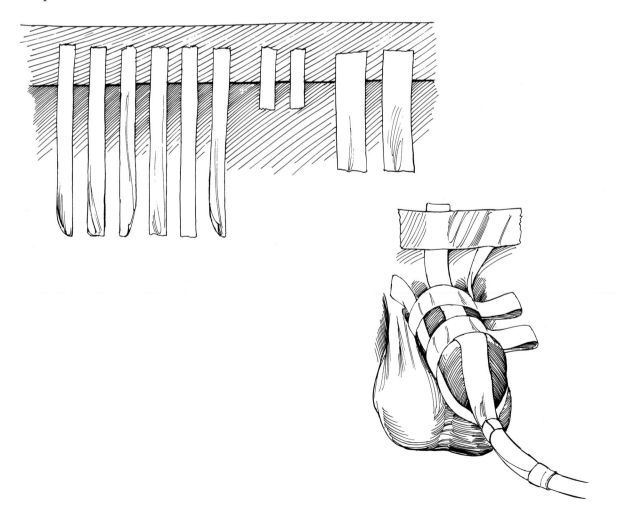

Balloon Catheter

The *balloon catheter* was invented by Frederic Foley primarily for the convenience of the physician, not because it is more physiologic than a straight catheter. In fact, it leaves about 6 ml of "residual" urine in the bladder, which becomes infected in a few days. Further, the balloon may injure the vesical neck if traction is applied inadvertently. Finally, for a given external size, a balloon catheter has a smaller drainage channel than a straight catheter.

Nondeflating Balloon Catheter. When filling a balloon catheter, use only fresh water or saline; irrigating fluid may contain particulate matter. Several methods are available for deflation. Overdistend the balloon with water. Fill it with ether to burst the balloon or with mineral oil to dissolve the latex. If those measures fail, cut the catheter proximal to the valve. If no water drains from the balloon channel, pass a guide wire through it to free it of obstructing debris. In men, if the balloon remains inflated, rupture it with a needle passed suprapubicly. Another method is to cut the catheter at the meatus and ligate it with a long strong suture, then push it into the bladder with a panendoscope, puncture it under vision, and withdraw it with the long suture (Bazeed, 1993). In women, insert a spinal needle vaginally alongside the finger while palpating the balloon. Alternatively, insinuate a 20-gauge 2-inch angiocatheter with the tip of the needle drawn back inside the sheath through the urethra beside the catheter until it impinges on the balloon. Advance the needle to puncture the balloon (Carr, 1995). Another method is to pass a ureteroscope beside the catheter and puncture the balloon under vision. All these methods carry the risk of leaving a fragment of the balloon that may subsequently form a stone; check it cystoscopically.

Securing Tubes and Catheters

4 Place a 2-0 braided silk suture through the skin and tie it loosely. Loop it once around the catheter, snug it up, and tie it. Loop and tie it once more.

Transvesical Anchor Suture
(see page 429)

If the bladder is open, an alternative to using a balloon catheter is to place a heavy suture into the end of a Robinson catheter with a large curved Keith needle, insert both ends of the suture in the eye of the needle, and run the needle through the bladder and body walls. Tie the ends together over a bolster.

Remember to attach the drainage tube to the catheter while the patient is still on the table to prevent contamination of the connector in the recovery room.

Suprapubic Drainage

Consider a suprapubic tube after operations on the bladder and urethra. It has several advantages over one inserted by the transurethral route. It allows cystography and a trial of voiding before it is removed. This type of drainage is preferred in a patient who may have difficulty emptying the bladder postoperatively. It provides superior drainage, especially if a 24 F Malecot catheter is used. Such a tube is less likely than a balloon catheter to become dislodged because it is routinely stitched to the skin. The disadvantages are the need to create a wound in the bladder and body wall and the tendency of the tip to irritate the trigone if it is not held up in the dome of the bladder.

Even if the bladder has not been opened, a suprapubic catheter can be placed during an open operation. Grasp the bladder between thumb and forefinger and insert a sharp clamp into the bladder on one side and out again on the other. Grasp the end of a balloon or Malecot catheter and pull it into the lumen, ducking it toward the trigone. Check that the catheter moves freely and that urine drains from it (Woo et al, 1996).

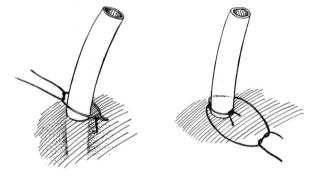

POSTOPERATIVE NERVE BLOCK

Even if the patient is operated upon under general anesthesia, blocking the site with the long-acting agent bupivacaine can reduce postoperative pain; this is especially useful in children who are not to be kept in the hospital. A caudal block with 0.5 ml/kg of 0.25 percent bupivacaine given just before making the incision continues to provide good analgesia to a child after the return home (see precautions described previously). For adults with flank wounds, inserting an infant-sized feeding tube in the posterior end of the wound and instilling no more than 20 ml of 0.5 percent bupivacaine during the postoperative period are effective in reducing pain. Take care not to enter the costal veins. Bupivacaine intravenously can cause cardiomyopathy with asystole, an effect that apparently is not dose related. Remember that properidol intraoperatively can decrease nausea and vomiting in patients who receive local anesthesia.

DRESSINGS

Avoid placing a truly occlusive dressing. Use one porous enough to allow skin products and wound secretions to move away from the wound.

Apply tincture of benzoin to the skin before placing adhesive tape. The tape adheres better and causes less irritation of the skin.

5 Montgomery straps are needed if appreciable drainage is expected and abdominal pads will have to be changed frequently.

Usually leave the dressing in place for at least 3 days. By that time the incision has sealed and is no longer susceptible to contamination.

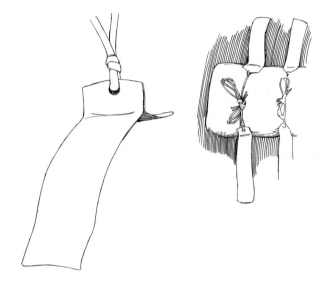

Postoperative Management

After complex cases, consider obtaining a plain x-ray film of the operated area on the way to the recovery room to be certain that sponges and clamps have not been left in the wound.

RECOVERY ROOM

In the recovery room use a postoperative checklist for orders, such as that outlined in Table 1, to avoid overlooking something important.

Monitor respiratory functions as listed in Table 2. For problems with acute renal failure refer to Table 3, and for septic shock use the lists in Tables 4 and 5.

Operative Report

Dictate the operative report yourself, not only for legal reasons but so that it will be useful in the follow-up of the patient and as a reference for future operations (or for a book you may write some day). Residents, be discreet but include all the facts to help you next time.

Operative records can be very valuable for a surgeon's education. It is a good idea to label 8 to 10 folders with the names of the various organ systems. After each operation, place a photocopy of your operative report in the appropriate folder, but only after making marginal notes about the objectives of the operation, what difficulties you might have expected, what steps were important, where you should have anticipated pitfalls, where you had to stop and make a key decision, and what you thought you did especially well. You can add a list of instruments you couldn't do without.

In addition, at the end of the procedure, draw a diagram of the patient in the chart, labeled to show the exit sites of the various tubes and drains for reference by house staff and nurses.

AVOIDANCE OF POSTOPERATIVE PROBLEMS

Expect that some of your patients will have complications, but many can be prevented if you are careful and think ahead as you work. *Prevention* is the purpose of the Death and Complication Rounds that are held at most hospitals. You can learn not only from your own mistakes but also from those of your colleagues. If you could just think of all possible untoward events, you could take measures to prevent most of them. In this atlas, most of the important postoperative problems are described at the end of the surgical protocols, although it may be too late to prevent them by the end of the operation. Therefore, be sure to review the possible complications before starting. With equally difficult case loads, the better surgeon has fewer postoperative complications.

Bleeding that occurs soon after the operation should have been controlled during it. If it appears later, it comes from

Table 1. Postoperative Checklist

1. Vital signs (every 15 min until awake; then every 4 hr; then as needed)
2. Mobilization (bed rest, up with assistance, turn and cough)
3. Intake and output
4. Pain and sleeping medication
5. Antibiotics
6. Diet (NPO; then clear liquids)
7. Laboratory orders
8. Nasotracheal suction, oxygen therapy
9. Care of catheters and drains
10. Monitor arterial and central venous pressure lines
11. Specific orders (wound monitoring; circulatory and neurologic checks)
12. Notification orders (hypotension, oliguria)

Table 2. Indications for Artificial Ventilation

		Normal Range
Tidal volume	<5 ml/kg	5–10 ml/kg
Respiratory rate	>35/min	12–20/min
Vital capacity	<15 ml/kg	65–75 ml/kg
FEV_1	<10 ml/kg	50–60 ml/kg
Force	-20 cm H_2O and above	-75 to -100 cm H_2O
PaO_2	<70 mm Hg (on mask O_2)	75–100 mm Hg (room air)
Alveolar-arterial gradient $P(A-aDO_2)$	>450 mm Hg	25–65 mm Hg
$PaCO_2$	>55 mm Hg	35–45 mm Hg
Deadspace (V_D/V_T)	>0.60	0.25–0.40

FEV_1, forced expiratory volume in 1 second; PaO_2, partial pressure of oxygen in arterial blood; $PaCO_2$, partial pressure of carbon dioxide in arterial blood.
Adapted from Fish D, Harp JR: Monitoring the critically ill urology patient. *In* Byrne JJ, Goldsmith HS (eds): General Surgery. Hagerstown, MD, Harper & Row, 1985, Ch 25, p 5.

Table 3. Checklist for Acute Renal Failure

1. Reduce fluid intake to measured losses plus 400 ml/day. Monitor intake, output, and body weight. Allow for small daily weight loss. Restrict sodium intake to measure losses. Remove potassium intake.
2. Treat elevations of plasma potassium above 5 mEq/L with sodium polystyrene sulfonate (Kayexalate) or hemodialysis.
3. Reduce protein intake but give 1200 to 1500 total calories per day.
4. Watch for acidosis. Give lactated Ringer's or sodium bicarbonate solution early.
5. Begin hemodialysis for weight gain, hyperkalemia, acidosis, and rising blood urea nitrogen levels.

Table 4. Checklist for Septic Shock

Findings:
  Reduced blood pressure and pulmonary capillary wedge pressure
  Greatly reduced peripheral resistance with increased cardiac output

1. Begin intravenous crystalloid fluids.
2. Install a pulmonary artery line (Swan-Ganz catheter). Measure right atrial, pulmonary arterial, and pulmonary capillary wedge pressures, as well as cardiac output.
3. Calculate hemodynamic variables.

	Normal Values
Arterial pressure	110–130/70–80 mm Hg
Mean arterial pressure (MAP)	82–102 mm Hg
Central venous pressure (CVP)	4–10 cm H_2O
Pulmonary artery pressure	25/10 mm Hg
Mean pulmonary artery pressure (PAP)	12–18 mm Hg
Pulmonary capillary wedge pressure (PCWP)	5–15 mm Hg
Right atrial pressure	1–10 mm Hg
Cardiac output (CO)	5–6 L/min
Stroke volume	60–90 ml
Total peripheral resistance $\dfrac{(MAP - CVP)}{(CVP)}$	11–18 U
Pulmonary vascular resistance $\dfrac{(PAP - PCWP)}{(CVP)}$	0.5–1.8 U

4. Start antibiotics.
5. Give vasopressors; consider naloxone.

Adapted from Fish D, Harp JR: Monitoring the critically ill urology patient. *In* Byrne JJ, Goldsmith HS (eds): General Surgery. Hagerstown, MD, Harper & Row, 1985, Ch 25, p 9.

Table 5. Treatment for Septic Shock

Antibiotic therapy
Surgical procedures (with radiologic guidance)
    Drainage of abscess
    Débridement
    Removal of foreign body
Therapy for shock and organ failure
    Correct cardiovascular derangement
    Correct metabolic derangement
    Correct fluid balance
    Give vasoactive and cardiovascular drugs

Consider organ-specific agents: anti-endotoxin, anti–gram-positive, and anti–fungal cell wall agents; non–organ-specific agents: antimediator/anti-inflammatory agents (anti–tumor necrosis factor, anti–interleukin-1, anti–platelet-activating factor).

Adapted from Sundaresan R, Sheagren JN: Current understanding and treatment of sepsis. Infections in Urology January/February, 1996.

disruption of part of a ligature or suture line and requires immediate intervention. Blood loss can be recognized by the clinical signs. Hematocrit determinations are unreliable and inappropriate to estimate acute blood loss. A patient who is cool and tachycardic is in shock and needs immediate transfusion. Septic shock produces a wide pulse pressure, an important differentiating point. The exception is the patient who is uremic or has received drugs like Motrin in whom bleeding can be controlled by administration of cryoprecipitate or desmopressin for immediate effect or conjugated estrogens for a more prolonged effect (Livio et al, 1986).

Peripheral ischemia must be watched for postoperatively by checking the femoral, popliteal, or dorsalis pedis pulse, by comparing pedal temperatures, and by inspecting skin.

FLUID REQUIREMENTS

Volume depletion is signaled in the recovery room by weakness, orthostatic hypotension, tachycardia, weak pulse, dry tongue, and poor skin turgor. The blood urea nitrogen level is disproportionately high in relation to the serum creatinine level. Replace half the estimated deficit in 8 hours and the other half in the subsequent 16 hours, in addition to giving maintenance fluids, while monitoring the CVP. Use hypotonic solutions in patients with elevated sodium levels and isotonic saline solution for the others. A fluid overload of 3 to 5 L causes edema, often accompanied by dyspnea, tachycardia, venous engorgement, and pulmonary congestion.

Hypotonic hyponatremia occurs in surgical patients after third-space losses and results in low urine volumes with high osmolarity. Replace the losses with saline solutions. Hypovolemic hypernatremia results from unreplaced renal or gastrointestinal water losses, producing thirst, hypotension, and lethargy. Use 5 percent dextrose in water to return the serum sodium level to normal over 24 hours, measuring it every 6 hours.

PAIN

Nerve Blocks

Postoperative pain may be aborted by bupivacaine nerve blocks and wound infiltration to provide enough time for the patient to start oral pain medication. Refer to Tables 6A and 6B, for available medications for mild-to-moderate pain and for severe pain.

Continuous epidural regional anesthesia is particularly versatile because it can be applied as the entire anesthetic and thus reduce the dose of general anesthetic. It can then be continued to provide pain relief postoperatively. Place the catheter through a needle at T7 to T9 for upper abdominal incisions and at T10 to T12 for those in the lower abdomen. Check by aspiration and by a 2-ml test dose of lidocaine. If negative, induce spinal block. Postoperatively, continue the infusion with an IVAC pump using morphine or a local anesthetic–narcotic combination such as morphine and bupivacaine in doses that produce a sensory but not a motor block. Bupivacaine is se-

Table 6A. Narcotic Analgesics for Mild to Moderate Pain

Name	Equianalgesic Dose (mg)	Starting Oral Dose (mg) (Range)	Comments
Aspirin	650	650	In combination not anti-inflammatory
Acetaminophen	650	650	
Motrin (ibuprofen)	ND*	200–400	Like aspirin
Nalfon (fenoprofen)	ND	200–400	Like aspirin
Dolobid (diflunisal)	ND	500–1000	Like aspirin
Naprosyn (naproxen)	ND	250–500	Like aspirin
Trilisate (choline magnesium trisalicylate)	ND	1500	No effect on platelets
Codeine	32–65	32–65	Impaired ventilation
Oxycodone	5	5–10	Like codeine
Demerol	50	50–100	Accumulates
Darvon (propoxyphene HCl)	65–130	65–130	
Talwin (pentazocine)	50	50–100	Combined with naloxone

*ND indicates not determined.
Adapted from Paulson DF: Management of postoperative pain in the urologic patient. Problems in Urology 3:219, 1989.

Table 6B. Narcotic Analgesics for Severe Pain

Name	Equianalgesic Intramuscular Dose (mg)	Intramuscular/Oral Potency	Starting Oral Dose (mg) (Range)	Comments
Morphine	10	3	30–60	Standard of comparison
Dilaudid (hydromorphone)	1.5	5	4–8	Shorter duration
Dolophine (methadone)	10	2	5–20	Good orally
Levo-Dromoran (levorphanol)	2	2	2–4	May accumulate
Heroin	5	(6–10)		
Demerol (meperidine)	75	4		Slightly shorter acting than morphine
Codeine	130	1.5		Orally for lesser pain
Talwin (pentazocine)	60	3		Orally for lesser pain
Nubain (nalbuphine)	10			
Stadol (butorphanol)	2			

Adapted from Paulson DF: Management of postoperative pain in the urologic patient. Problems in Urology 3:219, 1989.

lected because it produces the least motor block for the greatest sensory block.

Side effects are few: hypotension, pruritus, sleepiness, and weakness in the legs. Respiratory depression is uncommon, usually the result of overdosage. The benefits are many, including excellent pain relief, decreased analgesic requirements, and decreased nausea and vomiting, the three most common postoperative complications. The catheter is removed in 3 to 5 days or if any evidence of infection is seen. The result is earlier ambulation and discharge and more rapid return to normal activity.

Caudal block is useful not only in children for circumcision, hypospadias repair, hernia repair, orchiopexy, and hydrocelectomy, using 0.125 to 9.25 percent bupivacaine (0.5 to 0.75 ml/kg), but also in adults for a variety of operations on the lower torso. This block has an excellent safety record.

A *dorsal nerve block* of the penis, using 1 to 4 ml of 0.25 percent bupivacaine without epinephrine, is appropriate for many operations on the penis, although minor complications have been seen. Instillation of anesthetic locally or by topical application can also be a useful supplement. *Ilioinguinal/iliohypogastric block* (0.25 to 0.5 percent bupivacaine, up to 2 mg/kg) may be also effective for an inguinal incision.

Analgesics and Narcotics

An *oral analgesic* such as acetaminophen with or without codeine can be given if the pain is mild (see Table 6A). For pain control at home, elixir of Tylenol with codeine can be effective.

Intravenous Agents. If these measures are inadequate to control pain, supply drugs intravenously with agents such as morphine given at a rate of 0.05 mg/kg/hr or demerol given every 2 hours in a dose of 0.5 mg/kg. If the patient with severe pain cannot be given a local anesthetic for postoperative analgesia, a narcotic such as fentanyl (up to a dose of 2 μg/kg IV) is appropriate. *Patient-controlled analgesia* is preferable to the intramuscular administration of narcotics. The patient may receive up to 1 mg of morphine per hour intravenously, with a lock-out time to prevent overdosage. As a substitute, the nonsteroidal anti-inflammatory drug ketorolac has an analgesic potency equal to that of morphine and has fewer undesirable effects. Give a loading dose of 60 mg IV at the time of wound closure, then give 30 mg every 6 hours IV. Continue patient-controlled morphine on an "as-needed" basis. When bowel function returns and oral intake is possible, change to oral administration.

Postoperative Infections

Fevers occurring during the first or second postoperative day probably originate in the *respiratory tract*. Provide for coughing and deep breathing; ask the respiratory team for help. After the second day, look for infection in the urinary tract as well as for *abscesses* and *extravasation*. For invasive infections, supplement antibiotic therapy with nasal oxygen.

Wound infections are placed into three categories, depending on the type of wound from which they originate: from clean/uncontaminated wounds, from clean/contaminated wounds, and from frankly contaminated wounds. Postoperative infec-

tions are more common in neonates in all three categories, perhaps related to poor immunity and to the presence of the contaminated umbilicus. Other factors are undernutrition, diabetes, obesity, and hypoxemia.

For diarrhea postoperatively, examine the stool for *Clostridium difficile* toxin. If found, start metronidazole (Flagyl) at once.

WOUND MANAGEMENT

Even if the staples or stitches are removed on the seventh postoperative day, the wound may separate superficially. Apply sterile strips at the time of suture removal, and delay removal for 10 to 14 days in high-risk patients and in wounds on the back. Drainage of peritoneal serous fluid indicates fascial disruption and wound dehiscence. Mass closure techniques reduce the incidence of these complications, especially if buried retention sutures are used. Closing a midline transperitoneal incision (see page 867) with running No. 2 nylon or similar suture reduces the chance for wound infection and breakdown. Repair of late incisional hernias, related to weight gain and decrease in abdominal wall strength, may require application of synthetic mesh (see pages 908 to 909).

LATE COMPLICATIONS

Complications occurring late after surgery are discussed in the atlas after the appropriate operative descriptions. The alternatives available for reversing these complications have been assembled and are displayed in Table 7.

Table 7. Options for Correction of Specific Late Complications

Organ	Complication	Options
Ureter	Stricture or loss	Ureteroureterostomy
		Mobilization of kidney
		Psoas hitch; bladder flap; ileal ureter
	Dilation	Tailoring
Ureterovesical junction	Stricture	Reimplantation
	Reflux	Reimplantation
		Ileal nipple
		Others
Detrusor	Reduced compliance	Pharmacology
		Neural manipulation
		Hydrodistention
		Augmentation
		Vesicostomy
	Increased compliance	Intermittent catheterization
Outlet	Contracture	Dilation
		YV-plasty
	Incompetence	Vesical neck repair
		Sling with intermittent catheterization
		Artificial sphincter
		Closure of neck
	Dyssynergia	Sphincterotomy
		Intermittent catheterization

SECTION
2
The Urologist at Work

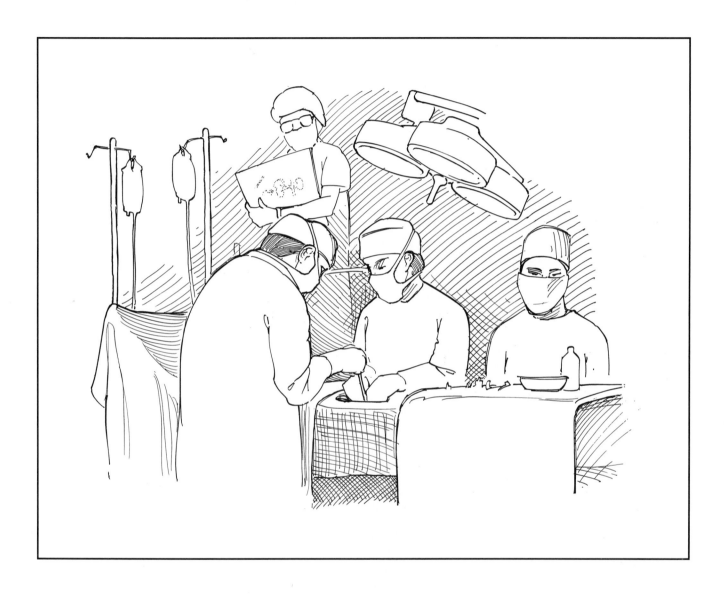

Basic Surgical Techniques

Those of us specializing in urology have need for skills and techniques common to all surgeons, especially in approximating tissue, anastomosing bowel, and closing wounds. We should come to the operating table armed with a set of general surgical procedures that we can apply in any urologic operation. These include the elements of suturing and plastic repair, the techniques of laparoscopy and microsurgery, and the methods for the repair of vascular or intestinal injuries.

Not only must we be able to use these basic techniques, but occasionally we must perform procedures that are not strictly in the field of urology. We may lacerate a spleen or injure a vessel, or we may need to form a gastrostomy for feeding during recovery or make a transverse colostomy for fecal diversion. Although a surgical colleague can help if available, we should be prepared for any emergency by having an adequate repertoire of suitable procedures in general surgery, and we should have the ability to do a few standard general surgical procedures without outside help. In this chapter the basic surgical techniques are described in detail so that they can be applied during any operation when required.

Basic Laparoscopy

TRAINING FOR LAPAROSCOPY

Urologists who perform laparoscopy have special training. The learning curve is steep, but once they master the basics, they continue increasing their skills if they expand their practice. On the other hand, urologists who do not have the training or do not have enough volume to keep in practice can be comfortable practicing standard urologic care without applying laparoscopic techniques.

CONTRAINDICATIONS TO LAPAROSCOPY

Transperitoneal laparoscopy is inadvisable in patients with abdominal wall infection, large abdominal hernias, extensive prior abdominal surgery, advanced intra-abdominal malignancy, intestinal distention and/or obstruction, appreciable hemoperitoneum, generalized peritonitis, abdominal wall infection, persistent coagulopathy, and shock. It is also a poor choice for patients with severe cardiopulmonary disease because pneumoperitoneum may reduce venous return to the heart. Chronic obstructive pulmonary disease may also be a contraindication. Patients who have large abdominal masses or aneurysms, who are extremely obese, or who have ascites are poor candidates.

Extraperitoneal laparoscopy (see page 994) and minilaparotomy (see page 995) are alternatives under certain circumstances.

MONITORING EQUIPMENT

Have available an electrocardiograph, a pulse oximeter, a blood pressure cuff, and a precordial or esophageal stethoscope. Have capnography available to follow CO_2 elimination, but take samples for blood gases in longer cases.

INSTRUMENTATION

Instruments include insufflator, imaging system with camera and monitor, puncture needles, and appropriately sized trocars with sheaths (either reusable or disposable). Laparoscopic instruments include a pair of 5-mm cutting-coagulating (endoscopic) scissors, two 5-mm coagulating-dissecting graspers, dissecting instruments, a needle driver, ligators, hemostats, stapling devices for vascular and tissue staples, a fan-type bowel retractor, a 10-mm spoon-shaped grasper, an ultrasonic attachment, baskets or entrapment devices with a tissue morcellator, a suction-irrigation device, monopolar or bipolar electrocautery, an argon-beam coagulator, and a disposable clip applier. In addition, it is well to have a robotic arm to hold intruments, an aquadissection system, and laser systems. For an extraperitoneal approach, prepare a balloon from a glove finger (see page 994), or obtain one commercially (Preperitoneal Distention Balloon System, Origin Inc., Menlo Park, CA).

A *standard laparotomy set* should be in the room on standby, ready to use if it becomes necessary to convert from a laparoscopic to an open procedure.

PREPARATION

Inform the patient of the nature and risks of the procedure and of the chances for resorting to open operation.

For major cases, provide a mechanical and antibiotic bowel preparation to reduce intestinal volume as well as decrease the ill effects of inadvertent bowel injury. For lesser operations, advise a clear liquid diet the day before and one packaged enema the night before. Type and screen (or cross-match for difficult cases) the patient for blood in case of hemorrhage. Give 1 g of cephazolin parenterally. Place compression stockings. Use endotracheal anesthesia.

Position the patient to contain the arms at the sides to prevent brachial or ulnar injury. Pad the elbows. Do not use arm boards; these impede the operators' access and the ability to move the patient into different positions needed to encourage the intestines to fall out of the field. Insert a urinary catheter and a nasogastric tube to empty the bladder and stomach. Except when performing orchiopexy, wrap the penis and the scrotum in Kerlix elastic tape to avoid pneumoscrotum. Prepare the skin from nipple to midthigh and from table top to table top; that is, have the abdomen prepared for an open operation if complications intervene. Take special care to clean the umbilicus. Drape the patient to leave the scrotum or vagina exposed, allowing manipulation of testes or uterus.

PNEUMOPERITONEUM

Check the pressure in the operating room CO_2 tank, and keep a spare tank in the anteroom. Place the patient in a 15-degree head-down position. Select the umbilicus as the site for induction of pneumoperitoneum: It is central, thin, and surrounded by few vessels, and the scar will be hidden. It does, however, lie directly over the sacral promontory and the aortic bifurcation or right common iliac artery. For insufflation, use the Veress needle or the open Hasson technique. The latter is safer. It should be used in children and in the presence of adhesions.

Veress Needle Technique

The Veress needle has an internal diameter of 2 mm and an outer diameter of 3.6 mm. It is available in lengths from 70 to 150 mm. The outer sheath has a sharp cutting edge. The inner obturator is blunt and retracts within the sheath during passage through the body wall but extrudes within the abdominal cavity to protect the bowel.

Make a short incision at the upper (or lower) rim of the umbilicus with a hooked (#11) blade. The peritoneal membrane is more firmly attached supraumbilically so that preperitoneal placement is less likely. If the patient has had a previous operation, select a site opposite that of the previous incision, placing the incision in the right or left upper or lower quadrant. In such cases, open insertion with the Hasson trocar is preferred.

1 **A** and **B,** Grasp and slightly elevate the adjacent skin in two towel clips to stabilize the anterior abdominal wall and draw it away from its contents. *Alternatively,* grasp the umbilicus in a towel clamp, and have the assistant grasp the lower abdominal wall. Hold the needle with its base in the palm and with the index finger along the shaft. Use the other hand as a brake. Let the edge of the hand rest on the abdomen to prevent inadvertent deep insertion. Keep the insufflation port toward the abdomen. Push the needle through the abdominal wall at a 60- or 90-degree angle, noting two successive planes of resistance as it passes first through the fascia and then through the peritoneum. Rotation of the needle aids its passage through the fascia.

C, Passage through the peritoneum is followed by a click as the obturator springs out to shield the sharp edge of the needle.

Confirm the position of the needle by aspiration. Do this by placing a 10-ml syringe containing 5 ml of saline on the stopcock, opening it, and simply aspirating. There should be no return: no blood, bile, intestinal contents, or urine. Such a return indicates injury to peritoneal contents and possibly warrants open laparotomy, depending on the surgeon's experience (see "Problems with Laparoscopy"). Instill 5 ml of saline; it should enter freely. Aspirate; there should be no return. Disconnect the syringe, and see that the drop remaining in the hub disappears. Advance the needle 1 or 2 cm deeper; there should be no resistance. The needle should rotate easily through a full circle.

Connect the insufflator to the stopcock, and read the intra-abdominal pressure. It should be less than 10 mm Hg and should fall when the abdominal wall is elevated. Start the flow of CO_2 at a low rate of 1 L/min, and check immediately to be sure that the pressure does not rise above 10 mm Hg. If it does, do not hesitate to replace the needle, inserting it several times if necessary until the proper parameters are achieved. Continue filling, now at an intermediate rate of 2 L/min (the maximum allowed by the caliber of the needle), until the pressure reaches 15 mm Hg in an adult (admitting between 5 and 7 L in about 5 minutes) or 6 mm Hg in a child less than 6 months of age. Percuss the liver for loss of dullness. A higher pressure, up to 25 mm Hg, can be induced during initial trocar placement but should be reduced to less than 15 mm Hg for the procedure itself to minimize the risk of gas absorption and hypercarbia, as well as reduced venous return secondary to compression of the vena cava and reduced renal function from compression of the renal veins. Impaired ventilation results from pressure on the diaphragm, requiring an increase in ventilatory pressure with its risk for pneumothorax. Turn off the flow, and remove the needle.

Error. Be alert that the needle may have been placed in the preperitoneal space because it was inserted at too great an angle. In this abnormal position, the abdominal enlargement during inflation appears asymmetric. When the trocar and laparoscope are inserted, the error is recognized because only fat is seen. To correct the error, open the peritoneum with laparoscopic scissors, and guide the trocar beneath it. Or aspirate the space with a needle and reinsert the Veress needle properly. An alternative is to proceed to an open operation.

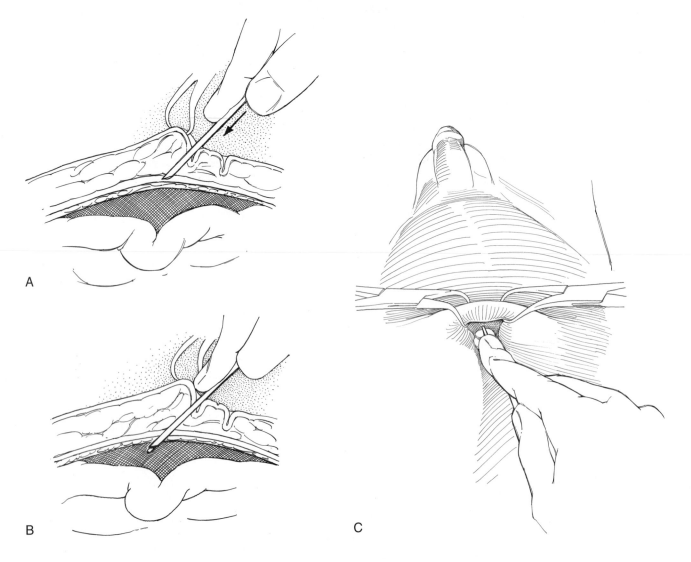

A

B

C

INSERTION OF PRIMARY PORT

2 Choose between (**A**) a reusable metal trocar (cheaper, but radiopaque) or (**B**) a disposable trocar (lighter, stays sharper, and has a safety shield that retracts on contact and springs forward and locks upon entry into the gas-filled abdominal cavity but costs more).*

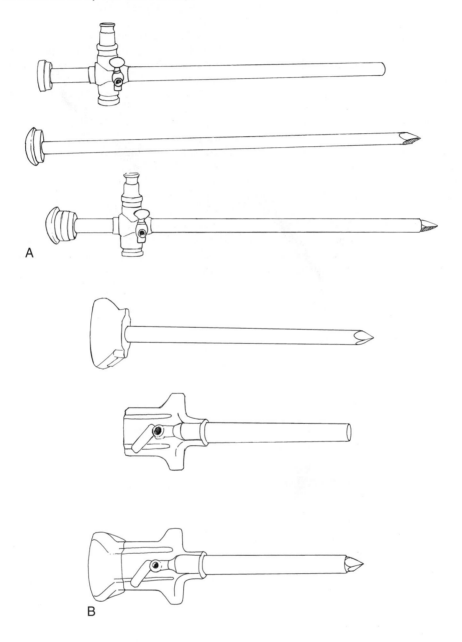

*Trocar, from Fr. *trois carre,* three sided. A surgical instrument traditionally used for drainage of body cavities. It consists of a pointed *obturator* (the trocar proper) enclosed in a *sheath* or cannula. The terms *trocar* and *trocar-sheath* are commonly (and properly) used to describe the combination of sharp obturator and *sleeve, sheath,* or *cannula,* and *port* is used for the sleeve. The use of the word *trocar* alone for the sheath can lead to confusion.

3 Select a 10-mm sheath (10 refers to inside diameter) with its contained sharp pyramidal trocar and retractable protective shield. Place the patient in a 15-degree head-down position. To insert the initial sheath and trocar, incise skin and subcutaneous tissue with a hooked blade transversely for a distance equal to slightly more than half the circumference of the 10-mm sheath (i.e., a little less than 2 cm). Make the incision either immediately above or, for pelvic procedures, below the umbilicus to the depth of the fascia at the linea alba, and spread it with a clamp to avoid injury to local vessels. Make a nick in the fascia with a #15 blade, taking care to include the peritoneum.

Place towel clips in the skin on either side of the incision to allow elevation of the anterior abdominal wall. This draws it away from the intestines and stabilizes it. Increase the intra-abdominal pressure to 25 mm Hg or greater. Hold the base of the trocar in the palm of the dominant hand while keeping the middle finger extended to prevent excessive penetration. Open the inflation valve. At first, hold the instrument vertically while penetrating the subcutaneous tissue. Then direct the trocar toward a point caudal to the sacral promontory (at a 60- to 70-degree angle for a pelvic procedure or toward the ipsilateral kidney for a renal procedure). Insert it into the abdominal cavity with a twisting motion of the wrist so that it does not suddenly jump through the wall. Resistance to the passage is felt at the fascial and peritoneal levels. As the peritoneal cavity is entered, see that the safety shield on the disposable trocar has descended by checking the indicator on the shield or by hearing the click as the shield descends to cover the trocar tip. (If the sheath descends prematurely, the trocar cannot be inserted; it must be withdrawn and the shield reset manually.)

As the trocar enters the peritoneal cavity, listen for the sound of gas escaping from the inflation valve. Remove the trocar from inside the sheath, and let the valve built into the sheath close the channel. Advance the trocar 1 to 2 cm. Connect the CO_2 tube, and set the flow control to maintain a pressure of 15 mm Hg.

Introduce a 10-mm laparoscope (endoscope) into the sheath with an attached focused and oriented full-beam videocamera. Monitor the area on the video screen placed at the foot of the table. First check immediately below the trocar to be certain no abdominal structures have been injured during needle or trocar insertion. Watch for blood running down the sheath, indicating an injured vessel in the body wall (see "Problems"). Gas leakage around the trocar site should not occur with a closed system but may require placement of a purse-string suture.

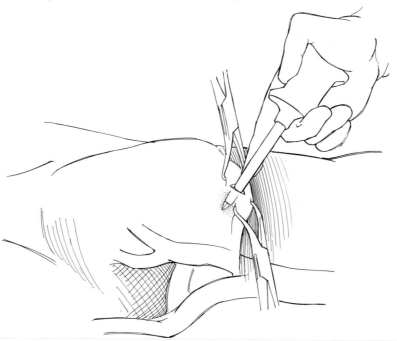

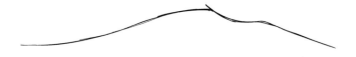

Open (Hasson) Technique

The open technique is safer. Even with injury to an adherent loop of bowel, the defect is immediately recognized and repaired. It is also better in obese patients. Its disadvantages are a slightly longer incision and more time for dissection, but this is compensated by the more rapid insufflation through the 10-mm trocar. It also permits removal of larger specimens, such as the kidney.

4 **A,** Make a 2-cm incision (longer in obese patients) in the midline above the umbilicus through skin to the level of the fascia while elevating the wall with towel clips. Place two heavy nonabsorbable sutures (NAS) in the tough periumbilical fascial fold, and incise it between them for 2 cm to reach the transversalis fascia and peritoneum. Pick up the peritoneum with forceps, and incise it under direct vision to enter the peritoneal cavity. Insert a finger to check for adherent bowel.

B, The Hasson cannula has a sleeve and a blunt-tipped obturator. Insert it through the opening in the peritoneum, and plug it firmly into the opening in the fascia. (An alternative is a screw-in port [Surgiport].) Wrap the fascial sutures around the wings to hold the occluding cone or sheath in place; they are used later to close the defect. Insufflate the peritoneal cavity at a rate of 6 to 8 L/min (insufflation can be faster than with the Veress needle). Insert the laparoscope with attached camera through the cannula.

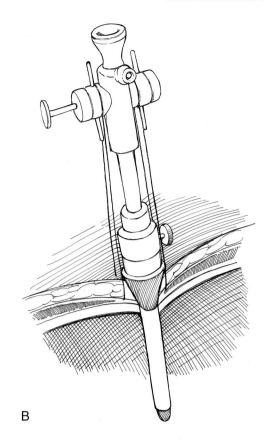

B

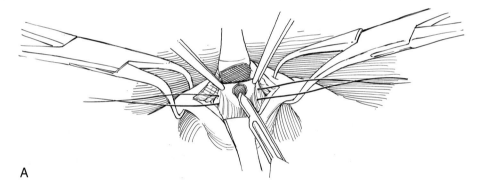

A

5 Systematically inspect the peritoneal cavity as for diagnostic laparoscopy.

A, *Male:* Note that the bladder terminates in the median umbilical ligament (urachus), which reaches to the umbilicus. The medial umbilical ligaments (obliterated umbilical arteries) lie parallel and lateral to it. More laterally, the inferior epigastric vessels may be seen through the peritoneal covering. Next, the vas deferens can be traced after it passes over the iliac vessels to its entrance into the internal inguinal ring with the spermatic vessels. The ureter crosses those vessels at a higher level and terminates behind the bladder, passing beneath the vas deferens and medial umbilical ligament. The sigmoid colon is evident on the left and the cecum and appendix on the right.

B, *Female:* The median and medial umbilical ligaments are seen, as are the round ligament entering the internal inguinal ring and the iliac and epigastric vessels. Below the bladder are the uterus, ovary, tubes, and round ligament.

C, In the upper abdomen, inspect the omentum for injury. Note the position of the spleen, stomach, gallbladder, and liver.

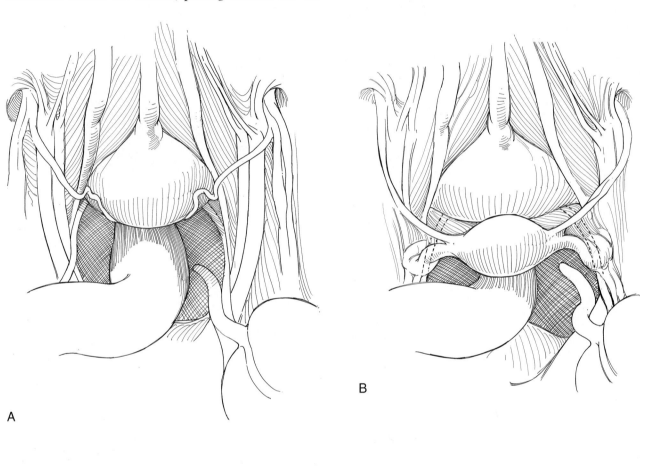

A

B

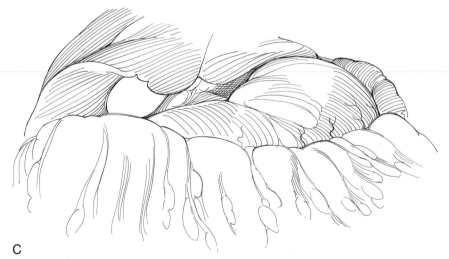

C

INSERTION OF SECONDARY PORTS

After the observation port is established below the umbilicus, select and mark appropriate sites for introduction of the instrument ports, depending on which area is to be treated. These trocars are 5 and 10 mm and do not need a safety shield, a sidearm for insufflation, or an elaborate valve. The larger 10-mm ports are placed either singly or in multiples, depending on the instrumentation to be used during the procedure (e.g., clip applier or entrapment sack). Placing a port too close to the operating site makes it difficult to manipulate such instruments as scissors and curved dissectors because of interference by the sheath. Placing it too far away creates a long fulcrum between the insertion site and the end of the instrument that, by exaggerating the movement of the tip, makes precise dissection difficult. Keep trocars away from bones and from each other. A few centimeters lateral to the border of the rectus muscle is usually a suitable site; beware of the inferior epigastric vessels.

Darken the room, and transilluminate the anterior abdominal wall to see the inferior epigastric and other vessels. Check to be sure that the pneumoperitoneum is complete at a pressure of 20 to 25 mm Hg. Insert the trocars required for the operation (see appropriate chapters). Under visual guidance, position them to form a circular array around the intended surgical site. Press on the abdominal wall with a finger, and note that the site of indentation is clear of vessels by placing the tip of the laparoscope against the site to define crossing vessels. Mark the size of the trocar by pressing the sheath on the skin, so that an incision of the proper size can be made, no larger than needed to allow admission of the particular trocar. With a clamp, open the incision to the level of the fascia to move significant vessels aside. Place each secondary trocar by pushing on the clamp again to view the site through which the trocar will pass to be certain that it is well removed from vessels or adhesions. Turn the laparoscope to bring the anterior abdominal wall into view. While illuminating the abdominal wall from within, insert the appropriate working ports, each with a twisting motion directed toward the area where the operation will be performed. Misdirected trocars are difficult to maneuver into proper alignment, and doing so may tear the peritoneum. Avoid traversing the inferior epigastric vessels, which can be seen by transillumination and by direct inspection.

If the trocar sheath has a detachable outer retentive groove, push the collar over the sheath until it extends 2 cm into the abdomen; then move the sheath back until it extends 2 cm beyond the collar, and tighten the retention bolt. With a spiral-grooved sheath, anchor it by screwing the spiral stability threads molded onto the sheath into the incision. The trocar sheath can also be held by heavy silk sutures in the skin, hooked over wings on the sheath to prevent displacement. If vessels in the abdominal wall appear too numerous to avoid, it may be possible to insert a floppy safety guide wire through a needle; remove the needle. Enlarge the tract with a fascial dilator; then introduce the trocar after the dilator has displaced the vessels. The fascial dilator is also useful for enlarging a 5-mm port to accommodate a 10-mm trocar.

Precautions are necessary to avoid injury to abdominal structures. Be sure to visualize the position of all instruments, and do not leave them unattended. Also, as soon as another port is placed, insert a 5- or 10-mm laparoscope through the port in order to examine the entry point of the primary trocar, thereby ruling out inadvertent bowel or omental injury.

LYSIS OF ADHESIONS

With laparoscopic scissors, divide only those adhesions that limit access to the operative site. Because most adhesions are related to previous incisions, make traction against the abdominal wall that has been elevated by the pneumoperitoneum, or have your assistant provide downward countertraction. Problems arise from injury to the intestine by the cautery and bleeding that may not be noticed. This is an ideal place to use only mechanical cutting or bipolar current; if monopolar current is used, be especially careful of injuries.

RETRACTORS

Graspers can often function for retraction. A solid metal bar with a rounded tip is useful for restraining bowel or the edge of the liver. A fan retractor has three flat blades that open into a fan shape for holding back a wider area. Likewise, the 5- and 10-mm expanding mechanical or balloon retractors are quite effective; the latter are atraumatic. Vein retractors are used to retract the external iliac vein.

IRRIGATION

With a combined aspiration/irrigation system, the aspiration channel is connected to the operating room vacuum system and the irrigation channel to a pressurized saline-heparin container. High-pressure irrigation can be used for some soft-tissue dissection.

DISSECTION

Pneumodissection with an instrument (Cook Urological) that delivers controlled bursts of high-pressure CO_2 allows the surgeon rapidly and bluntly to dissect along tissue planes without damage to adjacent organs.

SUTURING

Place sutures with a needle holder and graspers. Alternatively, apply an automatic device (Endo Stitch [Adams et al, 1995]) to insert the stitch and help tie the throw knots.

KNOT TYING

Polydioxanone Clip Technique

Draw the suture snug, and apply a synthetic absorbable clip (LapraTy, Ethicon) next to the tissue. Cut the ends of the suture. For securing a continuous suture, place a clip when the stitch is started and another at the end.

Fly-Casting Method (Kozminski, Richards)

First pass the needle through the tissue. Hold the free end taut with a clamp, and drop the needle over and behind it. Grasp the needle with a second clamp passed through the loop, and draw the needle through. Pull on both needle holders to draw the knot tight. Reverse the direction to form an opposite loop, thereby completing a square knot. Add additional loops to the knot, depending upon the suture material.

A similar knot can be placed using the automatic suturing device (Endo Stitch) to hold the end while a clamp manipulates the suture.

CLIPPING AND STAPLING

Clips are *occlusive* for securing blood vessels, *tacking* to approximate peritoneal surfaces (resurfacing), or *fastening* nonabsorbable mesh in place. Single-load appliers are cheaper in the long run, but multiple appliers save time, especially for operations involving numerous vessels or broad expanses of peritoneum, such as resurfacing the retroperitoneal space.

Staples (vascular or tissue load) are applied with a (disposable) stapler that inserts the staple and divides the tissue. They come in 3- and 6-cm lengths and usually place six rows of staples while simultaneously dividing the tissue between rows three and four. They are used, for example, to secure a cuff of bladder or, if applied successively, to occlude an isolated large vessel.

HEMOSTASIS

Accurate hemostasis is essential for laparoscopic surgery because any bleeding quickly obscures the field. When bleeding occurs, raise the pressure of the pneumoperitoneum to 20 mm Hg. Aspirate and irrigate the bleeding site. If the patient is otherwise stable, take some time to dissect the area around the bleeding site and precisely identify the source. If an artery has been injured, it can be seen spurting; if it is a vein, the increased intra-abdominal pressure tamponades it (this is true even for the inferior vena cava). If the injury is to a large artery, resort to an open laparotomy, vascular surgical consultation, and repair. If the bleeding vessel is isolated, apply the electrocautery or clip it. If important structures are adjacent, use the neodymium: yttrium-aluminum-garnet laser probe passed through the central channel of the suction-irrigation device. This not only restricts coagulation to a limited area but allows concomitant irrigation to cool the tissues. For parenchymal bleeding from the kidney, load 1 g of a microfibrillar collagen hemostatic substance (Avitene) into a 16-cm Teflon sheath with the aid of the butt end of an Amplatz dilator, and hold the resulting plug directly onto the bleeding surface for 3 to 5 minutes (Kerbl and Clayman, 1993). (A commercial device is available: Endo-Avitene, Med-Chem Products, Inc.)

ORGAN ENTRAPMENT

Introduce an impervious sack into the abdomen. Lead the whole organ into it and entrap it. Pull the drawstring to close the mouth of the sac, and deliver the string through a 10- or 12-mm port site. Fragment the contents with ring forceps, and remove the pieces to allow the sac to be withdrawn.

MORCELLATION

Although the size of the organ can be reduced in some cases with ring forceps or a Kelly clamp, a morcellator with a power-driven blade cuts the tissue and aspirates it into a trap in the handle of the instrument. The empty sack can then be removed.

LEAVING THE ABDOMEN

Lower the intra-abdominal pressure to 5 mm Hg. Inspect the operative site and each secondary trocar site. Remove the larger 10-mm sheath(s) first while the assistant holds a finger in the defect to preserve the pneumoperitoneum. Place two large skin hooks to catch the fascia on either side, and allow the fascial edges to be grasped in Allis clamps to maintain the pneumoperitoneum and also to facilitate placement of the fascial suture. Under observation from within, close the fascia from without with a 2-0 absorbable figure-eight suture swaged on a needle with an extreme curve (TT-3). Check the completeness of the closure by transabdominal inspection.

Irrigate the wound, and close the skin with a 4-0 absorbable subcuticular suture. Visualize the primary 10-mm trocar through a 5-mm laparoscope in a 5-mm port; remove the larger trocar, and close the fascia as described. Remove the smaller trocar sheaths in succession under vision while the assistant places a finger over each defect. Also under vision, withdraw the last trocar containing the 5-mm laparoscope. Manually decompress the scrotum. Release the fingers from the 5-mm openings, and allow the gas to escape. Apply sterile adhesive strips to all skin incisions

POSTOPERATIVE CARE

Remove the nasogastric tube and balloon catheter. Give two doses of a broad-spectrum parenteral antibiotic, and continue an oral antibiotic for the first 36 to 48 hours postoperatively. Start oral intake in the evening. Pain requiring parenteral analgesics suggests an underlying abdominal complication, such as a "missed" or "late" bowel leak.

LAPAROSCOPIC SURGERY IN CHILDREN

Laparoscopic procedures are somewhat different in children because the distance between the anterior abdominal wall and the great vessels is smaller and the organs are closer to the surface. Having shorter instruments, now under development, will help. In infants and small children, in whom the distance is extremely small, making a small paraumbilical incision first allows the insufflating needle to be passed by direct observation.

If the Veress needle is used, it requires less pressure because of the less-resistant fascia of the child; however, an open trocar insertion is safer. In the latter case, the peritoneotomy is sealed against the sheath with a purse-string suture. One new trocar has coarse threads and can be screwed into the abdomen through a small infraumbilical peritoneal incision. Less gas is needed to fill the small peritoneal cavity; it can be added at a slower rate. Transillumination of the abdominal wall is easy in children, a fact that helps placement of trocars to avoid vessels in the abdominal wall. Anatomic details are more clearly seen in children owing to the small amount of preperitoneal fat. This fact also reduces the chance for preperitoneal insufflation during insertion, but because the peritoneum is more loosely attached, it is more susceptible to emphysema. Also, the weak adherence to the abdominal wall makes the introduction of large cannulas difficult; an instrument introduced through a smaller port may be required to push upward on the abdominal wall to assist the entry of the larger-sized port.

Because children swallow air, it is important to decompress the stomach with a nasogastric tube and to leave it in place for extensive procedures.

Caution the parents that even though the operation is done through three to five small incisions, it is still a major surgical procedure because hemorrhage and bowel injury can lead to serious complications. Moreover, warn them that it may not be possible to complete the procedure through the instruments; an open operation may be necessary after all.

If adhesions are anticipated, prepare the bowel by both mechanical and antibiotic means. Give a broad-spectrum antibiotic parenterally preoperatively and postoperatively. Whether blood should be matched depends on the type of procedure and the risk of vascular injury, but blood should always be screened. As noted, it is mandatory to have a stand-by table with instruments ready for laparotomy in case of complications.

Use general anesthesia in children; the irritation of the diaphragm by CO_2 is painful, and any motion by the child is hazardous. Moreover, muscle relaxation is important because of the small intraperitoneal space with a greater liability for injury to intra-abdominal structures. Placement of a cuffed endotracheal tube is needed to ensure absence of voluntary respiratory movement and to allow mechanical assistance to respiration as the intra-abdominal pressure rises. Be aware that hypercarbia from absorbed CO_2 may be a problem during long procedures.

Compared with adults, the landmarks in children are readily palpated, including the aortic bifurcation and sacral promontory. The abdominal wall is thinner, and masses are easily felt. On the other hand, children have less space between abdominal wall and interior organs. They have an intra-abdominal bladder. Both bladder and stomach need to be decompressed before trocars are introduced. It is probable that children are no more susceptible to hypercarbia than adults because they have good lungs. Lower insufflation pressure (6 to 10 mm Hg) helps limit CO_2-related problems and the development of subcutaneous emphysema. The volume of CO_2 required to fill the peritoneal cavity varies from 0.5 to 3 L, depending on the age of the child.

For initial positioning, place the child supine. Give a parenteral dose of antibiotic. Induce anesthesia, and insert a cuffed endotracheal tube. Provide for pulse oximetry and for monitoring of end-tidal CO_2. Empty the bladder with a catheter, and leave it indwelling. Have the anesthetist place a nasogastric tube because a full stomach depresses the omentum into the route of the trocars. Determine by percussion that the stomach is empty. For orchiopexy and other pelvic procedures, insert a rolled towel under the lower back to create lordosis, and tip the table into a 10-degree head-down position to allow the intestines to drop out of the pelvis. Shift to a 30-degree head-down position for placement of the initial port. It can be helpful after the ports are inserted to tilt the table laterally 30 degrees to raise the involved side above the intestines. Prepare the entire abdomen in case laparotomy is required. Test all equipment before starting.

In infants less than 1 year of age, an open (Hasson) insertion is safer. For closed insufflation, it may be preferable to insert the Veress needle above the umbilicus in order to avoid the yet-undescended bladder. Begin insufflation with CO_2 at a rate of approximately 1 L/min until the pressure in a fully relaxed child reaches 15 to 20 mm Hg; then quickly withdraw the needle. Realize that some anesthetists do not immediately achieve relaxation.

The *primary port* is placed above or below the umbilicus. A 5-mm port may be large enough for infants but limits the types of instruments that can be used. As soon as the primary port is in place, reduce the intra-abdominal pressure to 10 to 15 mm Hg. *Secondary ports* are placed higher than in adults because a child has a smaller pelvis with generally shorter working distances. Therefore, place secondary ports at the umbilical level in infants and small children. The *physiologic effects* of laparoscopy on children include increased end-tidal CO_2, increased airway pressures, hyperthermia, oliguria, and mild renal tubular injury.

MINILAPAROTOMY

Operating through a limited incision is an alternative between open and laparoscopic surgery for node dissection and even for retroperitoneal nephrectomy. Make a short incision, place retractors strategically, and use standard operating room equipment. For a laparoscopically assisted retroperitoneal procedure, insert a trocar below the minilaparotomy incision and attach a video monitor so that the field can be viewed both through the incision and on the screen (Chung et al, 1995).

An alternative compromise is to make a short midline anterior abdominal incision. Place hooks under the edges of the wound to elevate the anterior abdominal wall, and allow air to fill the peritoneal cavity. Operate with laparoscopic instruments.

DIRECT EXTRAPERITONEAL ACCESS (Gauer)

Simple insufflation of the extraperitoneal space provides inadequate exposure because dissection is not uniform. By inflating a balloon just outside the peritoneum, the fibrous connections between it and the transversalis fascia can be separated, as is done with open extraperitoneal techniques of mobilization.

A balloon dissector is required. One can be made from materials available in the operating room (Gauer, 1992): A finger of size 7 surgical glove (washed) or latex balloon is tied over an 8 F red rubber catheter that is attached by a T to the pump of a sphygmomanometer and to a manometer to allow inflation and simultaneous observation of pressure. Alternatively, obtain a balloon dissector commercially.

For renal procedures, after the usual preparation and under general anesthesia, place the patient in the lateral position. Make a 2-cm incision through all layers just posterior to the tip of the 12th rib, in the superior lumbar triangle. With artery forceps on the finger, dissect a small space retroperitoneally. Grasp the knot at the tip of the balloon, and direct it into the retroperitoneal space. Place the balloon toward the area to be exposed: toward the umbilicus for exposure of the upper ureter, toward McBurney's point for exposure of the lower ureter and spermatic vessels, and toward the epigastrium above or below Gerota's fascia for renal exposure. Inflate it until a bulge on the abdomen can be seen. The balloon pressure varies from the 110 mm Hg needed to separate the transversalis fascia from the properitoneal fat to 40 or 50 mm Hg as the space is developed. Leave the balloon inflated for 5 minutes for hemostasis; then deflate and remove it. Insert a 10-mm Hasson-type laparoscopic sheath through the opening into the retroperitoneal space, and close the opening in the fascia and skin around it with a mattress suture. Insufflate in the usual way, holding the pressure between 5 and 10 mm Hg during the procedure. Insert a second 10-mm sheath posteriorly. A third may be placed in the anterior axillary line subcostally. If needed, place a fourth port above the iliac crest in the inferior lumbar triangle.

Proceed with laparoscopic dissection of the lower pole of the kidney, the ureter, the para-aortic lymph nodes, and the spermatic vessels, which now lie directly under the anterior lamina of Gerota's fascia. A drain can be inserted and left overnight or, for ureterolithotomy, for 5 days.

For discussion of retroperitoneal laparoscopic nephrectomy, see page 995, Figures 7 and 8.

For extraperitoneal exposure of the pelvis for pelvic node dissection, place the balloon just inferior to the umbilicus. For bladder neck suspension, place it midway between the symphysis pubis and umbilicus. Amplify the exposure by blunt dissection.

INTRAOPERATIVE PROBLEMS

Most complications occur during initial trocar insertion or during insufflation.

Preperitoneal emphysema from improper placement of the insufflation needle is heralded by scrotal emphysema early in the case. It makes identification of landmarks difficult. Alternatives include stopping the procedure, switching to the Hasson technique, or evacuating the insufflation and starting over again. Emphysema of the omentum causes it to obstruct the view. Leakage around a trocar sheath can cause emphysema; it usually resolves spontaneously. Emphysema may be an indication of malfunction of the insufflator, with resulting abnormally high pressures. *Pneumothorax* may result from defects in the diaphragm or from barotrauma from excessive positive-pressure ventilation. It can usually be treated expectantly, but needle aspiration followed by tube thoracotomy, placing a 12 F chest tube through the fourth intercostal space just behind the anterior axillary fold, may be needed.

Pneumomediastinum/pneumopericardium may be heralded by subcutaneous emphysema or pneumothorax. Consider stopping the procedure and allowing spontaneous absorption. Pericardial tamponade requires pericardiocentesis of the gas.

Barotrauma results from extended excessive intraperitoneal pressure, above 15 to 20 mm Hg in adults and above 10 to 15 mm Hg in children. The effect is a fall in venous return and in myocardial filling pressure that fosters hypotension. In addition, pneumothorax may result from alveolar rupture caused by increased ventilation pressures secondary to pressure on the diaphragm. High insufflation pressures suggest improper placement of the needle or a faulty CO_2 pump. Gas from the CO_2-cooled laser tip and the argon beam coagulator may also cause increased intra-abdominal pressure, requiring venting through one of the ports.

Extraperitoneal leakage of CO_2 from high filling pressures or from inadvertent external abdominal pressure usually clears spontaneously, although it can be evacuated with a needle by pressing the skin against the fascia. *Pneumomediastinum* is more serious; it can cause dyspnea and even cardiorespiratory failure. It requires immediate termination of the procedure.

Gas embolization has been reported with resultant cardiovascular collapse and pulmonary edema. A "mill-wheel" murmur may be heard over the heart, and the electrocardiographic tracing can become abnormal. Deflate the pneumoperitoneum at once, and turn the patient on the left side. Supply 100 percent oxygen and hyperventilate the patient. If possible, insert a central venous catheter and aspirate the gas. In severe cases, perform cardiopulmonary resuscitation. *Cardiac arrhythmia* is a common occurrence from the effects of hypercarbia (sinus tachycardia, premature ventricular contractions, and depression of the myocardium). The treatment is to reduce insufflation pressure, supply 100 percent oxygen and hyperventilate, and give appropriate cardiac medication.

Hypotension/cardiovascular collapse can result from hemorrhage, pneumomediastinum or pneumothorax, tension pneumoperitoneum, rupture of the diaphragm, vasovagal reflex, or gas embolus.

Injury of the *anterior abdominal wall vessels* leads to bleeding and formation of hematomas. It is more common with the Hasson technique but also is more readily managed because the wound is open. *Injury to the inferior epigastric vessels* by the sheath is recognized by blood dripping into the pelvis. Cauterize the route the vessels pass through with the aid of the laparoscope, or enlarge the incision and transfix the vessels with a suture above and below the puncture site. Alternatively, insert a balloon catheter, draw the balloon up against the vessel, and hold it on traction with a clamp at skin level while entering another site for the trocar. Maintain the tamponade for 24 or 48 hours (Morey et al, 1993). Another technique (Green et al, 1992) is to pass an NAS on a Stamey needle through the abdominal wall near the port responsible for the injury, remove the suture from the eye intra-abdominally, reinsert the empty needle nearer to the port to straddle the vessel, thread the suture in the eye, withdraw the needle, and tie the suture. Another alternative (Nadler et al, 1995) is to pass an angiocatheter through the subcutaneous tissue alongside the port. Loop a monofilament suture, and crimp the loop so that it will pass through the catheter. Remove the catheter, insert it on the other side, and introduce a single suture. Transabdominally pass a grasper through the loop of the first suture, and grasp the end of this second suture. Pull the looped suture to carry the first suture to the surface, where it is tied.

Vascular injury, including needle puncture of the abdominal aorta or other major vessel, is followed by a spurt of blood. Make a decision whether to withdraw the needle and reinsert it or to proceed directly to laparotomy. Usually the puncture site is small if the needle has not been moved, so intervention is not necessary. Minor injury to small vessels can be controlled with electrocautery. Application of clips or endoloops may be considered, but if accumulation of blood is marked and suction is inadequate, then open repair is necessary. Likewise, major bleeding uniformly occurs from trocar injury. Here, leave the sheath in place for tamponade and as a guide to the site of injury, and proceed with emergency laparotomy. Maintaining the pneumoperitoneum facilitates the subsequent exposure. Keep pressure on the vessel until the patient's blood pressure is stable.

Thermal injuries from the electrocautery occur when the unit is activated when the entire noninsulated portion of the tip is not in view or when a disruption occurs in the insulation on the shaft of the instrument. The injuries are more severe than they appear at first and often require open operation.

Puncture of a viscus with the Veress needle is usually not harmful, as long as the needle is not connected to the active CO_2 supply. Bowel penetration may be indicated when intestinal gas or cloudy fluid is aspirated or when the patient passes flatus or stool. Withdraw the needle, and insert a new needle in a better place. Inspect the site subsequently and, if necessary, repair it either laparoscopically or by open operation. Re-inspect the site at the end of the procedure. *Trocar injury* to the bowel is more serious but in some cases may be managed laparoscopically by closure in two layers using sutures or staples. Leave the trocar in place while the abdomen is opened to limit bleeding and localize the site of injury. Resection of a bowel segment or fecal diversion is seldom needed. The bowel may also be injured by the unipolar electrocautery, especially when it is inadvertently activated out of the field of view. If only a white area is seen, the injury usually heals spontaneously, especially in the large bowel. If the muscularis or submucosa is exposed, either laparoscopic repair or formal laparotomy is required. Cutting instruments may lacerate the bowel if they are allowed to stray outside the field or are passed into the field blindly. Bipolar electrocautery produces a more limited injury, but one that still may require repair. *Bladder laceration* is rare if the bladder remains deflated. It is managed either by continuing urethral drainage or by suturing either laparoscopically or through a small suprapubic incision. *Ureteral injury* requires stenting and possibly sutured closure.

Injuries to joints and nerves result from improper padding and, more often, from inadequate fixation of the patient during the movements (head-down and lateral rotation) required for the procedure. Guard against brachial nerve injury by limiting arm abduction and rotation. The ulnar and peroneal nerves must be padded. *Obturator nerve palsy* can occur during pelvic node dissection.

Deep venous thrombosis arises from poor venous return due to increased intra-abdominal pressure. Sequential pneumatic compression stockings and the usual early ambulation reduce the incidence. For long cases, minidose heparin may be advisable.

Overhydration is not uncommon because of the oliguria associated with the pneumoperitoneum and because the anesthetist automatically includes the insensible loss expected from the open abdomen. In an elderly patient, this may lead to congestive heart failure. Central venous pressure is not accurate because of the pneumoperitoneum and the position of the patient. If this information is needed, place a Swan-Ganz catheter into the pulmonary artery.

POSTOPERATIVE COMPLICATIONS

Bleeding is rarely seen if the operative and trocar sites have been closely inspected at low pressure (i.e., 5 mm Hg at the end of the procedure). *Dehiscence* through a large port or incisional hernias occur if the fascia is not closed.

Bowel injury must be suspected if nausea, vomiting, and ileus occur. Institute nasogastric suction; explore if improvement does not follow. *Ureteral injury*, especially from using electrocoagulation, may not be recognized at laparoscopy. It is suggested by flank pain from renal obstruction or development of a urinoma. Stenting may be tried; otherwise open repair and drainage are required. *Abdominal adhesions*, because not as much manipulation is involved, are less often found than after open procedures and are related to the extent of the dissection.

Severe pain should not persist for more than a few hours postoperatively. If it does, look for a rectus sheath hematoma producing an abdominal bulge, and confirm its presence with computed tomography (CT). The exception is shoulder pain secondary to irritation of the diaphragm by CO_2. This usually resolves in a day or two. If severe abdominal pain persists, rule out a bowel leak by CT scan. Similarly, pain increasing postoperatively indicates a bowel leak or hernia, the latter being localized to a specific port site.

Peritonitis occurring in the first 2 days is from mechanical injury of the bowel. The effect of electrosurgical injury appears later. Laparotomy must be done at once.

Commentary by Ralph V. Clayman

Laparoscopic urology offers the urologist the opportunity to enter an entirely new discipline of minimally invasive surgery. The demands of this new approach are significant owing to the confined working space and the loss of tactile feedback, three-dimensional vision, rapid blunt dissection, and customary suturing skills; meticulous attention to each detail of the procedure from "access" to "exit" is thus essential. All laparoscopic procedures consist of five basic components: insufflation (access), primary port placement, secondary port placement, the actual procedure, and exiting the abdomen. In reading the excellent text provided in this section on laparoscopy, only a few additional points come to mind.

With regard to "access," the current consensus is that open access is safer and does not add significantly to the length of the procedure. In the hands of experienced laparoscopists, the Veress needle has worked and continues to work well, provided that each of the tests is performed to ensure proper entry into the peritoneal cavity. I prefer to hold the Veress needle as though it were a dart, as I believe this imparts finer tactile control than the palm-held method illustrated. Veress needle passage and insufflation are the most dangerous parts of the procedure. It is the failure to properly obtain a pneumoperitoneum that leads to the life-threatening problems associated with passage of the first trocar. With regard to the pneumoperitoneum, the surgeon must be absolutely 100 percent convinced that a proper pneumoperitoneum has been obtained; if there is any doubt whatsoever, an open access should be pursued.

For "primary port placement," I prefer a 12-mm trocar with a safety shield; this is invariably a disposable trocar. A trocar with a clear plastic sheath is particularly nice, as it allows for proper positioning of the sheath with regard to the abdominal wall fascia. Prior to passing the initial trocar, we transiently raise the intra-abdominal pressure to 30 mm Hg in the belief that this presses the peritoneum more tightly against the anterior abdominal wall, thereby facilitating safe passage of the trocar. Once the peritoneal cavity has been entered, the pressure is lowered to 15 mm Hg. The primary port is affixed to the anterior abdominal wall with a 1-0 Prolene suture, so that the sheath cannot be inadvertently pulled out of the abdomen. All secondary ports are placed under direct endoscopic control. It is better to err on the side of placing a larger port if one is doing a major laparoscopic procedure, as this allows the passage of all types of instruments. Therefore, only 12- or 5-mm ports are used. Each sheath is again sewn to the abdominal wall with a

1-0 Prolene suture to preclude its premature removal. In exiting the abdomen, the importance of first lowering the pressure to 5 mm Hg cannot be overemphasized. Venous bleeding at times becomes manifest only with this maneuver. Also, for port closure, the technique that has gained the most favor at Washington University is use of the nondisposable Carter-Thomason device (Inlet Medical, Eden Prairie, MN). With this device, regardless of the size of the patient, 10-mm and larger ports can be reliably closed with incorporation of a broad expanse of fascia; in addition, a figure-eight suture or a suture to stop bleeding from a port site can be readily placed using this device.

Lastly, with regard to extraperitoneoscopy or retroperitoneoscopy, we too subscribe to the Gauer balloon technique. However, based on studies by Elspeth McDougall, we have been making a balloon by using the middle finger of a #8 Triflex latex glove affixed with 2-0 silk sutures to the end of a 16 F red rubber Robinson catheter. This balloon can be backloaded through a 30 F Amplatz sheath and introduced either directly through the wound during open access or through a 12-mm sheath if closed access has been used. The balloon is filled with saline, not air, to a volume of 800 to 1000 ml. If the balloon ruptures, a careful examination of the retroperitoneum must be done to seek out any pieces of latex that need to be removed. In general, balloon rupture is distinctly unusual in the unoperated retroperitoneum or extraperitoneal space.

For almost all ablative procedures and many reconstructive operations, laparoscopy offers the urologic surgeon the opportunity to achieve surgical success without the associated surgical morbidity. This situation applies to myriad procedures of increasing technical difficulty: abdominal exploration for the cryptorchid testicle, lymphocelectomy, varicocelectomy, pelvic lymphadenectomy, simple nephrectomy, adrenalectomy, radical nephrectomy, radical nephroureterectomy, bladder neck suspension, and possibly pyeloplasty, to name but a few of the more common applications. However, although the benefits to the patient are immediate and gratifying (less pain, shorter hospital stay, more rapid convalescence, improved cosmesis), the surgeon pays a high price owing to the shortcomings of operating at a distance via a television monitor. Nevertheless, the days of open surgery are likely numbered. For a society that succeeded in placing a man on the moon more than 25 years ago, it is indeed a sad commentary on the surgical profession that the best therapy we can offer our patients is performed through a large incision no different from the one made by our forefathers a century ago. In the late 1990s, there must be a better way!

Suture Techniques

The aim of suturing is to hold tissues together with the least interference with their blood supply. Apply the technique most suitable for the tissue, but try to use the smallest size and, for economy, the fewest types of sutures.

KNOT-TYING TECHNIQUES

1 Three basic knots are available—square, surgeon's, and double throw.

A, *Square knot.* The simple square knot holds in polyglactin and polyglycolic acid sutures if they are uncoated (Dexon).

B, If coated sutures (Vicryl and Dexon S) are used, an additional throw is needed. Care must be taken to lay each throw square to the last.

C, The *surgeon's knot* has the advantage of allowing the suture to hold the tissue without slipping after placement of the first throw but is no more secure than the square knot, requiring, except with Dexon, additional throws.

D, The *double-throw knot,* essentially a double surgeon's knot, has the greatest knot-holding ability for all suture materials. Only polydioxanone (PDS) and nylon (Ethilon, Dermalon) require an extra throw. Polyglyconate (Maxon) was found to be the best for knot-holding capacity and breaking force (Brown, 1992). To be absolutely safe, tie synthetic absorbable sutures (SAS) with three knots. Monofilament NAS may require six or even seven extra throws, all placed flat.

Tie a suture while holding it near its free end; the suture may thus be used twice, saving suture material and time. Instrument ties are somewhat slower to make but use appreciably less suture material.

SUTURES

Selection of Sutures

Individual surgeons have their own preferences for sutures, but two important variables must be considered: the persistence of strength and the degree of tissue reactivity. The initial strength is proportional to size, but the rate of loss of strength is a function of the suture material. The rate of absorption also depends on the suture material, but it is not directly related to the rate of loss of strength. In general, the strength of the suture is lost much more rapidly before it has been absorbed. A suture must maintain sufficient strength to ensure adequate apposition of tissue until the wound can withstand stress without mechanical support. Decrease in the strength of a suture during healing should be no more than proportional to the gain in wound strength. Relative absorption of suture material in the subcutaneous tissues: catgut—1 month; polyglactin (Vicryl)—2 to 3 months; polyglycolic acid (Dexon plus)—4 months; PDS—6 months; polyglyconate (Maxon)—7 months. Bladder regains 70 percent of tensile strength in 2 weeks, fascia 50 percent in 2 months, and skin 30 percent in 3 weeks.

Reactivity of the tissue to the foreign body depends on the size and type of suture material and the type of reaction it invokes. The larger the size, the greater the reaction.

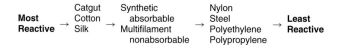

| **Most Reactive** | → | Catgut Cotton Silk | → | Synthetic absorbable Multifilament nonabsorbable | → | Nylon Steel Polyethylene Polypropylene | → | **Least Reactive** |

Absorbable and nonabsorbable sutures have different effects. Plain catgut (PCG) and chromic catgut (CCG) sutures, being absorbed by proteolytic enzymes, have quite a variable absorption time and incite the most reaction in the tissue. In addition, they vary in tensile strength, which is generally lower than that

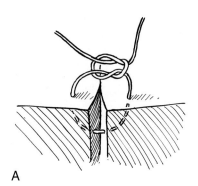

A

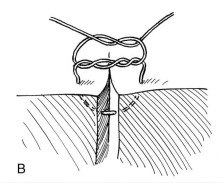

B

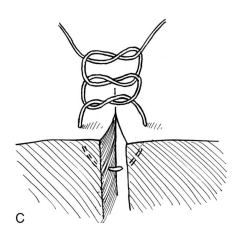

C

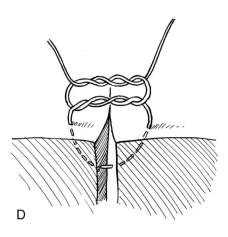

D

of synthetic sutures. SAS, in contrast, are removed by hydrolysis and have moderate tissue reactivity and predictable absorption times. Those made from polyglycolic acid (Dexon, Vicryl) retain 20 percent of their strength at 14 days, and those made from PDS retain 50 percent of their strength at 4 weeks, but neither is absorbed for several months. In infected urine, catgut sutures retain the most strength. NAS as monofilaments stimulate the least reaction in the tissues and have the least attraction for bacteria; when braided, they handle better and tie more securely. They are unsuitable in the presence of bacteria or urine. Silk and cotton rapidly lose their strength after the second month but probably are useful in the outer layer of an intestinal anastomosis and in the mesentery. Nylon is a polyamide; Dacron is a polyester; and polyethylene and polypropylene are polyolefins; of these, nylon loses its strength first.

Table 1 summarizes the characteristics of several sutures. In general, polyglycolic acid sutures are preferable to PCG or CCG for urologic surgery, except in cases of infected urine and for the skin. Because of expense, use as few different sizes and kinds of sutures as possible in a given case. Even though suture selection is a matter for the individual surgeon, certain practical guidelines can be given here.

Fascia

Regardless of what suture is used, the immediate strength of the wound is only 40 to 70 percent of the intact structure. With NAS, reduced strength persists at least for the 2 months or so that it takes for the wound to heal completely. For an absorbable suture, the initial strength is the same as that of a nonabsorbable one if an equivalent size is used, but in 1 or 2 weeks the strength declines appreciably. However, by that time, the wound itself has gained enough strength that it balances the diminished strength of the sutures. Thus, the wound is most vulnerable to separation during the second week. For this reason, NAS are often used for closure of wounds subjected to stress, such as those of abdominal and flank incisions.

For contaminated wounds, the process of absorbing the sutures stimulates macrophage activity with resultant low tissue oxygen tension. This activity also reduces endothelial migration and capillary formation, thus providing a suitable environment for anaerobic bacterial growth. Polyglycolic acid sutures foster the least inflammatory response of absorbable sutures, and the degradation products themselves may be antibacterial. Conversely, NAS, especially monofilaments, produce the least reaction, but once infected they may stay infected because they remain in the wound. Polypropylene is the best choice in contaminated wounds, much better than silk or cotton. For a debilitated patient, in whom poor healing is expected, use either an NAS or an absorbable suture that retains its strength the longest (i.e., PDS). Retention sutures of heavy nonabsorbable material (polypropylene or wire) may be needed in a debilitated patient, especially if the wound is contaminated. Bolsters cut from a red rubber catheter reduce damage to the skin.

Subcutaneous Tissue

This layer is the site of most wound infections because of the weak defense mechanisms in the fatty areolar tissue. Do not use sutures here unless really necessary, and then use the finest minimally reactive absorbable suture of polyglycolic acid. Avoid PCG or CCG.

Skin

Waterproof tape is best if it is not subjected to too much tension. Staples, if not too tight, are the next best choice because they do not penetrate the wound, but they cost more and are a nuisance because they require subsequent removal. A

Table 1. Suture Types

		Trade Name	
		Ethicon	*Davis & Geck*
Absorbable			
Synthetic braided			
Polyglactin	Coated	Vicryl	
	Uncoated		Dexon S
Polyglycolic acid	Coated		Dexon plus
Synthetic monofilament			
Polyglyconate			Maxon
Polydioxanone		PDS	
Gut			
Plain gut		Plain gut	Plain gut
Chromic gut		Chromic gut	Chromic gut
Nonabsorbable			
Synthetic braided			
Polyester	Uncoated	Merseline	Dacron
Nylon	Coated		Surgilon
Synthetic monofilament			
Nylon	Uncoated	Ethilon	Dermalon
Polypropylene		Proline	Surgilene

Adapted from Edlich RF, Rodeheaver GT, Thacker JG: Considerations in the choice of sutures for wound closure of the genitourinary tract. J Urol 137(3):373, 1987.

subcuticular stitch of monofilament nonabsorbable material leaves a better wound but must be removed. Polyglycolic acid sutures subcuticularly can remain until resorbed, at the same time producing little reaction. This material is not suitable when placed through the skin as interrupted sutures because it depends on hydrolysis for absorption, and so it persists on the dry surface.

Urinary Tract

Urothelium covers the suture line within 5 days. Ureteral and vesical wounds gain strength more rapidly than those in the body wall; normal strength is reached in 21 days. The type of suture material is not as critical here, but absorbable sutures cause less reaction than nonabsorbable ones in the long term. Although more subject to encrustation, absorbable sutures are usually gone before stones can form. Polyglycolic acid sutures are less reactive than CCG sutures, and they have a more predictable rate of absorption. Although polyglycolic acid sutures are not completely absorbed before 28 days, they are usually the better choice, with one exception. In the presence of *Proteus* infection, resorption is much too rapid and catgut should be used.

Intestine

Use interrupted NAS, reaching through the muscularis well into the submucosa. If a hemostatic layer is desired, place a running absorbable suture in the mucosa-submucosa. CCG is suitable for sutures penetrating the lumen; otherwise, use SAS. Controlled-release needles speed the process of suturing. In general, place continuous sutures if the tissue is of good quality and interrupted sutures if it is poor.

Vascular

Monofilament synthetic NAS are strongest and least reactive.

Size and Type

The size and type of suture and the appropriate needle for various structures are listed in Table 2.

Table 2. Suggested Type and Size of Suture for Various Tissues

Tissue	Adult		Pediatric	
	Type	*Size*	*Type*	*Size*
Skin				
Cosmetic closure	Absorbable	4-0	Absorbable	5-0
Noncosmetic closure	Staples		Nonabsorbable	5-0
	Nonabsorbable	4-0		4-0
		3-0		
Fascia	PDS	Zero	PDS	3-0
	Maxon silk	1-0	Maxon silk	2-0
Muscle	Absorbable	1-0	Absorbable	3-0
		2-0		3-0
Bladder	Absorbable	3-0	Absorbable	4-0
		2-0		3-0
Ureter-pelvis	Absorbable	5-0	Absorbable	5-0
		4-0		6-0
Urethra (vascular)	Absorbable	4-0	Absorbable	5-0
	(Maxon, PDS)	5-0		6-0
Bowel	Staples		Staples	
	Absorbable	3-0	Absorbable	5-0
	(inner layer)	4-0	(inner layer)	4-0
	Nonabsorbable	3-0	Nonabsorbable	4-0
	(outer layer)		(outer layer)	
Vascular	Nonabsorbable	4-0	Nonabsorbable	4-0
		5-0		5-0

Adapted from Foster LS, McAninch JW: Suture material and wound healing: An overview. AUA Update 11:86, 1992.

Commentary by Francis F. Bartone

Fascia. Suture strength is more important in fascial closure than in any other tissue. Therefore, NAS seem to be the most reliable. In the past, however, many of these sutures were braided and needed to be removed if the wound became infected. Many surgeons used absorbable sutures for this reason. With the advent of the synthetic monofilament sutures, especially polypropylene (Prolene), my preference has been to use Prolene exclusively for fascial closure. The suture causes little tissue reaction, has excellent long-term strength, and does not need to be removed in an infected wound. Although this material has been excellent in the vast majority of cases, in rare instances the suture extrudes through the wound or causes discomfort. An alternative might be PDS or glycolic acid–trimethylene carbonate (Maxon). The former suture holds its strength for an extended time period, but it is more difficult to handle than Maxon, which disintegrates more quickly. In the future, an absorbable suture of this type may be ideal.

Subcutaneous Tissue and Skin. The use of subcuticular sutures is well tolerated in the young but requires more time to place. For this use, polyglactin 910 (Vicryl) or polyglycolic acid (Dexon) has been useful in my experience. A thin Prolene suture may also be used but needs to be removed, and this causes discomfort. In penile skin where scarring is not a problem, CCG is the suture of choice because Vicryl and Dexon sutures are absorbed too slowly.

Urinary Tract. Dexon sutures are the best sutures for this site. I hesitate to use Vicryl because of some experimental work I did years ago. However, the work was done in only a few animals and may not be valid clinically. Although it is true that in the presence of *Proteus* infection, resorption of Dexon may be rapid, in a clinical situation the epithelium would rapidly cover the suture. In a storage organ like the bladder, a second layer of sutures may be necessary to be certain that this problem is obviated. In ureter, renal pelvis, and urethra, one layer is sufficient, and Dexon is my suture of choice. In situations where watertight closures are necessary (pyeloplasty), cutting-type needles should not be used because they allow fluid to seep through the needle holes.

Intestine. Dexon is my suture of choice for an inner layer because this suture is much better constructed than catgut. A second outer layer using monofilament NAS is my preference.

Vascular. A trend toward using an absorbable monofilament suture in vascular surgery is supported by experimental and clinical data. Large vessels with large lumina may have little need for absorbable sutures, but an increasing amount of data suggests that less reaction and greater lumen size occur in small vessels when a monofilament SAS is used. This is especially so in pediatric venous anastomoses. I really believe that the modern surgeon should abandon silk, cotton, and steel and use catgut only in areas where skin scarring is not important and when one does not wish to take the time to use a subcuticular suture. In the present or near future, different monofilament absorbable sutures causing little reaction and having variable strength and absorption rates may be all that is needed for all situations.

SKIN SUTURE TECHNIQUES

Alternatives include a subcuticular suture, interrupted sutures, staples, and tapes.

2 *Subcuticular closure:* Use a 4-0 SAS or a monofilament pull-out NAS.

A, Start the stitch from a buried knot at one end. Pull the subcutaneous tissue forward with a fine skin hook, and drive the needle point well into the dermis in a plane parallel to the surface, entering exactly opposite the exit site of the last bite.

B, To bury the last knot, place a deep stitch and, after tying it, bring the end out through the skin 1 cm from the wound. Cut the excess suture, and let the end retract. *Alternatively,* lock the suture at the start by passing back and forth at one end of the wound, having the needle enter exactly at the site of exit of the suture (Giddins). Do the same lock after the subcuticular suture line is completed. Another alternative is to apply inverted absorbable interrupted subcuticular sutures, thus burying each knot.

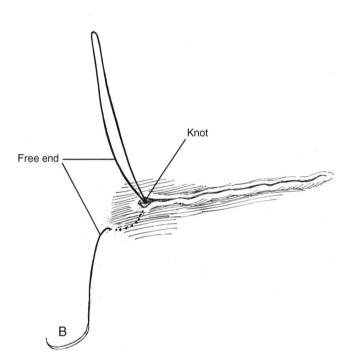

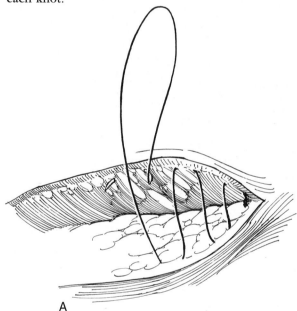

3 *Vertical mattress suture:* This suture is a double stitch that forms a loop around the tissue on both sides to produce eversion of the skin. Use monofilament NAS, and catch only the very edge of the skin in the second bite. Throw four or five knots.

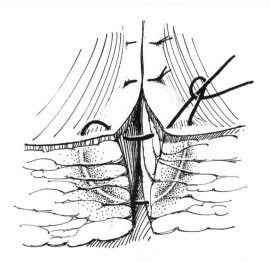

4 **A,** *Everting interrupted suture:* For plastic procedures, penetrate the skin close to the edge of the
incision; then encircle a larger amount of tissue beneath.

B, *Halsted mattress suture:* This suture inverts the
edge. Pass the suture into the skin, and have it pass out
again near the skin edge.

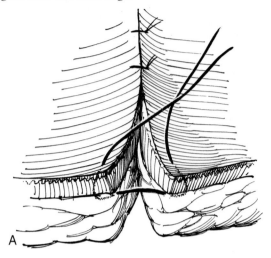

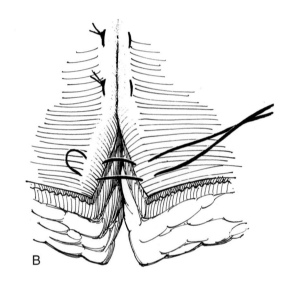

Far-and-Near Sutures

6 Place 2-0 SAS at 1-cm intervals, first deep on one
side and shallow on the other, then shallow on one
side and deep on the other.

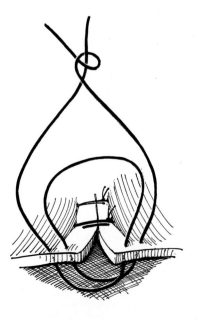

FASCIAL SUTURES

Interrupted Sutures

5 **A,** Place 2-0 synthetic absorbable or monofilament
sutures 1 cm deep and 1 cm apart (the "one-by-
one" rule).

B, Tie them only tight enough to bring the edges in
contact. Throw at least three square knots. Monofilament
sutures consist of only one strand, so they "can be inadvertently and easily damaged by any instrument, needle
or sharp-edged material that cuts or scratches its surface"
(Ethicon, Inc.). This risk is greater with running sutures
that depend on a single knot at either end. If the terminal
knot is tied with the so-called loop-to-strand knot, it may
pull out. Be sure in thin patients and in children that the
knots are buried to avoid wound discomfort.

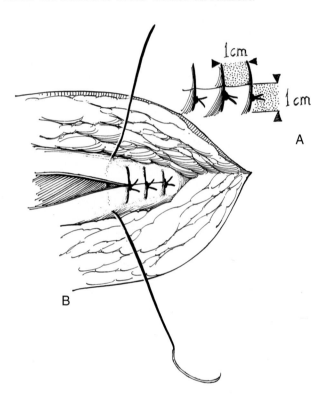

Skin Clips

Skin clips in an automatic dispenser are a rapid but relatively
expensive way of closing the skin. Partially squeeze the handle
to advance the staple into position. Hold the end of the stapler
loosely against the skin with the arrow in line with the incision,
and fire the staple. Clips require subsequent removal.

Other Types of Fascial Sutures

7 **A,** *Near-and-far suture* for mass closure of the abdomen. Use 2-0 NAS. Place the deep sutures first; then catch the edges with the shallower bites.

B, *Smead-Jones fascial closure technique:* Place 2-0 NAS 2 cm apart as figure-eight stitches, taking bites near and far.

C, *Vertical mattress suture* (sometimes called a Gambee stitch) incorporates both fascial layers. On the first side, pass the suture through the superficial and deep fascia and the peritoneum, then back through the peritoneum to exit from the muscle. Cross to the other side of the wound, enter the muscle layer, pass out through the peritoneum and deep fascia and then back through the peritoneum and both layers of fascia, and tie it subcutaneously.

The stitch was originally designed as a bowel stitch to prevent herniation of the mucosa (see Step 13). For application as a bowel suture, pass it through all layers on one side, then through the mucosa and submucosa on the opposite side, next through the submucosa to exit from the mucosa on the first side, and finally through all layers on the opposite side.

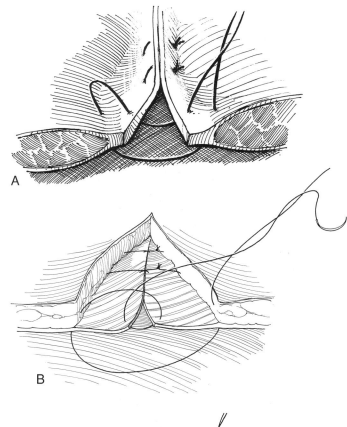

A

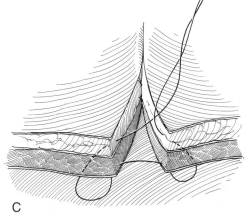

B

BOWEL SUTURES

Connell Suture

This is a continuous suture that inverts the inner wall of the intestine.

8 **A,** Insert the stitch so that it enters and exits the bowel on each side successively. It may include only the mucosa and submucosa. Use 3-0 SAS.

B, When passed from the inside to the outside, it is an especially useful technique for closing the angles of a bowel anastomosis.

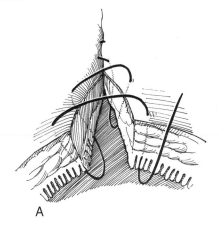

A

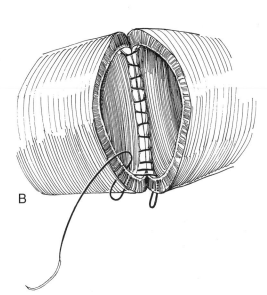

B

C

Lembert Suture

An inverting suture that produces serosal apposition, the Lembert suture includes the muscular layer and some of the submucosal layer. (No satisfactory form of intestinal anastomosis was available before the introduction of the Lembert suture.)

9 **A,** Place it as an interrupted suture. Insert each bite to reach into but not through the tough submucosal layer.

B, It may be placed as a continuous stitch. This stitch is useful for closing the end of the bowel or for anastomosis of two ends. Use 4-0 braided NAS. Be sure to catch the submucosa.

C, To close the end of the bowel, use interrupted Lembert sutures over a clamp (see page 660). Start by placing a traction suture at each end. Lay all the sutures. Hold the sutures on each side, and remove the clamp carefully. Tie each suture successively as the mucosa is inverted.

D, For a one-layer bowel anastomosis (see pages 650 to 651), place interrupted Lembert sutures on both sides; then have your assistant gently withdraw the clamps. Tie each suture successively, taking care that the ends are inverted.

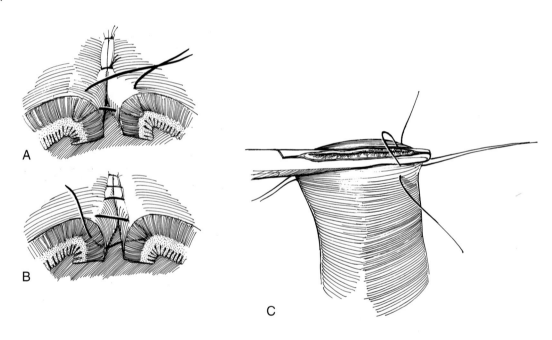

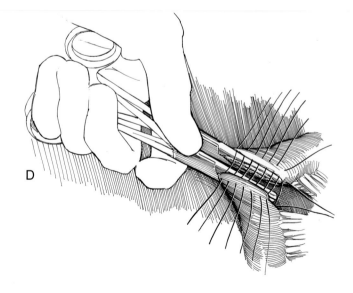

Parker-Kerr Suture

This inverting suture is used to close the end of the intestine. Place each stitch to reach the submucosa. It may be laid continuously or may be interrupted as a Lembert suture.

10 Use 4-0 NAS with bites taken parallel to the edge rather than across it, in contrast to the Lembert stitch.

Purse-String Suture

11 Place a continuous suture around a defect for inversion (appendix) or closure (hernia sac).

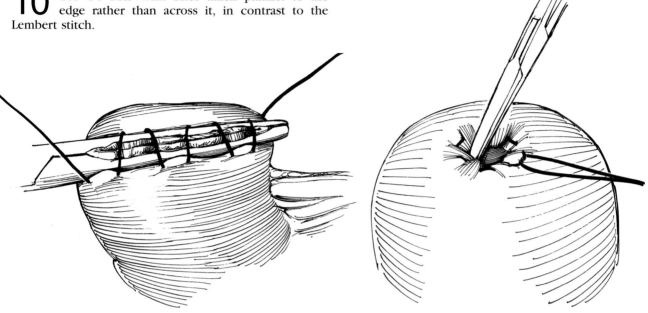

Lock-Stitch

12 This is a continuous suture used for mucosal edges. Pass every third or fourth stitch under the previous one. Select this stitch when puckering is to be avoided.

Figure-Eight Bowel Suture

13 This is an interrupted suture that approximates the mucosa independently from the muscularis and serosa. Pass the suture through all layers on one side, then through the mucosa and submucosa on both sides. Finally, bring it through all layers on the other side.

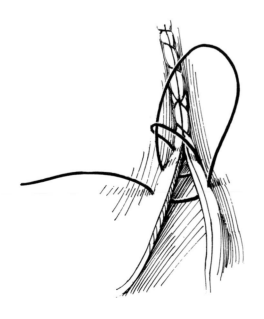

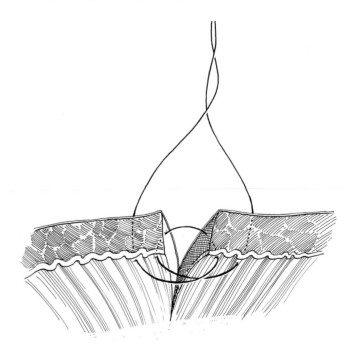

Gambee Inverting Intestinal Suture with Near-Far Suture

14 **A,** This through-and-through suture is used in a single-layer technique, with the sutures tied within the bowel. It helps to first place a Lembert suture (Step 8) at the mesenteric border of the bowel, and tie it to invert the edges of the mucosa. Insert the suture from inside the bowel through all layers, including the serosa on one side and back through the serosa and all layers on the other side. Tie it to invert the edge of the mucosa. Continue around the circumference of the bowel with sutures 3 mm apart.

B, *Near-far suture:* When the closure is almost complete, place the last stitch as a near-far suture from the outside, one that passes from the serosa into the lumen and exits from the lumen and through the serosa at a point closer to the edge, then re-enters and exits on the other side similarly. When tied, it inverts the edge.

Tissue Sealer

Tisseal is a protein-thrombin solution that produces stable fibrin on a dry, raw tissue surface. It can be useful for small defects or leaks remaining after suturing, such as in ureteral implantation and hypospadias repair, and for fixation of an ileal intussusception in conjunction with scarification of the opposed surfaces. Draw two solutions into a syringe, mix them, and inject the mixture through a blunt needle onto the surfaces to be glued together.

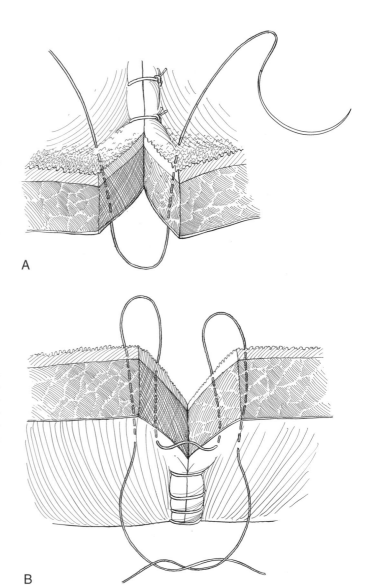

A

B

Commentary by Donald D. Trunkey

For subcuticular closure I prefer a 5-0 or 6-0 monofilament absorbable suture. Closure should be done with a cutting needle, and the dermis should be penetrated perpendicular to the skin margin while avoiding deep bites into the dermis. If deep bites are used, the dermis tends to pucker, resulting in a wave-like appearance to the final closure.

The vertical mattress suture is a particularly useful suture on wounds of the face, where geographic skin margins (such as the vermillion border of the lip) must be precisely approximated.

For fascial sutures, I prefer interrupted sutures in the young healthy male who is muscular or the patient who may be cachectic from cancer or malnutrition. In other patients a running absorbable monofilament (size 0) suture is acceptable. It must be emphasized that the fascia should be approximated, not strangulated. Fascial sutures that use near-far figure-eight–type stitches tend to strangulate one of the loops. The Connell suture is a particularly nice technique to use on each end of the inner layer of a bowel anastomosis. This stitch tends to avoid purse-stringing the lumen. Its disadvantage is that it is not a hemostatic stitch.

Plastic Surgical Techniques

Grafts, as free segments of skin, depend on support from the vascular bed onto which they are transferred. Flaps carry their blood supply with them or have it surgically re-established once transferred.

BLOOD SUPPLY TO THE SKIN

1 Blood is supplied either through a longitudinal artery arising dorsally that lies deep to the muscle or fascia, supplying perforators to the subdermal and intradermal plexus in the overlying skin, or through longitudinal vessels arising ventrally that lie superficial to the fascia, connecting directly to the plexuses in the skin. These systems are interconnected by a complex network of vessels of varying sizes. They are very delicate and cannot withstand compression in forceps, twisting, or undue stretching. Skin hooks and stay sutures are essential tools to preserve them.

Inferior epigastric a.
(from ventral segmental a.)

Perforating a.

Direct cutaneous a.

Branch of perforating a.

Superficial fascia

Cutaneous a.

Musculocutaneous a.

Perforating a.

Aorta

Dorsal segmental a.

GRAFTS

Grafts, bereft of central connections, must acquire nutrients from the bed for the first 24 to 48 hours (imbibition), then during the next 2 days must establish local vascular connections (inosculation). This requires that the graft remain immobilized and closely applied to the bed, which in turn must be well vascularized. Seromas and hematomas block these steps, as do infection and scar tissue.

Thickness of Grafts

2 Grafts may be full thickness to include the entire dermis to the adipose layer, or they may be split thickness.

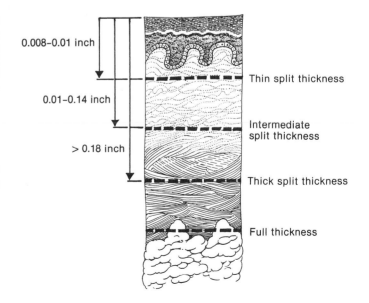

0.008–0.01 inch

Thin split thickness

0.01–0.14 inch

Intermediate split thickness

> 0.18 inch

Thick split thickness

Full thickness

Full-Thickness Grafts

Full-thickness grafts, made up of all skin layers, contract only 5 to 25 percent, provide a very durable skin covering, and are less likely than split-thickness grafts to become hyperpigmented, but they also carry the skin adnexal structures, making hair growth a potential problem. They take poorly more often than do split-thickness grafts, not only because they are thicker (bulkier) and thus require a greater supply of blood, but also because they depend almost totally on new vascular connections to the disrupted subdermal plexus, which characteristically has relatively fewer vessels available for the process of inosculation. The requirements for a "take" are an extremely well-vascularized bed and absolute immobilization. For urethral construction, if genital skin is not available, full-thickness grafts of bladder epithelium or buccal mucosa may be used.

3 Full-thickness grafts must be cleared of underlying fatty-areolar tissue to allow the vessels of the subdermal plexus direct contact with the new bed.

A good compromise for grafts from the lower abdomen may be a thick split-thickness graft (greater than 0.19 inch) because it has most of the favorable qualities of the full-thickness graft and little of the tendency to contract of thinner split-thickness grafts. Full-thickness grafts from the prepuce, the bladder, or the mouth, on the other hand, are thin and pliable and inherently have little subcutaneous fat. They too must have their deep surface meticulously prepared to expose the deep laminar plexus optimally.

Split-Thickness Skin Grafts

Split-thickness skin grafts may be thin (to include a minimal amount of dermis, from 0.010 to 0.015 inch), intermediate (approximately half the thickness of the dermis, from 0.016 to 0.19 inch), or thick (three quarters or more of the dermis, over 0.19 inch). Composed of only part of the dermis along with the epidermis, they take better than full-thickness grafts but provide a more fragile covering. They can contract about 50 percent, or even more in unsupported areas.

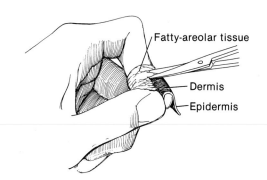

Dermal Grafts

Dermal grafts, cleared of both epidermis and fat, can be more elastic than full-thickness grafts and become vascularized on both sides. They are useful for replacement of deep structural layers such as penile tunica albuginea and fascia.

Application of Split-Thickness and Meshed Grafts

Meshing the graft in a meshing dermatome allows for expansion and provides greater coverage if necessary but, more importantly for the genitourinary surgeon, allows escape of serum and blood. However, such a graft may contract more. The graft must be placed with good hemostasis, be relatively free of contamination, and also be immobilized. Mesh grafts are placed with the slits parallel to the existing skin lines. They can be expected to contract 30 to 60 percent, except on the back of the hand and on genital tissue.

4 As a example of the use of meshed and unmeshed grafts, apply a nonmeshed split-thickness graft to a functioning penis because a meshed graft offers no advantages and can be expected to contract from 30 to 60 percent, creating a cosmetically unsightly appearance to the reconstructed penis. On the other hand, for reconstruction of the scrotum, the meshing allows for better contact with the underlying complex contours, avoids collections in the contour interfaces, and creates a cosmetically pleasing appearance, as the mesh scars are similar in appearance to the rugae seen in normal scrotal skin.

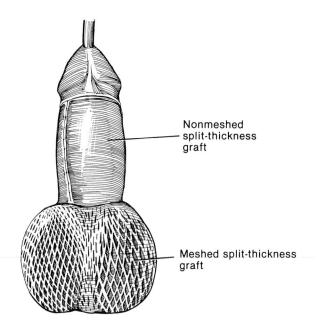

FLAPS

The deep surface of a cutaneous flap is composed of fat; a fasciocutaneous flap, of fascia; and a musculocutaneous flap, of muscle. Flaps may be used to cover (skin flaps), to provide structure and function and contribute to revascularization (muscle flaps), to provide sensation (sensible fasciocutaneous flaps), or for a combination of these purposes.

In contrast to grafts, flaps bring their own blood supply with them. Flaps can also be reattached directly to a new supply by microvascular techniques. They may be random pattern flaps for transposition, rotation and tube flaps, or axial pattern flaps. The classifications of random and axial depend on the inherent pattern of vascularity of the flap itself. Random flaps have no defined cuticular vascularity, and this varies from individual to individual, being somewhat undependable. In contrast, axial flaps have an organized, self-contained blood supply and defined cuticular vascular territories that vary little from one individual to another and thus are predictable and dependable. *Pedicle flap* is a redundant term because *pedicle* and *flap* mean the same thing.

Another approach to classifying flaps is to divide them into peninsular, island, and microvascular free transfer (MVFT) flaps. This classification deals with the design/shape of the flap itself. *Peninsula flaps*, as the name implies, are shaped like a peninsula, and thus both the cuticular and vascular portions of the flap remain attached to the "mainland" (body). A *random peninsula flap* (all random flaps are peninsula flaps by definition) is thus mobilized so that the skin survives on the random distribution of the skin plexuses. In the past, surgeons attempted to make random flaps more dependable by defining length-width ratios for the flap (i.e., if the flap was 3 cm long, its base needed to be 3 cm wide, for a 1:1 ratio). With experience, we now know that ratios are more limiting than useful, as clearly certain areas in the body with a 1:2 ratio or even a 1:3 ratio allow reliable survival. In other areas in certain individuals, a 1:1 ratio approaches the limit.

If in a peninsula flap the skin remains attached to the mainland, then in an island flap it does not. The term *island flap* implies that the cuticular continuity is interrupted but the vessels remain attached (the flap dangles on its vessels). If one goes a step further and detaches the vessels, then the flap becomes an *MVFT flap* or free flap.

The *musculocutaneous* or *fasciocutaneous flap* has come to be viewed as an island flap, but it is only truly an island flap if the muscle and/or fascia is totally detached, both origin and insertion, with the flap unit moved on the vessels from which it dangles. For most clinical uses, the muscle is left attached at the origin and transposed to the adjacent defect. To be accurate in both theory and semantics, the surgeon must view the muscle or fascia as the flap and the attached skin unit as a passenger on the flap. The proper term then is *skin island* or *paddle*. To use the gracilis as an example, the flap is properly thought of and termed "a gracilis flap with a skin island/paddle." Fascial flaps, almost by definition, cannot be elevated as islands. To use an example of a flap that has become almost common urologic terminology, the preputial/penile skin island flap should correctly be designated a dartos fascial flap with a preputial/penile skin island/paddle.

Flaps on the trunk are raised by dissection between the deep and the superficial fascias, a plane through which relatively few vessels cross. However, any vessel that is encountered needs to be controlled because hematoma formation may prevent graft adherence and cause interference with its circulation, fostering infection. Many flaps require removal of much of the underlying fat to make them suitable for the recipient site. In axial flaps, this can be done without jeopardizing the circulation because the vessels lie deep in the superficial fascia near the point of origin and become superficial to the fascia only toward the distal end of the flap. With magnification, the subdermal vascular plexus can be protected as the fat is dissected from the fat domes. At the same time, care must be taken not to disturb the deeper circulation arising from the axial vessels. In addition, fat at the edges of a flap may interfere with approximation by bulging into the suture line, a problem solved by trimming the edge obliquely.

The *musculocutaneous flap*, useful in reconstructive urology, is formed by elevating skin and muscle, together with their independent cutaneous vascular territory, on a single pedicle on the superficial inferior epigastric, superior epigastric, or superficial circumflex iliac artery.

Preparation of a Flap

Choose a flap with a size and ability to arc into place, with adequate vasculature, with accessibility, with proper composition, and with an acceptable donor site remaining. Outline the defect to be grafted with a marking pen; then quickly press a piece of glove-wrapper paper against it to obtain a pattern for the graft. Skin grafts and flaps are viscoelastic, so stretch the graft in place to overcome the elastic fibers in the skin. A pull for 10 or 15 minutes enlarges a flap, owing to stress relaxation and creep. However, a compromise must be made between proper tension and impairment of vascularity.

Secondary contraction occurs with maturation of the scar tissue, lying between the skin graft and its bed, beginning after the 10th day and continuing for 6 months. Thin grafts, flexible beds, and complete take all reduce the chances for contraction. Sensation begins to return to a graft in 3 weeks if dense scarring does not intervene. Skin grafts and flaps grow as the patient grows, stimulated by tension from the surrounding skin.

Avoid *marks in the skin* that result from tension on the sutures. Tie the suture just tight enough to approximate the edges and no tighter. Subcutaneous sutures reduce the tension, as does placing the incision parallel to the skin lines. The length of time the sutures remain is also a factor; 6 or 7 days are usually adequate, but allow 10 to 14 days for the heavy skin on the back. Small bites of tissue close to the edge are associated with less apparent skin marks; infection is accompanied by more prominent ones. Of course, a patient prone to keloid formation is at greatest risk.

Slight *eversion of the skin edges* results in a flat scar; inverted edges leave a depressed scar. In some areas, a vertical mattress suture (see page 35) is necessary to stabilize the skin edges. If skin clips are used, they should grasp the skin with equal bites and should be angled so that they slightly evert the skin. Microporous skin tape, used in conjunction with buried sutures, may be placed initially as primary skin closure or applied at the time of suture or clip removal. It helps adherence to wipe the skin with alcohol or acetone before application. Skin tapes have the advantages of quick application and avoidance of suture marks, and they do provide added tensile strength. Their disadvantages are that they do not evert the skin edges and they may come off prematurely.

Local Anesthesia

Use 1 percent lidocaine with 1:200,000 epinephrine; for a child, use 0.5 percent lidocaine with 1:400,000 epinephrine. Hyaluronidase may aid in diffusion of the agents. Inject it slowly while explaining the procedure to the patient. Stop for a minute if the injection is causing pain. Regional block often may be better than local infiltration.

Use of Langer's Lines

5 **A** and **B,** Make incisions parallel to Langer's lines. These are oriented at right angles to the line of maximal tissue extensibility. By orienting excisions or incisions with the lines, the wound tension (not to be confused with innate skin tension) is properly aligned.

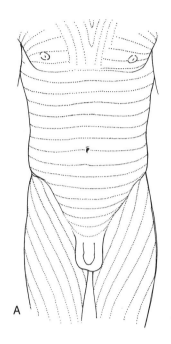
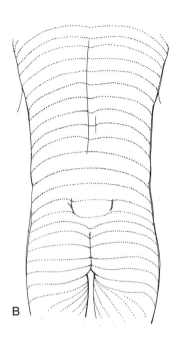

PLASTIC TECHNIQUES FOR SKIN

Z-Plasty
(Horner)

6 **A,** Make the central limb parallel to the contracture or scar. Cut at a 60-degree angle to this vertical limb at each end, rounding each incision at its angle. Cut all three incisions to the same length.

B, Elevate the two triangular flaps.

C, Transpose one flap (**a**) down and the other (**b**) up, and suture them in place. The central limb may now align with Langer's skin line, and the gain in length for a 60-degree Z-plasty is 75 percent. (Thirty-degree angles gain 25 percent; 45-degree angles, 50 percent.)

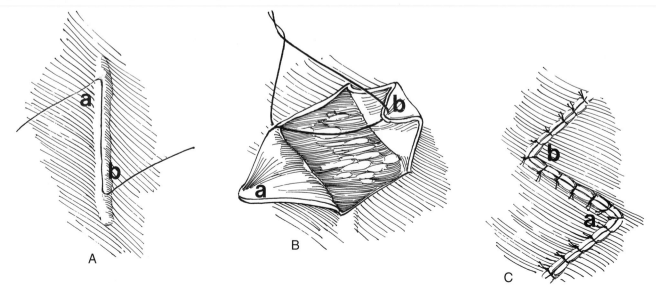

Four-Flap Z-Plasty
(Berger)

7 Place several smaller consecutive Z incisions to give a better cosmetic result, as there is more opportunity to align the central limbs with Langer's lines or other favorable skin lines.

A, Make the usual vertical incision and the two incisions angled at 60 degrees as described for the Z-plasty. Make two more incisions at 60-degree angles in the opposite direction.

B, Transpose the two triangular flaps on the left (**a** and **b**) down and the two on the right (**c** and **d**) up.

C, Suture them in place.

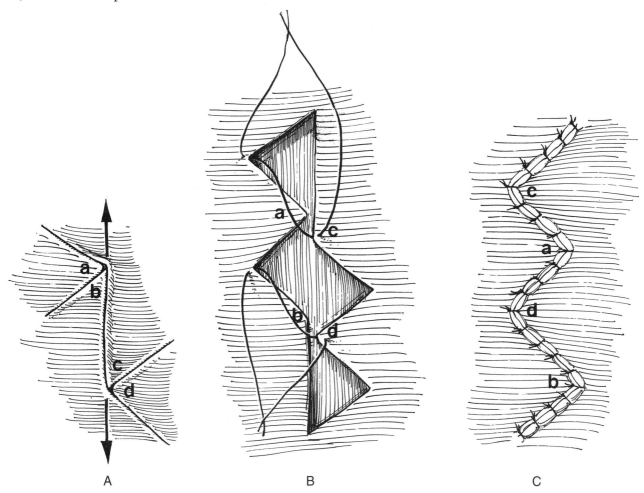

A B C

V-Y Advancement

V-Y advancement is used to *elongate an area* at the expense of narrowing the area immediately lateral (example: release of scrotal tethering).

8 A, Mark and cut a V in the line of relative shortening. It is well to round the tips of all V-shaped flaps.
B, The skin at the tip draws away.
C, Close the limb of the Y first.

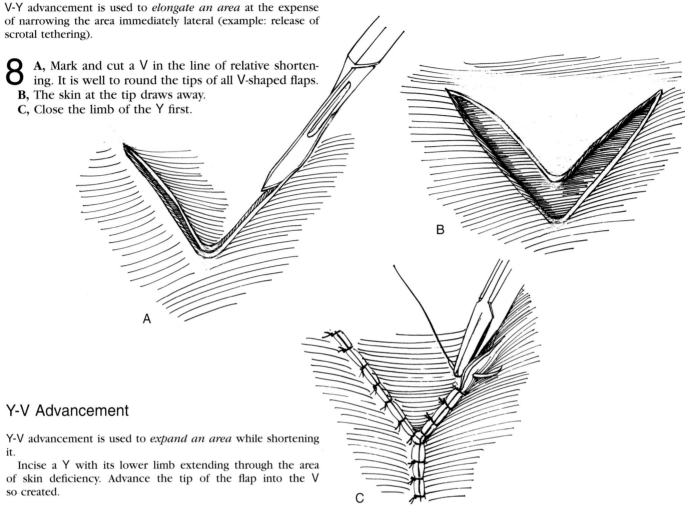

Y-V Advancement

Y-V advancement is used to *expand an area* while shortening it.

Incise a Y with its lower limb extending through the area of skin deficiency. Advance the tip of the flap into the V so created.

Rhomboid Flap
(Limberg)

The rhomboid flap is used to remove an area of excess skin.

9 Pinch the skin between the thumb and forefinger to determine in which direction the excess skin lies.
A, Mark and excise a rhomboid area formed with 60- to 120-degree angles across the excess skin. Draw a line perpendicular to the long axis of the defect equal to the length of one side of the rhomboid (**a** to **b**). Draw a second line at a 120-degree angle at (**a**) that is parallel to that side of the rhomboid. (The other three optional incisions are shown by dotted lines in the inset.)
B, Raise the flap, transpose it, and suture it in position.

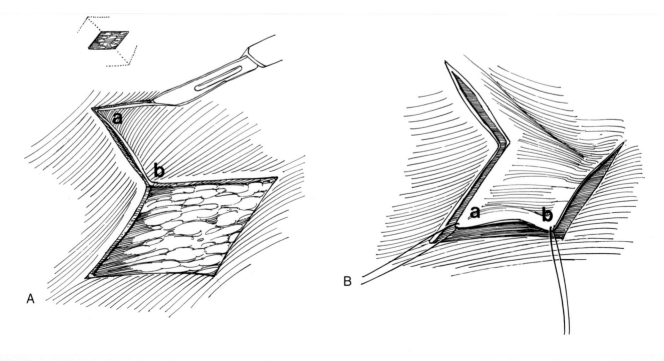

Flap Rotation/Flap Transposition

Use this technique for covering a small defect.

10 **A,** Trim a piece of glove-wrapper paper the size of the defect. Rotate it on the pivot point of the proposed flap (**a**) to be sure of its arc of rotation. Mark and incise the skin flap. Excise a small Burow's triangle at the base of the flap on the outside of the arc.

B, Raise and rotate the flap. *Note*: In many situations, the surgeon can visualize the needed cuts and rotations by cutting and manipulating a paper model of the defect before marking the skin.

Peninsula Flap

11 This flap, as a prototype of the random pattern flaps, is supplied only by branches of the residual perforating arteries that come from musculocutaneous/fasciocutaneous vessels at the base. When a peninsula flap is raised, the blood supply from three of its four sides and from its inferior surface is cut off, leaving it dependent on the randomly oriented vessels in the intradermal and subdermal plexuses that enter from the remaining side. Because of this vascular limitation, the ratio of length to width should be as low as possible. Tension on the flap readily distorts and compresses the small vessels in the plexuses, further limiting its viability.

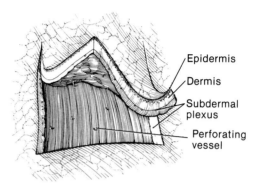

Epidermis

Dermis

Subdermal plexus

Perforating vessel

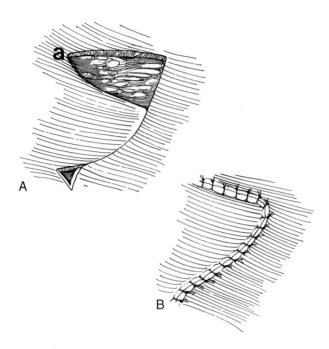

Flap Advancement by Excising Two "Burow" Triangles

Excising the triangles eliminates the dog ears.

12 **A,** Mark and incise two parallel lines extending from the edges of the defect, and two triangles with bases slightly shorter than the length of the defect. Excise the triangles.

B, Mobilize the flap and advance it over the defect.

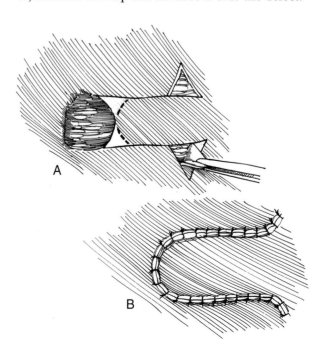

Flap Advancement by Pantographic Expansion/Cutback Incisions

Pantographic cutbacks work well for axial peninsular advances but must be used only with great caution in random peninsula advances because the incisions narrow the base and hence affect the length-width ratio.

13 **A,** Be certain that the base of the flap is wide enough to allow incutting. Mark and make two incisions as acute or preferably as curved (pantographic) cuts extending medially from the ends at **ac**.
B, Advance the flap to form triangular defects **abc**.
C, Suture it in place to close the gaps.

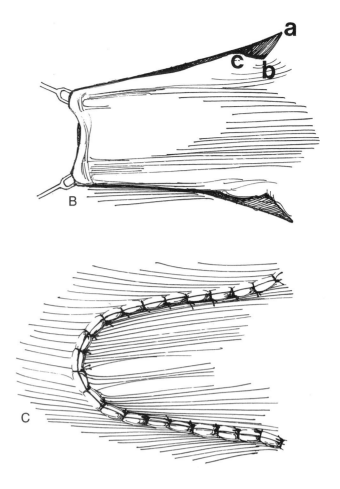

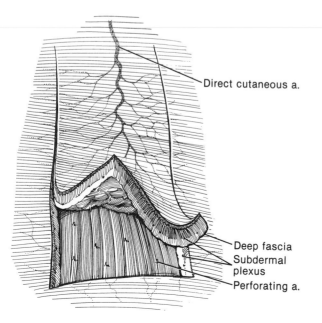

Axial Peninsula Flap

14 Elevate an axial peninsula flap to contain a branch of one of the direct cutaneous arteries (see Figure 1). Do this by incorporating the vessel in the full thickness of the subcutaneous tissue. Maintenance of a broad cutaneous attachment is also important. The flap depends primarily on the size and distribution of the artery, including its lateral random areas. Because these vessels often have a long distribution, the size of the cuticular vascular territory can be appreciable. With its organized self-contained blood supply, an axial peninsular flap may be converted to an island flap or made into a free flap by dividing the vessels and performing a microvascular anastomosis at the recipient site.

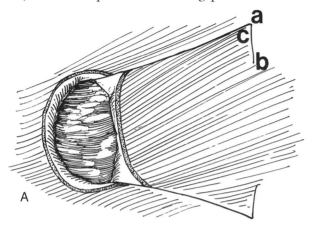

Island Flap

15 The island flap maintains all of the favorable vascular qualities of the peninsular flap but has the advantage of a maneuverable narrow vascular pedicle that contains the essential axial artery and vein. By completely severing attachments to the skin, the little blood supply lost from the random cutaneous vascular plexuses is made up by gain in greater mobility.

Choose a flap for size, ability to arc into place, and presence of adequate vessels. Although the island flap can be transposed much more easily than the peninsular flap, the vessels from which the flap dangles are fragile and easily injured. Flaps that can be transposed with much more freedom are the muscle flaps or fascial flaps and their respective skin island paddles.

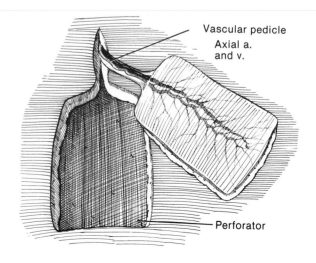

Correction of Dog Ear

16 **A,** Retract the center of the longer edge that remains beyond the last stitch.

B, Incise the skin in the line of the incision for a short distance on the opposite side.

C, Incise the skin on the redundant side, also in the line of the incision, to excise the flap of excess skin.

D, Close the remainder of the wound.

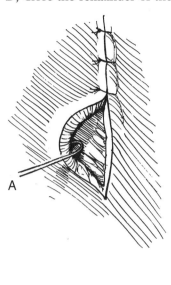

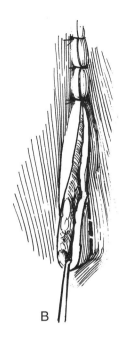

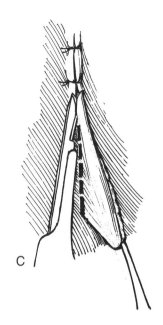

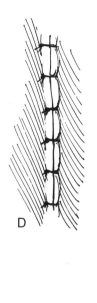

Release of Contracture
(Borges)

17 **A and B,** Mark and incise the length of the scar, and make a succession of staggered oblique cuts to form multiple small Z-plasties (**ab, cd,** and so on).

C, Transpose each pair of skin triangles.

D, Suture them in place.

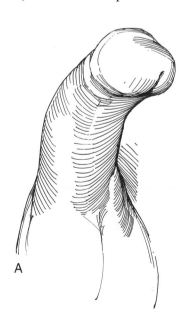

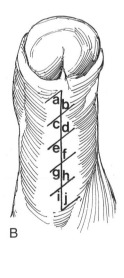

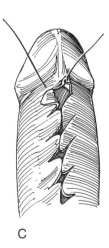

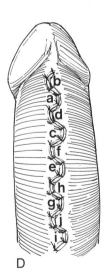

MUSCULOCUTANEOUS FLAPS

Elevation of muscle and the overlying skin on a single pedicle produces a musculocutaneous flap. These flaps are useful in the repair of urogenital defects, especially when based on the gracilis and inferior rectus abdominis muscles.

18 *Examples:* Muscles with perforators that supply the overlying cutaneous vascular territories suitable for formation of musculocutaneous flaps are shown. On the left are the deep inferior epigastric vessels supplying the *rectus abdominis muscle*. On the right is the median circumflex femoral artery to the *gracilis muscle*.

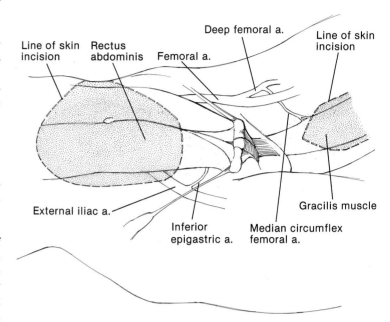

Gracilis Myocutaneous Flap

The gracilis flap is well suited for reconstruction of the perineum and genitalia, for pelvic fistulas, and for vaginal and phallic reconstruction.

19 The gracilis originates from the outer surface of the inferior pubic ramus and the ischial ramus and inserts on the medial shaft of the tibia below the medial condyle. These bony sites can be palpated very reliably. When the leg is abducted, the gracilis is the most medial of the superficial muscles of the leg, lying medial to and slightly behind the adductor longus, a relationship helpful in identifying it. The skin element of the flap lies behind a line drawn from the pubic tubercle to the medial tibial condyle.

The major vascular supply to the gracilis is the median circumflex femoral artery, a branch of the deep femoral artery. It enters the muscle about one third of the way (8 to 10 cm) from the proximal end, allowing the muscle to be transposed into the perineum, the pubic or ipsilateral inguinal area, or the ischial fossa.

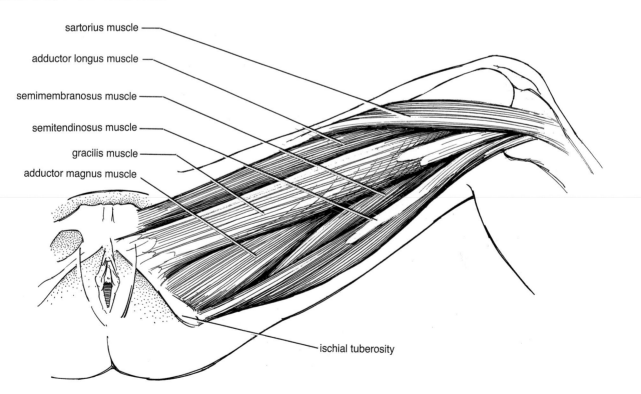

20 *Position:* Place the patient in the low dorsal lithotomy position, and establish the normal anatomic relationships before abducting the leg. Mark the pubic tubercle and the medial condyle at the knee. It is often useful for orientation to mark the line between the pubic tubercle and medial condyle while the patient's leg is flat and mildly abducted (*dashed line*) because the flap consists of the island of skin and the muscle posterior to the line between these two structures. Prepare the left (or right) leg from the lower abdomen to the midcalf. Also prepare and drape the vulva and vaginal area in the female.

Incision: The adductor longus tendon, inserting on the tubercle, is on tension as the leg is abducted, providing the key to locating the gracilis muscle that lies medial and posterior to it. Proximally, palpate the soft area below the pubic tubercle; the gracilis muscle originates there.

Then mark an ellipse 6 or 7 cm wide (it can be made as wide as the 12 cm needed for construction of a neo-vagina), beginning 10 cm below the tubercle and ending cephalad to the medial epicondyle about 18 cm distally. Take care in marking the ellipse to keep the skin of the thigh in its anatomic position because if it is redundant, it can sag posteriorly where it will no longer be supplied by perforators from the gracilis. This ellipse is made longer than required for the flap itself to allow for a tapering closure of the defect; the ends are trimmed later.

The circulation to the skin island overlying the proximal two thirds of the muscle belly is very reliable. Distally, it may not be consistently so. Therefore, if the distal portion of the island is needed for the repair, check the circulation in that portion of the flap with fluorescein after elevation.

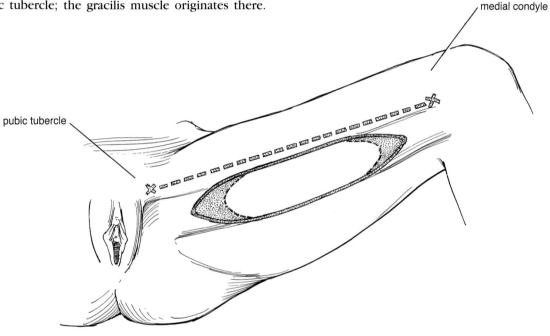

medial condyle

pubic tubercle

21 *First opening:* Make an incision at the medial condyle, and bluntly dissect the subcutaneous tissue until the tendinous insertion of the gracilis muscle is palpated where it lies under the sartorius and anterior to the insertion of the hamstring muscles (the semimembranosus and semitendinosus). Pass a right-angle clamp around the tendinous insertion of the gracilis, taking care to avoid the nearby popliteal artery. Pass a Penrose drain around the tendon, and hold it in a clamp.

Second opening: Tense the gracilis muscle by putting traction on the drain. Then palpate the origin of the muscle where it lies below the inferior pubic tubercle. Make an incision at this site. Dissect the subcutaneous tissue to locate the midpoint of the muscle belly.

Elevate the overlying skin if it is redundant and has slipped posteriorly; it should lie in an anatomic position over the muscle. A line connecting these two incisions identifies the midaxis of the muscle and its overlying skin paddle. Outline the paddle starting 4 to 6 cm from the origin to about 10 cm from its insertion. Usually a width of 7 to 8 cm is satisfactory.

Possible errors: The first is to elevate the sartorius instead of the gracilis. Avoid this mistake by recognizing that the insertion of the gracilis muscle is truly tendinous in consistency, whereas the sartorius is muscular. The other is mistaking the adductor longus for the gracilis. Although the adductor longus also has a tendinous insertion, it lies under the distal end of the sartorius, whereas the gracilis is generally posterior to the main belly of the sartorius. Thus, if the sartorius muscle belly must be retracted to dissect the distal end of the muscle, suspect that the muscle being elevated is the adductor, not the gracilis. You will not confuse the gracilis with the semimembranosus and semitendinosus muscles that lie behind because they are entirely tendinous.

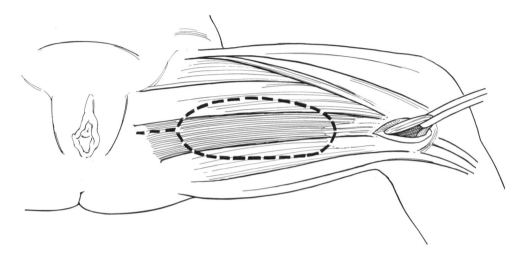

22 Divide the gracilis tendon with the electrocautery. Insert a silk traction suture, and lift the tendon from beneath the sartorius. Incise further along the sides of the skin paddle, at the same time tacking the island to the muscle as the incision progresses. Anteriorly, dissect the gracilis from the adductor. Preserve the two or three nondominant distal pedicles until the major pedicle has been identified. Place a bulldog clamp on each set of vessels, and check the vascularity of the distal limits of the flap with the Doppler probe. Continue to incise the lateral margins of the paddle. Adjust the margins to fit the orientation of the gracilis as it is dissected from the adductor longus anteriorly and the adductor magnus posteriorly and proximally. The saphenous vein is encountered. The branches from the saphenous vein to the gracilis can be divided. Divide the vein, keeping it anterior.

Continue dissecting on the medial side of the adductor longus, progressively exposing the belly of the gracilis muscle until the vascular pedicle of the gracilis muscle is approached. Locate the major pedicle that perforates from beneath the belly of the adductor longus muscle. If extra pedicle length is needed, the pedicle can be dissected back as far as the deep femoral artery.

Complete the elliptical incision over the belly of the gracilis, keeping the skin island attached to the muscle with sutures. Continue the dissection to the origin of the muscle, which usually does not need to be detached. Before removing the flap from its bed, place marking sutures at regular intervals along the muscle edges to prevent uneven tension when the flap is sutured in place.

The flap is now ready for rotation into a position as cover of a perineal defect or for vesicovaginal reconstruction.

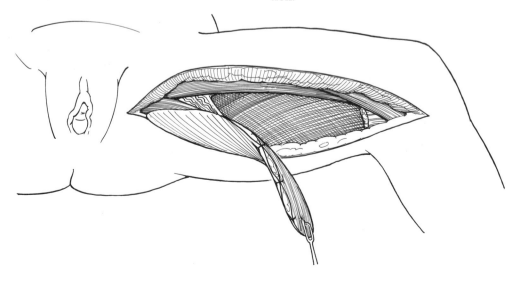

23 **A,** Tunnel under (or divide) the bridge of skin and subcutaneous tissue in the groin to provide a generous passageway. Transpose the flap clockwise (counterclockwise for the right gracilis). If there is any question about the size of the tunnel, divide the bridge and reapproximate it after the flap has been set in place.

B, Suture the muscle in position over the defect with 3-0 CCG sutures. Approximate the skin edges of the donor site over a drain.

For use for vaginal replacement, see page 231.

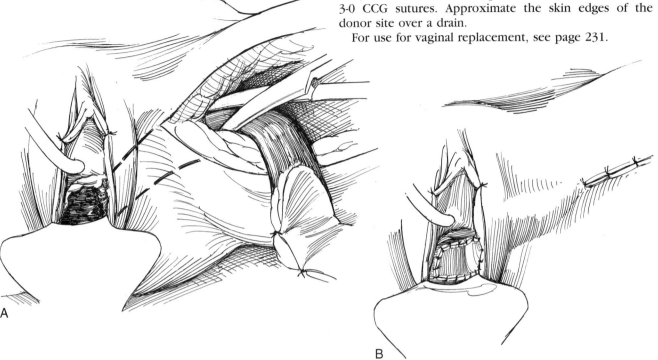

Gracilis Muscle Flap

24 **A** and **B,** For a muscle flap to fill a pelvic defect, raise the gracilis muscle as a flap as previously described but without including the overlying skin. Adduct the leg, pass the flap through a tunnel, and suture it in place. Fix the base of the flap to the adductor magnus. Detach the origin of the muscle to allow for more vigorous transfer. However, if this is done, take care to avoid tension on the vessels. In cases of aggressive transfer, obtain further freedom of the flap by dividing the profunda distal to the circumflex femoral vessel. Before doing this, be certain that the superficial femoral circulation is intact distally.

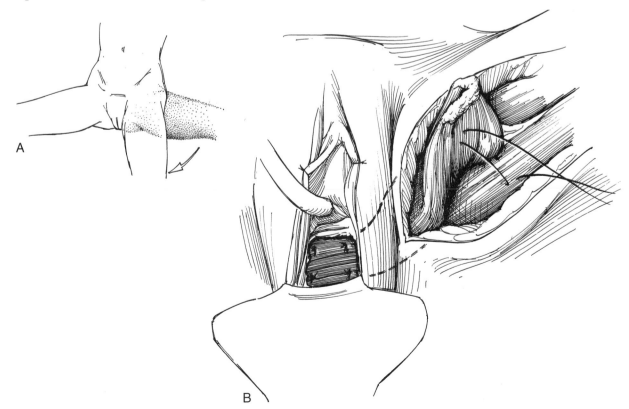

Inferior Rectus Abdominis Flap

Use for lower abdominal, perineal, and groin defects, for phallic and vaginal reconstruction, for vascular interposition in the deep pelvis, and for coverage of perineal defects.

The rectus abdominis is supplied inferiorly by the deep inferior epigastric artery and vena comitans, which are medial branches of the external iliac artery and vein. The supply from the superior epigastric artery is not necessary to maintain the caudal part of the muscle or the skin; that vessel can be sacrificed. However, the major perforators are periumbilical, requiring that skin islands include the periumbilical area to be reliably vascularized. Below the arcuate line, the muscle lies directly on the transversalis fascia and peritoneum; above that line, it lies on the posterior rectus sheath. The inferior epigastric artery provides a very flexible pedicle in most cases for placement of a musculocutaneous flap in defects around the genitalia. The vessels lie on the deep surface of the muscle almost to the level of the umbilicus in most individuals. Because the fulcrum of transposition is deep in the pelvis, in most cases the flap can be easily transposed. By dividing the attachment of the rectus to the symphysis, the muscle can be moved freely into place and can actually be used for coverage of the contralateral groin.

The donor site is readily closed. Either rectus muscle may be used, depending on the quality of the common femoral artery. The fulcrum of transposition of the flap allows placement into the perineum for reconstruction of the vagina and for repair of defects of the base of the bladder.

Prepare the recipient site first. If there is any question regarding the integrity of the common femoral artery on one side, use the contralateral rectus muscle. Also, if there is any question about the size or patency of the deep inferior epigastric artery, examine it by duplex ultrasonography. In addition, if desired, determine the relationship of the vessel to the muscle by the same modality.

25 **A,** Outline an asymmetric flap extending well below the umbilicus in order to include the perforating vessels that enter there. The width depends in part on the size needed for coverage of the defect and in part on the laxity of the abdominal wall for closure. The skin island can be oriented vertically, entirely transversely, or transversely with a vertical component. Incise the skin and subcutaneous tissue down to the rectus sheath. Circumscribe the umbilicus so that it may remain behind, adherent to a part of the rectus sheath.

B, Alternatively, incise beside the umbilicus for a better cosmetic appearance.

C, Elevate the skin edges.

D, Divide the fascia beneath the skin edges, beginning along the lateral border of the rectus. Leave 1 to 1.5 cm of the anterior sheath laterally for closure.

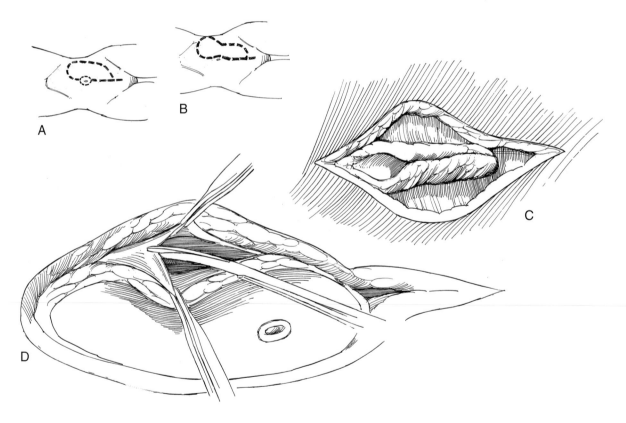

26 Dissect the rectus muscle from its sheath, again starting laterally, freeing its upper half to the midline posteriorly. The vessels usually enter the belly of the muscle at the level of the umbilicus and usually bifurcate there.

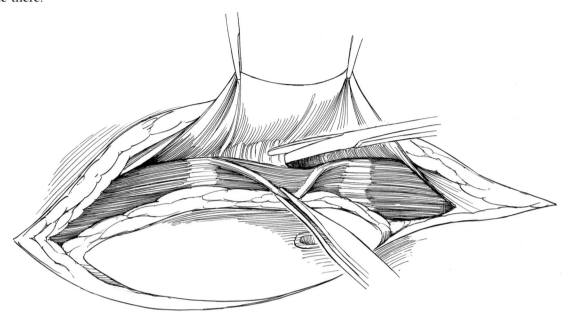

27 First dissect the anterior and then the posterior sheaths from the muscle. Inferiorly, below the arcuate line, the dissection is made directly on the peritoneum. Leave the major perforating vessels joining fascia to skin. Place silk tacking sutures to hold the skin edges to the muscle. During this dissection be cautious not to injure the muscle or small vessels; fortunately, the separation of muscle from sheath is usually not difficult except at the tendinous inscriptions.

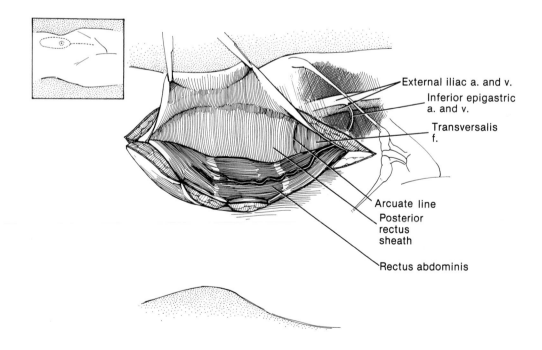

28 Divide the rectus muscle, even as far as its attachment at the xiphoid, and secure the superior epigastric artery. Insert a traction suture of 2-0 silk in the end. Continue freeing the muscle posteriorly, while dividing and clipping the segmental motor branches.

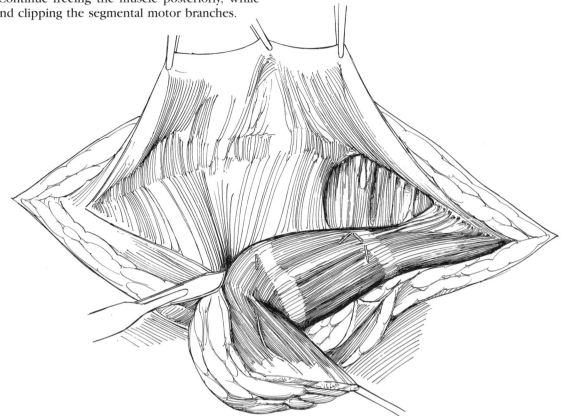

29 Approach the inferior end with care. The inferior epigastric vessels that make up the vascular pedicle arise somewhat laterally to enter into the lower fifth of the rectus muscle. Dissect these vessels, and encircle them with a vessel loop. The inferior end of the rectus muscle may be divided to allow the flap to rotate more freely and to reduce concern that it will be compressed when placed in a tunnel. Alternatively, leave that end intact to provide a margin of safety against harmful traction during placement. If divided, insert a stay suture in that end to aid in positioning.

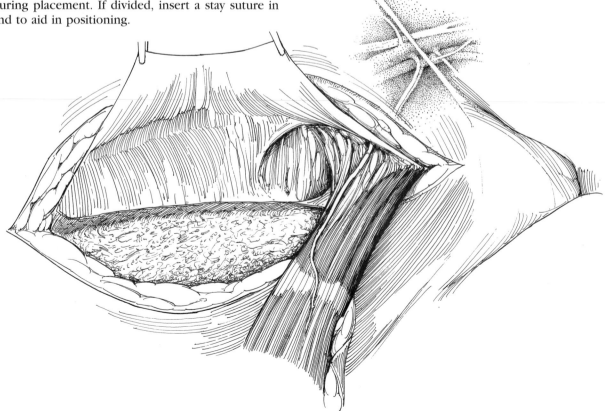

30 Tunnel the flap into position in the perineum or groin, making sure that the pedicle is not kinked or constricted, and fix it in place with two layers of sutures after inserting a suction drain beneath it. Close the rectus sheath with a running (possibly doubled) 0 nylon suture. Because the posterior wall is weak in the distal third where the posterior sheath is absent, a sheet of synthetic material (Gore-Tex) may be cut to size and sutured in place with heavy monofilament synthetic sutures tied with eight or nine knots. Insert a suction drain

within the rectus sheath because it often communicates with the perineal or groin defect, which may drain lymph. Close the subcutaneous layer with a running suture of 2-0 SAS and the skin intracuticularly with a 4-0 SAS on a PC-3 needle. Postoperatively, give two spaced doses of methylprednisolone (Solu-Medrol) to reduce the inflammatory reaction. The patient finds it difficult to walk at first but should not be allowed to sit for more than a few minutes and must either stand or lie down, perhaps on an air-cushioned bed.

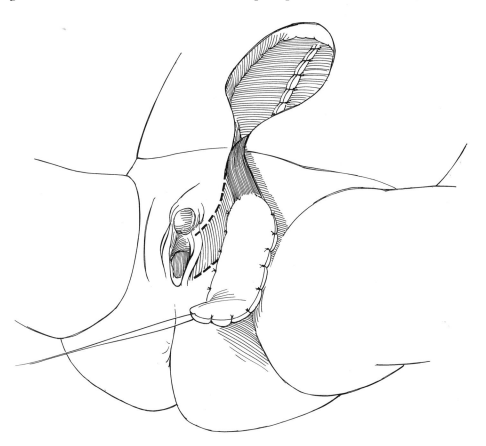

Other Musculocutaneous Flaps

Flaps useful in urologic repair: A *rectus femoris* flap can be used for reconstruction of the lower abdomen and groin but not the perineum. It is easy to raise and can fill large defects, but terminal knee extension may become limited. In most individuals, except those involved in very strenuous athletic activities, the muscle is dispensable. The *tensor fascia lata* flap, particularly when transposed with the vastus lateralis, can be used to cover large groin defects after radical inguinal lymphadenectomy and is useful in reconstruction of the lower abdominal wall. The *inferior half of the gluteus maximus muscle* not only can provide filling for closure of a vesicovaginal fistula but also can support the vaginal wall. A *gluteal thigh flap* (V-Y thigh flap) can perform much the same function. The *posterior thigh flap*, a fasciocutaneous flap, can cover large perineal defects as well as close defects of the lower abdominal wall.

Dressings for Grafts and Flaps

Fixation of the graft to the recipient site is essential to optimize graft apposition to the host bed. It depends on the quality of the dressing and the activity of the patient. Adhesive tape dressings, including sterile strips, adhere better if gum mastic (Mastisol) rather than tincture of benzoin is applied to the skin first. In the case of externally placed grafts, bolster dressings can help with this function. A misconception exists that bolsters prevent the accumulation of hematomas or seromas beneath the graft, but laboratory studies have shown that bolsters applied tight enough to prevent accumulations beneath the graft are also tight enough to interfere with the process of graft take. For grafts, the bolster serves as the graft dressing. Graft donor sites can be dressed with transparent adhesive dressings. Dressings are not usually needed for flaps. Antibiotic ointment can be placed on the suture line and sterile strips placed across it, but an occlusive dressing is usually not applied.

PROBLEMS AFTER GRAFT PLACEMENT OR FLAP TRANSFER

Loss of a skin graft results from factors that interfere with optimal graft take. Graft loss results from poor adherence, most often caused by hematoma, but incomplete immobilization of the graft is next in importance. Thus, perfect hemostasis and proper fixation are the keys to success. *Hematomas* and *seromas* separate the graft from the underlying recipient vessels. Hematomas can likewise interfere with the survival of flaps. They secrete substances that are vasospastic and can adversely affect a flap that has been aggressively transposed. Promptly drain a hematoma or seroma seen accumulating early in the area of the graft; it may be possible to salvage the graft. *Infection* beneath flaps and grafts can arise because of direct bacterial contamination during the transfer process or can represent seromas or hematomas that become infected. Not only do such *purulent collections* separate the graft vessels from the underlying recipient vessels, but the purulent reaction produces a direct toxic effect that interferes with endothelial migration.

A flap that is *too small* is usually the result of either improper selection of a flap or improper design of a skin island. Failure should never be the result of putting the graft on upside down.

Ischemia results in necrosis of the flap. This is in contrast to loss of grafts, which is the result of interference with the processes of graft take. It can come from surgical damage to the blood supply or from overstretching the vessels in the skin through failure to use a back cut or a long enough pedicle. *Tension* is especially harmful when the blood supply is marginal. Release a few of the sutures at once. It may be necessary, however, to redesign the closure or even put the flap back into its original position, to be remobilized at a later time. Inadequate blood supply is the principal cause of ischemia, usually from deficient arterial inflow, although venous congestion with stasis may be the initial event. As venous tension increases in the flap, flap perfusion suffers. Appropriate techniques during the procedure preserve the blood supply but do not completely eliminate the risk of ischemia. *Compromise of the vascular pedicle* can occur from passage through a tunnel that is too small, from stretching of the pedicle, or from blood and serum accumulation around the pedicle. In some cases, when the blood supply to the flap is tenuous, it may be necessary to open one aspect of the flap or the tunnel. These defects can be closed secondarily or grafted later. In the case of venous congestion, if the above measures are not successful, one may contemplate the use of medical leeches to salvage a flap.

Anticoagulation is seldom indicated, but aspirin in low doses may be helpful in improving survival of a flap. A number of drugs adversely affect the general circulation; nicotine from cigarette smoking is probably the substance most commonly encountered, and patients who smoke need to be so advised. Cocaine and cocaine-containing medications are also potent vasospastics and should not be used or administered following tissue transfer.

Commentary by Gerald H. Jordan

Improvements in tissue transfer techniques have revolutionized reconstructive surgery in general and genitourinary reconstructive surgery in particular. It is imperative for the genitourinary reconstructive surgeon to have a firm grasp of the techniques of tissue transfer as well as of the terminology associated with the techniques. The literature can then accurately reflect what is actually done. Terms such as *free grafts, pedicle grafts,* and *pedicle flaps* are all used in confusing ways. It is imperative that the terminology of grafts and flaps be reflective of the procedures done and that redundancies such as *free graft* (grafts are free by definition) be avoided.

Facility in the use of grafts comes from a recognition of the properties of the various graft units. Full-thickness grafts contract very little; however, they are fastidious in their take, both because of the nature of the subdermal plexus, which is composed of relatively large, sparsely distributed vessels, and because of the bulk of the graft itself. Split-thickness grafts, on the other hand, generally take readily; however, because they leave behind the reticular dermis, they contract significantly and tend to be brittle and somewhat fragile in the long term. Modern dermatomes allow grafts to be easily taken; their use merely requires practice.

The base of knowledge required for the successful transfer of flaps is very different from that required for grafts. Each flap has its own individual characteristics and its own quirks with regard to elevation, and it is necessary to have a knowledge that extends deeper than the sizes of the defect and the potential flap.

Axial peninsula flaps tend to be transferred very reliably; they suffer from the disadvantage of an attached base and hence are not usable in a number of situations. By dividing the cuticular adipose base and leaving the vascular pedicle intact, one facilitates transposition of the flap. The fragile, dangling vessels, however, are easily traumatized, possibly compromising the flap.

Microvascular free transfer flaps are obviously the most easily transferred in that the cuticular and the vascular bases are divided. However, an entirely new constellation of expertise is required to approximate the flap vessels to recipient vessels, to allow for flap survival.

For musculocutaneous or fasciocutaneous units, I have found it helpful to view the muscle or the fascia as the flap and the skin island or paddle as a passenger. Obviously, there are just so many seats in a car, and just so many ways that the skin paddle or island can be oriented on the muscle or fascial flap. One must have a firm knowledge of the relationship between the overlying skin island/paddle and the underlying muscle or fascia. This information is essential to the successful transfer of these musculocutaneous or fasciocutaneous units. For example, one might theorize that the inferior rectus abdominis skin island would be most reliable when oriented closest to the origin of the vascular pedicle. However, we know that the most reliable perforators are at the periumbilical area. Thus, the skin islands are most reliably oriented at that level and in essence paradoxically are on the "distal end" of the muscle. On the other hand, the gracilis skin island is unreliable on the distal tip, which in most cases receives its essential vascularization from the distal minor pedicle. In order to transpose the flap unit, this pedicle must be divided. Although the vascularity of the muscle is not affected, the distal tip of the skin island can become ischemic.

The literature reports a 40 percent loss rate for transfer of the gracilis musculocutaneous flap. However, at a number of centers, gracilis musculocutaneous units have been transferred for years with a zero loss rate. Ensuring that the skin island is accurately oriented over the muscle belly is paramount to successful transfer of the musculocutaneous unit. In the patient with redundant thigh skin, the skin that appears to be over the muscle belly indeed is in no way connected via perforators to the muscle. Thus, in that case, one could easily elevate a muscle with totally unrelated overlying adipose and skin tissues. The gracilis pedicle can be easily traumatized by tension. It is essential that the pedicle be optimally dissected to allow a smooth transposition of the flap unit. I prefer to elevate the muscle from distal tip to proximal origin. I believe that inclusion of the superficial fascia is important in making vascularity to the overlying skin adipose unit reliable. The flap appears to have a fasciocutaneous component, and inclusion of the lateral aspects of the fascia with the flap is, I believe, important. The major pedicle is reliably located in most individuals; however, it is not uncommon to find a major pedicle located somewhat distally. It is imperative to ensure that the "minor pedicles" are truly minor pedicles and that no pedicle is divided on the flap prior to encountering what appears to be the major pedicle and ensuring that it indeed provides vascularity to the distal tip of the muscle. In general, the nerve is always adjacent to the major pedicle. The course of the nerve to the gracilis is not, however, the same as the course of the vascular pedicle. Because the gracilis pedicle is located on the thigh, the applications of the gracilis muscle are somewhat limited. The muscle can be transposed into pelvic defects easily and can be used as a vascular interposition in the case of fistulas but is not very useful for defects of the lower abdominal wall. Application of the gracilis flap for lower abdominal wall defects or inguinal defects requires vigorous dissection and transposition.

On the other hand, the inferior rectus abdominis musculocutaneous flap can be used with great versatility in the pelvis, the lower abdominal wall, the groin, and the perineum. The vessels are situated low in the pelvis, the muscle origin is situated low in the pelvis, and the skin island is most reliable far distal on the muscle. The constellation of all of these attributes makes the flap extremely versatile.

The inferior rectus abdominis muscle can be very effectively used on its own to provide vascular interposition deep into the pelvis. Some patients are encountered in whom the omentum is unusable because of prior surgery; the inferior rectus abdominis muscle can be easily substituted in many of these cases. I have found it essential to define the relationship of the deep inferior epigastric vessels to the muscle and routinely screen all patients with duplex ultrasound examination in whom this flap is contemplated. The flow characteristics of the vessels can be easily assessed, and, as mentioned, the relationship of the vessels to the underlying muscle also evaluated.

The definitions of cuticular vascular territories, muscle, and fasciocutaneous vascularity have truly turned the entire body into a potential donor site. Whereas in the past we were virtually sentenced to addressing reconstructive problems via the reconstructive ladder approach, with reliable use of the large number of tissue transfer units now available we can select units that provide the optimal result. In the past, coverage was paramount, with all other functional aspects of the transfer secondary. Now the requirements for coverage can be combined with the need for improved vascularity in an area, sensibility to an area, and consideration of the eventual cosmetic result.

Microsurgical Techniques

INSTRUMENTS

Provide a nonlocking spring-handle needle-holder with a curved tip, long enough to fit in the hand like a pen; jeweler's #5 forceps for vascular work (padded so it can be rotated axially and with accurately aligned tips and checked under the microscope before starting work); both sharp-tipped and blunt-tipped slightly curved scissors; atraumatic vascular clamps both straight and curved, which may be mounted on a bar; a bipolar coagulator using low power; microsurgical sponges; a suction tip (3 F); a 30-gauge blunt-angled needle for delivery of heparin-saline irrigating solution; and plastic background material. For sutures, use 10-0 monofilament nylon on a triangular cutting needle. The CO_2 laser can be used for incising tissue by using a joystick that restricts the movement to the field of view, and the neodymium:yttrium-aluminum-garnet laser is useful for coagulation. Take special care of microsurgical instruments in washing and storing.

POINTERS ON TECHNIQUE

Position the patient so that the surgeon and assistant may put their knees under the table. This may require use of a table extension. Wear a custom-fitted $2.5\times$ surgical loupe in conjunction with a head light during exposure of the vessels, before moving the operating microscope into the field. Arrange the microscope so that it may be rotated over the site, and cover it. Place the instruments so that they can be picked up without moving the eyes from the field. Drip heparinized saline (100 IU/300 ml) from a syringe fitted with a fine blunt needle to keep the tissues moist and to allow blood to be drawn away by a pointed microsurgical sponge.

Place stitches with the needle entering perpendicularly to the vessel wall, and take equal bites on either side. Zoom to low power when drawing a stitch through the tissue to pull it in the long axis of the vessel to avoiding tearing or pulling it too far.

ARTERIAL ANASTOMOSIS

For arteries with diameters less than 2 mm, use the operating microscope. For larger vessels, a three- or four-power loupe may be adequate. Have your assistant sit opposite you.

Dissect the adventitia from the severed ends of the arteries adequately in both directions. Coagulate any fine branches with the bipolar current, and divide them 1 mm away from the vessel itself. Place a piece of blue background material behind the vessel. Looking through the microscope, carefully remove excess perivascular connective tissue by teasing it apart with jeweler's forceps and trimming it with scissors. Strip it back for a distance of 0.5 cm, but be very careful not to injure the vasa vasorum on the vessel wall. Reverse any vasospasm with a few drops of 1 percent lidocaine, and then keep the vessel moist with warm saline solution. Apply the fixed arm of the vascular clamp to the less mobile end of the vessel; then move the other arm to grasp the more mobile end, leaving them about 1 cm apart.

1 Cut the end of the vessel cleanly across. Flush the open end with saline solution, or bend it back over the clamp to express any debris. Pick up the adventitia at the cut end, and tease it out over the end in several places to form a stocking (circumcision technique). Trim this flush with the end of the vessel. Even a small tag projecting into the lumen can initiate a thrombus. Alternatively, carefully lift the adventitia from the vessel wall and trim it with the microscissors. Be very careful when cleaning the adventitia of small delicate vessels not to be too thorough and injure the vessel itself. Irrigate the lumen with heparinized saline again to clear it of blood. Repeat these steps on the opposite stump.

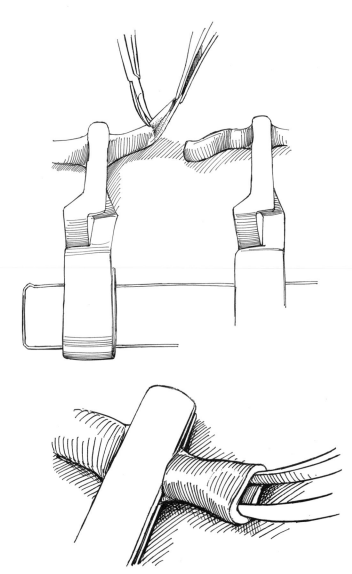

2 Dilate both lumina with #5 jeweler's forceps. Move the arms of the clamp to bring the two ends together until they lie about one vessel-diameter apart.

3 Grasp the outer coat with jeweler's forceps to steady the wall, and place the first guide suture (G1) of monofilament nylon through the vessel edge on the right at the 10-o'clock position. Grasp the needle again, pass it through the vessel to the left, and pull it until only 3 or 4 mm of suture remains free. Tie it by picking up enough suture on the needle end with the forceps to loop once, or preferably twice for a surgeon's knot, over the needle-holder that has already been aligned with the short end, and make the tie by drawing on the forceps and needle-holder simultaneously. Make the second loop in the opposite direction. If the knot is loose, tighten it by drawing on the short end, but do not make it so tight that it strangles the tissue. A third tie may be placed. Cut the short end near the knot; then cut the long end to a length of 1.5 cm, and grasp it with a clamp or loop it around the upper cleat in the vessel clamp. For small vessels, use 25× magnification for placing the sutures, decreased to 16× for tying.

4 Have your assistant put slight traction on the first suture (G1). Place the second guide suture (G2) one third of the way around. Tie, cut, and fix it in the same way as described in the previous step. Some models of clamps have a surrounding frame with cleats around which the long end of the stay suture can be looped. This serves to keep tension across the third of the circumference being sutured.

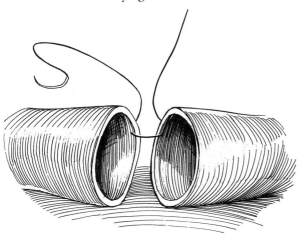

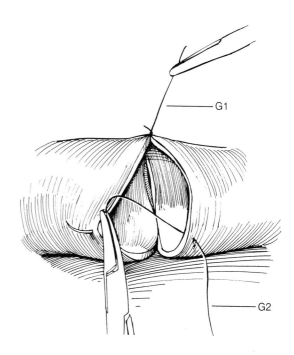

5 Place one or two approximating sutures (A1) between the guide sutures; use a single-throw technique, and cut both ends of the suture.

6 Invert the vessel in its holder, and inspect the interior transluminally for defects in the anterior suture line. Place the third guide suture (G3) equidistant from the other two.

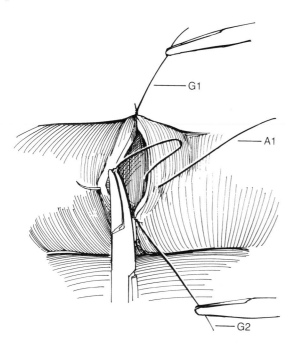

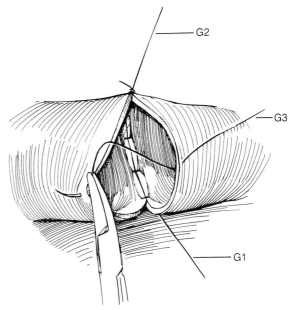

7 Insert one or two approximating sutures between G1 and G3 and between G2 and G3, having the assistant manipulate the guide sutures appropriately.

Remove the distal clamp first, and be sure that reverse blood flow immediately fills the entire segment; otherwise, the anastomosis must be revised. If the segment fills slowly, apply papaverine solution to release any factor of spasm. Release the proximal clamp, and observe for pulsation beyond the repair. Pulsation alone does not mean that the anastomosis is open. Look for lateral pulsations downstream that result from expansion of the vessel; longitudinal pulsations, in contrast, are associated with thrombosis. In doubtful cases, place a closed forceps beneath the distal vessel and gently raise it a few millimeters. As the lumen is progressively narrowed, flow becomes tenuous, and if the vessel is pulsating, jets of blood are seen to flick over the stenosis during systole. Doppler ultrasonography is an alternative method for assessing flow. Irrigate away any blood that leaks out to prevent initiation of a thrombus and to avoid spasm. Do not unduly manipulate the anastomosis. Bleeding at the anastomosis usually stops spontaneously or after applying some absorbable gelatin. If leakage persists, it is wise to replace both clamps and place a suture at the point to get a watertight seal.

In very small vessels in which the flow cannot be visualized, perform a patency test 20 minutes after completing the anastomosis by gently pressing the blood from a segment of vessel just below the anastomosis and ascertaining that it rapidly refills when the more proximal forceps are released. Be careful not to injure the intima by too much force. Do not hesitate to do the anastomosis over again if you are concerned about a technical detail because even a small error can result in failure.

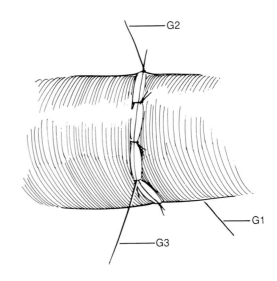

VENOUS ANASTOMOSIS

Use round-tipped microscissors to dissect a small vein to avoid damage to the media or inadvertent puncture. Avoid grasping the vein with forceps. Use maximum illumination. Place one arm of the vessel clamp on the body side first to avoid overstretching the vein. Clear the periadventitial tissue carefully with two pairs of #5 jeweler's forceps, working longitudinally. To see the lumen, float the walls open with saline irrigation. This visualization must be done with each stitch to keep from catching the opposite wall. The technique of suturing is the same as that for small arteries but requires constant visualization of the thin vessel wall and the tip of the needle to prevent incorporation of the opposite wall. Wrapping is not necessary. Release the proximal clamp, then the distal clamp, and perform a patency test.

Commentary by John S. P. Lumley

Irrigation with a heparinized saline solution is essential to all microsurgery to ensure that tissues do not become dehydrated. Blood can be diluted and washed away, allowing good visibility and preventing clotting within the anastomosis. Dissection is done by gently teasing tissues away from each other, using two jeweler's forceps, rather than sharp or vigorous blunt dissection.

When tying knots, gentle tension on the short end after the second throw allows a little tightening of the knot. Pulling on the long end locks the knot, and this is undertaken once the tension is appropriate. The use of a framed double clip allows tension to be maintained on a knot if one end of the suture is left long and hooked around a cleat: One cleat is situated on either side of an end-to-end anastomosis. Tension in the opposite direction by a second stitch, one third of the way around the circumference, enables easy placement of front stitches without risk of incorporating a lax posterior wall. The two long lengths are then released and used to rotate the vessel. This avoids endangering the anastomosis by rotating bulky vascular clamps.

With end-to-side anastomosis it may not be possible to rotate the vessels. The first stitch is, therefore, placed in the middle of the back wall and subsequent stitches are placed alternately on either side, proceeding around each corner to the front wall.

Establishing patency can be difficult, and flow rather than pulsation must be demonstrated. The most reliable technique is to use two jeweler's forceps. Gently occlude the vessel just beyond the anastomosis with the first forceps. The second is used to milk out the blood from a segment distal to the first. Gently maintain pressure to keep the segment empty, and then release the first forceps to see whether flow across the anastomosis fills the occluded segment. In the flicker test, partial occlusion of the distal vessel is obtained by angulation with a forceps. When the right tension is applied, blood flicks through the occlusion with each heart beat.

NEURAL ANASTOMOSIS

Microneurorrhaphy is more difficult than microvascular anastomosis. Practice is required to be able do it without hopelessly fraying the nerve ends.

Perform the nerve anastomosis last. Obtain hemostasis in the stump of the nerve with micro bipolar or ophthalmic hot-wire cautery, not with usual electrocoagulating current. Remove the adventitia from the nerve ends for a distance of 2 to 3 mm so that the fascicles may be easily visualized and the adventitia, like that of blood vessels, can be kept from becoming interposed. Too much excision removes intrinsic vessels and leaves the end hard to handle.

Examine the arrangement of the fascicles to allow proper alignment. Two elements are involved in repair: the epineurium encasing the bundle of fascicles and the perineurium encasing the individual fascicle. The objective is to incorporate both epineurium and perineurium in each stitch.

NERVE REPAIR

8 **A,** *Partial section:* Separate the cut portion from the remainder of the nerve by a vertical incision in the adventitial coat, the epineurium, and between the nerve bundles in the perineurium. Trim the nerve ends back to normal tissue with a razor blade, and approximate them with four fine NAS.

B, *Total section:* For small nerves (less than 3 to 4 mm in diameter), dissect the nerve free enough to allow approximation without tension, and place the nerve ends in a noncrushing approximation clamp (not shown). Cut the ends square with a razor blade. Under the microscope, align the fascicles that lie around the edge of the cut ends by rotating one end of the nerve. Place one or two 10-0 or 11-0 monofilament sutures in each peripheral fascicle, catching only the perineurium and epineurium, not the nerve matrix. Avoid tying the sutures too tight. Cut the suture ends short. For large nerves, split the fascicles into groups, and align and anastomose each group individually.

Microsurgical techniques *for vasovasostomy* and *vasoepididymostomy* are described on page 365.

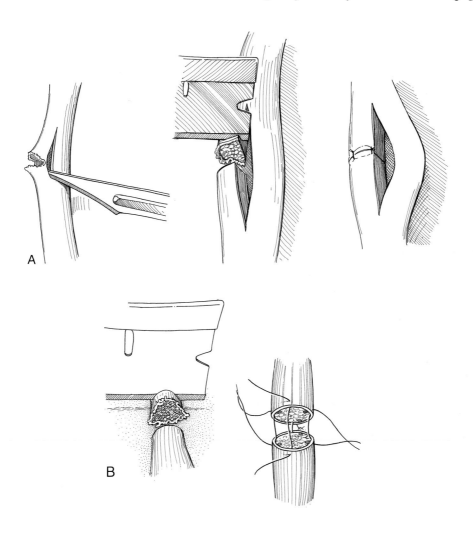

A

B

Bowel Stapling Techniques

Apply these techniques to noncontinent and continent diversion and to bladder augmentation and substitution (see Sections 15 to 18). Stapling for formation of an ileal conduit is described independently on pages 653 to 654.

Stapled anastomoses are less liable to leak than are sutured ones but are more likely to bleed because they do not devascularize the margins as thoroughly. Therefore, it is important to check the staple line for bleeding from both the mucosal and serosal sides, although it is not always possible to see the mucosal surface. Placement of a figure-eight stitch of 4-0 SAS usually controls the bleeding.

Absorbable staples may be preferable for bladder augmentation and substitution because they are not niduses for stone formation when chronically exposed to urine.

Several autostaplers should be available: TA 55, TA 30, EEA, and GIA.

END-TO-END ANASTOMOSIS

1 Clear the mesentery from the ends of the bowel for a distance of 1 cm (see page 683). Place a stay suture through the full thickness of both bowel segments at the mesenteric and antimesenteric edges. Grasp and elevate both adjacent walls together in the center with an Allis clamp. Place the jaws of the TA 55 stapler to include the bowel beneath the Allis clamp and the stay sutures. Approximate the blades by turning the thumb screw until the black lines on them are aligned. Push the pin firmly in place. Release the safety catch and fire the staples.

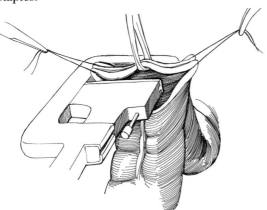

2 Shave off the excess bowel wall with a knife. Cut as close as possible to the anvil and cartridge to prevent retention of necrotic tissue.

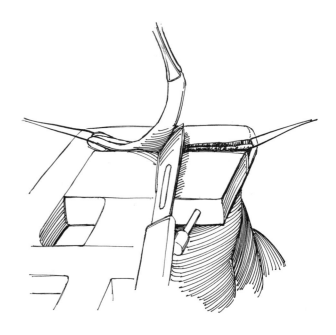

3 Insert everting stay sutures through the midpoint of both edges to triangulate the defects.

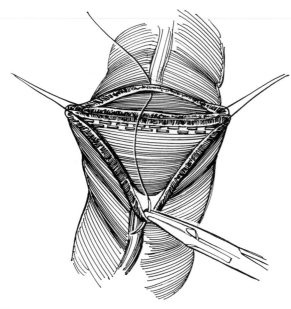

4 Place half of the remaining edges in the TA 30 stapler. Be certain to overlap the original row of staples at the angle. Push the pin in place and fire the staples. Trim the excess bowel wall, but preserve the central suture. Reinforce the mucosal edges with figure-eight sutures at any bleeding sites.

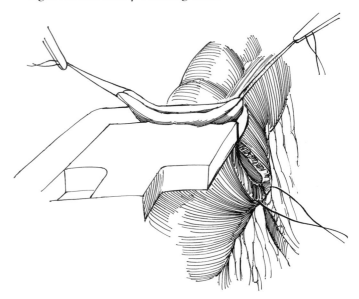

5 Staple the other half similarly, being sure that the rows overlap both in the center and at the angle. Shave the excess bowel. Check the anastomosis visually to be certain no gaps remain. Cut the stay sutures, and close the mesenteric defect.

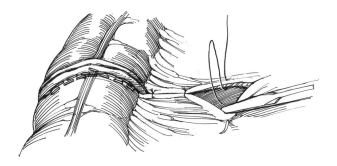

END-TO-END TRIANGULATION TECHNIQUE

6 Triangulate the bowel with three everting stay sutures. Staple the mesenteric border first with the TA 30 stapler; then staple one of the two sides of the triangle.

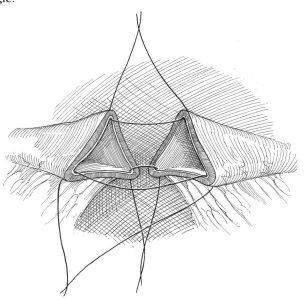

7 Staple the other side of the triangle. Take care not to catch the back wall. Be sure to incorporate the end of each previous line of staples.

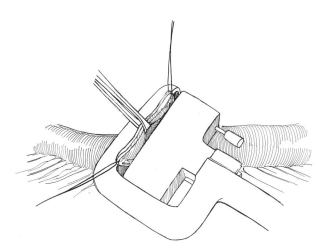

8 Check the staple line for bleeding; place a figure-eight stitch if necessary.

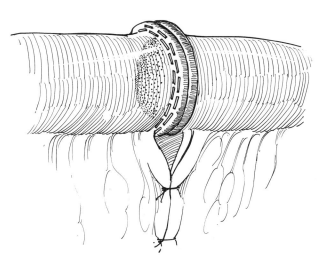

COLOCOLOSTOMY

9 Place a purse-string suture around the proximal end of the transected colon and a second one around the distal end. Make a short colotomy in the proximal end, and insert the EEA stapler. Tie the proximal purse-string suture around its shaft. Place three stay sutures in the distal end, and introduce the anvil, posterior lip first. Tighten and tie the purse-string suture. With traction on the handle, draw the bowel snugly against both anvils. Close and fire the stapler. Open the stapler. Place a traction suture on the staple line, and lift it to help negotiate the anvil back out through the anastomosis.

10 Close the colotomy with a TA 30 stapler.

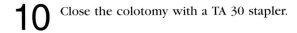

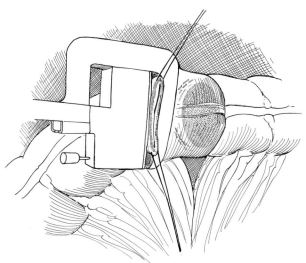

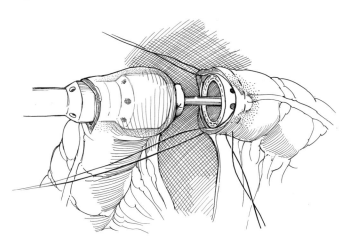

ILEOCOLIC END-TO-SIDE ANASTOMOSIS

The technique is similar to that described in Figures 9 and 10 for colocolostomy.

11 Spatulate the antimesenteric border of the ileum, and encircle it with a purse-string suture. Make a window in the antimesenteric wall of the ascending colon 3 cm above the end. Place a similar purse-string suture around the opening. Introduce the EEA stapler through the end of the colon and out the new opening. Advance the dome-shaped anvil, and tie the colonic purse-string suture around the shaft behind it. Grasp the ileum with Allis clamps and feed it over the anvil, unspatulated margin first. Tie the ileal purse-string suture. Close the EEA stapler loaded with 3.5-mm staples and fire the staples, simultaneously placing a double row of staples and cutting a stoma. Fold back the end of the colon to inspect the staple line, and add sutures for bleeding. Check the anvil to be sure the tissue button is complete.

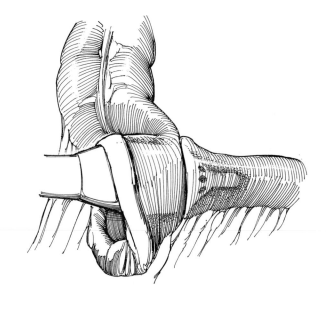

12 To close the end of the colon, place a stay suture in the mesenteric and antimesenteric borders. Apply the TA 55 stapler proximal to them. Turn the thumbscrew clockwise to approximate the blades so that the black lines are aligned. Release the safety catch and clamp the handles. Trim the excess bowel and close the mesentery. Reinforce the mucosal edges with figure-eight sutures at any bleeding sites. Check for viability because the blood supply may be attenuated there. This same closure technique can be used for ileum.

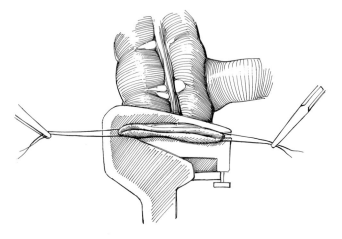

SIDE-TO-SIDE ANASTOMOSIS OF ILEUM

13 Clear the mesentery from the distal ends of the bowel for a distance equal to the length of the limbs of the GIA stapler.

A, Place stay sutures in the mesenteric and antimesenteric edges of both ends of the bowel to maintain alignment. Insert the limbs of the GIA stapler so that they lie in line with the mesentery. Lock the stapler blades, and push the driver to insert the staples and activate the knife.

B, Remove the driver, unlock the limbs, and remove the stapler. Check for viability of the distal mucosa and for hemostasis. Reinforce the serosal edges with horizontal inverting mattress suture of 4-0 silk as required.

14 Apply the TA 55 stapler to each side of the common opening as described in "End-to-End Anastomosis," Steps 1 through 5. Check for viability because the blood supply may be attenuated there. Close the mesentery.

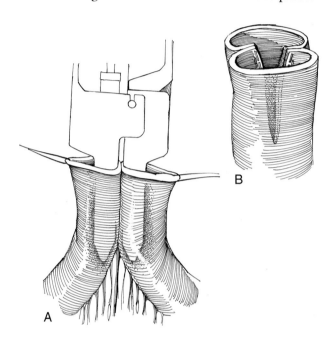
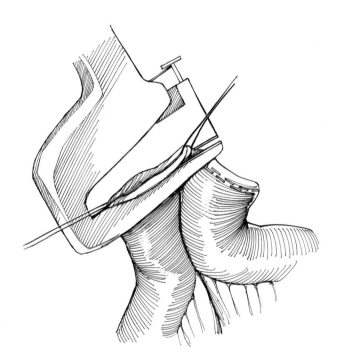

Commentary by Joseph A. Smith, Jr.

The advantages of a stapled bowel anastomosis are such that I rarely perform a hand-sewn anastomosis. With proper attention to technique, anastomotic leak or stricture is unusual. A stapled anastomosis can be completed more rapidly than a hand-sewn one, and the decrease in overall operating room time compensates for the expense of the devices.

I strongly prefer a side-to-side over an end-to-end anastomosis. The primary advantage is the larger lumen size with a side-to-side anastomosis. This is true whether it is an ileum-to-ileum or ileocolic anastomosis or a colocolostomy. Avoidance of tension on the anastomosis is a key technical factor. Although this is usually not a problem, a few maneuvers can be helpful in some circumstances. The mesentery should be divided for a sufficient length to allow mobility of the end of the bowel segment. It is important, however, to maintain good vascular supply, and incisions in the mesentery should not cross major vascular arcades. If there is a question of the viability of the end of the bowel segment, it should be excised and a portion either more proximal or distal used for the anastomosis.

A side-to-side alignment of the bowel sometimes places less tension on the anastomosis than an end-to-end one. Stay sutures of 3-0 silk in the seromuscular layer of the bowel help maintain alignment but also take tension off the anastomosis.

The technique I use for a stapled side-to-side bowel anastomosis is somewhat different from the one described. Figure 13A shows the anastomosis being initiated with open bowel segments. Bowel anastomosis is performed most often in urologic surgery after a segment of the bowel has been isolated for reconstruction of the urinary tract. During this process, I use a GIA stapler to divide the bowel. Therefore, the end of the bowel segment remains closed with the GIA staple line prior to the anastomosis. This helps avoid contamination. The ends of the bowel segments are positioned in a manner similar to that shown in the figure. This is where placement of the 3-0 silk seromuscular sutures is helpful for alignment. The bowel segments are approximated by passing two separate 3-0 silk sutures beneath the staple line at both the mesenteric and antimesenteric borders of the end of the bowel segment and tying them. Another 3-0 silk seromuscular suture is placed 4 or 5 cm farther down on the bowel away from the end at about the place where the tip of the GIA stapler will be. A corner segment large enough to accommodate a GIA stapler is excised from the antimesenteric border of the bowel using heavy staples. An Allis clamp can be used to grasp the bowel segment and help with the insertion of the GIA stapler. After the stapler is fired, a 3-0 silk suture is placed at the end of the staple line for reinforcement and to remove tension. A TA 55 stapler is then used to close the end of the bowel segment.

Sutures that reinforce the staple line generally are not necessary but can be comforting and may help prevent anastomotic leaks that occur because of small disruptions in the staple line.

A side-to-side anastomosis such as this can be performed with any bowel segment. No adaptation or change in technique is required even in the face of a disparity in the size of the bowel lumen. Thus, the technique is applicable for ileocolic anastomosis or when dilation of the small bowel occurs proximal to a point of obstruction. Closure of the mesentery is important to prevent an internal hernia. However, care should be taken to include only the peritoneal covering of the mesentery in order to avoid injury to a mesenteric vessel.

Ureteral Stents

An internal ureteral stent provides drainage for urine and a scaffold for reconstitution of the ureteral wall over defects. It should be made of a material that is smooth, resists breakdown in urine, discourages encrustation, and preferably is radiopaque. Insertion and reinsertion must be easy, and the stent must stay in place. Silicone has the least tendency to degrade or encrust, but it is very flexible and difficult to place and maintain in position. Hydrogel coating reduces reactivity for long-term use. More than 70 different stents are manufactured, and all are relatively expensive, especially compared with commercial silicone tubing.

INTRAOPERATIVE INSERTION TECHNIQUES

Double Pigtail Stent

1 Determine the length of the required stent by passing a calibrated ureteral catheter first to the renal pelvis and then to the bladder; add the length of the pigtails to the measured lengths. Most double-J ureteral stents are 26 or 28 cm long. Short patients may require a 22- or 24-cm stent, tall patients a 30-cm stent. The caliber should be one that fits easily inside the ureter without stretching it, usually 7 F or 8 F. A stent equipped with a 4-cm retrieval suture is easier to remove cystoscopically when the stent is not passed all the way into the bladder or when proximal migration occurs. Alternatively, attach a nylon loop to the end of a single-J stent, and string a 3-cm polyethylene tube on the loop to serve as an anchor to prevent migration and aid retrieval (Dauleh, Byrne, and Baxby, 1995). Magnetic retrieval devices are not practical.

Provide low-dose antibiotic coverage. Aspiration and irrigation may be used to prove that the tip of the catheter is in the pelvis and the bladder. Intravenous indigo carmine helps determine if the distal end of the stent has entered the bladder.

To place a stent, cut an extra hole in its midportion or gently enlarge a drainage hole with a mosquito clamp. Do not cut too large a hole, as this may allow the tube to kink or break. Insert a 0.035-inch guide wire, a size stiff enough to straighten the curl. Feed the stent into the renal pelvis and remove the wire. Repeat the process to pass the stent into the bladder. Alternatively, place two guide wires. Pass one wire into the bladder, and feed the stent over it; do the same for the renal end. For easy early removal in boys, make a small opening in the bladder, grasp the tip of the balloon catheter, and tie the stent to it. Close the cystostomy in two layers. In girls, use a stent with a retrieval string, or tie a long suture to the catheter, draw it out of the meatus, and fasten it to the labia. Close the ureterotomy and drain the area, or proceed with ureteral anastomosis if the ureter has been divided.

If the stent is to remain for a long time, check its position and possible associated obstruction occasionally by roentgenography or ultrasonography (the stent has a characteristic railroad track appearance), and follow with regular urine cultures. In a patient at risk for stone formation, change the stent at least every 2 to 3 months. When removing a stent, do not try to pull it out with sharp biopsy forceps; they may shear it off. Use appropriate grasping forceps.

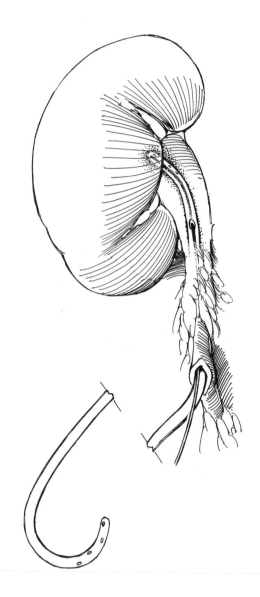

Straight Tubing

2 Use clear silicone-rubber tubing (5 F to 10 F) or an infant feeding tube (5 F and 8 F). Make extra holes in the wall but not so large as to compromise the integrity of the tube. Silicone tubing is more pliable, thinner walled, and better utilized in smaller sizes and is considerably less expensive than J-shaped stents. Insert the tubing through a short ureterotomy, and pass one end of the measured distance to the renal pelvis and the other to the bladder. Control advancement with a clamp placed loosely on the stent at the site of entry. Fasten the stent to the ureteral wall.

A, Run a 5-0 PCG suture (for shorter stay) or a 5-0 SAS (for longer stay) directly through the walls of the ureter and the walls of the stent, and tie it loosely on top of the ureter.

B, Alternatively, use a 2-0 NAS placed as in A, but bring both ends to the skin over a button. Later, cut the suture flush with the skin, and withdraw both the stent and suture through the bladder.

Stents for Ureteroureterostomy

For a description of ureteroureterostomy, see page 834.

3 Place a stent unless the ureters are of good caliber and well vascularized, with no constriction or tension anticipated at the anastomosis. Before completing the anastomosis, select a length of silicone-rubber tubing, an infant feeding tube, a double-J stent, or a pigtail catheter of a caliber that fits loosely in the normal ureter. Measure the distance to the donor pelvis and to the bladder with a 5 F angiographic exchange catheter or a ureteral catheter. If a feeding or silicone-rubber tube is used, cut holes in it at 1-cm intervals, and mark it with a removable suture at the length required to reach the pelvis. Cut the other end at the length needed to reach the bladder, but add 3 cm to this end so that it can be retrieved transvesically. Pass it up the donor ureter to the pelvis and down into the bladder. Fix it in place with a 5-0 CCG suture through the edge of the ureteral wall and through the tubing, tied loosely. Complete the anastomosis. If the recipient ureter is large, pass a second stent up and down it, as described previously for the pigtail and straight stents.

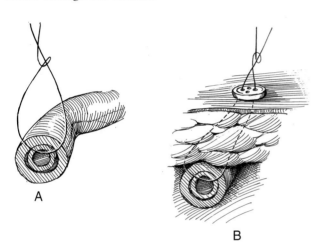

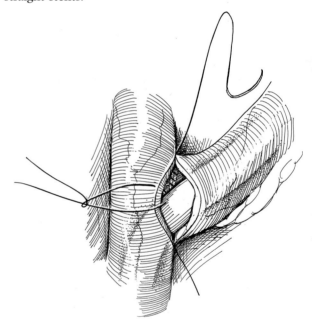

Alternative Technique. Pass the tubing with extra holes through the ureterotomy and up to the renal pelvis. Tack it to the exit site with a 4-0 absorbable suture through the ureteral edge tied around the tubing. Bring the stent retroperitoneally and out through a stab wound. If a stent is used with a nephrostomy, as in pediatric pyeloplasty, pass a length of fine-caliber silicone rubber tubing through a 10 F Silastic balloon catheter with the tip cut off, and fasten them together with an NAS.

Stent Replacement and Removal

Stents should be *replaced* every 3 to 4 months. In stone formers, the interval may need to be much shorter, as often as 6 to 8 weeks. The trick is to locate the end of the stent and feed a guide wire into it to straighten it. In women, grasp the end of the stent, move it to the urethral meatus, insert a guide wire under vision, and advance it under fluoroscopic control to straighten the stent. In men, bringing the end of the stent to the meatus is not practical because this frequently brings the proximal end into the bladder at the same time. Moreover, the stent may be partially obstructed by encrustations, and the wire may well exit through one of the side holes. A preferable method is to pass a guide wire alongside the stent into the renal pelvis, remove the stent with grasping forceps, being sure the guide wire is not accidentally removed along with it, and place a new stent over the guide wire.

Remove stents in adults under local anesthesia by passing grasping forceps through a flexible cystoscope. A stent can be retrieved blindly, especially in women, by passing a magnet on a probe if a metal rod has been built into the end of the stent (Mykulak et al, 1994).

PROBLEMS FROM STENTS

Dysuria, urinary frequency, urgency, and nocturia are common complaints, especially early after placement. In fact, these symptoms may be so severe that the patient may request that the stent be taken out. Give antispasmodic drugs and wait for subsidence of the symptoms; they frequently ease after a few days. *Flank pain* and pain in the lower abdomen are frequent complaints. *Reflux* sometimes results in flank pain during micturition, but the back pressure is buffered by leakage of urine through the side holes. Warn patients of this potential problem to limit the number of phone calls. Interrupting the urinary stream may relieve the pain. *Urinary tract infection* may intervene. It occurs less frequently if prophylactic antibiotics are given, especially in women, but chronic antibiotic administration is not advisable because it carries the risk of selecting for resistant organisms. Check the urine by culture at semimonthly intervals if clinically indicated. If results are positive and antibacterial therapy does not eradicate the infection, assess for evidence of obstruction with renal sonography and, if obstruction is present, change the stent and again provide culture-specific antibiotics.

Severe complications can evolve silently. *Obstruction* is a common and serious sequela, usually occurring 2 months or more after insertion. Scheduled replacement is a good practice in patients who form stones, especially if they have a solitary kidney. For others, checking regularly by renal ultrasonography and serum creatinine level determinations may be adequate. A program of regular replacement every 8 to 12 weeks may be safest, but the interval must be tailored to the conditions of the individual. *Distal stent migration* arises if the initial placement was faulty, the patient hyperextends the back, or the proximal end of a J stent has insufficient curvature once it is placed (less than 90 degrees or more than 270 degrees of curvature). *Proximal stent migration* is a greater problem, arising from insertion of too short a stent or one having an inadequate distal coil, or placing the proximal coil in an upper calyx. *Breakage* of a stent occurs with acute angulation during traction or from cutting the stent with the grasping (biopsy) forceps. The stent may also break from being left in place too long or from being exposed to extreme light or heat before insertion. If a stent is not easily withdrawn, do not continue to pull on it, but try again in 24 hours. Sometimes traction with a weak rubber band slowly withdraws a recalcitrant stent. *Fragmentation* can occur in stents left in place over several months. This type of accident requires cystoscopic, ureteroscopic, or percutaneous retrieval. Extensive encrustations may require intracorporeal or extracorporeal shock wave lithotripsy to allow removal of the stent. Unfortunately, the *forgotten stent syndrome* is well known; patients come in only when problems arise. Record the time for removal in a day book or computer, and review the entries at monthly intervals.

Commentary by Marshall L. Stoller

Placement of a ureteral stent can be frustrating. Contemporary double-J stents come prepackaged with hydrophilic coatings, appropriate wires (stiffness and length), pushers, and precut open-end edges. They are designed for endoscopic placement/replacement. When difficulties arise during endoscopic placement, a retrograde pyelogram helps delineate the anatomy, including a J-shaped distal ureter secondary to benign prostatic hyperplasia, or a severe kink that may require initial placement of a hydrophilic, coudé-tipped guide wire to negotiate the obstacle. An angiographic exchange catheter can be advanced over the guide wire and a stiffer, nonhydrophilic working wire exchanged to place the double-J catheter. Fluoroscopic guidance is critical in difficult cases. These aids are usually not available at the time of placement during open surgical procedures.

If one anticipates placement of a ureteral stent during open surgery, a preoperative imaging study of the upper tracts is helpful. An unappreciated distal ureteral stone makes intraoperative stent placement frustrating and dangerous. Preoperative assessment of the patient's height and prior double-J stent sizes helps selection of appropriate lengths. Placing a stent after an open ureterolithotomy or other procedures with associated long-standing edema or periureteral fibrosis may make identification of the ureteral lumen suboptimal. Care should be taken to ensure that wires and/or stents are not placed in a submucosal route. Gentle advancement rather than force helps prevent injuries. Smooth cut edges decrease resistance. Palpation of the renal pelvis helps ensure appropriate proximal placement, and intravenous methylene blue or indigo carmine helps you determine when the distal end enters the bladder. Pushing a kidney in a cephalad direction frequently straightens troublesome ureteral kinks. If the proximal or distal ends of the stents are not advanced into the renal pelvis or bladder, they do not ensure drainage and may create troublesome obstruction. A postoperative kidney-ureter-bladder film helps confirm appropriate stent location. A notification mailed to the patient helps eliminate the forgotten stent.

Most patients complain of irritative voiding symptoms and intermittent gross hematuria, and preoperative education of these potential problems alleviates many patient concerns and subsequent phone calls. Retrieval with a flexible endoscope eases the discomfort for the patient. Stiff-walled double-J stents are needed to bypass narrowed ureteral segments and help to ensure adequate drainage without extrinsic compression. Most stents cause passive ureteral dilation, which facilitates subsequent retrograde ureteroscopic manipulation if that is required. Endoscopic inspection immediately after stent removal reveals edema and makes identification of pathologic lesions difficult.

An appropriately placed double-J stent helps ensure drainage and a successful surgical procedure. On the other hand, a misplaced stent can lead to troublesome complications and turn a successful operation into a failure.

Mobilization of the Omentum

An omental flap should be applied to any area with a tenuous blood supply after anastomosis or repair. Before starting a complex reconstruction operation, plan the incision to allow access to the omentum in case an omental flap as wrap or interposition is needed. Children often have insufficient omentum to provide coverage.

1 Mobilization of the omentum based on the right gastroepiploic vascular pedicle in a left-to-right fashion is preferred because it is larger and more caudal in origin than the one on the left side.

Transilluminate the omentum. Note that the blood supply to the omentum comes from both the left and right sides. The larger right gastroepiploic artery is a branch of the gastroduodenal artery. The relatively small left gastroepiploic artery arises from the splenic artery. Together they form the gastroepiploic arterial arch.

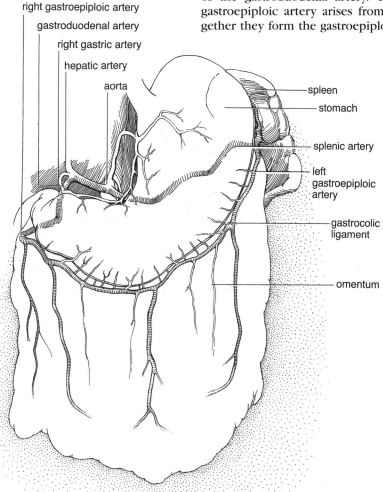

Certain anatomic facts are important:

1. The right gastroepiploic branch of the gastroduodenal artery supplies two thirds to three quarters of the apron. For placement of the omentum into the pelvis, it is always best to base it on the right gastroepiploic artery if it has not been damaged by previous surgery.

2. In one case in ten, the gastroepiploic arcade from left to right is deficient, usually near the origin of the left gastroepiploic pedicle. Basing a mobilized omentum on these smaller vessels may result in deficient vascularization.

3. The often-illustrated arcade running across the lower margin of the apron is of small caliber, if present at all, and can transport a minimal amount of blood.

4. Partial transverse division of the apron below the gastroepiploic arcade divides the vertical vessels and diminishes the circulation to the apron.

5. Because the origin of the right artery is lower than that of the left, a short apron mobilized on a full length of the gastroepiploic arcade can reach the pelvis. In fact, in one third of adolescents and adults, the lower margin of the omentum can be moved into a pelvic defect without mobilization. In these nonmobilized cases, however, the omentum should be separated from its natural adhesions to the transverse colon and mesocolic vessels to prevent its dislocation by postoperative intestinal distention. In another third of cases, division of the left gastroepiploic is all that is needed. In the remaining third, full mobilization on a right epiploic pedicle is required to achieve enough length.

2 **A,** Palpate the right gastroepiploic artery. Free the omentum from the transverse colon and mesocolon by dividing its avascular adhesion.

B, Trace the exposed gastroepiploic arch to the left.

C, When extra length is needed, divide and ligate the *left* gastroepiploic vascular pedicle at its splenic origin, although it is not necessary to divide it as high as shown.

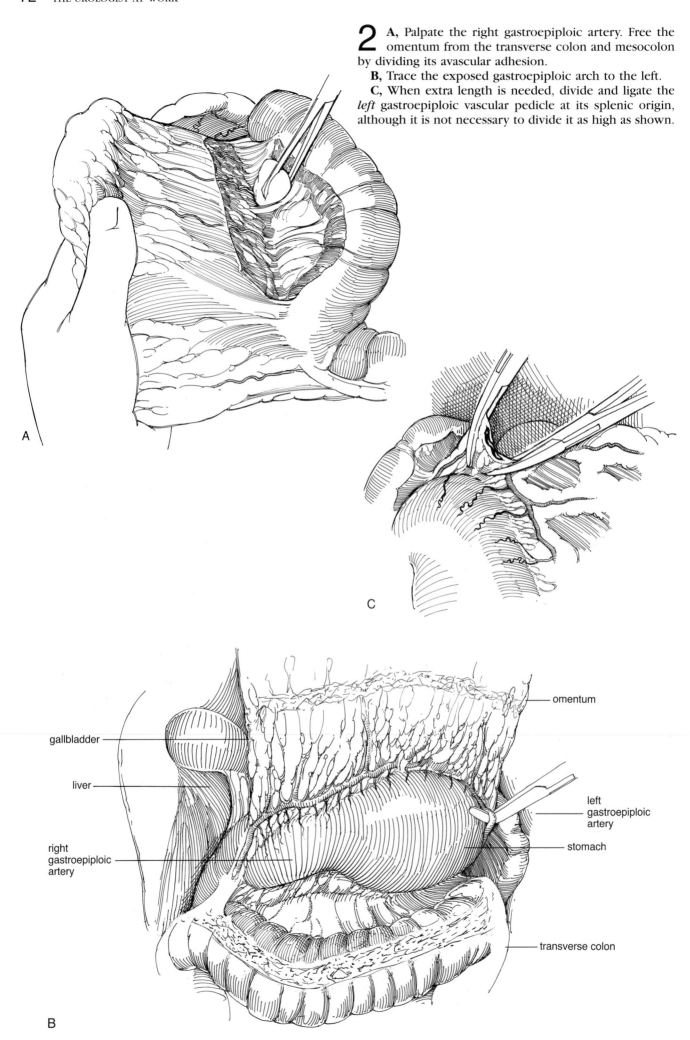

A

C

B

gallbladder

liver

right
gastroepiploic
artery

omentum

left
gastroepiploic
artery

stomach

transverse colon

3 **A,** Pass a Providence clamp through the omentum on each side of the first short gastric branch of the left gastroepiploic artery, elevate it, and draw a 4-0 SAS under it (NAS would foster infection and drainage in the recipient area). Tie the suture.

B, Clamp and divide the artery close to the stomach; then ligate the end of the vessel in the clamp. This technique of ligation avoids retraction of the proximal (omental) end that occurs when a hemostat ligation escapes and quickly produces a potentially harmful interstitial hematoma. An alternative and safer method is to pass and tie two sutures without clamping the vessel.

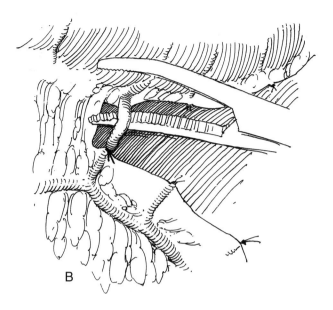

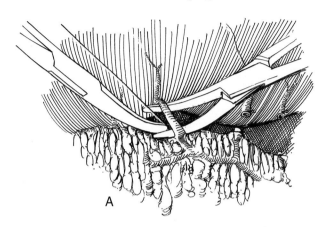

A

B

4 Continue dividing the remaining 20 or 30 branches individually to reach up to the gastroduodenal origin of the arch, carefully avoiding mass ligation that reduces the available length of the gastroepiploic arterial arch itself. An undivided branch is easily torn when the omentum is pulled into position. Preserve a 5- to 7-cm band of omentum intact at the right end to protect the vessels from avulsion.

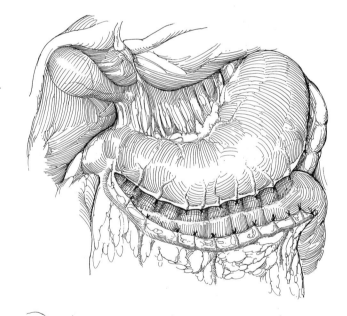

5 For use as graft or for interposition in the pelvis, mobilize the hepatic flexure and a section of the ascending colon to allow the omentum to lie in the paracolic gutter behind its mesentery. It is better not to pass the omentum over the transverse colon where it could be stretched by gas filling the bowel. Also, in females, it may interfere with ovum transport between ovary and tube.

In a complicated case with an extensively mobilized graft, place a nasogastric tube or, better, create a gastrostomy into the exposed stomach (see page 673). Use Penrose drains rather than suction drains, which tend to become clogged by the loose omental surface.

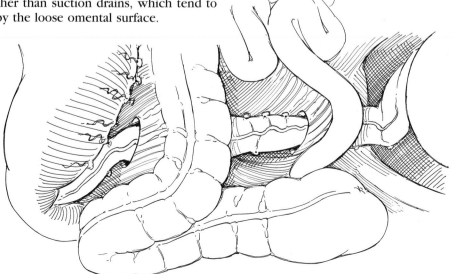

6 **A,** The patient is viewed from the flank.
B, For use as a wrap around the kidney or upper ureter, mobilization may not be necessary. Split the omentum and use only the ipsilateral portion.

C, Pass the hemi-omentum through a window in the colonic mesentery, and apply it over the defect.

POSTOPERATIVE PROBLEMS

Infection, abscess, and *persistent leakage* at the site of the repair can occur as a result of technical errors: damage to the blood supply during mobilization of the vascular pedicle; failure to make the tunnel behind the peritoneum large enough, compromising the omental blood supply; and failure to provide enough bulk of omentum to fill and cover. Ileus and abdominal distention can interfere with circulation to the graft only if it passes anterior to the bowel; it should always pass behind the hepatic flexure as the shortest and most protected route. Gastric suction is important prophylactically; a temporary gastrostomy may be more humane.

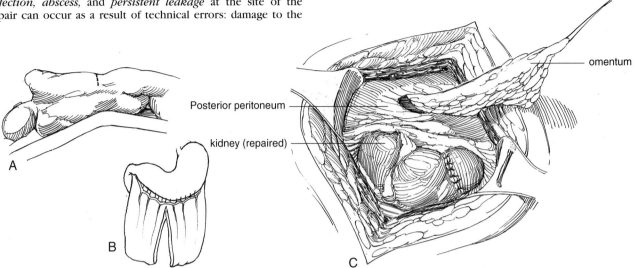

Commentary by Richard Turner-Warick

The "magic" of the omentum depends not only on its good blood supply but also on its excellent lymphatic drainage, which is the only route by which macromolecular exudates and inflammatory debris in the interstitial spaces can be absorbed. The real value of the omentum in the abdomen is illustrated by the fact that abscess formation in the peritoneal cavity is much more likely to occur in areas it cannot reach—under the diaphragm and in the pelvis.

Omental transposition for the support of complex reconstructive operations is often critical to their reliable success, especially (1) the replacement of a deficient bulk of pelvic, septal, or perineal tissue; (2) the vascular support of tissues compromised by previous surgery, infection, or irradiation; (3) the closure of complex fistulas; and (4) the preservation or restoration of urodynamic mobility of the urinary tract—an integral component of some functional reconstructions, such as urethral sphincteroplasty.

It must be remembered that there is only one omentum, and its loss, as a result of careless technique, can be a disaster for a patient whose reconstruction may be compromised by the lack of it. The preservation of the magic of the omentum during its surgical transposition is fundamentally dependent on preservation of the "pulsating efficiency" of its blood supply. In the 30 to 40% of cases (higher in children) in which full-length mobilization of its right gastroepiploic vascular pedicle is necessary, meticulous vascular technique is required to ligate and divide the 30 or so short gastric vessels. Fine curved-tip hemostats and fine (3-0) PGA ligatures are advised. Bunch ligation of several vessels should be avoided (this foreshortens the length of the pedicle and increases the risk of ligature escape). Individual in-continuity ligation of the proximal end of each vessel is advised to reduce the risk of hemostat pull-off and damage to the main gastroepiploic vessels. Once this is started, all the short gastric vessels should be divided, right back to the gastroduodenal origin (otherwise, traction on the pedicle may rupture the last undivided vessel). However, the bulk of the tissue around the root of the mobilized pedicle vessels should be carefully preserved because the lymphatic vessels run in it.

The use of Ligaclips is an inadvisable timesaver—they tend to catch on surrounding tissue and pull off the vessels, which are very delicate and easy to rupture. Similarly, diathermy coagulation is inadvisable (because each branch is surrounded by fat, the current tends to backtrack along it into its gastroepiploic parent vessel).

With regard to Step 4, after full-length mobilization of the right gastroepiploic pedicle of the omentum, we prefer to protect the extended route to the pelvis by mobilizing both the ascending colon and the hepatic flexure so that the slender vessels can be laid behind it, rather than bring it through the mesocolon where it is more likely to be divided in the course of any subsequent surgery.

We used to advise a prophylactic appendectomy to avoid the possibility that a subsequent appendectomy as an emergency might jeopardize the omentum (if one does this, it is most important to inform the patient so that an unnecessary subsequent exploration for suspected appendicitis is avoided). However, before proceeding to this, it is important to consider whether a retrieval procedure for the particular reconstructive endeavor might require it for Mitrofanoff self-catheterization.

A postoperative ileus lasting 1 or 2 days is not unusual after extensive mobilization of the right gastroepiploic omental pedicle from the stomach, and temporary gastric drainage may be advisable. When the stomach is exposed, a temporary gastrostomy is easy to insert and is a more humane procedure than a nasogastric tube (especially in children), but, to avoid the occasional complication of peritoneal leakage from the tract when the catheter is removed, it is advisable to achieve a self-sealing exit from the stomach with an imbrication tunnel of appropriate length.

Postoperative problems resulting from the redeployment of the omentum are rare, provided the anatomic principles of the mobilization of its vascularization are carefully followed. Some points are worth re-emphasizing. (1) The vertical omental branches of the gastroepiploic arch are virtually end vessels—there are almost no useful distal arcade collaterals. (2) Thus, the apron can often be divided between these (for ureteric wrapping) without having to ligate any vessel. (3) Mobilization of the apron by a transverse subgastroepiploic incision across some of the vertical vessels impairs the "pulsating efficiency" of its vascularization. (4) Because, in about 10% of patients, the right and left gastroepiploic vessels do not join together to form an arcade (easy to see if looked for), full-length mobilization of the pedicle of the omental apron on the basis of the smaller left gastroepiploic vessel impairs its distal blood supply in 1 of 10 cases. Finally, because the fenestrations of a suction drain tend to become clogged by "suck-in" of the supple mobilized omentum when surrounded by it, a Penrose drain may be preferable.

Methods of Nerve Block

Consider preliminary sedation. Guard against inadvertent intravascular injection; when aspirating, allow sufficient time for the blood to become visible in the syringe, and aspirate gently so that the vessel wall is not drawn and occludes the lumen. Also avoid an overdose of the anesthetic agent. If toxic symptoms appear, it may not be necessary to treat the reaction as long as respiration and circulation remain adequate. However, be prepared for reactions to the anesthetic agent, even though these are rare.

NECESSARY EQUIPMENT AND DRUGS

Seven items should be at hand before starting a nerve block: (1) a nasopharyngeal tube to relieve airway obstruction; (2) a bag and mask for assisted breathing; (3) a blood pressure cuff to monitor arterial pressure and pulse; (4) preparations for possible cardiopulmonary resuscitation; (5) diazepam in 2.5-mg doses or intravenous pentobarbital for convulsions; (6) antihistamines for mild allergic reactions and epinephrine for more severe ones; and (7) 5 to 30 mg of ephedrine for hypotension from cardiovascular depression, to be used in conjunction with elevation of the legs and administration of intravenous fluids.

Monitor the patient's blood pressure, and, when available, the electrocardiographic recording. Observations of color, pulse, respiratory pattern, and incidence of sweating are the most valuable monitors.

TOPICAL ANESTHESIA

Lidocaine and prilocaine hydrochloride bases in a 1:1 oil/water emulsion (EMLA) can be applied as a cream for topical anesthesia. It may be applied, for example, 1 hour before a meatotomy or release of labial fusion.

INTERCOSTAL NERVE BLOCK

1 *Anatomic relationships:* The intercostal nerves run segmentally under the respective ribs external to the endothoracic fascia. After passing the angle of the rib, the nerve continues below the artery and vein in the costal groove between the internal and external intercostal muscles.

Procedure. Place the patient in a lateral position with the ipsilateral arm extended over the head. Palpate the lower margin of the rib just beyond the angle. Insert a fine needle vertically until it touches the lower half of the rib. With the free hand, pull the skin with the embedded needle caudally until the needle point slips off the rib. Push it 3 mm deeper until a click is felt. Then angle the needle upward, and advance it 2 to 3 cm under the lower edge of the rib. Aspirate for air or blood. Inject 5 ml of anesthetic agent, preferably bupivacaine 0.5 percent, with epinephrine. Pneumothorax, even tension pneumothorax, can result if the rib is difficult to palpate and the needle is inserted too deeply.

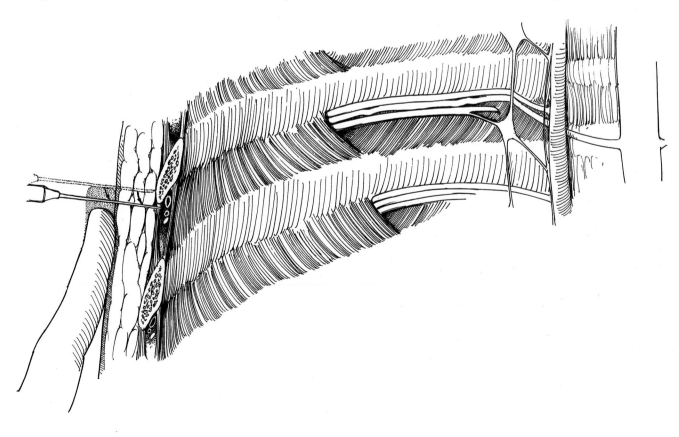

PENILE NERVE BLOCK

This is used for anesthesia for operations on the penis. The block also reverses intraoperative erections that occur under general anesthesia (Seftel et al, 1994).

2 The right and left dorsal nerves of the penis arise from the pudendal nerve, pass under the symphysis, and penetrate the suspensory ligament of the penis to run under the deep (Buck's) fascia.

Procedure. Palpate the symphysis pubis. Insert a short 22-gauge needle to one side of the midline at the 10-o'clock position to reach the caudal border of the symphysis. Withdraw it slightly, and move it so that it just misses the bone. Pop it through Buck's fascia. Aspirate and inject 10 ml of 1 percent lidocaine solution. Repeat the procedure at the 2-o'clock position.

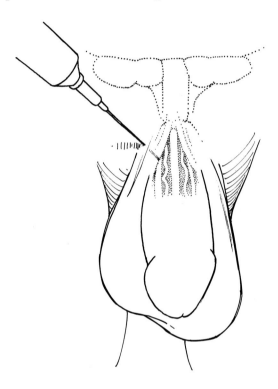

For *intracorporeal block*, apply a tourniquet to the base of the penis, and inject 20 to 25 ml of 1 percent lidocaine into a corpus through a butterfly scalp vein needle. Release the tourniquet after waiting 1 minute.

ILIOINGUINAL, ILIOHYPOGASTRIC, AND GENITOFEMORAL NERVE BLOCKS FOR ORCHIOPEXY AND HERNIA REPAIR

In general, select patients older than 16 years. Have the patient take nothing by mouth the previous 12 hours. If feasible, shave the area and inject the agent in the preparation room to allow time for the agent to work.

3 *Anatomic relationships:* The iliohypogastric nerve arises from T12 and L1 and exits through the transversus abdominis muscle just medial to the anterior superior iliac spine. It runs between the transversus muscle and the internal oblique muscle 2 to 3 cm medial to the spine. The ilioinguinal nerve from L1 arises slightly below and runs parallel to the iliohypogastric nerve and continues between the internal and external oblique muscles. The genitofemoral nerve from L1 and L2 runs over the surface of the psoas major muscle to divide just above the inguinal ligament into the genital and femoral branches. The genital branch enters the inguinal canal behind the cord.

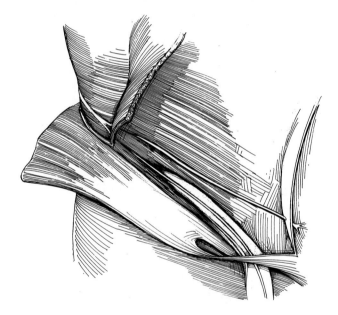

4 *Procedure:* To block the *iliohypogastric and ilioinguinal nerves* for operations on the scrotal contents, palpate the anterior superior iliac spine, and mark a point 2.5 to 3 cm medial and 2 to 3 cm caudal to it. Insert a 4-cm, 22-gauge needle to touch the inner surface of the iliac bone, and inject 5 to 7 ml of 1 percent bupivacaine (or a mixture of equal parts of 1 percent lignocaine and 0.5 percent bupivacaine). Inject as the needle is withdrawn. Repeat the procedure more medially, injecting 5 to 7 ml of solution just beneath the fascia of the three muscle layers.

To block the *genitofemoral nerve*, palpate the pubic tubercle and inject 5 to 7 ml of the anesthetic solution in the muscle layers laterally, cranially, and medially. Supplement the nerve block with subcutaneous injections fanned out to the inguinal fold laterally and the midline medially to reach the skin supplied by the pudendal nerve and perineal branches of the posterior cutaneous nerve of the thigh.

Alternatively, make an *iliac crest regional block* of the hypogastric and ilioinguinal nerves with 0.5 percent bupivacaine through a 22-gauge, 3.5-inch spinal needle. Inject 10 ml of anesthetic in the area of the internal ring, 2 cm medial and 2 cm caudal to the palpable anterior superior iliac spine. Push the needle down through the skin and deeper tissues until a pop is felt as the external oblique layer is penetrated. Aspirate to ensure that the needle in not intravascular. Place half of the anesthetic below the fascia and the other half above.

TESTIS NERVE BLOCK

Stand on the right side of the patient, and pull the testis down to relax the cremaster. Grasp the cord with the left hand, placing the thumb in front and the index finger behind the cord at the top of the scrotum. With the needle approaching the index finger, infiltrate the cord with 1 percent lidocaine solution without epinephrine through a 2.5-inch, 25-gauge needle. Alternatively, infiltrate the cord over the symphysis after it exits from the external inguinal ring.

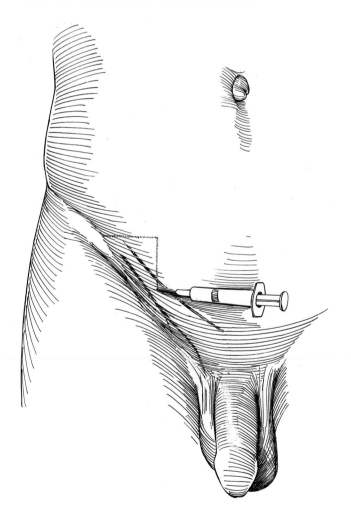

PUDENDAL NERVE BLOCK

5 *Anatomic relationships:* The pudendal nerve arises from S2, S3, and S4; runs laterally and dorsally to the ischial spine and sacrospinous ligament; and divides into the perineal nerve and the inferior rectal nerve. Aim to block the nerve as it passes the ischial spine.

6 *Procedure:* With the patient in the lithotomy position, insert an index finger in the rectum and palpate the ischial spine. Make a skin wheal 2 to 3 cm posteromedially to the ischial tuberosity. Insert a 12- to 15-cm, 20-gauge needle on a 10-ml syringe in a posterior and lateral direction to pop the needle through the sacrospinous ligament. Use the index finger as a guide to determine that the needle comes in contact with the bony prominence of the ischial tuberosity. Aspirate and inject 5 to 10 ml of local anesthetic laterally and under the tuberosity to anesthetize the inferior pudendal nerve. Move the needle to the medial side of the tuberosity, and inject another 10 ml after aspiration. Then advance the needle 2 to 3 cm into the ischiorectal fossa and inject 10 ml. Finally, guide the needle dorsolaterally to the ischial spine, and pop the needle through the sacrospinous ligament there. Aspirate for blood and inject 5 or 10 ml of the agent. Repeat the procedure on the other side.

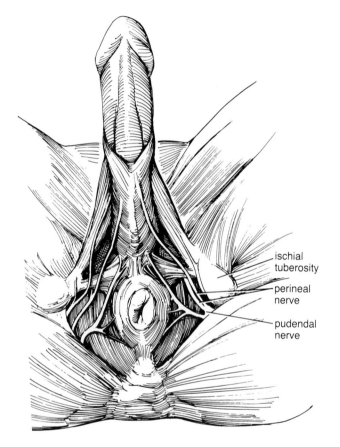

ischial
tuberosity

perineal
nerve

pudendal
nerve

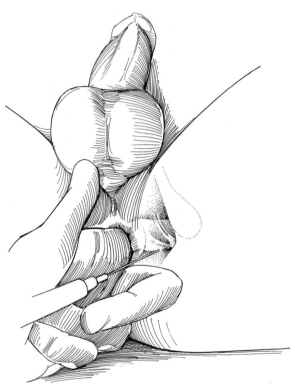

TRANSSACRAL BLOCK

7 *Anatomic relationships:* A layer of highly vascular fatty tissue lies between the two layers of the sacrum. This continuation of the lumbar epidural space contains the posterior primary divisions of the sacral nerve, which exit through the posterior foramina to supply the buttocks, and the anterior primary divisions, which exit through the ventral foramina to innervate the perineum and part of the leg.

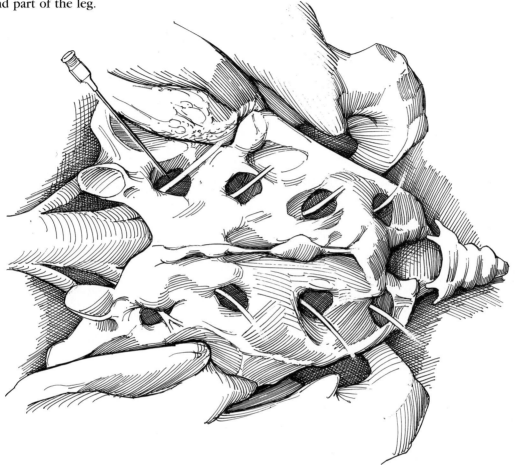

8 *Procedure* (see page 617 for placement of a vesical pacemaker): Place the sedated patient prone with a pillow under the hips. Palpate and mark both posterior superior iliac spines. Mark a point 1.5 cm medial and 1.5 cm cephalad to the posterior superior iliac spine to locate the first sacral foramen. Draw a line from this point to the lateral surface of the sacral cornua. Mark points 2 cm apart below the first foramen for the other three foramina.

Inject the agent subcutaneously to raise wheals. Insert a 12-cm, 22-gauge spinal needle containing a stilet perpendicular to the surface to contact the rim of the selected foramen. Move the rubber marker on the needle to a point 1.5 cm from the skin surface. Withdraw the needle slightly, and angle it 45 degrees caudally and 45 degrees medially to insert it into the foramen up to the marker, a depth of 1.5 cm. Inject 1.5 to 2 ml of anesthetic agent. For total caudal anesthesia, inject 15 to 25 ml. Hazards include producing a subarachnoid block and injecting the agent intravascularly in the large venous plexus.

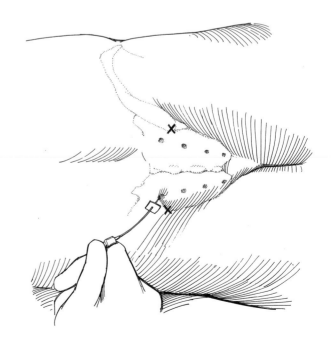

PROSTATIC NERVE BLOCK UNDER ULTRASOUND GUIDANCE
(Nash and Shinohara)

9 *Anatomic relationships:* The neurovascular bundle reaches the prostate at its base posteriorly at the 5- and 7-o'clock positions.

Procedure: Place the patient in the left lateral decubitus position. Load a 10-ml syringe with a 50:50 mixture of 1 percent lidocaine and 0.5 percent bupivacaine. Inject through a 7-inch, 22-gauge spinal needle. Under the guidance of a biplanar variable-frequency rectal probe, insert the needle and inject the solution into the region of the neurovascular bundle at the base of the prostate, just lateral to the junction of the prostate and the seminal vesicle on each side.

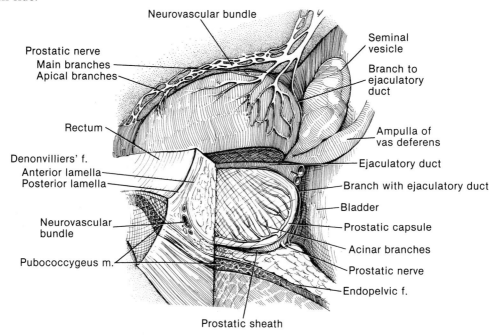

Commentary by Warren R. McKay

This concise and readable passage provides us with information that can be difficult to discover in a single text. Specifically, the discussions of anatomy in the genitourinary system are generally not mentioned in most pain texts in regard to nerve blocks. It is becoming increasingly apparent that nerve blocks for operative procedures with local anesthetics not only provide pain relief during a procedure but also provide long-lasting relief postoperatively. Evidence is now mounting that nerve block procedures may actually prevent severe pain from ever occurring after operative procedures. This likely results from the inhibition of the "wind up" that occurs in the dorsal horn of the spinal cord during nociceptor input, which then gives way to spinal cord memory for pain. The more one uses nerve blocks for operative procedures, the more one becomes aware that patients appear to have a better postoperative period in terms of comfort than do their counterparts done with a more general block of the central nervous system, that is, by inhalation anesthetics. Clinical literature now supports the fact that patients with regional nerve blocks using local anesthetics do have less pain postoperatively and for days afterwards, resulting from the disruption of the nociceptor response to surgery.

One pearl that I might add has to do with preblock procedures, specifically, infiltration of the skin before the nerve block is performed. One way to increase your patient's confidence in your skill and also to increase the chances of a successful nerve block is to make the first skin puncture painless. I approach this problem by using the smallest gauge needle available (e.g., a 27- or 30-gauge needle) and adjusting the pH of the local anesthetic. If lidocaine is the chosen local anesthetic, then 1 ml of sodium bicarbonate (standard 1 mEq/ml) can be used for every 10 ml of local anesthetic. This cannot be performed with bupivacaine because the local anesthetic precipitates when sodium bicarbonate is added. One way to get around this is to use lidocaine that has been pH adjusted for infiltration and then perform the procedure with bupivacaine.

Repair of Vascular Injuries

Control the bleeding with digital pressure. Immediately dissect to increase the exposure; obtain blood; set up a second intravenous line and second suction set; obtain appropriate instruments and sutures; and get assistance.

VENOUS INJURIES

Laceration of the Vena Cava

Have your assistant compress the vessel digitally at the site of injury. Inform the anesthetist, and have the nurse open a vascular pack.

1 Free the vena cava from the surrounding tissues both above and below the laceration. Have your assistant block the flow above and below with stick sponges. Small lacerations may be closed with fine silk figure-eight sutures or with a continuous suture placed under the surgeon's controlling finger. Alternatively, apply a Satinsky clamp and oversew it with a continuous suture (see page 1033). For larger tears, a more formal method is required, which includes greater mobilization of the vena cava.

2 Grasp both edges of the laceration with several fine Allis clamps to control bleeding and allow further dissection for better exposure. Run a 5-0 or 6-0 vascular suture down the laceration, inserting the needle and drawing the suture up as the clamps are successively removed.

For large defects, dissect the vena cava and cross-clamp it. If bleeding continues, also clamp the entering lumbar vein. Place a saphenous vein patch graft (see page 953), cut to size, suturing it in place with a 5-0 or 6-0 running vascular suture. If both anterior and posterior walls are damaged, close the defect in the posterior wall first, working through the defect in the anterior wall. If a saphenous vein patch graft is not available, cut a synthetic graft of polytetrafluoroethylene (PTFE) or Gore-Tex, a nonporous material that does not require preclotting, and suture it in place with a 5-0 or 6-0 monofilament vascular suture.

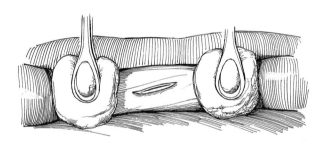

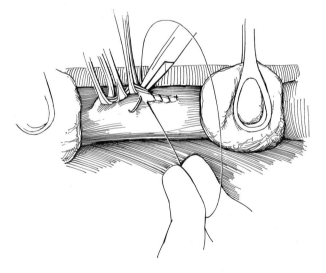

Pelvic Venous Plexus Injury

3 Immediately pack the area with moist sponges. Do not clamp blindly. Attach shoulder braces, and place the patient in a steep Trendelenburg position to empty the pelvic veins. Orient yourself to the anatomic distribution of the pelvic veins before attempting repair. Slowly remove the pack. Clamp and tie the bleeding vein. Or compress it with a stick sponge distal to the tear, and suture it with a 5-0 arterial monofilament suture (Prolene). Blind suture ligation can result in an arteriovenous fistula. If exposure is still not adequate, expose the ipsilateral internal iliac artery, and clamp it with a vascular clamp at its origin from the common iliac artery. You may have to temporarily clamp both internal iliac arteries. Slowly remove the pack, and suture the vessel. If control still is not obtained, it is possible to place some large packs wrapped inside a rubber dam and remove them 48 hours postoperatively. The rubber dam reduces traction on the vessels as the packs are removed, decreasing the chance for rebleeding.

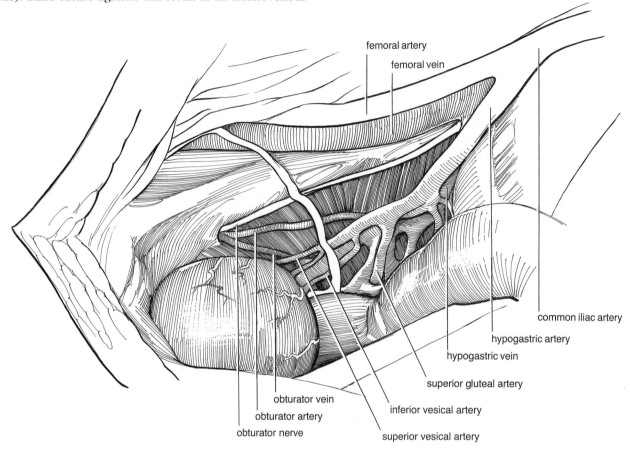

femoral artery
femoral vein
common iliac artery
hypogastric artery
hypogastric vein
superior gluteal artery
inferior vesical artery
superior vesical artery
obturator vein
obturator artery
obturator nerve

Injury of the Common and External Iliac Veins

Maintain direct pressure over the site. Visualization is facilitated by the more superficial location of these veins compared with the hypogastric and pelvic veins, so that Trendelenburg tilt and proximal occlusion of the common iliac artery are usually not needed. Obtain proximal and distal control of the vessel with vascular clamps.

4 After longitudinal or transverse laceration or complete division, if tension and venous constriction can be avoided, proceed to repair the vein. Carefully suture the edges of the defect with a running 5-0 or 6-0 monofilament suture. Place a continuous over-and-over stitch, taking small bites (1 to 2 mm deep and 1 mm apart). Inspect the vein for constriction.

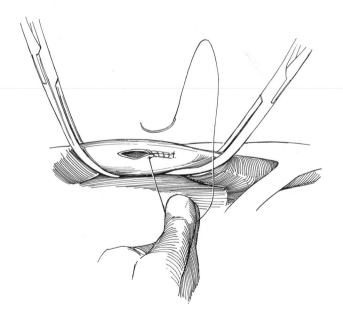

5 **A,** When the caliber of the vein would be significantly reduced by simple closure, substitute a venous patch graft. Expose the saphenous vein in the opposite leg (see page 953). Resect a suitable length of vein; open it longitudinally and excise the valves. Trim one end of it to fit the defect. Manipulate the patch by the edges that will be trimmed to avoid intimal trauma and later platelet deposition and thrombosis. Suture the trimmed end to an end of the defect with a double-armed 5-0 or 6-0 monofilament mattress suture.

B, Fasten the midportions of the patch to the corresponding part of the laceration with monofilament sutures. Trim the distal end, and coapt it with a second double-armed mattress suture. Complete the anastomosis by running the two mattress sutures, starting at each end and tying them to each other in the middle on each side. Release the vascular clamps one at a time.

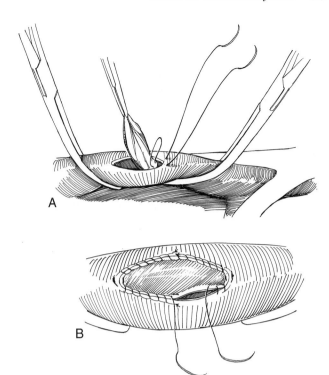

6 **A,** For repair after transection of a vein, trim the ragged edges obliquely, but do not spatulate them. Mobilize the vein proximally and distally so that the ends come together without tension. If tension is inevitable, one can try an interposition graft of saphenous vein or a synthetic graft.

B, Place two double-armed 5-0 monofilament sutures.

C, Run one down each side.

In order to enhance venous flow to maintain patency of a synthetic graft, a small arteriovenous fistula can be constructed in the groin, usually between the superficial femoral artery and the common femoral vein. In some patients, ligation of the vein may be necessary in conjunction with postoperative heparinization and a transition to warfarin for 3 to 6 months. Compression hosiery is used until sufficient venous collaterals have developed to prevent chronic venous insufficiency in the leg.

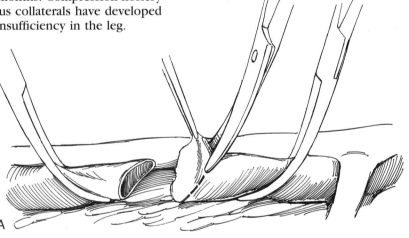

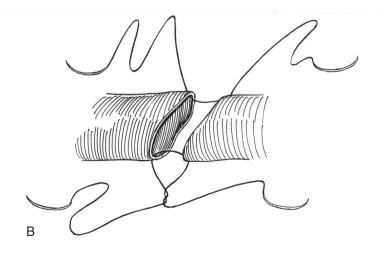

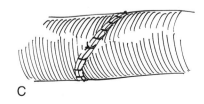

7 **A,** If near-total venous occlusion of the iliac vein is present, as after disruption of pelvic collaterals, with the possibility that the limb may be lost, a saphenous tube graft may be attempted, although subsequent thrombosis is highly likely. Obtain a vein graft 6 or 7 cm long from the opposite saphenous vein (see page 953, Step 43), one large enough to allow for contraction of the vein and to permit it to be used doubled. Mark the proximal end with a suture to indicate the direction of the valves. Trim the saphenous vein to a length twice that of the defect. Open the vein longitudinally with Potts scissors, and cut it in half transversely.

B, Suture one side of each half together with a running 5-0 monofilament suture.

C, Place the combined segments over a catheter of the same size as the iliac vein to be replaced, maintaining the correct orientation. Trim the other side, and suture the graft around the catheter. Cut the catheter next to the graft, and gently slide the graft free.

D, Suture the graft in place as for an end-to-end anastomosis (see Step 6).

As an alternative, use an appropriately sized synthetic graft as described above, providing a small distal arteriovenous fistula to enhance flow.

Note: Collaterals are numerous and can dilate in a few days after acute occlusion of a major vein.

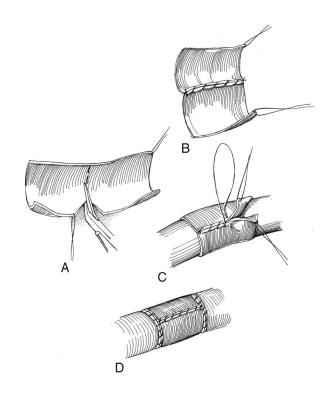

Injury of a Lumbar Vein

8 While slowly removing the pack, gently grasp each end of the lumbar vein with an Allis clamp and occlude it. Suture-ligate the ends with 6-0 monofilament sutures. If the cut end retracts into the intervertebral space, pack the site until the bleeding stops. Then expose the area and sew over the end of the vein.

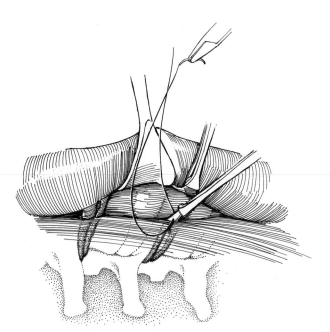

ARTERIAL INJURIES

Aortic Laceration

9 Control proximal flow by quickly preparing two stick sponges to hold a tightly folded (4 × 8) sponge between. Have the assistant apply firm pressure with the gauze pad without entering the field. Control backbleeding yourself with digital pressure. Suture the laceration with a 4-0 or 5-0 mattress suture. Teflon pledgets can be used on both sides of the mattress suture to avoid further tears in the aorta as the suture is tied.

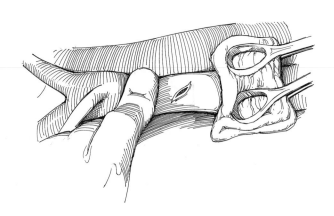

Laceration of the Branches of the Internal Iliac Artery

10 Temporarily occlude the abdominal aorta just above its bifurcation with one hand to reduce the bleeding. Clamp and ligate the cut artery. This can be done without risk of ischemia. Alternatively, maintain pressure on the bleeding point with a stick sponge while you free up the artery proximally and distally for several centimeters. Apply an arterial clamp proximally only tight enough to stop blood flow; be wary of dislodging a friable arterial plaque. Divide and ligate the vessel. When diffuse pelvic bleeding is present, consider ligation of the internal iliac artery on one side of the pelvis as a hemostatic measure.

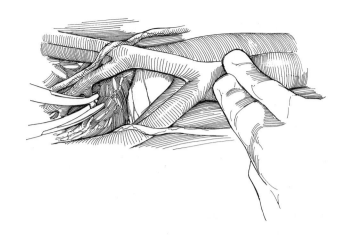

External Iliac Artery Laceration

11 **A,** Maintain compression over the defect with a stick sponge or fingers. Free the vessel proximally and distally. Apply vascular clamps, minimally closed. Place a running, over-and-over 5-0 monofilament suture.

B, If the laceration is tangential or irregular, divide, trim, and reanastomose the artery. Up to 1 cm can be lost without consequent tension. Check the anastomosis for a strong pulse and absence of a thrill. Otherwise, redo the anastomosis. One can insert an arterial graft, although this is seldom necessary in the external iliac arteries.

When a major artery is clamped, the clamp should be briefly released to allow injection of heparinized saline into both ends of the artery to prevent local thrombosis.

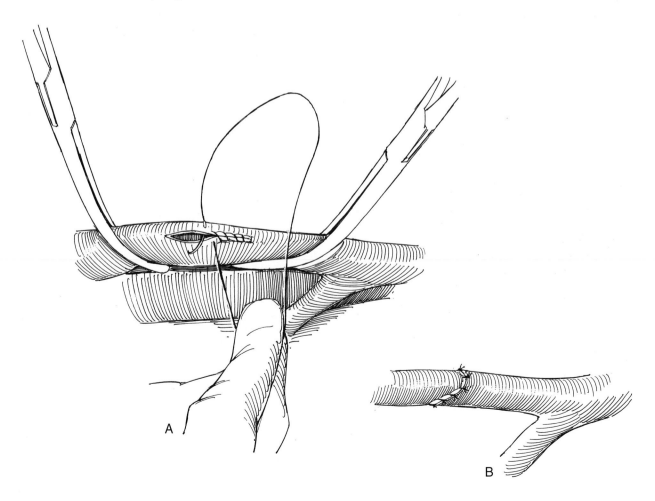

A

B

Loss of Control of a Renal Artery

12 **A,** With loss of control of the left renal artery during flank nephrectomy, especially during donor nephrectomy when a long segment of artery is removed, compress the pedicle area. Expose the aorta just below the diaphragm and compress it. Identify, clamp, and suture-ligate the stump of the artery.

B, Control the stump with stick sponge or digital pressure while freeing the aorta over the vena cava. Clamp and suture-ligate the stump. During a difficult nephrectomy, before placing a clamp on the *right* renal artery, it may be advisable to dissect the vena cava away from the aorta above and below so that, in an emergency, the aorta itself may be clamped.

Necessary Arterial Resection

Remove the segment of a major vessel involved in the disease process after controlling blood flow proximally and distally. A vascular surgeon should then be called for assistance.

13 **A,** If the wound is not infected, select a knitted Dacron graft of a size similar to that of the artery, place it in a sample of the patient's blood, and allow clotting. Aspirate the intraluminal clot before use. Anastomose it to the less accessible end first with a 4-0 or 5-0 monofilament continuous suture. Stretch the graft to flatten the crimps, and trim it to length. Alternatively, use a PTFE graft for this repair.

B, Begin the second anastomosis on the back side, and run it up both lateral walls with a double-armed suture. Before the last sutures are placed and tied, release the proximal clamp to flush the graft with heparinized saline. Complete the anastomosis and release the distal clamp, followed by release of the proximal one.

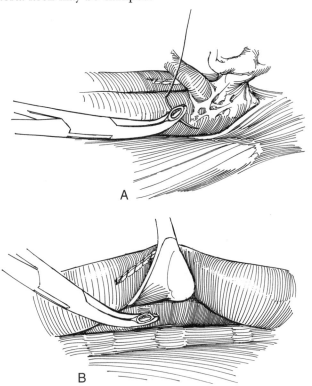

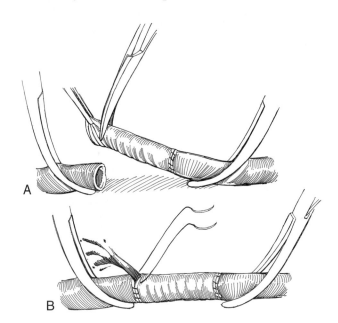

Commentary by Ralph A. Straffon

Urologic surgeons should have some training in vascular surgery and be familiar with vascular instruments. If a vascular injury occurs during a surgical procedure, the first objective is to control the bleeding, which can usually be done by applying pressure to the area. This allows the surgeon time to evaluate the injury and prepare to ligate or repair the blood vessels involved.

The hemodynamic status of the patient should be checked, and, if needed, blood replacement ordered. At least two suctions should be obtained to keep the field dry. Vascular instruments, if not on the surgical table, should be obtained and should consist of: (1) vascular needle holders with a fine tip and diamond-coated jaw for gripping small vascular needles; (2) vascular forceps, which allow the surgeon to grasp the wall of the vessel without damaging it; (3) vascular clamps, which are used to occlude blood vessels without damaging the wall; (4) special scissors such as a fine Metzenbaum, Strully, and Potts; and (5) surgical loupes, which may be useful when repair of a blood vessel is planned.

Special vascular sutures are used to repair blood vessels. These should be monofilament sutures, size 5-0 and 6-0, with both ends swaged on needles. A three-eighth's to one-half circle needle is preferred. When tying monofilament sutures, at least six knots should be used to prevent the suture from coming untied. Siliconized silk vascular sutures are much easier to use and tie and may be used in certain repairs.

Once the patient is stable and all equipment is available, the bleeding site should be exposed by slowly releasing the pressure. With the aid of two functioning suckers, the bleeding point can usually be identified and exposed for repair or ligation.

In general, if the bleeding is from an artery, it should be repaired unless it is simply too small and does not supply a vital area. These small vessels can be ligated. Larger vessels should be clamped with vascular clamps and the area carefully exposed to allow repair of the vessels as described in the text. A dilute heparinized saline solution should be used to flush the vessel to remove any clots and prevent thrombosis.

Venous bleeding from major vessels such as the vena cava or iliac vein should be repaired. Small veins such as lumbar veins or veins in the pelvic area can simply be ligated or suture-ligated with a figure-eight stitch. Remember that venous bleeding can usually be controlled by pressure, which should be applied for several minutes. In rare cases of significant venous bleeding in the pelvis, leaving a pack in place for 48 hours as described is an excellent choice.

Vascular surgery is not difficult if you have the proper equipment to deal with the problem. Control the bleeding by pressure, and avoid blindly clamping in a pool of blood. Also remember that Ligaclips are available in various sizes and are particularly useful for control of bleeding deep in the pelvis where ligation of the vessel is planned.

RECTAL INJURY

For a small injury occurring during retropubic prostatectomy, complete the operation before repair. Trim devitalized edges. Close the rectal defect transversely with interrupted 3-0 SAS. Apply a second layer of mattress sutures. Tack any adjacent fat over it. Thoroughly irrigate the wound. Mobilize the omentum (see page 71), and cover the defect. *Alternatively,* incise the endopelvic fascia on either side of the pelvis anterosuperiorly for a distance of 5 to 10 cm, and make two perpendicular incisions to form two fascial flaps (Brawer and Defalco, 1993). Fold one flap over the rectal defect, and tack it to the rectal wall. Cover it in double-breasted fashion with the flap from the other side.

Overdilate the anal sphincters digitally. Irrigate the pelvis copiously, and place drains to the area. Consider a diverting colostomy if the repair is tenuous or the injury is related to prior irradiation.

Repair of rectal injury occurring during perineal surgery is described on page 476.

Commentary by Thomas R. Russell

During abdominal pelvic surgery for urologic conditions, it is not uncommon for bowel injuries to occur. Injury is often related to previous surgery and adhesions and/or to prior radiation therapy. The most important thing is to recognize an injury so that it can be repaired. In addition, one must assess the degree of damage in order to plan the appropriate repair. Simple lacerations, as demonstrated in the illustrations, can frequently be repaired with simple interrupted NAS, approximating the serosa and submucosa to each other in an inverting fashion. These Lembert sutures predictably allow the bowel to heal. Frequently when injury occurs, there is a more significant laceration than depicted, with significant contusion, hematoma, and vascular impairment of the bowel. In situations of this sort, a simple repair of the laceration may not heal, often owing to ischemia of the tissue, resulting in contamination postoperatively and leakage that leads to intestinal contamination, abscess, and perhaps fistula formation. In such cases of significant injury to the bowel, the most conservative procedure to perform is a resection of the small bowel and/or colon with a primary anastomosis approximating healthy, viable bowel to other healthy, viable bowel.

The techniques of intestinal anastomosis are multiple. Rectal injuries represent a more complicated situation owing to their location deep in the pelvis. As is known, the rectum is an extraperitoneal structure, and mobilization may be extremely difficult. Again, if the laceration is simple and clean, one can repair it with interrupted sutures as illustrated. More frequently the injury is more complicated, and resection may be necessary with primary anastomosis and/or a colostomy with repair at a later time. In approaching patients who are undergoing difficult pelvic surgery and in whom bowel injury may occur, it is often useful to prepare the colon preoperatively with laxatives to decrease the fecal mass. Such preparation results in less contamination during surgery and aids in the repair if injury occurs. Prior to repair, particularly of the colon and rectum, one must be able to mobilize these structures in order to adequately see the injury, assess it correctly, and carry out the appropriate repair. Injuries that are not repaired correctly often leak, leading to catastrophic complications and the need for additional surgery.

Vascular Access

PERCUTANEOUS CEPHALIC VEIN CANNULATION

Use plastic cannulas with an inner metal needle stilet (Medicut) to facilitate access to the antecubital vein of the forearm or the dorsal surface of the hand in infants.

Place the arm on a padded board held with roller gauze to hyperextend it, and tape the board to the mattress. Apply a Penrose drain as a tourniquet. Wipe the site and your palpating finger with antiseptic solution; then dry the area. Use an 18-gauge needle to make an initial puncture 1 cm proximal to the vein; then insert the cannula very slowly with the bevel down, at the same time palpating it and the vein with a finger of the other hand. Slowly advance it toward the vein while aspirating with the syringe. When blood appears in the chamber, aspirate a small amount into the syringe; then reinject it to dilate the vein ahead of the needle while at the same time advancing the cannula. Withdraw the stilet and advance the cannula until the hub meets the skin. If blood does not flow, slowly withdraw the cannula until it does; then rotate and advance it. Fix the cannula permanently with waterproof tape over tincture of benzoin, and fasten the arm firmly to the armboard so that flexion is not possible.

CUTDOWN PERIPHERAL VEIN CATHETERIZATION

With the development of percutaneous techniques of venous catheterization, an open procedure is rarely used. However, if other methods fail, cutdown catheterization of the cephalic vein may be required.

1 Sit down so as to be able to rest your arms on the bed. Place the forearm in the prone position, tape it to a padded arm board, and prepare it to the elbow. Clip the drapes to the armboard. Place a venous catheter on the drapes, attached to a sterile syringe of saline. Identify the anatomical snuffbox. The cephalic vein is found crossing the center of the snuffbox and the styloid process of the radius as it runs up the lateral side of the elbow. Locate it visually or by palpation. If that is not possible, use your knowledge of local anatomy that it lies dorsal and proximal to the radial styloid.

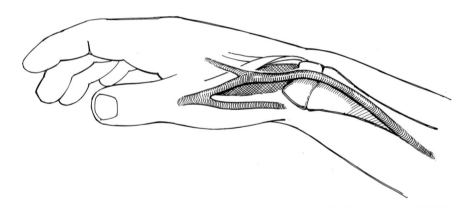

2 Make a short vertical (not transverse) incision, so that it can be extended proximally if the vein becomes injured.

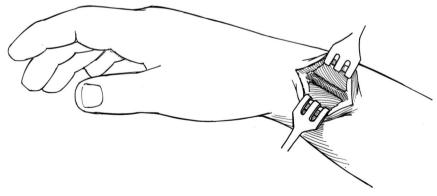

3 **A,** Grasp the vein with fine forceps, and ligate it with a fine absorbable suture. Encircle it proximally with a second suture to aid in manipulation; it will be used to ligate the vein around the catheter before closure.

B, Elevate the vein and cut it on a tangent with fine scissors.

C, Insert the tips of the scissors, or use a plastic catheter introducer if the hole is too small. Grasp and insert the catheter without taking your eyes off the ve-

notomy. Slowly infuse saline as you advance the catheter. Tie the vein over the catheter proximally with the loop suture. Close the incision with a running fine SAS, and fix the catheter and tubing with sterile tape.

Percutaneous subclavian vein puncture done by an interventional radiologist does not require administration of a general anesthetic but carries a slightly higher risk of pneumothorax or arterial puncture than an open method.

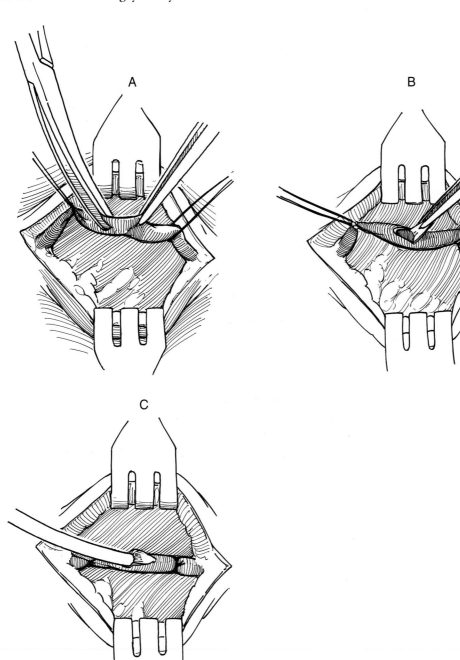

CENTRAL VENOUS CATHETERIZATION

A central venous catheter can be placed either by cutting down on the basilic vein in the antecubital fossa or by the standard procedure described here, entering through the jugular veins in the neck, usually the deep jugular vein or percutaneously. Almost all central venous access is now performed percutaneously.

4 With the patient under general anesthesia, placed in a 20-degree Trendelenburg position to eliminate the possibility of introducing air, elevate the shoulders and extend the neck to the left. Prepare the neck, chest, and upper arm. Make a 1.5-cm transverse incision above the clavicle over the right external jugular vein (*black dashed line a*). If this incision is not adequate, usually because of previous utilization, extend the skin incision medially to expose the internal jugular vein between the heads of the sternocleidomastoid muscle. The anterior facial vein, an excellent alternative, is reached through an incision 1.5 cm below the angle of the jaw over the medial border of the sternocleidomastoid. Make a second transverse incision on the chest below (*white dashed line b*).

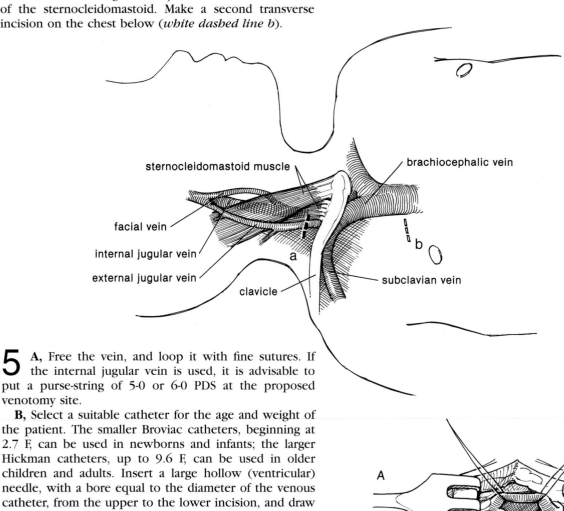

5 **A,** Free the vein, and loop it with fine sutures. If the internal jugular vein is used, it is advisable to put a purse-string of 5-0 or 6-0 PDS at the proposed venotomy site.

B, Select a suitable catheter for the age and weight of the patient. The smaller Broviac catheters, beginning at 2.7 F, can be used in newborns and infants; the larger Hickman catheters, up to 9.6 F, can be used in older children and adults. Insert a large hollow (ventricular) needle, with a bore equal to the diameter of the venous catheter, from the upper to the lower incision, and draw the tip of the catheter up through the tunnel. Position the monofilament knitted polypropylene cuff 2 to 5 cm deep to the site of entry. Trim the catheter to the appropriate length to lie at the junction of the superior vena cava and right atrium. Estimate the length by following the external landmarks.

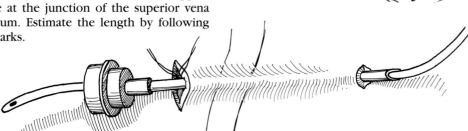

6 Elevate the vein and cut it on a tangent with fine scissors. Flush the catheter with heparinized saline (100 units/ml), and insert the tip of the catheter into the vein. (A small vein introducer may facilitate this maneuver.)

Advance the catheter into the superior vena cava toward the right atrium. The position of the catheter can be checked fluoroscopically. Be sure the catheter can be irrigated freely and that blood can be readily withdrawn. Ligate the vein above with the upper suture, and tie the catheter in place with the lower one. Infuse the catheter with heparinized saline solution, and cover the end with the Luer-Lok cap.

7 Suture the catheter to the skin, and cover it with sterile strips.

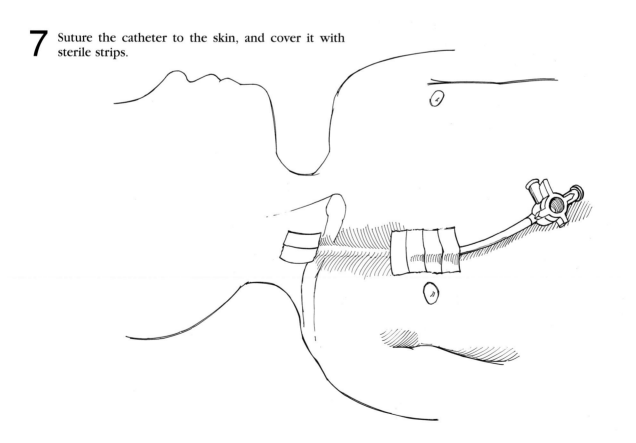

Commentary by Donald C. Martin

Percutaneous access: The use of a small volume of lidocaine without epinephrine administered through a small (tuberculin) syringe and a fine-gauge (#25 to #28) needle at the site of skin puncture aids in patient comfort and cooperation.

Central venous catheterization: The placement of a Broviac or Hickman catheter is useful for prolonged intravenous alimentation or chemotherapy, providing a reliable access for repeated use.

Percutaneous techniques are most frequently used for short-interval treatment or monitoring of central venous pressure. They are performed with a kit that uses the Seldinger technique of passing a catheter over a guide wire. Local anesthesia is used in most patients for the percutaneous procedure.

Percutaneous techniques are associated with many potential complications, including inadvertent arterial puncture, pneumothorax, hemothorax, and air embolism. The use of steep Trendelenburg position is extremely important to reduce the risk of air embolism. Placement of catheters into the chambers of the heart can be associated with cardiac arrhythmias so that electrocardiographic monitoring is necessary.

Scrupulous adherence to aseptic technique is essential, as the most frequent complication of vascular access procedures is local and/or systemic infection.

SECTION

3

Penis: Plastic Operations

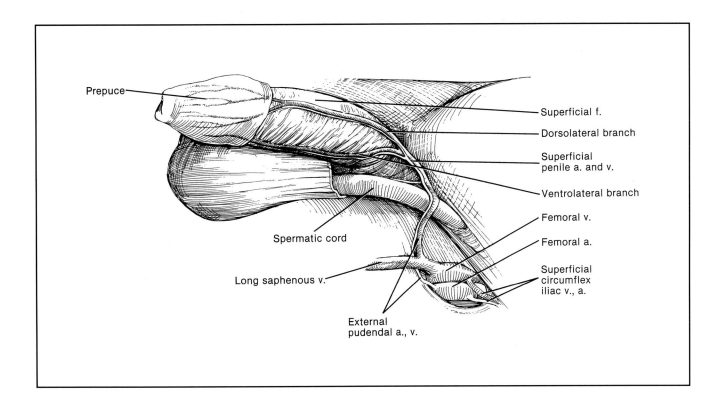

Prepuce

Superficial f.

Dorsolateral branch

Superficial penile a. and v.

Ventrolateral branch

Femoral v.

Femoral a.

Superficial circumflex iliac v., a.

Spermatic cord

Long saphenous v.

External pudendal a., v.

Basic Instructions for Hypospadias Repair

OBJECTIVES OF HYPOSPADIAS REPAIR

The aims of repair are to relieve the chordee completely and allow unrestricted erection; to bring the urethra to the tip of the penis; to form a urethra free of hair, stricture, or fistula; to effect a solid stream with no splattering, splashing, or backflow on micturition; to render the external surface of the penis symmetric with no abnormal tissue tags or fistulas; and to allow the patient to be able to have normal sexual function. Remember, a one-stage procedure is best, but performing a staged procedure is better than being forced to redo the initial procedure.

Success appears to be directly related to the experience of the surgeon. For a successful result in hypospadias repair, the penile tissues must be handled with great care under optical magnification. Experience in mobilizing and rotating skin flaps is needed, as in the detail involved in plastic surgical techniques. A two- or three-layer closure with fine suture material is necessary so as to avoid crossing suture lines. It is not enough to review pictures and follow descriptions; training in the techniques is essential. Knowledge of a few methods is not enough, because the one used must be the best for the individual boy.

AGE FOR OPERATION

With modern techniques, restoration of the penis to normal appearance and function can be done early in one stage with few complications. Select an age for operation between 6 and 18 months, within the window of least damage to the infant's psyche (Schultz et al, 1983). Infants do not remember, and they are also easiest to manage in diapers. Some pediatric urologists prefer a time between 4 and 12 months; others prefer to operate after 24 months, when the boy's penis is larger and he can be kept amused in the hospital.

Intramuscular depot testosterone (25 mg testosterone propionate and 110 mg testosterone enanthate may be administered at a dose of 2 mg/kg at 5 and 2 weeks preoperatively to increase the size of the glans and make it more suitable for glanuloplasty. It may also increase the size and vascularity of the prepuce (Davits et al, 1993). The surgeon and nurse should give considerable support to the parents and their need to know what to expect.

OUTPATIENT REPAIR

An uncomplicated hypospadias operation can be done without hospital admission; the exception is a repair involving free grafts or a redo. Have the parents and child visit you sometime before the date of surgery for the purpose of giving a history and having an examination, as well as to obtain instructions in feeding and preoperative care. You can explain the procedure, hand out suitable booklets for details, and obtain the most informed consent possible, given the difficulties of explaining procedures to parents and your need to adapt the operation to the tissues available. Also schedule an appointment for a complete blood count, urinalysis, and any other test suggested by the history. Arrange for the anesthetist to evaluate the child, especially if any problems are anticipated. Preputial adhesions may be separated at this time, preferably 1 month before operation, to allow maturation of the inner face of the prepuce.

The day before the procedure, have one of the outpatient staff call the parents to be sure everything is clear to them. Ask that the patient and family arrive 2 hours before the scheduled time of the operation to complete the final details. Obtain consent if that was not done on the initial visit. Arrange for the parent and child to meet the anesthetist and surgical nurses outside the operating room.

Premedicate the infant or child according to orders by the anesthetist. Halothane is a good agent for induction, and isoflurane is suitable for maintenance. Monitor the patient with a precordial or esophageal stethoscope, a Doppler blood pressure recorder, and a rectal temperature probe. Add bupivacaine for regional block, and consider its use as a caudal block for postoperative comfort. It is good to have someone informing and reassuring the family as the operation progresses.

At the end, place the child in the postanesthesia care unit for a short time before he returns to the holding area and his parents. Discharge the child when he is fully awake and able to take fluids. Tell the parents how to care for the indwelling catheter, be sure you or an associate is available around the clock for questions or emergencies, and have a bed available if it is needed. Make a telephone call to the parents the next day to check on progress.

Prophylactic Antibiotics

A broad-spectrum antibiotic administered intraoperatively, although not essential prophylactically except with salvage repairs, may be wise. Start it at the beginning of the procedure and continue it for 1 week postoperatively or until the tube is removed.

Preparation of the Genitalia

Use povidone-iodine soap, but do not apply any substance like povidone-iodine solution that stains the skin and so could obscure its vascularity. If a skin graft in older boys is planned, do not shave the genitalia until you have identified a hairless area for grafts or flaps.

Selection of the Operative Technique

Reclassify the degree of hypospadias after mentally correcting the chordee but before deciding on the particular technique you plan to use (Table 1). The shape of the glans helps in the decision (Snyder, 1991). In general, a cone-shaped glans usually is accompanied by a fibrous urethral plate requiring division, followed by a tubed transverse island flap (see page 134) and a tunneled glanuloplasty. With a flat glans, the plate usually is normal and may be preserved for application of an onlay flap with the glans folded over it.

Choices for Repair

Several procedures are available: coronal repair, meatal advancement and glanuloplasty (MAGPI), perimeatal flap (Mathieu)

Table 1. Selection of Technique

Distal Hypospadias	
No chordee, mobile urethra	MAGPI (p 116)
Megameatus variants	Pyramid (p 120)
Immobile/dysgenic urethra	Revise and reclassify as proximal hypospadias
Chordee after skin takedown	Revise and reclassify as proximal hypospadias
Proximal Hypospadias	
No chordee	Onlay island flap (p 130)
Persisting chordee	Transverse preputial island flap (p 134)

Adapted from Keating MA, Duckett JW Jr: Failed hypospadias repair. In Cohen MS, Resnick MI (eds): Reoperative Urology. Boston, Little, Brown & Co, 1995, p 187.

Table 2. Algorithm for Distal Hypospadias

Clear Superficial Chordee
Penis straight
Normal
MAGPI
Pyramid
Fixed urethral plate
Onlay flap

technique, perimeatal tube (Mustardé), onlay and tubed preputial flap, a double-faced flap, a ventral tube (Thiersch-Duplay), or a tube graft. Application of bladder epithelium or buccal mucosa may help. With their abundant dorsal vasculature, island flaps laid on as patches have become increasingly popular as the poorer vascularization associated with the Mathieu and flip-flap procedures has been recognized. Much depends on the position and characteristics of the meatus. The MAGPI technique corrects a coronal defect and achieves a normal-appearing reconstruction. If the meatus on the glans is abnormal (e.g., fish-mouth), turning a flap over from the shaft, as in the Mathieu or the flip-flap technique, replaces it. If the meatus is in midshaft without chordee—not a common situation, an onlay island flap without tubularization of its inner face or a perimeatal-based tube repair (Mustardé) is needed.

With mild distal chordee, a MAGPI procedure may be possible, but a type of Mustardé procedure may be better. With ventral deflection and some fibrous chordee, an onlay island flap may suffice. If the chordee is fibrous and extensive but the meatus lies on the distal portion of the shaft, a mobilized transverse island flap (Duckett) is most suitable. However, if the meatus is more proximal, a two-stage repair is advisable. Beware of penile rotation during the second stage of such a repair. For salvage, a double-faced island flap (Asopa) may work best. A dorsal relaxing incision (Denis Browne) should not be used. In summary, the vast majority of cases can be managed by a MAGPI, a perimeatal-based flap (Mathieu), an onlay flap, or a tubularized island flap

Tables 2 and 3 present algorithms for distal and proximal hypospadias that relate the type of repair to the method of correction of the chordee.

One-Stage Operations. Operations completed in one stage are preferable to two-stage operations, not only for the avoidance of further surgery but also for the use of virginal skin. In any case, do not promise the patient or parents that only one stage is necessary.

Two-Stage Repair. The swing transition to one-stage procedures is now complete, and two-stage repairs are returning for special cases. The versatility of a two-stage repair recommends it as the procedure of choice for urologists for whom hypospadias surgery is a small part of their practice. One straightforward and reliable technique can be applied. Children with scrotal or perineal hypospadias with severe chordee and a small phallus especially deserve a two-stage procedure (Byers, Belt-Fuqua, Durham Smith).

Default Two-Stage Repair. If during a planned one-stage procedure, you question the viability of the skin, fall back to a two-

stage procedure. At the first stage, take down the shaft skin to correct the chordee. In these extreme cases, dorsal plication may be needed to straighten the penis. Open the glans in the midline. Unfurl and transfer the prepuce to the ventrum (Byers). At the second stage, done 6 to 12 months later, make two parallel incisions 1.5 cm apart on the ventrum (Thiersch-Duplay, see page 140). Carefully mobilize the edges and fold them in to form a tube that can be advanced into the glans groove. Cover the tube with subcutaneous tissue or with a pedicle graft from the adjacent tunica vaginalis, and suture the shaft skin over it.

Secondary Operations. Apply an island flap if the prepuce is still available after initial failure. Otherwise, you may have to use a free tube graft, obtained from preputial tissue remaining on the shaft. If that is not available, take tissue from the buccal mucosa, bladder epithelium, or nongenital skin, in that order of desirability. Remember that penile skin itself has a random blood supply (Step 1), but the vessels in the dartos fascia that supply it run axially from the superficial external pudendal arteries, with one or the other side usually dominant, a fact that can be determined by transillumination. The dorsal surface of the corpora cavernosa has a meager blood supply; if a split-thickness graft is applied, it must be thin to encourage the entry of new vessels. In all cases, try to provide an intermediate layer between the new urethra and the skin. One way is to remove the skin from one edge of the preputial or penile flap and bring the subcutaneous dartos layer across (Durham Smith, 1973). A flap of scrotal fatty subcutaneous tissue, or a mobilized flap of tunica vaginalis (Snow, 1986; Snow et al, 1995), can be used for the same purpose, as can the subcutaneous tissues of the prepuce after mobilization on a short pedicle. To cover a large defect, place a meshed split-thickness graft over the tunica vaginalis flap (Ehrlich and Alter, 1996). Anyone performing hypospadias repair must be fully able to perform most of the many good procedures that have been developed to fit the procedure to the boy's defect. One operation does not fit all.

PREOPERATIVE INVESTIGATIONS

Urologic investigation is required in boys with a history of infection or a family history of urinary disease, for whom renal ultrasonography and intravenous urography may be needed. Endocrinologic and genetic investigation is indicated in a boy with perineal hypospadias, severe chordee, and bifid scrotum to detect intersex states. These abnormalities make for a poor prognosis.

Instruments

Select instruments for delicate handling of tissues. A full list includes genitourinary fine and micro sets, fine Allis clamps, two pairs of Bishop-Harman forceps, jeweler's forceps, sharp tenotomy scissors, iris scissors with the tips ground down, McPherson-Vannas scissors, blunt Castroviejo scissors, four small two-prong skin hooks, two small one-prong skin hooks, plastic scissors, a peanut dissector, and plastic Castroviejo needle holders. Bend the tips of neurosurgical forceps for bipolar electrodes.

Also include the following: infant sounds; a set of bougies á boule size 8 F to 14 F for calibration before, during, and after repair; fine lacrimal probes; grooved tunnel sounds if perineal urethrostomy is contemplated; 8 F, 10 F, and 12 F Robinson catheters; 5 F and 8 F infant feeding tubes; a pediatric stilet; Dow Corning 8 F trocar catheter (Cystocath); lubricant; rubber bands; a marking pen; a 23-gauge butterfly needle and syringe; microsponges; a #15 blade knife; #39, 64, and 69 Beaver blades and handle; Andrews and Frazier suction tips; and ophthalmic bipolar electrocautery. Have appropriate fine sutures at hand (synthetic absorbable suture [SAS], nonabsorbable suture [NAS], plain catgut [PCG], and chromic catgut [CCG] in small sizes). A three-power optical loupe or commercial magnifying visor is essential; an operating microscope is optional except that it does allow use of 7-0 and 8-0 sutures.

Table 3. Algorithm for Proximal Hypospadias

Clear Superficial Chordee
Penis straight
Onlay flap
Penis not straight
Divide urethral plate
Penis straight
Onlay flap
Penis not straight
Dorsal plication
Penis straight
Transverse preputial island flap
Staged repair

NERVE BLOCK

Use long-lasting bupivacaine (0.5 percent) mixed with quick-acting lidocaine (1 percent) in a volume of 3 to 4 ml or marcaine (0.025 percent) in a dose of 1 ml/kg to a maximum of 5 ml. Either inject it through a 1.5-inch 22-gauge needle (see page 76) as a ring block at the base of each crus just below the symphysis or inject it vertically in the midline deep to the notch of the symphysis. When placed at the beginning of the operation in the morning, it not only reduces the amount of general anesthesia required but also provides pain relief well into the postoperative period in the afternoon. A caudal block is good as an alternative or a supplement to local block. Continuous epidural anesthesia postoperatively is complicated and expensive, although it reduces the need for pain medication.

ARTIFICIAL ERECTION
(Gittes-McLaughlin)

Place a rubber band or red rubber catheter around the base of the penis and secure it with a hemostat. Introduce a butterfly needle through the glans into one corpus cavernosum. (Direct puncture into a cavernous body may cause a hematoma.) Distend the penis with normal saline solution (approximately 10 ml). Avoid overdistention. The erection may be maintained during dissection of the chordee; repeat the erection to check that the chordee has been corrected.

PENILE BLOOD SUPPLY

Blood Supply to Glans and Frenulum
(see page 95)

The dorsal artery of the penis, after giving off a few cortical branches and circumflex arteries to the corpus spongiosum, reaches the glans. There it turns ventrally to enter the glans near the coronal sulcus, a site where it may be injured during dissection. The frenulum has a separate blood supply from the dorsal artery.

Preputial Blood Supply

1 The superficial penile arteries, arising from the inferior external pudendal arteries, divide into anterolateral and posterolateral branches. The terminal branches turn circumferentially as they approach the coronal sulcus.

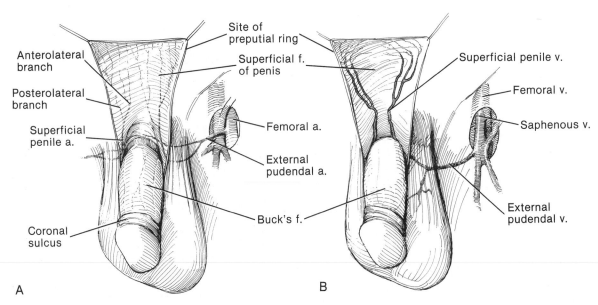

SURGICAL TECHNIQUE

The tissue must be viewed with magnification and be handled delicately if the operation is to succeed. Use traction sutures and fine skin hooks rather than forceps for a minimal-touch technique. The surgeon must know how to mobilize skin flaps while preserving all their vasculature and tissue viability. It is a good idea, when starting out, to "intern" with a pediatric urologist with a good referral practice to see (and help with) these complex procedures. The diagrams of the operative steps can only be reminders. Magnification is necessary. Use a 2.5× or 3.5× loupe or the operating microscope, and use microsurgical instruments and sutures.

As confidence is gained, magnification becomes a boon, especially because the goal of repair is the placement of two layers of sutures. Apply pinpoint monopolar electrocautery during dissection, but do not use it on flaps that will be used in reconstruction. Handle the tissues with microhooks—never with forceps. Crushed tissue does not heal primarily. Approximate layers with precise suturing. Use 6-0, 7-0, or 8-0 sutures. Avoid strictures by providing adequate spatulation; ensure good blood supply and avoid tension. For traction to support the penis, insert a 4-0 silk or CCG suture on a tapered needle vertically in the tip of the glans, not transversely on the dorsum, where it leaves two disturbing scars.

Stretch a rubber band around the holding clamp, and fasten

it to the drapes to maintain the position of the penis during ventral dissection. Press a finger under the shaft and use skin hooks to immobilize the penis during this dissection. Clamp traction sutures to the drapes to avoid false rotation. Close the edges of grafts with running, inverting locking sutures to prevent reefing. Do not close glans flaps too tightly over the new urethra; make these flaps very loose. The width of the graft in millimeters is equal to the French size of the resulting tube.

Place subcutaneous sutures where possible to take tension off the skin closure. Inject methylene blue–tinted saline into the urethra through a Christmas tree adapter to test for leaks. The possibility of ischemia is reduced if the connective tissue layer underlying a flap is preserved and approximated and if the flaps are not made too long. Of course, suturing under tension impairs the blood supply. Fluorescein is rarely helpful; it shows inflow of blood but not outflow. Sometimes the flap or adjacent skin can be salvaged: Excise the ischemic portion, remove the subcutaneous tissue, and reapply the skin as a full-thickness graft. Avoid "lily gilding" procedures; however, trimming skin tags is worthwhile. If intradermal suture tracts form, they can be opened in the office under local anesthesia.

When placing a circumcising incision, make it at the original site of circumcision even if that is well down the penile shaft. This ensures that the blood supply then enters both distally and proximally. A ventral vertical incision at the penoscrotal junction contracts and forms a drawstring; a Z-incision can be used instead (see pages 44 and 49). Fistulas may be avoided by not superimposing suture lines and by interposing at least one layer of healthy tissue between the neourethra and the skin, tissue obtained from the preputial pedicle or from de-epithelialized shaft skin (Step 12). Repeated calibration with bougies à boule during formation of the neourethra is essential to be certain that it is of uniform caliber, without wide areas suscepti-ble to formation of a diverticulum or narrow areas in the glans channel at the meatus. Topical irrigation may be done during the procedure with a kanamycin-bacitracin solution, alternating with Normosol-R.

HEMOSTASIS

To reduce bleeding, inject a solution of 1:100,000 epinephrine in 1 percent lidocaine through a 27.5-gauge, 1.5-inch needle around the corona, meatus, and chordee area. Wait 7 minutes for it to take effect. Although this injection makes dissection less bloody and does away with the need for a tourniquet, rebound vasodilatation can be expected if the operation is prolonged beyond 90 minutes. Venous bleeding may be increased toward the end of a long operation by a full bladder, which restricts venous return. Avoid electrocoagulation; if it is necessary, use it sparingly. There is disagreement about which is better—a low-current monopolar unit with a needle point for the electrosurgical unit, which provides exact coagulation with low current, or a bipolar electrode, which, although it adheres to the tissue, produces less heat around it. Once the skin flaps are applied, bleeding seems to stop, and a pressure dressing completes the hemostasis. Evacuate a hematoma and insert a miniature suction drain (Step 11) if necessary.

A gauze-covered finger held behind the penis over the dorsal artery provides hemostasis along with support during dissection of chordee. During the operation, a tourniquet can be placed at the base of the penis. After the penis has been degloved, apply the tourniquet directly to the corporal bodies. If it is used, release it every 20 to 30 minutes, although considerable oozing occurs with its release. For this reason, if a tourniquet is used, fulguration must be aggressive.

CHORDEE

2 **A,** Normal corpus spongiosum. **B,** Fan-shaped fibrous tissue causing chordee. A major cause of chordee is adherence of the ventral skin and dartos fascia to Buck's fascia and the tunica albuginea of the corpora, not necessarily accompanied by shortening of the urethral plate. Corporal disproportion, in which the tunica albuginea is shorter on the ventral aspect than on the dorsal, is not uncommon. Hypoplasia of the urethra and corpus spongiosum distal to the meatus is the third most common cause. This tissue has the shape of a fan, with its apex surrounding the now proximally situated urethral meatus and the undersurface of the glans (Devine and Horton, 1973). The severity of chordee roughly parallels the degree of hypospadias, except for infrequent cases of chordee without hypospadias. For example, the majority of boys with the meatus at the corona have at most a glanular tilt; however, as many as one in three has significant chordee. In a few cases, the curvature corrects itself with age, but surgical repair is usually necessary. If chordee persists after ventral skin release or after dividing the hypoplastic urethra, it is caused by corporal disproportion that can be corrected only by dorsal tucks. Experience teaches that chordee must be corrected at the first stage and that the artificial erection is a boon in ensuring complete straightening.

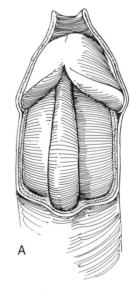
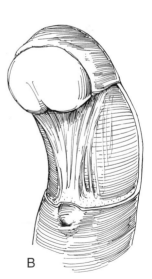

A

B

Dissection of Chordee

Circumcise the corona proximal to the meatus, and deglove the shaft to expose the tunica albuginea of the corpora cavernosa. Dissect in a proximal direction against the tunica. Stay under both the skin and the fibrous dartos layer that forms part of the chordee, but preserve the urethral plate. Use small, blunt-tipped, curved scissors, cutting back and forth as you move proximally superficial to the urethral plate to whatever length the dysplasia dictates, even beyond the penoscrotal junction. If necessary, dissect well around the lateral aspects of the glans and remove any fibrous tissue distal to the meatus.

Produce an artificial erection in order to see and clear any remaining fibrous tissue. If any chordee persists because the urethral plate is too short or there is corporal disproportion, it may be corrected by incising the intercavernous septum longitudinally on the dorsum and rotating the corpora by placing transverse dorsal plicating sutures that bridge the neurovascular bundle (Snow, Koff, see page 133) or by making dorsal Nesbit-type tucks (the tunica albuginea plication [TAP] procedure of Baskin and Duckett, see page 132) to correct it. The urethral plate is preserved to receive an onlay flap. Avoid dissecting under it. Transect it only for very severe chordee without hypospadias, in which case it is necessary to place a tubed flap to complete urethral construction (see page 134). If the curvature is greater than 20 to 30 degrees, the ventral tissue may have to be incised-excised and patched with tunica vaginalis or vein.

Chordee Without Hypospadias

The cause for the chordee may be a short hypoplastic urethra or a normal urethra and corpus spongiosum with abnormal development of the corpora cavernosa (corporal disproportion). Once the penis has formed with a curvature, it remains curved throughout development.

Dorsal Tucks. Make a circumferential incision in the coronal sulcus and reflect the skin of the shaft. Dissect the dysgenetic tissue on the ventral side of the corpora cavernosa from the tunica albuginea and mobilize the corpus spongiosum. To demonstrate the site of the curvature, create an erection by injecting saline intracorporeally distal to a tourniquet or by injecting papaverine, augmenting it with saline if needed. For detumescence, inject 500 μg of neosynephrine. Place dorsal tucks (see page 130). Replace the skin over the shaft.

If the chordee is released by incision-excision of the ventral tunic, perform ventral dermal grafting (Devine): Mark a 2 × 3 cm ellipse of skin in a hairless region near the anterior superior iliac spine. Trim the epidermis from the marked ellipse in situ with a sharp scalpel. Remove the graft from its site and defat it. Close the deep layer of the dermis with interrupted sutures and the skin with a subcuticular running NAS with occasional stitches crossing over the surface to facilitate later suture removal. (An alternate method to secure the graft: Incise and raise a book flap of epidermis with the assistant holding the adjacent skin taut. Harvest a patch of dermis from beneath it and replace the flap.) Drop the meatus back by elevating the urethra, and make transverse incisions in the ventral tunica albuginea bilaterally at the site(s) of maximal bend. Divide the graft and trim it to fit the resulting ellipses. Suture each of them in place with four quadrant and one subcutaneous 5-0 SAS. After placement of the appropriate number of grafts, proceed with a transverse island flap repair (see page 130) or rotate the prepuce ventrally to cover the shaft preparatory to a subsequent two-stage repair. Immobilize the area for at least 2 days.

For severe curvature requiring partial urethral replacement, straighten the penis by shortening the dorsum or releasing the ventrum before constructing the urethra.

Spontaneous Erections

Have the anesthetist give nitroglycerine sublingually or break a 0.3-mg ampule of amyl nitrite into the breathing bag. If necessary, inject 0.2 ml of a 1:100,000 solution of epinephrine in normal saline into one corpus through the butterfly needle used for artificial erection.

SUTURES

For the skin and subcutaneous tissues, absorbable sutures are best because they do not require general anesthesia for removal. If possible, place sutures subcuticularly with inverted knots. Useful is 7-0 CCG (colored ophthalmic sutures on a cutting needle are handy). Although catgut sutures are absorbed most rapidly, they maintain their strength the longest when exposed to urine. Monocril sutures lubricated with glycerine may be substituted for catgut. Polyglycolic acid sutures are not as good as polyglactin 910 (Vicryl) and polydioxanone sutures (PDS); they last too long and may promote fistulas. Place vertical mattress or subcuticular sutures in the skin if necessary to avoid overlapping or inverting the edges. Fine (4-0) running nylon sutures that can be pulled out provide the greatest strength and least reaction. They also avoid the "blackheads" created by epithelialization of suture tracts.

For deep sutures, PDS has the disadvantage that it loses strength most rapidly when exposed to urine, especially infected urine; polyglycolic acid sutures are better in this respect. Coat the synthetic suture with mineral oil to allow easier passage through the tissues. Tissue glues (Tisseel) may have a place in skin closure.

BUCCAL MUCOSAL AND BLADDER UROTHELIAL GRAFTS

For the complicated case in which sufficient preputial skin is not available, buccal mucosa or bladder urothelium with its lamina propria may be substituted.

Buccal Mucosal Graft

Grafts from the mouth are preferred over those from the bladder because the mucosa is thicker and the lamina propria is thinner and well-vascularized, conditions that make for rapid revascularization by imbibition. Grafts from the bladder are also less desirable because of greater difficulty in harvesting and greater chance for late failure. Buccal grafts have the additional advantage that they do not create a sticky protruding meatus. Cheek grafts are preferable to those from the lip because a strip can be harvested wide enough to be tubularized. Two grafts as large as 6 cm can be obtained, one from each cheek. The edges of cheek grafts provide a better edge at the meatus. Large grafts from the lower lip may distort the lip. Moreover, the lip mucosa contains glands and must be left open, in contrast to the cheek wound, which may be closed with inverted sutures for less painful healing. Give the patient penicillin G for 48 hours.

Intubate the child with an endotracheal tube (a nasotracheal tube is not necessary) to maintain anesthesia. Have a second team and separate instruments for the harvesting and the grafting.

3 Use the thumb and forefinger to flex and insert a lip-cheek retractor (**A**) ("A" Company, San Diego, CA) or a Steinhauser mucosal retractor (**B**) (Lorenz Surgical, Jacksonville, FL). Stuff rolled 4 × 4 gauze pads between the cheek and the lip. Inject a mixture of 1 part epinephrine and 100,000 parts of 1 percent lidocaine beneath the mucosa to facilitate dissection and reduce bleeding. Identify the parotid (Stenson's) duct. Sponge the surface and outline the graft with a marking pen.

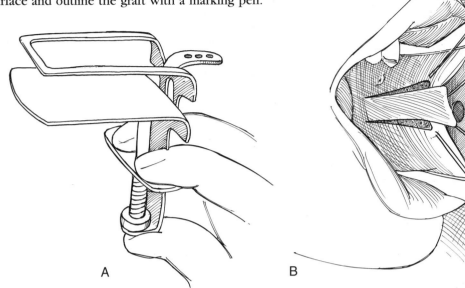

A   B

4 **A,** On the the lip, mark a flap up to 4 cm long and 1.3 cm wide. **B,** On the cheek the flap may be wider, extending from the parotid duct orifice to the inferior vestibular fold, but in practice it is seldom longer than 5 or 6 cm. Both cheeks may be used if a large graft is required. In any case, two strips may be sutured together side to side to make a wider graft or end to end to make a longer one. Make the graft only slightly larger (10 percent) than the defect; shrinkage will be minimal. To obtain the graft, place four fine sutures at the corners of the proposed graft to manipulate the edges so that the mucosa is not traumatized with forceps. Incise the margins on either side with a #15 blade. Before dividing the ends, dissect just beneath the submucosa to avoid obtaining too thick a graft, and watch out for the parotid duct in the cheek opposite the second molar tooth. The buccal neurovascular bundle lies in the buccinator muscle, and the facial nerve runs beneath it, so the muscular

layer should not be entered. Divide the ends of the graft and remove it. Obtain hemostasis with pressure, aided by pin-point electrocoagulation; bleeding postoperatively may be controlled by internal pressure and external ice packs.

Close the cheek wound with an inverted running 5-0 CCG. The defect in the lip does not require closing; instead, apply benzocaine (Orabase). Start feeding with soft foods the following day.

Pin the graft on a board. These grafts are thick, so it is important to thin them. Wearing a loupe, defat the graft by pinning it on a board and removing the fat and subcutaneous tissue with a scalpel to foster quick imbibition. The lip graft is thicker and consequently stiffer than the cheek graft. If it is too thick, try to remove some of the submucosa, although this may be difficult. Two grafts may be joined end to end for a long graft. To form a tube, suture them side by side.

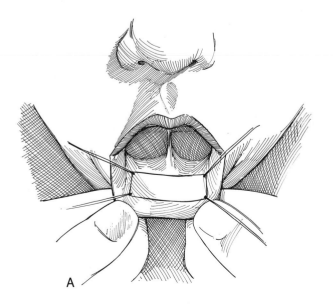

A

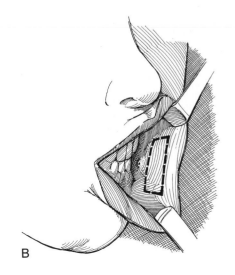

B

5 To form a urethral tube, apply the graft with the mucosa inside to a catheter of suitable size (usually 18 F) pinned to a box. Run a locked 5-0 SAS to approximate the edges, with interrupted sutures at the end to permit trimming. Do not place sutures too close to the ends, to allow for an oblique anastomosis. Trim the stump of the urethra on the dorsal and lateral sides to allow an inverted oblique epithelium-to-epithelium anastomosis (Mollard et al, 1989). Orient the suture line on the graft dorsally. Suture the proximal end to the urethral stump with interrupted fine sutures, keeping the mucosa inverted. Tack the urethra at the site of the anastomosis to the corpora to prevent redundancy.

Split the glans and form generous glans wings to be able to cover the graft with two flaps of vascularized tissue and skin. Alternatively, tunnel the graft through the glans by removing adequate glans tissue. In either case, be sure the channel is large enough. If you are concerned about meatal stenosis, insert a dart of glans tissue or make the meatal anastomosis oblique. Undermine the edges of the glans around the meatus to invert the meatal skin to make it flush with the graft, and suture it with CCG. This reduces the chance for stenosis. Cover the defect with previously mobilized penile skin.

Drain the bladder with a catheter in the urethra, or place a suprapubic tube and insert a well-lubricated fenestrated catheter to a point below the sphincter, sutured at the glans. It may be wise to insert a small suction drain (Step 10) (Winslow et al, 1986).

Dress the wound carefully with a compressive occlusive dressing. Keep the patient as immobilized as possible for 2 or 3 days to prevent shearing of the graft. Amyl nitrite inhalation may help reduce erections. Do not replace the drainage tube if it becomes displaced.

Provide antibiotic coverage. A diet of soft food (ice cream for babies) and daily cleansing of the mouth with povidone-iodine solution are advised. Leave the stenting catheter in place 7 to 10 days. Teach the patient or his mother to dilate the meatus daily for 6 months.

Complications include damage to the buccal neurovascular bundle by dissecting the buccinator (damage to the facial nerve that lies deep to the buccinator is highly unlikely). Postoperative bleeding from the graft site is corrected by resuturing the wound under local anesthesia. For infection, usually in a hematoma, remove the sutures to drain the area and give antibiotics to control the infection. Continuation of soft food and daily cleansing of the mouth with povidone-iodine solution are advised.

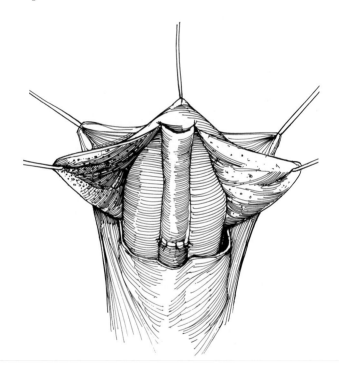

Bladder Urothelial Graft

Harvesting bladder epithelium with its lamina propria is straightforward, but the application of the resulting thin graft may be more difficult than application of skin or buccal mucosa. These grafts are suitable for midurethral repair not extending to the tip and also for complete substitution. In that case, it is advisable to attach a 1-cm preputial skin tube to form the terminal part to prevent weeping and stenosis, problems that may require regular self-dilatation for 3 or 4 months postoperatively. The bladder must be large enough to allow the harvest of adequate urothelium for the graft.

6 Carry the correction of the hypospadias as far as possible before obtaining the graft so that it may be placed immediately in the bed. Insert a catheter or place a perineal urethrostomy tube. Distend the bladder with saline solution or air. Make a transverse lower abdominal incision (see page 490), and retract the rectus muscles. **A,** Make a vertical incision in the exposed anterior surface of the bladder, deep enough to reach the underlying urothelium. **B,** Peel the muscle from the urothelium with scissors and a peanut dissector to expose an area of suitable size for the graft. Mark the outline of the graft with a skin marking pen before the bladder is entered *(dashed line)*. Make the outline wide to allow for loss during suturing, usually 10 percent longer and 20 percent wider than needed, but realize that, in contrast to skin grafts, it does not shrink appreciably after placement. Place traction sutures at the four corners. Excise the graft with scissors along the marks. Keep it moist. Alternatively, harvest the graft transvesically.

Proceed at once to roll the graft around a 12 to 14 F silicone tube stent, and suture it with an inverting running lock stitch of 7-0 SAS. Be sure to have the scrub nurse keep the graft constantly moist. Invert the catheter and graft, and insert the catheter into the stump of the urethra. Anastomose the graft first to the glans and then to the spatulated urethral stump, trimming it as required.

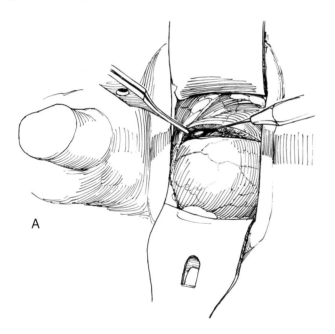

A

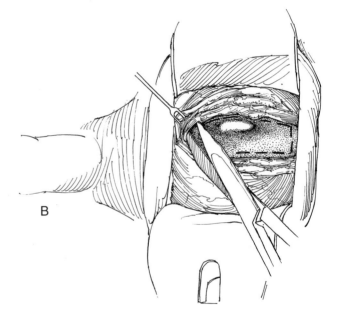

B

7 Insert a Malecot catheter in the bladder, and bring it out through a stab wound. Close the bladder in one layer; do not attempt mucosal approximation. Place a Penrose drain. Have your assistant close the wound while you apply the graft. Dress the penis, and immobilize it with an appropriate dressing.

Do not remove the stent earlier than the 10th postoperative day because the healing process takes considerably longer for this delicate graft than for a buccal graft. Sponge the meatus with neosporin before the boy makes the first void. If voiding is then satisfactory, remove the cystostomy tube on the same day. In most cases, the parents need to dilate the meatus at home with a tapered nozzle.

Complications include stenosis of all or part of the graft, diverticula, and proximal and distal strictures at the sites of anastomosis. Fistulas are uncommon, but protruding bladder urothelium has been a problem; it is reduced by stretching and trimming the graft at the meatus before suture. Regular meatal dilation for 6 months reduces the chance for meatal eversion or stenosis.

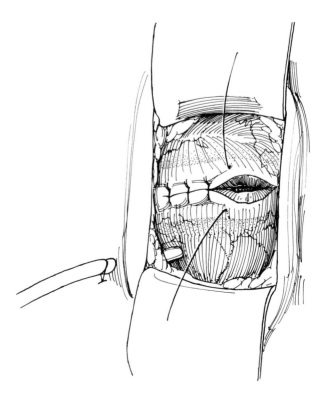

SKIN COVERAGE AFTER URETHRAL REPAIR
(Byers Flaps)

Translocate the dorsal preputial skin by incising the opened prepuce dorsally, swinging the resulting flaps around ventrally, and applying them to the ventral surface as Byers flaps. After opening the flaps, fix the apex of the split dorsally to the coronal sulcus. Suture the preputial edges to the coronal skin edge. Place a suture ventrally to draw the edges together, and trim the excess skin.

TESTING THE REPAIR

Test a repair before closure of the skin. Fill the bladder and press on the abdomen. Alternatively, instill dilute methylene blue into the meatus with a blunt-tipped syringe while compressing the urethra proximal to the repair.

8 **A,** Another testing technique is to introduce an 18-gauge angiocatheter percutaneously into the tip of a suction tube in the urethra at the level of the penoscrotal junction. Withdraw the suction tube and remove the trocar of the angiocatheter, leaving the plastic angiocatheter in the urethral lumen. **B,** Attach a 20-ml syringe and inject saline to test the integrity of the repair. The addition of a little methylene blue to the saline helps detect tiny fistulas.

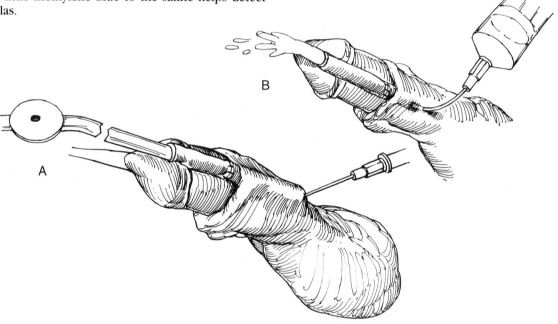

DIVERSION OF THE URINE

Select the type of urinary drainage suitable to the site of repair and the age of the child, so that no voiding takes place through the neourethra during the early postoperative period. Distal repairs probably do not require diversion. Diversion of urine away from the suture lines has always been a problem because tubes induce bladder spasms. Many techniques have been tried to minimize spasms. For infants, insert an infant feeding tube that terminates in the prostatic urethra and suture it to the glans. A catheter ending in the posterior urethra is not acceptable to older children because it causes pain on voiding. Yet a catheter ending in the bladder, especially one with a balloon, stimulates bladder spasms that force urine out around it and harm the repair. Whatever system is used in infants, collect urine in a double diaper.

The simplest method of diversion is to cut the butt end from an 8 F infant feeding tube and make extra side holes in the distal end. Make the overall length enough to extend 3 cm into the bladder. Insert a 3.5 F infant feeding tube inside it to help guide the now blunt end into the bladder. Fix the funnel end to the glans with a suture through the tube and let it drain into the diaper. The built-in funnel helps prevent retraction into the meatus.

Another method combines stenting with drainage: Obtain a fine silicone tube, such as 6 F neurosurgical shunt tubing (Kluge-Firlit) with its wandlike end, or a newer form of tubing made with a ball near the outer end that both prevents upward migration and provides a site for suturing it to the glans. Insert it into the bladder through the urethra until it just starts to drain, then push it 3 cm farther to place the tip within the bladder (or measure double the distance to the penoscrotal junction and add 3 cm). Fasten the catheter or ball to the glans in two places with polyglycolic acid sutures that will dissolve in 6 to 8 days. For the tube without a ball, leave a long stay suture on the end to be taped to the abdomen as extra protection against upward migration. This technique does carry a risk of damage to the repair if the catheter is handled carelessly. Let the tube drip into the diaper.

For still another method of drainage, use a 7 F Jackson-Pratt drain that is fenestrated all the way to the bladder. Tie it in place with a traction suture in the glans.

9 **A,** The Splent. As an alternative to diversion, make a tube from a length of silicone tubing (Dow Corning, size 132) long enough to reach from the meatus to a point 1 cm above the repair by cutting a longitudinal strip from it that removes one fourth of the tube's circumference (Mitchell and Kalb, 1986). Trim both ends obliquely. **B,** Insert the tube while it is compressed with neurologic forceps, cut it flush, and suture it loosely to the meatus with two fine NAS. Test for patency by passing a 5 F or 8 F infant feeding tube through it. Let the stent drain into a double diaper. Remove it in 5 to 9 days.

TISSUE DRAINS

Use a drain only if hemostasis is unsatisfactory and a hematoma appears imminent.

10 It is possible to make a suction drain from a butterfly needle with the adapter cut off and holes cut in that end. Insert the tubing subcutaneously, and place the butterfly needle into a sterilized vacuum blood collection tube, as shown. Miniature suction drains (TLS drains) are commercially available.

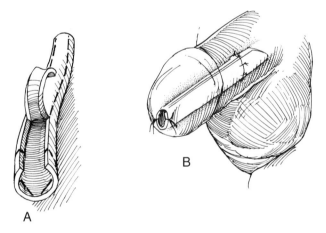

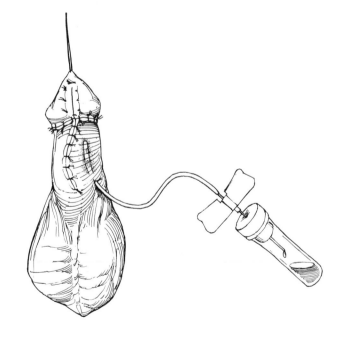

Avoid using a balloon catheter. It promotes infection and does not allow for a trial of voiding. The balloon usually rests on the trigone and produces excessive bladder spasm, whether it is used for perineal, urethral, or suprapubic drainage. Also, its lumen is small compared with that of a straight catheter, especially a plastic one. Because the smaller tube tends to be obstructive, a suprapubic trocar cystostomy, although not as secure as open cystostomy, provides better drainage than the catheter. Use an 8 F Cystocath and allow it to drip in an outer diaper. Perineal urethrostomy (see page 630) is rarely needed.

Bladder spasms can disrupt a repair. To prevent them, insert one third of a methantheline bromide and opium (B & O) rectal suppository every 8 hours. Give methantheline bromide (Banthine) by mouth in doses of 12.5 mg four times daily to an infant under 1 year of age, with a gradual increase to 25 mg four times daily after that. For older children, the dose can be as much as 50 mg four times daily. For pain, give acetaminophen, plain for infants or with codeine for older children.

DRESSINGS

Before placing a dressing, grip the penis firmly in a gauze pad to arrest all oozing. It may be helpful before placing a dressing to add support for the incision by applying sterile strips over a coating of tincture of benzoin or similar substance (Mastisol) to the penis.

Apply a dressing to immobilize the area and reduce edema and hematoma. An improper dressing can cause the best operation to fail. Two types are in use—concealing and nonconcealing. In any case, mineral oil applied to the skin reduces adherence of the dressing and facilitates its removal. Concealing dressings immobilize the area, provide some pressure, and are comfortable, but they prevent inspection. They may be partially or totally concealing, depending on the layers and the taping.

1. A simple dressing is formed from impregnated (Xeroform) gauze covered with fluffs held in place with elastic adhesive (Elastoplast).

2. A nonadherent pad (Telfa) may be applied and covered with a folded 4 × 4 gauze sponge that does not encircle it completely but compresses it against the abdomen. Hold it in place with 2-inch elastic adhesive tape splayed out dorsally to adhere to the pubic area, which is prepared with tincture of benzoin.

3. One effective modification consists of covering the repair with Telfa, firmly wrapping a foam-backed karaya pad (Duo-Derm) around the penis, overlapped. Apply absorbent transparent plastic film (Tegaderm) over it, and use it to anchor the dressing to the abdomen and scrotum.

4. Another popular modification merely uses an absorbent transparent plastic film (Tegaderm or Op-site) applied over Telfa gauze or tincture of benzoin.

5. Another simple nonconcealing dressing is the direct application of a plastic semipermeable dressing (Bioclusive) around the penis. The glans can be left exposed for inspection, although this probably is not necessary.

Before the child is brought in for removal of the dressing in 2 to 7 days, have the parents soften the dressing by applying baby oil or by soaking the child in the bathtub. After removal of the dressing, depending on the state of healing, it may be advisable for the parents to apply Neosporin ointment during diaper changes. Check the child's status in 6 weeks and 6 months, having the parents pay special attention to the quality of the urinary stream and the orientation of the penis on erection.

POSTOPERATIVE CARE

For postoperative analgesia, consider providing a caudal block with bupivacaine at the end of the operation, although a penile block with the same agent may give comparable analgesia. Give analgesics, such as acetaminophen, and antispasmodics, such as meperidine (Demerol) with promethazine (Phenergan). Bladder spasms are not common if the stent does not press on the trigone and, if they do occur, may be reduced with oral medication (methantheline bromide, propantheline bromide, or oxybutynin) and rectal insertion of one third of a belladonna-opium suppository.

To avoid infection in patients with a catheter, trimethoprim (Septra) may be given for 3 days. To avoid meatal stenosis, one may need to ask the parents to insert the nozzle tip of a small ophthalmic ointment tube into the meatus daily. Although one can calibrate the urethra with a small-caliber sound or a bougie à boule in the office in 2 weeks, this is a painful procedure; a proper repair should maintain caliber without interference.

After the dressing has been removed, have the child soak in the bathtub daily. If the child is sent home with a stent in place, instruct the parents in its care and make an appointment for return in 10 to 14 days for stent removal. If a suprapubic tube was necessary, remove it in 14 days. At 1, 2, 4, and 6 weeks, and then in 6 months, 1 year, 3 years, and 6 years, check the repair and observe the stream. It is seldom necessary to actually measure the flow rate, but it is a good way of detecting asymptomatic obstruction.

Commentary by R. Lawrence Kroovand

The issue of whether residents should learn how to perform hypospadias repair is one that I have been wrestling with for a long time. I think that many residents who have trained at a variety of programs over the past 5 to 10 years believe that they can perform practically any type of urologic procedure. As far as hypospadias repair is concerned, in many programs the pediatric urologist may draw out the flaps and allow the resident to perform most or all of the dissection and place most of the sutures. This practice clearly gives a resident a sense of having performed the hypospadias repair itself, when in reality he or she probably does not understand many of the nuances involved in the surgical procedure. Thus, in a urology residency, I think it is appropriate for residents who are interested in going into pediatric urology or who are technically adept to perform parts of hypospadias repairs, but I do not think that they should be allowed to be misled into thinking that they have the judgment and experience necessary to perform these repairs on a regular basis.

EARLY POSTOPERATIVE PROBLEMS

Not only do bladder spasms cause a child to move about with pain, but the accompanying straining forces urine through the repair. Remember to stop antispasmodic drugs before removing the catheter. Do not reinsert the catheter if it falls out; if necessary, insert a cystostomy tube percutaneously. Constipation may result from the antispasm regimen and lead to straining and urine leakage. It is important to prescribe stool softeners and a suitable diet.

Bleeding is not a common problem. At the end of the operation, if hemostasis is seen to be incomplete, insert a miniature vacuum drain and apply a mild occlusive dressing to control the ooze. Be sure to evacuate any hematoma first, and do not apply the dressing too tightly. Hemorrhage usually can be arrested by compression but may require reopening the wound. Infection begins after injury to the tissues; therefore, be gentle during the operation. Preoperative genital scrubs, perhaps perioperative antibiotics, and washing with povidone-iodine solution in the operating room help, but the basic cause is ischemia. If the operated area appears inflamed, tub baths are helpful. Edema is inevitable but may be reduced by a compressive dressing left in place for 2 days.

Ischemia with devitalization of skin flaps is more serious but may not result in failure if the underlying structures are well vascularized. Ischemia of skin flaps results from taking too small a flap to cover the defect, thus creating tension, or from attenuating too much of its underlying support and blood supply. Look for blanching during suturing as tension is applied and for absence of bleeding from the cut edge, a situation that leads to local necrosis. The area usually granulates and becomes covered with fairly normal-appearing skin. Take special care with the wings of the split glans; any separation of them creates a fistula. Avoid excessive compression from the dressing. Fistulas are the most troublesome problem in hypospadias repair. Acutely, treat a fistula as you would a wound separation. Use sterile adhesive strips. Later, try breaking a piece of silver nitrate from a stick and applying it to the fistula to destroy the epithelium. If small, fistulas usually close spontaneously. If wound separation occurs on removal of the dressing, reapproximate the edges with sterile adhesive strips, although a later repair is usually necessary. Edema from rough handling of the tissues is the usual cause and could have been avoided. An erection in a postpubertal patient is a problem that is best controlled with amyl nitrite inhalers and administration of diazepam. Diethylstilbestrol is of no value.

LATE POSTOPERATIVE PROBLEMS

Strictures

Although urethrocutaneous fistulas account for most of the late problems after hypospadias repair, strictures do occur, often in relation to a fistula. Proximal strictures, usually at the site of the proximal anastomosis, should be dilated early. For those strictures not responding to dilation, make one attempt with direct-vision internal urethrotomy and stenting. Excision and anastomosis are seldom applicable because of the difficulty of dissecting the neourethra and the chance for chordee. Marsupialize the area and repair it later as a fistula, usually with an island flap. Alternatively, close it by the Johanson technique (see pages 279 to 280).

For residual hair, usually accompanied by infection, it may be possible to depilate transurethrally with a laser if the hairs are few. For stones with hair, seen at the penoscrotal junction, open the urethra and excise that section of the urethra and replace it with a flap or buccal mucosal graft.

Meatal Problems

Stenosis at the meatus results from local ischemia or improper construction. Have the parents dilate the urethra daily with small plastic sounds or the tip of an ophthalmic ointment tube. If this fails, incise the meatus either dorsally or ventrally, depending on its situation on the glans, and close the incision transversely (Heineke-Mikulicz). If the entire distal glanular urethra is stenosed, divide the glans, advance a vascularized flap, and cover it with glans wings. Alternatively, split the terminal urethra ventrally, applying the MAGPI technique (see page 116).

A retrusive meatus may be corrected by a perimeatal-based flap, by a perimeatal-based tube, or by an onlay flap. Ectropion of the meatus can occur with a bladder epithelial graft and requires resection of the redundant tissue, although stenosis may follow. Balanitis xerotica obliterans may occur as long as 15 years after repair. It usually requires meatoplasty by excision of the distal urethra and replacement with a graft, although steroid injection and self-dilatation may be tried.

URETHROCUTANEOUS FISTULAS

Fistulas may be caused by distal obstruction; check for strictures first with bougies à boule. Strictures may be secondary to impaired vascular supply to the neourethra, use of NAS material in creating the neourethra, crossing of suture lines, use of poorly vascularized skin flaps to cover the neourethra, postoperative wound infection, or urinary extravasation.

If obstruction is found, it must be corrected, in which case divert the urine to prevent blowout of the fistula closure caused by edema at the site of stricture repair. A stent is indicated if a distal repair has been done in addition to closure of the fistula. Because of these many factors, closure of a fistula is not always successful, and the success rate falls with the number of attempts.

Before resorting to surgical repair, try to apply part of a silver nitrate stick to the opening. If that fails, try trimming the epithelium from a small fistula and inverting it with a loosely applied Michel clip. Wait 2 months before attempting repair.

Conduct all repairs under at least loupe magnification; the microscope may be better. The basic principles for repair include trimming all the involved tract and inverting the epithelium with fine sutures, bringing in a vascularized layer if possible, closing the subcutaneous layer with a fine running absorbable suture, and swinging in new skin and closing it with a running subcuticular suture.

Simple Procedures for Fistula Repair

Place a traction suture in the glans. Calibrate the urethra with bougies à boule to detect strictures distal to the fistula. If any are detected, correct them before tackling the fistula. Compress the bulbar urethra and inject dilute methylene blue into the meatus through a blunt adapter on a 10-ml syringe to inflate the urethra. This may detect more than one fistula, some being very small. If multiple large fistulas are found, do not attempt to close them individually because each closure interferes with the adjacent repair by inducing tension that interferes with the blood supply. Rather, join the tracts and treat the resulting fistula with an onlay flap.

Be aware that fistulas may pass diagonally; insert a lacrimal probe through the fistula to determine its track. If the urethra is dilated around the fistula, repair it as a diverticulum (see page 226). After repair of larger fistulas, consider placing a silicone catheter through the urethra to protect the suture line. Fistulas near the meatus or in the coronal sulcus, where the tissue is poorly vascularized, respond poorly to the methods described subsequently. Instead, incise the meatus down to the fistula and repair the defect with perimeatal tubularization (see page 126) or with an onlay flap from the prepuce or shaft (see page 130).

Simple Advancement Flap Closure

11 **A,** Mark the proposed incision to encircle the fistula on one side and extend it widely laterally on the other side to outline a flap of the loosest nearby skin. Do not be afraid to make an extended incision. Inserting a 3 F catheter into the fistula and suturing it to the rim may help elevate the edge for circumcision. **B,** For a larger fistula, raise a flap from the ventral skin and, after excising the fistula, rotate it into position. For subcoronal fistulas, make a transverse incision (Step 14A and B); for those on the shaft, make a longitudinal incision. **C,** While wearing a loupe, elevate the skin edge around the fistula with fine double-pronged skin hooks and dissect widely with tenotomy scissors. **D,** Free the skin to the edge of the tract and continue the dissection around the fistula to its base. Use a needle electrode delicately on the bleeders. Divide the fistula 1 or 2 mm from the urethral lumen, which is identified by the indwelling catheter. **E,** Run a 6-0 or 7-0 SAS across the fistula or, if it is very small, place two or three interrupted sutures to invert the fistula into the urethra. Start and end the suture well away from the fistula. If possible, mobilize subcutaneous tissue to cover the repair. **F,** Incise and raise a generous skin flap. **G,** Advance and fasten the flap to the deep tissue at the far side of the defect with two subcutaneous 4-0 or 5-0 SAS. If at all possible, interpose subcutaneous tissue. Check for leaks by injecting saline into the meatus while compressing the bulbar urethra. **H,** Close the skin edges with a 5-0 SAS running subcuticularly around the perimeter. Remove the catheter. Apply a collodion or Superglue dressing (being certain to let it dry before contact with the adjacent skin), and allow the child to return home. For more secure coverage, a rotation flap may be applied (see page 47).

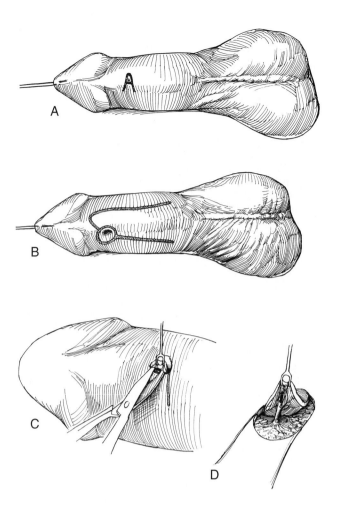

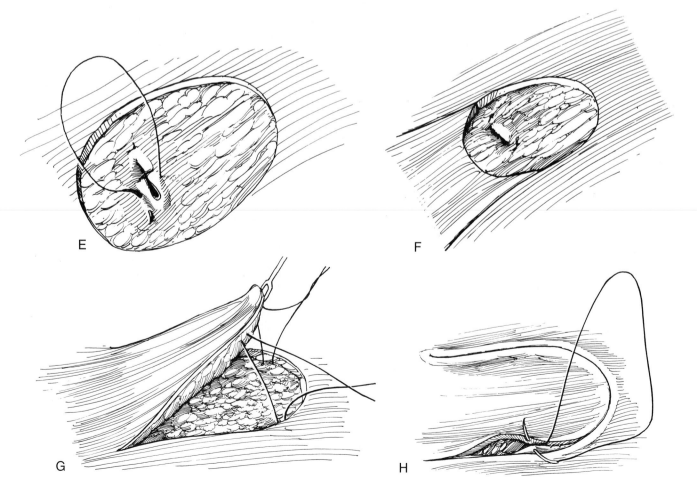

De-epithelialized Flap Closure
(Durham Smith)

12 **A,** For greater security against fistulization or refistulization, interpose a de-epithelialized flap. Incise the skin ventrally in the midline. Make it somewhat longer in order to undermine the skin flaps laterally, keeping close to the corpora to preserve blood supply. Close the fistula transversely. Raise a skin flap on one side and remove an ellipse of epithelium to leave a dermal flap. Place this flap across the fistula and suture it under the base of the opposite flap. **B,** Suture the free skin edge to the line of de-epithelialization on the opposite side.

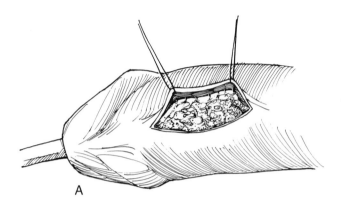

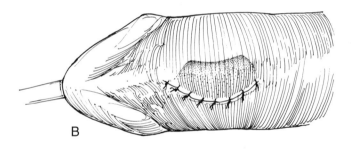

Repair of Coronal Fistula

13 **A,** Excise the tract through a transverse incision. Free the lateral and proximal skin widely. **B,** Remove the epithelium from the margin of the glans distal to the fistula. Invert the fistula with fine interrupted sutures. **C,** Place a row of 6-0 SAS to bring the subcutaneous tissue onto the glans over the fistula. **D,** Suture the proximal skin edge to the edge of the denuded glans with 6-0 interrupted SAS. Apply a light dressing, and remove the catheter. *Alternative*: Incise the skin bridge between the fistula and the meatus to connect the fistula with the meatus. Repair the defect by the pyramid procedure (see page 120) or an onlay flap (see page 130).

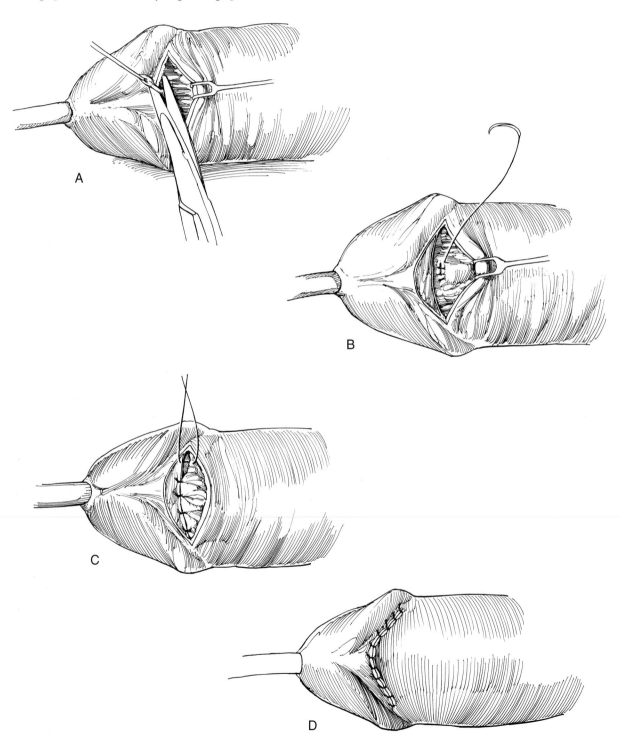

Repair of Scrotal and Perineal Fistulas

Place the patient in the lithotomy position. Inject dilute methylene blue via the meatus. Press on the bulb to force the dye through one or more fistulas to identify them. Place a metal sound in the urethra.

14 **A,** Mark and incise an eccentric ellipse of skin around the fistula. **B,** With traction on the skin edges around the fistula, dissect the tract down to the sound.

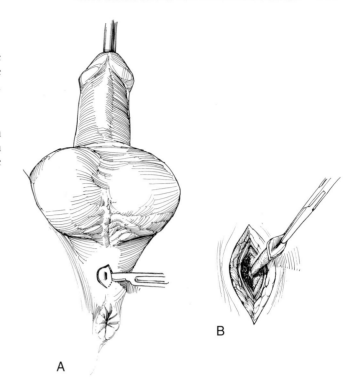

15 **A,** Trim the fistula almost flush with the urethral wall, leaving only enough cuff to allow inversion. **B,** Invert the urethral epithelial edge with a running 6-0 SAS placed as a subcuticular inverting stitch, so that the remains of the fistula are flush with the urethral lining. **C,** Free enough subcutaneous tissue on one side to cover the defect without tension, and approximate it with 5-0 or 6-0 SAS. Close the skin with interrupted 6-0 SAS. If the urethral defect was large, place a 22 F silicone balloon catheter into the bladder. **D,** When tension is present after repair, it may be relieved with mattress sutures bolstered with beads.

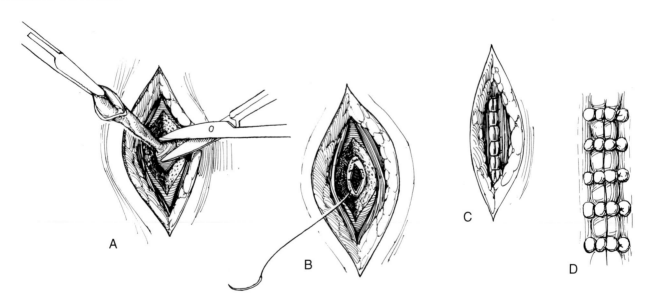

Repair of Large Defects

Larger fistulas, either primary ones or those that arise secondarily after combining multiple fistulas, require a more extensive procedure like a Johanson second-stage urethroplasty (see page 279), taking care not to narrow the channel. For very large fistulas use an onlay flap, an island flap based on a fasciocutaneous pedicle of penile shaft skin (Orandi), or a fasciocutaneous pedicle flap from preputial skin (McAninch, see page 289).

Scrotal Dartos Flap for Complex Repairs

Multiple attempts at repair of hypospadias may leave persistent fistulas, strictures, and diverticula. The bed must be revascularized by bringing in fresh tissue. Mobilize a generous fibrofatty vascularized dartos flap from the area between the subcutaneous tissue of the scrotum and the tunica vaginalis, somewhat like a labial flap (see page 590). Tunnel beneath the skin between scrotum and penis, and interpose the flap before closing the skin over the defect (Churchill et al, 1995).

Excision of Urethral Diverticulum

If the neourethra is made too wide, even slight distal stenosis induces it to distend during urination because it is unsupported by the corpus spongiosum, allowing urine to drip after voiding. This is especially a problem of repairs with bladder epithelial grafts. It is also possible that an initial leak from the inner suture line may create a pool that subsequently is re-epithelialized as a diverticulum.

Hair in the urethra alone, a consequence of earlier techniques of repair, usually is not a problem (other than requiring occasional trimming), but if it lies in a pool of urine in a urethral diverticulum, it fosters the formation of stones. The treatment consists of exposing and excising the diverticulum, with depilation while the remaining surface is exposed.

For repair, fill the diverticulum retrogradely to determine its dimensions. For the simplest procedure, make a longitudinal incision through skin and urethra, excise the excess urethral and penile skin asymmetrically, and close the defect in three layers over a stent. For a more secure technique, if the ventral skin is free, deglove the penis before incising the diverticulum and urethra. Resect the diverticulum. Insert a catheter or stent. Close the edges of the diverticulum with fine inverted interrupted SAS. Close the subcutaneous tissue with a vest-over-pants technique, and reapproximate the skin with a fine subcuticular suture. For repair of bulbar diverticula, see page 226.

Persistent Chordee

Persistent chordee, like chordee without hypospadias, may require only dorsal tucking (see pages 132 and 133). If it is severe and the meatus is short, wait until the child is older. At that time, free the shaft skin at the corona and release the neourethra from the corpora; then excise the chordee. Mobilization of the urethra is difficult, and if a short urethra is responsible for the chordee, it often must be replaced or supplemented with buccal mucosa or bladder urothelium. Secondary scarring can be treated with Z-plasty. In two-stage procedures, watch for penile rotation.

REPEAT REPAIR

For reoperation after multiple previous failures, observe the following five precepts: (1) obtain wide exposure; (2) excise all abnormal tissue remnants, including the old urethra; (3) look for and use the best-quality skin that is available, and plan for skin cover at the outset; (4) correct the chordee first, then reconstruct the urethra; and (5) if possible, correct all the problems in one stage. However, do not hesitate to completely revise any part that proves inadequate by resorting to a second stage. Too often, the complex of fistula, stricture, and chordee is the result of the many previous minor attempts at correction. For these difficult cases, it is best first to re-create the deformity without worrying too much about loss of part of the repair from taking it apart, and then set about putting it back together.

Several options are available for secondary repair: For the persistently hypospadic meatus, if skin is available for mobilization, use a perimeatal flap (see page 124) or an onlay island flap (see page 130). It may be best to incise the glans deeply and thin out the spongy tissue so that the glans is flat. Cover the raw undersurface, inserting a graft if necessary. Use subcuticular sutures. If placed as a continuous stitch, Prolene sutures are easier to pull out than nylon sutures.

For the second stage, consider a tube graft tunneled under the new skin cover, or form a tube from the bed and cover it with the glans wings. Always use suprapubic diversion. If the defect is in midshaft, apply the ventral tube technique (Thiersch-Duplay, see page 140) or an onlay island flap (see page 130). Shaft skin is usually available but is not necessarily adjacent to the defect. It must be deployed as an onlay island flap over the (usually intact) urethral plate. This technique is suitable to correct a urethral stricture or bring a retracted meatus to the tip of the glans, as well as to bridge the defect between a proximal meatus and an adequate urethra in the glans.

When shaft skin has already been depleted, use a buccal mucosal graft. A graft from the cheek brings sturdy new tissue to the site (Steps 6 and 7). Prepare a bed for it before harvesting the graft. Deglove the penis and resect all of the abnormal urethra. Before proceeding with insertion of a buccal graft, check the vascularity of the bed. If it would not support a free graft, redistribute the skin of the shaft, close the wound, and return after 3 to 6 months for insertion of the graft.

For severe defects after multiple procedures, it is usually necessary to use a staged procedure. Take the repair down in a first stage, and apply a meshed graft (see page 290), a pedicle flap from the tunica vaginalis, or both to the resulting defect. Then at a second stage, put the elements together again.

PSYCHOSOCIAL MALADJUSTMENT

These patients regard their genitalia more negatively than normal subjects to a degree related to the severity of the hypospadias and the age at repair (the older the patient, the greater the problem). This is especially true in cultures in which circumcision is rare. A third of patients were found to desire functional or cosmetic improvement (Mureau et al, 1995), especially improvement in penile size. They also may be inhibited in seeking sexual contacts, but they adjust similarly to normal men, achieving a normal adult sexual life.

Commentary by Alan B. Retik

We usually repair hypospadias between the ages of 4 and 12 months. Very little penile growth occurs between the ages of 6 months and 3 years. If a phallus is of reasonable size, we operate early. If it is small, we often pretreat with 5 percent testosterone ointment applied to the shaft of the penis twice a day for 3 weeks prior to surgery. I do not find it necessary to separate preputial adhesions 1 month prior to surgery. This is done in the operating room at the time of the procedure.

In general, most cases of hypospadias can be corrected in one operative procedure. The procedures that I use for distal hypospadias are the MAGPI, perimeatal-based flap (Mathieu), Duplay tube for a gaping urethral meatus, and in some instances an onlay flap. Recently, we have used the Snodgrass procedure (incision of the posterior wall of the urethral plate with a Duplay tube). Catheters are not routinely used following surgery for distal hypospadias. The dorsal relaxing incision of Denis Browne should never be used because of the tendency to produce an unsightly and in some instances painful scar.

We do two-staged repairs infrequently in the infant with severe hypospadias (perineal or proximal scrotum) whose penis is small with little growth following testosterone administration. It is important at the first stage to incise the glans in the midline deeply with a slight dorsal extension in order to bring enough foreskin on the glans for the creation of a urethral meatus at the tip of the penis at the second stage.

In most instances, imaging of the upper urinary tract is not necessary preoperatively. However, in a boy with a documented urinary tract infection, voiding cystography and renal ultrasonography should be done.

For traction on the glans, I use a 5-0 Prolene suture on a fine tapered needle. Reapproximation of the glans over a newly constructed urethra should be done loosely in two layers. In order to accomplish this, the glans should be incised deeply and reapproximated with 6-0 Vicryl over a sound inserted between the glans and the urethra to avoid making the glans too tight.

An alternative to ventral dermal grafting for persistent chordee is the use of a tunica vaginalis graft. In the harvest of a bladder mucosal graft, I do not use cautery to incise the bladder wall for fear of damaging the mucosa. The distal portion of the graft should consist of a small segment (approximately 5 mm) of skin or buccal mucosa to avoid prolapse at the meatus, which is commonly seen.

I use a #7 Jackson-Pratt catheter sewn to the glans with two 5-0 Prolene sutures draining urine into a double diaper. In the correction of urethrocutaneous fistulas, my limited experience with the early application of silver nitrate has been uniformly unsuccessful. I usually wait 6 to 12 months rather than 2 months following the original repair to close a fistula. It is important to excise a rim of the fistulous tract and mobilize the surrounding tissues widely. The fistula is closed with a subcuticular inverting stitch. Coverage is with multiple layers of mobilized adjacent tissue. The de-epithelialized flap technique of Durham Smith is very effective. It is not necessary to drain the bladder with a catheter following fistula repair.

Commentary by Charles J. Devine, Jr.

The dressing, the use of stents, and the techniques of urine diversion have evolved greatly within recent years. Using these simpler modalities has markedly shortened the hospital stay of these children. Originally we used urinary diversion (first perineal, then suprapubic) with a stent (first red rubber, then soft silicone). Later we placed a soft silicone stent into the repair and passed a silicone feeding tube through it to divert the urine for a day or two. When this tube was removed, the patient would void through the stent for the rest of 3 weeks.

Currently, we place the "drippy tube" that my associate Boyd Winslow, M.D., improved by securing it through the bladder to a button on the abdomen. In all patients with hypospadias we perform a cystoscopy as the first step in the repair, as we have occasionally found more proximal significant urethral anomalies, such as valves. This allows, under cystoscopic control, introduction of nylon sutures through a hollow needle passed into the bladder dome to be withdrawn through the urethra. At the conclusion of the repair they are fixed to the tip of a 6 F Kendall polyurethane pediatric Ultramer catheter that is drawn into the bladder and fixed in place by tying the sutures over a button on the abdomen. The tube is left in place for about 3 weeks and easily removed by cutting the sutures at the button.

We have always used drains postoperatively. First, they were simply sterile rubber bands cut and tucked into the wound as it was closed. Today we use suction drains; once we made them from "butterfly" needles and blood collection tubes, but now TLS drains are readily available. We use these in all of our reconstructive surgery, placing one or two within the repair and removing them when they are no longer productive, one on one day and the other on the next. We have not used a compression dressing for years.

We cover the penis with a single layer of Johnson & Johnson's Bioclusive dressing. The sticky side of the plastic material is applied to the ventrum of the penis. It is then brought around the penis loosely, and the two sticky surfaces are stuck together on the dorsal side, forming something like a keel. This furnishes adequate pressure and, being clear, allows observation of the status of the penile skin. The adhesive material loosens in a week or so, after which the dressing can easily be peeled off. *Note:* Other wraps, such as Tegaderm or Op-site, have a different consistency and have not been satisfactory for this.

Meatotomy

VENTRAL MEATOTOMY

No-Suture Method for Infants

1 **A** and **B,** Instill 1 percent lidocaine through a 25-gauge needle passed through the meatus and directed into the frenulum. Alternatively, apply 2.5 ml of Emla cream (2.5 percent lidocaine and 2.5 percent prilocaine) and hold it in place for 1 hour with a Tegaderm wrap.

2 **A,** Clamp the ventral meatal lip with a fine clamp. Insert it deeply, as healing reduces the depth of the cut. **B,** Divide the thinned tissue, now rendered avascular, with scissors.

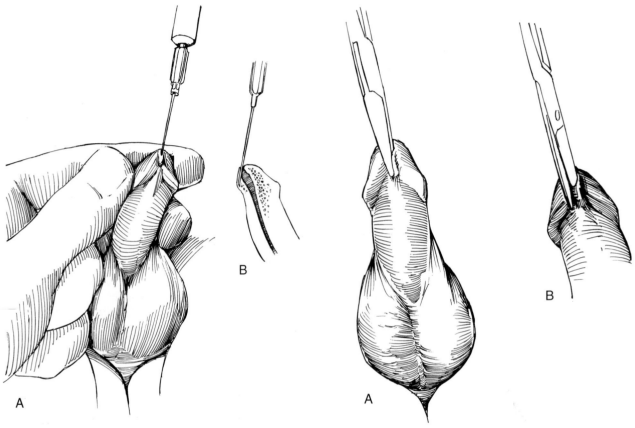

3 Spread the edges and apply petroleum jelly (Vaseline) or ophthalmic antibiotic ointment to the cut edges with a proximal wiping movement. Instruct the parent to do the same at home by inserting the tip of the ointment tube or an infant feeding tube three times a day for a day or two to keep the edges from resealing. The parent should check the caliber occasionally for at least 3 months.

Suture Method for Older Boys

4 **A,** Instill 1 percent lidocaine through a 25-gauge needle passed through the meatus and directed into the frenulum. Alternatively, impregnate the area with 2.5 ml of Emla cream. Incise the ventrum with scissors, creating a V-shaped defect. Take care not to create hypospadias. Calibrate with a sound of appropriate size. **B,** Place up to five 3-0 or 4-0 PCG sutures or SAS to approximate the edges of the V.

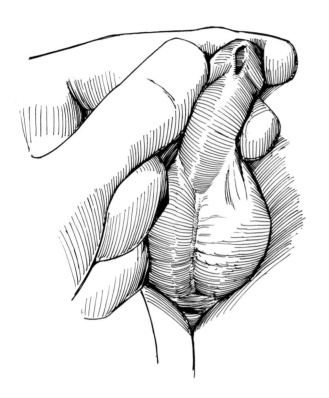

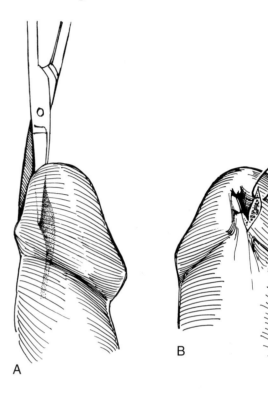

Commentary by Jeffery Wacksman

We have used Emla cream to accomplish meatotomies. This is something that readers may wish to undertake.

With regard to the suture methods for older children, I advise using a 5-0 CCG suture on a C1 needle rather than the 3-0 or 4-0 PCG, which I believe is too large a suture. We usually suture the opening in the glans so that it stays open during healing. I think this provides a much better overall result.

DORSAL MEATOTOMY

5 Dorsal meatotomy is used for narrowing the fossa navicularis in adults. It is very useful prior to urethral instrumentation, especially transurethral prostatic resection, and protects against meatal strictures.

Insinuate a #10 Bard-Parker knife blade into the meatus, cutting edge up. Withdraw the knife while applying moderate upward pressure to incise the roof of the fossa navicularis and meatus. Repeat until a lubricated sound of appropriate size passes readily.

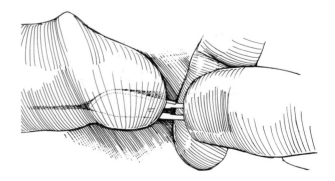

Meatoplasty and Glanuloplasty (MAGPI)
(Duckett)

MAGPI works best for correction of distal hypospadias without chordee. The principal goal is to provide good support for the glans, so that it remains elevated with the meatus at the tip. The meatus should be no more than 1 cm proximal to the glans for the MAGPI procedure to be applicable. The skin on the ventrum proximal to the meatus should be thick and mobile enough to be lifted off the urethra so that it can be moved distally. If the perimeatal skin is of poor quality, resort to an onlay repair. Do not try to extend the indications for the operation. It is not suitable if the meatus is fixed without the typical bridge of tissue between meatus and glans. For a wide-mouth, flat, fixed meatus that cannot be moved into the glanular groove, a Mathieu procedure (see page 124), an onlay island flap (see page 130), or, probably best, a pyramid procedure, described subsequently, is more appropriate.

Operate at 6 months of age; if necessary, the repair can be revised 6 months later. This is an outpatient procedure performed under general anesthesia. Insert a vertical traction suture in the glans. Infiltrate the subcoronal area and glans groove with 1 percent lidocaine containing epinephrine 1:100,000 to improve hemostasis. Blocking the dorsal penile nerves with 0.25 percent bupivacaine hydrochloride (see page 76) decreases the need for intraoperative anesthesia and decreases pain postoperatively. A Scott retractor can be helpful.

1 Make a circumferential incision in the ventral skin proximal to the coronal sulcus and the meatus.

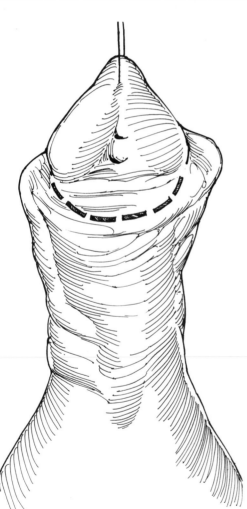

2 Mobilize the skin of the shaft proximally as a sleeve, taking care not to injure the delicate urethral wall. Free the skin to the penoscrotal junction. Clear from the corpora all tissue that is causing tethering. Ascertain that the penis is straight by creating an artificial erection. Any residual curvature is probably caused by corporal disproportion and can be corrected by dorsal tucks (see page 132).

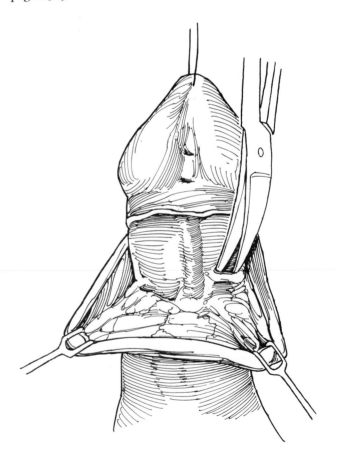

3 Make a deep vertical incision starting inside the dorsal margin of the meatus and extending to the distal end of the glanular groove. This vertical cut widens the dorsal meatal margin even when meatal stenosis exists. Occasionally it may be desirable to excise a wedge if the bridge of tissue is prominent distal to the meatus.

4 **A** and **B,** Suture the edges of the meatal V to the groove in the glans with fine sutures as a Heineke-Mikulicz transverse closure to advance the meatus and flatten the groove.

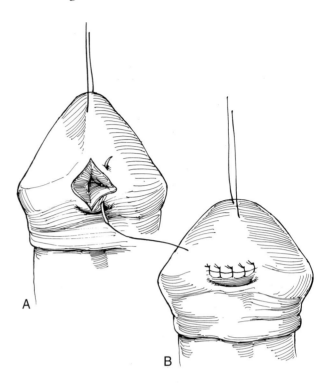

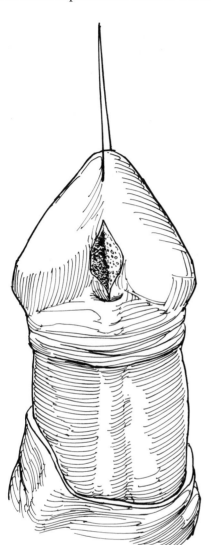

5 **A,** Lift the proximal edge of the meatus with a skin hook or traction suture, pulling it toward the tip of the glans to form an inverted V. Excise the glans tissue *(dashed lines)* on the medial margins of these glans wings to allow them to come together to provide support for the glans. **B,** Approximate the deep glans tissue with one or two layers of 5-0 SAS. Do not place them so deeply that they compromise the urethral lumen. Test the caliber of the meatus repeatedly with a bougie à boule. Trim excess glans epithelium and approximate it with sutures of fine CCG. Correct any persistent ventral tilt of the glans by tacking the dorsal coronal edge of the glans to the dorsal tunica albuginea on either side with two fine NAS. *Alternative:* Make a dorsal vertical incision proximal to the glans and close it transversely (Heineke-Mikulicz). Avoid the midline structures. **C,** Align the median raphe and trim the excess preputial skin at a point proximal to the wrinkled portion. Suture the edges with 6-0 CCG sutures or with fine subcuticular sutures, trimming the skin edges as necessary to improve appearance.

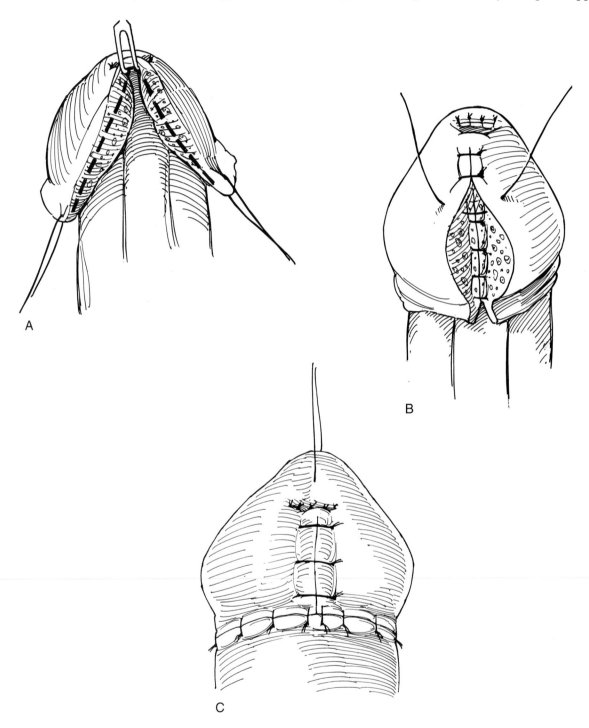

6 **A,** If the ventral skin is deficient, split the preputial skin dorsally. **B,** Tack the apex to the dorsal edge of the coronal sulcus. **C** and **D,** Bring the edges around as Byers flaps. Trim the flaps *(dashed line)* to preserve symmetry and approximate them in the midline. Dress the penis with Tegaderm. In some cases it may be desirable to insert a catheter or a stent.

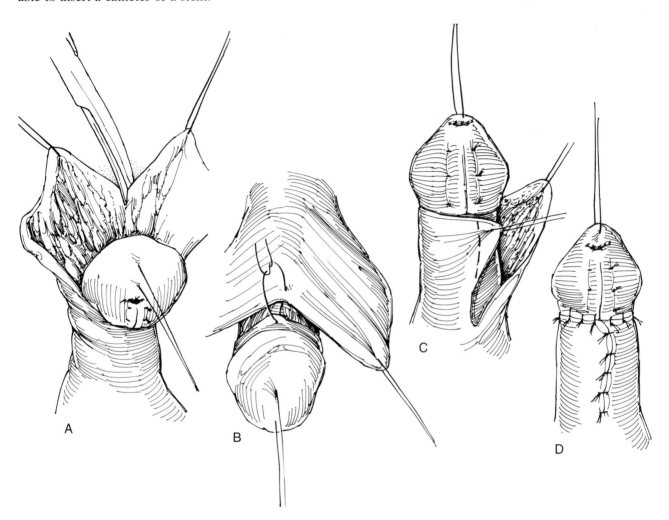

POSTOPERATIVE PROBLEMS

Meatal stenosis is the result of an inadequate meatoplasty. The dorsal vertical incision did not open the meatus widely and/or did not adequately deepen the urethral groove. *Meatal regression* results when the glans wings are not firmly coapted ventrally to provide support for the glans. To correct it, repeat the steps of the original operation. For greater degrees of retrusion, place an onlay flap (see page 130) or tubularize the plate (Thiersch-Duplay, see page 140).

MODIFIED MAGPI REPAIR
(Arap)

An alternative to the MAGPI, the Arap procedure advances the ventral aspect of the urethra and extends the application of the operation to patients with distal hypospadias. Such patients may not have a dorsal lip of tissue in the glanular groove that allows a Heineke-Mikulicz maneuver. If the urethral plate is flat, it is more suitable for an onlay island flap or, if the distance is short, for a Mathieu repair. In any case, the distal urethra must be mobile after release of the skin and dartos fascia. The ventral skin along the urethra may be thin, requiring cutting back to normal urethral spongiosum and thereby leaving a gap too great to bridge.

Advance the meatus as described for the MAGPI operation by a longitudinal incision in the glanular groove with transverse closure (Steps 3 and 4). Make a circumferential incision proximal to the corona and deglove the shaft.

7 **A,** Place traction sutures on the ventral skin on either side of the midline, 1 to 1.5 cm apart. **B,** Pull these sutures distally to create two flaps. **C,** Suture the flaps together in the midline, thus forming a floor for the glanular urethra. Suture the deep tissue of the glans together in the midline and approximate the epithelium of the glans. Close any ventral defect with Byers flaps or as a single pedicle flap; trim excess skin. Drainage tubes are not necessary.

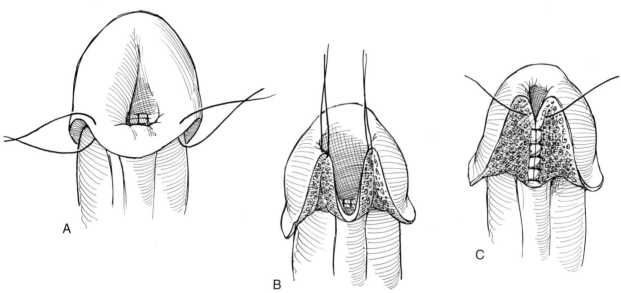

PYRAMID PROCEDURE FOR REPAIR OF MEGAMEATUS–INTACT PREPUCE HYPOSPADIAS VARIANT
(Duckett)

In this variant, the large meatus is found concealed beneath an intact prepuce with a deep cleft forming the glanular groove. Techniques such as the MAGPI or Mathieu repair do not correct the large meatus. The pyramid procedure (so called because placing two traction sutures at the coronal sulcus and a third at the frenulum forms a pyramid with the base located distally) exposes and allows excision of the excess tissue in the terminal urethra, with reconstitution of the meatus to a proper size while bringing it to the tip of the penis. The procedure or its modifications may be applied to other cases of subcoronal hypospadias and, if combined with a de-epithelialized flap, allows release of the shaft skin before a choice is made among a perimeatal-based flap, a preputial flap, or a modified pyramid repair.

Place three traction sutures in addition to the one on the tip of the glans: one on each side of the meatal base near the coronal sulcus and one in the midline at its ventral margin. After infiltration with lidocaine-epinephrine to reduce bleeding, make a tennis-racquet incision in the glanular groove that extends around the meatus. With iris scissors, mobilize the urethral cone (pyramid) proximally until it becomes normal in size. Develop glans wings on either side. Remove a wedge from the excess ventral urethral tissue, and approximate the edges with a continuous 7-0 SAS to provide a normal caliber to the urethra (Thiersch-Duplay). Bring the wings together with two layers of fine interrupted sutures, and place 7-0 interrupted CCG mattress sutures in the skin. *Alternative* (Hill et al,1993): Reinforce the midline suture line by de-epithelializing a strip of shaft skin and covering the suture line with it before approximating the glans flaps. After closing the skin, test the urethral caliber with a 10 F or 12 F bougie à boule; observe the quality of the stream by applying pressure over the bladder. Follow the repair with a circumcision if desired.

GLANS APPROXIMATION PROCEDURE (GAP)
(Zaontz)

This procedure is designed for the repair of glanular and coronal hypospadias in the presence of a wide and deep glanular groove with a noncompliant or fish-mouth meatus, based on the Thiersch-Duplay principle.

8 **A,** Incise the cleft in the glanular groove if it is present. Close the defect by slightly advancing the dorsal side of the meatus and suturing it with fine sutures to form a smooth urethral plate. Mark the glans wings in a thick U around the meatus with a marking pen, and excise a band of epithelium with tenotomy scissors, including the marked line. Approximate the inner, urethral edges first, with a running suture of 7-0 CCG placed subcuticularly. For an improved cosmetic effect (applicable to all repairs), form a *mucosal collar* (Firlit) by raising V-shaped flaps *(dashed lines)* from the inner preputial lining on both sides. **B,** Approximate the outer edges of the glans with interrupted imbricating stitches (it is not necessary to form glans flaps). Complete the collar by bringing the inner V-flaps together in the midline. Close the remainder of the defect by approximating the preputial tissue ventrally.

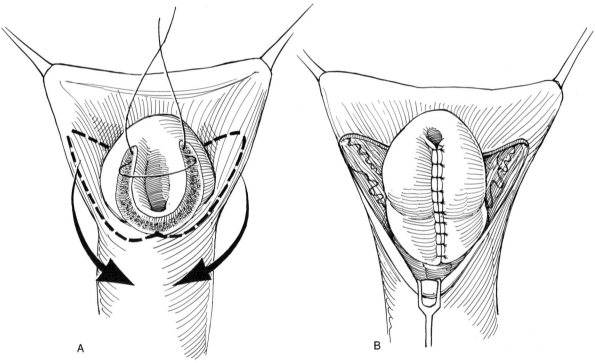

A   B

GLANULAR RECONSTRUCTION AND PREPUTIOPLASTY (GRAP) PROCEDURE
(Gilpin)

As the name suggests, this one-stage procedure, suitable for outpatient surgery, leaves the penis with an uncircumcised appearance. It is not suitable when chordee is present.

9 **A,** Mark, incise, and raise the margins of skin and glanular epithelium on either side of the glans groove, forming a U around the meatus. **B,** Close the skin as a tube with 8-0 SAS. Test the suture line to be sure it is watertight. Place a catheter in the neourethra. Raise glans flaps and close them over the neourethra with two layers of 7-0 SAS. **C,** Hold the prepuce up with two stay sutures placed far enough apart on the preputial hood that when they are approximated ventrally the distal margin of the prepuce forms a preputial ring of adequate diameter to prevent phimosis. Make a Y-extension from the original incision along the margin between the inner and outer preputial surfaces, almost to the stay sutures. Close the inner preputial edges vertically in two layers with 7-0 SAS to cover the neourethra. Confirm that the prepuce is fully retractable. This leaves a vertical defect on the ventrum that is closed as a Z-plasty *(dashed lines)* to allow the prepuce to extend over the glans. Expect marked edema of the prepuce initially that resolves with time.

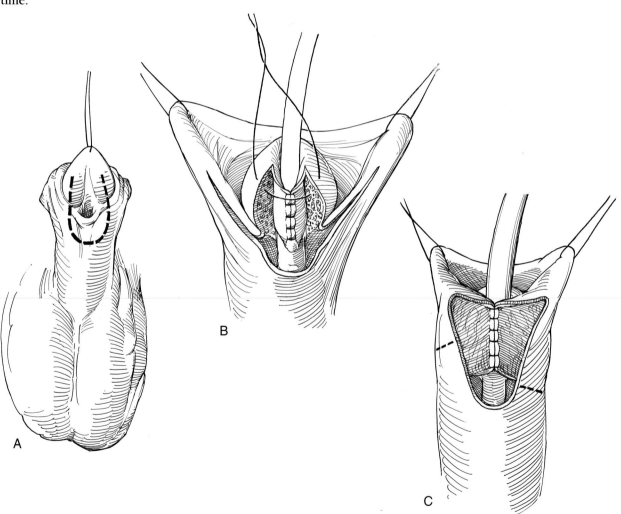

POSTOPERATIVE PROBLEMS

Glans breakdown and meatal retraction are the principal reasons for failure (Duckett). It is most important to bring the glans wings together in the midline, excising excess skin on their medial edge and approximating two layers of deep glans with a superficial epithelial layer. This firm, conical reconfiguration of the glans avoids meatal regression. It is important to excise these glans skin edges in order to approximate glans tissue primarily with the ventral meatal edge brought well forward.

Commentary by Barry A. Kogan

Only in recent years have repairs for distal hypospadias been performed with consistent techniques. Because the lesion is not associated with major abnormalities of urinary or sexual function, the problem is primarily one of appearance and the related psychological ramifications. Hence, in an era in which significant complications were associated with repairs, it was quite reasonable not to operate on these minor lesions. Today, however, a number of approaches are associated with minimal morbidity and a high success rate, so these lesions are commonly repaired.

There are innumerable published and unpublished accounts of hypospadias repairs. Were that not enough, there are any number of variations of them as well. These attest to the fact that no one repair is optimal, and each has advantages and potential risks. The procedures used in the majority of instances include the MAGPI or the Mathieu procedure. We have used these for outpatient repairs with a very high rate of success and very few complications. For those patients with a deep glanular groove, however, we currently use the GAP procedure, as the cosmetic results are unsurpassed.

The use of lidocaine with epinephrine is controversial for these repairs. It may distort the tissues more than is desirable; a tourniquet is a reasonable alternative to maintain hemostasis for distal repairs. Because distal repairs are rarely absolutely necessary, complications are particularly annoying.

It is critical that the correct repair be applied to the patient's anatomic defect. To avoid fistulas, I use a de-epithelialized flap (Hill) to cover the repair whenever possible. I believe that the cosmetic effect is enhanced by using a mucosal collar (Firlit) in nearly all cases. Apply either no dressing or a simple Tegaderm covering. A catheter is generally not needed in children less than 18 months of age. For postoperative pain control, instill lidocaine jelly intraurethrally, or better, create a caudal nerve block.

Perimeatal-Based Flap Repair

(Mathieu)

The Mathieu or flip-flap procedure is suitable for hypospadias with minimal chordee. Glanular tilt and limited distal chordee may be corrected easily by dorsal tucks. The glanular urethral groove forms the roof of the distal urethra, and a meatal-based flap is the floor. It also allows reconstruction of the split prepuce, if the uncircumcised state is desired. However, the vascular supply to the flap may be tenuous, and, because it is not defatted, it cannot acquire a good local blood supply as a graft. Thus, late meatal stenosis is not uncommon. Keeping the dartos tunic attached to it improves the vascularity. The Barcat modification (Redman, 1987) provides a better cosmetic result with fewer complications by relying on more extensive mobilization of the glanular urethral plate and the formation of a matching flap from the shaft to bury the meatus at the tip of the glans. The Mustardé repair (see page 126) is similar but tubularizes the meatal-based flap. Consider a vascularized preputial flap as an onlay (see page 130), especially if the perimeatal skin is thin. Do not use the Mathieu technique for secondary repairs.

Create an artificial erection to evaluate chordee.

DISTAL MEATUS WITH MINIMAL CHORDEE

1 Insert a monofilament synthetic NAS swaged on a fine tapered needle in the glans for traction. Mark lines for the glans flap on either side of the glanular groove, 6 to 8 mm apart and extending from the tip of the penis to the meatus. The final dimensions of the flap should provide an adequate distal urethra but at the same time not result in a patulous, flaccid pocket. As continuations, mark the incisions for the proximal urethral flap, but make them farther apart (12 to 15 mm). Infiltrate the subcutaneous tissue with 1:200,000 epinephrine in 1 percent lidocaine (optional). Incise along the marks. For valuable additional blood supply, lift up the skin edges, divide the dartos layer with tenotomy scissors, and free it proximally from the skin of the shaft to provide a pedicle for the flap (DeJong and Boemers, 1993). Incise the prepuce circumferentially 1 cm proximal to the coronal sulcus.

2 Dissect in the plane between the corpora cavernosa and the glans cap to develop the lateral portions of the glans as wings. Raise the flap from the shaft, taking care to preserve the attached subcutaneous tissue with its blood supply. The vascular supply is most tenuous at the hinge of the flap. Avoid the base during dissection in order to preserve the adventitial blood flow. Fold the flap over the distal urethra in the glans, and approximate it on either side with interrupted 5-0 SAS. Take care to invert the edges of the neourethra proximally to avoid dog ears, which contribute to fistula formation. Alternatively, place one layer of suture continuously, adding a few interrupted sutures at the neomeatus, and place a second running suture for the adventitia. Tack the subcutaneous tissue of the flap to the deep tissue of the glans. Test for a watertight suture line by injecting saline into the meatus. Correct leaks with additional sutures.

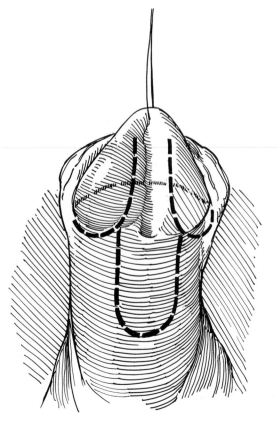

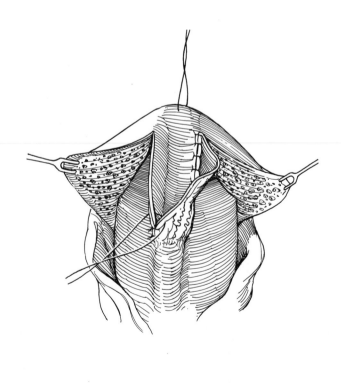

3 Approximate the glans flap with fine interrupted sutures. If necessary, undermine the flaps to avoid tension. Keep a large sound in the meatus while suturing it to prevent constriction.

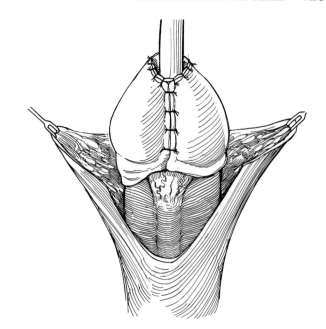

4 Draw the shaft skin around to the ventrum as Byers flaps. Close the circumcision defect. Trim excess skin, and close the ventral defect. Use the best-looking flap to cross the midline, or close like a Z-plasty to avoid having the suture lines converge as shown in the figure; this leads to fistula formation. A running suture is preferable to interrupted sutures. Skin may have to be trimmed later.

To retain the prepuce: Do not make a circumcising incision at the outset, then reconstruct the prepuce ventrally.

Alternative covering 1: Raise a vascularized dartos subcutaneous flap from the dorsal surface of the penis, rotate it ventrally, and suture it in place to cover the urethral flap (Retik).

Alternative covering 2: De-epithelialize a portion of one of the Byers flaps and bring it around to the ventrum to provide a cover of dermis for the repair.

Finally, calibrate the urethra with a bougie à boule or curved sound corresponding to the size of a normal urethra for the age of the child. Pass an 8 F silicone catheter into the bladder and tether it to the penis by a traction suture, which should remain a day or two. Alternatively, omit a catheter. Provide a penile nerve block with bupivacaine (see page 76).

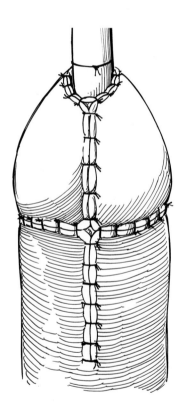

Mobilization of the Distal Plate (Barcat Technique)
(Redman)

Adjust the urethral meatus with Heineke-Mikulicz cuts (see page 117). Outline the urethral plate in the glans groove and draw a matching proximal meatal–based skin flap on the shaft. Each should be about 8 mm wide. Incise and elevate the proximal flap first, then raise the distal flap by making deep incisions on either side of the plate in order to obtain full thickness. Undermine the urethra to gain enough length for the flaps to reach the end of the glans. Apply a tourniquet and undermine the glans to form glans wings. Approximate the two flaps

with 7-0 SAS to form a tube, placing interrupted sutures terminally to allow for trimming. Tack the tube to the end of the glans with a fine suture. Cover the neourethra with subcutaneous and lateral spongy tissue (Koff et al, 1994) and approximate the glans flaps. Suture the glans edges to the end of the neourethra to provide a caliber of 20 F. Insert a 5 F feeding tube, which should remain for about 5 days.

Salvage repair: For the abnormally positioned meatus persisting after a previous repair, a perimeatal-based flap or an island flap can be successfully raised and placed as a secondary procedure, even though the skin had been previously mobilized, but a de-epithelialized flap must be interposed.

Perimeatal-Based Tube Repair

(Mustardé)

This procedure is intended for mild chordee that requires separation of the meatus from the coronal sulcus. A perimeatal-based tube repair makes a tunnel in the glans rather than a V-flap like the Mathieu procedure (see page 124) and avoids splitting the glans. The technique is not suitable for repeat operations because it requires good vascularization of the flap.

Placing the single suture line dorsally against the corpora may reduce the risk of fistula formation.

Insert a Prolene stay suture vertically in the glans. If the meatus is small, incise it laterally.

1 Mark and incise a skin flap 1.5 to 2 cm wide (equivalent to 15 F to 20 F) on the shaft proximal to the meatus. Make it long enough to reach the distal end of the glans. Excess skin can always be trimmed later.

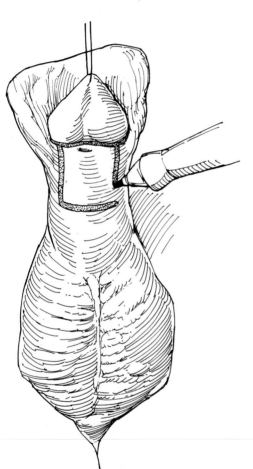

2 With a #15 blade, incise the prepuce circumferentially 0.5 cm proximal to the corona. At the midline, direct the blunt tips of dissecting scissors beneath the skin to develop a space as they are spread apart. Avoid cutting, but do transect any fascial bands distal to the meatus that produce chordee and tilt the glans. Bleeding should be controlled by bipolar cautery applied precisely to individual vessels.

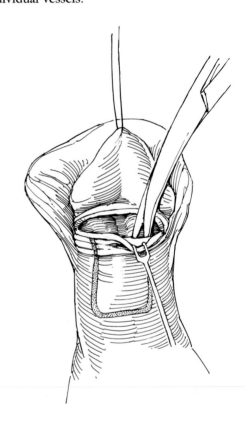

3 **A,** Tunnel through the glans by first directing fine tenotomy scissors to separate the undersurface of the glans from the underlying corpus on each side. Usually this space can be developed by spreading the tips of the scissors. If the midline contains residual fascial tissue, create a separate tunnel over each corporal tip, and divide the septum between them. Alternatively, if the glans is flat, open it widely to form two glans flaps. **B,** Direct the scissors horizontally to reach the apex of the glans. Lift the glanular tissue with toothed forceps, and remove a generous divot of skin and glanular tissue. This opening must be tubular, not tapered. Use compression to stop the bleeding. Bring the scissors out through the tip, and spread the blades to make the tunnel wide enough to easily admit the double-thickness skin of the flap. Alternatively, incise the site of the new meatus as a V so that it can be laid into the distal end of the new urethra that was not completely closed.

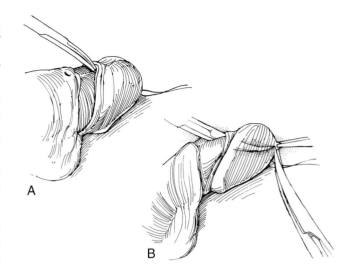

4 **A,** Recheck the outlined length of the flap to be sure it is still adequate. Incise the margins of the flap. Place stay sutures in the four corners and free the flap from the corpora, leaving as much adventitial tissue on it as possible to preserve the blood supply. Free the lateral skin margins remaining on the shaft generously. Carefully place one or two 6-0 or 7-0 SAS subcuticularly at the junction of the flap with its base. Start the tubularization over a catheter-stent. **B,** Continue the closure skin edge to skin edge with an interrupted inverting subcuticular 6-0 or 7-0 SAS. Too many sutures can devitalize the edges of the flap. The suture line lies deep in the wound, free of pressure from the urinary stream, and a loose fit is all that is necessary.

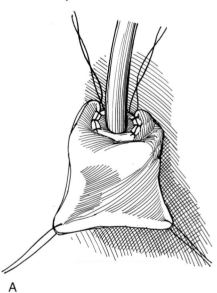

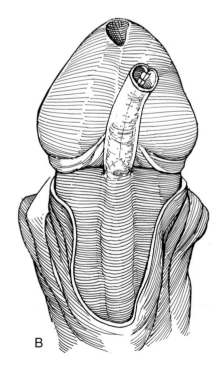

5 Draw the skin tube and stent through the glanular tunnel. Suture the two peripheral corners together, and attach them to the dorsal end of the opening in the glans (stent not shown).

6 Trim the end of the flap to conform to the opening; cutting it obliquely makes the lumen larger. If a V-flap was formed at the meatus, fix it into the end of the suture line of the tube. Suture its edges accurately to the glans with interrupted 6-0 SAS.

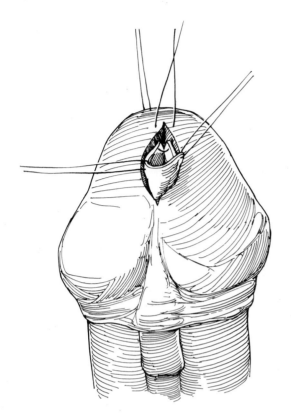 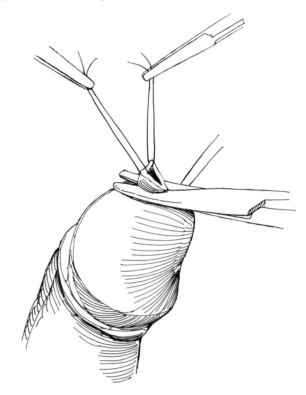

7 **A** and **B,** Open the prepuce by incising it vertically, and bring the wings around to cover the defect on the shaft. It is possible to de-epithelialize the distal part of one flap and pass it over the urethra into the tunnel to provide a second layer of coverage. Excise excess skin to achieve a good appearance, and approximate the wings so that the suture line lies in the midline. **C,**

Although not as good cosmetically, a buttonhole may be made in the prepuce to bring it over the glans. Insert a stent and fasten it to the glans with the stay suture. Loosely apply a Bioclusive dressing to remain until it loosens and can be taken off. If the "drippy tube" is used for diversion, remove it in 3 weeks.

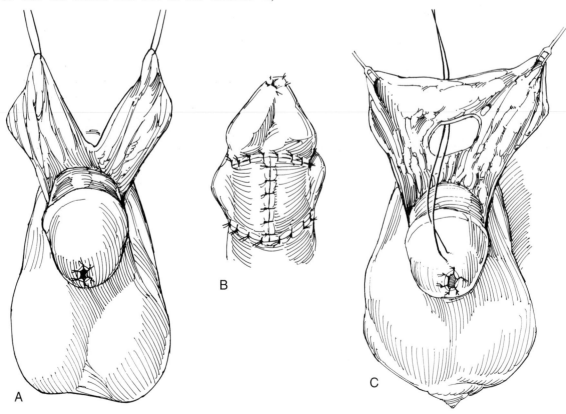

Urinary Diversion

The *drippy-tube method* (Winslow) (not shown) may be used. Fill the bladder through an 8 F infant feeding tube in the urethra. Place an 18-gauge spinal needle suprapubically, and pass a Prolene suture through it into the bladder; retrieve it transurethrally with an alligator forceps through a small panendoscope. Repeat the maneuver with a second suture. The sutures are now available for fastening to the end of a stenting catheter to be drawn into the bladder through the repair. The end is then cut off so that drainage is free and no penile suture is needed to hold it.

Commentary by Charles J. Devine, Jr.

By now the Mustardé operation is probably an anachronism. If any significant amount of chordee is present, distal hypospadias can be reconstructed in better ways. The flap is a random flap; it has no major artery, and maintaining its vascular integrity during its elevation can be difficult. Yet, when no chordee is present, it can be used to advance the meatus into the tip of the glans; alternatively, if the vascularity of the ventral skin is excellent, that skin could be applied when previous surgery has not brought the urethra as far distally as we and the patient or his family think it should be. (Some surgeons who fix hypospadias continue to believe that a subcoronal meatus is an excellent result.)

When the flap is mobilized, dissection must be precise. After the skin incision, the tips of the dissecting scissors should be introduced beneath the flap and spread apart, separating but not cutting the tissues of the dartos fascia and preserving the delicate vessels within it. Any bleeding should be controlled with a fine-tipped bipolar cautery applied to the vessel at a low power setting. Heat generated is confined to the tissue between the tips and is not transmitted to other vessels within the pedicle, as would happen with a unipolar cautery. Indeed, because of this effect, the bipolar cautery should be the only fulgurating instrument used in any penile reconstructive surgery.

In these illustrations, the constructed tube is narrower than it should be. In the past we have used 6-0 CCG sutures to construct this tube and to close the skin. However, Ethicon "Monocryl" synthetic sutures are hydrolyzed in the process of absorption and leave no marks. The skin edges should be loosely approximated using intermittent rather than running sutures. This allows the tube to be shortened without having to retie the suture. Also, it facilitates opening the most distal section of the tube to allow a V-shaped tongue of glans epithelium to be set into the meatus. I prefer this to cutting a plug of tissue from the glans, as it can prevent stenosis and obstruction caused by contraction of the anastomosis. During creation of the tunnel through the glans, the tips of the scissors should be kept against the tunica of the corpora cavernosa. Here again, the dissection should be carried out by spreading the tips of the scissors rather than by cutting in this loose tissue layer. Buck's fascia inserts into the undersurface of the glans at the coronal margin, and no large vessels are present in this space.

When significant chordee is present with hypospadias, we undertake a more extensive dissection and excise the fibrous tissue under and distal to the urethral meatus. This is the dysgenic residuum of the mesenchyma that would have formed the structures surrounding the urethra if it had developed normally. In almost every case, its resection releases the penis and corrects the chordee. Extension of this dissection involves mobilization of the tissue of the glans penis to form two flaps that are lifted off the tips of the corpora. These flaps are closed in the midline to cover the reconstructed urethra. Urethral construction depends on the skin available. If the dissection has created a midline strip of skin extending from the meatus to the tip of the penis, the strip can be covered with an "onlay flap" derived from the preputial skin on the dorsum of the penis. If no midline strip remains, the flap from the dorsum can be formed into a tube to cover the defect.

One school of pediatric urology denies the significance of this residual fibrotic tissue and does not attempt to resect it. For them, the procedure of choice is to mobilize the skin on the ventrum of the penis while maintaining a midline strip of the skin and the underlying fibrous tissue distal to the meatus, which they call the "urethral plate." They then apply an onlay flap to complete the urethroplasty, closing the glans over this neourethra. Before approximating the skin, they demonstrate the residual chordee with an artificial erection and straighten the penis by shortening the dorsal aspect of the shaft with tucks. I hope that these young men do not develop recurrent chordee during puberty.

A number of the young adult men we have seen with chordee without hypospadias had a normal penis with straight erections during childhood yet developed penile curvature as they went through puberty. This curvature was caused by inelasticity of the tissues in the ventral aspect of the tunica albuginea of the corpora cavernosa and in the adjoining layers of Buck's and dartos fascias, but not in the corpus spongiosum or the urethra. These dysgenic changes are a result of the failure of normal growth and maturation of these structures during puberty. Suggestive but not yet conclusive evidence indicates that this results from a deficiency in 5α-reductase in these tissues; we do not know about the occurrence of this enzyme in hypospadias.

More recently we have taken advantage of the normal elasticity in the urethra proximal to the hypospadic meatus to extend the urethra to the tip of the glans without using a flap. We excise the deficient portion of the urethra and the fibrous bands that cause the chordee. We mobilize the sheath of skin to the base of the penis and dissect free the full length of the urethra. The end of the urethra can then be stretched forward, placing the meatus in the glans. To ease the tension on the urethra, several sutures are placed, tacking the corpus spongiosum along its length to the tunica of the corpora cavernosa.

Onlay Preputial Island Flap

(Duckett)

An island flap taken from the prepuce and placed as an onlay on the preserved urethral plate is the preferable technique for boys in whom no or only minimal chordee persists after takedown of the ventral skin but in whom either the meatus remains too proximal for a perimeatal flap (Mathieu) or the quality of the ventral skin is too poor to use for such a flap. Onlay flaps are suitable not only for distal hypospadias but also for mid and proximal hypospadias because a long horseshoe-shaped graft may be taken from the prepuce. The residual chordee found in one fourth of the cases may be corrected by dorsal (tunica albuginea plication [TAP]) tucks (Step 5). Reserve a tubed transverse island flap (see page 134) for those patients with greater degrees of chordee requiring division-resection of the urethral plate.

1 Place a stay suture on a tapered needle in the glans. Infiltrate the ventral meatal area with 1 or 2 ml of 1:100.000 epinephrine in 1 percent lidocaine solution and wait 7 minutes. Using a magnifying loupe, mark and incise the coronal sulcus circumferentially 8 mm from the glans, and extend the incision as two parallel cuts 8 mm apart down the shaft, continuing around the meatus as a U *(dotted lines)*. Release the tethering skin and dartos fascia, but leave the urethral plate intact. Mobilize the skin and superficial fascia from the proximal urethra with dissection around the lateral aspects of the shaft and distally into the glanular tissue. This may be enough to correct the chordee. If possible, avoid dissecting behind the plate. If the quality of the skin over the urethra is poor, do not hesitate to open the urethra proximally into a region of good spongiosal tissue. Test by artificial erection. If chordee persists, mobilize the urethral plate (see subsequently) or plicate the dorsal tunica albuginea by the TAP technique (Step 5). For cases of perineal or scrotal hypospadias for which plication is not sufficient, divide the plate and fashion the preputial flap with a midsection 1.5 cm wide. Roll the expanded portion into a tube to join the ends of the urethral plate (Flack and Walker, 1995).

Dissection Behind the Plate. Freeing the plate may be necessary if chordee persists (Mollard and Castagnola, 1994). Place the parallel incisions on the ventral shaft at least 8 mm apart to leave a sufficiently wide strip because it will become narrower as it is stretched. Excise the dysgenic fibrous tissue that extends in a fan shape to the undersurface of the glans, freeing it from the corpora and the skin. Cut through Buck's fascia to allow dissection on the distinctive tunica albuginea, thus releasing the plate.

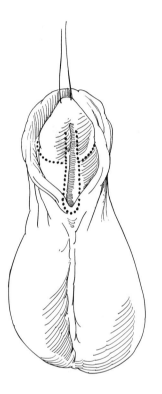

2 Develop glans wings by extending onto the ventrum of the glans parallel incisions that continue out to the end of the glanular groove. Mobilize them by dissecting in the plane between the glans and the tips of the corpora. If a lip is present in the glans groove, correct it with a longitudinal incision and transverse closure as in the MAGPI technique (see page 116). Take a wedge *(dotted lines)* from the urethra proximal to the meatus to cut it back into well-developed spongy tissue, and trim any excess thin urethral epithelium to provide a clean edge for suturing. Place four traction sutures in the opened prepuce to fan out the ventral surface. Mark the skin for the flap *(dashed lines)*, making it larger than necessary. Incise along the marks. Develop a plane well down to the base of the penis between the flap and the dorsal skin to form a substantial pedicle. Take great care not to devascularize the flap while raising it.

3 Rotate the flap ventrally. Suture the edge nearest the pedicle (the right edge in this case) to the urethral plate, starting at the tip and using a continuous 7-0 SAS. Trim the skin generously because only a portion of it is needed to form a 12 F to 14 F urethra when it is combined with the urethral plate. Discarding excess skin ensures adequate blood supply to the remaining strip. Continue with interrupted sutures around the native meatus and with continuous sutures up the left side of the shaft. Turn the pedicle back to the right for cover of the anastomosis. Check with bougies à boule to be sure that the new urethra is neither too narrow nor too wide and thus exposed to diverticular formation. Bring the glans flaps together in the midline over the onlay, trimming any excess, and suture them with a deep layer of interrupted SAS and a superficial running CCG suture. Check for leaks by overfilling the urethra with saline. Spread the pedicle over the anastomosis and tack it in place. If it is too thick, trim it carefully so as not to injure the vessels.

De-epithelialized Flap. To buttress the repair, divide the dorsal skin deeply. With tenotomy scissors, de-epithelialize the preputial flap on one side to provide a pedicle of subcutaneous tissue (Durham Smith, 1973). Cover the neourethra with this tissue.

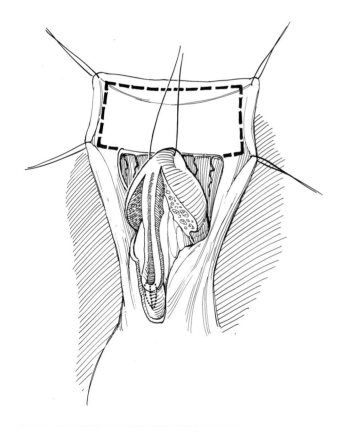
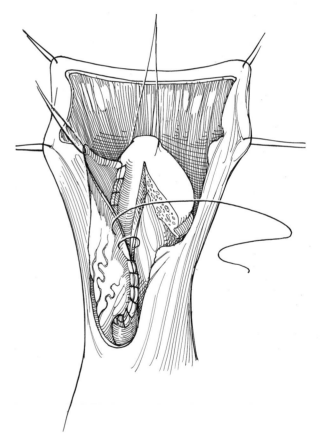

4 Bring the remainder of the preputial flaps around to the ventrum. Trim their ends aggressively to provide a fit around the corona. Reapproximate the skin ventrally with CCG horizontal mattress or running sutures to cover the repair. Insert a 6 F urethral stent (a Kendall catheter with extra holes works well) into the bladder, and withdraw it until it just stops dripping. Suture it to the glans and trim it to drip in the diaper. Apply a dressing of Telfa and biofilm, then fold the penis back on the abdomen. Let the dressing remain 3 to 4 days.

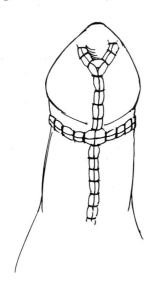

ONLAY ISLAND FLAP URETHROPLASTY
(Perovic)

Mobilize the urethral plate without dividing it to release the chordee. Create a strip of skin 2 cm wide as an island flap from the dorsal penile skin, preserving the redundant subcutaneous tissue. Buttonhole the pedicle and bring the strip onto the ventrum. Suture it to the urethral plate, and cover the suture lines with the vascularized tissue of the pedicle. Bring the remainder of the dorsal skin ventrally to close the defect.

TUNICA ALBUGINEA PLICATION PROCEDURE
(Baskin-Duckett)

The TAP procedure, a modification of the Nesbit operation (see page 174), can correct penile curvature secondary to corporal disproportion. Preservation of the urethral plate, which may be short even though fibrous tissue has been resected, may leave some chordee. More commonly, the chordee is caused by corporal disproportion. Use artificial erection to determine how much dorsal tucking is needed.

5 Before skin closure, determine the site of maximal curvature by artificial erection. Put traction on the glans and elevate Buck's fascia at the 10- and 2-o'clock positions on either side of the midline to elevate the neurovascular bundle. Make two parallel incisions approximately 4 to 6 mm apart and 8 mm long through the tunica albuginea on one side of the midline at the site of maximal curvature. Bring the two incisions together with inverted NAS, starting from inside out at the proximal cut and outside in at the distal cut, thus drawing the two openings into apposition while ducking the intervening bridge. Repeat the procedure on the other corpus. Check by artificial erection. If correction cannot be obtained by tucks, incise the ventrum and place a tunica vaginalis graft.

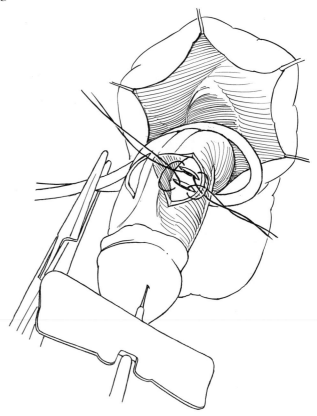

CORPORAL ROTATION
(Snow, Koff)

For persistent chordee after clearing the chordee on the ventrum (as described on page 99), rotate the corpora by transverse corporal plication, an alternative technique to dorsal plication, which avoids injury to the neurovascular bundle. Make a midline incision on the ventrum between the corpora cavernosa that extends from the coronal sulcus to the meatus and halfway to the dorsum. Insert inverted interrupted 5-0 NAS through Buck's fascia on either side to pass over the neurovascular bundle. Place the first suture over the area of greatest curvature, and add sutures as needed to straighten the penis, as determined by artificial erection. *Alternative*: Make two longitudinal incisions 1.5 to 2 cm long just through Buck's fascia on the dorsum over the area of chordee on either side of the neurovascular bundle, and rotate the corpora by approximating Buck's fascia.

POSTOPERATIVE PROBLEMS

Fistulas are the most common problem. Unless they are very tiny, do not attempt closure for 6 months (see pages 107 to 111). *Strictures* are not rare and usually result from kinking from overlap of two suture lines or from ischemia. Open repair usually is needed. *Meatal stenosis* may require meatoplasty (see pages 114 to 115). A very wide urethra, resembling a *diverticulum*, necessitates open excision of the extra skin. If chordee is present after repair, resort to dorsal tucks.

Commentary by John W. Duckett

We must first define *urethral plate* because it has different meanings for embryologists than for hypospadiologists. I have used the term to define skin, and the spongiosal tissue beneath, that lies distal to the urethral meatus in hypospadias and goes out onto the ventral glans. This tissue is often very pliable and healthy. It is not "fibrous chordee," as described by Mettauer. Preservation of the urethral plate makes reconstructive surgery most useful in hypospadias.

Tubed Preputial Island Flap

(Hodgson III–Asopa–Duckett)

If division of the urethral plate is required to correct the chordee, the missing portion may be bridged with a tube of preputial skin raised as an island flap. It does require a circular anastomosis, putting it at risk for fistula, stricture, and formation of a diverticulum. Even penoscrotal defects can be bridged because a long horseshoe-shaped graft may be taken from the prepuce (Duckett, 1995). If the plate can be preserved, even by making dorsal tucks, place an onlay graft rather than a tubed flap.

1 Mark and incise the dorsal and lateral coronal sulcus almost circumferentially 4 mm from the glans *(dashed lines)*. Extend the incision ventrally down the shaft and around the meatus as a narrow U *(dashed lines)*, leaving the ventral plate intact. Mobilize the skin and fascia from the proximal urethra laterally and dorsally, effectively degloving the shaft. Obtain hemostasis with a low-temperature ophthalmic cautery. Test by artificial erection. If the chordee can then be corrected using dorsal tethering sutures, the urethral plate can be preserved and reconstruction performed with an onlay repair, as described on page 130. If the chordee persists, excise the urethral plate and any fibrotic tethering tissue with it. Trim poor-quality skin from the meatus.

2 Place four fine traction sutures in the inner prepuce to fan out the ventral surface of the prepuce transversely as much as 5 or 6 cm. Mark the skin for the neourethra *(dashed lines)* to provide the length needed to bridge the gap and a width of 1.2 to 1.5 cm. If it is too wide, it acts as a diverticulum even if the meatus is of good caliber. Incise along the marks through the subcutaneous tissue, at the same time preserving the cutaneous supply to the dorsal skin (see page 98).

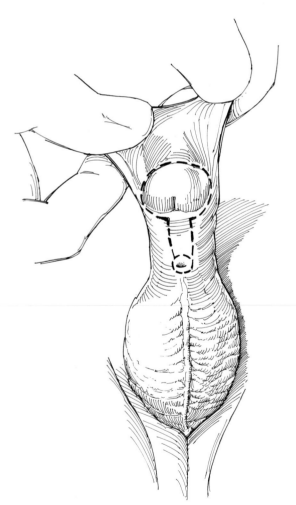

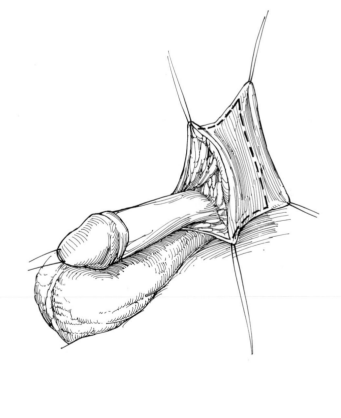

3 With fine scissors (McPherson-Vannas micro iris ophthalmic scissors held by thumb and index finger), develop a plane deep to the superficial vascular supply well down to the base of the penis between the flap and the outer prepuce to form a substantial pedicle. The vasculature of the pedicle usually is obvious, but take great care not to interfere with the vessels to either the flap or the dorsal preputial skin.

4 Roll the flap over a 12 F catheter and invert the edges with a running subcuticular 6-0 or 7-0 SAS. Approximate the subcutaneous tissue as a second layer over the suture line with a continuous 7-0 SAS. Place interrupted sutures at the ends to allow trimming. Examine the ends of the flap for ischemia and trim them appropriately. Remove the catheter and test the caliber of the tube with a 12 F bougie à boule.

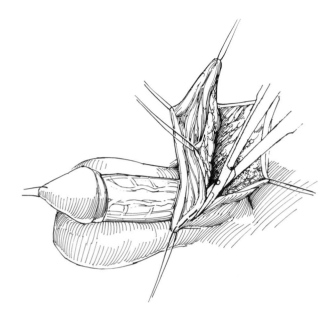

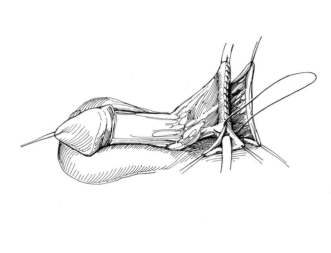

5 Rotate the tubularized flap around the right side of the penis so that its right side may be anastomosed to the native urethral meatus. Avoid torsion by freeing the base of the pedicle adequately. Trim the urethra into good spongiosum and spatulate it ventrally. Suture the flap to the tube so that the suture line of the flap lies dorsally against the corpora. Use 7-0 interrupted SAS placed with the knots outside. Include the tunica albuginea in the three most dorsal sutures to fix the anastomosis to the shaft.

Place a red rubber catheter as a tourniquet (not shown) around the shaft distal to the anastomosis to enable bloodless coring of the glans channel. Insert plastic scissors flat against the corpora cavernosa in the plane between the cap of the glans and the corpora, and snip a path to the tip of the glans. Remove a large plug of glans (0.2 × 1.5 cm), and reach inside the meatus to excise excess glanular tissue and provide a wide channel, at least 18 F in size. It must be large enough not to compress the vessels in the tube. Check with bougies à boule. If the tunnel is not adequate, split the glans and form glans flaps.

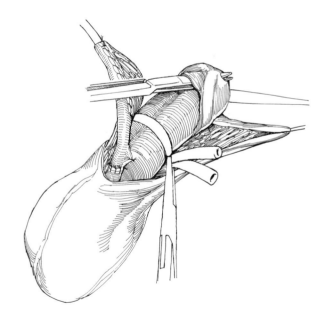

6 Remove the tourniquet and pull the tubed flap through the glans channel, keeping the suture line against the corporal bodies. Straighten it so that no redundancy remains; then trim the excess length. Suture the tubed flap to the new meatus carefully with interrupted 7-0 SAS. Fix the tube to the corpora along the shaft to prevent kinking of the anastomosis. Instill saline to check for leaks; place extra sutures as needed. Check to be sure that an 8 F infant feeding tube passes easily. Insert a 6 F silicone tube as a stent 1 to 2 cm proximal to the anastomosis, allowing the tip to protrude 0.5 cm from the neomeatus. Suture the end to the glans with two interrupted 4-0 NAS. Cover the anastomosis with pedicle tissue, tacked in place to cover the whole repair, being careful not to interfere with its vascular supply. Check for torsion of the penis. Remember that if the flap appears to have been devascularized, it can be defatted and converted into a graft.

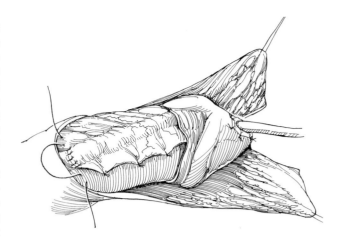

7 Divide the dorsal prepuce in the midline, rotate the flaps ventrally, and trim them appropriately for skin coverage. The blood supply may be tenuous because the majority of it has been diverted to the flap. If insufficient vascularized skin remains, it is possible, although not advisable, to make a relief incision in the dorsal skin. Empty the bladder with a small feeding tube passed through the silicone tube so that the boy awakens with an empty bladder. Place a circumferential Tegaderm dressing. Instruct the parents to aim the penis toward the chest with each diaper change. Begin 5-minute tub baths daily after 4 days. The dressing will come off by itself. Remove the silicone tube in 1 week.

Alternative: To keep the repair in the midline, form a *longitudinal island flap* (Chen et al, 1993). Make a coronal incision and free up the turned-back prepuce. Make a vertical incision in its pedicle similar to that done for coronal repair, and pass the glans through it, moving the open prepuce to the ventrum. Make two parallel incisions in the preputial skin, form a tube from the intervening skin, and attach it to the urethra proximally and to the glans distally. Bring the portions of prepuce remaining on either side together in the midline as cover. For long defects after division of the urethral plate, place a preputial flap cut with a wider midportion that is tubularized to bridge the defect in the plate and the ends laid as an onlay (Perovic and Vukadinovic, 1994; Flack and Walker, 1995).

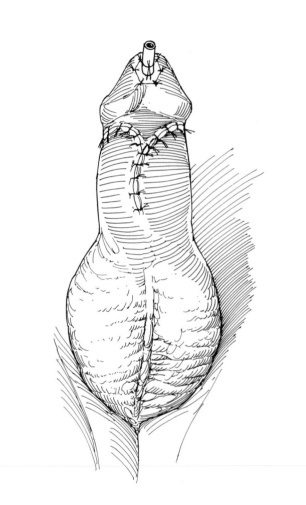

Commentary by Ronald Rabinowitz

In my experience with proximal hypospadias, it is much less common to be able to preserve the urethral plate and use the transverse island onlay technique. The degloving technique is readily accomplished with a low-temperature ophthalmic cautery. When separating the dorsal shaft skin from the underlying vascular pedicle to the transverse island flap, remember that the blood supply to the flap is more important than the dorsal skin. When anchoring the proximal anastomosis, use the anastomotic stitch passed through superficial tunica. The tourniquet is helpful in making a precise glans channel in a bloodless field. It is released just as the neourethra is passed through the glans channel. It is of utmost importance that the completed repair be straight and taut to avoid kinking. Rather than passing the silicone tubing into the bladder, I prefer to leave it only as a splint across the repair. This eliminates bladder spasms. It is important to drain the bladder just prior to completing the anesthetic so that the boy does not awaken with a full bladder. The Tegaderm dressing covers the shaft and glans, with only an opening for the silicone tube. This ensures that the dressing does not roll back to the base of the penis and act as a tourniquet. I do not use antibiotic ointments. Once the Tegaderm comes off, a small amount of petroleum jelly applied to the inside of the diaper prevents sticking.

Double-Faced Transverse Island Flap

(Hodgson XX–Asopa)

By using both sides of the prepuce, this procedure brings more skin to the area for urethral construction and coverage, but it is harder to distribute in a cosmetic fashion and its circulation may be more tenuous. A pedicle is formed from the prepuce on the penile branches of the superficial external pudendal system to supply both the tubularized flap and the covering flap.

1 **A,** Make a submeatal circumcising incision, and retract the edges of the prepuce *(dashed lines)*. Make a V-shaped incision onto the glans *(dashed lines)*. **B,** Encircle the meatus and tack its dorsal wall to Buck's fascia at the corners. Free the glans wings from the corpora after incising a wedge in the ventrum of the glans and folding it between the edges of the wings. Also tack it to the corpora. At this point, decide whether a transverse island flap, a free graft, or a perimeatal flap is preferable. The last may be satisfactory if a well-vascularized flap with an adequate attached dartos can be fashioned. Otherwise, choose one form of island flap, the double-faced transverse island flap theoretically being the most anatomically sound because it does not split the pedicle.

137

2 Incise the prepuce vertically at a site dictated by transilluminated axial vessels to form asymmetric flaps. Mark and incise an island on the inner preputial fold of the smaller flap, and excise and discard it. Mark and incise a larger measured island on the larger flap, leaving it attached to the flap in a transverse or oblique direction.

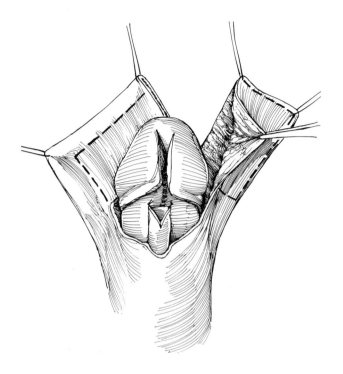

3 Roll the inner layer of the larger flap into a tube over a 12 F catheter and suture it with interrupted or continuous 5-0 SAS.

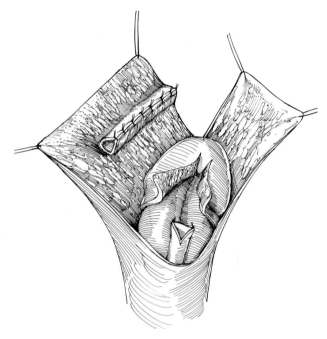

4 Rotate the tube, and suture it proximally to the spatulated urethra and distally to the V-flap at the meatus, using 6-0 or 7-0 CCG sutures. The shaft skin must be freed to the penopubic angle to prevent rotation of the penis after application of the flap. Tack a second layer composed of dartos tissue on the pedicle to cover the anastomotic suture lines.

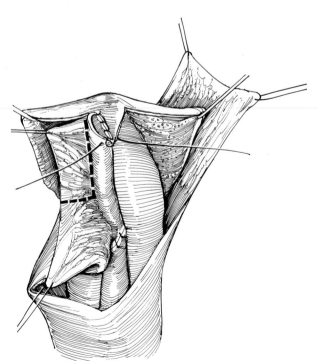

5 Bring the glans flaps over the new urethra. This flap can provide additional dartos tissue to cover the suture lines. Trim the smaller preputial flap to fit. Draw the rest of the larger flap across to cover the repair. Insert a 6 F silicone tube into the bladder. Apply a Tegaderm dressing over tincture of benzoin.

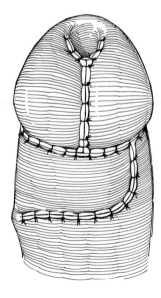

Commentary by Norman B. Hodgson

As can well be imagined, description of the variations on a two-faced flap have caused me considerable difficulty over the years. Time has shown that a glanular split is preferable to a V-flap in avoiding secondary meatal stenosis.

The many numbered flap techniques were chosen methods for depicting what, in reality, were a series of experiments. The initial goal was to complete the repair of hypospadias defects in a single operation and to achieve a cosmetically satisfactory or superior result. As time passed, the Hodgson II and III techniques fell into disuse. They were double-pedicle flaps to enhance the healing process, but they left a considerable bundle of tissue on the ventrum and have since been replaced by more versatile techniques. The Hodgson III has little applicability for the longer defects because of the relative paucity of available skin in that area to accomplish the new urethra. Perovic and Vukadinovic (1994) has recently renewed interest in this. In addition, the limitation of glanular advancement by the Denis Browne denudation has been replaced by various glans-split or glans-wing mobilization techniques, all of which have more nearly approximated a normal glans configuration.

Although these procedures (i.e., I, II, and III) had some merit in the earlier phases of one-stage repairs, they have been replaced by the current assortment of procedures, such as the Hodgson XX or mobilized transverse island flap (Duckett). I do not disown types II and III, but their place is historical, not current. (The appellation *Hodgson XX* was picked randomly because I had difficulty conveying the earlier nuances, and so each modification got a new number up to XIII; at that point a sudden jump was made to XX, for no other reason than it looked good and reflected the 20 years of discovery.) This is a commentary on the Hodgson XX procedure.

It is crucial that the reader distinguish between a mobilized and a nonmobilized rotated inner face flap. The essence of the healing process lies in the preservation and protection of trauma-free axial superficial external pudendal vessels. The Hodgson XX has the merit of a nonmobilized tangential inner face preputial flap rotated to the ventrum through a dorsal cutaneous releasing incision, which protects the integrity of the superficial external pudendal vascular system. The definition of that vessel system was not fully known until 1982 (Quartey), although Standoli, Duckett, Quartey, and Hinderer had each emphasized the ability to exploit and utilize those vessels when they had gained some character. The main benefit of the Hodgson XX lies in the rotated nonmobilized superficial external pudendal vascular system that allows ventral presentation of the inner face of the prepuce for urethral patching.

The initial incision in one-stage repairs circumscribes the shaft, leaving skin collars (width of surgeon's discretion) at the coronal margin. The shaft skin is mobilized. The surgeon encounters some perforators communicating with the deep vessels, and almost routinely these have to be sacrificed.

At this point, the entire shaft skin is a pedicle dependent on the anterior and posterior branches of the superficial external pudendal system. The quality and distribution of the vessels can be established by direct observation and transillumination.

The defect to be repaired is measured. The measurement is transposed to the available preputial skin, which dictates the donor site and angle. Ordinarily the transverse inner face may have 3 or 4 cm available for choice. The verge usually offers the greatest length. A tangential island is limited to 2 or 3 cm.

Vascular preservation and nonmobilized epithelial strips (islands) have been the defining features of the repairs I have described and advocated. It has been my position that creation of a pedicle from dorsal branches of the pudendal vessels (Duckett) supports the inner face island but jeopardizes the outer face and shaft skin because of the marginal quality of the intracuticular vessels. I am not a believer in a true splitting of the pudendal axial vessels.

The outer face releasing (skin deep only) incision (which can be vertical, horizontal, or tangential) eliminates the tension of the rotation. This presents the prepuce on the ventrum and provides the surgeon with a choice of nonmobilized islands to complete the repair. A verge island is realized by excision of a parallel narrow (2 mm) marginal skin strip.

The well-vascularized dartos layer, tacked properly, secures the suture line. Healthy shaft skin is approximated in two layers (deep Monocryl and superficial 6-0 chromic).

Utilizing these precepts, we have encountered a 4 percent fistula rate, a 1 percent incidence of glans separation, and no meatal stenosis. Ballooning of the neourethra has also occurred rarely.

The current environment stipulates minimal or no hospitalization, with a home care setting, freedom from discomfort, and markedly diminished complications and healing defects. Much of the current success has been the result of new materials, such as 7-0 Vicryl or Dexon S sutures, or the occasional use of PDS. The move has been away from CCG because of tissue reactivity. Dissection is commonly done with magnification and pinpoint electrocautery. Tissues are handled with microhooks, all with the goal of primary healing. The tubes are created with delicate suturing and are anastomosed over wide spatulations. Drainage of the neourethra is accomplished with Kluge-Firlit tubes, and dressings are commonly elastic membranes, such as Tegaderm. The recent addition of Telfa padding beneath the Tegaderm has protected the healing process.

Urine ordinarily is collected in a double diaper. The surgery can be accomplished on an outpatient basis or with a 24-hour stay, and subsequent wound care is managed in an office setting. For severe hypospadias persisting after multiple repairs or a perineal defect underendowed with appropriate vascularized flaps, my preference has been free grafts of bladder epithelium or (even better) buccal mucosa, which create their own set of problems, but have, on the whole, been rewarding.

We now have plenty of choices among the MAGPI, Mathieu, Hodgson XX, mobilized inner face flap (Duckett), external face flap (Standoli), one of the Hinderer perimeatal flaps, and free grafts of skin (Devine-Horton) or bladder epithelium.

Ventral Tube Repair

(Thiersch-Duplay)

Ventral tube repair may be useful when previous procedures have failed, but it may also be applied as a second stage after correction of chordee when it was not possible to complete the procedure in one stage.

1 Mark a V-incision on the glans, as for a perimeatal-based procedure (see page 124). To form the urethral tube, mark two parallel lines on the ventrum spaced suitably for the age of the patient (i.e., 1.5 cm apart in infants, 2.5 cm in children, or 3 cm in adults). Place these incisions more to one side so that the urethral suture line at closure does not coincide with that of the skin. Incise along the marks. Begin with a knife, then proceed with blunt-tipped scissors to cut an edge in the skin at right angles to the surface. Mobilize the edges of the strip minimally (the drawing exaggerates the dissection). Insert a small silicone tube into the bladder (not shown).

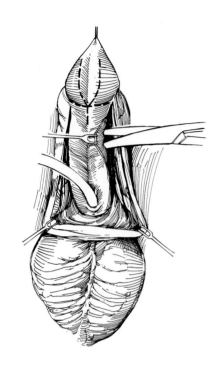

2 Form a V-shaped glans flap and glans wings. Mobilize and incise the distal end of the ventral strip vertically in the midline to receive the V-shaped glans flap, and suture the flap in place with 6-0 CCG sutures.

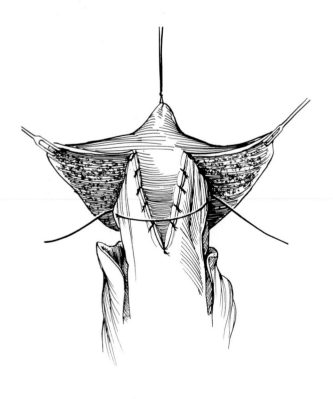

3 Elevate the edges of the strip with skin hooks and tack them together in three or four places. The suture line will lie to one side. Run a 6-0 PDS subcuticularly from end to end. Close the glans with a layer of deep SAS, adding fine interrupted sutures on the surface.

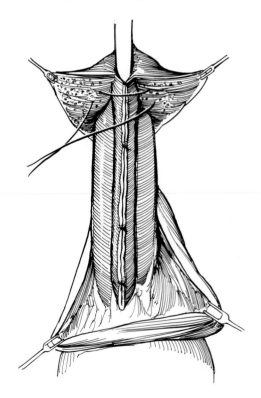

4 Make a Z-plasty if the skin is scarred and tight. A dorsal relaxing incision, covered with a split-thickness graft, is a last resort. Place some subcutaneous sutures, and close the skin eccentrically with either a running subcuticular suture or interrupted sutures. Dress the penis appropriately. Remove the catheter in 7 to 10 days.

For *two-stage repair* for extreme proximal hypospadias accompanied by a small phallus and chordee, apply the ventral tube technique. Correct the chordee in the first stage, as described on page 99, placing a ventral dermal graft or tunica vaginalis graft to correct the chordee. Split and bring the preputial flaps around to cover (Byers flaps). After 6 to 12 months, proceed with formation of a ventral tube, as described above.

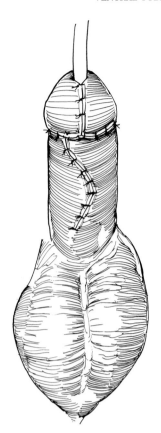

Commentary by George W. Kaplan

There are a number of technical nuances to this operation. In estimating the size of the neourethra, I have used the caliber of the native urethra (as determined with bougies à boule) and then added 2 mm as a "fudge factor." Hence, if the child's urethra is calibrated as 14 F, I would outline a 16-mm strip. Additionally, I no longer bother to offset the suture lines because I have found that the longer side often does not come across without mobilization, and I would prefer not to mobilize that strip. I usually divert the urine with a small silicone Foley catheter, although silicone tubing as a splint is perfectly acceptable.

I no longer use the type of glansplasty shown in Figure 2 but, rather, have employed a modification of the Barcat repair in which the distal portion of the strip (which usually is redundant) is mobilized, and after the urethroplasty is completed, the distal portion of the urethra is laid into a deep groove in the glans and sutured thereto. I usually use slightly finer suture material (usually 7-0 or 8-0 Vicryl), but 5-0 Vicryl is used to reapproximate the glans subcutaneously.

In the formation of the urethra in Step 3, I prefer to use a complete resutured urethra. The curve of the U-incision that passes proximal to the native urethral meatus is relatively closely applied to the meatus (perhaps 2 mm from the ventral edge of the meatus). The entire epithelium is inverted into the lumen of the neourethra, and the suture line is continued out to the end as a subcuticular closure. The urethra is then tacked to the split in the glans dorsally, and after the glans is reapproximated, the neourethra is tacked to the glans circumferentially. I believe that it is important to bring some subcutaneous tissue over this closure to minimize fistula formation. This subcutaneous tissue can be obtained by using Durham Smith's technique of de-epithelializing one edge of the skin (see page 109), provided that sufficient skin is available to do so. If not, a flap of subcutaneous tissue can be rotated up from the scrotum to cover the urethral closure and then tacked over the closure with fine absorbable sutures.

I prefer to close the skin with interrupted sutures so that I can better tailor the closure. I really do prefer to avoid relaxing incisions. If I recognized preoperatively that a relaxing incision would be necessary, I would probably choose a free graft of bladder epithelium, which I would then tunnel under the tissue between the native urethral meatus and the corona. I often attempt to use a Z-plasty closure to avoid contraction of a midline scar. Last (based on our experimental observation of urethral wound healing), I tend to leave the catheter for only 7 days, because urethral re-epithelialization is complete by that time and I believe that the presence of a foreign body beyond the time of urethral re-epithelialization acts as a nidus for urethritis rather than assists in wound healing.

Free Tube Graft and Partial Island Flap

TUBE GRAFT
(Devine-Horton)

1 **A,** Insert a cystostomy tube (see pages 625 to 627). Place a traction suture in the glans. Mark a V-shaped incision on the glans, and run it around the meatus. Infiltrate the area with 1 ml of 1:200,000 epinephrine solution in 0.5 percent lidocaine. Incise the coronal sul-

cus. **B,** Elevate the wings of the glans with skin hooks, and begin dissection of the ventral tissues that produce chordee. Continue freeing behind the meatus and urethra until the penis can be shown to be straight by artificial erection. Trim and discard the thinned tissue from the terminal urethra, and notch it on the ventral edge. Separate the glans from the corpora. Cut the glans flaps (see pages 104 to 105) and excise the bulged tissue at their base.

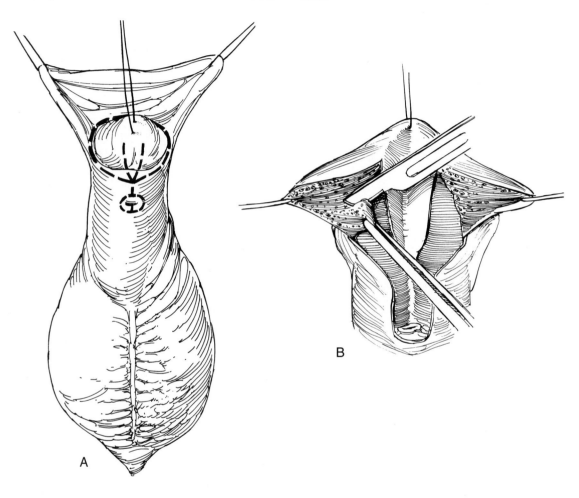

2 **A,** Unfold the dorsal prepuce and place four stay sutures in it at least 1.4 cm apart, because 75 percent circumferential shrinkage of the graft is expected, and at a length 10 percent longer than that needed to replace the urethra. **B,** Cut the graft from the inner face of the prepuce. Defat it over the index finger (see page 42) or on a board coated with double-surfaced derma- tome tape. **C,** Attach the full-thickness, fat-free graft, with the skin surface inside, to a catheter of the size of the normal urethra. Use interrupted 5-0 or 6-0 SAS. Cut both ends of the graft obliquely. Remove the graft from the larger catheter and thread it onto a catheter of slightly smaller size, place the distal end of the catheter in the bladder, and move the graft to the proper position.

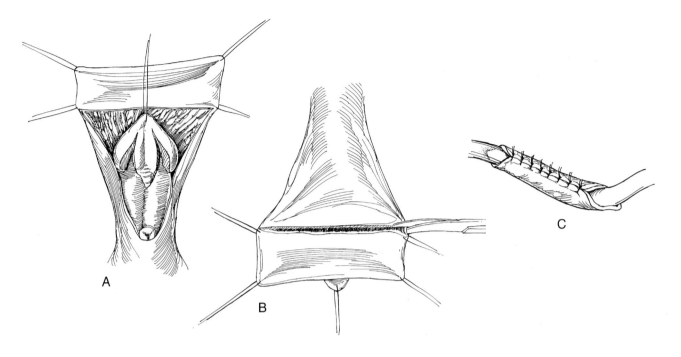

3 Suture the dorsal side of the proximal end of the graft to the spatulated end of the urethra with 5-0 SAS, and continue suturing around to the ventrum. Place a suture from the tip of the glans flap through the apex of the oblique cut in the graft.

4 Complete the approximation of the graft to the glans flaps.

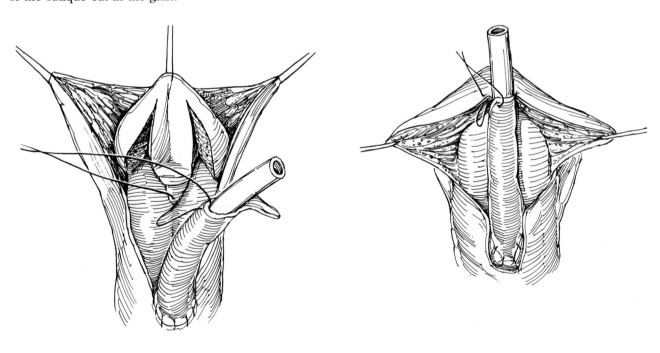

5 Close the glans flaps over the graft with three or four 5-0 SAS, and suture the graft to the edges of the glans at the new meatus with 5-0 CCG sutures. Approximate the glans flaps with two layers of sutures.

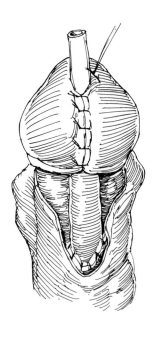

6 If possible, bring in a layer of subcutaneous tissue to cover the proximal anastomosis. Split the remaining prepuce, and approximate it ventrally, trying to keep from superimposing suture lines. Suture the cut-off catheter to the meatus and leave it in place for 10 days.

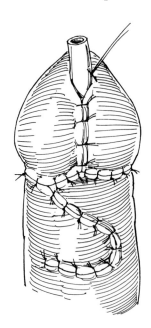

COMBINED TUBE GRAFT AND ISLAND FLAP

7 **A,** For longer and more proximal defects, incise the hairless skin around the proximal end of the defect and partially raise the edges to form a proximal tube from adjacent skin. **B,** Close the proximal skin tube over a catheter (Thiersch-Duplay, see page 140). Open the prepuce between stay sutures and cut a rectangular graft. Trim it to size.

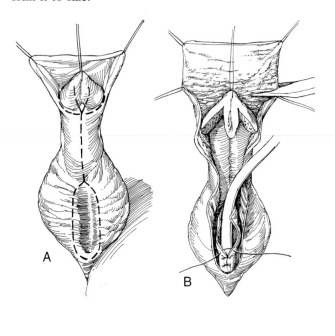

8 **A,** Tubularize the graft, invert it so that the suture line is dorsal, and anastomose it to the end of the proximal skin tube. **B,** Suture the distal end of the graft to the glans flaps. Place several anchoring sutures to the tunic. Split and approximate the residual preputial flaps ventrally.

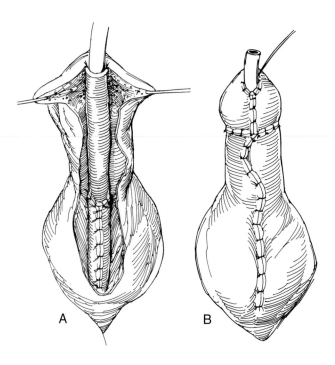

PARTIAL ISLAND FLAP
(Kaplan)

The partial island flap is an alternative to applying the skin as a double-faced island flap (see page 137).

9 **A,** Open the prepuce and resect the inner preputial skin. Clear the skin of fat, form it into a tube, and place it as a free graft. **B,** Cover the ventral defect by rotation of the remainder of the island flap, formerly the outer layer of prepuce, on its dartos pedicle.

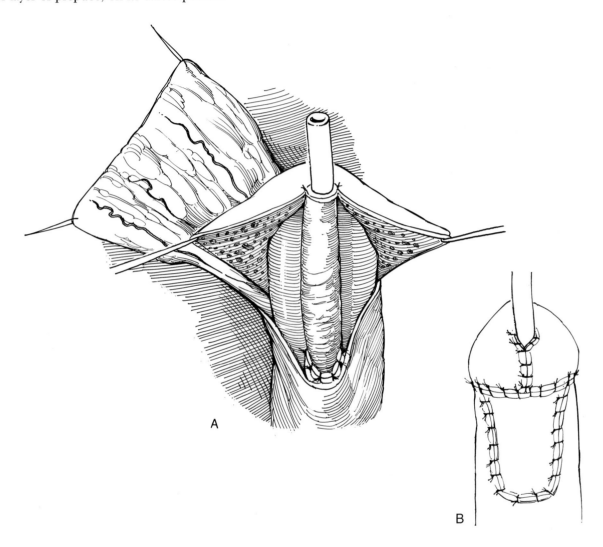

Commentary by Ahmed Shafik

The important aspect of the operation is that it represents the modern trend in managing first- and second-degree hypospadias in a one-stage procedure. The results are successful in more than 75 percent of the cases. Preputial skin is most suitable as a urethral graft because it is hairless and pliable. Other sites such as the groin and medial aspect of the arm are suitable donor areas only in circumcised males. Full-thickness grafts take (revascularize) mostly through their edges and less through the bed. It is to be noted, however, that the vascularized preputial skin technique represents a natural progression of this technique with a much lower complication rate.

The size of the graft taken should accurately correspond to the length of the deficient urethra. The width of the graft should equal the circumference of a catheter with a diameter comparable to that of the proximal urethra, although it is preferable that the graft be stented over a catheter with a smaller diameter. This allows easier manipulation of the graft and lessens the danger of too much pressure by the catheter on the suture line. Skin closure is preferably achieved by transverse mattress sutures, which allow eversion of the edges. The sutures should be loosely tied to allow for postoperative edema because, otherwise, necrosis may develop at the suture line. The technique of suturing and handling should be very meticulous, making use of the finest adaptable suture material. We use 7-0 Vicryl or PDS for the edges of the graft and urethra, placing the sutures under magnification. Sutures preferably are applied through the dermis of the graft and urethral submucosa. This makes the suture line slightly inverted to the inside. This tip allows better watertight healing of the suture line.

The beveling of the mouths of the tube graft and urethra provides a longer graft edge for anastomosis; thus, the chance for revascularization increases and stenosis is avoided. The preputial grafts, in particular, offer the advantage of greatest adaptability, hairlessness, and matching to the edges of the urethra, with an infection rate lower than with buried skin grafts.

Nevertheless, the hypothetic advantage of reconstructing any length of defective urethra by tube grafts is counterbalanced by the high rate of complications. We have met with dehiscence, infection, fistula formation, and stenosis. The indication for tube grafts is relevant in circumcised patients, and in these vesical mucosa is better than skin for the graft.

Preputial pedicled flaps have superseded grafts (Duckett). They are more dependable in terms of survival and safety; they fit well and have fewer complications, such as the one small fistula we have seen that was easily closed secondarily. The Asopa modification gives even more security to the preputial island by including the top layer of the skin island with it, thereby safeguarding its vascularization and covering as a patch without a superimposed suture line. This is my preferred and dependable technique for proximal hypospadias. For the distal one, the Mathieu or flip-flap technique is satisfactory. In scrotal hypospadias with vulviform scrotum, a combination of Duplay urethroplasty and Duckett's technique advances the urethra to the forepart of the penis, with safety not being at the mercy of graft take.

I am not in favor of diversion through a Cystocath or cystotomy because these are not devoid of complications and they prolong the discomfort of the patient. Although perineal urethrotomy may be an alternative to cystotomy as a method of urinary diversion, the latter has the advantage of allowing testing of the repair (usually after 1 week). If leakage occurs, the period of diversion can be prolonged. We depend on indwelling urinary catheter diversion in proximal hypospadias; the catheter should be smaller than the caliber of the urethra so as not to be irritating (6 F to 8 F) and is usually left no longer than 3 to 5 days.

I depend more on a safe anastomosis, which is tested for watertightness during the operation by injecting saline through the neomeatus and sealing any leakage at the suture line by additional sutures. In my opinion this is the best safeguard against fistula. The catheter, if left for longer periods, hinders lining epithelialization and may be the cause of unsatisfactory results. In tube grafts, it entails longer periods of diversion amounting to 2 weeks. Silicone catheters are preferred because they are less likely to obstruct. In case of blockage or dislodgment, no attempt should be made to reposition for fear of disrupting sutures. Instead, a Cystocath is indicated if diversion is still needed.

SECTION

4

Penis: Excision

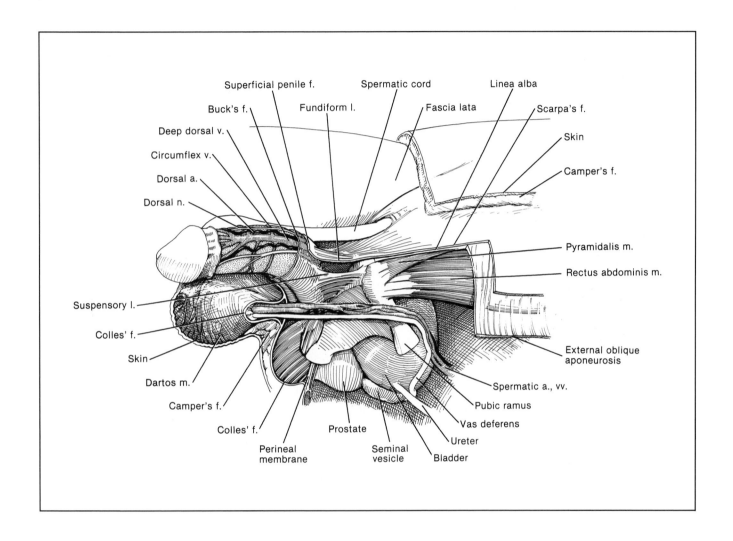

Anatomic Basis for Penile Excision

Circumcision may be adequate treatment for a few cases of carcinoma of the penis, and laser therapy also has a role for superficial lesions. Small cancers are candidates for fresh tissue chemosurgery (Mohs). Reserve partial amputation for larger tumors near the glans because recurrences in the stump are not common and the patient will be able to stand to void. Larger and more proximal lesions require total penectomy. The lesion typically has destroyed the overlying skin and is usually infected because of tissue necrosis, with bacteria invading the lymph nodes. This often renders the nodes palpable, making the distinction between inflammation and neoplasm difficult. The presence of infection also makes adequate antibiotic treatment mandatory before amputation and especially before the decision is made to perform lymphadenectomy.

1 Anatomically, the ilioinguinal area is covered by a superficial fatty layer (Camper's fascia), beneath which is a deep fibrous layer (Scarpa's fascia) extending over the lower abdomen to fuse with the fascia lata. Camper's and Scarpa's fascias fuse to cover the scrotum as the dartos fascia and the perineum as Colles' fascia. The vascular supply to this area is provided by the superficial epigastric, superficial circumflex iliac, and superficial pudendal arteries, but collateral vessels enter at either side from the thigh and abdominal wall.

Approximately 8 nodes (range 4 to 25) lie in the fatty tissue of the membranous layer of the superficial fascia overlying the fascia lata. The central zone of nodes lying at the junction of the long saphenous vein with the femoral vein is the principal drainage zone of the penis.

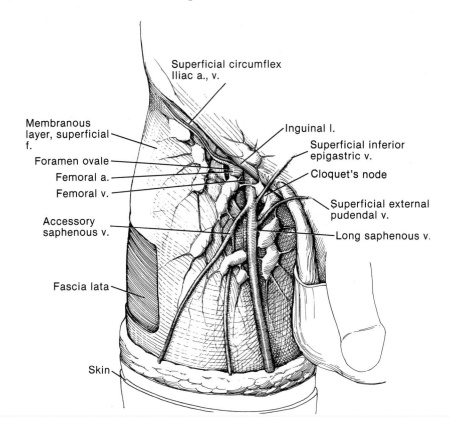

2 The adductor longus muscle, the inguinal ligament, and the sartorius muscle form the femoral triangle. The triangle lies over the iliopsoas and pectineus muscles and under the fascia lata and contains deep nodes that require removal. Cloquet's node lies just medial to the femoral vein at the femoral canal. The superficial nodes lie between the fascia lata and Camper's fascia. For iliac node dissection, the obturator artery is the medial margin. The lymphatic drainage of the penis is bilateral; thus, dissection of both sides may be indicated.

The nodes of the deep drainage system form a chain along the femoral artery and femoral vein in the femoral triangle under the fascia lata. The chain runs under the inguinal ligament through the femoral septum in the femoral canal to connect with nodes around the external iliac vessels, eventually to reach the pelvic nodes on the sides of the external, internal, and common iliac nodes.

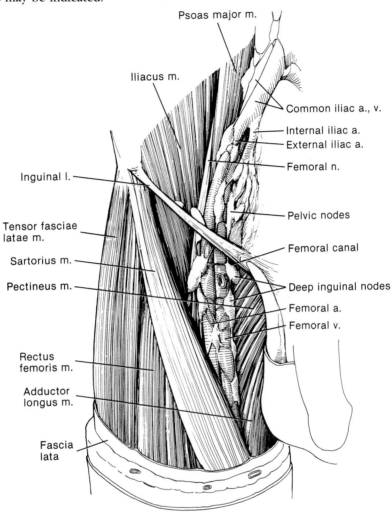

Partial Penectomy

For small lesions on the glans (stages T1 and small T2), use CO_2 or neodymium:YAG laser microsurgery or microscopically controlled zinc chloride chemotherapy (Mohs) to minimize functional loss. For lesions on the prepuce, circumcision (see page 167) may appear to provide an adequate margin, but it does not always prevent local recurrence.

Evaluate the edges of the lesion prior to partial penectomy to be sure that a 2-cm margin can be obtained that will at the same time leave at least 3 cm of shaft. If not, proceed with total penectomy (see page 154) because voiding an undirectable stream from a stump is less acceptable than urinating through a perineal urethrostomy. Palpate the inguinal nodes. Obtain sonograms and computed tomograms of the pelvis, as well as bone scans, an intravenous urogram, and a chest radiogram. Obtain biopsy of the lesion by scalpel or dermal punch to confirm the diagnosis. Also obtain tissue from the normal-appearing lateral and deep margins. Close the biopsy defects with fine chromic catgut (CCG) sutures.

Urethral Carcinoma. Perform panendoscopy and retrograde urethrography. Obtain tissue for cytology or do a transurethral biopsy. For a *tumor at the meatus*, resect it transurethrally or perform partial penectomy. If the tumor is in the *pendulous urethra,* remove part or all of the penis and provide a perineal urethrostomy plus superficial inguinal lymphadenectomy. For *proximal tumors,* resect the genital area and perineum en bloc and proceed with both superficial and deep node dissection bilaterally as well as removal of the external iliac, obturator, and internal iliac nodes.

Culture the tumor for bacteria and give appropriate preoperative antibiotics for at least 3 days, in addition to perioperative antibiotics. If nodes are palpable and inflamed, give antibiotics postoperatively and observe the patient for several weeks after penectomy. If the nodes remain enlarged in spite of adequate therapy, proceed with node dissection (see page 158).

1 *Position:* Supine. Use the lithotomy position if a total penectomy may be necessary. Drape the anus from the field. Prepare the penis with povidone-iodine solution, and isolate the tumor in a condom or rubber glove sutured in place. Apply a tourniquet at the base of the penis, using a 20 F red rubber catheter or a Penrose drain. *Incision:* Mark an elliptical incision on the skin 1.5 to 2 cm proximal to the lesion, and incise the skin circumferentially. For dorsal lesions, the incision may be made more obliquely, leaving more ventral skin to form a flap for coverage (Step 6A and B). Divide and ligate the superficial and deep dorsal veins. Incise Buck's fascia onto the tunica albuginea of the corpora.

2 Divide the corpora cavernosa, leaving the corpus spongiosum intact. Temporarily release the tourniquet to clamp and ligate the central arteries. Obtain tissue from the stump for frozen section analysis. If insufficient penile length (less than 3 cm) remains to allow for directed voiding, lengthen the remaining stump by dividing the suspensory ligament and splitting the ischiocavernous muscle to free the crura from the pubic rami.

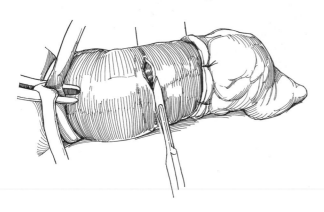

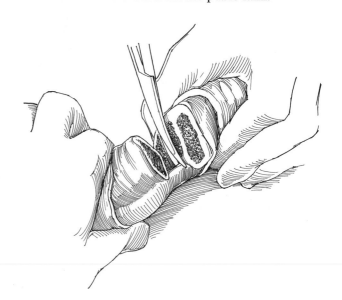

3 Dissect the urethra in the corpus spongiosum distally for at least 1 cm to facilitate formation of a stoma; then transect it. Spatulate the urethra on its dorsal surface.

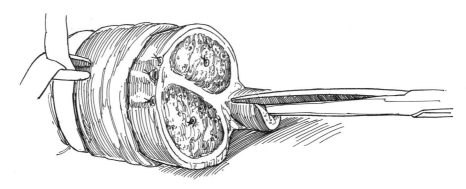

4 Close the ends of both corpora with a series of interrupted 2-0 synthetic absorbable sutures (SAS) that include the septum. Place two sutures in the corpus spongiosum around the urethra. Remove the tourniquet and secure hemostasis as needed. Residual bleeding from the spongy tissue is controlled by sutures during the cutaneous anastomosis.

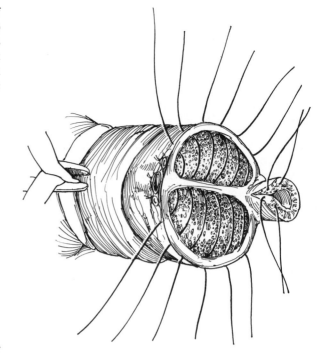

5 **A,** Begin skin closure ventrally. With 4-0 CCG sutures, approximate the spatulated urethra to the penile skin to form an oblique meatus, open side up. **B,** Suture the remainder of the skin dorsally, taking care to include the apex of the urethral V. Place an 18 F 5-ml silicone balloon catheter. Dress with nonsticking 4 × 8-inch gauze and elastic adhesive tape.

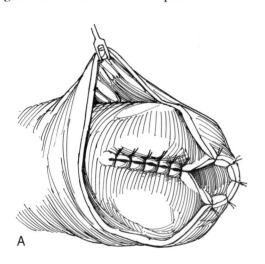

A

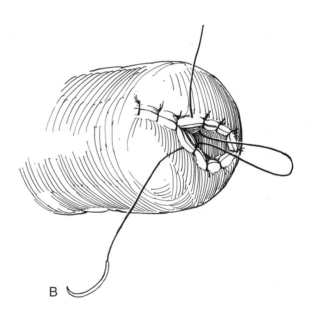

B

FLAP CLOSURE

6 **A,** If the initial skin incision was made obliquely and redundant skin remains ventrally, draw the flap over the end of the stump. **B,** Make a slit in the skin and anastomose the end of the urethra to it (see page 215).

Alternative (McLoughlin): Tack the adventitia of the protruding urethra circumferentially to the skin at its base. Incise one side of the urethra, fold it back upon itself, and suture the edge to the skin peripheral to the first ring of sutures. The technique is similar to that for an ileal stoma (see page 656, Step 21).

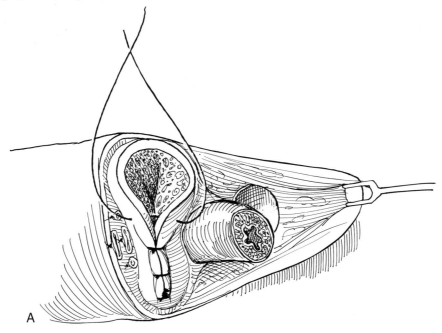

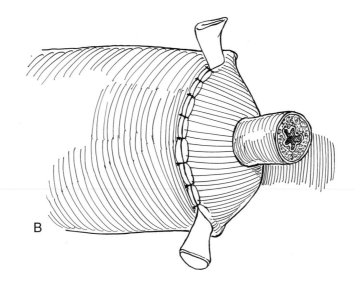

POSTOPERATIVE PROBLEMS

Infection and *tumor spillage* can occur, but the chances are reduced by isolating the lesion in a rubber glove during preparation. *Urethral meatal stenosis* is not uncommon but is less likely if a long elliptical suture line is created. After adequate follow-up, consider *penile lengthening*: Invert the penile skin and make numerous transverse incisions in the tunica albuginea. Insert a semirigid prosthesis to keep the tunic expanded.

Commentary by Joe Y. Lee and Alexander S. Cass

The goals of penile-sparing surgery for primary penile cancer are eradication of local disease and preservation of sufficient tissue for directed micturition and coitus. A phallus of at least 3 cm is required for directed micturition and coitus. Premalignant lesions and carcinoma in situ are well treated with conservative penile-sparing procedures. Circumcision alone is best reserved for small preputial penile cancers in which a wide margin is obtainable. Failure rates for circumcision in lesions of the proximal prepuce are as high as 50 percent. Therefore, proximal preputial lesions warrant a more aggressive circumcision or a partial penectomy.

Mohs microscopic controlled surgery is well suited for small lesions of the glans. The lesion is surgically excised. The base of the lesion is treated with dichloroacetic acid and fixed with a zinc chloride paste. Successive layers are excised at intervals of 4 to 24 hours until the base of the lesion is free of tumor. Poorly differentiated (grade 3) lesions and lesions larger than 3.0 cm, however, tend to recur locally and therefore may not be suited to Mohs surgery. Microscopic outgrowths can occur in an unpredictable pattern. Partial penectomy for larger lesions requires a margin of 2 cm of grossly normal tissue to ensure eradication of local disease. Microscopic examination of the margins and close follow-up are required in all penile-sparing procedures.

Urethral carcinomas may present as unexplained penile abscesses. Upon drainage of the abscess, one must obtain biopsies of any suspicious lesions. Carcinoma presenting as a penile abscess usually represents a widely invading cancer and requires extensive surgical excision.

Total Penectomy

Obtain histologic confirmation by biopsies that include adjacent tissue. Culture the surface of the tumor and begin appropriate antibiotic coverage at least 3 days before operation.

Consider adjuvant chemotherapy for a patient with a poor prognosis, such as one with multiple involved lymph nodes, followed by surgery at a later time.

1 Isolate the penile lesion with a condom or rubber glove firmly affixed with sutures. *Incision:* Make an elliptical incision around the base of the penis with an extension for a short distance both inferiorly along the scrotal raphe and superiorly in the midline.

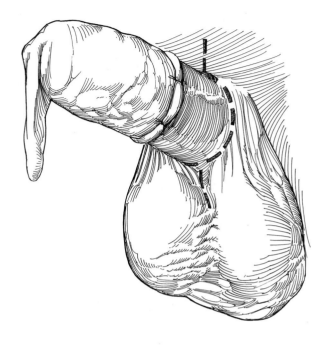

2 Divide the fundiform and suspensory ligaments, and ligate the exposed superficial and deep dorsal vasculature. Dissect and include the prepubic fat and prepubic lymph nodes with the specimen.

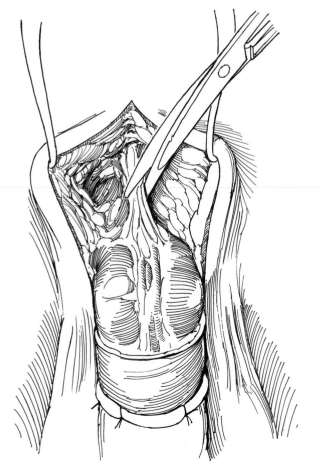

3 Open Buck's fascia ventrally. Dissect the urethra free from the corpora cavernosa in the distal bulbar region and divide it, leaving it long enough to reach the perineum.

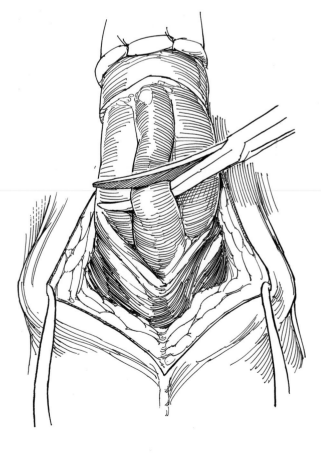

4 Continue the dissection of the urethra proximally, freeing it from the crura of the corpora cavernosa. Clamp and divide the crura at the pubic rami, oversewing the ends with 3-0 SAS. Provide at least 2 cm of grossly tumor-free margin. Remove the specimen.

5 Grasp the skin overlying the perineal body and cut a 1-cm ellipse from it. Make a tunnel bluntly with a curved clamp so that the urethra will not be angulated. Draw the urethra into the perineal incision.

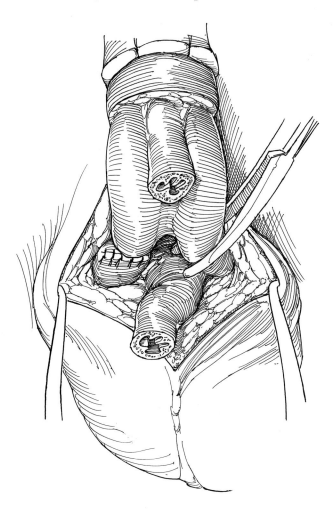

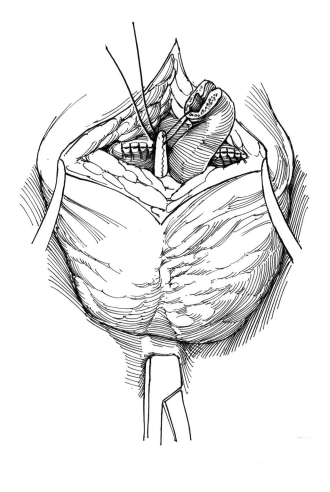

6 Spatulate the urethra dorsally. Place an indwelling 18 F 5-ml balloon catheter. Suture the urethra to the skin with 3-0 CCG sutures. Use a water-tight technique to prevent urinary leakage under the flap. Place two Penrose drains in the scrotal wound unless node dissection is to follow immediately. Close the scrotum transversely to elevate it. Remove the drains in 3 days and the catheter 2 days later.

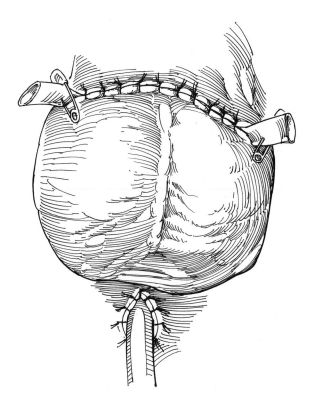

PERINEAL APPROACH

7 *Position:* Lithotomy. **A,** *Incision.* Make an inverted
U-shaped perineal incision across the urethral bulb,
with a distal extension over the scrotum. **B,** Place traction
on the skin flap and dissect the surface of the bulbospongiosus muscle all the way back to the perineal body.
Open that muscle and strip it from the corpus spongiosum. Free the corpus spongiosum from the corpora cavernosa. Divide the corpus spongiosum and urethra; leave

enough length to reach the skin of the perineum. Dissect
the stump back to the urogenital diaphragm to ensure a
straight run to the perineum. Then incise the scrotum to
and around the base of the penis. Divide the suspensory
ligament of the penis, and dissect the corpora to the
beginning of the crura. Place clamps on the corpora,
divide them, and oversew the ends. Make a buttonhole
incision in the perineum, attach the urethra to the skin,
and close the wound transversely around drains.

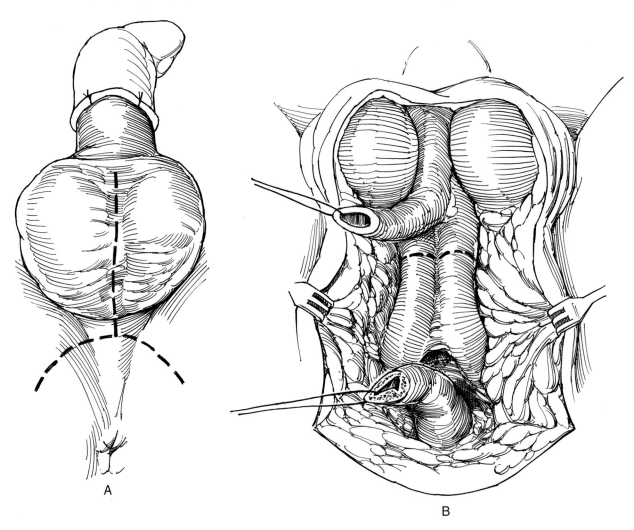

A

B

EXTENDED EXCISION

For local control, advanced cases may require excision of
the scrotum, the pubic arch, the urogenital diaphragm,
and even the bladder. First, mobilize the bladder transabdominally. Make an inverted U-shaped perineal incision
as for perineal prostatectomy (see page 446). Mobilize an
anterior perineal flap laterally to the attachment of the
adductor musculature to the inferior pubic rami. Free the
penis as described previously, at least to the penoscrotal
junction; if necessary, divide the scrotum and excise appropriate portions.

URETHRECTOMY

Excision of the urethra for urethral carcinoma or as an adjunct
to radical cystectomy is described on page 513.

POSTOPERATIVE PROBLEMS

Oozing from the cut end of the stump secondary to erections
can be controlled by oversewing the end under penile block
anesthesia, if pressure applied by the patient does not stop it.
Meatal stenosis is not an uncommon complication. Self-dilatation should be started as soon as the patient notices any diminu-
tion of stream. Do not be concerned if the urethra seems too
long; it will retract appropriately.

Commentary by E. David Crawford

The surgical therapy of penile cancer dates back to the first century, when it was recognized that excision of a presumed cancerous lesion with a margin of healthy tissue resulted in local control. Little has changed in the surgical management since that time, with the exception of marked refinement in the technique. Even though radical penectomy remains the cornerstone of therapy for many penile cancers, it is mutilating; therefore, alternative therapies are constantly being sought. Primary radiation therapy and chemotherapy for these cancers have not become popular in the United States. Interest has been evolving in the Nd:YAG laser as a less aggressive form of management, as well as local excision and Mohs micrographic surgery for management of penile tumors.

Total penectomy is the method of choice for local control and perhaps cure of more proximal invasive penile cancers. It is performed where an acceptable penile stump cannot be achieved with partial amputation. Prior to the surgical excision, it is imperative that preoperative antibiotics be given, particularly in patients who have extensive necrotic lesions. The operative procedure is relatively straightforward and has few complications and little risk. It is important that the corpora cavernosa be divided proximal enough that they are well beneath the covering scrotum. Prepubic lymph nodes are present, and at the time of the penectomy the adipose tissue of the suspensory ligament should be removed.

Ilioinguinal Lymphadenectomy

First clear the skin of rashes and infection, although cleanliness of the inguinal skin folds is difficult to achieve, especially in obese patients. Measure the leg for an elastic stocking. Give appropriate antibiotics perioperatively and postoperatively. Administer warfarin sodium (Coumadin). Prepare the bowel. For palpable nodes, treat with antibacterial agents for 4 to 6 weeks. After resecting gross inguinal metastasis, consider a myocutaneous flap to repair the defect (see page 50).

Select unilateral dissection if ipsilateral nodes are detected late after penectomy; perform bilateral dissection for most patients.

Instruments. Include a marking pen, skin hooks, loop retractors, vascular clips, closed suction, and a dermatome.

UNILATERAL DISSECTION

Inguinal Component, Modified Technique

The modified lymphadenectomy described here has a lower complication rate than the standard operation.

If the nodes taken from the inguinal dissection are negative, do not proceed with the abdominal component.

1 Note distribution of lymph nodes and extent of exposure through an inguinal incision. The black node is the sentinel node. This node, usually the first to be involved with penile carcinoma, corresponds to the lymph nodes associated with the superficial epigastric vein and lies no more than 1 cm away. In some cases, more than one lymph node is found in this group. In this situation, all nodes should be removed, but the sentinel node is always the larger and more medially situated (Cabanas, 1992; Cabanas and Whitmore, 1981).

Sentinel Node Biopsy. Although the routes of lymphatic spread are legion, biopsy of the so-called sentinel node has been advocated, even though a negative node does not rule out nodal spread. Proceeding directly to node dissection, even without evidence of nodal involvement, is advocated with increasing frequency because 20 percent of patients with metastasis have no external evidence of involvement of the nodes.

To biopsy the sentinel node, make a 5-cm incision two

fingerbreadths lateral and two fingerbreadths inferior to the pubic tubercle, positioning it over the junction of the saphenous vein with the femoral vein. Insert the index finger under the flap in the direction of the pubic tubercle and palpate and remove the node or nodes near the superficial epigastric vein.

It is usually better to perform biopsy and frozen section examination as a step in the lymphadenectomy rather than as a separate procedure. If the biopsy results are positive from the nodes in the tissue at the fossa ovalis between the superficial epigastric and superficial external pudendal veins, proceed with lymphadenectomy. Biopsy of the sentinel node as an isolated procedure is indicated in cases of penile carcinoma localized to the prepuce or in patients who refuse lymphadenectomy. During modified lymphadenectomy, perform a biopsy of the sentinel node first; if it is negative and no nodes are palpable, consider stopping further dissection and observing the patient closely instead.

If a biopsy has been done, incise the tissue widely around the site and include the skin in the specimen.

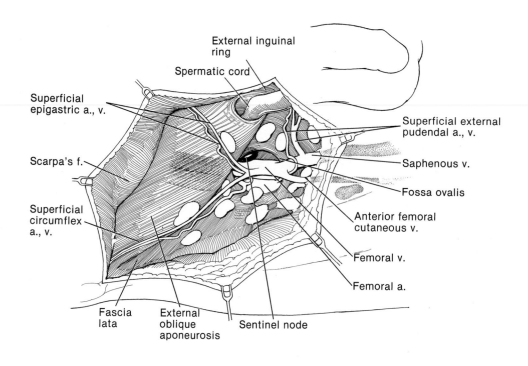

2 *Position:* Abduct and externally rotate the thigh, and place a small pillow under the knee. Anchor the foot to the opposite leg. Put the elastic stocking on to the level of the knee; after the operation, extend it to the thigh. Drape to expose the umbilicus, pubic tubercle, anterior superior iliac spine, and anterior thigh. It may be advisable to insert an 18 F silicone balloon catheter through the penile stump. Suture the scrotum to the opposite thigh. Mark the extent of the tissue to be excised with a marking pen on the skin. Place a line in the groin crease 1 cm above and parallel to the inguinal ligament, starting at the pubic tubercle and running 12 cm laterally. Run a perpendicular line 20 cm long medially and a 15-cm line laterally, and close the quadrangle with a fourth line.

Incision: Incise the skin obliquely from the anterior superior iliac spine to the pubic tubercle, running it below and parallel to the groin crease. If a biopsy specimen was obtained, excise a strip of skin to include that site; if not, and the nodes are not palpable, excise one of them for biopsy and obtain a frozen-section diagnosis. If the biopsy specimen is positive, proceed to the next step.

Important: To prevent lymphoceles, control all subcutaneous lymphatics at the periphery of the dissection and institute Jackson-Pratt suction drainage.

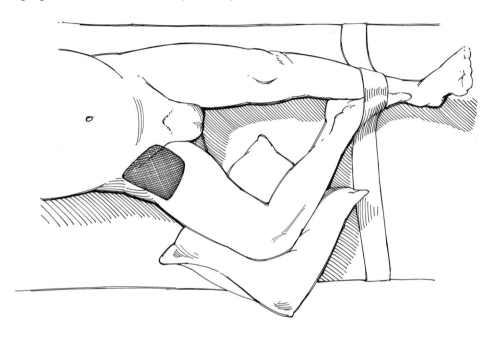

3 Fashion skin flaps above and below by sharp dissection, extending to the marked margins and to the depth of the fascia lata. Leave them adequately covered by 2 to 3 mm of Camper's fascia with its attached subcutaneous fat. Use skin hooks, stay sutures, and retractors. Handle the flaps gently, and keep them covered with saline-moistened sponges. Mobilize to the premarked margins but not beyond. If skin is involved with tumor, excise it and subsequently place a graft.

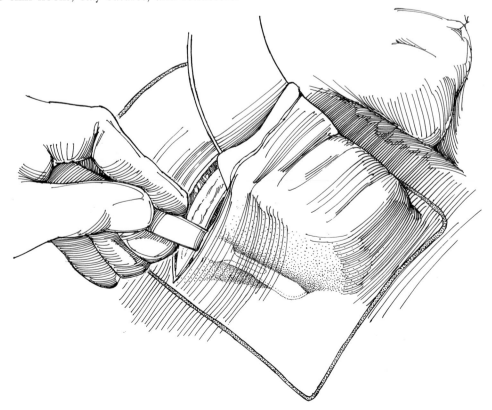

4 Begin at the upper margin of the incision to expose the external oblique fascia, and clear the superficial fascia and areolar tissue downward over the inguinal ligament to the fascia lata of the thigh.

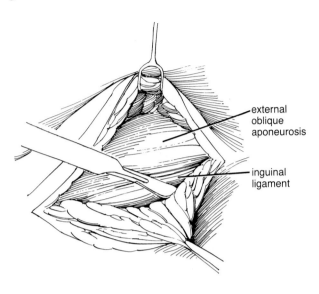

external oblique aponeurosis

inguinal ligament

5 Start incising the fascia lata just below the inguinal ligament along its lateral margin over the sartorius muscle, dividing the tissue between clamps and ligating it with fine SAS. Avoid lymphatic leakage by clipping all identifiable vessels.

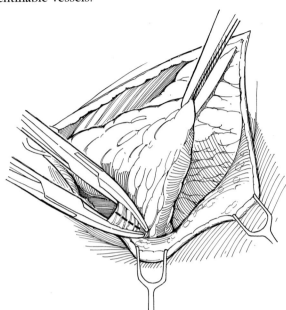

6 Free the deep lateral and medial margins by dissection and ligation. When the greater saphenous vein is reached inferomedially, dissect around it but preserve it to reduce edema of the leg postoperatively. With bulky disease, the vein may require sacrifice. Avoid dissection inferolaterally to the fossa ovalis.

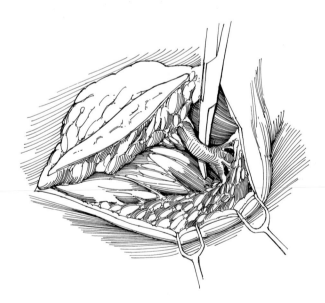

7 Mobilize the mass by blunt and sharp dissection from the lateral to medial side, over the branches of the femoral nerve and then over the femoral sheath. Preserve the motor nerves but sacrifice the cutaneous nerves, and divide those branches of the femoral vascular system supplying the overlying subcutaneous tissue.

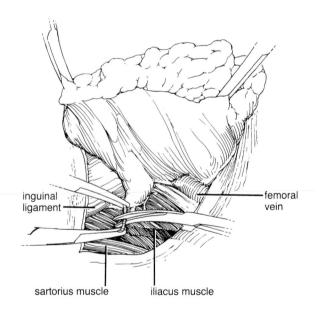

inguinal ligament

femoral vein

sartorius muscle

iliacus muscle

8 Mobilize the deep fascia medially from the adductors to the femoral sheath and excise the fascia.

9 Skeletonize the femoral vasculature medially and anteriorly in the femoral triangle. Avoid dissection lateral to the femoral artery below the fossa ovalis, but ligate all the branches, thus freeing the deep inguinal nodal mass.

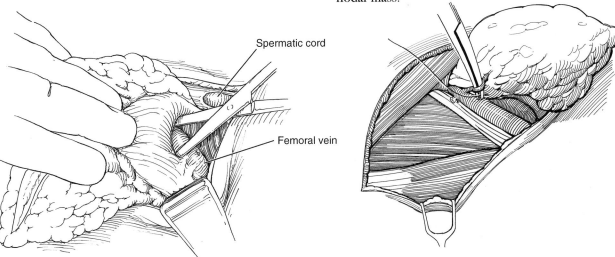

Spermatic cord

Femoral vein

10 Preserve the greater saphenous vein. Dissect it free, leaving an empty fossa with the nodal mass attached only at the femoral canal. Send suspicious nodes for frozen-section diagnosis.

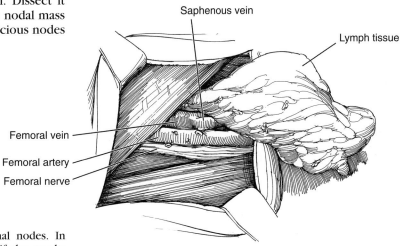

Saphenous vein

Lymph tissue

Femoral vein

Femoral artery

Femoral nerve

Pelvic Component

Obtain frozen-section examination of the inguinal nodes. In general, do not proceed with pelvic dissection if the results are negative.

11 Incise and divide the external oblique fascia about 3 cm above the inguinal ligament in the direction of its fibers for the length of the wound. Open the internal oblique muscle and the transversalis fascia.

12 Dissect deeply and laterally, exposing the peritoneum; bluntly separate it from the lateral pelvic wall. The ureter ascends with the peritoneum. The crossing of the ureter at the bifurcation of the common iliac artery marks the upper end of the dissection. Begin iliac dissection from above downward.

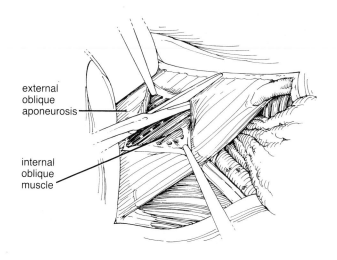

external oblique aponeurosis

internal oblique muscle

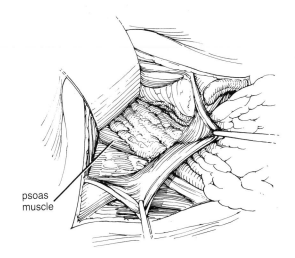

psoas muscle

13 Identify the genitofemoral nerve lateral to the iliac vessels through the endopelvic fascia and divide the fascia just medial to it, reflecting the fascia laterally off the psoas muscle. For the lateral iliac chain, roll the external iliac artery medially after entering its adventitia, and dissect between the artery and the muscle. Continue between and over the iliac vein, transecting the inferior epigastric vessels again at the lower end of the dissection. Divide the lymph cord at the common iliac bifurcation, using clips to occlude the lymphatics. For the medial iliac chain, retract the external iliac vein laterally to clear its undersurface, exposing the external obturator muscle. Open the plane next to the muscle, exposing the obturator veins, which are easily torn and then difficult to control.

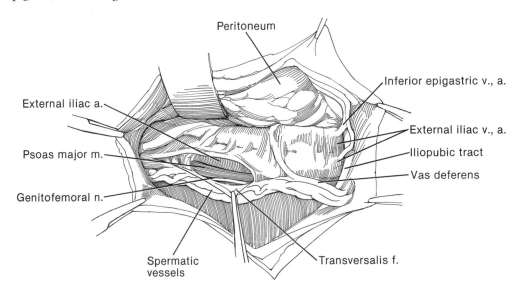

14 Locate the obturator nerve as it exits under the medial border of the psoas muscle, passing beneath the iliac vessels near the bifurcation of the common iliac vein. Dissect the nerve free and hold it laterally. Divide the cord as it becomes attenuated on the inner surface of the internal obturator muscle. Free the lymph cord medially and pass it through the femoral canal, or divide it and submit it to the pathologist separately. Mark it for identification appropriately with tags on the pelvic and inguinal components.

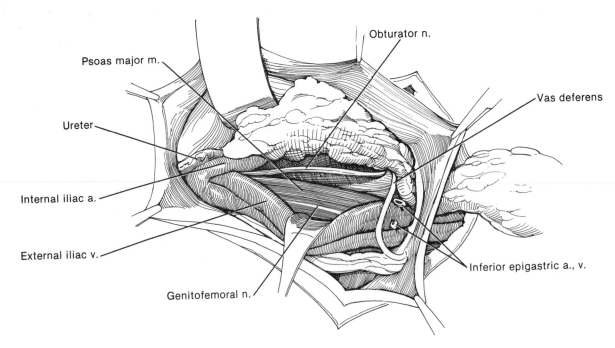

BILATERAL DISSECTION

Make a midline abdominal incision first, and perform a pelvic node dissection, as described on page 517. If the nodes are negative for tumor, make an inguinal incision 2 inches below and parallel to the inguinal ligament. The palpable femoral artery is in the middle of the incision. Proceed as for the previously described "Unilateral Dissection, Inguinal Component," stopping the dissection before incision of the external oblique fascia. Repeat the procedure on the opposite side.

CLOSURE
Coverage with Sartorius

15 Divide the sartorius muscle where it joins the anterior iliac spine. Place it over the femoral nerve and vessels. Suture it to the reflection of the inguinal ligament, tacking it laterally as well. Check the skin margins, especially the lower margin, and excise any nonviable edges. If necessary, apply a split-thickness skin graft, which is preferable to having a slough later.

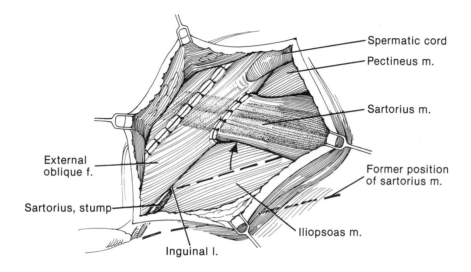

Coverage with Rectus Abdominis Myocutaneous Flap

16 An *inferior rectus abdominis myocutaneous flap* may be applied in patients who have extensive unilateral inguinal node metastasis with disruption of the overlying skin or who required extensive dissection for inguinal metastasis with consequent postoperative skin breakdown and wound infection. Raise a flap from the contralateral rectus muscle (see page 54). Include an ellipse of skin unless the flap is to be covered with a split-thickness graft. Move the flap anterior to the ipsilateral rectus muscle, and pass it through a subcutaneous tunnel into the groin defect. Place a suction drain in the abdominal defect before closure, as well as one in the groin area.

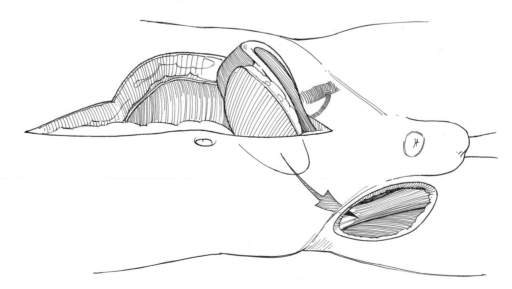

17 Insert suction drains through nondissected areas, placing the tubes on both sides of the sartorius muscle. Close the skin with absorbable subcuticular sutures. Apply collodion but do not apply compression. Raise the elastic stocking to the thigh level. Continue antibiotics. The patient should be kept constipated. Position the patient in bed with the foot of the bed slightly elevated for 5 to 7 days, and have him do toe-heel exercises frequently to promote venous circulation. Remove the drains at the time of ambulation. Warn the patient about sitting with the thighs flexed and about the need for wearing the stockings. With this regimen, delayed skin grafting is seldom necessary.

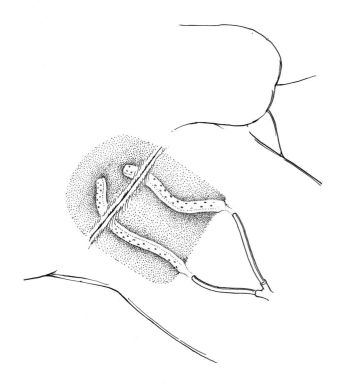

INTRAOPERATIVE PRECAUTIONS

Avoid *venous bleeding* by careful dissection. Do not clamp blindly. Do not place clamps on the thin-walled pelvic veins; rather, isolate and pass ligatures or use medium-size surgical clips. If a vein is torn, control bleeding with sponge sticks placed above and below the rent to allow suturing with swaged 5-0 arterial silk suture as the rent is progressively exposed. For veins that are avulsed flush with apertures in the pelvic wall, apply sponge pressure. Because these veins cannot be clamped, use a 3-0 silk suture swaged on an intestinal needle to oversew the site.

POSTOPERATIVE PROBLEMS

Necrosis of the edges of the skin flaps is not uncommon, usually because insufficient subcutaneous tissue with its capillaries remained. Small defects may be debrided and allowed to heal by second intention. Later application of split-thickness skin grafts may be necessary. *Wound infection* begins in areas of devascularization and in dead spaces; it is difficult to really cleanse the bacteria from the skin in this area. *Seromas* are not rare. *Lymphoceles* can form but are inhibited by ligating all lymphatics and by tacking the skin flaps down to the muscle, providing adequate suction drainage, and placing proper dressings. Treat them with intermittent aspiration or by continuous closed percutaneous aspiration. *Lymphorrhea*, however, is rare. Early cautious mobilization of the patient can reduce the chance of deep vein thrombosis without jeopardizing the healing of the wound. Minidose heparin can reduce the incidence, but prolonged lymphatic drainage may be a problem. *Lymphedema* of the leg is to be expected, and waist-high elastic stockings should be fitted before the patient begins ambulation. Have him keep the leg elevated when sitting or and when in bed. Diuretics may help. Paresthesia medial to the operative site can also be expected but is not disabling.

Commentary by Perinchery Narayan

We recommend the three-incision technique advocated by Elwin Fraley, which allows for an inguinal lymphadenectomy followed by a pelvic lymphadenectomy without the line of the incision traversing the femoral triangle. This incision has significantly reduced the incidence of wound complications. Inguinal lymphadenectomy was formerly associated with a significant number of complications related to several factors—the technique of surgery, the need to do extensive dissection, and the lack of adequate prophylaxis for deep vein thrombosis and its associated complications. The most significant complications noted in the literature have been skin necrosis (60 percent), lymph under the flap (5 to 23 percent), wound dehiscence and infection (2 to 20 percent), lymphedema (20 percent), and need for secondary skin grafts (20 percent). Hemorrhage from femoral vessels, deep vein thrombosis, and pulmonary embolism have also been reported as significant complications, although the percentages are low.

At least three significant changes in technique and postoperative management have helped reduce these complications. The most important is the preservation of the saphenous vein and all of its tributaries. Fraley was one of the first to recognize this problem, and several other authors have subsequently reported

a lower incidence of lymphatic complications of the extremities following preservation of the saphenous vein and its tributaries as far as feasible.

A second important means of preventing serum and lymph collection under the flap is the practice of meticulously ligating all of the subcutaneous lymphatics under the flap and at its edges using 3-0 and 4-0 Dexon or similar absorbable sutures. This region is richly supplied by lymphatic channels, and meticulous ligature of these vessels significantly reduces incidence of lymphoceles and resulting complications of flap necrosis. Meticulous suturing is preferable to cauterization because use of compression stockings and movement result in lymphatic collections when only cauterization is used to control lymphatic leakage. Meticulous ligation of lymphatics should be combined with suction drainage and compression dressing.

The third major advance in recent years has been adequate prophylaxis for deep vein thrombosis by use of both sequential compression stockings and warfarin. Warfarin is less likely than heparin, at least in our hands, to cause either bleeding or complications secondary to deep vein thrombosis and pulmonary embolism. The use of heparin, still favored by many, is associated with a significant incidence of prolonged lymphatic drainage.

SECTION
5
Penis: Correction

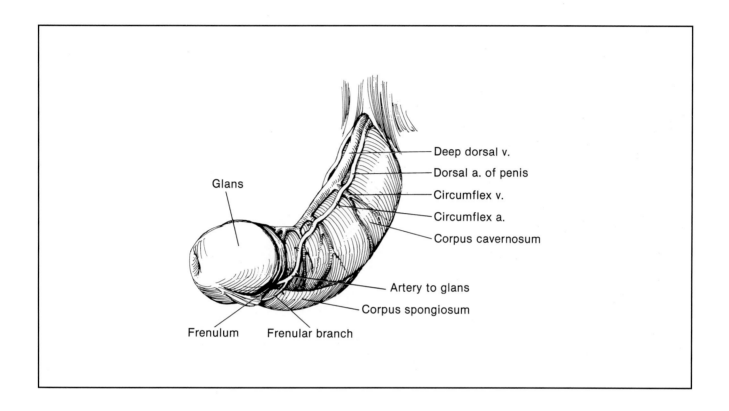

Glans

Deep dorsal v.

Dorsal a. of penis

Circumflex v.

Circumflex a.

Corpus cavernosum

Artery to glans

Corpus spongiosum

Frenulum   Frenular branch

Correction of Penile Defects

STRUCTURAL LAYERS OF THE PENIS

Understanding the anatomy of the penis helps in the correction of deformities of the penis.

1 **A,** The skin over the penis is distensible, has good vascularity, and is available. It adapts readily to prolonged contact with urine, making it suitable material for urethral replacement. The superficial fascia of the penis or dartos fascia, as a part of Colles' fascia, is useful as secondary reinforcement. Embedded in it are the superficial penile arteries and the superficial dorsal vein, the

vessels that supply the skin of the penis. Beneath them lies a very thin connective tissue layer, the tela subfascialis, which covers the extracorporal segments of the cavernous arteries, veins, and nerves. Deeper is Buck's fascia, a heavy elastic layer that not only encloses the two corpora cavernosa and the corpus spongiosum but also encases the deep dorsal vein, the dorsal arteries, and dorsal nerves. **B,** The tunica albuginea is the deepest layer around the corpora cavernosa and the corpus spongiosum. It has an outer longitudinal coat and an inner circular coat. Internally, the two corpora cavernosa are separated in the sagittal plane by a dense tunica albugineal layer, the intercavernous septum.

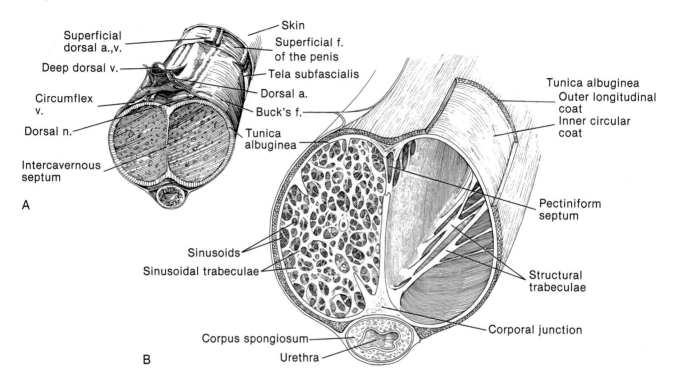

During erection, when the tunica albuginea becomes distended with blood, its two layers of fibers, running at right angles, like those in an automobile tire, limit expansion and provide the necessary longitudinal rigidity at full erection. Because the tunica is then under tension, it is subject to flexion injury, either a fracture or a lesser injury that, if repeated, may result in a deforming scar in susceptible men (Peyronie's disease).

PROCEDURES ON THE PENIS

The most common reasons for correction of structural defects of the penis are a redundant or phimotic prepuce and curvature of the penis, which usually is first noticed at puberty. Circumcision in childhood is readily performed with a clamp device; in adults, a plastic surgical excision is necessary. Ventral penile curvature, congenital in origin, can be corrected by shortening the dorsum or lengthening the ventrum. The former is the simpler procedure and results in minimal reduction in the overall length of the penis.

166

Circumcision

Circumcision, because it is a procedure performed on an organ important to the individual, must be done with precision, especially in adults. The newborn should be mature and in good health, and the parents must give informed consent. Preputial plasty has been suggested as an alternative (Persad et al, 1995).

Prepare the penis with iodophor solution. Infiltrate the base of the penis with 1 ml of 1 or 2 percent plain lidocaine (Xylocaine) or 0.25 or 0.5 percent bupivacaine hydrochloride through a 26-gauge needle. In older boys, general anesthesia may be needed to supplement the local block. For techniques requiring an incision, a tourniquet may be applied at the base for initial hemostasis, although it is rarely necessary.

DOUBLE-INCISION TECHNIQUE

This technique is preferred for older children and adults.

1 **A,** Mark the site of the coronal sulcus onto the unretracted prepuce with a marking pen. **B,** On the ventrum, opposite the frenulum, provide a V extension.

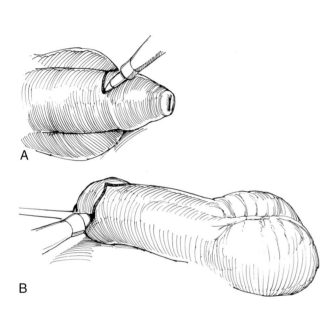

2 Retract the prepuce. Mark a second incision 0.5 to 1 cm proximal to the sulcus to leave enough membrane for suturing. Make it either straight across the base of the frenulum, as depicted, or dipping proximally as a V to leave a major portion of the frenulum. Identify the urethral meatus. *Alternative:* Make the inner preputial incision before the outer incision. Pulling down the prepuce while making the outer incision reduces bleeding from the inner incision.

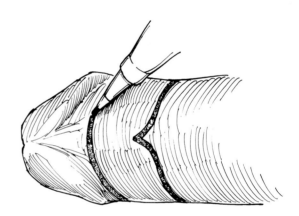

3 **A,** Incise along the marked lines proximally. A knife leaves a cleaner edge than scissors. **B,** Draw the prepuce back and incise distally. A traction suture in the glans leaves a mark; it is usually not helpful.

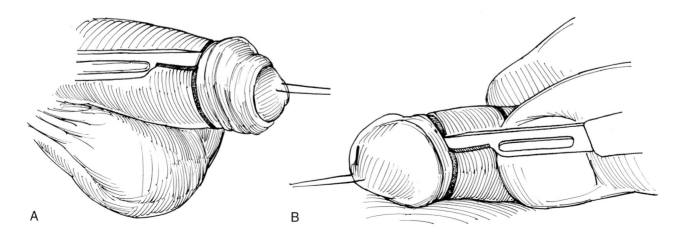

4 On the dorsum, divide the ring of skin with scissors.

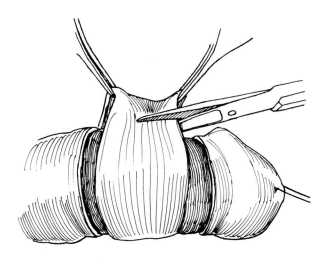

5 Lift the edges of the skin and free the skin from the dartos layer. Fulgurate bleeders, or tie the larger ones with 5-0 plain catgut (PCG). Inspect the frenular area, and secure and ligate the frenular artery or arteries. Release the tourniquet, and complete the hemostasis with the electrocautery.

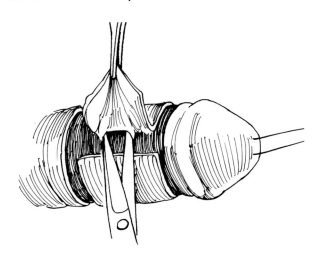

6 Place 4-0 PCG sutures through the skin of the shaft and corona in each of the four quadrants. Leave them long, holding them in mosquito clamps. Place two or three sutures between each pair, plus two more to approximate the V at the frenulum. End-on mattress sutures may be needed at the frenulum. Try to take small bites in the skin, catching more subcutaneous tissue to roll out the skin edges and leave fewer suture marks.

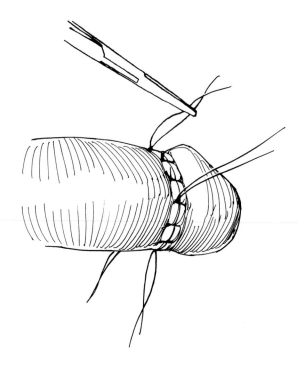

7 Take a 1-inch strip of gauze impregnated with petroleum jelly (Vaseline) and coil it on itself by rotating the clamp as if waving a flag; pull the free end to form a helical tube.

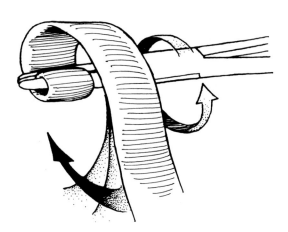

8 Tie the tube successively into the four quadrant sutures. Leave enough slack between sutures to avoid constriction should erection occur. Trim a 4 × 4-inch gauze square, wrap it around the tube, and encircle it with plastic tape that extends onto the pubis.

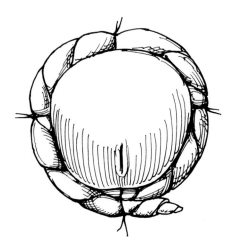

ALTERNATIVE TECHNIQUE

This technique is preferred for small boys in whom it is not possible to retract the prepuce.

9 After anesthesia has been induced, retract the prepuce, freeing it completely from the glans using a mosquito clamp while maintaining traction on the glans with moist gauze held over the thumb and fingertips. Clear the lumps of smegma. Check for hypospadias. Mark the skin at the coronal level with the prepuce in place. Make a dorsal slit to the mark, and grasp the edges. Avoid getting too close to the coronal sulcus.

10 Divide both layers of the prepuce circumferentially on the marked line with scissors.

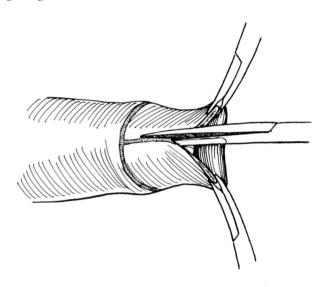

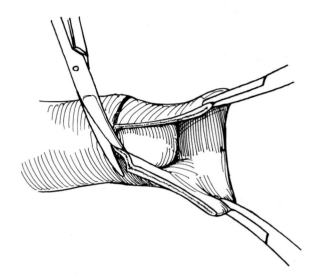

11 At the frenulum, cut a V, leaving the frenulum in place. Reapproximate the edges as described in Steps 6 to 8.

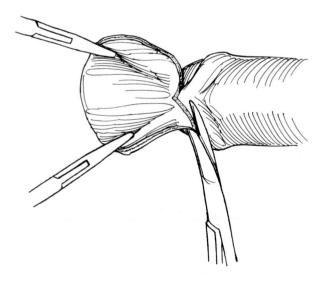

PLASTIBELL TECHNIQUE

This technique is intended for infants. Wait 24 hours after birth. Obtain informed consent from the parents. Before starting the procedure, reread the printed instructions accompanying the Plastibell device. Identify the baby and place him firmly in papoose restraints. Prepare and drape the penis. Be strict about aseptic technique.

Local Anesthesia. Anesthesia should be used even in infants; a sugar teat may supplement it. Palpate the inferior border of the symphysis pubis with the index and middle fingers of one hand. With the other hand, insert a needle under the symphysis pubis and aspirate and inject 1.0 to 1.2 ml of 1 percent lidocaine *without* epinephrine from a 3-ml syringe. Redirect the needle toward Alcock's canal to infiltrate the pudendal nerve plexus. Again aspirate carefully to avoid accidental intravascular injection, and inject the agent. Withdraw the needle, and repeat insertion and injection toward the opposite side. Inject the remaining anesthetic in the ventral surface of the scrotum around the base of the penis.

12 **A,** Mark the location of the coronal sulcus on the skin of the shaft with a marking pen. **B,** Dilate the preputial ring with a hemostat and identify the urethral meatus. Place straight hemostats on the prepuce at 10 o'clock and 2 o'clock, taking a shallow bite of skin 0.5 cm deep. Tease the preputial surface off the dorsum of the glans. Clamp the prepuce in the midline, one third of the distance to the corona, with a straight hemostat for 10 seconds. Divide the crushed groove with straight blunt-tipped scissors to allow the prepuce to be retracted. Free the prepuce from the glans with a flexible probe until it can be completely retracted and the sulcus exposed. Look for hypospadias.

13 **A,** Select the correct size of Plastibell from the three sizes available. The arrows point to the groove that receives the suture. **B,** Choose the size that allows the bottom edge of the bell to completely cover the corona. The prepuce should appear slightly distended as it is drawn down over the bell and glans. Continue to pull the prepuce over the bell until the skin mark at the coronal sulcus lies over the groove in the bell.

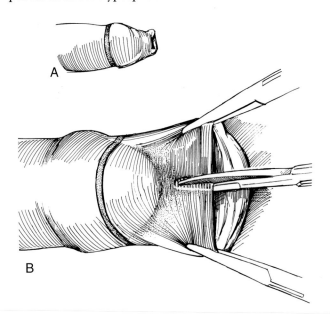

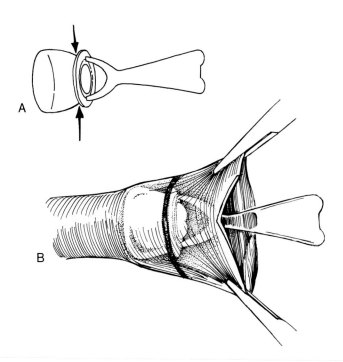

14 Tie an absorbable suture as tightly as possible in the inner groove of the device, and cut the prepuce off with scissors just past the outer groove. Do not use electrocautery. Break off the handle. Discharge the child, telling the parents to expect the bell to fall out in a few days. If it does not, have them return the child for division of the ring with bone-cutting forceps.

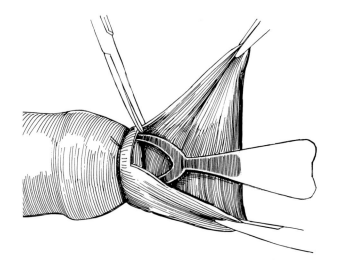

GOMCO CLAMP TECHNIQUE

Select the correct size of Gomco bell and place it as described for the Plastibell in Step 13. Pull the prepuce over the bell and through the plate and yoke portions of the clamp until the skin mark at the coronal sulcus lies at the level of the top of the clamp. Be certain that the bell is not skewed so that an uneven amount of skin is included. Screw the clamp down onto the bell as tightly as possible and keep it in place for several minutes. Cut the prepuce off right next to the top of the plate. Remove the entire clamp and bell, together with the excised prepuce. If it is necessary to control bleeding, apply interrupted 5-0 synthetic absorbable sutures (SAS) to the cut edge. If bleeding starts after removal of the clamp, separate the cut skin edges, fulgurate the bleeding vessels, and suture the skin edges. *Caution:* Never use electrocoagulation while the metal device is in place.

REVISION OF CIRCUMCISION

Prepuce redundant: Excise the redundancy as a sleeve (Steps 2 to 8).

Penis concealed: Incise the distal cicatricial ring deep enough to retract the remainder of the prepuce back over the glans. Excise the redundancy as a sleeve (Steps 2 to 8).

Prepuce and shaft of disparate size (Redman): Place a traction suture in the glans and stretch the penis. Pull the skin of the shaft distally and hold it out with thumb forceps. With a skin pen, mark the proposed incision on the skin at the coronal margin. Incise the outer leaf through the dartos tunic; then incise the inner prepuce 0.5 cm from the coronal sulcus. Start suturing the edges from the dorsal surface. This leaves the redundancy ventrally in the form of a dog ear. Excise it as described on page 49, and close the ventrum with 5-0 chromic catgut (CCG). Apply a light compression dressing, to remain overnight.

Phimosis: A dorsal slit is the simplest procedure but the least cosmetically satisfactory. A circumcision is an alternative, but a Z-*plasty* gives the best appearance without loss of the foreskin. Retract the prepuce and make a diagonal incision across the constricting ring. Make two more diagonal incisions, one from each end of the original incision, and extend them into normal skin. Elevate the Z-flaps with stay sutures and dissect them free. Transpose them as for a Z-plasty (see page 44), and approximate the edges with 4-0 CCG sutures.

POSTOPERATIVE PROBLEMS FROM CIRCUMCISION

Skin necrosis may occur if epinephrine is used in the local anesthetic. Avoid electrocoagulation; *necrosis of the shaft* and even sloughing may result. If coagulation is used, keep the penis grounded by applying a saline-soaked sponge around it

and holding the organ against the body. *Necrosis of the glans* results from application of a constrictive bandage or from using a Plastibell that is too small. *Laceration* or *amputation of the glans* results from using a blind technique. Immediate reanastomosis of the glans is usually successful. *Bleeding*, usually on the ventrum and more often with the Gomco clamp than with other methods, can be stopped by local pressure but may require application of a hemostat and tie or a suture ligature. Take care not to enter the urethra when placing the stitch. *Infection* is occasionally seen, more commonly with the Plastibell than the Gomco clamp, and is managed with hot tub soaks and topical antibiotics. Severe infections, such as necrotizing fasciitis with systemic spread, are rare, but any infection should be treated immediately with antibiotics. *Separation of the shaft skin* at the corona heals spontaneously and rarely needs treatment.

For *excessive removal of skin*, if limited to one area, simple re-epithelialization may be adequate. If excision has been extensive, apply a petrolatum dressing and wait for healing by second intention.

Commonly the skin edges come together during healing. Immediate skin grafting is both unwise and unnecessary. Should the result be a buried penis, correct that abnormality. Often only shaft skin has been denuded; the prepuce remains for later repair. The situation is similar to that in which too much prepuce remains attached to the glans while too much skin has been removed from the shaft (the shaft, not the prepuce, has been circumcised), so that the penis becomes "buried." After healing, it can be released by circumcising the junction and covering the defect with the excess preputial tissue that was left behind. Seldom is a skin graft needed. With *inadequate removal of skin*, phimosis may reoccur as the suture line contracts. A very redundant residual prepuce may require recircumcision.

Dense adhesions from adherence of the inner preputial skin to the glans resulting from an inadequate circumcision may require surgical division and suturing of the defect in the glans and the shaft with fine sutures. *Chordee* is secondary to inflammation on the ventrum with delayed healing, or less often on the dorsum after circumcision. Infection and separation may result in *lymphedema* that may need revision and/or skin grafting. *Bivalving the glans* either dorsally or ventrally can occur during the dorsal or ventral slitting of the prepuce, fostered by inadequate separation of the prepuce from the glans. *Skin bridges* that appear late usually can be divided with small scissors without anesthesia. If they are large, anesthesia may be needed for their division and suturing. *Inclusion cysts*, from inversion of the skin, require shelling the cyst out with its wall.

Glanular necrosis may result from contact of the cautery with a clamp. *Total ablation* may necessitate raising the boy as a girl. *Urethral injury* results from sutures hurriedly placed to stop bleeding. A *urethrocutaneous fistula* may appear after Gomco or Plastibell circumcision or may be secondary to hemostatic sutures placed in the frenular area. Delay repair for 6 months. When located at or below the coronal margin, the fistula can be repaired by splitting the glans, forming a ventral skin flap (Mathieu, page 124), and wrapping the glans wings around the neourethra (Baskin). *Urinary retention* can occur later with secondary phimosis or immediately with a dressing that is too tight.

The worst complication results from *not recognizing hypospadias* before circumcision; the resultant loss of preputial skin makes subsequent hypospadias repair more difficult.

DORSAL SLIT FOR PARAPHIMOSIS

15 **A,** Make a vertical dorsal incision sharply, centered over the junction of the shiny inner and the duller outer skin. After releasing the constriction, manipulate the prepuce over the glans to be sure that the dorsal incision is long enough for easy passage. **B and C,** Approximate the longitudinal cut transversely with interrupted 5-0 PCG sutures. **D,** Replace the prepuce around the glans, and cover it with a medicated gauze dressing. *Alternative:* Proceed with circumcision before suturing.

Alternative to dorsal slit for paraphimosis (Ohjimi et al, 1995): Make a vertical incision through the constricting ring and close it transversly. To remove the resulting excess skin, excise a wedge of skin dorsally at the base of the penis, leaving 2 cm of a skin bridge ventrally. Draw the shaft skin proximally and close the defect.

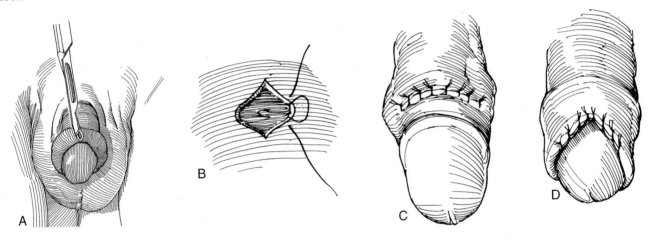

FRENULOPLASTY

For a short tethering frenulum, incise it transversely at the base. Traction on the gland disposes the incision longitudinally. Trim the resultant dog ear. Close it with fine PCG sutures.

UNCIRCUMCISION
(Lynch and Pryor)

16 **A,** Circumscribe the base of the penis down to Buck's fascia. Slide the shaft skin distally and hold it with four stay sutures. Make three or four short circumferentially oriented incisions in the distal end and close them transversely to narrow the new prepuce. Mark a midline full-thickness flap from the scrotum of the same size as the defect on the shaft and depilate it. Raise the flap, basing the pedicle on the dartos layer. **B,** Rotate the flap and suture it into the defect. Insert a 16 F balloon catheter and tape the stay sutures to it, to remain 5 days.

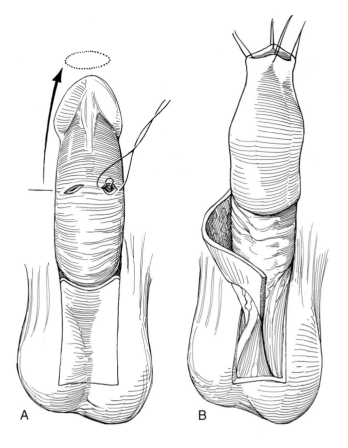

A   B

Commentary by Stuart B. Bauer

Circumcision, often relegated to the least-experienced member of the surgical team, is actually a delicate procedure that demands skillful and careful technique. It will receive close attention from the boy's parents and a more critical inspection from the patient when he grows up. In newborns, complications arise primarily because too little skin has been removed or the operator fails to recognize that a prominent pubic fat pad will cause the penis to be buried or concealed as the shaft retracts below the incision line, unless measures are taken to prevent it. Failure of parents to retract the shaft skin below the glans after the initial healing phase may result in adhesions between the shaft and the glans.

In the last several years, children undergoing circumcision beyond the newborn period have had bupivacaine injected locally at the beginning of the procedure to decrease the amount of general anesthetic required and to reduce both the level of discomfort and the amount of oral analgesics needed in the early postoperative period. The narcotic is injected below the pubic symphysis and along the inferior aspect of each pubic ramus near Alcock's canal, where the pudendal nerve exits. When planning the circumcision incisions, it is important to leave an adequate amount of mucosa below the coronal margin as well as to keep the frenulum intact. I tend to make the distal circumferential incision first. Then I pull the foreskin up over the glans, allowing it to fall in place naturally. The more proximal incision line is marked out over the impression of the coronal ridge. The orientation of the incision line is slightly closer to the base on the dorsal than the ventral side of the penis. Marking and cutting this more proximal circumferential incision is made easier because bleeding from the first incision does not interfere with grasping and manipulating the penis, as might occur if the order of the incisions were reversed. I then remove the isolated circumferential strip of skin and subcutaneous tissue, avoiding injury to the dorsal neurovascular complex and urethra.

Before suturing the skin edges together, I allow the cut edges to fall in place once again and the penis to lie naturally. If the penile skin does not align itself properly with the mucosal edge, more shaft skin is trimmed. In addition, a meticulous search for all bleeding points is mandatory to reduce the chance of delayed postoperative bleeding. Sutures are placed to evert the skin edges and minimize the amount of epidermal surface to be incorporated in the ligature. Once tied, there is a broad edge of tissue for adherence and only a minute area for cross-hatching impressions to develop in the skin.

A satisfactory dressing is as important as the procedure itself. Benzoin is painted on the penile shaft skin, glans (avoiding the meatus), and pubic and scrotal regions. A strip of Telfa padding, cut as wide as the penis is long, is wrapped around the shaft and held by Steri-Strips. A Tegaderm dressing is placed around the penis, attaching it to the pubic and scrotal areas, while leaving the meatus uncovered. At times, a conforming occlusive dressing is wrapped around the penis to reduce the risk of postoperative bleeding. This aids in preventing adhesions from forming and in helping to keep the penis partly erect so that it does not retract into the pubic fat and become secondarily concealed. In teenagers and young adults, instructions are provided to minimize the incidence of postoperative erections.

Penile Curvature

For correction of minor chordee during hypospadias repair in which the urethral plate is left intact, see page 130.

RELEASE OF DARTOS AND BUCK'S FASCIAS
(Devine)

Have the patient take a lateral Polaroid photograph of the erect penis to demonstrate the degree of curvature. Instruct him to shower preoperatively with antiseptic soap.

Position: Supine. Create an artificial erection to estimate the degree of curvature.

Incision: Make an incision around the shaft at the site of the circumcision scar, and dissect the shaft skin back to the base of the penis.

Elevate the dysgenic dartos and Buck's fascias that are concentrated on either side of the corpus spongiosum. In rare cases, the corpus spongiosum and urethra may have to be mobilized to resect all the fibrous tissue. Repeat the erection. If curvature remains, proceed to elliptical excisions on the dorsum (Step 1 and following).

ELLIPTICAL EXCISION TECHNIQUE FOR VENTRAL CHORDEE
(Nesbit)

With the penis erect, measure the length on the ventrum and dorsum with a tape. The difference in length determines the number and width of the ellipses to be removed. Most often, excision of only one ellipse on each side is required. Alternatively, remove a 1-mm width of ellipse for each 10 degrees of curvature.

1 Incise Colles' fascia longitudinally. Mobilize the dorsal neurovascular structures dorsomedially along with Buck's fascia from each side. The bundle may be elevated with a vessel loop. Remove the ellipses from each side as shown in the figures (the vascular bundle may be elevated and the incisions carried from one side to the other).

Clamp Technique

2 Grasp the tunica albuginea with Allis clamps, and excise the ellipses that are elevated. Check by penile inflation to gauge if sufficient tissue has been excised, remembering that 2 mm are needed for placement of the sutures. Close the defects with inverted interrupted SAS.

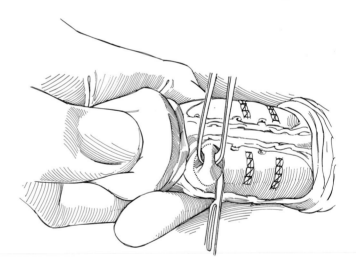

Open Technique

3 **A,** Mark 1-cm ellipses on the tunica albuginea on each side of the neurovascular bundle with a marking pen. Incise the ellipses. **B,** Remove the ellipses. Try to keep the depth of the excision just superficial to the endothelial layer. **C,** Approximate the edges of the defects successively as each ellipse is removed, using two or three interrupted size 0 polydioxanone sutures (PDS). Invert the sutures to bury the knots. A running suture of the same material may be placed to ensure a smooth surface. **D** and **E,** Alternatively, close the tunica with a running fine nonabsorbable sutures (NAS) supplemented by interrupted plicating sutures to achieve a smoother surface (Kelami, 1987). Test for straightness by artificial erection, and excise further ellipses if necessary. Be sure the erection is symmetric.

Alternative 1: Form *orthoplastic dorsal tucks* (page 132) instead of excising ellipses. Make two parallel transverse incisions in the tunica albuginea on each side of the midline approximately 8 mm apart. Place inverted sutures of NAS material, starting from inside out at the proximal cut and outside in at the distal cut, to draw the two openings in apposition and bury the bridge of tissue between.

Alternative 2 (Lue): Instead of excising ellipses, place two or three paired size 0 braided NAS vertically into the tunica albuginea on both sides of the dorsal vein, displacing the neurovascular bundle to either side.

Alternative 3 (Yachia): Apply an Allis clamp to gather the tunica vaginalis appropriately, remove the clamp, and incise the tunica albuginea vertically between the marks left by the clamp. Insert a skin hook on either side of the incision at the midpoint and convert it into a transverse opening (Heineke-Mikulicz). Close the incision with a continuous locked 3-0 PDS. If necessary, place plicating sutures at either end to smooth the bulge.

Alternative 4 (Goldstein and Blumberg): Remove ellipses from the convex side and insert them in slits on the concave side.

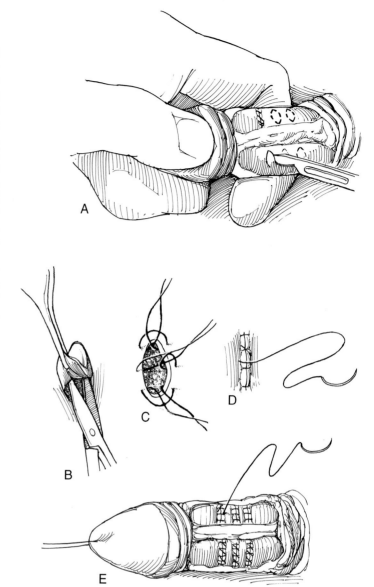

4 Reapproximate Buck's fascia and subcutaneous tissue with 5-0 SAS, and reapproximate the skin at the coronal sulcus with 4-0 CCG sutures. If the patient has not been circumcised, trim redundant distal skin to avoid postoperative edema. A suction drain is probably not needed. Dress with Tegaderm. The palpable ridges from the sutures will subside.

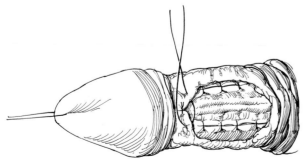

Commentary by John P. Pryor

I do not personally bother with a preoperative photograph. The patient is able to demonstrate with a finger the extent of the deformity; if there is any doubt I prefer to give an intracavernous injection of prostaglandin E_1. For congenital curvatures, I raise the dorsal neurovascular bundle and place a sling around it. I then inflate the penis; I believe that it is a mistake to use a tourniquet around the base. I apply Allis forceps, pinching 1 mm for every 10 degrees of curvature, but allow 2 mm extra for the sutures when excising the ellipse. I then check inflation before excising the ellipse. I think that a strong NAS should be used, such as size 0 PDS, because the tunica albuginea is essentially fibrous tissue and does not heal well. Use of absorbable sutures or failure to tie the knots properly gives rise to an "aneurysm" and recurrence of the deformity. I use interrupted sutures with knots on the inside, placing the end sutures wider to prevent a dog ear. I then check the inflation again. If the penis is not quite straight, I then take an additional ellipse or plication if necessary.

In Peyronie's disease, I carry out a similar technique but mobilize the corpus spongiosum off the corpora cavernosa. If the bend is 90 degrees or more, I do not go for complete correction; stopping at 10 to 20 degrees of residual curvature prevents too much shortening but restores function.

SECTION

6

Penis: Reconstruction

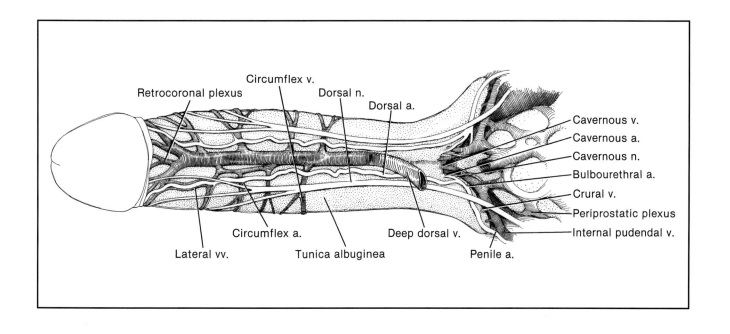

Principles for Penile Reconstruction

Advances in our understanding of the structure and function of the internal components of the penis have permitted more direct approaches to erectile dysfunction. This is particularly true for the penile vascular system. Treatment of erectile failure has changed markedly and can be expected to continue to advance. Implantable devices with separate elements are being displaced by self-contained units. Both may be needed less as other methods of therapy, such as injection and revascularization, are perfected.

Arterial Supply. The penile artery exits from the urogenital diaphragm and divides into three branches. The most important is the cavernous artery (deep artery of the penis), which runs lateral to the cavernous vein along the dorsomedial surface of the crus of the corpus cavernosum to enter the erectile tissue where the two corpora fuse and then continues in the center of the corpus almost to its tip.

The termination of the penile artery is the dorsal artery of the penis. It runs over the respective crus and then along the dorsolateral surface of the penis as far as the glans between the deep dorsal vein medially and the dorsal nerve of the penis laterally.

Venous Drainage. Multiple superficial veins run somewhat randomly on the dorsolateral surface of the penis under the superficial penile fascia to join a single or double superficial dorsal vein that drains into either saphenous vein.

The deep dorsal vein and the circumflex veins form an intermediate drainage system, draining the glans penis, the corpus spongiosum, and the distal two thirds of the corpora cavernosa. The cavernous veins, the bulbar veins, and the crural veins constitute the deep drainage system, collecting blood from the sinusoids by the emissary veins that drain directly into cavernous veins at the periphery of the corpora cavernosa. The cavernous veins unite between the crura into one or two large thin-walled main cavernous veins that lie under the cavernous arteries and nerves, making them less readily accessible for surgical ligation. A few crural veins arise from the dorsolateral surface of each crus, and the bulb itself is drained by the bulbar veins, which empty into the prostatic plexus.

Based on new knowledge of the structure of the penis, not only erectile dysfunction but priapism as well can be treated more directly, as can injury and the fibrous distortion of Peyronie's disease.

Insertion of Flexible Prosthesis

For a single-component prosthesis, select a Dynaflex, Dura II, AMS 600, Mentor Malleable or AccuForm, OmniPhase, or Dura-Phase (Table 1). The last may be the most generally useful. Have proper sizers and sizes available and sterile, either in a sealed package or soaking in an erythromycin solution (500 mg in 500 ml of saline). To reduce infection, try to have the patient first on the operating list.

Approaches for Insertion. Although the subcoronal, penoscrotal, and infrapubic approaches are most commonly used, suprapubic, dorsal and ventral midline, and perineal approaches have advocates. For the average patient, the penoscrotal incision is probably best. Implantation by the perineal approach takes longer and increases the risk of infection because of proximity to the anus. The dorsal penile incision may be followed by penile edema from obstruction of the dorsal lymphatics. Partial sensory loss into the glans can occur after making a distal penile incision, even though the midline dorsal nerve is avoided. A circumcision probably is not necessary, and it increases the risk of infection.

Preparation. Start parenteral broad-spectrum antibiotics the day before the operation and continue them for 3 days postoperatively. Gram-positive bacteria are the main concern. Have the patient scrub his genitalia in the shower for 10 minutes with povidone-iodine solution the night before and the morning of surgery and insert antibiotic cream into the nares every 4 hours. Shave or depilate the genital area in the operating room and scrub for 10 minutes with povidone-iodine. Instill 3 ml of bacitracin-neomycin solution into the meatus and hold it with a penile clamp. Give antibiotics intravenously at the start of the procedure.

Put warning signs on the door to limit traffic in the operating room. Wear surgical hoods and paper gowns and use waterproof paper drapes. Irrigate the wound frequently with antibacterial solution, and consider instilling gentamicin into the corpora after corporotomy and dilation.

Table 1. Available Penile Prostheses

Name	Manufacturer
Nonhydraulic	
AMS malleable 600	American Medical Systems
Dura-II	Dacomed
Mentor Malleable	Mentor
Mentor AccuForm	Mentor
Unitary hydraulic	
DynaFlex	American Medical Systems
Two-piece hydraulic	
Mark II	Mentor
Ambicor	American Medical Systems
Three-piece hydraulic	
AMS 700CX	American Medical Systems
AMS 700CXM	American Medical Systems
AMS 700 Ultrex	American Medical Systems
AMS 700 Ultrex Plus	American Medical Systems
Mentor alpha 1	Mentor
Mentor inflatable	Mentor

Adapted from Montague DK: Penile prosthesis implantation. *In* Marshall FF (ed): Operative Urology. Philadelphia, WB Saunders, 1991.

Instruments: Provide a Basic set; Hegar dilators; small Deaver, thyroid, and Richardson retractors; male sounds; an 18 F 5-ml silicone balloon catheter with 12-ml syringe; plug and lubricating jelly; a small Penrose drain; bacitracin-neomycin irrigant; and heparin irrigant (500 units in 500 ml of saline).

If an inflatable penile prosthesis is to be replaced with a flexible one, infiltrate the base of the penis with lidocaine. Sever the tubing and remove the old prosthesis through incisions in the corpora at the penoscrotal junction. Make an incision in the scrotum after infiltrating it with local anesthesia and remove the pump. Leave the reservoir in place. Proceed as described subsequently.

VENTRAL PENILE APPROACH

1 *Anesthesia:* Local anesthesia is effective. Make a cutaneous penile block with lidocaine (see page 76). After placing a tourniquet around the base of the penis, instill 20 to 25 ml of 1 percent lidocaine, with or without epinephrine, into one corpus through a butterfly needle. Release the tourniquet so that the proximal rami are filled.

Incision: Make a 4- to 5-cm incision in the midline raphe in the penile shaft distal to the penoscrotal junction. Draw the incision distally to expose the dartos and Buck's fascia in midshaft. An alternative is to make the incision transversely. Grasp the subcutaneous tissue with mosquito clamps to act as retractors; hold it with vein retractors or place a Scott ring retractor. Expose the urethra and corpus spongiosum and select an insertion site to one side. Fulgurate any superficial vessels. If the corpus spongiosum is nicked, close it with a figure-eight 4-0 synthetic absorbable suture (SAS).

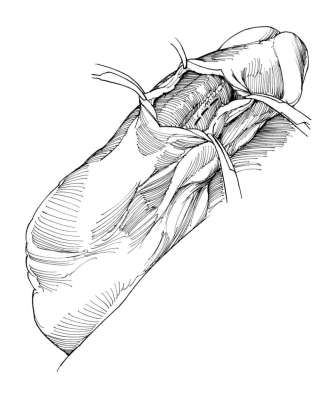

2 Place two stay sutures in the tunica albuginea and make a 3-cm incision between them into the corpus, beginning 0.5 cm from the distal end.

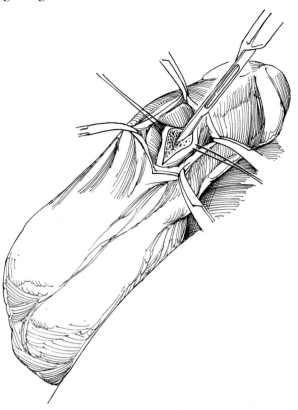

3 **A,** Stretch the corporal incision and insert a 10-mm Hegar dilator (or an AMS Dilamezinsert instrument, if available) until it fits well beneath the glans. Progress through larger dilators, pointing the curve laterally, to 12 or even 14 mm, depending on the type of prosthesis. **B,** Sponge forceps may help the dilation under the glans. **C,** Insert an 8- or 10-mm dilator proximally, taking care not to perforate the crus. Stop when the dilator is held up at the ischial tuberosity. It is unnecessary to use larger dilators there because the prosthesis is tapered proximally.

Difficulty with dilation, as after trauma, priapism, or Peyronie's disease, may require use of long Metzenbaum scissors to cut through the fibrotic cavernous tissue, followed by the dilators. An Otis urethrotome may be used if the blade is kept away from the inferior quadrant of the corpus cavernosum, thus avoiding the urethra. If that fails, peel back the penile skin, incise the corpora, and cover the defect with a Marlex mesh patch. Terminate the procedure if the urethra is accidentally perforated, place a balloon catheter to remain for 10 days, and wait for 6 weeks to reoperate. If the septum is breached with the dilator, it is felt beneath the opposite side of the glans. Go to the second side and dilate the corporal body, insert the prosthesis on that side first, then return to the first side to redilate and implant. If the crus is perforated, continue dilating but be careful not to make the hole larger. If the crus does not support the prosthesis, fold, stitch, and trim an 8 × 3-cm piece of absorbable synthetic mesh or a length of size 12 or 14 vascular graft to fit over the proximal end as a buttress. If necessary, the mesh or graft may be sutured to the pubic rami. Irrigate liberally with antibiotic solution. Irrigate the corpora in both directions with the antibiotic solution.

Change gloves before handling the prosthesis. Accurately measure the length needed for the prosthesis.

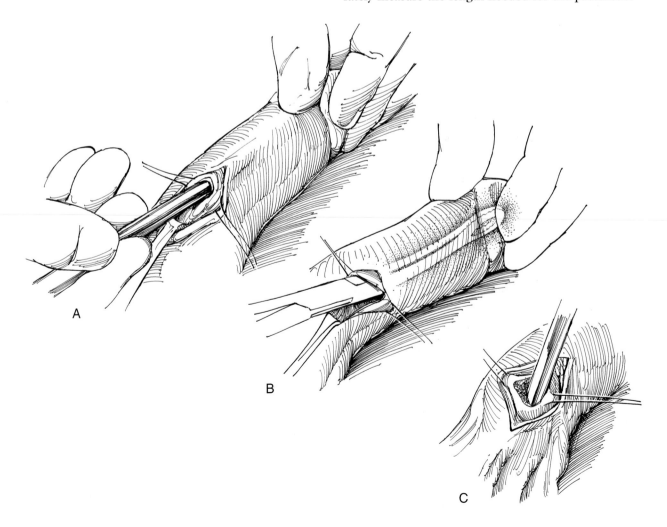

A

B

C

4 Insert the proximal end of the prosthesis first.

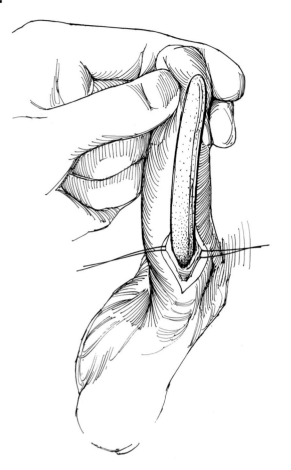

5 Bend the distal end into a loop or circle. Enlist the aid of your assistant to slip it into the corpus. It may be necessary to open the tunic a little more to get it in. A vein retractor can be inserted like a shoehorn to lift the distal end of the corporotomy over the end of the prosthesis (Mulcahy). Check for length. If the prosthesis bows the corpus, remove it and trim off 1 cm more. If it is too short and the glans droops downward, add appropriate rear tip extenders. Irrigate the wound with bacitracin-neomycin solution. Perform the same procedure on the other side.

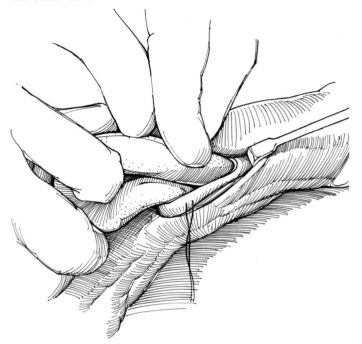

6 Close the tunica albuginea with a running 3-0 SAS. Check the position of the paired prosthesis and irrigate the wound again. Close the subcutaneous tissues with 4-0 SAS, and approximate the skin with 4-0 SAS placed subcuticularly.

Continue antibiotic coverage, and caution the patient to obtain coverage at future manipulations or operations.

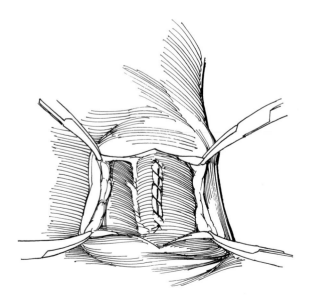

PERINEAL APPROACH

7 *Anesthesia:* General.
Position: Lithotomy. Exclude the anus from the operative field by a sterile plastic drape securely cemented and sutured to the skin (not shown).

Incision: Make a midline or inverted U-shaped incision. Expose the bulb of the urethra in the midline, and free its lateral attachments so it may be swung to one side and the other. Expose the crus of each corpus cavernosum by bluntly separating the ischiocavernosus muscles in the direction of their fibers. Laterally, each crus is fused to the ischial tuberosity, providing a useful landmark. Incise each crus with a #10 blade for a distance of 2 to 3 cm, entering the cavernous tissue. Place a 2-0 silk suture through each edge for traction and localization. Proceed as for the penoscrotal approach.

SUBCORONAL APPROACH

8 This approach is suitable for the AMS 600, Mentor Malleable and AccuForm, and Dura II prostheses. This approach can at times cause a partial sensory loss into the glans.

Position: Supine. For local anesthesia, infiltrate 10 ml of 0.25 percent lidocaine subcutaneously around the base of the penis under the dartos layer and 5 ml subcoronally. Compress the base of the penis against the symphysis and inject another 5 ml into a corpus cavernosum.

Incision: Make a dorsal transverse skin incision 1 cm proximal to the coronal sulcus. Alternatively, through a circumcising incision, retract the penile skin to midshaft. Expose the corpora. Mobilize the dorsal neurovascular bundle medially. Stay sutures may help exposure. Incise each corpus transversely, making a 1-cm cut (*dashed line*).

Alternative: Make the cuts longitudinally (*dotted line*) to avoid the neurovascular bundle. Place stay sutures on both sides of each incision. Dilate and measure appropriately, as described in Step 3. Insert the prosthesis proximally first, then bend the distal end to insert it (Steps 4 and 5). Instead of bending the prosthesis, use a vein retractor to lift the distal end of the corporotomy over the end of the prosthesis. Conclude the operation (Step 6). When local anesthesia is used, the patient may be treated in the same-day surgery unit.

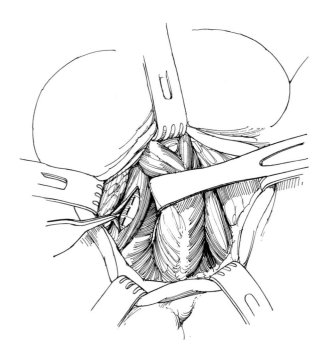

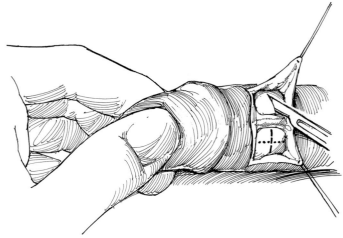

DORSAL PENILE SHAFT APPROACH

This approach is not as suitable for the Dura II prosthesis. It may result in penile edema because of obstruction of the dorsal lymphatics.

9 *Position:* Supine.
Incision: Make a single incision on the dorsum near the proximal end of the penis. Dissect down to the tunica albuginea, avoiding the neurovascular bundle. Retract the skin, and place a pair of stay sutures in the tunica albuginea on each side of the proposed incision.

10 Incise the tunics individually. Measure and insert the prosthesis proximal end first. Complete the operation as described previously.

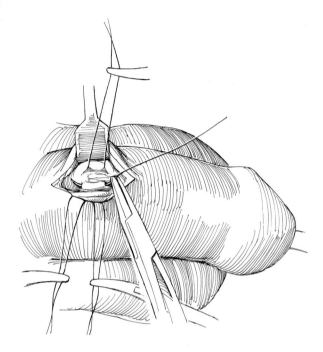

VENTRAL APPROACH
(Mulcahy)

Block the penile nerves with 1 percent lidocaine (see page 76). Apply a tourniquet to the base of the penis, and inject 20 to 25 ml of lidocaine into the corpus through a butterfly scalp vein needle. Release the tourniquet.

Make a 4- to 5-cm midline ventral incision over the proximal shaft. Open the dartos and Buck's fascia over the corpus spongiosum. Expose the tunica albuginea of the corpora on either side. Draw the penile skin distally with a vein retractor, place stay sutures, and incise the tunic for a distance of 2 to 3 cm beginning 0.1 cm from the distal end. Proceed as described in Steps 2 to 6, using a vein retractor to "shoehorn" the distal end into the cavernous space.

PUBIC APPROACH
(Kelami)

11 *Position:* Supine.
Incision: Make a transverse incision just above the inferior border of the symphysis pubis. Expose the dorsal surfaces of the corpora cavernosa under Buck's fascia and the associated connective tissue over each corpus, uncovering the shiny, tough tunica albuginea. Avoid the midline neurovascular bundle. A rake retractor helps expose the bases of the corpora. Complete the operation as previously described.

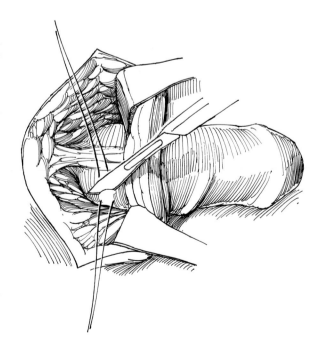

POSTOPERATIVE PROBLEMS

Ventral sagging of the glans (SST deformity) results from inadequate dilation under the glans and placement of a short prosthesis. It requires redilation and placement of a longer cylinder or insertion of a dorsal tuck (see page 174).

Erosion of the corpus cavernosum may result from overdilation. Urethral premature intercourse may cause erosion. Tell the patient to wait 4 weeks before starting sexual activity. *Prolonged pain* or *bowing of the penis* is caused by an implant that is too long.

If endoscopy becomes necessary, use a flexible cystoscope or insert a resectoscope through a perineal urethrostomy (see page 630) to skirt the problem of penile rigidity.

Infection is the most serious problem, usually appearing in the first few weeks and requiring removal of the prosthesis. Try incision and drainage and give antibiotics both orally and as wound irrigants, but do not persist too long before removing the prosthesis. Remove infected components one at a time through separate noncontaminated incisions (pump via scrotal incisions, reservoir via inguinal incision, and cylinders through the incisions used in their placement).

Flush the spaces with antibiotic solution through drains (Jackson-Pratt or Hemovac) to irrigate the wounds each 8-hour shift.

A new component could be placed after 3 days of irrigation or, for more severe infections, after 1 year. At the time of reimplantation, allow cultures to incubate for 48 hours to be certain that bacteria are sensitive to the antibacterials used in the irrigant. Infection may appear after a long interval, the bacteria borne by a hematogenous route from infection elsewhere in the body. Antibiotic prophylaxis during dental repair or other sources of bacteremia is needed, especially a cephalosporin effective against staphylococci.

Urinary retention is not common and can be managed with catheterization and administration of an alpha-blocker. *Paraphimosis* may be seen in a patient with a short foreskin that cannot be kept over the glans; it may require an in situ dorsal slit. *Pain* with or without intercourse occurs occasionally but rarely necessitates removal of the prosthesis. Patients often notice that the glans feels cool in the winter.

Pre-existing scarring secondary to *priapism* or *scleroderma* may make proper insertion of dilating sounds impossible. In such a case, insert a flexible prosthesis between Buck's fascia and the tunica albuginea. Alternatively, perform cavernosal reconstruction: Incise the scar tissue, lay the prosthesis in the resulting trough, and rebuild the outer wall of the corpus cavernosum using a synthetic material such as Gore-Tex or Dacron.

Commentary by John J. Mulcahy

This class of prostheses is important in the armamentarium of penile implants. Ease of insertion and, in most cases, ease of operation are their advantages. The malleable and mechanical rods (AMS 600, Mentor Malleable and AccuForm, and Dura II) are easy to operate and are indicated in situations of impaired manual or mental dexterity. This group is most easily inserted via a ventral penile or subcoronal incision, where the proximal part of the cylinder is inserted first and the distal portion of the corporotomy is lifted over the distal end of the prosthesis with a vein retractor. This avoids the need to bend the device, which would require a longer corporotomy and, in the case of the Dura II, might stress the mechanical parts. The ventral penile incision offers more abundant subcutaneous tissue for layered closure and avoids overlapping suture lines.

These implants come in a choice of widths. Prior to opening the presterilized packages, the appropriate width is determined by placing two Hegar dilators of the smaller width into each corporal body side by side, first proximally and then distally.

The operator then apposes his thumb to index finger between the dilators. A slight separation or movement of the dilators between the fingers indicates an ideal fit. No movement is a tight fit. If the thumb touches the index finger, a loose fit is present and the wider cylinders should be chosen. In selecting an appropriate length, cylinders 0.5 cm shorter than the measured total corporal length allows the device to bend more freely with less spring-back and bowing. The Dynaflex, the only hydraulic prosthesis in this group, can easily be placed through any of the incisions described in the text. It is still somewhat difficult to inflate, although the deflation technique is much simpler than that of its predecessor, the Hydroflex. Tips on length and width sizing are the same as for the other unitary prostheses. If mechanical malfunction occurs with any of these devices, they can simply be removed and new cylinders inserted via the original implanting incision using a penile block as for a circumcision. Anesthetizing the corporal bodies is unnecessary.

Insertion of Inflatable Prosthesis

At present, several types of prosthesis are available (see Table 1). The choice lies among (1) the single-component prosthesis, either nonhydraulic or hydraulic, which has the advantage of being quicker to install and less prone to failure, but does not increase in girth or length, does not become as flaccid as two-piece prostheses, and costs more; (2) a two-piece hydraulic prosthesis; and (3) a three-piece hydraulic prosthesis. In the two- and three-piece devices, a combination of scrotal pump and reservoir provides increased girth during inflation. The technique for insertion of the AMS 700CX is described. For penile straightening in cases of Peyronie's disease (see page 201), this is the best selection.

Either a pubic or a penoscrotal approach is satisfactory for insertion. The perineal route is no longer used, but if a perforation of the crura occurs when placing the cylinders, a perineal approach allows closure. Consider a simpler prosthesis (semi-rigid or malleable, see page 179).

Preparation. Perform urine cultures several days before operation and treat infection if a culture is positive. Have the patient arrive 2 hours before surgery. Obtain a urine specimen for a second culture.

1. Start broad-spectrum intravenous antibiotics (an aminoglycoside and cephalosporin) immediately before operation, and continue them for 2 to 7 days. They should cover both *Staphylococcus epidermidis* and gram-negative organisms.
2. Have the patient take a povidone-iodine shower.
3. Shave the operative site in the operating room area.
4. Perform a 10-minute skin and hand scrub.
5. Wear a hood (optional) and use lint-free drapes.
6. Limit operating room traffic.

Instruments: Provide a GU Fine set, Hegar or Pratt uterine dilators, Furlow sizer and cylinder insertion tool, 2.5-inch Keith needle, four straight and four curved Providence Hospital clamps shod with clear tubing, Babcock clamps, perineal ring retractor (Turner-Warwick or Scott), two small Deaver retractors, two thyroid retractors, AMS tubing passer, appropriate prostheses of all sizes, Jackson-Pratt drains (7 mm), 22-gauge angiocatheter, 12 F silicone balloon catheters, and irrigation solution of bacitracin 50,000 units and neomycin 1 g in 500 ml of normal saline. Sutures include 2-0 polydioxanone (PDS), 0 PDS, 3-0 plain catgut (PCG), and 4-0 Maxon or Vicryl.

Premix 75 ml of iothalamate meglumine (Cysto-Conray II) solution (60 ml contrast solution with 15 ml sterile water).

PUBIC APPROACH

Inserting the AMS 700CX Prosthesis

1 *Anesthesia:* General or regional.
Position: Supine. Insert a 12 F balloon catheter.
Incision: Make a transverse incision across the midportion of the symphysis.

Reservoir Implantation

2 Incise the rectus sheath horizontally or vertically to expose the prevesical space. Evacuate the bladder. Develop a pocket digitally for the reservoir under the rectus muscle to the left or right of the midline. Be sure to make it large enough to accommodate the reservoir and so avoid the complication of reservoir trapping and subsequent spontaneous erections. Remove the packaged solution from the reservoir with a blunt-tipped needle and a 60-ml syringe. Clamp the tubing with a mosquito clamp that has been shod with some excess silicone tubing.

Alternative (Hirsch): Insufflate the prevesical space with a 200-ml balloon through a laparoscopy trocar. Remove trocar and balloon and insert the reservoir.

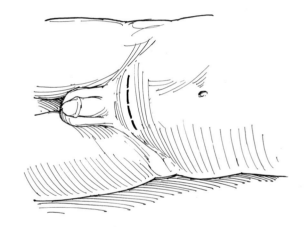

3 Irrigate the prevesical space with antibiotic solution. Place the reservoir in the space and bring the tubing out midway between the rectus muscles. Check to be sure that the pocket is large enough. Close the rectus sheath with 2-0 interrupted SAS. Fill the reservoir with the appropriate amount (65 or 100 ml) of sterile saline. Clamp the tubing with a shod mosquito clamp.

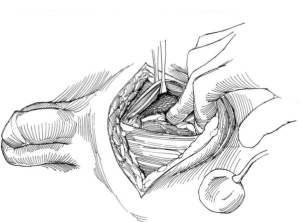

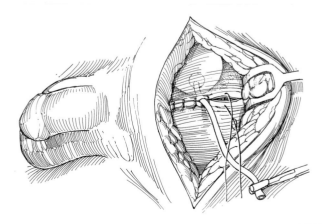

Cylinder Insertion

4 Expose the base of the penis by retracting the lower margin of the wound. Clear the dartos and Buck's fascia over each corpus cavernosum down to the tunica albuginea. If the operation is done under local anesthesia, consider injecting 10 ml of 1 percent lidocaine with epinephrine into a corpus and waiting 5 minutes. Place stay sutures bilaterally and make a 2-cm incision in the right (or left) corpus as proximally as convenient, avoiding the midline neurovascular bundle.

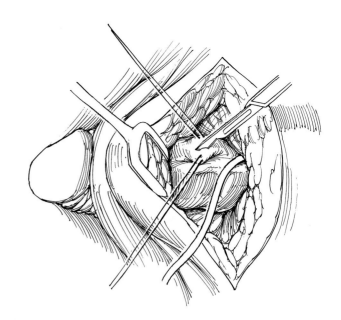

5 **A** and **B,** Initiate dissection within the corpus with Metzenbaum scissors followed by gentle dilation by a sequence of uterine dilators, 8 to 13 mm in diameter (Hegar sizes 7 to 13, Pratt sizes 25 to 33), distally and proximally. Dilate to one Hegar size larger than the cylinder diameter, making certain that the dilation is complete to the tip of the penis, well under the glans. Keep the curve of the dilator laterally. Take care not to perforate the septum between the corpora cavernosa nor to damage the urethra, especially when inserting the smaller dilators. Palpation of the dilator through the cavernous wall with traction on the penis facilitates distal dilation and reduces the chance of perforation. If a perforation is recognized, direct the dilator laterally and place the implant so that a sheath forms around it. For *distal perforation,* usually into the urethra, close the defect and abandon implantation, placing a balloon catheter and reoperating in 3 months. If the perforation is only through the tunica and the correct space is subsequently found, usually no repair is needed. *Proximal perforation* is recognized by the dilator not seating solidly in the crus on the periosteum or by an abnormally long corporal measurement. In rare cases it may need to be treated by direct perineal repair or by application of a synthetic cup. In general, if you can re-enter the appropriate proximal corporal space, no repair is necessary because the exit tubing holds the proximal portion of the prosthesis in place until healing occurs.

An *SST deformity* occurs when the end of a cylinder is not properly situated in the subglanular region, usually due to inadequate dilation. In some cases the corpora do not extend distally enough under the glans; this situation requires a dorsal tuck (Ball procedure).

Fixation of the glans can be done if the glans appears to be too mobile after the cylinders are implanted and the glans does not adequately cover the lateral surface of the tip of the cavernous bodies (de Stefani et al, 1994). Fully inflate the cylinders and make a small transverse subcoronal incision. Dissect on the tunica albuginea lateral to the urethra under the glans cap to mobilize the glans wings. Place a horizontal mattress suture of 3-0 SAS or nonabsorbable suture (NAS) material to attach the anterolateral surface of the glans wings to the tunica albuginea of the corpora. Avoid puncture of the tip of a cylinder with the needle. Tie the suture to bring the glans wings over the tip of the corpora. Close the subcoronal incision with a fine running subcuticular suture.

If the corpora are involved in *cavernous fibrosis,* try the routine method of insertion first, but if this fails, proceed at once with cavernosal reconstruction. Incise the penile skin circumferentially in the coronal sulcus and peel it back. Starting proximally, open the corpus 1 cm at a time to be able to divide it in half. It may be necessary to excise some of the fibrous tissue during this process. With persistence it is usually possible to dilate the corpora proximally. Once adequate space has been developed, lay the prosthesis in the defect and cover it with synthetic mesh (Gore-Tex), held in place with a running 4-0 Prolene suture.

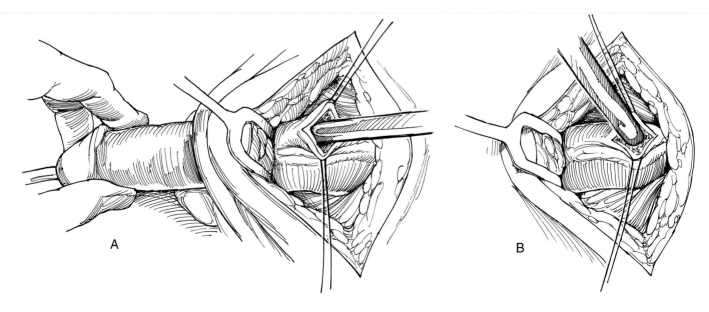

A

B

6 Measure the length needed for the prosthesis with the cylinder insertion tool. Ultrex cylinders are provided in 12-, 15-, 18-, and 21-cm lengths with one, two, or three rear tip extenders available. Select the appropriate cylinder length, with or without rear tip extenders, to adequately fill the corporal space without buckling of the prosthesis. Take care in the measurements because the prosthesis must fit completely within the corpora and the tubing must exit from the corporal space without buckling of the prosthesis to prevent kinks and wear. Avoid oversizing, especially with the Ultrex prosthesis; when 0.5-cm measurements are obtained, reduce the total length to the next smaller size.

7 Empty the cylinder and refill it to capacity with normal saline. Implant the cylinder using the Furlow cylinder insertion tool (FIT). Double-thread a suture on a Keith needle, and draw it back into the slot in the tip of the FIT. Be sure that the needle is completely retracted before insertion.

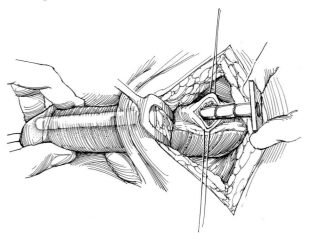

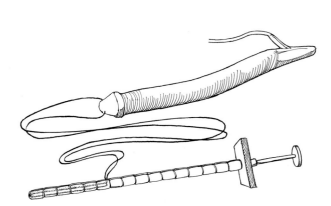

8 Pass the FIT to the distal end of the corpus and eject the needle through the dorsal glans at the tip of the corpus cavernosa, usually about 1 to 2 cm lateral and 1 cm proximal to the meatus. Grasp the needle with a clamp and remove the FIT. Pull the needle the rest of the way out and clamp the suture.

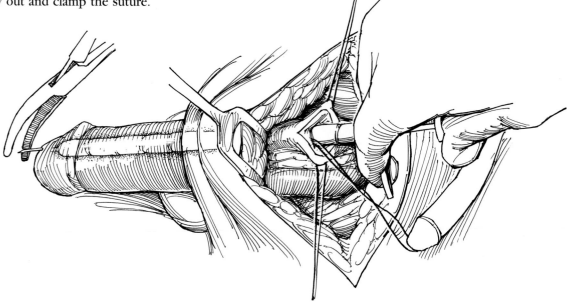

9 Pull the cylinder into the corpus by traction on the suture, being sure that its tip rests at the extreme tip of the corpus, well under the glans, and that the cylinder is not kinked within the corpus.

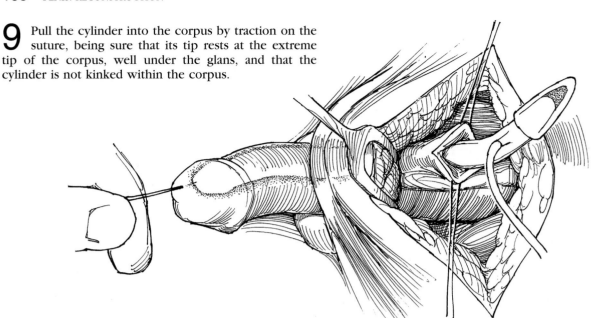

10 Partially deflate the cylinder. Pass the proximal end with or without a rear tip extender into the proximal crus. Proper position can be checked by palpation along the outer surface of the crus. It may help to insert the rear tip extender first, then insert the rear tip itself. If the crus was inadvertently perforated, either make a Dacron sock to cover the rear tip extender or approach the area perineally and close the defect. Close the tunica albuginea with interrupted 2-0 SAS that include the previously placed stay sutures. Repeat the procedure on the other side. Take care not to cross over when ejecting the needle and thereby puncture the opposite prosthesis. To avoid this, you may place both traction sutures before drawing the cylinders into the penis. Test the cylinders by simultaneous inflation with normal saline to be certain that they are correctly placed and that a symmetric erection is produced. Clamp only with plastic-shod clamps and never overinflate the cylinders, which could lead to an aneurysm or rupture. After inflation, remove the fluid and clamp the tubing with shod clamps.

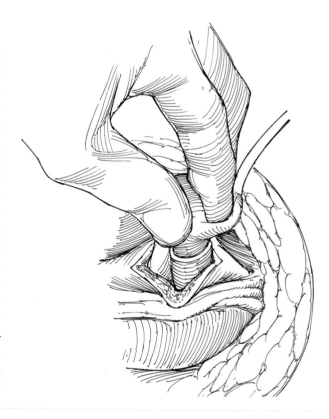

Because the most common cause of a leak is wear of the input tubing to the cylinder where it makes contact with the inflated cylinder, placement of a rear tip extender can provide a direct line for the tubing to exit from the tunica albuginea.

Insertion of the Pump

Have the scrub nurse remove air from the pump by compressing it sequentially while the reservoir tubing is submerged in normal saline. This is an important step to prevent air locks in the pump.

11 Either digitally or with a large Hegar dilator, create a scrotal pouch beneath the dartos layer lateral to the testicle and the spermatic cord. Be certain that the pouch is large and deep enough to allow the pump to lie in the most dependent portion of the scrotum, well below the penoscrotal junction. The pump should be placed in the right or left hemiscrotum, depending on the patient's preference, whether the patient is right- or left-handed, and whether previous scrotal surgery has been performed.

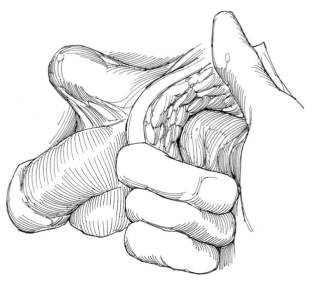

12 Irrigate the pouch with antibiotic solution and insert the pump, placing the deflation button and the reservoir tubing anterolaterally.

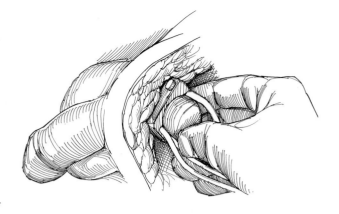

13 Hold the pump in place with a single click of Babcock clamps around the tubing above the pump. Clean the tubing and cut it; trim it to correct lengths with dry scissors. First join the tubing from the pump to the reservoir. Use a straight plastic quick connector: Insert the locking rings over the ends of the tubing. Insert the central connector in one end, flush the tubing, and insert it in the other end. Lock the rings and connector with the assembly tool. Be certain that the pump has been pulled down into the scrotum so that neither tension nor redundancy occurs. Then join the tubes from each cylinder to those from the pump with right-angle plastic connectors in a similar manner (straight connectors may be required on occasion to prevent kinks). Remove all clamps. *Note:* If a single component is being replaced because of a fluid leak, use standard connectors with reinforcing 4-0 Prolene sutures rather than quick connectors.

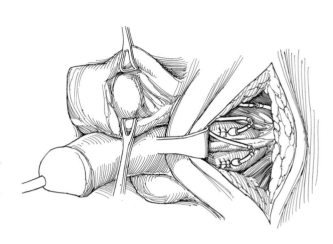

Testing the Prosthesis

Inflate the prosthesis several times to be sure that the tubing is not obstructed and that the cylinders inflate symmetrically, are in proper position, and deflate properly. Remove the traction suture in the penis by cutting one segment at the glans and pulling the other free. Close the wound in two layers over the tubing, with 3-0 plain suture in the subcutaneous tissue and a 4-0 subcuticular SAS for the skin. Place a 3.2-mm diameter Jackson-Pratt drain in the subcutaneous tissue and dependent portion of the scrotum, bringing it out through a separate stab wound and securing it to the skin with 2-0 silk. Leave the drain for 24 to 48 hours postoperatively, to prevent scrotal swelling that might make manipulation of the pump difficult. Place a 12 F balloon catheter in the bladder, to remain overnight, particularly if spinal anesthesia has been used.

Maintain the penis on the abdomen as much as possible during the healing phase and have ice packs applied for 24 hours. Avoid immediate inflation of the device.

Commentary by William L. Furlow

There are very few hard-and-fast rules pertaining to the implantation of the inflatable penile prosthesis, Model AMS 700, using the pubic approach. In my opinion, the ideal incision for the pubic operation is a transverse one made over the midportion of the symphysis because this avoids any extension of the scar onto the shaft of the penis at its base. Once the reservoir is placed in a space paravesically, the kink-resistant tubing can be passed through the midline between the rectus muscles and through the incision in the rectus sheath without fear of a kink developing as a result of angulation.

The most critical part of the operation is the accurate development of cavernous tunnels for measurement and cylinder placement. The key point to keep in mind is that when an inflatable cylinder is to be positioned in the cavernous body, the number of rear tip extenders to be used should be kept to a minimum. This necessitates placing the cavernotomy incision as far proximally as possible. In my experience, the average total length of rear tips to be added to the proximal end of the inflatable cylinder rarely exceeds 3 cm. When measurements suggest the need to add 5 cm of rear tip extender to a certain length of prosthesis, the solid portion of the device may be projected forward onto the shaft of the penis, where it is palpable and where it can cause a "water-hydrant" type of erection. Whenever the proximal measurement suggests the use of 5 cm of rear tip extender or even 4 cm, the surgeon should assess the possibility of extending the incision proximally for 1 or 2 cm more, to reduce the size of the extender to be added. A reduction of the size of the extender in turn increases the length of the inflatable cylinder to be implanted, a more optimal situation.

Great care should be taken not to oversize the total length of the prosthesis. This problem can be avoided by making measurements through a small, 1- to 1.5-cm cavernotomy incision before enlarging the incision. Measurements in 0.5 cm (e.g., 17.5 or 18.5 cm) should be reduced to the next smaller even size for total length. Oversizing carries a significant risk of penile curvature and the buckling phenomenon. Undersizing by 1.5 to 1 cm with the inflatable penile prosthesis rarely if ever results in an SST deformity but it significantly minimizes or eliminates any risk of buckling or penile curvature.

PENOSCROTAL APPROACH

Position: Modified lithotomy.

Anesthesia: General anesthesia or local anesthesia by infiltration of the inguinal area, including the subcutaneous tissue, external ring, and cord with 1 percent lidocaine. Insert a 12 F balloon catheter.

Cylinder Insertion

14 Incise vertically in the midline for 3 cm at the penoscrotal junction, then divide the subcutaneous tissue and dartos fascia lateral to the urethra. Use the urethral catheter to identify the course of the urethra. Place stay sutures not more than 2 to 3 mm on either side of the corpus spongiosum. Open the tunic of each corpus cavernosum between stay sutures well posteriorly so that the input tube remains as far proximal as possible in the scrotum. This also prevents the junction of the distensible and nondistensible portions of the cylinder from being felt by the patient and ensures that the joint is proximal to the hinge of the penis. Proper cylinder sizing and selection of appropriate rear tip extender results in the tubing exiting from the tunica albuginea at a right angle. Tunnel and dilate as described for the pubic approach; measurement is done in the same way. Insert the cylinder distally with the Furlow insertion tool; add the rear tip extender and insert this end proximally. Close the incision around the tubing with a 2-0 PDS suture.

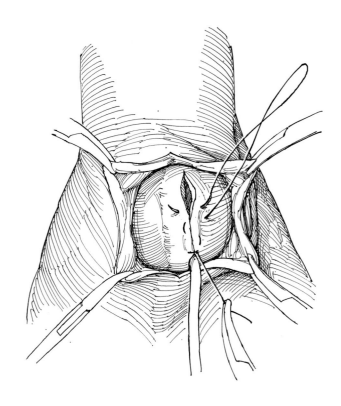

Reservoir Insertion

15 Evacuate the bladder. Palpate the pubic tubercle with a finger through the scrotal incision, and feel for the external ring.

16 Pass the closed blades of Metzenbaum scissors through the thin transversalis fascia below and medial to the cord. Enlarge this opening with the tip of the index finger and develop a pouch behind the symphysis and anterior to the bladder.

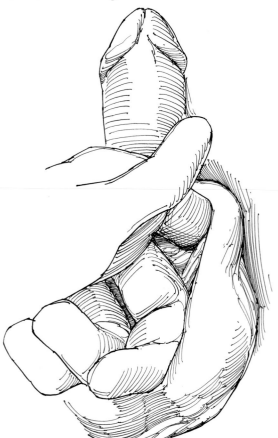

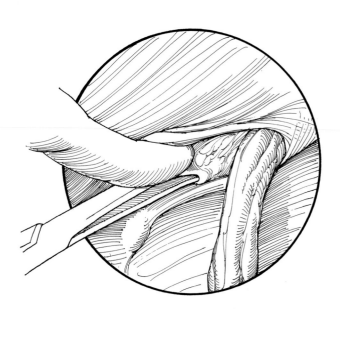

17 Insert the reservoir on its insertion tool through a long-nosed nasal speculum and fill it with an appropriate amount of sterile saline. Whether the reservoir space is too small can be determined by watching for back pressure on the syringe when the reservoir is filled to the proper amount. *Note:* If, after filling the reservoir with the syringe connected, the syringe begins to refill, the space that has been created is not adequate.

18 Pull on the tubing to set the reservoir against the floor of Hesselbach's triangle. Close the defect with one or two stitches if the opening is so large that the reservoir bulges into subcutaneous tissue of the inguinal region.

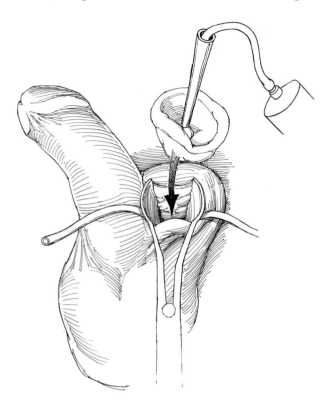

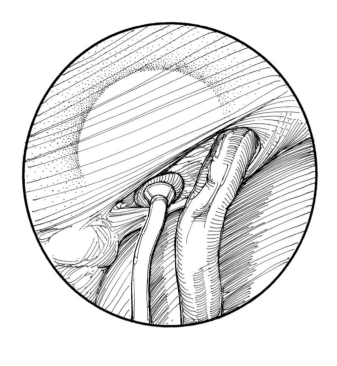

Pump Insertion

19 Insert the pump in the scrotum and connect the tubing using quick connectors. The tubing from the pump to the cylinder in the opposite hemiscrotum should pierce the scrotal septum to hold the pump in an inferior position and prevent its rotation. Test the connections by gentle traction, and cycle the prosthesis to determine if it inflates and deflates properly. Close the wound in two layers. Leave the cylinders deflated.

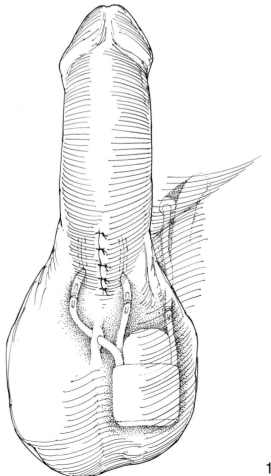

POSTOPERATIVE CARE

Provide a scrotal ice pack. Keep the patient head down for a day, and maintain catheter drainage overnight. Keep the penis against the abdomen with jockey shorts to prevent scar fixation in a nonerect position. Continue antibiotic prophylaxis for the first week. Check the position of the pump daily. After 5 days, instruct the patient how to keep the pump in position and how to manipulate it. He should perform progressive inflate-deflate exercises during the first month, and daily thereafter for at least 6 months.

Warn the patient of the risk of infection. Have prophylactic antibiotics provided for any procedure, such as dental manipulation, that carries a risk of bacteremia.

POSTOPERATIVE PROBLEMS

Delayed climax and ejaculation result from too little emotional input during "mechanical" intercourse. *Failure to meet expectations* can be a serious complication. Possible causes are inadequate counseling preoperatively, unreasonable expectations of the patient, and not involving the sexual partner in the discussion.

Spontaneous erections can be problems with inflatable prostheses. If a prosthesis is not kept deflated, the empty reservoir may become encased in scar. Too small a space may have been provided for the reservoir, or it may have been placed too near a muscle. In some muscular patients, during the Valsalva maneuver or straining, intra-abdominal pressure rises above 30 cm H_2O and an erection results. *Loss of glans sensation* may result from pressure from a dressing, from injury to the dorsal bundle, from placement of a subcoronal incision, or from infection.

A *high-riding pump* may be the result of tight clothes and neglect by the patient to pull it down into the scrotum several times a day. Rarely does it require reoperation. An *aneurysm* may rarely form in the cylinder from overinflation or inadequate closure of the incision in the corpus. It requires replacement of the cylinder with or without a synthetic patch to reconstruct the corpus. An *S-deformity* may result if cylinders that are capable of expanding in length (Ultrex) when placed are slightly too long because of inexact sizing. Remove that cylinder and substitute an AMS CX or Mentor prosthesis (Wilson et al, 1996).

Mechanical complications occur less frequently with the new devices. *Failure to inflate* can be the result of air or blood in the system. *Leaks* can occur from any area in the device, but most commonly they occur from the cylinders. When the device fails to inflate, reoperation is required. At exploration, open one of the connectors and connect an ohmmeter to detect loss of resistance. If this does not localize the leak, expose and disconnect all three connectors, then test each component separately. If the leak is in a cylinder, replace both of them. Use the electrocautery to dissect along the tubing until the cylinder is exposed, being careful not to injure the urethra.

Infection involving the prosthesis usually requires its removal, although salvage is sometimes possible. First determine if the problem is actual infection or ischemic necrosis because salvage is more likely with the latter. Usually this is obvious at the operating table. Administer vancomycin and an aminoglycoside until cultures are able to identify the organism, then switch to the appropriate antibiotic. In the vast majority of cases, if infection is present, the device must be removed and the scrotum and corpora irrigated with an antibiotic solution (gentamicin 80 mg, neomycin 500 mg, and polymyxin 100 mg in 1 L of saline) through fenestrated suction drains for 6 or 8 hours a day for a week. Irrigation is important to decrease the intracavernous fibrosis that will be encountered when replacement is attempted later.

Immediate replacement (Brant et al, 1996). Whether the device should be removed before irrigating is a matter of judgment, although success as high as 91 percent has been reported with complete removal of the infected device and its replacement at the same operation in favorable cases (no necrotic tissue, slowly developing infections not associated with bacteremia, and freedom from urethral erosion). With this technique, clear the spaces of all foreign material. Through a red rubber catheter, systematically and thoroughly irrigate the corpora, reservoir pocket, and pump pocket using 80 mg/L kanamycin and 1 g/L bacitracin solution first, followed in succession by half-strength hydrogen peroxide, half-strength povidone-iodine solution, pressure irrigation with 5 L of normal saline containing 1 g vancomycin and 80 mg gentamicin, half-strength povidone-iodine solution, half-strength hydrogen peroxide, and finally kanamycin-bacitracin irrigation. Change gloves and add fresh drapes. Insert a new prosthesis. Continue ciprofloxacin for 1 month.

Erosion of a cylinder into the urethra is less common with inflatable prostheses than with semirigid ones. Erosion distally is the result of impaired sensation caused by the presence of a balloon catheter or implantation of too long a cylinder. The infrequent proximal erosion is usually the consequence of unrecognized perforation at the time of implantation. Erosion, especially into the balloon, does not usually require removal of the prosthesis, but the chance of salvage is reduced if it is accompanied by infection. Impending distal erosion should be treated immediately with removal of the prosthesis and repair of the distal tunica with or without placement of synthetic material. If the device has eroded through the urethra, it must be removed and drains must generally be placed to irrigate the corpus cavernosum with antibiotic solution in anticipation of later replacement with a cylinder of the proper size.

REOPERATION

Make every effort to avoid the risk of a *two-stage procedure*, with its attendant chance for infection. If a second operation is done, insert a prosthesis 1.67 cm longer.

Reoperation after the corpora have become fibrotic can be very difficult. If you wait an extended period for the inflammation to subside, fibrosis will be extremely dense. Therefore consider immediate salvage after the prosthesis has been removed and the infection cleared.

Selection of an incision or combination of incisions is critical. If a degloving incision is necessary, a circumcision should be done at the same time. Occasionally a perineal incision may be needed to allow multiple corporotomy incisions in order to dilate the corpora adequately. Proximal dilation is significantly easier than distal dilation, and it is usually during distal dilation that urethral injury occurs. Bivalve the corpora and core out the fibrous tissue, doing it 1 cm at a time. After coring, cover the device with a Gore-Tex patch held in place with a running 4-0 Prolene suture. The chance for urethral injury is appreciable.

Commentary by Ralph C. Benson, Jr.

The choice of incision for implantation of an inflatable penile prosthesis is certainly one of surgeon preference, but I personally believe that the infrapubic approach is the most versatile and complication free. A transverse incision and not a longitudinal incision over the pubis should be made, as this prevents the possibility of longitudinal scarring and subsequent penile tearing. Although rare, a penoscrotal incision can result in ventral chordee and significant penile deformity, necessitating revision. In addition, the infrapubic approach allows for performance of a Sabrini procedure or a UY-plasty for penile lengthening (primarily in patients with scarring secondary to previous surgery). An infrapubic incision also presents easy access to the paravesical space for reservoir placement and for easy removal of the reservoir if necessary in the future. Placement of the reservoir within the inguinal canal through a penoscrotal approach often results in difficulty removing the reservoir if revision is necessary.

Certainly, one of the most critical parts of the operation is accurate development of cavernous tunnels for measurement and cylinder placement. After a corporotomy incision is made, many surgeons try to carefully pass closed Metzenbaum scissors proximally and distally to judge not only distance but also the possible presence of corporal fibrosis. Dilation with Hegar dilators is usually possible. However, in the very obese patient, Mentor offset dilators occasionally facilitate this process. The corporotomy incision should be placed as far proximally as technically feasible. If there appears to be need for more than 3 cm of rear tip extender, the corporotomy incision may be too far distal. I believe that sutures should be placed around the corporotomy incision prior to insertion of the cylinders. This obviates possible cylinder damage when one closes the corporotomy incision after placement of the cylinder and also allows the procedure to be done more expeditiously; if the sutures are not pre-placed, use great care and a cylinder protection tool in order not to violate the cylinder.

It is most important not to oversize the total length of the prosthesis. This problem can be avoided by making measurements through a small, 1- to 1.5-cm cavernotomy incision before enlarging the incision so that measurements are more accurate. Measurements ending in 0.5 should be reduced to the next smaller size. This is especially important with placement of the Ultrex prosthesis, which elongates when inflated and adequately fills the corpora cavernosa.

Although surgeons do not agree as to whether or not drains should be used in penile prosthetic surgery, I routinely do so. A small round drain is placed adjacent to the pump and brought out through a separate stab wound on the opposite side of the incision. Although in the past these drains were periodically irrigated with antibiotic solution, that is no longer my practice. The drain is left for approximately 24 hours and then removed if drainage is not excessive. No evidence indicates that placement of drains increases infection rates in patients undergoing penile prosthesis implantation, and they appear to reduce scrotal edema and shorten hospitalization time.

Certain controversial issues arise when discussing complications during implantation and also during redo implantations. The usual advice given when urethral perforation has occurred during corporeal dilation is to abandon the procedure and return at a later date for implantation. Certainly, this is a reasonable approach. However, when the urethral perforation is identified and easily accessible and is not particularly extensive, immediate urethral repair and implantation of the device are often successful. If the existing device eroded distally to the urethra, device removal and later implantation are advisable. If distal erosion of the corpora cavernosa has occurred, whether the erosion has been through the urethra or not, an Ultrex prosthesis should not be reimplanted because this cylinder may exert undue distal pressure during elongation.

If immediate infection requires removal of a prosthetic device, the usual procedure is to remove the entire prosthetic device (I would advise against retaining any component, if possible) and to place drains within the corpora cavernosa, scrotum, and paravesical space for irrigation with antibiotic solution for a period of time. After adequate healing has occurred, the patient should be instructed to use a vacuum suction device once a day to attempt to maintain the distal corporeal space. I have found that this practice markedly facilitates subsequent implantation.

Alternatively, if immediate infection is noted, under certain circumstances a salvage procedure can be performed. The infected device should be removed, drains placed, and the infected space irrigated over several days. Frequently, one can then place a semirigid rod prosthesis to maintain the corporeal space until reimplantation of an inflatable device can be performed 3 or more months later. Although the possibility of a lingering infection is always a concern in these patients, this approach is often necessary and successful in the patient who has had multiple previous operations.

Penile Arterial Revascularization

Revascularization can be done by several techniques, all of which have limitations. The operation that has been most successful connects the inferior epigastric artery to the dorsal artery.

In a selected group of patients under the age of 60, make the diagnosis of reduced arterial inflow by the intracavernous injection and stimulation (CIS) test and by duplex ultrasonography. Use color Doppler imaging to detect communications between the dorsal and cavernous arteries and the direction of blood flow. Locate the site of the block by phalloarteriography, and be sure that a segment of the penile artery communicating with the cavernous artery is patent. Rule out psychogenic impotence by performing a nocturnal penile tumescence test and venous leakage by cavernosometry.

Instruments: Provide the following: a Basic set, a GU plastic set, a GU micro set, a special hook made by bending the end of a blunt-tipped knitting needle upon itself 180 degrees, an Andrews suction tip, a bipolar hand electrode, a microscope and drape, a bulb syringe, Weck spears, microwipes, visibility background, vascular loops, vessel clips, a skin drill, a three-power loupe, vascular sutures, a padded adjustable stool, a 7-mm Jackson-Pratt drain, 2 percent lidocaine, a 12-ml syringe with blunt 18-gauge needle, heparinized saline in a 6-ml syringe with a 20-gauge angiocatheter sheath, 9-0 Dermalon sutures with an LE-100 needle, and 10-0 Dermalon sutures with a TE-100 needle.

Position: Place the patient supine, and prepare the area with organic iodine solution. Place a balloon catheter.

SECURING THE EPIGASTRIC ARTERY

Obtain the artery after preparing the bed into which it will be placed to shorten its warm ischemia time.

1 **A,** Stand on the left side of the table. Make a vertical lower abdominal incision two fingerbreadths from the midline. Alternatively, make an oblique incision in Langer's lines. **B,** Incise the anterior rectus sheath over the center of the muscle, open the sheath with scissors, and retract it laterally with Kocher clamps.

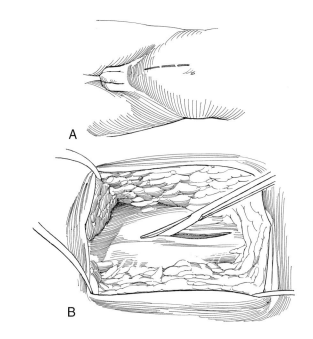

2 Expose and dissect the inferior epigastric artery, including its two accompanying veins, from the connective tissue underlying the muscle and hold it in a vascular tape. Continue dissecting cephalad for 15 to 16 cm to free two major branches; clip and divide them 2 to 3 cm from their bifurcation. This allows selection of the branch of the same size as the dorsal artery for the arterial anastomosis. Divide and ligate other, more proximal vascular branches. Apply papaverine hydrochloride topically to reduce arterial spasm.

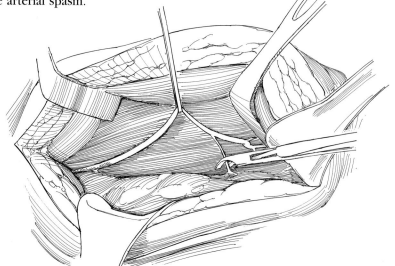

EXPOSURE OF THE PENILE VASCULATURE

3 **A,** Make a hockey-stick incision at one side of the base of the penis, beginning at the pubic tubercle and extending into the upper portion of the scrotum through the fundiform ligament (avoid dividing the ligament) to Buck's fascia at the depth of the neurovascular bundle. (Do not use a subpubic incision.) **B,** Expose the base of the penis and drag the shaft out of the wound.

Join the two incisions by digital dissection under the fundiform ligament. Obtain vascular control of the epigastric artery with a microvascular clamp at its proximal end, and occlude the distal end with clips. Divide the artery distally and draw the proximal end through the tunnel with a long curved clamp. Watch out for twisting and tension. Apply a microvascular clamp to the free ends and remove the one placed at the proximal end after placing a vessel loop to allow reapplication if needed later.

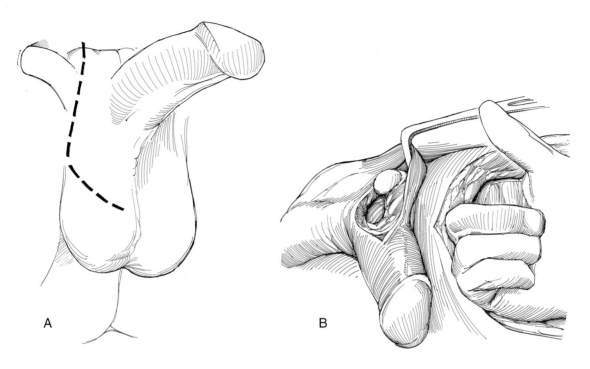

A

B

The surgeon has several choices for utilization of the epigastric artery, depending on the findings of arterial occlusion. The best solution usually is to connect the epigastric artery to the divided dorsal artery with an anastomosis of a branch both distally and proximally. Anastomosis to a segment of the deep dorsal vein, with or without an additional anastomosis to the dorsal artery, is an alternative.

EPIGASTRIC ARTERY–DORSAL ARTERY ANASTOMOSIS
(Michal)

4 *Arterial anatomy:* The internal pudendal artery, becoming the penile artery, passes through the urogenital diaphragm and along the medial margin of the inferior ramus of the pubis. As it passes the bulb, it divides into three terminal branches—the bulbourethral, the dorsal, and the cavernous arteries. The bulbourethral artery enters the bulb of the urethra. The dorsal artery of the penis runs along the dorsum of the penis between the deep dorsal vein lying medially and the dorsal nerve lying laterally to it. It divides into a number of circumflex branches that course with the corresponding veins to supply the corpus. The cavernous artery enters the corpus cavernosum at the base of the penis and runs to the tip, giving off the multiple helicine arteries in the cavernous spaces. Crural arteries, small branches of the main penile artery, supply the crura on both sides.

5 Position the microscope over the field. Expose one dorsal penile artery, a vessel that communicates with the cavernous artery. Free 3 cm of the artery proximally, avoiding the adjacent nerve fibers. Divide it and dilate the lumen of each end. Be very careful to avoid injury to the endothelium. Irrigate with papaverine solution. Clear the adventitia for a distance of 1 cm. Use bipolar coagulation for control of bleeding. Remove the microvascular clamp to check the flow in the epigastric artery. Place two small microvascular clamps on the dorsal penile artery, and transect it between them. Clear the adventitia and anastomose the distal end to one branch of the inferior epigastric artery by a microvascular technique (see page 60), using 12 or more sutures. If the vessels are different sizes, tailor them before anastomosis. Placement of a stent may prevent backwalling; take the stent out before inserting the last 4 sutures. Anastomose the second branch to the proximal end of the dorsal penile artery. Alternatively, insert each branch of the inferior epigastric artery into one of the dorsal arteries by an end-to-side technique.

Approximate the rectus sheath with interrupted sutures, allowing the artery to exit freely at the inferior end, and close the abdominal wound in the usual fashion. Bring Buck's fascia carefully over the artery and close the infrapubic skin defect.

Anticoagulation is not indicated. Discharge the patient the following day. Instruct the patient to avoid all sexual activity for 4 to 6 weeks. Remove the sutures in 7 days. Retest the patient with Doppler ultrasound recording in 6 weeks, and perform a more complete impotency evaluation at 6 months.

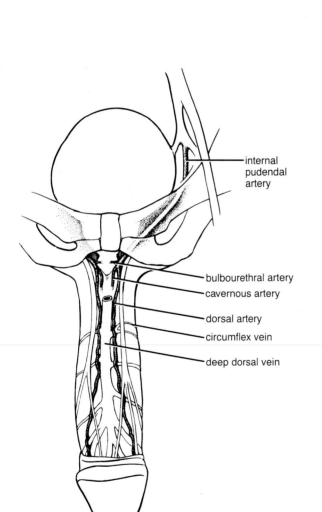

- internal pudendal artery
- bulbourethral artery
- cavernous artery
- dorsal artery
- circumflex vein
- deep dorsal vein

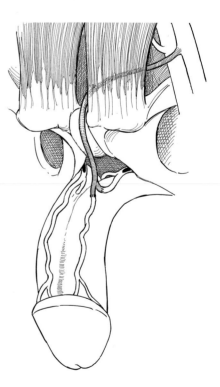

Other Procedures. Anastomosis of the epigastric artery directly to the cavernous arteries can be done (Crespo), but it is a technically difficult procedure. The second branch of the epigastric artery may be inserted into the opposite dorsal artery. Or the donor artery may be anastomosed end to side to one dorsal artery, then the artery swung across and connected end to end to the other dorsal artery. A length of greater saphenous vein may be used as a connection between the femoral artery and the cavernous artery (Crespo II). For younger men who have suffered injuries, the inferior epigastric artery may be inserted end to side in one dorsal artery (Michal II). Less effective is the earlier Michal I procedure that directly anastomosed the inferior epigastric artery to the corpus. In addition, the epigastric artery may be anastomosed to the dorsal vein (Goldstein).

EPIGASTRIC ARTERY–DORSAL VEIN ANASTOMOSIS
(Goldstein)

This technique is less effective than anastomosis of the epigastric artery to the dorsal artery.

Two centimeters lateral to the base of the penis make a curved incision that extends from the pubis to the scrotal raphe on the opposite side, from which the epigastric artery will be harvested. Through the dartos fascia, bluntly dissect proximally on the tunica albuginea to the level of the ischiopubic ramus and distally along the shaft to allow its extrusion. Preserve both the fundiform and suspensory ligaments by dissecting laterally, and make an opening between them to accommodate the epigastric artery. Expose the neurovascular bundle and deep dorsal vein. Divide and ligate the deep dorsal vein beneath the symphysis between the suspensory ligament and the urogenital diaphragm. Divide the valves with a 2-mm Leather valve cutter introduced from the distal part of the dorsal vein. Divide and ligate the vein.

Harvest the inferior epigastric artery with its vena comitans (Steps 2 to 4), and deliver it to the base of the penis between the suspensory and fundiform ligaments. Control the vein with vessel loops distally and proximally. Remove the adventitia for a distance of 2 to 4 cm. Make a dorsal venotomy and a similar arteriotomy, and anastomose the vessels with 8-0 nylon sutures. Release the vessel loops and observe blood filling the epigastric artery. Remove the clamp on the artery and observe venous pulsations.

Anastomose the second branch of the epigastric artery to the dorsal artery (Step 5).

POSTOPERATIVE PROBLEMS

Recurrent erections, occurring as often as 9 or 10 times a day, can endanger the anastomosis. Amyl nitrite inhalation may be helpful. *Disruption* of the arterial anastomosis can follow early sexual activity.

Commentary by Tom F. Lue

I prefer to confirm the diagnosis with a CIS test followed by duplex ultrasonography. A color Doppler scan is preferred because of its ability to detect communications between the dorsal and cavernous arteries and blood flow direction. Psychogenic impotence and venous leakage are ruled out with a nocturnal penile tumescence test and cavernosometry, respectively. The objectives of pharmacologic phalloarteriography are (1) to locate the site of blockage, (2) to confirm the presence of communications between the dorsal and cavernous arteries, and (3) to ensure that both the donor (the inferior epigastric) and recipient (dorsal) arteries are healthy.

I prefer a midline abdominal incision because it provides access to both epigastric arteries in case the first artery is not suitable for the intended surgery.

An adequate pressure gradient between the epigastric and dorsal arteries is critical to the success of the anastomosis. Therefore, I do the following before performing the anastomosis: Request the anesthesiologist to set up an arterial line. Puncture the dorsal artery with a 25-gauge angiocatheter to measure the arterial pressure by inserting the plastic sheath of the angio-catheter directly into the lumen of the transected artery. A pressure gradient of more than 15 mm Hg should exist to allow adequate flow through the anastomosis. If the gradient is less than 10 mm Hg, anastomosis to the dorsal vein is performed instead. I like to pass the epigastric artery through the inguinal ring, not through the inferior end of the rectus sheath, to avoid the possibility of kinking at the fascial level.

In the postoperative period, I prefer to start mini-heparin (5000 units subcutaneously every 12 hours for 2 days) after the anastomosis is completed, followed by daily baby aspirin or dypyridamole (Persantine) for 3 months.

The most dreadful complications are priapism (after epigastric artery–corpus cavernosum anastomosis) and glans hyperemia (epigastric artery–dorsal vein anastomosis). The former surgery is no longer performed. To prevent glans hyperemia, all the venous channels distal to the epigastric artery–dorsal vein anastomosis should be ligated to prevent overperfusion of the glans. Visualization of these channels can be facilitated by injecting saline with methylene blue into the dorsal vein before anastomosis is performed.

Correction of Penile Venous Leakage

Select patients with good arterial inflow and normal cavernosal tissue.

Consider the anatomy of the venous drainage from the penis.

It follows three pathways: (1) superficial, (2) intermediate, through the deep dorsal and circumflex veins, and (3) deep, through the cavernous and crural veins.

1 The *superficial system*, between Colles' and Buck's fascias, drains through a superficial dorsal vein into the saphenous vein. In the *intermediate drainage system*, one portion starts from many small veins that run from the glans into a single vein or multiple deep dorsal veins and then into the periprostatic plexus. Another portion arises from the more ventral aspect of the corpus spongiosum and from minute emissary veins emerging from the lateral and dorsal surfaces of the corpora cavernosa, which, combining as the circumflex veins, course around the lateral surfaces of the glans and also empty through common channels into the deep dorsal vein. The *deep system* drains from the proximal third of the penis as emissary veins, joining one or two cavernous veins buried in the septum. These veins enter the pudendal vein, which passes between the bulb and the crus of the penis. In addition, several small crural veins join together to run to the internal pudendal vein. Thus, it is evident that surgically occluding penile outflow is a complex problem.

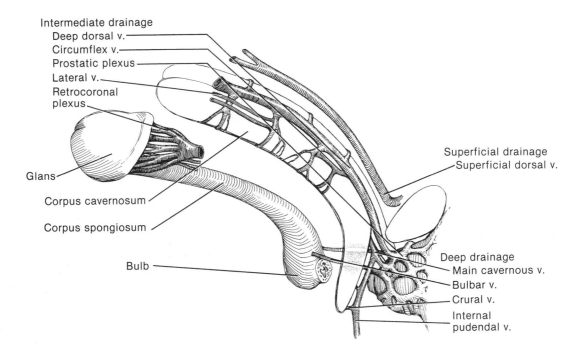

Intermediate drainage
Deep dorsal v.
Circumflex v.
Prostatic plexus
Lateral v.
Retrocoronal plexus
Glans
Corpus cavernosum
Corpus spongiosum
Bulb
Superficial drainage
Superficial dorsal v.
Deep drainage
Main cavernous v.
Bulbar v.
Crural v.
Internal pudendal v.

Select patients who do not respond to intracorporeal injections (papaverine, 40 to 60 mg, and phentolamine, 1 mg) and who have few risk factors for vasculogenic impotence. Check with a color Doppler examination, followed by infusion pharmacocavernosometry and cavernosography.

Instruments: Provide a Basic set, Gelpi and Weitlaner retractors, medium vascular forceps, three-power loupes, a butterfly needle, and a syringe filled with methylene blue well diluted with saline (2 ml methylene blue to 250 ml saline). Have the films from the contrast cavernosography study at hand. Give prophylactic antibiotics before and again after the operation.

Place the patient in a low lithotomy position.

198

2 **A,** Make a 3-inch oblique incision along the course of the spermatic cord at the upper scrotum, 1 inch lateral to the base of the penis. **B,** Bluntly dissect the root and pendulous part of the penis, and extrude the entire penile shaft into the wound (Lue). Detach the suspensory ligament from the pubic bone and the upper half of the crura from the ischium.

Insert a 19- or 21-gauge butterfly needle into one of the corpora and tie it in place with a purse-string suture, passing the ends of the suture around the cut-off wings of the needle for fixation. This allows evaluation before and after venous ligation. Inject 30 mg of papaverine through the butterfly needle. Wait 10 minutes and follow with 180 ml of the dilute methylene blue solution to determine the degree of tumescence before vein ligation and to detect small collateral veins.

Open Buck's fascia vertically. Identify the deep dorsal vein and circumflex veins. Dissect, doubly clamp, divide, and ligate any large veins that are seen draining into the external pudendal veins from the lateral surface of the tunica albuginea. Look for a direct communication between the tunica albuginea and these veins. If one is found, close it with a running suture of chromic catgut (CCG). Dissect along the deep dorsal vein, and pick up and individually ligate close to the tunica albuginea all the circumflex and emissary veins entering the dorsal vein.

3 Stay exactly in the midline during dissection of the deep dorsal vein to spare the neurovascular bundle. Stop short of the glans distally where the nerves running with the short glanular branches could be injured, but ligate each of the venous branches individually. The resection of the deep dorsal vein should continue up under the pubic bone; catch all the circumflex and emissary veins that are encountered. Ligate the dorsal vein proximally and distally, using silk or 2-0 SAS for ligation, and resect between the ligatures. (Nonabsorbable suture on the shaft may cause discomfort later, but silk can instigate granulomas.)

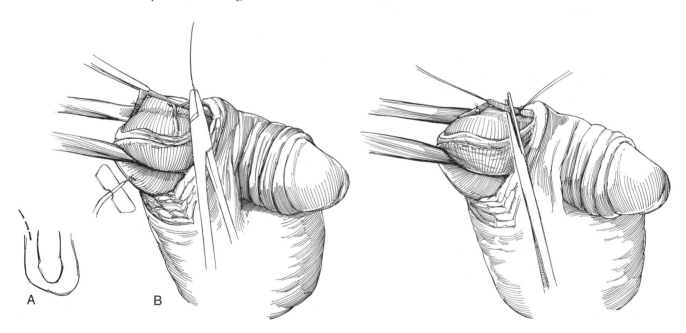

4 Divide the suspensory ligament to draw out the base of the penile shaft. Don three-power loupes or use a 5× operative microscope. Expose but do not dissect out the three or four cavernous veins; rather, ligate them carefully in situ with 2-0 silk ligatures swaged on needles, then divide them. Do the same for the crural veins. Use great skill to avoid the fine cavernous nerves and arteries.

Repeat the papaverine–methylene blue insufflation to allow detection of small collaterals, and review the cavernosogram to be sure all branches are ligated.

For *closure*, put traction on the penis and attach the suspensory ligament at a more proximal site on the shaft to add length to the penis. To prevent tethering, be sure to separate the body of the penis from the pubic arch by suturing a tongue of areolar tissue between them. Approximate Buck's fascia carefully to prevent adherence of the penile shaft to the skin, and close the wound by the usual technique, either without drainage or with a small Jackson-Pratt suction drain placed subcutaneously. Place a balloon catheter in older patients, to be removed the next morning. Use a very light elastic adhesive compression dressing on the shaft to reduce edema, and apply a scrotal support. (Check the glans every 3 to 4 hours to be sure compression is not excessive.) Remove the dressing in 5 days.

Other techniques have been used to correct venous leakage. The internal iliac vein may be tied; the crura may be ligated by a perineal approach; and detachable coils can be inserted or the associated veins embolized via the deep dorsal vein.

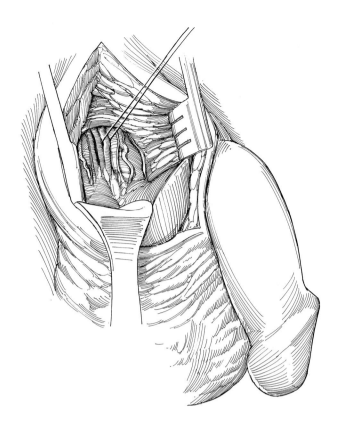

POSTOPERATIVE PROBLEMS

Penile edema is expected, but it usually resolves in 1 to 2 weeks. *Shortening* of the penis does not occur if the enumerated precautions are taken. *Hypesthesia* of the glans is the result of dissecting too distally on the dorsum.

Commentary by Eric Wespes

The technique described is the resection of the venous drainage in patients with venous leakage. The technique is described exactly as I performed it in the past.

Currently, I do only deep dorsal vein arterialization with ligature of the proximal part of the deep dorsal vein and of the distal part just close to the glans. I do this surgery in place of a complete resection because I believe that the results depend on the percentage of smooth muscle cells in the penis (Wespes et al, 1994).

The trouble that can occur with deep dorsal vein arterialization is formation of a slight hematoma and edema of the penis, but the most dangerous problem is hypervascularization of the glans. For this reason, I ligate the distal part of the deep dorsal vein.

Procedures for Peyronie's Disease

Wait until the patient has experienced no increased pain for at least 6 months and he reports that the curvature has stabilized but he still has difficulty with intercourse because of the curvature. Three procedures are available for correction: (1) For a short penis or one with an hour-glass deformity with adequate erectile function, apply a dermal, a synthetic, or, preferably, a venous graft; (2) for a penis of adequate length and function, tuck the tunica albuginea either ventrally or dorsally, depending on the angle of curvature (see page 174); and (3) for curvature associated with severe erectile dysfunction, place an inflatable prosthesis (see page 173) and then forcibly straighten the penis to break the plaque.

Be sure that the patient has a realistic expectation of the outcome. Evaluate the erectile function with duplex ultrasonography after intracavernous injection of 30 mCi of prostaglandin E_1. Have the patient supply a lateral Polaroid photograph of the erect organ.

GRAFT TECHNIQUES

Instruments: A GU plastic set, a 19-gauge butterfly scalp needle with a high-flow pump and 1-L bags of injectable normal saline solution, skin hooks, Bishop-Harman forceps, and a 0.5-inch Penrose drain. *Position*: Supine.

1 Prepare the genital area. Inject saline with a butterfly scalp needle into a corpus cavernosum through the glans and produce an artificial erection. A tourniquet at the penile base (shown) is not needed if a high-flow pump is used.

Alternative: Inject 1.5 to 2 ml of papaverine into the corpus cavernosum. Supplement this with compression of the crura or saline injection if rigidity is not adequate. Assess the deformity.

2 *Incision:* Make a circumcision incision, especially if the patient wishes to be circumcised. If he is already circumcised, cut through the easily visualized scar; it may be nearly at midshaft. Deglove the penis by dissecting in the layer between the deep dartos and Buck's fascia.

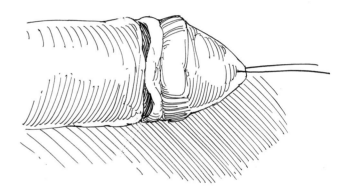

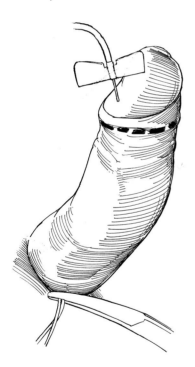

3 Elevate Buck's fascia beginning just lateral to the corpus spongiosum. Dissect with scissors against the tunica albuginea on either side of the corpus spongiosum. For congenital cases (ventral curvature), elevate the dorsal nerves and vessels and displace them first to one side and then to the other.

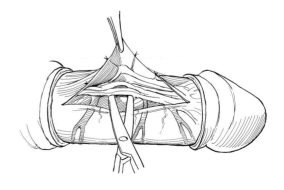

4 Place 3-0 NAS in the tunic on either side of the plaque. Mark the extent of the plaque with a marking pen. Create an artificial erection at this time to judge the effect of the plaque on the curvature.

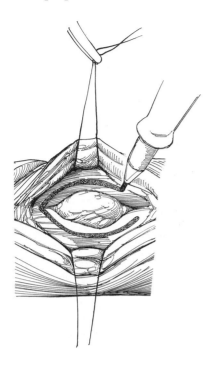

5 Using a #10 or 12 knife blade, excise the plaque by an incision that encompasses all of the identifiable scar and extends just through the tunica albuginea. Then elevate one edge of the plaque to allow careful dissection against the plaque, preferably using a knife. Do not include any of the spongy tissue beneath the plaque.

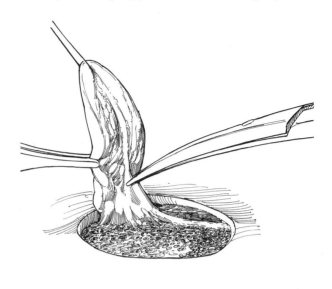

6 Make stellate relaxing incisions in the normal tunic surrounding the plaque. Place four fine nonabsorbable stay sutures at the four quadrants, well away from the line of incision. Measure the corporotomy defect both longitudinally and transversely by stretching the penis straight with the stay sutures.

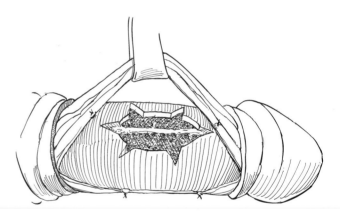

Dermal Graft Technique
(Devine)

7 **A,** Mark an ellipse of skin on the lower flank over the iliac crest lateral to the hairline, and remove the epidermis either free hand or with a dermatome set at approximately 0.012 inch. Then excise the dermis and close the donor site in two layers. Remove the subcutaneous tissue from the graft. **B,** Tack the graft to the inner edge and ends of the defect with four fine absorbable monofilament sutures; then run a suture along the entire inner edge, locking every third stitch. Fold the graft back and run a suture down the center of the graft, fixing it to the septal fibers in the midline. Place two more tacking sutures, and run a suture down the outer edge. Make sure the suture line is watertight by repeating the artificial erection, a maneuver that also proves that the deformity has been corrected. If it has not, further excision of the plaque is required.

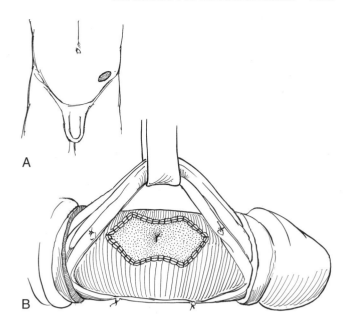

Incision and Vein Graft Technique
(Lue)

A segment of vein makes a more physiologic patch than dermis.

During erection, measure the length of the normal and diseased sides of the penis to determine the length of vein required. Proceed through Steps 1 to 4. Expose and take a segment from the deep dorsal vein. Alternatively, make a supramalleolar incision at the ankle, and obtain a segment of the saphenous vein.

8 **A,** Make an H-shaped relaxing incision through the plaque. Do not attempt to excise it. The CO_2 laser may be used to thin the plaque by evaporation (hold it parallel to the surface, set it at 5 watts, and apply 0.5-second bursts), but this may result in a venous leak because the tunica becomes paper thin after the evaporation. **B,** Open a segment of vein. If the defect is wider than the circumference of the vein, divide the vein segment and, with the aid of a loupe, suture two (or even three) open sections side by side with a continuous 4-0 monofilament SAS. Apply the patch to the defect endothelial side down with a continuous 4-0 monofilament

SAS. If multiple individual relaxing incisions were made, suture an open segment of vein into each of the defects (Moriel). Cover the graft as much as possible with Buck's fascia. Test with saline inflation for elimination of the curvature. If the curvature is overcorrected or if lateral curvature persists, place plication sutures in the ventral aspect of the penis without excision of an ellipse of the tunica albuginea (Step 9B). Close the wound with 4-0 CCG sutures and wrap the penis in a lightly compressive dressing, checking the glans after an hour to be sure the dressing is not too tight. Change the dressing in 24 hours, and instruct the patient in daily changes for 10 days. Intercourse is permitted in 6 weeks.

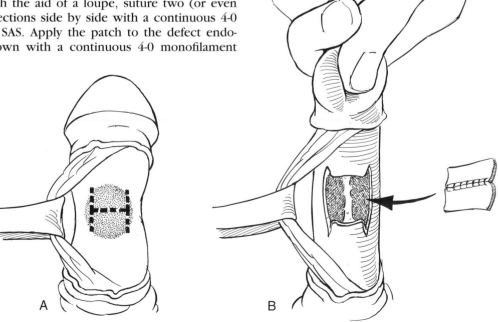

Synthetic Graft Technique
(Ganabathi et al)

Deglove the penis and apply a tourniquet at the base. Create an artificial erection through a butterfly needle, and mark the site of maximal deflection. Mobilize and retract the neurovascular bundle. Expose the plaque. Rather than excising the plaque, incise it transversely and open it widely. If necessary, make more than one slit in the plaque. Lay a 0.55-mm Gore-Tex graft into each defect and trim it to size. (Temporalis fascia has also been used.) Suture the graft in place with 3-0 braided synthetic NAS. Check the correction by reinflating the corpora.

Alternative: Mobilize a flap of tunica vaginalis through a separate incision at the neck of the scrotum (Helal et al, 1995). Bring it subcutaneously through the dorsal penile incision to cover the defect.

PLICATION TECHNIQUES

Ventral Tuck Technique
(Nesbit, Pryor-Fitzpatrick)

Create an artificial erection by rapid infusion of normal saline through a scalp needle with a pump or by applying a tourniquet and filling the corpora with a syringe, recognizing that a tourniquet distorts the configuration. If this procedure is done under local anesthesia, block the nerves at the base of the penis with 0.25 percent bupivacaine.

9 Incise the penile skin and dartos fascia circumferentially 1 cm from the coronal sulcus, and deglove it back to the base. Replace the tourniquet. Dissect the corpus spongiosum from the corpora cavernosa and retract it with a Penrose drain. Excise ellipses from Buck's

Approximate Buck's fascia with 4-0 monofilament SAS, and close the skin with fine interrupted or subcuticular sutures. Insert a miniature suction drain (see page 105). Remove the drain in 1 to 2 days. Place a Bioclusive dressing. In some cases a mildly compressive Kling dressing is advisable for 4 hours, but be sure to check the circulation in the glans every 30 minutes.

During the first 3 months, a dermal graft may contract. At 2 weeks, ask the patient and his sex partner to massage and gently straighten the erect penis to counter this tendency. By 6 to 8 weeks, intercourse should be safe and beneficial to healing. By 3 months, the dermal graft starts to soften, and erection should become straighter again. If potency does not return, this procedure does not interfere with insertion of a penile prosthesis at a later date. Before proceeding with prosthetic insertion, be certain that the impotence has an organic cause.

fascia and the tunica albuginea at a point exactly opposite the site of greatest concavity. Alternatively, the corpus spongiosum can be left in place, with the tucks taken on both sides of it. For a deformity of 45 degrees, make the ellipses about 0.5 cm wide, encompassing one third of the circumference of the corpora cavernosa. For 90 degrees of curvature, increase the maximum width to 0.8 cm. Close the defects with interrupted 3-0 NAS with the knots buried. Alternatively, merely take multiple bites with each NAS without excising ellipses. Remove the tourniquet and reinstitute the erection, looking for leaks and persistent curvature.

For leakage, add sutures; for curvature, insert another tuck with or without excision of an ellipse. Tack the bulbospongiosus and urethra back in place with fine sutures; they may be somewhat redundant. Replace the penile skin and suture it as in a circumcision. If a catheter was used, attach it to drainage and remove it as soon as the dressing is taken off.

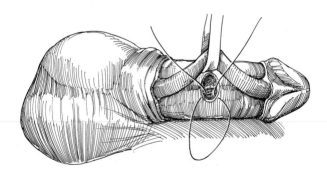

Alternative Methods for Plication

Simple Plication. Excision of an ellipse of tunica vaginalis may not be necessary if heavy braided or monofilament NAS are placed symmetrically through the tunica albuginea.

10 **A,** For ventral curvature, place 1-0 braided NAS (usually three) in the tunica albuginea on the dorsum just lateral to the dorsal vein on both sides, at sites between the vein and the dorsal artery and nerve. Tie them with surgical knots. **B,** For dorsal curvature, place the sutures on the ventrum immediately lateral to the corpus spongiosum. **C,** For a more secure approximation, place the sutures as a figure-eight (Klevmark et al, 1994). Insert two modified figure-eight 2-0 monofilament NAS at the sites illustrated in **A** and **B,** using the configuration shown in this diagram. The portion of the suture indicated by the dotted line is within the tunica albuginea. Limit the width of the stitch to 5 mm to avoid constricting the corpora; the length determines the amount of correction (1 cm = 30 degrees). Tie the sutures five or six times and bury them in the tunica. Cut the ends as short as possible to avoid local irritation at intercourse.

Heineke-Mikulicz Incision and Closure Technique (Sassine et al, 1994). Make 1-cm longitudinal incisions in both sides of the tunica albuginea, and close them transversely with interrupted 3-0 SAS.

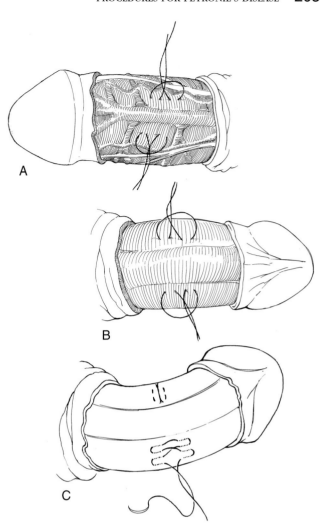

PROSTHESIS IMPLANTATION

For impotent patients requiring penile straightening for Peyronie's disease, it is not necessary to take tucks or excise the plaque. Rather, place an inflatable prosthesis and forcibly straighten the curvature. The AMS 700CX is the best device because it provides the best rigidity, although the Mentor Alpha generates more force to disrupt the plaque. The technique for insertion of a prosthesis is described on page 185.

After implantation of the prosthesis, partially inflate it to the point where curvature is noted, then forcibly straighten the penis until a cracking sound is heard (Wilson and Delk, 1995). Repeat this maneuver until the prosthesis is fully inflated and the penis is as straight as it can be made. Alternatively, make relaxing incisions in the tunica albuginea to allow the penis to be straightened. Check that the corporotomies for cylinder insertion remain sutured. If curvature persists, expose the plaque and make transverse incisions through it, taking care not to injure the cylinders. The defect in the corpus does not need to be covered if an AMS 700CX cylinder is used.

POSTOPERATIVE PROBLEMS

It is not necessary for the patient to be concerned about having *erections* postoperatively because they may improve the straightening. Sexual play, however, is discouraged for 1 month, and intercourse is proscribed for 2 months. After the tucking procedure, intercourse is less risky than after grafting. *Hematomas* occur if hemostasis was inadequate or the dressing was displaced; they may require evacuation. *Infection* can result in loss of the graft and need for a repeat procedure. Alternatively, a chronic sinus may result, requiring removal of the graft and its sutures. *Pain* is not a problem after the period of healing. *Edema* is reduced by cold saline soaks after removal of a moderate compression dressing. *Anesthesia of the glans* may occur after extensive mobilization of the neurovascular bundle. *Skin loss* can result from too tight a dressing. For *impotence* not diagnosed before operation, the patient should be worked up in the standard way; some may require a prosthesis at a second operation. *Return of curvature* after dermal grafting may be seen a month or so later as a result of contraction of the graft, but after 3 to 6 months this secondary deformity usually resolves. The disease may recur on the opposite side.

Commentary by Gerald H. Jordan

Peyronie's disease may result from trauma to the tunica albuginea during intercourse, particularly at the insertion of the midline septal fibers, perhaps associated with either acute or subtle buckling. It seems to occur when erections are beginning to diminish, yet the libido remains "young." It may be fostered by certain positions at intercourse that stress the penis. The partner-superior position is used by more than 70 percent of our patients. Devine's theory of microvascular injury is that the penis buckles during intercourse, disrupting the insertion of the midline septal fibers. Dorsally, the tunica albuginea is bilaminar, with an outer longitudinal layer and an inner circular layer. The septal fibers interweave with the inner layer, and, in some cases, the septal fibers probably shear their connection to the lamina of the tunica albuginea. In other cases, there may be a delamination of the two layers. The anatomy of the tunica albuginea is different ventrally. There the outer longitudinal layer is typically attenuated as a monolayer. Patients who have ventral Peyronie's disease appear either to have sheared the septal fibers from the circumferential layer or to have had significant breakdown of the fibers of the single ventral layer. Ventral Peyronie's disease is a very different disease from the dorsal form, and surgical correction such as by excision and grafting is far less successful.

After trauma in a susceptible individual, a scar develops in the tunica albuginea. The disease process then is self-limited as the scar matures. No acceptable double-blind studies have shown that any treatment to modulate the course of the disease is effective. Modalities that are not harmful to the patient may reassure him while nature takes its course. Because the disease is a self-limited maturation process, surgery to straighten the penis should not be undertaken until the scar in the penis is indeed mature. Surgery should also be undertaken in patients in whom the distortion of the penis precludes intercourse. A subset of Peyronie's patients exists in whom the distortion does not preclude intercourse but rather is caused by their progressive erectile dysfunction. Whether the disease causes erectile dysfunction or erectile dysfunction causes the disease, it is my opinion that the vast majority of patients have a background of erectile dysfunction that contributes to the chance for injury from either acute or subtle buckling. Thus, one must evaluate the patient's erectile function before advising surgery. If erectile function is severely abnormal preoperatively, it will clearly be dismal postoperatively, and these patients will fail therapy.

A number of options are available for the correction of curvature of the penis. Very large series from overseas and in this country report successful use of plication techniques, in some cases combined with excision. Plications do not appear to break down with time, probably because most patients cannot develop high intracavernosal pressure. Some patients are correctly treated with plication; in fact, for some patients it probably represents the optimal form of therapy. We see a number of patients who have long penises that are relatively unaffected by shortening. Many of these patients have good erectile function and are very concerned about anything that might interfere with erectile function. Many patients have decided that they will never accept a prosthesis. Those patients are optimally managed with a plication technique, as the risk of surgery having ill effects on their erections is probably less.

Plication should not be applied to all patients. There are patients who are concerned about the length of their penis, which may already be shortened because of the scarring process. These patients are very reluctant to accept anything that might further shorten the penis; they choose incisional or excisional techniques, which offer the advantage of maintaining penile length. Clearly, however, these techniques do not reverse the shortening that has already occurred with the scarring process. These techniques all require surgery on the tunica albuginea, exposing the underlying erectile tissue, and all require management of the corporotomy defect. Some cases can be managed by placing incisions through the plaque, as opposed to totally excising the scar. In most cases incisions correct the deformity. Plaques that are severely calcified are usually managed at our institution by total excision.

The Peyronie scar involves only the tunica albuginea of the corpora cavernosa. Any scar present in the deeper layers occurs because the septal fibers become thickened. In some patients the thickening descends into the midline between the corporal bodies. It is not necessary to remove these thickened septal fibers, and it is absolutely unnecessary—and potentially harmful—to dissect or remove any of the spongy erectile tissue of the corpora cavernosa. The plaque can be elevated off the spongy erectile tissue successfully in all cases.

A number of graft materials have been proposed for management of the defect: dermal graft, tunica vaginalis, temporalis fascia, and vein. The use of synthetic material for management of the corporotomy defect is not recommended. We have seen far more failures due to placement of synthetic material than we have ever seen successes.

For a dermal graft, the corporotomy defect must be measured and the graft then made oversized by approximately 30 percent in all dimensions. The graft material must be properly tailored to the corporotomy defect, thus avoiding both redundancy and any potential re-creation of deformity because the graft is too small. The preferred area for harvesting the dermal graft is the hairless area overlying the iliac crest because the thickness of the dermis is rather uniform in this area from individual to individual and the behavior of the graft is therefore predictable. We use dermal grafts to fill the corporotomy defects.

Prosthetic implantation may be proper treatment for some patients, but this is not the only option and can be considered an admission of failure. In order to assess the results of Peyronie's surgery, one must establish criteria for successful surgery. At our center, we consider a successful reconstructive procedure for Peyronie's disease to be satisfactory straightening of the penis so that any residual curvature does not interfere in any way with intercourse. The second criterion is that the patient can resume intercourse using natural erections. This means that the patient who requires injections postoperatively in order to have intercourse would be considered a failure; likewise, all prosthetic patients are by definition failures. Again, this does not condemn the use of prostheses for selected patients, but it is our opinion that many options other than prosthetic placement are available to Peyronie's disease patients. Using these criteria of success in patients who have undergone excision of the plaque with dermal grafting, we find an overall success rate of approximately 70 percent. Success clearly depends on the patient's background erectile function. Those with demonstrably good erectile function as measured on vascular testing, with good accumulated intracorporal pressures, do much better than those with demonstrably poor erectile function. Early in our experience, it appeared that good erectile function preoperatively virtually guaranteed a successful result, but, as numbers have accumulated, we have found that some patients with nearly normal erectile function preoperatively have deterioration of their erectile function postoperatively. However, those with good erectile function have a success rate in excess of 90 percent. In the group with fair erections, the success rate drops to the middle to upper 70 percent range. In patients with demonstrably poor erectile function, defined by us as accumulated intracorporal pressures of less than 30 mm Hg, results are inevitably unsuccessful. These patients should be told that the best option is prosthetic placement with penile straightening at the same time.

Avoid overdependence on vascular function testing (Duplex/ DICC). These studies are based on the fact that the patient's erectile tissues normally dilate in response to the injected agents. We routinely use high-dose combination papaverine/ Regitine/prostaglandin E_1 and find that most patients dilate maximally in response to those agents. However, if all other portions of the evaluation (i.e., history, sexual history, photos, history from partner) do not support the results of vascular testing, further evaluation by a sleep laboratory or with Rigi-Scan must be done.

It is a misconception that Peyronie's surgery makes subsequent prosthetic placement difficult, if not impossible. This is not necessarily the case. In our patients who had secondary placement of prostheses after the primary procedure to straighten their penis using an excisional technique with grafting, we found that the complication rate was no greater than in the population at large receiving prosthetic surgery.

Peyronie's disease is a devastating disease for most men. However, it does not have to spell the end of their sex lives. Moreover, it is a disease with a pattern of evolution, and the time to undertake surgery is when the disease is no longer evolving. For couples dealing with Peyronie's disease, who are in a fair amount of distress, waiting is not easy. They must be supported through the waiting stages.

Operations for Priapism

Measure blood gases to distinguish the usual *ischemic* low-flow venous priapism due to pharmacologic or neurogenic causes, a hematologic disorder, or idiopathic cause from the less common *nonischemic* high-flow arterial priapism due to vascular trauma, surgery, intracavernosal injection, or idiopathic factors. Obtain a complete blood count and hemoglobin determination. Stop suspected medications; treat hematologic or malignant disease. Aspirate the cavernous space and send for a blood gas determination. Intracorporal blood gases of pH less than 7.25, Po_2 less than 30, and Pco_2 greater than 60 indicate ischemic, low-flow priapism. (For high-flow, nonischemic priapism, the findings are pH greater than 7.5, Po_2 greater than 50, and Pco_2 less than 50, and shunts are contraindicated.)

In black patients, order electrophoresis for sickle cell anemia. If the disease is detected, hydrate, alkalize, oxygenate, relieve pain with analgesics, and hypertransfuse or perform erythrocytapheresis. If these measures fail, proceed with alpha-adrenergic injections, irrigation, and ultimately shunting.

Nonischemic Priapism. Confirm the diagnosis by detecting high flow with color Doppler imaging and minimal changes in blood gases. Embolize the ruptured cavernous artery angiographically, or ligate the arteriosinusoidal fistula surgically.

ISCHEMIC PRIAPISM

If the patient is seen within 4 hours, inject 100 μg phenylephrine. If this fails, try aspiration and irrigation of the corpora cavernosa with a large-bore needle through the glans to avoid a hematoma on the shaft. Lidocaine injected into the region of the plexus of Santorini between the penis and the symphysis pubis may relax and open venous channels. Administer intermittent phenylephrine irrigations (1 mg in 1000 ml of saline) of the cavernous bodies (insert one needle on a syringe into one corpus for aspiration and disposal into a liter bag and another needle and syringe into the other corpus for injection of dilute phenylephrine solution (Futral and Witt, 1995).

After 36 hours, do not delay diversion because fibrosis will intervene. Evacuate the clot and perform a distal shunt: distal glandulocavernous shunt (Ebbehoj, Winter, Goulding, Datta, El-Ghorab, Kinlinc, or Hashmat-Waterhouse). If a unilateral shunt fails, perform a bilateral shunt. If there is still no response, place a proximal shunt: cavernosospongiosum (Quackels), cavernososaphenous (Grayhack), cavernous vein–dorsal vein (Barry), or cavernosospongiosum with saphenous vein patch (Odelowo), each done first unilaterally, then bilaterally if necessary.

Resort to penile implants if fibrosis with impotence results.

Before starting treatment, make sure the patient understands both the odds for successful reversal and the chances for subsequent impotence.

DISTAL SHUNTS

Glans–Corpora Cavernosa Shunt (Winter)

1 Inject lidocaine into the glans. Aspirate one corpus cavernosum with a large-bore needle passed through the glans (to avoid a hematoma of the shaft) in the midline and irrigate with saline solution through one corpus.

Insert a biopsy needle (Travenol Tru-Cut) through the glans in the midline dorsal to the meatus. Pass the obturator through the septum to enter the right corpus cavernosum. Push the sheath home; rotate the needle 360 degrees and withdraw the needle. Repeat the maneuver to obtain two cores from the septum between the glans and the corpora on each side. Close the puncture site with a figure-eight 3-0 CCG suture. Have the patient squeeze the penis every few minutes to keep it empty for the next 12 hours. If partial (up to 50 percent) erection persists, repeat the procedure or resort to an alternative shunt. Intracorporal pressure monitoring may help evaluate the effectiveness of any of these procedures.

Alternative Methods. *Method 1* (Goulding): Through a stab wound on one side of the glans made with a pointed knife, insert a Kerrison rongeur into the corpus cavernosum and take a wedge of tissue from the septum on that side. Repeat the procedure quickly on the corpus on the other side before the penis deflates. Close the defect in the glans with 3-0 CCG sutures. *Method 2* (Datta): For a larger shunt, insert a skin biopsy punch through a 0.5-cm incision into the glans, and rotate it firmly against the tunica albuginea of the corpus cavernosum to cut a circular piece from it. Pull the piece out with a clamp and trim it free. Close the glans with a running 5-0 SAS. *Method 3* (Kinlinc): Insert a special trocar through the glans to permit drainage of blood between the side holes. *Method 4* (El-Ghorab): This method opens both corporal tips. Apply a tourniquet. Make a 2-cm transverse incision on the dorsum of the glans 1 cm distal to the coronal sulcus. Separate the tips of the corpora from the glans, transfix them with heavy sutures so that they do not withdraw during detumescence, and sharply excise a segment of tunica albuginea 5 mm in diameter from each. Close the skin of the glans with 3-0 SAS.

Do not place an indwelling catheter or a pressure dressing. It is possible to have the patient manually compress the penile shaft. Follow the course of the condition with penile blood gases. Provide antibiotics.

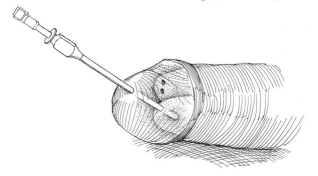

PROXIMAL SHUNTS

Cavernosospongiosum Shunt
(Quackels)

After failure of distal shunts, make a shunt more proximally where the circulation is better.

Place an 18 F 5-ml balloon catheter in the bladder.

2 Incise the skin of the penis vertically on the undersurface 1 cm off the midline, just distal to the penoscrotal junction. Instead of placing the incision on the shaft, it may be made more posteriorly where the substance of the corpus spongiosum is greater. Incise Buck's fascia, and mobilize 3 cm of both cavernous bodies to create a groove between the corpus cavernosum and the corpus spongiosum.

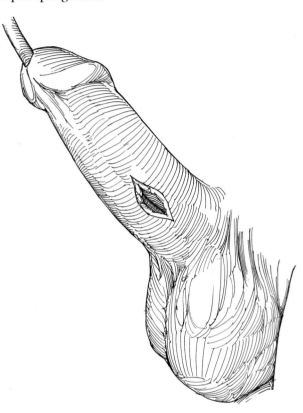

3 Suture the walls of these structures together with a running 5-0 NAS.

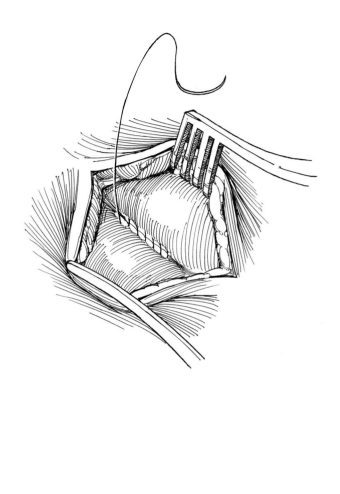

4 Excise an ellipse 1 cm long from both structures. *Caution*: The spongy tissue of the corpus cavernosum is thin and the urethra is easily entered.

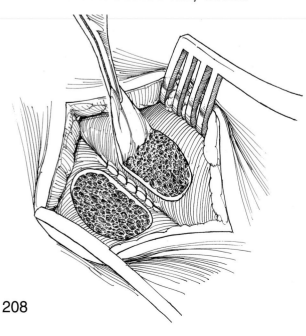

5 Anastomose the two structures with running 5-0 NAS, beginning at both ends of the defect. Close the subcutaneous tissues and skin.

If detumescence is not satisfactory, repeat the procedure at a different level on the other side.

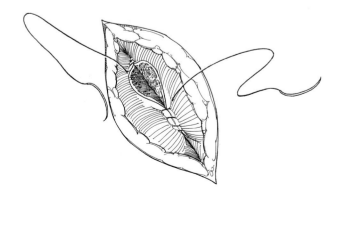

Cavernososaphenous Shunt
(Grayhack)

6 Incise the skin of the penis at the base and expose the tunica albuginea of the corpus cavernosum. Palpate the femoral artery, and make an oblique incision over it 3 or 4 cm below the inguinal ligament. Expose the saphenous vein for a distance of 10 to 12 cm. Divide the vein distally so that it is long enough to reach the penis, and tie the distal end with 3-0 SAS.

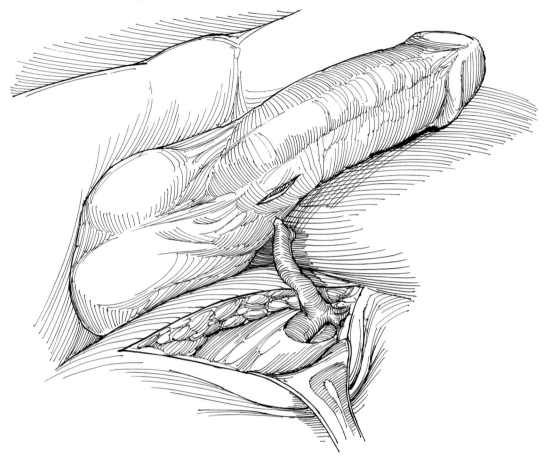

7 Burrow beneath the skin with the index finger to join the two incisions.

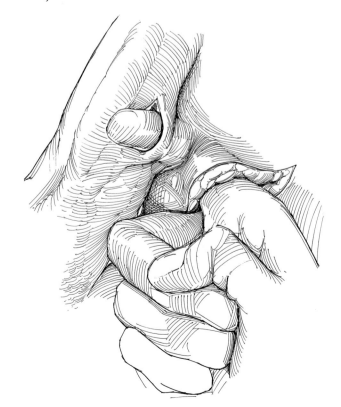

8 Excise an ellipse of tunica albuginea about 1 cm long. Insert a needle through the glans, and thoroughly irrigate the corpora cavernosa to obtain a flow of bright red blood.

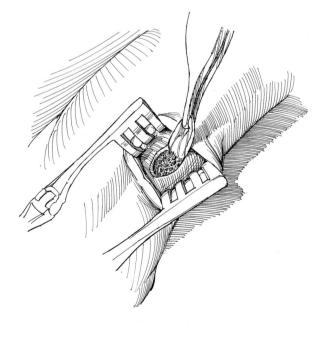

9 Insert a clamp through the skin tunnel and draw the vein into the penile wound. Cut the vein obliquely and spatulate it. Place and tie a 5-0 NAS at each end of the cavernous defect, leaving the ends long. Suture the back walls together, then complete the front walls.

10 Close the subcutaneous tissues with 4-0 SAS and the skin incisions with 4-0 subcuticular SAS. Apply a dry dressing. Proceed with intermittent squeezing as previously described.

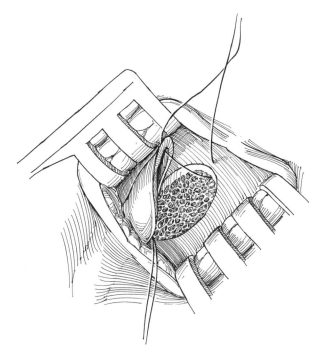

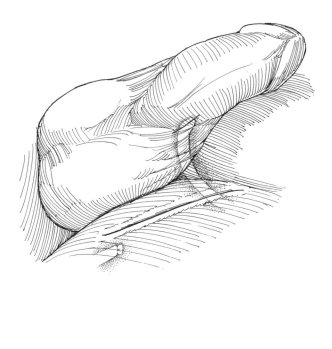

Cavernous Vein–Dorsal Vein Shunt (Barry)

11 Make a circumcising incision and deglove the penis. In midshaft, open the superficial fascia and incise Buck's fascia. Dissect the dorsal vein from its bed, taking care not to injure the dorsal artery or nerves. Tie it distally with an SAS. Make an incision in the tunica albuginea of one corpus opposite the proximal end of the vein, and anastomose the vein to the corpus end to side with a running 7-0 NAS. Replace the penile skin and suture it at the corona. Do not place a compression dressing.

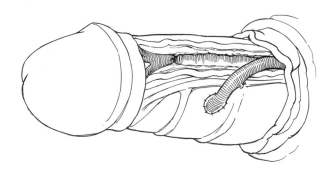

POSTOPERATIVE PROBLEMS

Impotence follows priapism in as many as half the cases. It is due to edema and resulting fibrosis of the cavernous septa, more so if treatment is delayed. Implantation of a flexible, not inflatable prosthesis may be indicated.

Commentary by John P. Blandy

In practice, *nonischemic* priapism is very rare and is always associated with a history of trauma. There is no hurry about making the diagnosis. If available, a Doppler study confirms the high flow. Operation should be planned on the basis of really good selective angiography. Embolization is all very well, but surgical correction is more precise and certain. Most cases, however, fall into the category of *ischemic* priapism, and here the most important thing is not to waste time with futile "noninvasive" procedures. The second most important thing is to explain to the patient (and give him the explanation in writing) the risks of subsequent impotence no matter how diligent treatment has been. This is a medicolegal minefield. Whatever you do, even if it is nothing at all, that will be assumed to be the cause of the impotence.

In my experience, these procedures have never worked. Perhaps this is because I did not do them right; more likely, it seems to me, is that none of them is any good. Note the large number of "alternative methods" that are reported when they work, but not when they do not. My advice is to try one or two of them, but do not delay making a better opening between the distended cavernosa and the flaccid spongiosum if the other methods do not immediately succeed. Above all, take care not to enter the urethra: Extravasation of urine complicating priapism is a recipe for the disaster of Fournier's gangrene. Cavernous vein–dorsal vein shunts are tricky operations that must be done perfectly if they are not to clot up and fail. They do not always work. The patient must be warned of this, or he will sue.

Repair of Genital Injuries

AVULSION OR BURN INJURY OF PENIS AND SCROTUM

For major injury of the genital skin, as after a third-degree burn, débride virtually all of the skin and provide wet-to-dry dressings to complete the débridement. It is seldom necessary to put the testes in thigh pouches as a first stage. Rather, apply a split-thickness graft on the shaft and a meshed graft on the scrotum when the bed is ready.

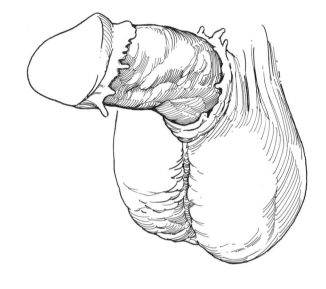

1 *Avulsion injury:* Repair the defect at once, at least within 8 to 12 hours. Remove distal skin remnants from the penis; they lose their venous drainage and so are subject to prolonged edema. Cleanse the denuded area thoroughly with saline. Remove foreign bodies and hematomas. Achieve hemostasis, although bleeding usually is minimal after this type of injury.

Burn Injuries. For thermal burns, apply a 0.5 percent silver nitrate dressing immediately and wait for separation of the eschar. For chemical burns, flush the wound thoroughly with normal saline (or neutralizing solutions when the agent is known). With electrical burns, it is difficult to assess the severity and extent of burn immediately because of dissemination of the current through tissue, and coagulation necrosis occurs beyond the obvious limits of the burn. Wait until demarcation between viable and nonviable tissue is obvious, then excise devitalized tissue and proceed with split-thickness skin grafting unless secondary infection has occurred.

Remove all the skin from the shaft distal to the injury to avoid subsequent lymphedema. Do it at once before infection can set in. It is not necessary to wait for separation of the eschar to see how much skin remains because the small amount of skin that could be saved in that way is easily replaced by a graft. Treat the area with whirlpool baths, soap and water soaks, and antibacterial topical dressings until the eschar has separated completely and clean granulation tissue remains, ready for skin grafting.

Split-Thickness Graft Technique

2 Tack both coronal and proximal skin edges to the shaft with 4-0 SAS placed subcutaneously. Wait for formation of a well-vascularized bed.

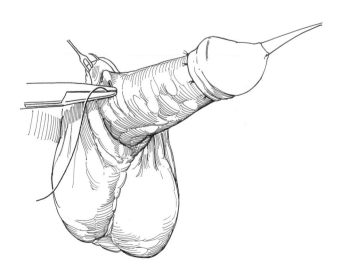

3 With an electric dermatome, obtain a medium split-thickness skin graft from the lower abdomen or the inner or outer aspect of the thigh from areas with the least hair. For primary grafting, make the graft 0.020 to 0.024 inch thick; for grafting after the bed has been infected, raise a thinner graft, 0.012 to 0.016 inch.

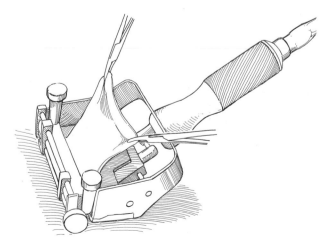

4 **A,** Wrap the graft around the shaft, placing the suture line ventrally to mimic the raphe. Trim the edges of the graft and approximate the edges with a running 5-0 SAS. Bank the excess skin. Insert a balloon catheter of suitable size. **B,** To reduce the risk of chordee, incise the skin vertically in two or three places to lengthen the suture line (Z-plasty). Suture the skin to the corona and to the edge of the scrotal skin with interrupted 4-0 CCG sutures. Suture the graft proximally and distally with 4-0 SAS. Leave these sutures long.

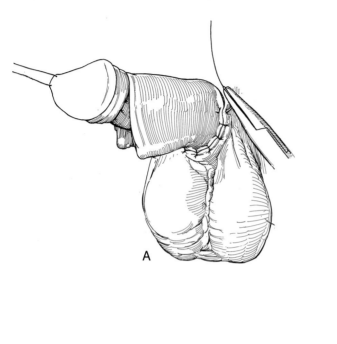

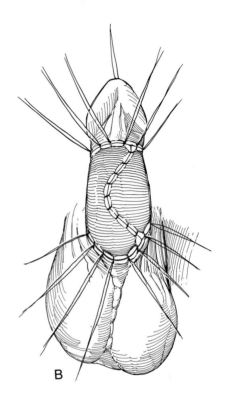

5 Apply cotton wool impregnated with glycerin around the penis, and anchor it by tying the sets of long sutures together. The graft must be immobilized. Cover the wool with gauze and elastic adhesive tape. Apply tincture of benzoin and fix the tape to the pubic skin.

6 **A** and **B,** Suspend the penis inside a section removed from a plastic bottle that has been cut appropriately and padded with adhesive foam padding.

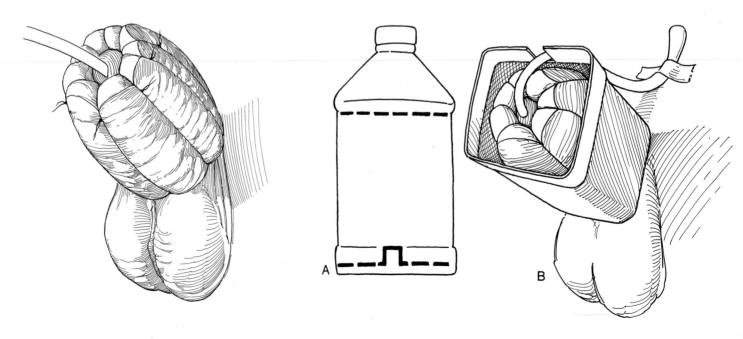

PENILE FRACTURE

Choose operation over conservative management and operate as soon as possible. Look for blood at the meatus or have the patient void and examine the first part, looking for evidence of urethral laceration. If urethral injury is suspected, check by urethrography and repair it with fine absorbable sutures. Cavernosography is not necessary. Insert an 18 F 5-ml silicone balloon catheter.

7 *Incision:* Make a circular incision 1 cm proximal to the corona; peel back the shaft skin and evacuate the hematoma. Trim the edges of the tear through the tunica albuginea into the corporal tissue. Although the tear is semicircumferential, the neurovascular bundle is dorsal to it. Close the tunica albuginea with interrupted 3-0 SAS, inverted so that the knots are not palpable.

8 Replace the shaft skin and suture it to the coronal margin with interrupted 3-0 PCG sutures. Avoid placing a constricting dressing. Leave the catheter in place overnight. Give prophylactic antibiotics. Complications are rare.

For urethral involvement, delay insertion of a catheter that might extend the tear. Close the urethral defect accurately with 4-0 CCG sutures, and leave an indwelling catheter for 2 weeks. For severe trauma to the urethra with apparent devitalization, resect the affected segment of urethra, mobilize it both proximally and distally, and perform an elliptical anastomosis (see page 273).

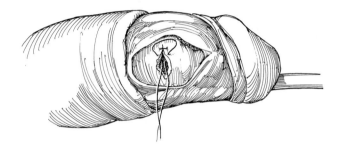

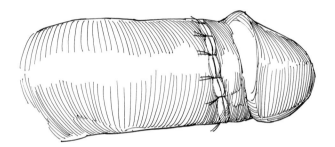

PENILE REIMPLANTATION

Have the recovered segment of penis placed in a bag containing cold saline or lactated Ringer's solution within a second bag containing iced slush. This should permit reattachment up to 24 hours after injury.

Instruments: Use an operating room microscope or optical loupe and microsurgical instruments. For position, see page 365.

Insert a urethral catheter and fill the bladder. Proceed with suprapubic cystostomy. Remove the urethral catheter. If possible, place a tourniquet (24 F Robinson catheter) around the base of the remainder of the penis and débride the raw edges.

9 Identify the ends of the deep dorsal veins on each cut surface, noting the largest vein that is exposed. Ligate any extra veins. Ligate the deep dorsal arteries with a 2-0 SAS, but do not ligate the cavernous arteries.

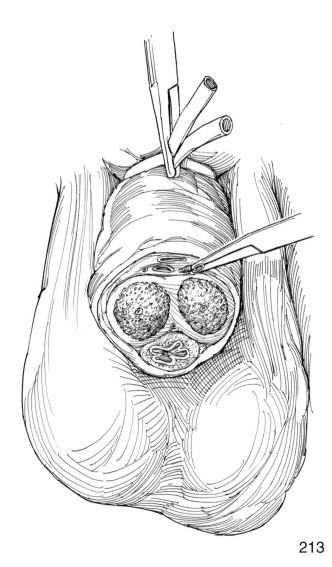

10 Release the tourniquet temporarily and insert a 16 F 5-ml silicone balloon catheter retrogradely through both portions of the penis. Mobilize and anastomose the urethra and corpus spongiosum with an inner layer of interrupted 6-0 SAS, tied with the knots inside the lumen. Place a second row of interrupted sutures through the tunic of the corpus spongiosum and include its enveloping Buck's fascia.

11 Approximate the tunica albuginea of the corpora cavernosa starting at the septum, using interrupted 3-0 SAS, placed with the knots on the inside. Insert the final sutures on the dorsum, but do not tie them.

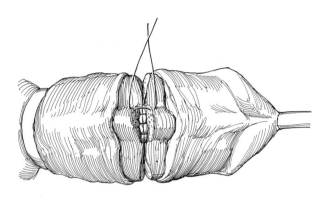

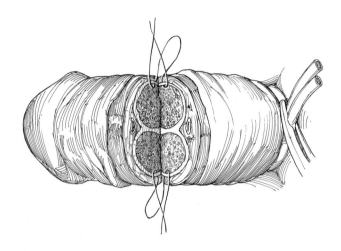

12 Using the operating room microscope or a loupe, spatulate the proximal end of the selected deep dorsal vein on the dorsal aspect and its distal end on the ventral aspect. Anastomose the vein by the single-stitch, double-swaged method of microvascular repair (see page 60): With double-armed 9-0 nylon NAS, place a continuous everting row in the posterior half of the anastomosis; draw on the ends to pull the edges together.

13 Continue as a normal everting stitch while keeping tension off the anastomosis. Tie the free ends.

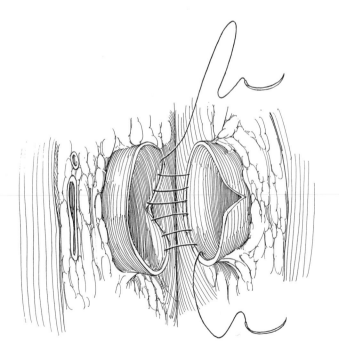

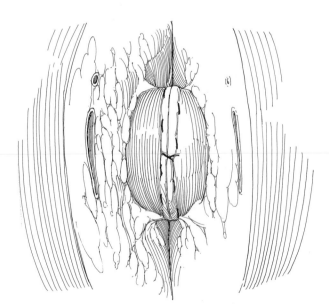

14 *Alternatively*, use a single-stitch method by inserting the suture on one side and tying it, then running it down and around the back wall and finally across the front.

Under magnification, approximate the epineurium of the dorsal nerves with 9-0 NAS (see page 63). Anastomose the dorsal arteries with 10-0 NAS (see page 60). It is not necessary to anastomose the corporal arteries. Complete the closure of the tunica albuginea by tying the remaining sutures.

Close Buck's and Colles' fascias with 3-0 interrupted SAS to relieve tension. Approximate the skin with 4-0 PCG sutures and apply a nonconstrictive dressing. *Note:* If there is redundancy of skin on the proximal shaft, trim some skin from the distal segment to prevent overlap of suture lines and also to reduce the amount of distal skin exposed to ischemia and edema.

Postoperatively, provide hemodilution, dextran infusion, and heparinization to reduce the incidence of thrombosis. Give broad-spectrum antibiotics. Periodically aspirate the sludged blood from the distal segment. Monitor revascularization with Doppler ultrasonography. Perform voiding cystography in 2 weeks, and remove the cystostomy tube if no extravasation is seen. Check the skin distal to the suture line for viability; it may require débridement and replacement with a split-thickness graft (Step 21).

REPAIR OF PARTIAL AMPUTATION OF THE PENIS

Cleanse the area with iodine compound. Lavage the wound thoroughly with 0.9 percent saline solution. Apply a 24 F Robinson catheter around the base as a tourniquet. Loosen the tourniquet and ligate bleeding vessels.

15 *Incision:* Mark a dorsal flap that extends to the margin of healthy skin. Make it 0.5 cm longer than the width of the penile stump (see page 150).

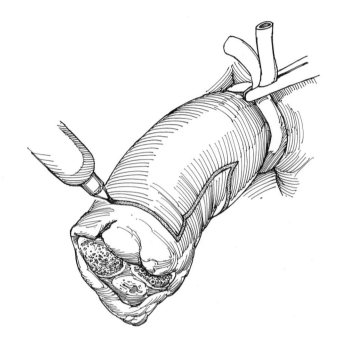

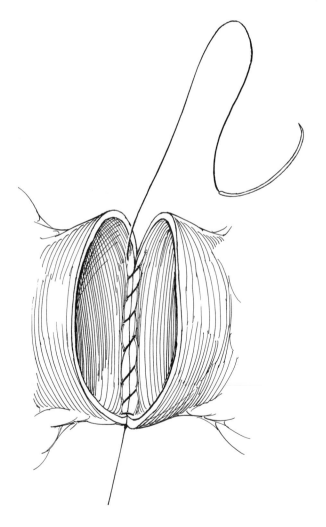

16 Trim the corpora cavernosa back to leave the corpus spongiosum and contained urethra exposed for a distance of 1 cm.

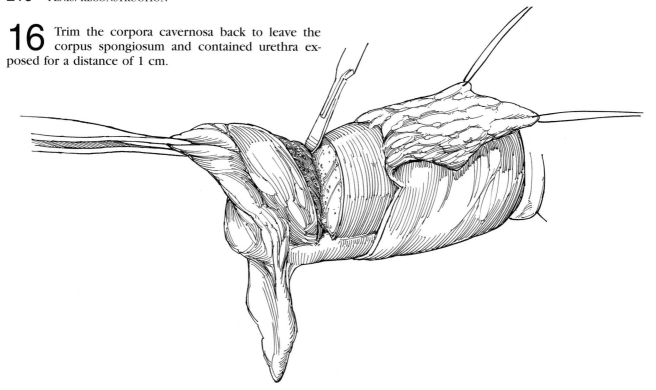

17 Close both corpora together with interrupted 1-0 SAS that pass from one side through the septum to the other side. Trim the end of the urethra back to normal tissue, and cut a 0.5-cm slit in the roof.

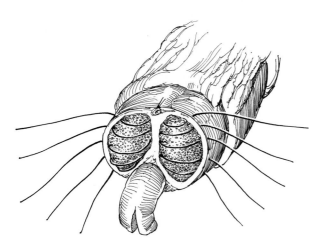

18 Mark and cut a 1-cm buttonhole with a V-projection in the dorsal flap at the site corresponding to the new meatus.

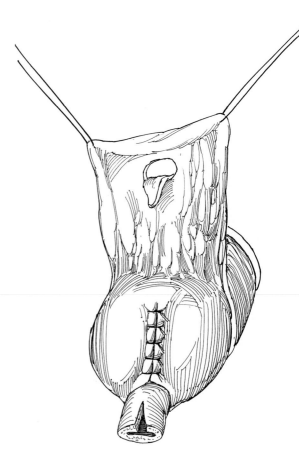

19 Suture the flap to the meatus and to the ventral skin with 4-0 CCG sutures. Place an 18 F 5-ml balloon catheter and dress the wound as previously described.

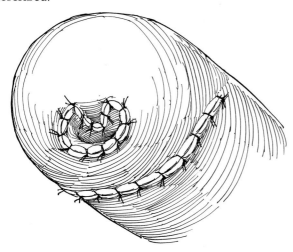

REPAIR OF AVULSION INJURY OF PENIS AND SCROTUM

Repair the injury at once, at least within 8 to 12 hours. Place a 20 F 5-ml balloon catheter in the bladder.

20 Make a circumcising incision, and excise and discard the skin remaining on the shaft of the penis to prevent prolonged disabling edema. Cleanse the denuded area thoroughly with saline. Remove foreign bodies and hematomas. Achieve hemostasis; bleeding is usually minimal after this type of injury.

Methods for protecting the testes until the time for scrotal reconstruction are split-thickness skin grafts, meshed grafts, thigh flaps, and thigh pouches. Alternatively, the testes may be wrapped in wet-to-dry gauze coverings without scrotal débridement. This may suffice if the patient is not septic or burned until he can be subjected to grafting—within 1 week.

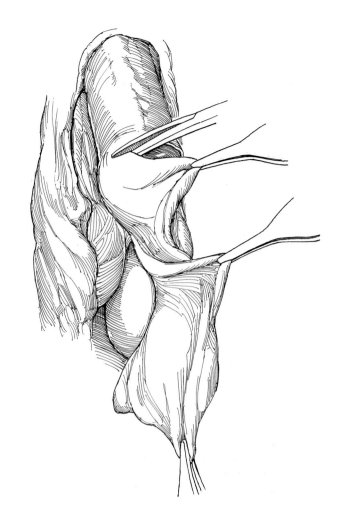

Split-Thickness Skin Graft

21 Obtain a 10 × 20-cm split-thickness skin graft from the inner thigh, as previously described. For primary grafting, cut the graft 0.020 to 0.024 inch thick; for grafting after the bed has been infected, obtain a thinner graft, 0.012 to 0.016 inch. The thicker graft experiences less contraction. Wrap the graft around the shaft, placing the suture line dorsally or placing it ventrally to mimic the raphe. Incising the skin edge vertically in two or three places lengthens the suture line and reduces the risk of chordee. Suture the skin to the corona and to the scrotal skin with interrupted 4-0 CCG sutures, and incorporate the dressing by tying the sutures over it. Cover the testes with residual scrotal skin if possible. Even though the skin may appear to be under tension, the testes are accommodated in time.

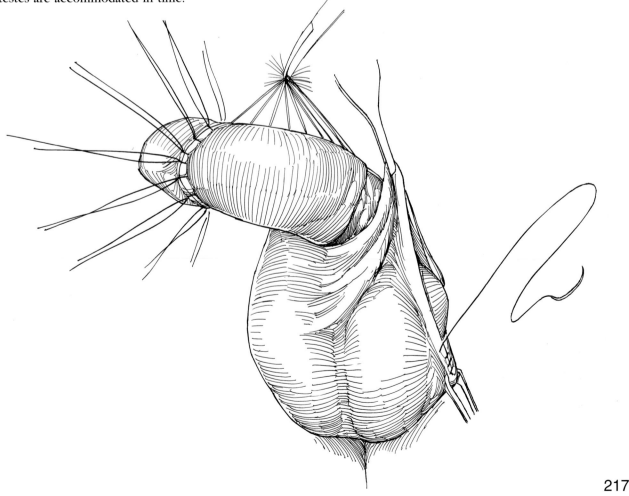

Meshed Grafts

When the condition of the patient allows it, dissect the testes free and cover even large scrotal defects with meshed split-thickness skin grafts. Meshed grafts are not suitable for covering an active penis because they contract more than an unmeshed graft, but they are adequate for scrotal coverage and also for coverage of the penis in men who are impotent.

22 **A,** Cut a 0.015-inch-thick split-thickness skin graft from the thigh and place it in a meshing dermatome containing a meshing sheet with an expansion ratio of 1.5:1. Be generous with the size of the graft so that it does not have to be stretched when placed in the defect. **B,** Lay the graft on the scrotum with minimal expansion and suture it in place. The principal purpose of the mesh is to provide drainage and encourage angiogenesis—not to allow the use of less skin.

Tissue Expansion

A two-compartment scrotum can be formed by using the technique of tissue expansion (Still and Goodman). Place a 200- to 250-ml tissue-expansion balloon in the perineum on each side and lead the filling tubes into the inguinal region. Gradually fill the balloons over a 2- to 3-month period. When the skin has reached an adequate dimension, remove the balloons, mobilize the testes, and insert them on each side.

Thigh Flaps

Flaps raised from the inner thigh provide coverage but require a major procedure. Mobilize the testes, and suture them together in the midline. Raise a broad-based flap from each inner thigh based in the inguinal region. Include the fat and cutaneous vascular supply. Rotate the flaps medially, and suture them together over the testes.

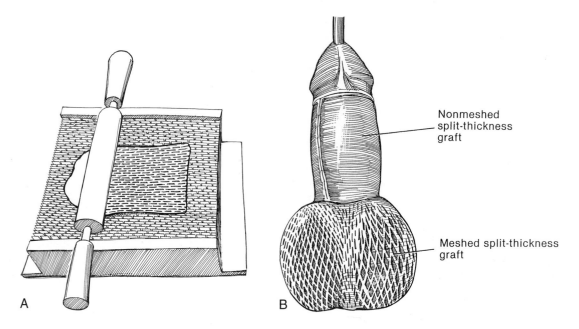

Nonmeshed split-thickness graft

Meshed split-thickness graft

Thigh Pouches

23 Thigh pouches are seldom necessary and require a second-stage operation. Raise symmetric skin flaps from the inner aspect of each thigh to include little subcutaneous tissue. The skin must be loose enough that the donor defects can be closed; thus, the method is more appropriate for older patients.

Construct thigh pouches as far posteriorly as possible by digitally burrowing subcutaneously down the inside of each thigh. Gently press one testis into its pocket; an anchor suture is not needed. Place the second testis at a slightly higher level to allow the patient to cross his legs without contact.

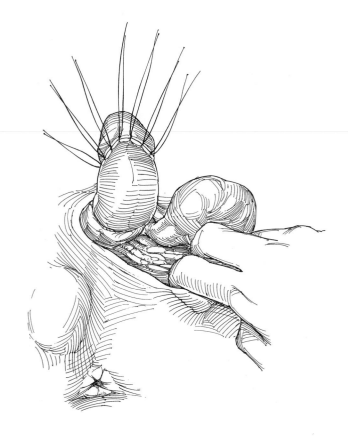

RUPTURE OF THE TESTIS

Ultrasonography may assist in the diagnosis by demonstrating a hematocele, a finding diagnostic of rupture. It may even show the disruption of the tunica albuginea. Consider torsion in the differential diagnosis.

24 **A,** Expose the testis by incising the scrotum transversely into the traumatic hydrocele, evacuate the blood, then extrude the testis. Examine the testis for ischemia from injury of the cord. Inspect the wound, and clamp and ligate any bleeding vessels. Even if the testis is fragmented, resect as little tubular tissue as possible. Close the tunica albuginea over the extruded tubules with a continuous 3-0 SAS. **B,** Leave the tunica vaginalis open, or cover the defect with a graft from the tunica vaginalis. Close the dartos layers hemostatically around a Penrose drain that is led through a stab wound, then close the skin. Give antibiotics. Remove the Penrose drain in 3 or 4 days, when the drainage has stopped.

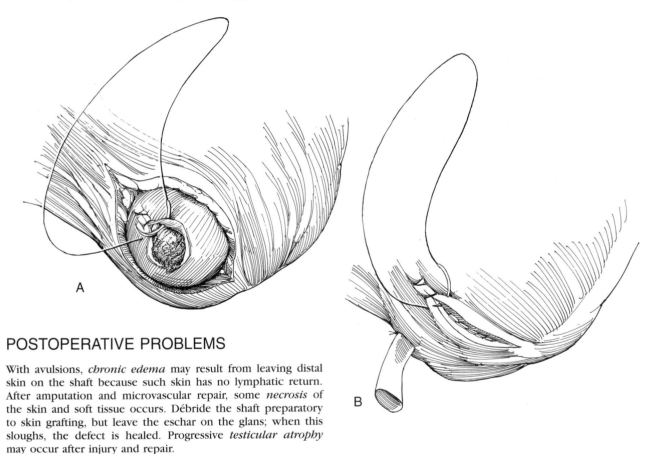

POSTOPERATIVE PROBLEMS

With avulsions, *chronic edema* may result from leaving distal skin on the shaft because such skin has no lymphatic return. After amputation and microvascular repair, some *necrosis* of the skin and soft tissue occurs. Débride the shaft preparatory to skin grafting, but leave the eschar on the glans; when this sloughs, the defect is healed. Progressive *testicular atrophy* may occur after injury and repair.

Commentary by Joseph N. Corriere, Jr.

I agree with most of the surgical techniques described in this chapter. There are, however, three injuries that I handle a bit differently.

First, I think the use of thigh flaps or thigh pouches to cover denuded testicles after loss of scrotal skin, for example, as the first stage of a two-stage reconstruction, is an unnecessary extra step (Step 23). Moreover, thigh flap scrotal reconstruction is usually cosmetically unacceptable. The use of wet-to-dry dressings wrapped around the exposed testicles is more comfortable for the patient, performs daily débridement when the dressings are changed, and allows for more rapid resurfacing. The exposed genitals can be observed during the dressing changes and usually in a week are ready for covering by primary scrotal closure or skin grafting.

Second, I do not think mesh grafts are necessary in the creation of a new scrotum. We have always used unmeshed grafts with good cosmetic and functional results.

Finally, I think the technique described to repair a partial amputation of the penis will lead to a bothersome incidence of meatal stenosis (Steps 15 to 19). I prefer to make a circular skin incision approximately 2.5 cm behind the severed end of the urethra and carry it down through the corpora cavernosa. I leave the urethra and corpus spongiosum 2.5 cm longer than the cut stump to cover the end of the penis. I close the corpora cavernosa with a running transverse suture line of 3-0 Vicryl for hemostasis and then bevel the urethra on the ventral surface. The beveled urethra is then turned back and sewn to the skin edge with interrupted 3-0 Vicryl sutures. The meatus so formed does not stenose, and the patient can direct his stream without difficulty.

Construction of Penis

RADIAL FOREARM FLAP
(Chang and Hwang)

The radial forearm flap has been the most successful form of construction. An ulnar forearm flap, based on the ulnar artery and the superficial veins of the forearm with innervation from the medial cutaneous nerve, avoids the hair present on the radial side but has a more tenuous venous drainage. The donor site requires split-thickness skin grafting in either case, with a resultant scar on the arm. Less satisfactory alternatives are lateral upper arm flaps, the dorsalis pedis flap, and the island groin flap.

Organize two surgical teams, one to prepare the forearm skin flap and the other to cover the donor site with a skin graft from the thigh; prepare the recipient site; mobilize the inguinal or femoral recipient vessels; and perform a suprapubic cystostomy. Consider placing pneumatic pressure devices on both legs.

1 **A,** Make certain that the dominant blood supply to the hand is from the radial artery. If it is from the ulnar artery, adapt the procedure by forming the larger flap medially (Section A in Fig. 1*B*). With the patient in the frog-leg position, place the nondominant arm on an arm board and prepare the arm, the lower abdomen, and the genital areas. Palpate and observe the position of the pertinent vessels on the forearm. **B,** *First team:* Outline a skin flap on the radial side of the forearm 12 to 14 cm long and 14 to 15 cm wide, the dimensions being dependent on the size of the patient. With a marking pen, mark three sections: Section A, a wider section on the radial side from which to construct the penis itself; Section B, a 1-cm strip, de-epithelialized to increase the area of tissue contact for the prosthesis; and Section C, a smaller section on the ulnar side 3.5 to 4 cm in width which will become the new urethra. Provide a tongue of skin 1 cm in length on Sections A and B to shape the glans. **C,** The flap as it appears after mobilization.

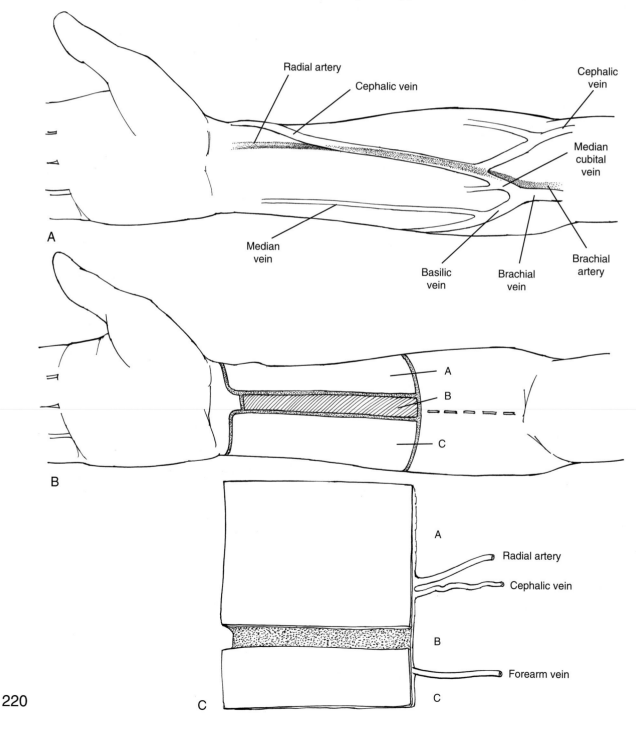

2 Partially exsanguinate the forearm with an Esmarch bandage, and apply and inflate a sterile tourniquet to 250 mm Hg. Raise a full-thickness flap beginning distally, taking with it the subcutaneous tissue down to but not including the epitenon over the distal forearm tendons and the six or seven arteriolar branches of the distal third of the radial artery, as well as the venae comitantes. (The epitenon is preserved as a bed for the subsequent skin graft.) If the superficial radial nerve becomes involved, repair it to prevent distressing symptoms in the hand. The vascular pedicle contains the radial artery and its venae comitantes, the cephalic vein, and another forearm vein and should be at least 10 cm in length proximal to the flap. It also contains the medial and lateral antebrachial cutaneous nerves. Release the tourniquet and secure hemostasis. De-epithelialize the center Section B. Roll the narrow Section C into a tube around a 16 F silicone balloon catheter, and suture it closed with two layers of interrupted 3-0 SAS.

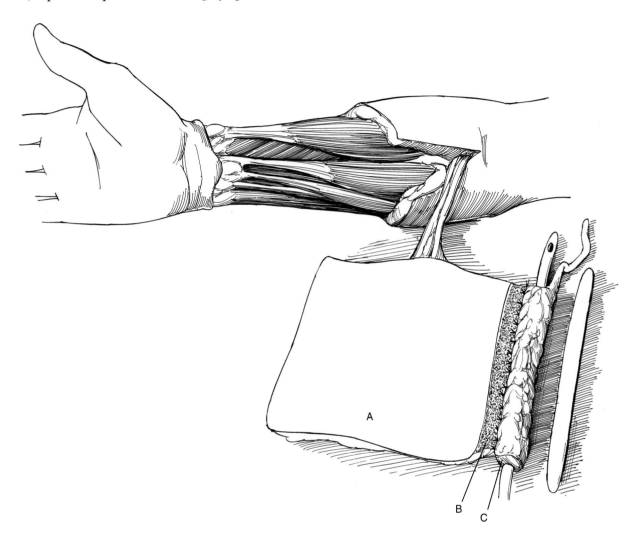

3 Cover both the neourethra and the raw area with the larger Section A. Closure may be difficult because of protrusion of fat. Mold the extensions to fit the meatus, and mold the distal portion into a glans. Insert a Silastic catheter into the bladder to act as a stent. This figure and Figure 2 show a prosthesis, but do not place the prosthesis at this step because the new phallus will not have protective sensation and erosion will occur. Wait 6 to 12 months for sensation to return.

Second team: Cover the donor site with a split-thickness skin graft harvested from the thigh.

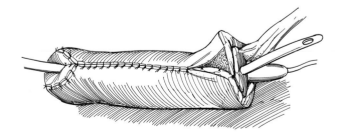

4 *First team:* Divide the vascular pedicle along with the antebrachial nerve(s) (not shown), and tunnel it subcutaneously under the inguinal region. Using the operating room microscope, anastomose the cephalic vein to the greater saphenous vein or to the femoral vein by a saphenous vein interposition graft. Anastomose the superficial veins in the flap to the saphenous veins on both sides. It is usually possible to create a third anastomosis between a vena comitans and a saphenous branch. Join the radial artery to the inferior epigastric artery, the circumflex femoris lateralis, or the profunda femoris. Anastomose the lateral antebrachial nerve to the erogenous pudendal nerve or the dorsal nerve of the penis (or clitoris in transsexuals). Make the connection epineurium to epineurium with 10-0 monofilament sutures (see page 63). Alternatively, use the pudendal nerve with a sural graft or one from the ilioinguinal nerve.

Second team: Create a widely spatulated two-layer anastomosis for the urethra with interrupted 4-0 CCG sutures. It is not advisable to place a prosthesis at the first stage; wait until the phallus has protective sensation. Approximate the skin circumferentially around the base of the new penis.

Closing the defect in the arm may result in an unsightly scar, especially in heavy patients. Instead, cover the donor site with a medium split-thickness skin graft (0.014 to 0.016 inch) taken from the thigh. A full-thickness graft from the anterior thigh provides an even better appearance. Immobilize the arm at the elbow and apply a compressive dressing to it.

Postoperatively, after removal of the arm from the splint, continue with a compressive sleeve for 3 months. Leave the penile urethral stent in place for 2 or 3 weeks. Perform retrograde urethrography through a small catheter alongside the stenting catheter 3 to 4 weeks postoperatively. If extravasation is not seen, remove the stent. Clamp the cystostomy tube and observe voiding. If it is satisfactory, remove the tube.

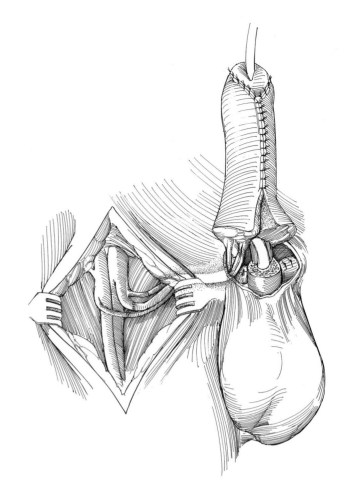

Alternative Flap Design (Gottlieb and Levine)

5 Mark and incise a 15 × 17-cm flap. If the native urethra ends in the perineum, increase the length of the neourethra to 25 cm by forming a proximal extension to just above the antecubital fossa. De-epithelialize two strips, each 1 cm wide, on either side of the neourethra, from the proximal edge to within 2.5 to 3 cm of the distal portion. Raise the flap as described in Step 2, from distal to proximal and from the radial and ulnar border to the thin intramuscular septum containing the septocutaneous perforating vessels. Identify and preserve the superficial branch of the radial nerve as it pierces the brachioradialis tendon and courses close to the cephalic vein at the wrist. The dissection is made beneath the deep fascia of the forearm over the flexor musculature and tendons.

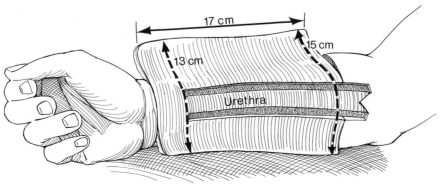

Make the proximal incision with care to identify and preserve the cephalic vein. Identify the medial and lateral antebrachial cutaneous nerves and dissect them an additional 3 to 4 cm proximal to the skin paddle. Tag and divide them. Elevate the radial artery and its venae comitantes from the bed from distal to proximal until the bifurcation of the brachial artery is encountered. Continue dissection of the proximal venae comitantes until the two veins merge into one. Proceed more proximally. It is frequently necessary to make an incision in the antecubital fossa skin to allow the coalesced venae comitantes to join the cephalic vein. This extra dissection makes it possible for one large vein to drain not only the superficial cephalic system but also the venae comitantes, providing for a single venous anastomosis (Step 6). Create the distal neoglans flange with full-thickness transverse incisions to the central neourethra. The flap is then attached only by the radial vascular bundle proximally and distally. Check for adequate ulnar blood supply to the hand before clamping, ligating, and dividing the distal radial vascular bundle.

"Tube" the neourethra over a 12 F catheter with a four-layer closure. Turn the flap over and close the dorsal skin in two layers.

Trim the wings of the neoglans to the appropriate shape and roll them back on the shaft. De-epithelialize the distal portion of the shaft that will be under the rolled-back neoglans.

Formation of a Corona: Leave the constructed neophallus on the arm attached to its vascular pedicle while the recipient site is being prepared.

Harvest approximately 20 cm of saphenous vein from the thigh, and leave it attached to the femoral vein at the fossa ovalis. Anastomose the divided end of the vein graft to the femoral artery, creating a saphenous vein loop arteriovenous fistula. Isolate the dorsal penile branches of the pudendal nerve. If no nerves are apparent, continue dissection toward the perineum, where the pudendal nerves can be identified as they emerge from Alcock's canal and travel along the inferior pubic ramus.

Before ligating and dividing the proximal radial artery, give 5000 units of heparin intravenously. Secure the neophallus with tacking sutures before performing the microvascular anastomoses.

Make a primary end-to-end two-layered spatulated urethral anastomosis first. Divide the saphenous vein loop and anastomose the cephalic vein end to end to the venous limb of the saphenous loop with 8-0 nylon. Anastomose the radial artery to the arterial limb of the saphenous loop end to end. Perform neurorrhaphies as an epineural repair (see page 63). Close the remaining wounds of the proximal shaft, the neophallus, and the femoral vessels. Avoid tunneling the flap or saphenous loop vessels; instead, make connecting incisions between the proximal femoral vessels and the recipient site. Dress the phallus postoperatively to support it in an upright position and avoid damage at the hinge site. Close the forearm defect with a split-thickness skin graft.

Placement of Prosthesis

Wait 6 to 9 months for protective sensation to return by finding the glans to be half as sensitive as the index finger when tested for vibratory sensitivity by biothesiometry. If sensation is not adequate, avoid a noninflating prosthesis.

Make a transverse low suprapubic incision and dissect to the base of the penis, staying close to the symphyseal periosteum. Dilate a space proximally for 8 cm for the prosthesis, starting with scissors and proceeding with long clamps and Hegar dilators on the side opposite that of the vascular supply. Create a tunnel in the neophallus that remains 1 to 1.5 cm beneath the skin distally. For an inflatable prosthesis, create a second tunnel between the suprapubic incision and one made over the ischial tuberosity, keeping the dilation against the inferior ramus of the pubis. Prepare a single-cylinder inflatable prosthesis, preferably an AMS 700CX (two cylinders can rarely be accommodated and may lead to loss of sensation), by covering it with a 14-mm sleeve of vascular stretch polytetrafluoroethylene (Gore-Tex). After insertion, suture the sleeve to the symphysis. Implant the pump and reservoir (see page 189), making a thigh pouch for the pump if scrotum is not available or delay its implantation until a scrotum is formed at a later procedure. Wait 6 to 8 weeks before cycling the prosthesis.

POSTOPERATIVE PROBLEMS

The incidence of *fistula* is very high, occurring usually ventrally at the base (the site of the hinge). Primary interposition of a gracilis flap may prevent breakdown in this area. Perform fistula repair after tissues are fully healed (at least 3 months), using primary local skin flaps, full-thickness skin grafts, buccal mucosa, or bladder epithelium. *Urethral loss* can be corrected by applying a bladder epithelial graft, a buccal mucosal graft, or a full-thickness skin graft. *Strictures,* if anticipated, may be prevented by having the patient use balloon dilation at home. *Erosion* and *extrusion* can be a problem after placement of a prosthesis.

Commentary by Laurence A. Levine

Until recently, the reconstructed phallus was considered simply a symbol of masculinity for the unfortunate male who had lost his penis as a result of devastating illness or injury. As a result of free tissue transfer and microsurgical techniques, one-stage total phallic construction is now possible, offering a functionally and psychologically satisfying neophallus.

The radial forearm free flap phallic construction, first proposed by Chang and Hwang in 1984, has undergone several refinements and modifications, including neurorrhaphies of the sensory nerves in the flap with the pudendal nerves, providing restoration of erogenous sensibility as well as protective sensation in the neophallus.

The radial forearm flap as originally designed for phallic construction is limited in size and has the propensity to develop meatal stenosis. In an attempt to eliminate the meatal suture line and its potential to cause stenosis, the radial forearm flap was modified into the shape of a cricket bat. The major disadvantage of this design is that it significantly limits phallic length.

Gottlieb and Levine redesigned the radial forearm flap by including a centrally located neourethra that is connected to a neoglans (Step 5). With this technique, meatal stenosis was eliminated, adequate phallic length was maintained, and the esthetic result was improved by the incorporation of a neoglans.

It is imperative that all patients who are candidates for this procedure undergo a comprehensive psychological evaluation. Allen's test for radial or ulnar patency (digitally compress the radial or ulnar artery after having the patient clench his fist to evacuate the blood; failure of the blood to return is evidence of occlusion of the noncompressed vessel) is performed on both hands preoperatively. A patient with an equivocal Allen test is referred for noninvasive duplex Doppler imaging of the vasculature of the hand. Arteriography is generally not necessary. The nondominant forearm is typically chosen. We have found that the 13-cm width initially described for this flap reconstruction is inadequate for "tubing" and for closure without tension. Also, the 10-cm length is usually unsatisfactory for successful intromission; therefore, in most cases, the flap dimensions should be at least 15 × 17 cm. If the native urethra ends in the perineum, the length of the neourethra may be safely increased to 25 cm by designing a proximal extension to just above the antecubital fossa.

In the new design, two strips, each 1 cm wide, on either side of the neourethra are de-epithelialized from the proximal edge to within 2.5 to 3 cm of the distal portion. The technique of forming the flap is described in Steps 5 and 6.

The forearm muscles in the bed of the flap donor site are approximated over any exposed tendons to minimize contour irregularities. The donor site is covered with a split-thickness graft. Although the donor site remains a cosmetic concern, this can be addressed in the postoperative period with tissue expansion techniques. Considering the high quality of phallic construction possible with the radial forearm flap, the resultant donor site scar is usually well tolerated by patients.

Sexual function of the reconstructed penis has been less than satisfactory until recently. We strongly believe that primary prosthesis placement is not advisable because of the increased pressure with ischemia, which increases the risk of erosion or extrusion secondary to pressure necrosis. The use of a neuro-sensory flap was a critical step that made possible functional

and safe placement of a prosthesis. Innervation of the neophallus allows for erogenous sensitivity and, in addition, protects against ischemic damage within the flap from chronic pressure and sheer forces. The development of adequate protective sensation takes 6 to 9 months from the time of initial construction of a neophallus, after which a prosthesis may be placed and unrestricted sexual activity becomes possible.

Successful prosthesis placement has been accomplished in 14 patients with a mean follow-up period of more than 4 years. If no proximal corpora remain, so that it cannot migrate, the prosthesis is secured by forming a sleeve from the 14-mm diameter Gore-Tex vascular graft material, as described previously.

Postoperatively, intravenous antibiotics are discontinued on the second day following the procedure and replaced with suppressant oral antibiotic coverage, which is continued until all catheters are removed. Low-dose aspirin is continued indefinitely. Physical therapy for the donor arm begins when the initial dressings have been removed, 7 to 10 days postoperatively. With this modified radial forearm flap technique, meatal stenosis has been eliminated. Although proximal urethral stricture is not uncommon, typically at the anastomosis, all patients have ultimately been able to stand to void.

Although refinements in the radial forearm flap have allowed a one-stage functional total phallic construction, this procedure is best performed by two teams, incorporating the reconstructive skills of a plastic surgeon and a urologist. It typically takes 16 to 20 hours to complete.

SCROTAL FLAP RECONSTRUCTION WITH BACULUM
(Bissada)

6 **A,** Outline a scrotal skin flap that encompasses the scrotal urethrostomy. Make it 10 cm long with a 10-cm base tapering to 8 cm. Dissect it with a generous amount of fatty subcutaneous tissue. **B,** Expose the stumps of the corpora cavernosa. Inject normal saline into them and make a 1-cm incision in each. **C,** Flatten the distal ends of two small (8 × 9 mm) flexible rod penile prostheses, and insert the tapered proximal ends into the corpora. Measure their length in relation to the scrotal flap, and trim the proximal taper accordingly. Wrap the distal two thirds of each in Marlex or polyglycolic acid mesh to form an implantable baculum.

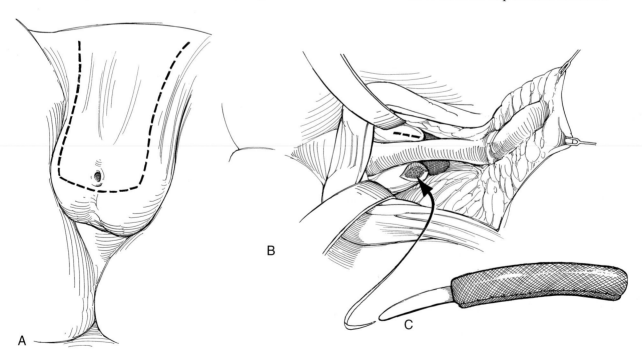

A

B

C

7 Insert the proximal ends into the corpora, trim excess mesh, and suture the mesh to the tunica albuginea with 3-0 SAS.

8 Close the scrotal flap ventrally.
Urine exits from the previously placed perineal urethrostomy. If a urethra-sparing penectomy has been done, place the urethra under the folded scrotal flap.

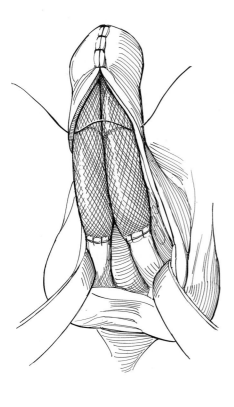

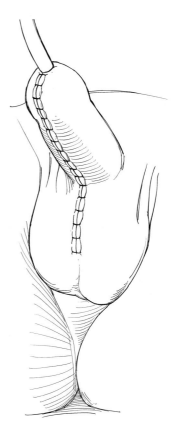

VASCULARIZED EXTENDED GROIN FLAP RECONSTRUCTION
(Perovic)

Raise a combined groin and lower abdominal flap based on the superficial iliac and inferior epigastric system.

Form the flap in two parts: a medial narrow hairless part for the new urethra and a medial wide part for shaft reconstruction. De-epithelialize the base for a pedicle. Place the urethral portion inside the larger portion of the flap. Transfer the pedicle to a site below the symphysis, and anastomose the new urethra to the stump. (This may be done at a second stage.)

Excision of Male Urethral Diverticulum

In the adult male, diverticula are secondary to distal stricture (see page 271) or result from a periurethral abscess. In boys, they are a complication of hypospadias repair, usually secondary to a more distal stricture or application of too large a patch. They also occur at the penoscrotal junction associated with anterior urethral valves.

The repair of urethrocutaneous fistulas is described on pages 108 to 111, Steps 11 to 15. For an abscessed diverticulum, open and trim it and tack its edges to the penile skin as part of a staged linear urethroplasty.

Clear urinary tract infection if possible and provide perioperative antibacterial coverage. Suprapubic urinary diversion may be indicated.

1 *Position:* Lithotomy. Examine the patient with a bougie à boule and a cystoscope to be sure that the caliber of the urethra is normal distal to the diverticulum. For a small diverticulum, insert a sound or bougie (or a Fogarty catheter) into the diverticulum. Inject dilute methylene blue into the meatus to fill and stain the diverticular lining. Insert a 20 F 5-ml silicone balloon catheter into the bladder.
Incision: Incise vertically in the midline or make a Y incision over the diverticulum. Dissect the walls free laterally as much as possible. For diverticula in the pendulous urethra, deglove the penis.

2 Open directly into the exposed diverticulum with a longitudinal incision. Place stay sutures.

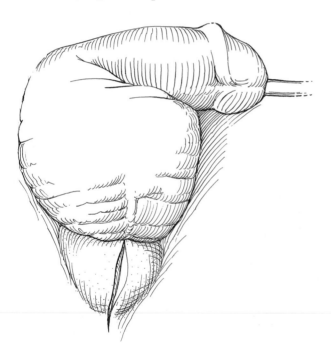

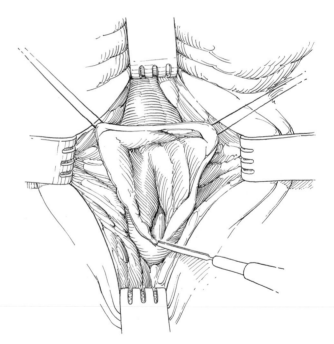

3 Before trimming the walls, plan urethral closure to leave a urethral strip 3 cm wide in an adult in order to provide a urethral caliber of 30 F. If hairs are present, depilate. Trim the excess lining asymmetrically to avoid overlapping suture lines. Insert a 20 F balloon catheter. If a distal urethral stricture was found, use part of the diverticulum, either by making a Y-V incision or by rotating a diverticular flap.

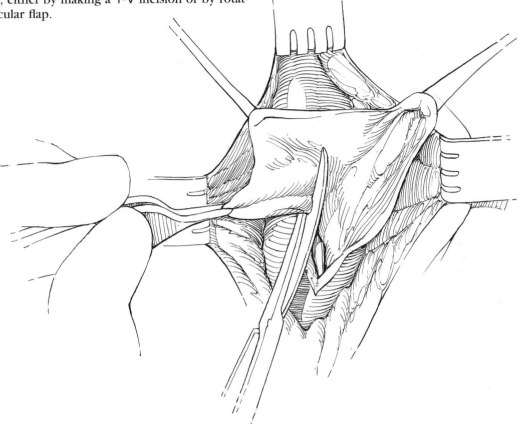

4 **A,** Invert the mucosal edge over the catheter with a running submucosal 3-0 CCG suture. Close the remainder of the defect with interrupted 3-0 CCG sutures. Because synthetic material such as PDS is absorbed more slowly, it should not be used, as stone formation may occur on the exposed sutures. It can also serve as a nidus for persistent infection. **B,** Approximate the fascia and subcutaneous tissue in as many layers as possible with 4-0 CCG sutures, avoiding overlapping suture lines, and close the skin with interrupted catgut sutures or with a fine running subcuticular SAS. Drainage is rarely needed, but a piece of a Penrose drain may be inserted and sutured to the skin. Leave the catheter in place for 10 days. Check for leakage with retrograde urethrography at the time of catheter removal.

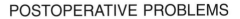

A

B

POSTOPERATIVE PROBLEMS

Urethrocutaneous fistula can be treated by prolonging catheter drainage. A *fistula* suggests distal obstruction, as does recurrence of the diverticulum. *Strictures* require dilation, urethrotomy, or even urethroplasty. For repair of urethrocutaneous fistulas, see pages 108 to 111.

Excision of Utricular Cyst

The most direct route to a utricular cyst is the transtrigonal approach. Another direct route is the transrectal posterior sagittal approach of deVries and Peña. The transabdominal and perineal approaches used for exposure of the seminal vesicle can also be applied to utricular cyst excision (see page 481).

Position: Supine. Insert a urethral catheter. *Incision:* Make a transverse (see page 490) or vertical (see page 487) lower abdominal incision.

TRANSTRIGONAL APPROACH
(Monfort)

1 Open the bladder and place a Denis Browne retractor to expose the trigone. Insert infant feeding tubes into the ureteral orifices. If possible, insert a balloon catheter through the ostium of the cyst to aid in the dissection. With the cutting current, make a vertical incision through the trigone and posterior bladder wall that approaches the vesical neck, and hold it open with stay sutures (not shown). Dissect down to the utricle with tenotomy or Lahey scissors under direct vision while pushing the peritoneal fold cephalad. Avoid the urethral wall and sphincters; identify their location by the urethral catheter. Dissect and displace the vasa deferentia laterally.

Expose the anterior wall of the cyst. Remove the retractor blade at the inferior end of the bladder incision to expose the bladder neck. Dissect the cyst to its contact with the posterior urethra as low as possible. Remove the cyst and close the defect at the urethra.

Close the trigone in two layers with 3-0 SAS. Insert a cystostomy tube, to remain for 1 week. Close the bladder in layers. Place a Penrose drain in the retropubic space.

The same approach can gain access to the refluxing residual ureteral stump after heminephrectomy for an ectopic ureter, an approach less formidable and damaging than extravesical dissection.

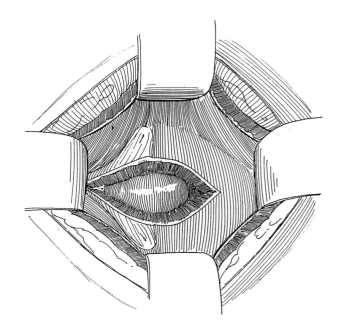

POSTERIOR SAGITTAL RESECTION

The posterior sagittal approach (deVries and Peña) is well suited for excising müllerian duct cysts and cysts of the seminal vesicle. Visualization for excision and for closure of the defect in the urethra is excellent.

Commentary by Jack S. Elder

Utricular or müllerian duct cysts are most common in boys with penoscrotal or perineal hypospadias and in those with intersex conditions. These cysts vary in size and usually are asymptomatic. However, some individuals may experience dysuria, perineal discomfort, urinary tract infection, epididymitis, lower abdominal mass, obstructive symptoms, hematuria, incontinence, reduced semen volume, or oligospermia. By definition, these cysts should communicate only with the prostatic urethra. The literature, however, reports müllerian duct cysts that communicate with the vasa deferentia. These latter cysts are more appropriately termed *genital duct* or *ejaculatory duct cysts*.

Utricular cysts often are palpable on rectal examination. They are usually apparent on an imaging study, such as transrectal ultrasonography, retrograde urethrography, or voiding cystourethrography. One of these studies should be done to evaluate the size of the cyst. Endoscopy is indicated to determine whether the ostium of the cyst is narrow. In addition, a small ureteral catheter should be inserted into the cyst and contrast injected to determine whether the vasa deferentia enter it. In selected patients, it is necessary to perform vasography to learn whether there is communication with the cyst.

Although the ostium of the cyst may be incised endoscopically, signs and symptoms often are not relieved. Consequently, an open surgical approach usually is necessary. The perineal approach should be avoided because of the risk of iatrogenic impotence.

The transtrigonal approach provides the best exposure. After the bladder is opened, a Denis Browne retractor is placed. Ureteral catheters or pediatric feeding tubes should be inserted into the ureteral orifices. The trigone is then incised in the midline with the cautery. Stay sutures should be placed in the edges of the trigone. The utricle should be immediately apparent and can be dissected out with tenotomy scissors. Extreme care should be taken to avoid the vasa. The cyst may be dissected to its communication with the urethra. At times, opening the cyst is helpful in its mobilization. The cyst may be intubated with a balloon catheter, which facilitates access to the retrovesical margin of the cyst.

The urethra should be closed over a urethral catheter with a fine running imbricating polyglycolic acid stitch for the inner layer and interrupted sutures for the outer layer. Generally, no drainage of the retrovesical space is necessary. The trigone should be closed in two layers with polyglycolic acid sutures. It is preferable to leave ureteral catheters for 2 to 3 days and a urethral catheter and suprapubic tube for 7 to 10 days postoperatively.

If the vasa enter the cyst, they need to be transected. Ideally, they should be implanted into the bladder; usually this can be accomplished in a nonrefluxing manner. However, subsequent fertility seems unlikely, even with current methods of retrieving sperm from the bladder.

Although this approach has been used mainly for genital duct cysts, it also may be used in excising remnants of fistulous tracts in children born with high imperforate anus.

SECTION

7

Female Genitalia: Reconstruction

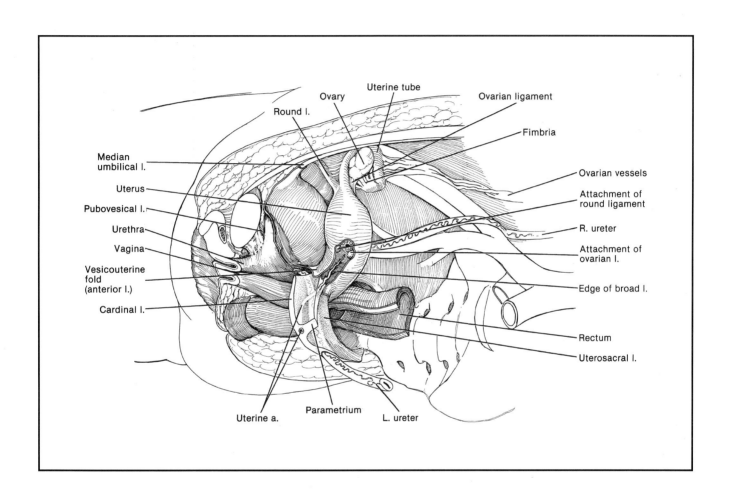

Reconstruction of the Female Genitalia

Vaginal construction can be challenging, but several options are available. Fistulas between the urethra and the vagina are usually complicated by loss of part of the urethra and thus require considerable reconstruction. Formation of a new urethra may be necessary. Diverticula of the female urethra may be difficult to define and completely excise. Appreciation of the technique of hysterectomy, although it is not strictly a urologic procedure, can be useful in operations in the pelvis.

Vaginal Reconstruction

Tissues from several sites have been used for replacement of the vagina: skin expanded locally, split-thickness skin grafts, full-thickness skin grafts or flaps after skin expansion, and segments of bowel.

Evaluate the anatomic and functional arrangements preoperatively, using ultrasonography, voiding cystourethrography, and endoscopy. Urodynamic studies may be indicated; spinal cord disease must be detected before repair. Computed tomography and magnetic resonance imaging may also give useful information.

Make every effort to complete the procedure in one stage. Include vaginal reconstruction in the same procedure as correction of anal anomalies. Be prepared for major revisions of the urinary tract. The follow-up of these patients is most important to ensure that the new vagina maintains an adequate size.

FORMATION OF PERINEAL CAVITY FOR NEOVAGINA

Before a vagina can be formed, a space must be created for it. With *congenital gynetresia*, locate the hymenal dimple and make a short transverse incision that passes between the urethra and the perineal body. Carry the incision in the midline as far as the rectovesical pouch, and extend it laterally by blunt dissection. For the congenitally short vagina, begin the dissection at the apex of the vagina. In infants, dilation with a Hegar dilator may be adequate.

After previous surgery, and especially after radiation therapy, the dissection is much more difficult. Start with a median episiotomy and develop the space occupied by scar tissue, although the dissection risks entering the rectum or, when continued higher, the bladder. If the rectum is injured, close the defect and delay insertion of flaps or grafts, but pack the space to allow formation of granulation tissue. The ureters may have been displaced by previous procedures; preliminary insertion of ureteral catheters is advisable in these cases.

SKIN GRAFT INLAY (Abbé-McIndoe)

Be certain that the patient is well motivated. If possible, have her meet a patient who has had a similar operation. Provide showers and antibacterial soap, a low-residue diet, and a bowel preparation. Give perioperative antibiotics.

Instruments: Provide a dermatome with cement, a vaginal conformer (Heyer-Schulte prosthesis), condoms, three narrow Deaver retractors, mineral oil, and liquid thrombin.

Position: Low lithotomy. Thoroughly prepare the lower abdomen, upper legs, and perineum, and drape the perineum and one thigh. Insert a 24 F 5-ml balloon catheter in the urethra, fill the bladder, and insert a 24 F Malecot cystostomy tube (see pages 625 to 628). Place traction sutures to hold back the labia.

1 *Incision:* Make an X-shaped incision in the anterior perineum in the mucosal plaque, with the crossing of the X below the urethra to create four symmetric mucosa-like flaps. This allows four cutaneous flaps to be infolded into the vaginal canal to reduce circumferential scar contraction.

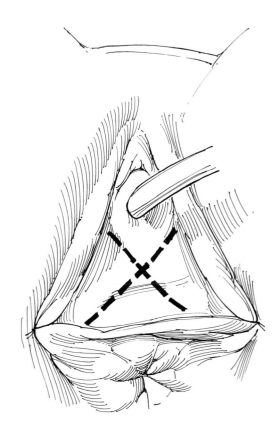

231

2 Don a second left glove, and place the left index finger in the rectum. Inject the proposed flaps and urethrorectal septum with a solution of 0.5 percent lidocaine (Xylocaine) with 1:2000 dilution of epinephrine to aid dissection and improve hemostasis. With the right index finger and the knife handle, bluntly dissect cephaloposteriorly between the rectum and the urethra on alternating sides of the median raphe to form a tunnel on each side. Divide the now-conspicuous raphe with Metzenbaum scissors, keeping the division closer to the rectum than to the bladder. Identify the anterior rectal wall so that accidental perforation can be avoided. Take care that the blunt dissection does not force the raphe to tear the rectum. If that occurs, stop the operation, repair the tear, and reoperate several months later. Make the pocket much deeper and wider than needed (in an adult it should be 21 cm deep and 17 cm wide) because it will contract. Pack the pocket with 2-inch roller gauze to achieve hemostasis. Turn the patient on her side. Obtain partial-thickness skin grafts from the upper thigh with a dermatome (see page 211). More than one sweep usually is needed. Alternatively, full-thickness grafts may be obtained bilaterally from the groin, lateral to the hair line. These leave less scarring in the donor site than the split-thickness grafts and contract less during healing.

3 **A** and **B,** Trim a piece of foam rubber larger in diameter than the proposed stent but of appropriate length, at least 10 cm. Compress the foam into a cylinder 3 or 4 cm in diameter, and tie it with a series of 3-0 synthetic absorbable sutures (SAS). Cover the cylinder with two or three washed condoms preparatory to suturing the graft to it.

Alternative: Inflate a commercial vaginal conformer with air and coat it with mineral oil. The advantage of the inflatable conformer is that it may be deflated and removed painlessly, but it may be too short. Another disadvantage is that the patient may decide to remove it and then become lost to follow-up, with subsequent failure of the repair. Fit the sheets of skin on the stent or conformer with the raw side out, and suture their edges to each other with running 5-0 SAS, placing the knots against the mold.

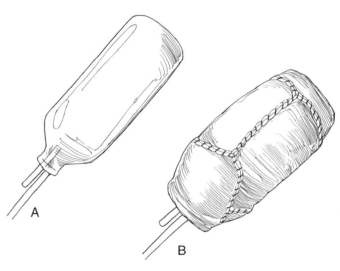

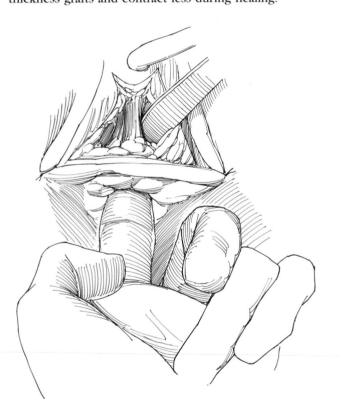

4 Check hemostasis in the rectourethral defect, then coat the walls with liquid thrombin. Ease the stent covered with the grafts into the canal over three narrow Deaver retractors. Seat it well in the depths. If an inflatable stent is used, partially deflate it while measuring the amount of air withdrawn, so that the air may be accurately replaced after insertion.

5 Make notches in the graft. Insert the four flaps from the X-shaped skin incision and fasten them with interrupted 4-0 SAS to provide a noncircumferential suture line. Put two or three restraining sutures across the vestibule (not across the vulva) to hold the stent in place. Remove the urethral catheter. Place coated gauze and fluffs held with elastic tape to compress the perineum. Postoperatively, order the patient to remain at bed rest. Give stool softeners or mineral oil, 30 ml orally three times a day, on the first postoperative day; then maintain a low-residue diet for several days. Thereafter, have the patient keep the bowel movements loose by taking petroleum agar and stool softeners for 1 to 2 weeks. On the seventh or eighth day, provide sedation, remove the introital sutures, and deflate and gently withdraw the stent. If it hangs up, inject mineral oil around it through a small, soft catheter. Cleanse the perineum. Wash, lubricate, and replace the stent, and hold it in place with a perineal binder. Educate the patient on its regular removal and reinsertion. It must be retained day and night for at least 3 months, then at night for 3 more months, because split-thickness grafts readily contract.

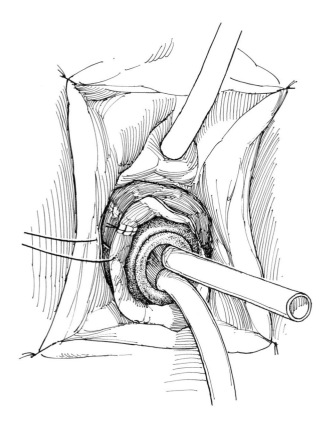

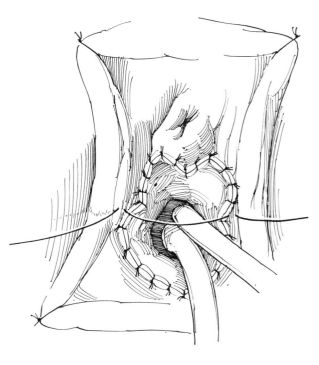

PUDENDAL THIGH FLAP VAGINA
(Wee and Joseph)

6 **A,** This technique depends on blood supply from the posterior labial arteries arising from the perineal artery, but also from anastomoses with the deep external pudendal artery, medial femoral circumflex artery, and anterior branch of the obturator artery.

Position: Lithotomy with the legs in stirrups. Place a balloon catheter in the bladder. Insert a Hegar dilator in the rectum to develop a plane between it and the base of the bladder large enough to accommodate the new vagina (Steps 1 and 2). **B,** *Incisions:* Mark two slightly curved and tapered flaps on either side of the vulva, centered on the crease of the groin. The base in an adult is 6 cm wide, and the length may be up to 15 cm, placing the tip over the femoral triangle.

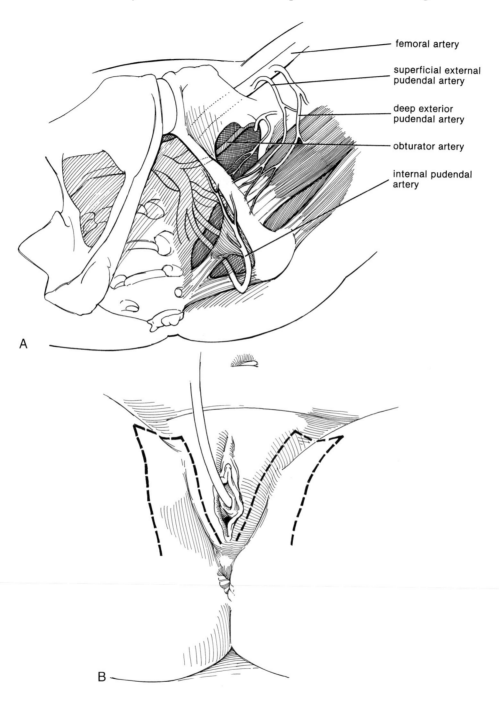

femoral artery

superficial external pudendal artery

deep exterior pudendal artery

obturator artery

internal pudendal artery

A

B

7 Incise down to the deep fascia, beginning at the end of the flap, and raise it, taking care to include the perimysium of the adductor muscles to avoid damage to the nerves in the flap. At the base of the flap, divide the skin through the dermis to a depth of 1 to 1.5 cm (*inset*) to allow freedom for the flap to be depressed for passage under the labium.

8 Form tunnels under the labia by dissecting them from the pubic ramus. Pass the flaps under the labia. With the flaps everted, suture the pairs together in the midline to close the posterior wall of the new vagina.

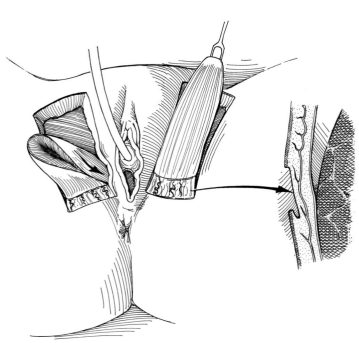

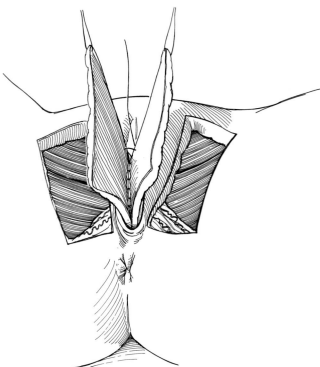

9 At the apex, continue suturing to approximate the anterior wall by bringing the lateral borders together to form the vaginal tube. Invert the tube, and fasten the apex to the posterior bladder wall. Close the lateral defects from the graft site. Insert a loose pack over gauze impregnated with petroleum jelly. As an alternative, a *free flap* of full-thickness hairless skin can be obtained from the scapular region (Johnson) and connected to the external pudendal vessels.

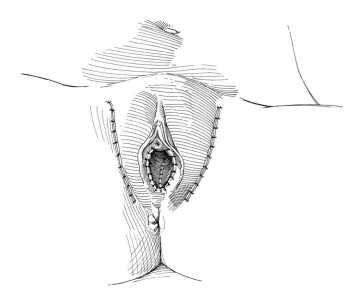

VAGINA FROM LABIA MINORA FLAPS
(Flack)

Start an M-shaped incision transversely beneath the urethral meatus, then incise upward on either side along the medial border of the labia minora. Continue the incision caudally between the labia majora and minora. Suture the paraurethral flaps together to form the floor of the new vagina, then approximate the caudal flaps to form the roof. Rotate the pocket so formed into a cavity created

in the perineum. Begin dilations with lucite dilators and bicycle-seat dilation (Ingram) as early as 3 weeks.

VULVOVAGINOPLASTY
(Williams)

To form a simple superficial copulating pouch, make a U incision down the labia majora and around the posterior vulva and perineum. Free up the edges on both sides of the incision. Approximate the medial edges with two or three layers of sutures and cover with the lateral edges.

TISSUE EXPANSION TECHNIQUE
(Patil and Hixson)

Make a right inguinal incision, and digitally dissect a pocket in the right labium majus. Select a tissue expander of suitable size; 250 ml is suitable for an adolescent. Insert the tissue expander in the labial pocket, and place the filling port subcutaneously in a (future) hair-bearing area, where it can be felt through the skin. Every 2 weeks add up to 20 ml of normal saline through a 25-gauge needle, the volume being dependent on the tolerance of the girl.

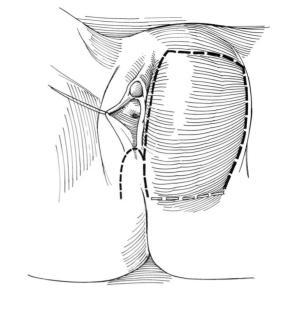

10 When an adequate size is reached (in approximately 6 weeks), mark and raise a 7.5 × 10-cm flap on the expanded labium with an incision that circumscribes the area of expansion and also crosses the perineum posterior to the introitus. Remove the expander, but preserve the new vascularized sheath that has formed beneath it.

11 Rotate the flap and suture the proximal end to the stump of the vagina with 2-0 SAS. Because it does not reach completely around the vaginal opening, leave a 1-cm gap at the junction with the vagina to epithelialize.

12 Suture the distal end to the skin. Insert the initial posterior perineal flap to fill the outer portion of the posterior gap in the tubed flap. Close the labial defect.

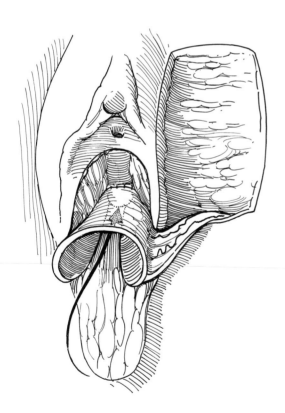

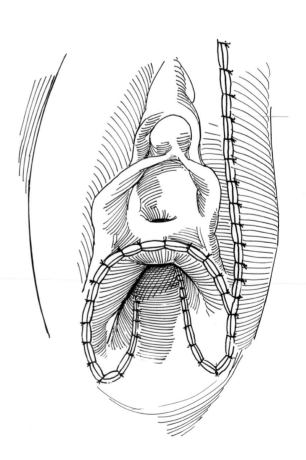

BILATERAL GRACILIS
MYOCUTANEOUS FLAP VAGINA

A myocutaneous flap may be needed if the vaginal defect is large and the tissues are in poor condition.

13 Raise a gracilis flap from each leg (see pages 50 to 51). Form a tunnel to connect the flap incision with the vagina under the intact perineal skin, as described on pages 590 to 592 for closure of a vesicovaginal fistula.

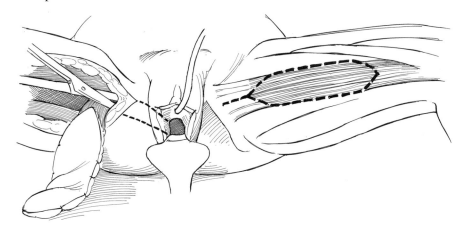

14 A and B, Rotate and draw the flaps gently through the tunnels. Suture the two flaps together with 3-0 SAS, first in the midline and then peripherally to form a tube. Insert the distal end of the tube through the introitus into the prepared area in the perineum. Fix the muscle to the levator ani muscle and to the periosteum of the symphysis with interrupted 3-0 SAS.

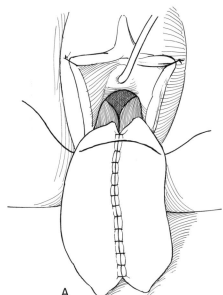
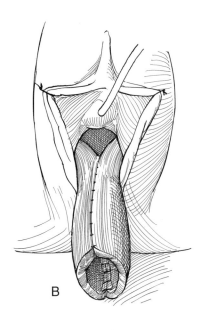

A

B

15 Trim the proximal end of the flap and suture it at the introitus with 3-0 interrupted SAS. Close the incisions in the fascia lata with 2-0 interrupted SAS. Insert suction drains bilaterally. Close the subcutaneous layer with 3-0 sutures and the skin with 4-0 subcuticular sutures.

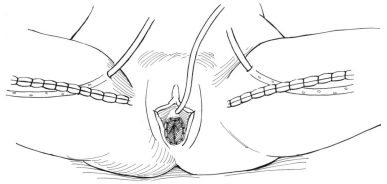

POSTOPERATIVE PROBLEMS WITH GRAFTS AND FLAPS

Contraction of the graft is the greatest problem. It is usually caused by poor compliance by the patient in keeping the new vagina dilated. For this reason, careful selection of candidates and persistent long-term follow-up are crucial. In some patients, bowel that does not require dilation may be a better choice. The vagina may be too short, resulting in dyspareunia. *Necrosis* and sloughing of some of the edge of the graft are usual, but major loss is uncommon. With healthy perineal tissue and good quality skin, *infection* is unusual. Estrogen suppositories may be used to keep the neovagina supple.

CECAL VAGINA

Although placement of a cecal vagina may be used as a primary procedure, usually one resorts to intestinal segments to substitute for a vagina when previous procedures have failed and have left the area scarred or involved in fistulas. The procedure is useful in infants and children because it does not require postoperative dilation.

Provide preoperative bowel preparation and prophylactic antibiotics. Insert a nasogastric tube.

Position: Supine, with the legs slightly flexed and widely abducted and the head tilted down. Prepare and drape a single abdominoperineal field. Insert a urethral catheter.

16 *Abdominal team:* **A,** Make a lower abdominal incision, either vertical or transverse. Mobilize the posterior wall of the bladder and urethra. **B,** Incise the peritoneum along the white line to free the cecum and ascending colon, and continue the release around the hepatic flexure to allow the subsequent anastomosis of ileum to colon. Locate the ileocolic artery by transillumination to determine that the segment will be adequately vascularized and that the ileocolic vascular pedicle will allow the colon to reach the perineum.

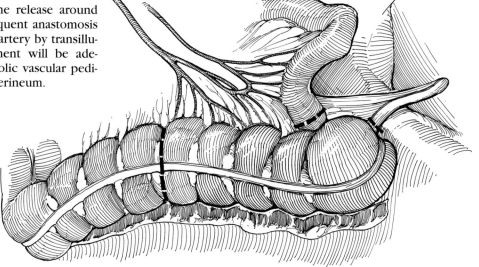

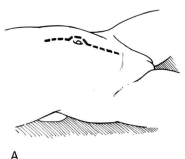

A

B

17 Divide the colon and the terminal ileum, spatulate the ileum, and perform an ileocolic anastomosis (see page 744). Close the mesentery. Irrigate the segment with saline through a balloon catheter. *Optional:* Perform an appendectomy (see pages 675 to 676). Rotate the cecum 180 degrees counterclockwise (*arrows*).

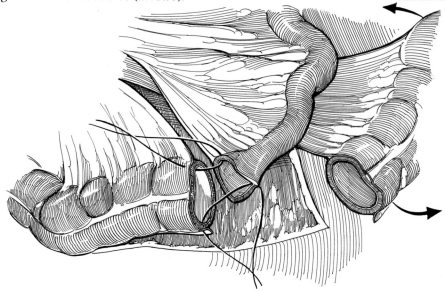

18 If the lower part of the new vagina is short or sacculated, incise the antimesenteric border for a distance of several centimeters and close the mesenteric border for a similar distance. A transverse incision in the peritoneum of the mesentery may allow additional length (see page 742). If high insertion of the ileocolic artery prevents inversion and descent, open the cecum and close the colonic end. If the cecum still does not reach, create a cuff from a U-shaped piece of ileum to attach to the colon distally.

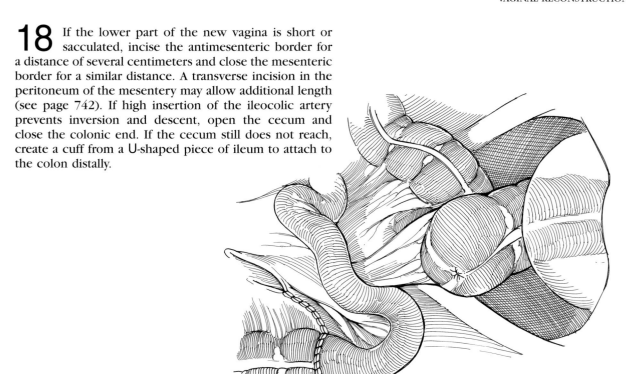

19 **A,** *Perineal team:* Make an H-shaped incision. In some male pseudohermaphrodites raised as females, the perineum is flat without an introital appearance, so that larger flaps are required. **B,** With blunt and sharp dissection, create a canal to the level of the vesicorectal pouch. The new canal should accommodate three fingers in the adult. Pull the bowel through the perineal tunnel. *Abdominal team:* Anchor the neovagina to the lateral abdominal wall or sacrum, insert a vaginal drain, and close the abdominal wound.

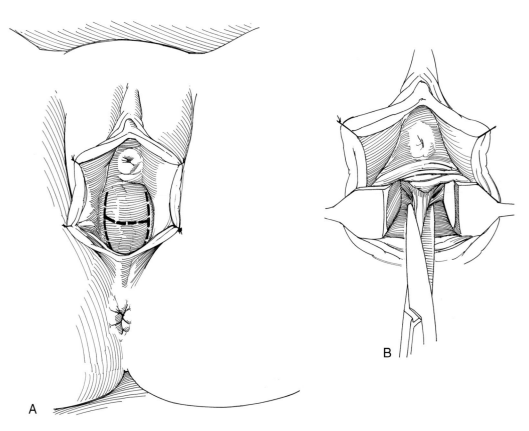

A

B

20 Suture the margin of the colon to the vulva with 3-0 SAS. Attach the posterior flap of perineal skin first, tying the sutures with the knots inside. Connect the anterior flap by placing all the sutures and tying them after placement. Place a vaginal pack coated with petroleum jelly in the new introitus. After 1 week, examine the perineum under anesthesia to separate accumulated synechiae. At 3 weeks, have the patient start daily dilation for 5 or 10 minutes twice a day, continually increasing the size of the dilator. Dilations must not be stopped until coitus is begun.

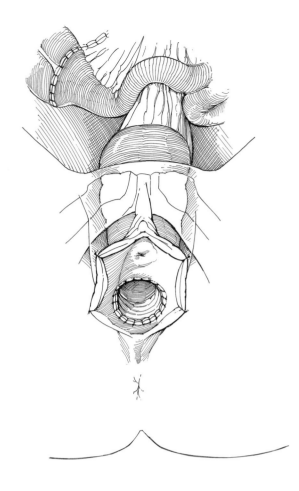

SIGMOID VAGINA

The sigmoid colon may be a better choice for a vagina than the cecum. The techniques illustrated in the previous section on cecal vagina are similar and adaptable.

Through a transverse lower abdominal incision, take a sigmoid segment between noncrushing clamps based on the left colic or, better, the superior hemorrhoidal artery (see Step 6A) and reanastomose the bowel with staples (see page 66). Close the proximal end of the segment with two layers of 3-0 SAS, and bring the distal end to the perineum (see Figure 20). Rotate it 180 degrees if necessary because of limitation from the length of the mesentery. If a portion of the vagina is present, have an assistant push it into the pelvis with a large Hegar dilator; grasp it with clamps. Open the residual vagina widely for anastomosis. If the vagina is absent, create an adequate space for passage of the bowel, so that its vasculature is not compromised, and fasten it directly to the perineum, making use of the anterior and posterior perineal flaps (Step 1). For 5 days provide a stent formed from the barrel of a syringe covered with Xeroform-impregnated gauze or from a polyvinyl foam bundle. If stenosis is found at 3 weeks, dilate the vagina under anesthesia.

Ileal Vagina. A segment of the ileum can be used in cases of congenital vaginal absence. Fifteen to 20 cm of ileum is opened, folded once, and sutured into a tube, leaving a V-shaped slot to accommodate the inverted V-shaped perineal flap after the segment is tunneled into the perineum. This alternative may be less acceptable to a fastidious patient because of soiling from mucus.

Postoperative Problems with Bowel Substitution

Avoid *ileus* by continuing nasogastric suction for 4 or 5 days. Intercourse is proscribed for 6 weeks. Manage *mucous accumulation* by prescribing douching or simply by having the patient open the introitus while in the bath. Treat *redundancy* of the neovagina by circumferential trimming.

PERINEAL PRESSURE TECHNIQUE (Frank-Ingram)

For the short blind vagina found with the androgen insensitivity syndrome, this technique is effective in the hands of some experts working with well-motivated patients. Start by pressing vaginal dilators in the dimple and progress to pressure applied to the perineum 2 hours a day by a bicycle-seat stool that holds a plastic dilator. This technique can indent enough skin to form a functional vagina.

Commentary by John P. Gearhart

The subjects of vaginal construction are usually male pseudo-hermaphrodites who are being raised as females or females with müllerian duct anomalies requiring vaginal construction. Any associated anomalies are corrected before vaginal construction is done. Certainly, none of the procedures described here should be undertaken until the patient has achieved full growth. For practical purposes, this typically means waiting until the later teen years.

Skin Inlay, Abbé-McIndoe Procedure. It is important initially to make a cruciate incision on the perineum, so that the plane between the urethra and the anterior rectal wall can be entered and dissected without injury to either of these structures. I have had only limited experience with the procedure but have been involved in revision of a number of them. Reoperation was needed for correction of three problems: (1) The four perineal flaps were not made large enough to avoid contracture of the introitus; (2) the graft was brought too far distally in the perineum so that it did not appear as a mucosal opening; and (3) the entire graft contracted. As mentioned in the text, contracture of the graft is usually caused by poor compliance of the patient in keeping the vagina dilated with dilators used regularly or with frequent intercourse. Male pseudohermaphrodites, I have found, do better long term using estrogen suppositories on a regular basis because this seems to keep the graft and introitus supple and aids in preventing contracture.

Cecal Vagina. Although several authors have recommended the use of cecum to create a neovagina, I have found that it may be difficult to rotate the cecum downward enough to reach the perineal flaps. I prefer the modified Wagner-Baldwin technique, utilizing the sigmoid colon, because it usually is redundant and close to the operative field. When the sigmoid colon is used, I typically bring the omentum down to cover the colonic anastomosis and to separate the anastomosis from the superior suture line of the sigmoid vagina. Also, Step 19 should show the sigmoid well secured to the presacral area to prevent prolapse of the neovagina. Whether cecum or sigmoid is used, the difficulties typically lie at the introitus. Although Step 19 shows an H-type incision, with the labia majora and minora present, many male pseudohermaphrodites raised as females have a very flat perineum without an introitus. In that case, both a large perineally based flap and a flap based cephalad are necessary to suitably exteriorize the neovagina. A vaginal pack of iodoform gauze impregnated with vaseline placed for 2 days postoperatively has proved worthwhile. Although the anastomo-

sis between the perineum and the bowel-vagina usually is quite capacious, care must be taken in the postoperative months to make sure that stenosis does not occur.

Pudendal Thigh Flap Vagina. Although I have not had personal experience with this procedure, I am a bit concerned about the postoperative appearance of the junction between the upper thigh and the perineal area. This procedure requires removal of a large mass of tissue. I would have to see postoperative pictures before I would be convinced that it is superior to bowel interposition.

Tissue Expander Technique. Certainly tissue expanders have made an impact in reconstructive urology in boys with failed hypospadias repairs and in those with epispadias-exstrophy. It is truly amazing what a few weeks of tissue expansion does to increase the availability of local skin. I think the wide-based perineal flap shown in Step 10 certainly will help to prevent stenosis of the neovaginal orifice, and I believe that the amount of redundant tissue present will allow tension-free closure of the ipsilateral labia majora area.

Bilateral Gracilis Myocutaneous Flap Vagina. After pelvic surgery and/or radiation therapy when large amounts of new tissue are required and bowel cannot be used, this technique continues to be our preference.

In summary, although all of the techniques described certainly are helpful in creating a neovagina, application must be dictated by the surgeon's ability and experience. Hensle has reported excellent results using colonic segments in male pseudohermaphrodites raised as females and in those with vaginal agenesis. My results mirror those of Hensle, and I believe that a bowel segment is the best substitute for a vagina and that the sigmoid colon segment is superior to the cecal segment because the larger diameter of the colon permits anastomosis of the distal end of the straight segment to the perineum, requiring less mobilization of the mesentery than with the cecal procedure. Lastly, the colon segment offers the following advantages over the other techniques described, all of which require mobilization of large amounts of skin in the perineal area: (1) The procedure is technically simpler; (2) there is no uncertainty about "take" of the graft; (3) molds are not required to maintain patency; (4) colonic mucosa is more resistant to trauma; (5) adequate spontaneous lubrication is present for sexual intercourse without excessive mucus discharge created by small bowel; and (6) most pediatric urologists are quite familiar with using bowel segments for reconstructive procedures and thus have basic familiarity with the technique.

MALE-TO-FEMALE GENDER TRANSFORMATION

Raise a broad flap from the scrotum, and form a flap by an incision on the ventrum of the penis (the two will be combined to line the neovagina). Enter the perineum as for perineal prostatectomy (see page 452) to provide a bed for the vagina. Open the bulbospongiosus muscle and divide the urethra at the midpoint in the perineum.

Dissect the penis from the pubis; transect and close the crural stumps with sutures. Bring the urethra through a slit in the penile skin flap. Suture the end of the penile flap to the end of the scrotal flap and close the combined flaps as a tube, skin side out. Invert the tube into the perineal space and close the introital defect, sacrificing scrotal skin edges if necessary for a cosmetic result. Insert a vaginal pack by forcing it over a traction suture previously placed at the apex of the vagina. Tie the suture to hold the pack in place.

Urethrovaginal Fistula Repair

Perform urethrocystoscopy and vaginoscopy. Rule out an associated vesicovaginal fistula by voiding cystography. If necessary, obtain a urethral pressure profile, looking for the site of pressure drop.

Techniques available to close those fistulas not amenable to simple excision and closure include flap closures from the vagina or perineum. A fistula extending through the bladder neck requires excision and then careful approximation of the vesical neck musculature. If incontinence is due to associated vesicourethral incompetence, cystourethropexy may be combined with closure of the fistula or a sling may be applied. Apply a gracilis muscle flap if the urethral defect is large or the tissues are fibrotic as a result of prior operative procedures or radiation.

EXCISION AND CLOSURE OF URETHROVAGINAL FISTULA

Culture the urine and give appropriate antibiotics.

Instruments: Basic set, GU fine set, Turner-Warwick instruments, fiberoptic suction, medium vascular forceps, tenaculum, weighted posterior retractor with deep blade, punch cystostomy set, 24 F 5-ml silicone balloon catheter, and adrenaline 1:200,000 with syringe.

Position: Lithotomy. Insert a suprapubic punch cystostomy. (Alternatively, place the patient prone in the jackknife position, so that the urethra lies directly in view.) Prepare the lower abdomen, vagina, and perineum. Examine the area cystoscopically to visualize the defect and, in suitable cases, to attempt passage of a catheter through the fistula. Suture the labia laterally. Insert a silicone balloon catheter into the bladder, and place a weighted posterior retractor in the vagina. Infiltrate the vaginal mucosa with epinephrine diluted in saline to reduce bleeding during the dissection.

1 *Incision:* Place multiple fine holding sutures around the fistula for traction (for clarity, the sutures are not shown). Incise the vaginal mucosa around the fistula, and continue proximally on one side of the midline.

2 Dissect the fistula laterally with Lahey scissors, using sutures for traction. Mobilize a margin of pubocervicovesical fascia asymmetrically. Excise the margins of the fistula back to normal urethral tissue.

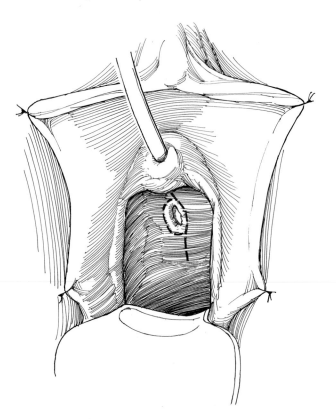
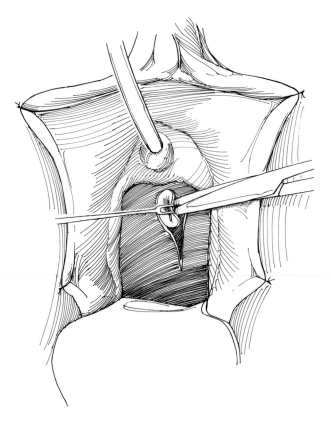

3 Close the defect in the urethra transversely with interrupted subepithelial 5-0 SAS. Bring the pubocervicovesical fascia over the defect asymmetrically with 4-0 SAS. Trim the vaginal mucosa on the opposite side to fit (*dashed line*).

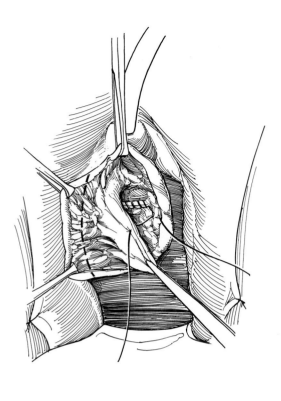

4 Bring the vaginal edges together with 4-0 SAS. Place a vaginal pack for 24 hours. Tape the catheter firmly to the abdomen to avoid traction on the repair and connect it to sterile drainage, to remain for 7 days. If a cystostomy tube has been placed, remove the urethral catheter.

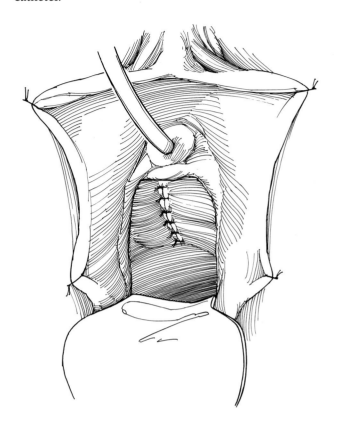

BULBOCAVERNOSUS MUSCLE AND FAT PAD SUPPLEMENT
(Martius Flap)

Locate the bulbocavernosus muscle and its associated fat pad by palpating it between the index finger placed just inside the hymenal ring and the thumb on the labium majus.

5 After repairing the fistula but before closing the vaginal mucosa, make a vertical incision in the groove between the labium majus and labium minus.

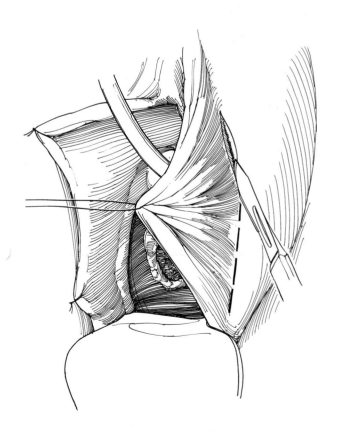

6 Expose the fat pad and underlying bulbocavernosus muscle. Dissect the muscle free with the fat pad surrounding the muscle. Take care not to disturb the blood supply, which comes from the deep perineal branch of the external pudendal artery and enters the muscle posteriorly close to its origin. Ligate the tip of the muscle and divide it anteriorly.

7 With a Mayo clamp, develop a tunnel starting near the repair, extending laterally under the labium minus, and ending near the dissected muscle. Enlarge it with the left index finger positioned against the tip of the clamp as it is withdrawn.

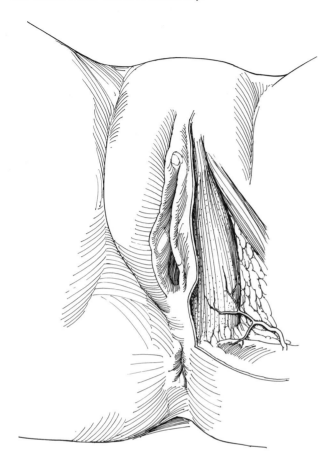

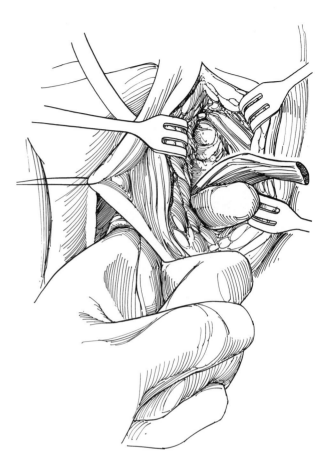

8 Grasp the tip of the muscle and pull it through the tunnel. Suture it over (around) the defect with interrupted 3-0 SAS.

9 Approximate the vaginal mucosa after trimming it asymmetrically, and close the lateral labial defect with a subcuticular 4-0 SAS.

Alternative: If less tissue supplementation is needed, instead of mobilizing the bulbospongiosus muscle itself, dissect through the subcutaneous fat to reach the labial fat pad that overlies the muscle. Preserve the blood supply that enters the pad posteriorly. Create a tunnel under the lateral vaginal wall. Rotate the fat pad under the skin bridge and fasten it over the repair with interrupted 4-0 SAS. Close both incisions.

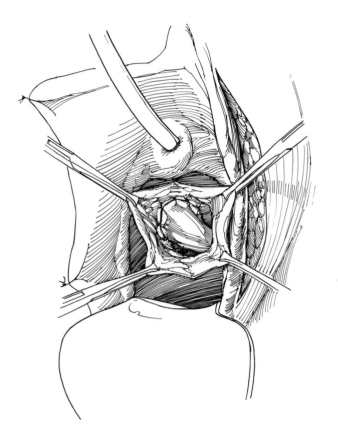

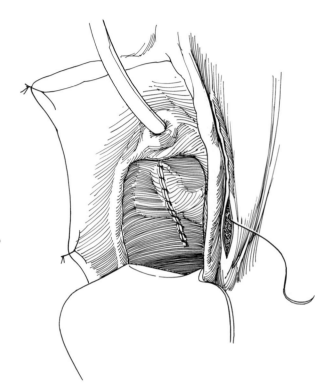

POSTOPERATIVE PROBLEMS

A *hematoma* may form following premature removal of the vaginal pack. A *fistula* may develop if tension persists after repair, if the balloon catheter is forcibly displaced, or if infection supervenes.

Commentary by Jerry G. Blaivas

This technique is suitable for fistulas that are not associated with significant loss of urethral or vesical neck tissue. With significant loss of tissue, it is usually necessary to reconstruct the vesical neck and urethra using vaginal flaps. When sphincteric incontinence or significant urethral hypermobility is present or an extensive dissection beneath the vesical neck is necessary, I favor a fascial pubovaginal sling with a Martius flap interposed between the sling and vesical neck. In my personal series of 49 urethral reconstructions, standard cystourethropexy procedures have had a 50 percent failure rate, whereas pubovaginal sling procedures have produced uniform success.

I use a slightly different technique to obtain a labial fat pad graft. A vertical incision is made at the crest of the labium majum parallel to the introitus. The incision is carried down just beneath Camper's fascia and the fat pad without any muscle isolated, as described by Dr. Hinman. If the dissection is begun too superficially, significant bleeding from barely visible, flat veins on the undersurface of the skin is often encountered. I leave a 0.25-inch Penrose drain at the lower margin of the wound.

Female Urethral Diverticulectomy

Diverticula may be treated by transurethral unroofing, but for more definitive treatment either marsupialize the diverticulum into the vagina or excise and repair it.

The diverticulum may often be palpated vaginally as a tender mass from which pus, blood, or urine extrudes on digital pressure. Voiding cystourethrography under fluoroscopic control, preferably with the patient standing, may fill the diverticulum so that it can be seen on the postvoid film. Intravenous urography may be needed to rule out upper tract duplication with ectopic ureterocele. Do retrograde positive-pressure urethrography with a double balloon three-way (Trattner) catheter if the voiding films are not diagnostic. Perform cystourethroscopy with a 30- or 0-degree lens, looking for the diverticular orifice. Vaginal pressure on the diverticulum may cause its contents to be extruded into view. Performing endoluminal ultrasonography at the time of surgery more clearly visualizes the diverticulum and may help to achieve complete excision.

If incontinence is part of the problem, study the patient appropriately and correct the incontinence at the same time the diverticulum is excised.

TRANSURETHRAL UNROOFING
(Lapides)

Insert a knife electrode through a panendoscope into the orifice of the diverticulum (or if that cannot be located, into the adjacent roof of the urethra) and incise the length of the diverticulum, staying in the midline.

MARSUPIALIZATION TECHNIQUE
(Spence-Duckett)

This technique is appropriate for diverticula that open below the continence mechanism. The result is a shortened urethra, which can be a factor in urinary incontinence following childbirth. It leaves a patulous intravaginal urethral meatus, which can cause spraying of the urinary stream and vaginal voiding with postmicturition incontinence, as well as difficulty with catheterization.

Retract the labia majora with traction sutures and insert a weighted speculum. Insert traction sutures on both sides of the meatus.

1 A and B, Identify the orifice of the diverticulum with the panendoscope. Insert Mayo scissors into the meatus and cut the urethra, urethrovaginal septum, and anterior vaginal wall from the meatus to the diverticular orifice, including the wall of the diverticulum itself, to saucerize the sac.

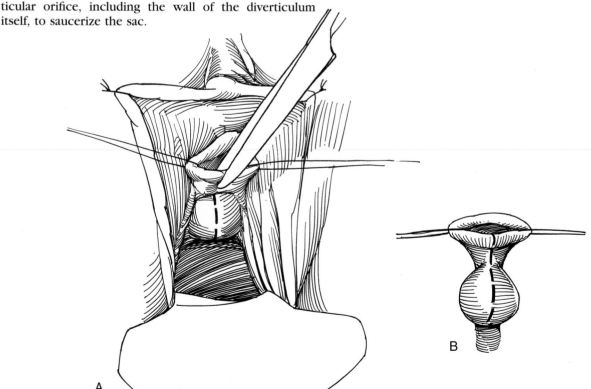

2 Trim the edges of the sac if they are redundant.

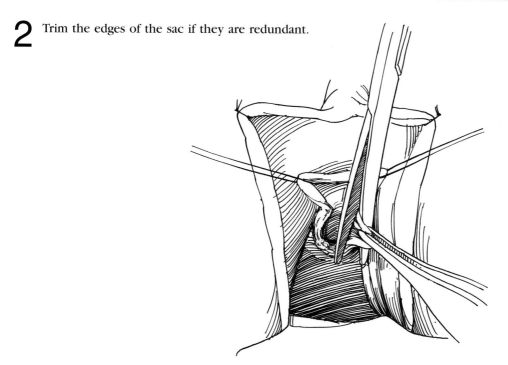

3 **A,** Run a 3-0 chromic catgut (CCG) suture in a continuous lock stitch to join the vaginal and diverticular edges. **B,** Place a 24 F 5-ml balloon catheter. Pack the wound with iodoform gauze and the vagina with roller gauze. Remove the catheter and the pack in 2 days.

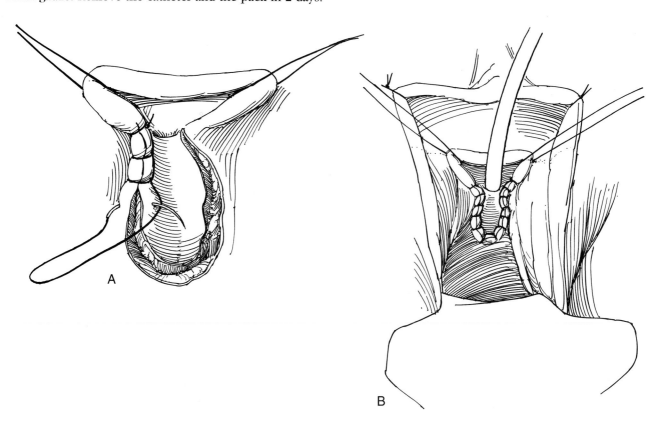

TRANSVAGINAL EXCISION

Delineate the diverticulum as described above. Attempt to sterilize the urine preoperatively and provide prophylactic antibiotics.

Instruments: Include a probe, urethral sounds, tenotomy scissors, a 5-ml balloon catheter, a Fogarty vascular balloon catheter, and methylene blue.

Perform vaginal preparation and drape the rectum from the field. Place 2-0 silk stay sutures in the labia, and suspend them over curved clamps or sew them to the skin of the thigh. Insert a urethral catheter. Consider placing a cystostomy catheter (see pages 625 to 627). Insert a weighted posterior speculum. Inspect the urethra with a panendoscope. If possible, insert a vascular balloon (Fogarty) catheter through an endoscope into the orifice and inflate the balloon. Coagulum mixed with the dye may be instilled via an angiocatheter inserted transurethrally or transvaginally. If it has not been filled with a balloon, instill methylene blue into the meatus to fill and stain the diverticulum, especially if the diverticulum appears complex by radiography. Be careful not to spill the dye. Insert a 22 F 5-ml silicone balloon catheter through the urethra into the bladder.

4 *Position:* Exaggerated lithotomy. The operation can also be done in the jack-knife position (see page 593), with the advantage that the operation is done at eye level. Draw the area into view with an Allis clamp placed at the meatus. Place another clamp in the vaginal wall just beyond the diverticulum. In older patients, draw the cervix down with tenaculum forceps or heavy traction sutures. If possible, place a Fogarty catheter transurethrally or fill the diverticulum with stained coagulum.

Incision: Make a stab wound into the diverticulum. If the size of the diverticulum can accommodate it, insert an 8 F balloon catheter with the tip cut off and inflate it to fill the diverticulum.

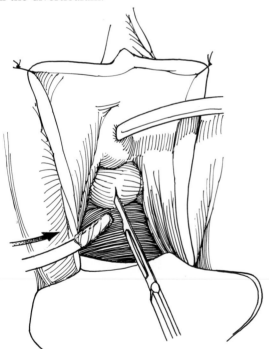

5 **A,** Place a purse-string suture around the catheter in the mucosa of the vagina, taking care not to perforate the balloon. Incise the vaginal mucosa elliptically and eccentrically over the length of the mass, and dissect it back to form vaginal flaps. Next, dissect the cervicovaginal fascia back from the surface of the diverticulum. In difficult cases, the entire distal urethra may be opened, to be closed later with subepithelial and epithelial sutures (Kropp technique). **B,** Alternatively, turn back a U-shaped vaginal flap.

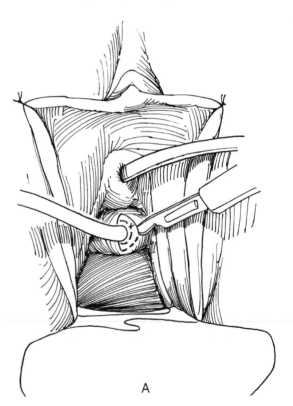

A

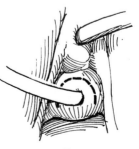

B

6 Dissect against the epithelial wall of the diverticulum with Lahey scissors using a separating motion while pulling the 8 F balloon catheter from side to side to reach the neck of the diverticulum. If the urethra is opened during the dissection at a site other than the neck of the diverticulum, close the urethra transversely with a fine absorbable suture.

7 Divide the neck of the diverticulum transversely on the urethra. Traction on the balloon catheter draws the area down for better visualization. Alternatively, open the diverticulum, remove the balloon catheter, and trim the diverticulum to its junction with the urethra, aided by the methylene blue stain. If possible, progressively transect it while successively placing interrupted 4-0 CCG sutures transversely in the urethral edges. Alternatively, place a purse-string suture around the defect after the neck has been transected. Two layers are desirable because a watertight closure is important.

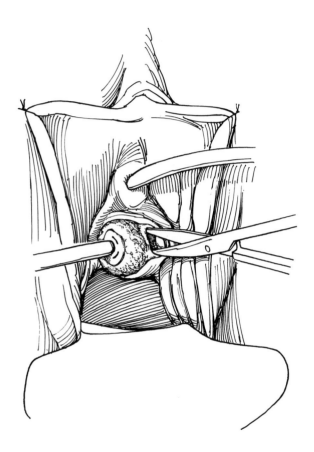

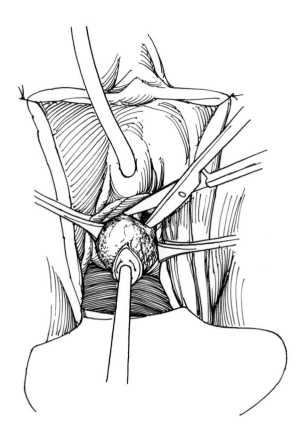

8 Draw the cervicovaginal fascia medially and approximate it with interrupted 3-0 CCG sutures. For better buttressing, reach laterally and bring the pubococcygeus muscle and fascia together. Consider interposing a labial fat pad or the bulbospongiosus muscle (see pages 243 to 245).

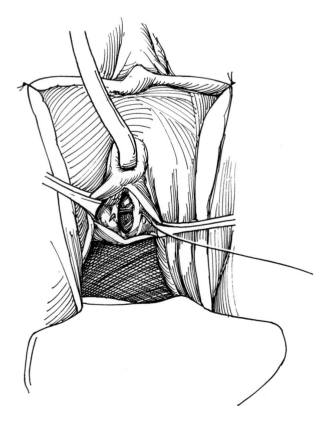

9 Excise any redundancy of the vaginal mucosa and close it at right angles to the previous suture line. To provide additional security, de-epithelialize a vaginal strip on one side of the incision, and lap the mucosa from the opposite side. If a U incision was used, the flap covers the deeper suture lines.

10 Insert two right-angle retractors covered with strips of petroleum jelly gauze into the vagina anteriorly and posteriorly, and pack it loosely with 2-inch roller gauze between the retractors before removing them. Tape the suprapubic and urethral catheters to the abdomen and thigh, respectively. Provide anticholinergic medication. Remove the pack in 1 or 2 days, and leave the catheter in for 7 to 10 days after aspirating it for urine culture and sensitivity testing. Start antibiotics and obtain a voiding cystourethrogram. For women with concomitant stress incontinence, place sutures to suspend the bladder neck first and tie the sutures after the diverticulum has been excised.

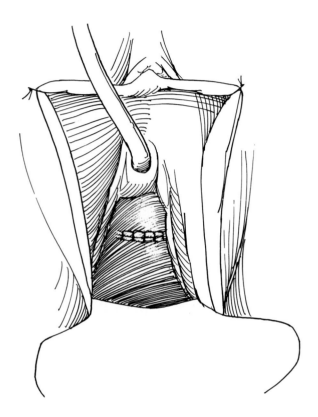

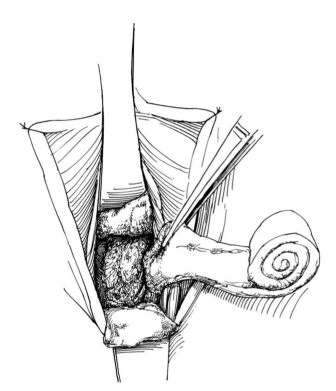

Commentary by Etienne Mazeman

Transvaginal excision is the most appropriate technique for treating female urethral diverticula. Even when diverticula are located in the distal urethra, we do not use endoscopy or marsupialization because there is a low risk of incontinence.

In most cases we prefer the prone position rather than the exaggerated lithotomy position. It has the advantage that the operative field is below the surgeon's eye level, compared with the gynecologic position, in which the field is above eye level. It facilitates access to the diverticulum and enables cystourethroscopy when indicated. The prone position does create two inconveniences: It requires general anesthesia and intubation, and it prevents suprapubic access in cases requiring concomitant bladder neck suspension during the same operation.

An inverted U-shaped vaginal incision helps maintain alignment of sutures. Multilayered sutures are desirable because a watertight closure lowers the risk of urethrovaginal fistula and of recurrent diverticulum. If urethral reconstruction is difficult, thereby increasing the risk of complications, the Martius procedure of interposing a labial fat pad may be very useful.

In patients treated for a urethral diverticulum who later develop stress urinary incontinence requiring surgery, the dissection may not be easy. Combining a bladder neck suspension with the diverticulectomy may be recommended in cases of severe stress urinary incontinence, although it does add significant morbidity.

Neourethral Construction

After the distal urethra has been lost or when a distal urethro-vaginal fistula persists, the urethra may be lengthened by forming a tube from vaginal flaps.

U-FLAP RECONSTRUCTION

Develop a U-shaped flap proximal to the end of the defect. Carry the incision alongside the urethra. Suture the flap to the vaginal wall to form the back wall of the urethra. If possible, bring in a layer of fascia to cover. Undermine the vaginal flaps and approximate them in the midline.

For losses of a greater part of the urethra, roll a flap of labia minora or vagina into a tube extending distally from the recessed urethral opening. Cover it with deep tissue that includes the bulbocavernosus muscle and with lateral vaginal flaps. The gracilis muscle may also be mobilized for support (see pages 50 to 51).

LATERAL FLAP RECONSTRUCTION
(Symmonds-Hill-Blaivas)

1 *Position:* Lithotomy. Prepare the vagina and perineum. Suture the labia laterally. Insert a silicone balloon catheter into the bladder, and place a posterior retractor in the vagina. Infiltrate the vaginal mucosa with epinephrine diluted in saline to reduce bleeding during the dissection.

Incision: Make a U-shaped incision in the distal vagina proximal to the urethral meatus. Undermine the vaginal flaps enough medially to allow their edges to meet. Mark an inverted U incision in the vagina proximal to the first incision *(dashed lines).*

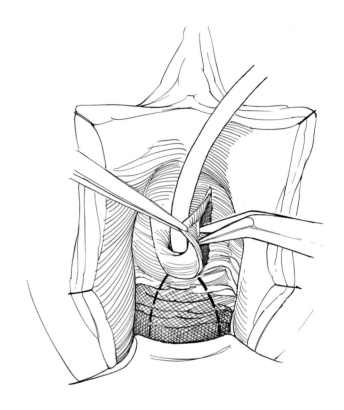

2 **A,** Approximate the flaps on either side of the meatus in the midline with 3-0 CCG over a 24 F catheter. Bring the submucosal connective tissue together to cover the suture line. For added security, cover the suture line with a bulbocavernosus muscle supplement (see pages 243 to 244). Incise along the proximal inverted U shape marked in the vagina and raise a second vaginal flap. **B,** Bring the proximal vaginal flap forward and suture it with 3-0 CCG to cover the new urethra. Place a vaginal pack for 24 hours. Tape the catheter to the abdomen to avoid traction on the repair, and connect it to sterile drainage for 7 days.

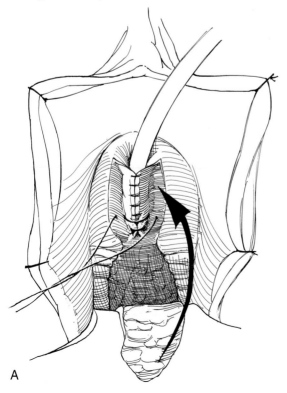

A

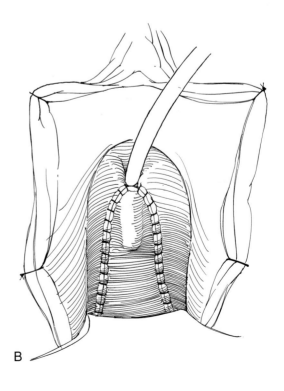

B

Excision of Urethral Caruncle and Urethral Prolapse

URETHRAL CARUNCLE

Differentiate a caruncle from carcinoma. If it is small, consider coagulation or laser excision.

1 *Position:* Low lithotomy. Place three stay sutures through the mucosa of the urethra at the meatus, one on either side and one posteriorly.

Incision: Incise the mucosa posteriorly from 3 to 9 o'clock with a #10 scalpel blade, staying outside of the stay sutures; then progressively cut the submucosa posteriorly and posterolaterally with the cutting current as the floor of the urethra is drawn out.

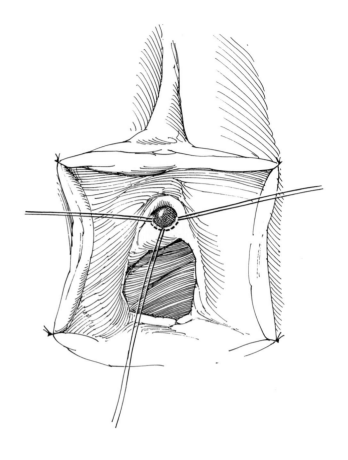

2 Start to transect the posterior wall of the urethra just proximal to the caruncle, and place a 4-0 SAS to approximate the lateral urethral edge to the margin of the meatus.

3 Continue alternately cutting and suturing until the posterior mucosa, including the caruncle, is excised and the defect is closed. Insert a 24 F 5-ml balloon catheter and apply petroleum jelly gauze.

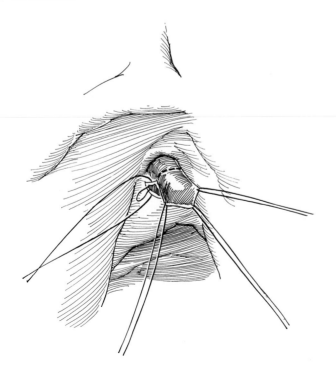

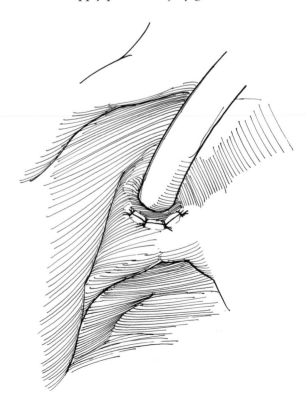

URETHRAL PROLAPSE

Treat the acute phase conservatively and wait for the swelling to abate.

Place four stay sutures peripheral to the extrusion. Incise the epithelium at the junction of the urethra and vagina to the level of the muscularis and catch the urethral epithelium circumferentially in small Allis clamps. First incise one margin vertically and then trim the excess circumferentially. Place a series of 3-0 CCG sutures around the defect to attach the urethral wall to the surrounding vaginal epithelium.

POSTOPERATIVE PROBLEMS

Urethral stricture may result from excessive fulguration. Retention and incontinence are rare.

Commentary by Winston K. Mebust

Putting stay sutures into the mucosa posteriorly and bilaterally allows the surgeon to place gentle traction on the caruncle to expose the normal mucosa. The caruncle can be excised with cutting cautery, as described, or with delicate sharp scissors (e.g., iris scissors), coagulating as necessary. As you transect the mucosa proximal to the caruncle, it is critically important to suture the mucosa to the meatus, in an alternate cut-and-sew technique, to avoid retraction of the mucosa deep into the urethra. If, by accident, the posterior urethra is torn completely across, the surgeon can usually insert a nasal speculum into the urethra and identify the retracted cut mucosal edge. The edge can then be brought to the meatus using a suture with a short arc needle (such as the Davis-Geck TT-2).

If the caruncle completely surrounds the meatus, one can place another stay suture at the 12-o'clock position and excise it, as described. Although I prefer stay stitches, one can accomplish the same thing by grasping the caruncle with Allis forceps.

Using a catheter postoperatively is not mandatory, but without a catheter, the patient could suffer urinary retention as a result of acute postoperative swelling. Therefore, I usually use a catheter as a safety device.

I do not use petroleum jelly on the suture line but rather apply topical antibiotic ointment and then use a petroleum emulsion gauze (such as Adaptic) or simply plain gauze. The caruncle is usually infected, and whether the topical antibiotics actually reduce postoperative infection is debatable. However, I consider this another safety measure.

Hysterectomy

VAGINAL HYSTERECTOMY

If necessary, sew the labia minora to the thighs. Insert a weighted speculum posteriorly and a right-angle retractor anteriorly. Place tenaculum forceps on the cervix.

Vaginal Incision

1 It may be helpful to inject hemostatic solution in the vaginal mucosa around the cervix in the line of incision. Make a full-thickness incision starting in the anterior vaginal wall and circumscribe the cervix, but defer dissection laterally and posteriorly until the uterus is to be removed, when it can be done retrogradely. Push the mucosa off the cervix anteriorly and posteriorly.

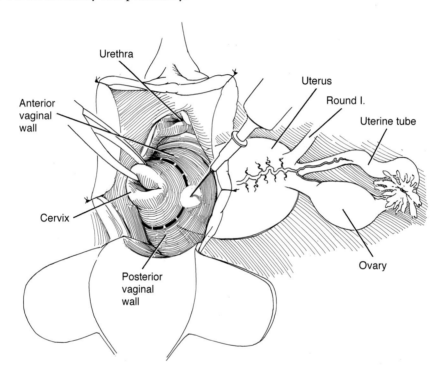

Incision of the Peritoneum in the Vesicouterine Pouch

2 Dissect along the cervix to mobilize the bladder and elevate the peritoneal vesicouterine fold that lies anteriorly. Take care to stay in the proper plane; excessive bleeding indicates that the dissection is too close to the cervix and lower uterine segment. Incise the peritoneum to allow entry into the peritoneal cavity in the vesicouterine pouch. Insert right-angle retractors, and spread the opening to displace the ureters laterally.

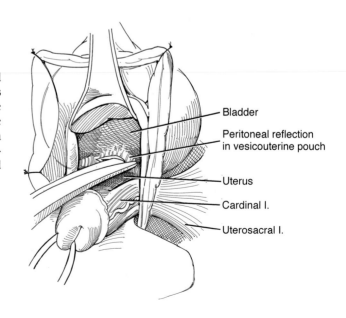

Entry into the Cul-de-sac

3 Elevate the cervix to expose the rectouterine pouch at the peritoneal reflection. Pick it up in forceps and incise it transversely. Digitally explore the pelvis.

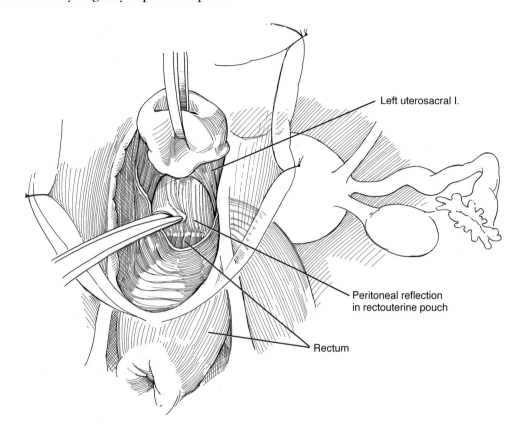

Left uterosacral l.

Peritoneal reflection in rectouterine pouch

Rectum

Uterosacral and Cardinal Ligaments

4 Push the tissue laterally to displace the ureter. Divide the uterosacral ligament serially along with the cardinal ligament, staying close to the uterus to avoid the ureters. Suture-ligate the ligament as the first bite. Hold these sutures to be tied outside the vaginal cuff at the end of the procedure for pelvic support. It will be used to suspend the vaginal cuff. If there is any chance that the ureter has been compromised, insert a cystoscope and pass a catheter up the ureter. If there is a problem, correct it and replace the catheter with a stent.

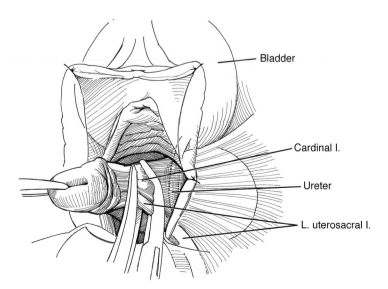

Bladder

Cardinal l.

Ureter

L. uterosacral l.

Uterine Pedicle

5 Clamp, divide, and doubly ligate the uterine pedicle.

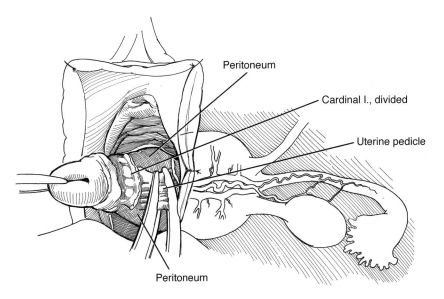

Broad Ligament

6 Grasp the uterine tube and broad ligament in clamps and divide them. After dividing the ovarian ligament, deliver the fundus through either the anterior or posterior peritoneal openings. Cut the cornual angles and remove the uterus. *Alternatively,* if the ovaries are to be removed, grasp the ovary with a Babcock clamp and clamp, cut, and ligate the infundibulopelvic ligament.

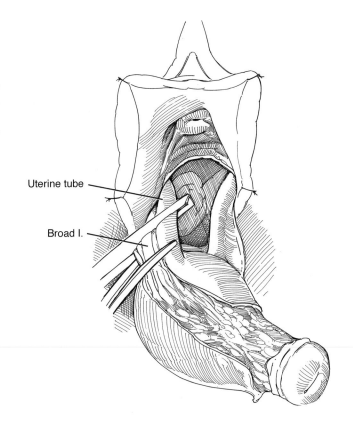

Support and Reperitonealization

7 Pass a suture through the anterior leaf of the perito-neum; then include in it the round ligament, ovarian ligament, and uterosacral ligament. Complete the reperi-tonealization of the pelvis with a running suture. Closure of the vaginal vault may be performed in a way that can correct both cystocele and rectocele (not shown). Bring the uterosacral sutures into the posterior vagina and tie them together across the midline.

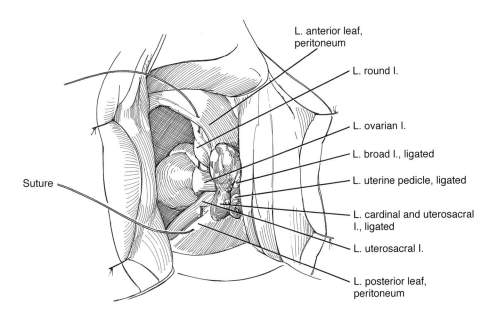

L. anterior leaf, peritoneum

L. round l.

L. ovarian l.

L. broad l., ligated

L. uterine pedicle, ligated

L. cardinal and uterosacral l., ligated

L. uterosacral l.

L. posterior leaf, peritoneum

Suture

ABDOMINAL HYSTERECTOMY

Position: Supine. Insert a balloon catheter and drain the bladder.

Incision: Make a lower midline transperitoneal inci-sion. Alternatively, a Pfannenstiel incision may be ade-quate (see page 490). If malignancy is suspected, make a vertical incision to allow the necessary access to explore the upper abdomen for staging. Systematically explore the abdominal viscera. Insert a self-retaining retractor, and place the patient in 45-degree Trendelenburg posi-tion. Pack the intestines superiorly. You and your assistant should be alert to the importance of traction and rotation of the uterus for exposure.

Round Ligament

8 Place curved Kocher clamps at the uterine cornu to include the round ligament, tubes, and utero-ovarian vessels. Elevate the uterus up and to the left. Divide the round ligament on the right and ligate it, tagging the suture with a clamp, which hangs over the edge of the wound to maintain exposure of the area beneath. Enter the avascular space in the broad ligament.

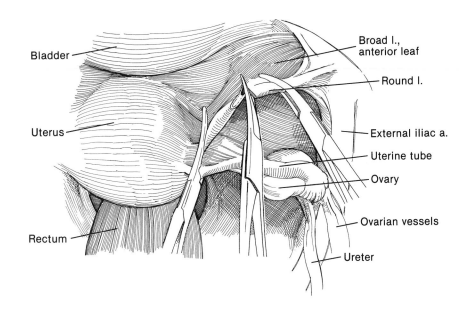

Bladder

Uterus

Rectum

Broad l., anterior leaf

Round l.

External iliac a.

Uterine tube

Ovary

Ovarian vessels

Ureter

Broad Ligament

9 Separate the leaves of the broad ligament to allow the bladder to be freed, and divide the anterior leaf. Identify the ureter on the peritoneum medially. Place a clamp across the tube and the ovarian ligament if the ovaries are to be preserved. Cut and tie. If the ovaries are to be removed, clamp the infundibulopelvic ligament behind the ovary while directly visualizing the ureter and cut and doubly tie it.

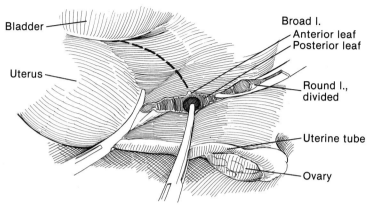

Uterine Tube and Ovarian Ligament

10 Divide the uterine tube and ovarian ligament. Open both leaves of the broad ligament down to the region of the parametrium and the cardinal ligaments.

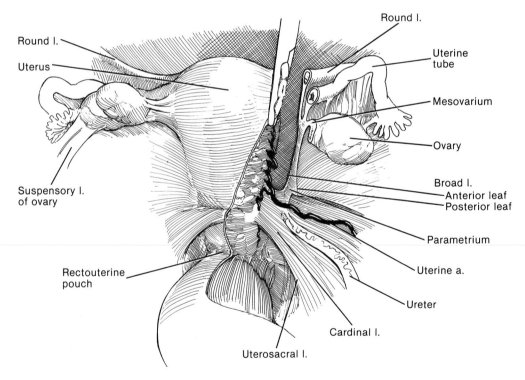

Uterine Vessels

11 Triply clamp and divide the uterine artery and veins (*white dashed line*) as well as part of the cardinal ligament. Secure them with suture ligatures.

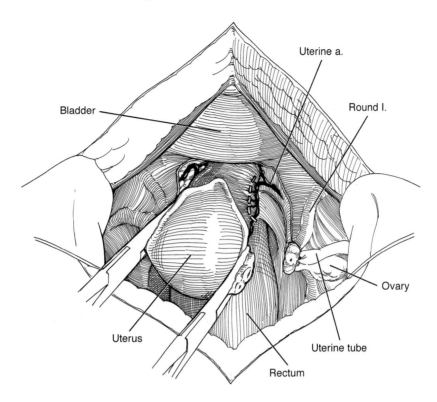

Bladder · Uterine a. · Round l. · Ovary · Uterus · Uterine tube · Rectum

Uterosacral Ligaments

12 Cut the posterior leaf of the broad ligament to expose the uterosacral ligaments, which are then divided. Push the bladder from the cervix and upper vagina, and clamp and cut the cardinal ligament and parametrium and paracolpium on both sides. Secure them with suture-ties. Divide the pubocervical fascia.

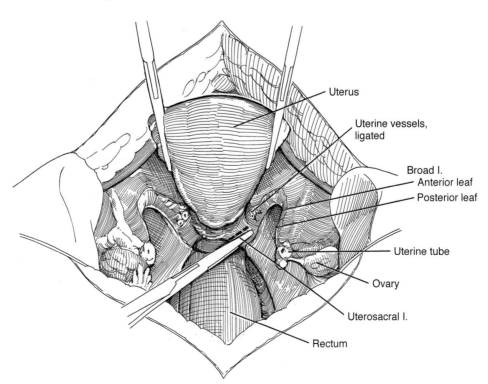

Uterus · Uterine vessels, ligated · Broad l. Anterior leaf Posterior leaf · Uterine tube · Ovary · Uterosacral l. · Rectum

Vagina

13 Incise into the vaginal vault anteriorly close to the cervix. Transect the vagina with curved scissors as close to the cervix as possible and remove the specimen. Suture the vaginal angles to the stumps of the uterosacral and cardinal ligaments. Close the vagina with figure-eight sutures to the muscularis. The pelvis does not need to be reperitonealized.

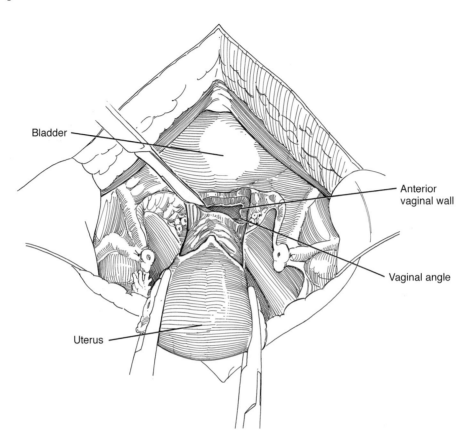

INTRAOPERATIVE PROBLEMS

Hysterectomy places the *pelvic (inferior hypogastric) plexus* at risk. The main branches may be injured during division of the cardinal ligament where the nerves pass under the uterine arteries. Injury to the nerves may also occur during dissection of the uterus and cervix from the bladder base and also during extensive dissection of the paravaginal tissues on the lateral aspect of the vagina. Dysfunction of the bladder can result.

The *ureter* lies against the peritoneum within the intermediate stratum of the retroperitoneal connective tissue, so it can be seen transperitoneally along most of its course. Only after it passes under the medial umbilical ligament (obliterated hypogastric artery) does it disappear from view. The ureter is vulnerable during salpingectomy as it crosses the ovarian ligament under the site of entrance of the ovarian vessels into the uterus. It can also be injured during hysterectomy. After going over the iliac vessels, it swings under the uterine artery, where it lies within 2.5 cm of that vessel. It passes through the cardinal ligament enclosed in the uterine venous plexus, where it lies within 1.5 cm of the cervix.

SECTION

8

Urethra: Reconstruction

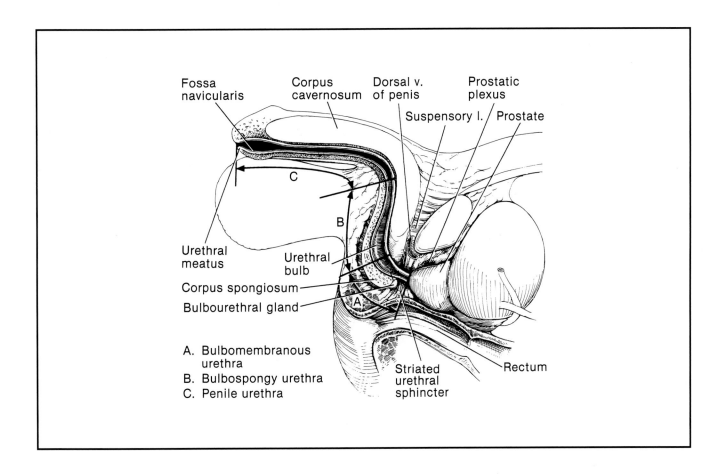

Fossa navicularis
Corpus cavernosum
Dorsal v. of penis
Suspensory l.
Prostatic plexus
Prostate

C

B

Urethral meatus
Urethral bulb
Corpus spongiosum
Bulbourethral gland

A

Striated urethral sphincter
Rectum

A. Bulbomembranous urethra
B. Bulbospongy urethra
C. Penile urethra

General Considerations for Urethral Strictures

SELECTION OF OPERATION

The urethra can be reconstituted by *regeneration* after urethrotomy and stenting, by *excision and anastomosis*, and by using *tissue transfer techniques* (grafts or flaps). Of the three, anastomosis gives the best long-term results, but substitution techniques must be used when the defect is too long. In general, repair in one stage is better than in two stages.

The region of the urethra involved affects the choice of the procedure. The penile urethra presents little difficulty, but the bulbar urethra, because of the critical importance of its surrounding spongy tissue, is much more challenging. Reconstruction of the prostatomembranous urethra is the most difficult, not only because of problems of access, but because the sphincteric mechanisms are involved. Factors impacting the selection of the procedure are the cause of the stricture (traumatic strictures are easier to repair than inflammatory ones), its length, the extent of spongiofibrosis, and associated adverse features such as local fibrosis, fistula, and infection (Table 1).

Repair *pendulous urethral strictures* in one stage. Because reanastomosis usually leads to chordee and free full-thickness skin grafts may do the same, a vascularized island flap is usually the best choice. The placement of a coil spring is a possible alternative in selected cases but often results in chronic pain.

For short *bulbospongiosus urethral strictures* secondary to trauma, end-to-end anastomosis is preferred. Longer strictures require a free full-thickness graft or a pedicled flap. If the stricture is secondary to inflammation, place a full-thickness skin graft, or better, a vascularized island pedicle from the prepuce. A staged inlay procedure may be necessary for long bulbar strictures, particularly those associated with infection or watering-pot perineum.

Bulbomembranous urethral strictures after pelvic fracture injury are usually less than 2 cm long and, if correctly managed at the time of injury by suprapubic urinary diversion, can be treated by reanastomosis in a delayed one-stage perineal repair. Abdominoperineal transpubic procedures may be needed in a few cases. Reanastomosis is the best solution; grafts take poorly in this region. A vascularized island flap is used when reanastomosis is not possible. Revert to a two-stage procedure when the penile urethra cannot be mobilized sufficiently and the defect is long.

If the stricture does not involve the membranous urethra, try dilations, then direct-vision internal urethrotomy. Realize that each deep urethrotomy incision itself initiates some spongiofibrosis that may make later repair more difficult. Consider open repair after two such failures. For long or multiple strictures, open operation is the first choice.

After injury, allow adequate time for healing and provide for drainage of urine away from the site. Strictures occur in the spongy urethra because the urethral lining itself is very thin and easily injured. This allows an irreversible diffuse fibrous reaction in the vascular tissue of the corpus spongiosum, the spaces of which become filled during urination. The contraction of this scar produces the stricture. During repair, take care not to incorporate areas of incipient fibrosis ("gray urethra") because the result will be eventual contracture.

Counsel the patient about potency, especially with bulbomembranous strictures.

Instruments

Supply a cystoscope, a flexible ureteroscope, GU fine and GU plastic sets, a Turner-Warwick set, small skin hooks, an Andrews suction tip, Cushing forceps (2), DeBakey forceps (2), fine Allis clamps, a needle electrode, a Scott retractor and two packages of large stays, curved van Buren sounds, pediatric sounds, bougies à boule, an Air Brown dermatome with components and two tongue blades, a dermacarrier with four 25-gauge needles, adhesive drape, a syringe and Christmas-tree Luer connector, silicone balloon catheters, methylene blue and saline mixed 1:1 and a syringe, antibiotic solution, a skin pen, and a soft chair. Bipolar cautery is preferred to monopolar, being less damaging to the small vessels of flaps and grafts.

Sutures: 2-0 silk CE-6 for drapes and drains, 3-0 T-16 synthetic absorbable sutures (SAS), 4-0 T-31 SAS, and 6-0 monofilament polydioxanone sutures (PDS), which are strong and have a low volume.

TECHNICAL CONSIDERATIONS

Preoperative studies: Obtain a cystogram and retrograde urethrogram to detect pockets and fistulas.

Instrumentation: Avoid instrumentation or dilation of the urethra preoperatively; this renders the surface unstable, making it very difficult to identify the extent of the stricture at operation.

Epilation: At a separate sitting, mark the area of skin to be used. Epilate it as needed to extend the areas of non–hair-bearing skin. Under an operating microscope, insert a 30-gauge needle held on a hemostat into each hair follicle with one hand and apply low-power coagulating current to it with the other. Extract the hair with its attached follicle. Apply antibiotic ointment. Assess the results in 4 to 6 weeks. If only a few hairs remain, they can be epilated at the time of the repair.

Urethral staining: Instill methylene blue, realizing that it does not warn of deeper involvement. When laying open the diseased area, carry the incision well into healthy tissue. If you have any doubt, extend the urethral incision or excision. Look for gray urethra (spongiofibrosis). Be able to pass a 30 F bougie à boule (in adults) both ways after excision of the stricture.

Obtain good exposure: This is particularly important for operations on the perineum. Place the patient in the exaggerated lithotomy position with the feet in boot-type stirrups. Be sure that the feet are well seated in the boots and nothing is pressing on the calf area.

Avoid nerve injury: Acute flexion of the thigh against the groin, especially in an obese patient, can compress the obturator nerve after it exits through the obturator foramen and starts dividing in the upper thigh. Injury results in weakness or paralysis of the adductors of the thigh. Such acute flexion also can compress the femoral nerve against the pubic ramus, resulting in an abnormal gait. Compression of the knee against the knee brace can injure the saphenous nerve and cause loss of sensation in the medial aspect of the leg. Compression of the lateral aspect of the knee affects the peroneal nerve, resulting in instability of the foot and foot drop.

Use magnifying loupes: Loupes are especially helpful in operations on children (2.5 or, better, 3.5 power).

Table 1. Applicable Procedures for Urethral Strictures

Meatal strictures	Full-thickness graft
	Rotation flap
Penile strictures	
Short inflammatory	Free patch graft
Long inflammatory	Island flap
Bulbospongy strictures	
Short traumatic	Excision and reanastomosis
	Free patch graft
Short inflammatory	Free patch graft
	Island flap
Long inflammatory	Preputial pedicle flap
Severely infected	Staged mesh repair
Bulbomembranous strictures	
Uncomplicated	Excision and reanastomosis
Complicated	Perineal excision and rerouting

Fixation: Place stay sutures through the entire thickness of the urethra and erectile tissue and hook them over the rings of the self-retaining retractor to keep the urethra open and reduce bleeding. A Robinson catheter passed in the meatus and out of the defect can be grasped with a clamp for traction to aid in visualizing the deeper urethra.

Tissue mobilization: Widely mobilize the tissues to be sutured into the defect. Proximal mobilization of the urethra and gouging out of the inferior ramus of the pubis help. Tension cannot be tolerated.

Use bipolar electrocautery: Monopolar current may damage the deeper tissues.

Provide a well-vascularized bed: Use bulbar spongy tissue if at all possible. Mobilize the spongy tissue so that it may be brought over the repair or flap for nourishment and support. For massive defects or those associated with injury of the bladder neck, use an abdominoperineal approach, and fill the defect with omentum.

Tissue closure: Use fine absorbable sutures. Make exact skin-to-epithelium anastomoses to avoid granulation tissue and scarring. Do not overlap suture lines.

Form the neourethra with a uniform caliber; avoid both sacculation and constriction. Make the repair watertight; test it by instilling water or very dilute methylene blue before closing the wound. Provide wide lateral separation and interpose connective tissue. Support the neourethra with adjacent tissue, such as that from the corpus spongiosum (tight approximation) and the bulbospongiosus muscle (loose approximation to allow drainage of blood and serum).

Spontaneous erections: Erections can be a problem but usually subside after the anesthetist gives nitroglycerine sublingually or breaks an 0.3-mg ampule of amyl nitrite into the breathing bag. If that is not effective, inject 0.2 ml of a 1:100,000 solution of epinephrine in normal saline into one corpus.

Catheters: A urethral catheter left indwelling can be damaging; it moves up and down in the repair when the patient is ambulatory. If a catheter must be used, choose a small size to merely divert the urine. It may also support a flap and prevent adhesions. Fenestrations in the catheter may improve local drainage. It is best to divert the urine suprapubically away from the repair. The following is a rule of thumb for the length of time needed for a leakproof repair with an indwelling urethral catheter: end to end, 10 days; island flap, 16 days; and full-thickness graft repairs, 21 days. If a suprapubic tube is used instead of a urethral catheter, these times may be reduced by one third.

Drainage: Provide drainage by a miniature suction drainage device unless hemostasis is excellent.

Ambulation: Allow the patient out of bed only after the graft or flap is firmly adherent.

DIVERSION AND STENTING

Pendulous strictures that do not require diversion may be stented with a 14 F silicone tube that does not reach the sphincter, held in place by a meatal suture.

For extensive repairs, both stenting and suprapubic diversion are usually needed until the epithelial lining has sealed. Fill the bladder and insert a suprapubic cystostomy trocar two fingerbreadths above the symphysis. Use an open technique if the patient has had previous surgery (see pages 625 to 627). Fasten the catheter to the skin with a silk suture and tape it as well. In older patients, drainage by perineal urethrostomy (see page 630) may be preferable. If a urethral catheter is placed, periodically clear the meatus of encrustation to prevent accu-

mulation of urethral secretions that are not only irritating but also may produce a meatal stricture.

Before discontinuing diversion, instill contrast solution through the suprapubic tube to detect leakage and test by having the patient void.

POSTOPERATIVE PROBLEMS

Bleeding from the corpus spongiosum usually can be controlled by digital pressure over sponges. *Secondary strictures* from the presence of the catheter can occur, but the use of a small-caliber (less than 20 F), nonreactive silicone catheter reduces their incidence. Keep the shaft of the catheter at the meatus clear of encrustation. *Restenosis* at an anastomotic site arises from a circumferential suture line, in contrast to an oblique anastomosis. If a stricture develops, revise the repair in 4 to 6 months. Also, de-epithelialized surfaces may cross-adhere. *Ventral chordee* is uncommon, but patients may describe ventral tightness.

Fistulas are rare. *Sacculation* from construction of too generous a urethra with a variable diameter in the bulbospongiosus region, especially after repair with scrotal pedicle grafts, not only fosters urinary dribbling but may lead to infection and stone formation. An important factor in preventing this complication is the provision of adequate supporting bulbospongiosus connective tissue and muscle over the repair. Reoperation may be required (see page 226).

Hair balls become a problem in adulthood when hair-bearing skin was used for constructing the urethra, especially if the passage is sacculated and persistently contains infected urine. The hair can be dissolved by filling the bladder with water, instilling thioglycolic acid lotion in the urethra and leaving it for 10 minutes, and thoroughly washing it out as the patient voids. However, the hair does regrow. Epilation by electrolysis is impractical, and electrocautery damages the lining. The neodymium:YAG laser applied through a panendoscope either directly to the hair or, better, at an angle without contact, destroys the follicle and allows the hair to float free (Finkelstein and Blatstein, 1991).

Infection leads to fistulas and is to be avoided by perioperative antibiotics and skin preparation. Strangulated and traumatized tissue lies behind infections, so be gentle. *Necrosis* of the edges of the patch or graft is not serious if the suture lines are not superimposed and if a connective tissue layer intervenes. *Hematomas* can be a problem if hemostasis, especially of the cut edges of spongy tissue, is not secure.

Incontinence may follow overdilation of the intrinsic sphincteric mechanism in the membranous urethra. Furthermore, loss of this mechanism during repair of posterior urethral stricture must be balanced by the presence of a competent vesical neck. Uninhibited detrusor contractions open this mechanism and cause leakage; they may be prevented with anticholinergic medication.

Impotence seldom is caused by repair of the urethral stricture but is associated with the pelvic fracture itself. Many branches of the erector nerves are present at this level, especially in children, so that some may be divided without ill effect. If the original injury tore the nerves, orgasm may be normal, and erection can be provided later with a prosthesis. Emission may be ineffective because too large a urethral caliber was left after a vascularized flap repair. If it is necessary to mobilize the prostate during repair, take care to avoid the neurovascular bundles (see page 435). Furthermore, fibrosis inside the posterior extensions of the corpora cavernosa can cause venous leakage, and arterial injury is not rare. Either may contribute to impotence.

IMMEDIATE URETHRAL REALIGNMENT

1 **A,** *Position:* Prone with the legs spread.
Incision: Make a lower midline incision, evacuate the pelvic hematoma, and obtain hemostasis. Note elevation of the prostate. **B,** Make a short cystostomy and insert an 18 F silicone catheter down through the prostate. Pass a second catheter through the urethra and suture it to the first. Do not use a balloon catheter because of the risk of damaging the bladder neck if traction is inadvertently applied. Pull the urethral catheter into the bladder and secure it with a suture passed through the anterior abdominal wall and tied over a bolster.

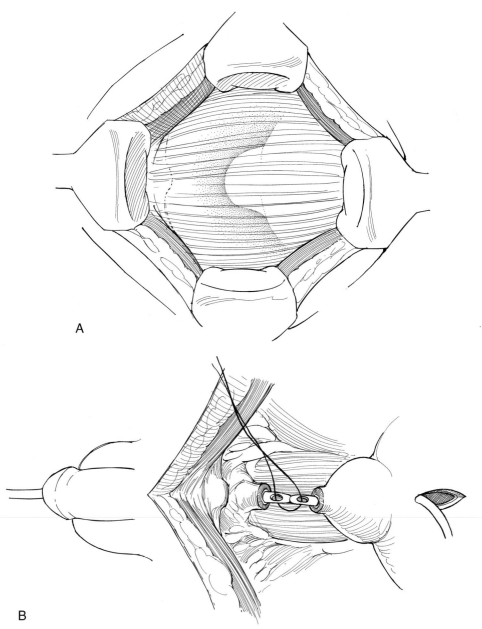

A

B

2 Place a nylon traction suture through the base of the prostate, taking care not to angulate it (Vest suture, see page 462). Pass each end of the suture through the perineum on a Keith needle. Tighten the suture until the prostate reaches the pelvic floor and tie it over a bolster. Insert a cystostomy tube. Drain the pelvis with suction drains and close the wound. Cut the traction sutures in 5 to 7 days. Make a urethrogram after 3 to 6 weeks with the urethral catheter in place; remove it when extravasation has ceased. Have the patient start voiding, but leave the cystostomy in place for a few more weeks to be sure a stricture does not immediately develop.

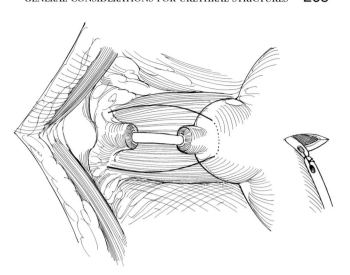

Commentary by Jack W. McAninch

Prostatomembranous disruptions: Consider immediate realignment when the patient is hemodynamically stable and no major associated injuries to the abdomen and lower extremities are present. Otherwise, suprapubic diversion provides the most appropriate management.

Delayed repair of posterior urethral rupture defects: Before repairing the urethral rupture defect, associated injuries should have healed and the patient should be rehabilitated. At least 2 months should pass between the initial injury and the repair.

Cut-for-the-light urethrotomy procedures provide inconsistent results owing to residual scar tissue. The open procedure should begin through a perineal incision, and in 90 percent of cases successful end-to-end anastomosis can be accomplished through this route. Partial pubectomy can be accomplished from the perineum, although a lower abdominal incision is needed. The key to success is complete excision of the scar at the prostate apex and adequate mobilization of the bulbar urethra to provide a tension-free mucosa-to-mucosa anastomosis of the bulbar urethra to the prostatic urethra. I use 5-0 PDS.

Optical loupes should be used at all times. I place a suprapubic catheter and a stenting silicone 16 F urethral catheter in all cases for 3 to 4 weeks.

Anterior urethral strictures: I use sonourethrography to determine stricture length as an aid to selecting the appropriate procedure. Strictures less than 2.0 cm can be repaired by excision of the scar, mobilization of the urethra, and end-to-end anastomosis. Longer strictures when the bulbar urethra is involved and minimal fibrosis is present in the spongiosum should be repaired using grafts. Buccal mucosa and penile skin are the best sources. Long, dense, fibrotic strictures are best repaired by using penile flaps of hairless skin. Mobilization of the pedicle vasculature using Buck's fascia ensures preservation of the blood supply and thus flap survival. Onlay repair should be done using a running suture of 6-0 PDS, carefully approximating skin to urethral epithelium. Optical magnification is essential. I use a 16 F silicone catheter to divert urine and stent the urethra, leaving it for 3 weeks. A suprapubic catheter is not used routinely.

Strictures of the Fossa Navicularis

The fossa navicularis is essential for producing a normal urinary stream. It is compromised by ischemia during transurethral prostatic resection or by balanitis xerotica obliterans (BXO). In contrast, meatal stenosis in children, secondary to diaper irritation, is limited to the meatus itself and therefore can be treated by simple meatotomy (see page 114).

SKIN FLAP TECHNIQUE
(Blandy-Tresidder)

This procedure leaves an open but somewhat hypospadic meatus.

1 **A,** Place a traction suture in the glans, using a tapered needle. Make a single-throw knot in the suture to help control the bleeding from the needle hole. Mark a chevron-shaped incision on the ventrum, and raise a flap proximally. Because it is an axial flap, include the underlying dartos fascia. **B,** Incise the entire fossa navicularis into normal urethra with scissors or with a knife over a grooved director.

2 **A,** Suture the apex of the flap to the apex of the penile incision with fine chromic catgut (CCG) sutures. **B,** Continue to fold and suture the flap into the defect. Placing the stitches advances the flap distally and inverts the tip. Approximate the residual cut edges at each margin of the glans. Divert the urine with a small silicone balloon catheter for 2 days.

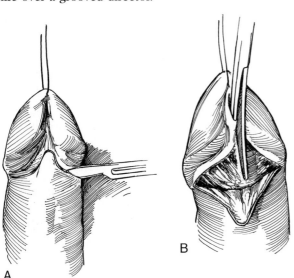
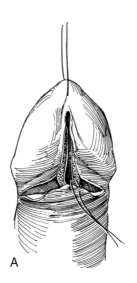
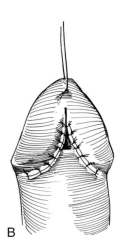

SKIN GRAFT TECHNIQUE
(Devine)

This is a method for opening and resurfacing the stenotic fossa navicularis with skin. It may fail in cases of BXO. If local skin is not suitable, use a buccal mucosal graft (see pages 100 to 101) or place a flap that is vascularized (Steps 9 to 12).

3 **A,** Place a traction suture in the glans. Mark a ventral vertical line on the glans and a circumcising line on the shaft at the corona. **B,** Open the fossa navicularis with scissors as far as the normal urethra. Excise any diseased mucosa from the glans and form glans flaps. Mobilize and spatulate the normal urethra. Mark and excise a strip graft on the ventral skin, extending half way around the shaft. Alternatively, harvest a buccal mucosal graft.

4 **A,** Suture one edge of the strip to cover the distal area of the opened glans and the other edge to the new meatus. Use 4-0 CCG sutures. Place several quilting sutures to hold the graft to the glans tissue. **B,** Insert an 18 F 5-ml silicone balloon catheter into the bladder. Attach the graft to the ventral rim of the new meatus, and form a tube by approximating the edges of the graft with fine sutures in the dermis in the midline. Close the glans flaps over the graft.

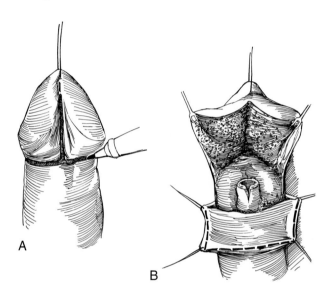

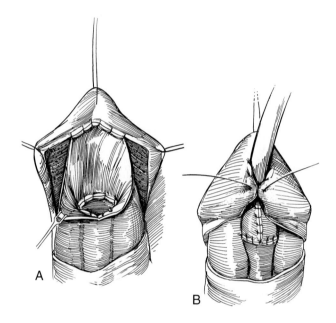

5 Complete the closure of the glans flaps over the graft, and approximate the skin of the shaft. Apply a loose fluff dressing over an absorbent layer held with elastic tape. Leave a short silicone stent, and consider punch suprapubic drainage.

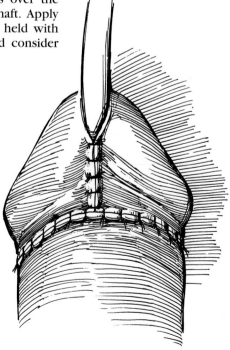

ROTATION ONLAY FLAP

Glans Tunnel Technique
(McAninch)

6 Make a short transverse incision on the ventrum 0.5 cm proximal to the coronal sulcus or proximal to the circumcision scar (the skin distal to the circumcision scar may not be adequately vascularized). Lift the wings of the glans, and dissect in the plane between the glans and the tips of the corpus spongiosum to the site of the meatus. Incise the glans distally, ventral to the meatus, and enter the suburethral plane to connect with the proximal dissection over the corpus spongiosum. Open the strictured fossa navicularis by dividing the ventral margin with a hooked blade, working from both the proximal and distal ends. Outline a ventral transverse flap of skin approximately 3 cm wide to provide a 30 F meatal channel after patching.

7 Raise the ventral flap on a dartos pedicle.

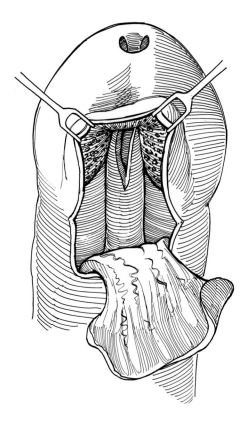

8 Invert the flap and draw it into the defect. Suture it in place at the meatus with interrupted sutures. Working from the proximal end, run a submucosal suture of 4-0 CCG to complete the urethral closure. Approximate the incision at the coronal sulcus with a fine subcuticular suture.

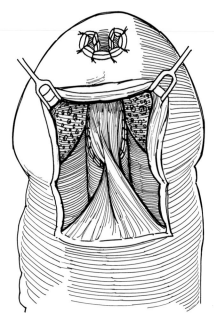

Glans Split Technique
(Jordan Flap)

Splitting the glans allows adequate incision of the stricture and mobilization of the glans wings from the corpora and also avoids having to suture inside a tunnel.

9 Place a traction suture. Mark a ventral vertical line on the glans. Make a short circumcising line on the shaft 0.5 cm proximal to the corona. Elevate the skin with the accompanying dartos fascia to expose the distal urethra.

10 Insert a grooved director into the fossa navicularis and incise it with a knife. Extend the incision 1 to 1.5 cm into the normal urethra, as demonstrated by a bougie, thereby spatulating it. Mark and incise a flap on the ventral skin of a length equal to the meatal defect and of a width that, when combined with the residual urethra, forms a 30 F tube (about 3 cm). Take care to incise only through the skin on the proximal aspect of the flap to avoid interference with the blood supply beneath it in the fasciocutaneous dartos pedicle.

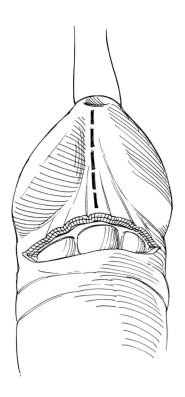

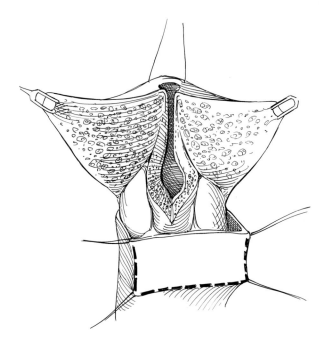

11 Raise the flap on a broad dartos pedicle immediately superficial to Buck's fascia, invert it, rotate it 90 degrees, and suture the now proximal end to the spatulated urethra. Fix the distal end of the flap to the site of the new meatus with two inverted 5-0 CCG sutures. Attach the flap to the ventral rim of the meatus on each side with a running 5-0 or 6-0 SAS. Test the neourethra for watertightness by injecting saline through the new meatus. Mobilize the lateral wings of the glans off of the tips of the corpora generously, as much as is needed to approximate them over the graft without tension. Control bleeding with bipolar electrocautery forceps.

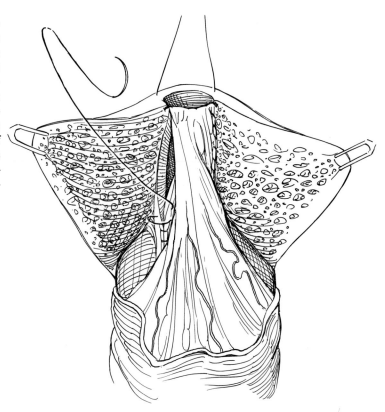

12 Insert a 26 F or 28 F sound into the urethra to prevent constriction during closure. Approximate the wings with fine SAS, and close the skin with CCG, taking care to fashion a meatus of a suitable diameter. Close the donor site with transposed preputial skin. If necessary, trim the dog ears with excision of a Burrow's triangle (see page 49). Place a balloon catheter, or use a suprapubic catheter to allow a later trial of voiding. In children, insert an 8 F prepared Silastic splent (see page 105), and apply a loose fluff dressing over an absorbent layer held with elastic tape. For longer strictures, form a longitudinal skin island flap (Orandi, pages 275 to 278). Elevate it sufficiently on a dartos pedicle so that it can be advanced into the meatus. The skin from the dorsum may also be transposed as a transverse skin island to the ventrum on a dartos pedicle.

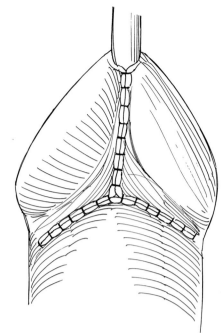

Commentary by Gerald H. Jordan

True strictures of the fossa navicularis represent a unique challenge to the reconstructive surgeon. Although all strictures of the anterior urethra require careful attention for good functional results, reconstruction of the fossa navicularis requires attention for excellent cosmetic results as well.

Strictures of the fossa navicularis, particularly those associated with BXO, rarely respond to dilation, internal urethrotomy, or aggressive meatotomy. To correct the fibrotic process associated with a stenosis of the fossa navicularis, one must interpose nonfibrotic vascularized tissue to prevent recurrence.

Because "conservative" techniques generally do not yield good results in these strictures, one should proceed early with an open reconstruction. We are fortunate now to have a number of procedures at hand that allow for good functional correction of the stenotic process, with good to excellent cosmetic results as well.

Cohney in 1963 described a penile flap procedure using a circumferentially elevated random flap. The flap left the patient with a retrusive meatus. Because it was a random flap, one wonders also if flap reliability was not a problem. In 1967, Blandy and Tresidder devised a flap for reconstruction of the fossa which could be elevated based on the vascularity of the dartos fascia. This flap provides excellent functional results but also leaves the patient with a retrusive meatus. In an effort to improve the cosmetic result, Brannen et al (1976) described a modification of the Blandy flap in which the flap was much more aggressively elevated and advanced onto the glans. Because of the significant amount of advancement required, the meatus again often became retrusive and offered little improvement with regard to cosmetic results. De Sy (1984) reported further modification of the Blandy-Brannen flap in which a skin island is carried on the dartos fascial pedicle. Again, in this procedure, significant advancement is required to invert the skin island into the urethrostomy defect. De Sy, however, reports excellent results in a relatively large series of patients. Jordan (1987) described a procedure in which a ventral transverse preputial or penile skin island is carried on a broad ventral dartos fascial pedicle. His series now has 18 patients, 16 of whom have more than a 1-year follow-up. In that series, there have been no recurrences of stricture, no fistula, and essentially no complications. Although the procedure is best suited for isolated strictures of the fossa navicularis, Jordan has used the procedure in one patient in whom the stricture extended from the meatus proximally for a distance of approximately 4 cm, hence requiring a 5- to 6-cm skin island.

The advantage of Jordan's procedure is that minimal advancement is required to transpose and invert the skin island into the urethrostomy defect. By orienting the skin island transversely, the transposition in essence advances one end of the skin island to the proposed site of the neomeatus. Because the dartos fascial pedicle is based entirely on the ventral dartos fascia, it is imperative that the ventrum of the penis have a reliable fascial blood supply. Hence, the procedure may have minimal application in the hypospadias patient. The flap is based on the distal arborizations of the superficial external pudendal vessels. In the hypospadias patient, the arborizations dorsally are far more reliable than the ventral arborizations because of the defect of ventral fusion, which can involve all layers. Circumcision in no way contraindicates the use of the flap; however, the skin island must be elevated proximal to the circumcising incision in those cases because the preputial skin may not be reliably vascularized by the proximal dartos fascia. Additionally, the patient who has had multiple operations may not have a reliable ventral dartos fascial blood supply.

It is essential to raise the glans wings broadly. This can be accomplished in the plane between the tips of the corpora cavernosa and the overlying spongy erectile tissue of the glans penis. This is a relatively avascular plane, and any bleeding can be controlled easily with bipolar electrocautery forceps. It is essential that the scar associated with the fossa stricture be divided completely. Elevation of the glans flaps allows for this and further allows for refusion of the glans without the potential for restenosis after placement of a relatively bulky flap into the meatus. The ventral glans is easily fused by the use of subcuticular monofilament absorbable sutures and absorbable sutures placed to reappose the skin edges. As mentioned, in the series thus far, fistula has not been a problem.

McAninch has modified the procedure by leaving the ventral glans intact. Although this may be of use in some patients, in patients in whom the fibrotic process is deep into the overlying spongy erectile tissue of the glans penis, incomplete division of the fibrotic process may not be accomplished. Additionally, I have found elevation of the glans off the tips of the corpora to be somewhat more difficult with the ventrum of the glans intact.

Some patients with meatal stenosis have experienced flattening of the glans. Leaving the ventrum of the glans intact does not allow for sculpting of the glans. With wide mobilization of the glans wings, a portion of the proximal glans can be excised, re-establishing the more normal conical shape of the glans penis. Devine's procedure, which he terms resurfacing of the fossa navicularis, yields excellent cosmetic results. The procedure may be of limited application in the patient afflicted with BXO. Evidence suggests that the BXO process can "invade" or involve grafts in general, and specifically grafts coapted to skin already affected by the inflammatory process.

As initially described by Devine, the tubularized full-thickness skin graft was placed with the graft suture line ventrally. However, in later cases, the graft suture line was rotated dorsally. That maneuver still allows for the placement of quilting sutures and allows one to avoid a situation of overlying suture lines. I have applied the procedure in a limited number of patients. It must be noted that fistulas, no matter where the suture line is placed, have not been a problem in that limited series.

Strictures of the Penile Urethra

Determine the length of the stricture by combining retrograde with voiding urethrography. Estimate the depth and extent of involvement of the spongy tissue by ultrasonography (Table 1).

Strictures in the pendulous urethra are simple to repair compared with meatal and bulbar strictures. *Excision* and *reanastomosis* are best if they do not shorten the penis. Efforts should be made to keep the urethra in continuity. Chordee limits how much urethra can be excised. If excision and reanastomosis are not possible, form a tube of uniform caliber that will not be prone to restricturing.

Because the overlying penile skin and adjacent prepuce are hairless, well vascularized, and adaptable to a wet environment, these surfaces can be rolled in or transported from the prepuce as an *island flap*. If penile skin is not available, the alternatives are bladder epithelium or, better, buccal mucosa (see pages 100 to 101) placed as *patch grafts*. Make the repair over a 16 F catheter and leave it in place for 3 weeks. If the bed is of very poor quality, a long stricture can be repaired in two stages by inserting a *mesh graft* at a first stage and forming the urethral tube later. Short, dense strictures that involve the spongy tissue can be managed with patch grafts or with island flaps, a technique that also may involve resection and partial reanastomosis with the flap acting as a *roof strip*. Because it is desirable to remove the stent as soon as possible, vascularized flaps have advantages over free grafts.

Table 1. Management of Penobulbar Strictures

Type of Stricture	Treatment
Diaphragm	Internal urethrotomy
Mucosal involvement	Internal urethrotomy; end-to-end spatulated anastomosis, penile urethra; augmented roof-strip graft, penile urethra; transverse island flap (Duckett); longitudinal island flap, pendulous urethra (Orandi)
Spongy involvement	End-to-end spatulated anastomosis, bulbar urethra; patch graft, bulbar urethra; tubed patch graft, bulbar urethra; longitudinal/transverse preputial island flap (Quartey)
Outside spongy tissue	Preputial island fasciocutaneous flap (McAninch); flap roof strip (Turner-Warwick); Quartey procedure; staged procedure
Complicated stricture	Quartey procedure or island flap; meshed graft, two-stage procedure

VASCULAR CONSIDERATIONS

1 The penile artery, arising from the internal pudendal artery, branches into the cavernous artery and the artery to the bulb and terminates as the dorsal artery of the penis. The artery to the bulb forms an important *proximal* blood supply to the bulbar and pendulous urethra. The vascular spaces of the corpus spongiosum allow blood to communicate along the urethra in both directions, making devascularization during repair unlikely. The dorsal artery also provides circumflex arteries that run with corresponding circumflex veins to supply the corpus spongiosum and contained urethra. It turns ventrally as it approaches the glans, where it terminates after giving off a frenular branch. This terminal portion supplying the glans is an important *distal* source of blood for strictures of the pendulous urethra. The superficial penile fascia (penile dartos) is continuous with the dartos layer of the scrotum and becomes Colles' fascia posteriorly over the ischiocavernosus and bulbospongiosus muscles. Buck's fascia covers the tunica albuginea of the penile bodies, including the crura. Proximally it extends to the perineal membrane and distally to the coronal sulcus. Buck's fascia encloses the corpora cavernosa in one compartment and the corpus spongiosum in another. It fuses with the superficial fascia at the coronal sulcus. The ischiocavernosus and bulbocavernosus muscles lie beneath the superficial penile and Colles' fascia but superficial to Buck's fascia.

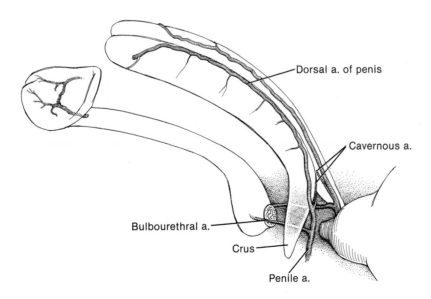

END-TO-END SPATULATED ANASTOMOSIS, PENILE URETHRA

Excision and anastomosis are the most direct method of repair, but if the defect is more than 1 cm in length this method is not suitable in the pendulous urethra because end-to-end repair of longer gaps results in penile shortening with chordee. In children, because of the inelasticity of the urethra, only very short strictures are suitable for treatment by this method.

Position: Supine. Instill diluted methylene blue to stain the diseased epithelium. The dye helps define the extent of mucosal involvement, not the extent of the spongio-fibrosis. If spilled on the skin, the dye can make the evaluation of skin flap viability difficult. Insert a sound to the level of the stricture but do not push it through.

2 *Incision:* Make a longitudinal incision slightly to one side of the midline with its distal end just beyond the tip of the sound. A circumcising incision followed by mobilization of the skin of the shaft has advantages of avoiding overlapping suture lines (*dashed line*). Expose the urethra by dividing the spongy tissue. Starting proximal to the stricture where dissection is easier, mobilize the urethra enough to allow a 1- to 1.5-cm overlap of the ends after resection of the stricture. The urethral bulb is the most fixed area; it must be freed to obtain adequate length for anastomosis.

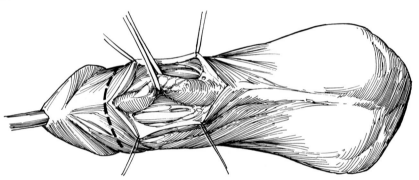

3 **A,** Insert a stay suture in the normal distal urethra and incise it transversely just distal to the tip of the sound. **B,** For better control, incise over the tip of the sound with a hooked #12 blade. Make the incision longitudinally to expose the entire length of the stricture into normal urethra.

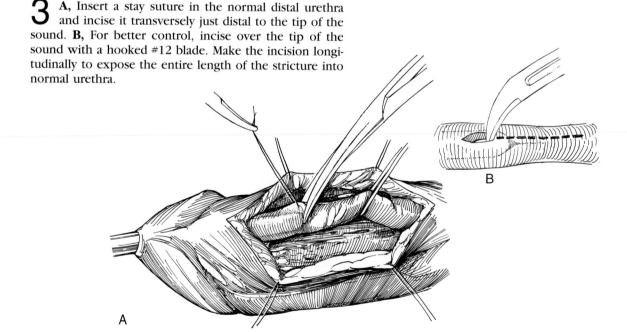

4 Excise the strictured section. Examine the proximal and distal ends to be certain that all the spongio-fibrosis has been removed.

5 Spatulate the distal end on the ventral aspect and the proximal end on the dorsal side to minimize incision into the bulbospongiosus muscle.

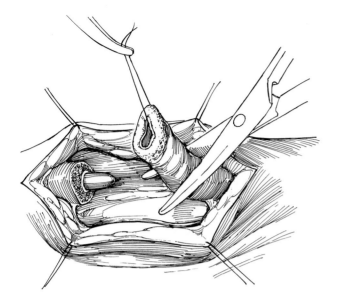

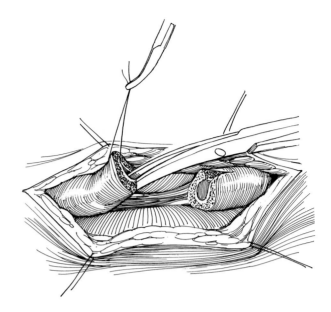

6 Place two interrupted 5-0 monofilament SAS through all layers except the urethral epithelium in the dorsal V cut. Tie the knots on the outside. Continue to approximate the urethral epithelium with watertight stitches. Close the adventitia of the corpus spongiosum as a second layer.

7 Approximate as much of the subcutaneous tissue as possible, using fine interrupted sutures, and close the skin with a running 5-0 SAS or CCG subcuticular suture.

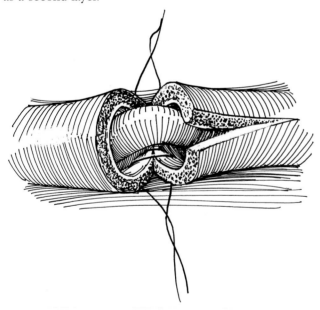

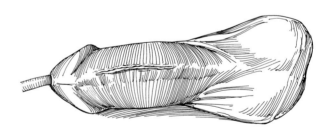

AUGMENTED ROOF-STRIP GRAFT, PENILE URETHRA

For dense strictures of the pendulous urethra, expose the urethra by degloving the penis.

8 Open the urethra over the stricture well into normal tissue. Mobilize the urethra and resect all tissue involved with spongiofibrosis. Free the urethra thoroughly posteriorly to see if a primary end-to-end anastomosis is possible. If it is seen that chordee would occur with erection, proceed to apply a roof strip.

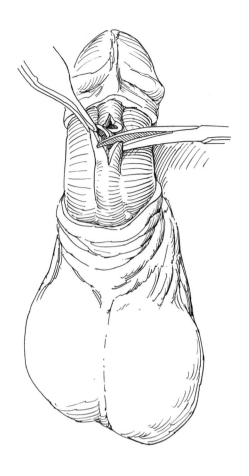

9 Incise both ends of the urethra ventrally. Place 4-0 SAS in the distal dorsal periurethral tissue and suture them to the corpora cavernosa for fixation.

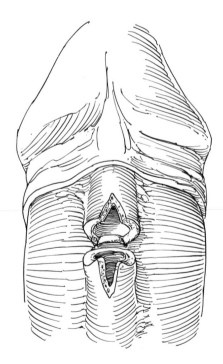

10 Complete the repair of the dorsal half of the urethra with interrupted 4-0 SAS. Insert a 5-ml silicone balloon catheter of suitable size, usually 18 F.

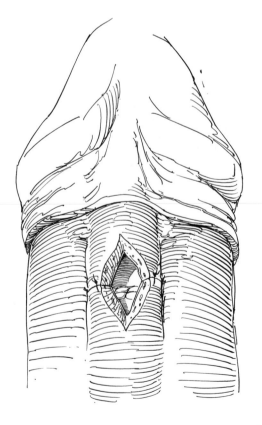

11 Measure the remaining defect. Secure and apply a defatted patch graft, usually taken from the prepuce. Do not make the patch too large; it should fit snugly around a suitably sized sound—24 F in the adult. Suture it in place with continuous 5-0 SAS. Replace the penile skin, and approximate it with 4-0 catgut sutures to the corona. Dress the wound and remove the catheter in 8 to 10 days. *Alternative (rotation) technique* to avoid overlapping suture lines (Barbagli et al, 1996): If spongiofibrosis is moderate, rotate the urethra 180 degrees and incise it longitudinally on its dorsal aspect throughout the stricture and beyond. Cut a patch graft from the edge of the prepuce to the proper size and tack it to the underlying tunica albuginea opposite the urethral defect, using stay sutures. Rotate the urethra into its normal orientation and suture the edges of the defect to the patch. With larger defects, a free tube graft may be substituted. This rotation technique may also be applied for roof strips.

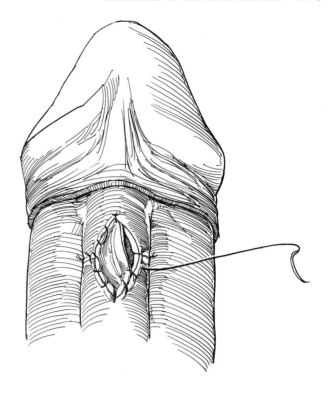

TRANSVERSE ISLAND FLAP, PENILE URETHRA
(Duckett)

See illustrations of this technique on pages 130 to 132, Steps 1 to 4.

After measuring the defect, mark an island on the dorsum of the prepuce, as is done for hypospadias repair. Deglove the shaft and open the stricture longitudinally. Resect part of the wall if it is diseased or excise a section of urethra and form a floor for a roof strip (Steps 8 to 11). Apply the flap to the defect or tubularize it to replace a section of the urethra.

LONGITUDINAL ISLAND FLAP, PENILE URETHRA
(Orandi)

Use an island flap based on a fasciocutaneous pedicle for dense recurrent strictures of the pendulous and bulbar urethra. For long strictures, the flap may be placed distally where the blood supply is less plentiful and a full-thickness skin graft placed proximally where the bed is better vascularized. The flap can be tubularized if necessary, or if the local tissue has been damaged, it may be applied in a two-stage procedure, involving preparing a bed at the first stage with a meshed split-thickness graft (see page 291).

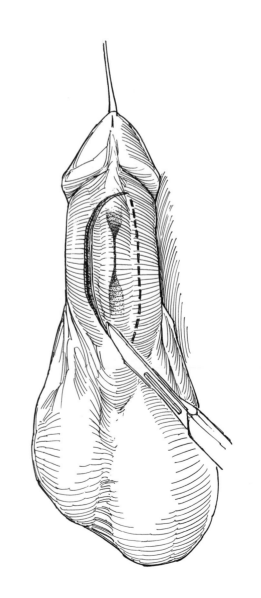

12 Incise the skin on one side of the midline on the ventral shaft through the dartos layer and Buck's fascia onto the tunica albuginea of the right corpus cavernosum. Elevate the edge and dissect across the midline over the left corpus (*dashed line*), exposing the diseased urethra.

13 Incise the urethra on the left side throughout the stricture and at least 1.5 cm beyond. If necessary, excise the entire circumference of the urethra.

14 Incise the skin longitudinally on the opposite side of the penis at a distance equal to the measured width of the urethral defect. For long strictures, raise two separate flaps and combine them. Application of too long a full-thickness flap that is not adequately perfused from the dartos layer may result in chordee.

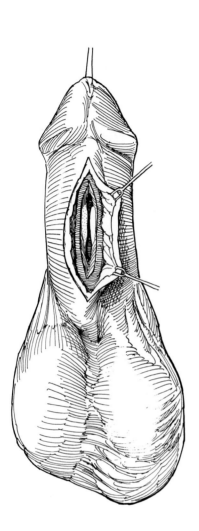

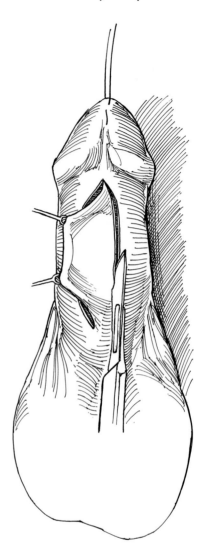

15 Elevate the edge and mobilize the skin flap. Avoid damaging the dartos pedicle beneath it. Undermine the skin lateral to it to preserve as much of the subcutaneous tissue and fascia as possible for the pedicle, realizing that the skin here has a random blood supply. If the entire circumference of the urethra has been excised, make a wider flap and tubularize it.

16 Tack the medial edge of the flap to the adjacent edge of the urethra (i.e., the right edge of the flap to the left edge of the urethra) with a few fine SAS and complete the closure with a running subcuticular 5-0 SAS. Insert a 14 F silicone balloon catheter to serve as a stent and to provide urinary drainage. Alternatively, place a suprapubic tube with a separate stent for the urethra.

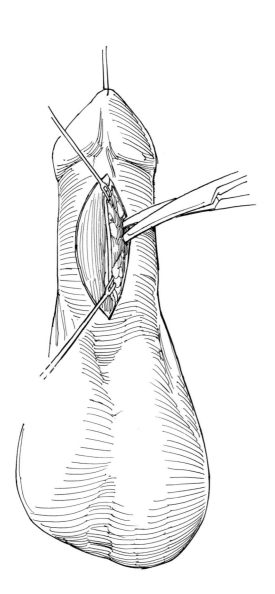

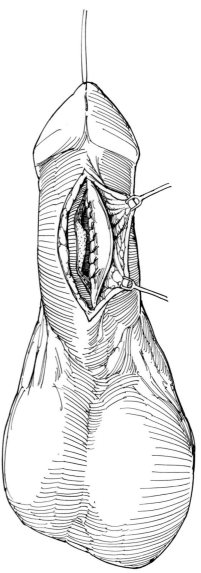

17 Invert the flap and tack its previously lateral margin to the far (right) side of the defect with fine CCG sutures. Complete the approximation with a continuous layer of fine subcuticular SAS.

18 Close the skin with interrupted 4-0 subcutaneous SAS, with a continuous 4-0 CCG subcuticular stitch for the skin itself. Apply a suitable compression dressing. After 10 days, obtain a voiding cystourethrogram with the stenting catheter in place. If no leakage occurs, remove the stent.

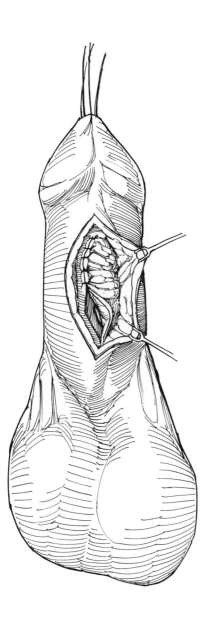

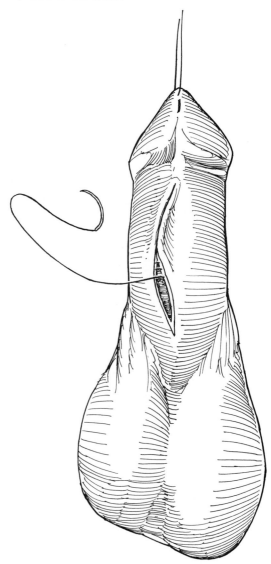

STAGED LINEAR URETHROPLASTY
(Johanson)

This technique may be used for extensive, scarred strictures of the pendulous urethra.

First Stage

19 Incise the ventral skin and expose the normal distal urethra. Incise the urethra and insert a blade of the scissors into the opening. With the scissors, divide the urethra through the entire length of the stricture into normal tissue.

20 A and **B,** Coapt the skin edges to the edges of the urethral wall with interrupted 4-0 CCG sutures. *Alternatively,* obtain a skin graft, divide it in two longitudinally, and apply it on either side of the defect to cover the raw areas. Insert an 18 F 5-ml silicone balloon catheter. Dress with prepared gauze, 4 × 8 inch elastic gauze, and elastic adhesive tape.

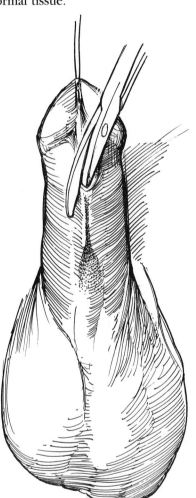

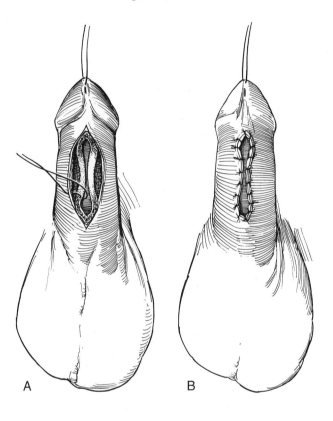

A   B

Second Stage

21 **A,** Incise the skin to encompass the two urethral openings, making an asymmetric incision 2.6 cm wide. **B,** Mobilize the skin edges both medially and laterally, using skin hooks and fine scissors. Dissect just enough to allow tubularization. Place a 16 F 5-ml silicone balloon catheter via the meatus in the glans. **C,** Close the urethra with a running subcuticular suture of 4-0 SAS. Approximate the subcutaneous tissue with 4-0 SAS if possible. **D,** Close the skin with a running subcuticular 4-0 SAS. Note that the suture lines are not superimposed. A dorsal longitudinal relaxing incision may be required to prevent tension.

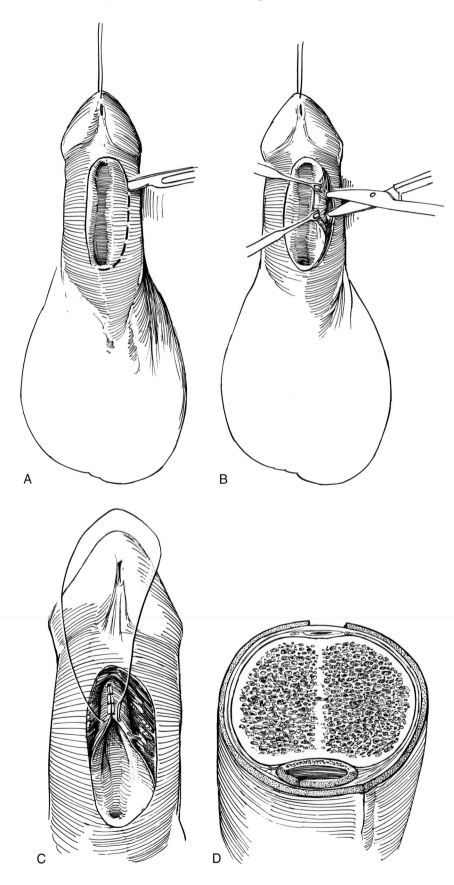

A

B

C

D

Commentary by J. Edson Pontes and René Frontera

The type of procedure to be used in repairing a urethral stricture is dictated by two basic considerations: (1) location and (2) the anatomy of the stricture. Location is important because of the propensity for development of chordee in a pendulous urethral stricture and its less generous vascularity compared with more proximal strictures. Location also influences the type of local flap used. Accurate determination of the anatomy of a stricture is of paramount importance, and this includes length and degree of spongiofibrosis. A urethrogram, whether antegrade or retrograde, is essential to define the stricture. Other techniques, including an ultrasound study of the urethra or a spongiosogram, have been used in an effort to determine the extent of fibrosis and therefore the adequacy of the urethra's vascular supply. This is of great importance because poor vascularity is probably the most important factor determining the likelihood of recurrent stricture formation, degree of contracture, and graft take. Although these diagnostic techniques have been reported to be of help, the ultimate determination is made during exploration, and therefore the actual length of the stricture is best determined at the time of surgery.

Although the one-stage end-to-end urethroplasty is the simplest and most reliable type of repair, its use in the penile urethra is limited to the occasional very short, mildly fibrotic case. Generally, for strictures of the pendulous urethra, skin island flaps used as a patch or tube give the best results for one-stage procedures. Multistage procedures should be used only in cases of refractory strictures that have failed previous repairs for which no local skin is available to be used in the repair. However, most of the time penile skin can be used even in circumcised patients. When exploring a penile urethral stricture, it is therefore advisable to make a longitudinal incision in the urethra. This has several advantages over a transverse cut. Mainly, leaving the stricture in situ minimizes further compromise to the blood supply and chordee formation. Second, it allows evaluation of the proximal and distal extension of the fibrosis. Third, by tailoring an onlay patch over the full length of the stricture, one avoids the risk of developing chordee. It is helpful to place a small catheter or filiform through the stricture so as not to lose the lumen and dissect into spongiosum. Finally, for mild-to-moderate-caliber strictures in the penile urethra, an Orandi flap is ideal. However, in very tight and long fibrotic strictures, this may compromise skin closure and require dorsal skin incision and grafting. Here, a complete or partial distal circumferential preputial island flap is ideal because it may be dissected to reach up to the deep perineum and it heals with excellent cosmetic results. Depending on the caliber of the stricture, these circumferential flaps may be obtained, even in circumcised patients, with excellent take and minimal contracture, thus avoiding staged procedures.

Strictures of the Bulbar Urethra

Strictures in the posterior pendulous and bulbar urethra can be repaired by one of four procedures: internal urethrotomy, excision and reanastomosis, grafting, and insertion of flaps.

An *internal urethrotomy* in anticipation of urethral regeneration is simple to perform, but the recurrence rate is high. *Spiral stents* are an extreme alternative.

The most straightforward method is the *excision and reanastomosis method,* which has the greatest success. Its use is limited to short traumatic strictures. It is less applicable in children, in whom most strictures are inflammatory, and the part involved in the spongiofibrotic reaction is relatively long. Thus, only the very short traumatic stricture that results from a minor straddle injury is suitable for reanastomosis in a child. In adults, the lesions may be traumatic or inflammatory, with the latter seen less often. The size of the defect cannot be any longer than the elastic lengthening obtained by mobilizing the bulbar urethra proximal and distal to the stricture, and this carries the danger of devascularization if it is extensive. Consequently, few bulbar strictures can be repaired this way.

Grafts are not uniformly successful, but because they are free patches, they may be the only solution. When skin grafts are used for urethral reconstruction, any failure of graft take results in stricture, a risk that rises in proportion to the size of the graft. Originating from the preputial skin, they are more adaptable to a wet environment than skin from other sites. *Full-thickness grafts* are better than *split-thickness grafts* for strictures, and, when placed within healthy, well-vascularized spongy tissue, they most nearly imitate the normal urethra. Bladder epithelium, or better, buccal mucosa (see pages 100 to 102), is reserved for cases in which skin is not available.

A *vascularized flap* is much more trustworthy than a graft because it carries its own blood supply. Even though a patient has been circumcised, a sufficient patch of skin from the penis is usually available. Although scrotal skin is relatively easy to form into a graft, it should be avoided because it is more subject to irritation when constantly wet, and, because it is hair bearing, it can cause distress if the graft becomes sacculated. If it is used, careful depilation is important. A random flap can be raised on a pedicle as an island flap. Such an island flap from the ventral portion of the penis or from the inner surface of the prepuce can be invaginated to fill the urethral defect and then covered with previously separated spongy tissue. Vascularized flaps do not require the well-vascularized bed that is needed for free grafts. If skin had been mobilized and transposed in an initial surgical procedure, it becomes revascularized and can be reused as a flap.

Because replacement of an entire segment of urethra by a flap is more susceptible to restenosis at one of the two sites of anastomosis, a *roof strip* can be added after overlapping the remaining portions of the urethra, which is stitched flat against the corpora to maximize its width as the floor for the repair. The graft or flap is then sutured to the edges of the strip. Even if the flap fails, re-epithelialization can occur and bridge the gap. If the quality of the tissues is in doubt, choose a staged procedure.

SUPERFICIAL PERINEAL ANATOMY

1 Colles' fascia as the penile dartos covers Buck's fascia over the penis, with a thin layer of connective tissue—the tela subfascialis—between Colles' fascia enclosing the bulbocavernosus and ischiocavernosus muscles in individual compartments, and it forms the roof of the superficial perineal space. Its major leaf is the partition between the superficial perineal space and the scrotum.

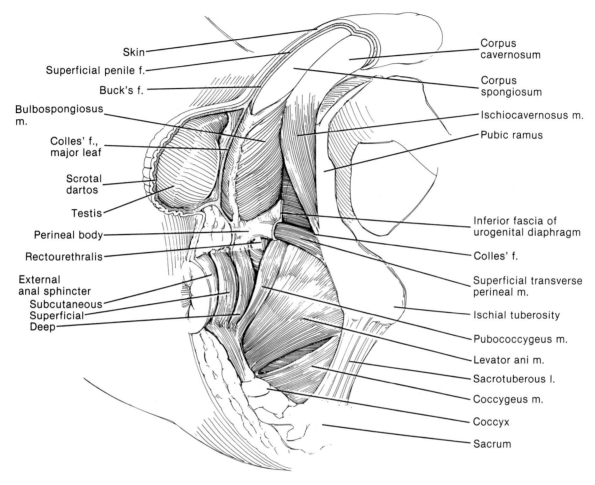

EXPOSURE OF THE BULBAR URETHRA

Preparation: Give a Fleet enema the evening before surgery to prevent soiling and avoid the need for a bowel movement in the immediate postoperative period while the patient is on bed rest. Give prophylactic antibiotics intravenously 1 hour before surgery, and repeat 8 hours postoperatively. Start trimethoprim-sulfamethoxazole suppression, and continue until all drainage tubes are removed.

Instruments: Provide a Scott ring retractor or the Turner-Warwick perineal retractor, skin hooks, and curved sounds.

2 *Position:* Exaggerated lithotomy.
Incision: Make a vertical perineal incision, extending from the penoscrotal junction to the anus or alongside the anus within 3 cm (*dashed line*). For more exposure, form the incision into an inverted Y by carrying the wings to a point medial to the ischial tuberosities (*dotted line*).

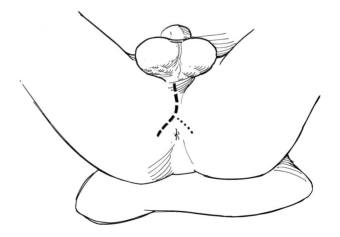

3 Expose Colles' fascia and open it in the midline. **A,** Expose the bulbocavernosus muscle and its midline raphe. Dissect distally to reveal the uncovered corpus spongiosum. **B,** Burrow under the bulbocavernosus muscle with scissors to separate it from the bulb of the urethra. **C,** Incise the bulbocavernosus muscle in the midline, and retract it laterally to expose the bulb. **D,** Free the bulb laterally and posteriorly, keeping close to the corpora cavernosa dorsally. For some strictures the muscle needs to be freed only on one side, but for extensive disease both of the arteries to the bulb may have to be divided.

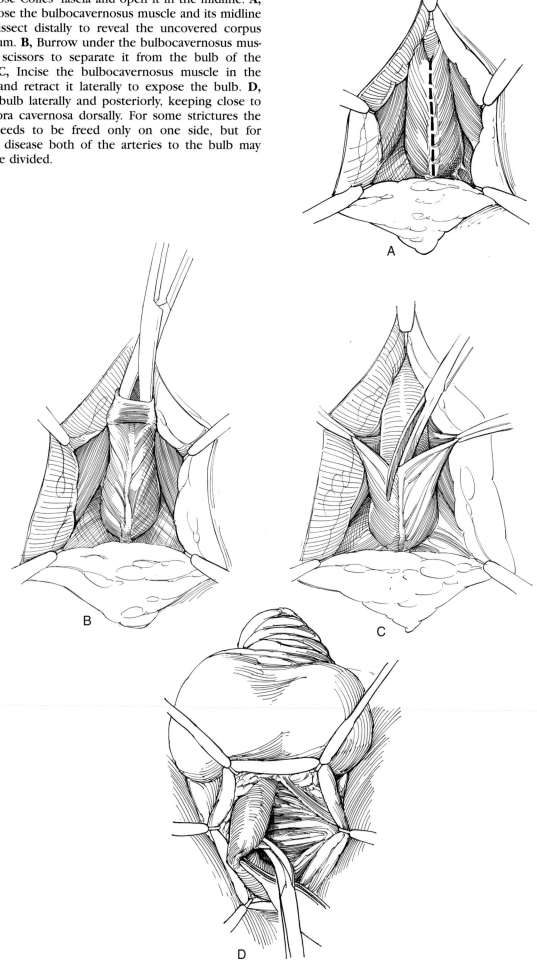

END-TO-END SPATULATED ANASTOMOSIS

The excision and anastomosis method is a technique used for severely fibrotic strictures of the bulbar urethra. The excision must be no more than 1.5 cm in length to avoid shortening the penis and creating chordee.

4 Expose the bulbar urethra as shown in Steps 2 and 3. Pass a van Buren sound into the urethra to rest against the stricture. Do not force it and tear the mucosa and spongy tissue. Palpate the tip of the sound, and cut directly through the scar upon it to reach the urethra.

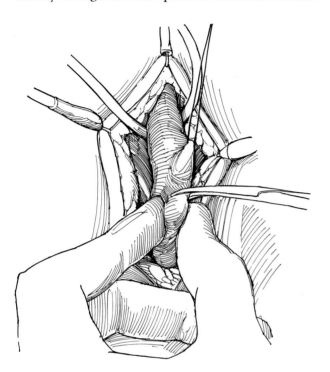

5 Cut the bulb and urethra transversely, both proximal and distal to the stricture.

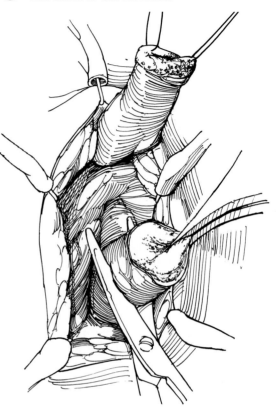

6 Place hemostatic traction sutures in the proximal cut end. Incise the urethra distally on the ventral (superficial) side well beyond the stricture. Do the same for the proximal urethra on the dorsal (deep) side. Look carefully for gray urethra, indicating spongiofibrosis, which must be excised. If tension on the suture line is anticipated, consider leaving only a roof strip and covering the floor with a patch or pedicle graft.

7 Place 5-0 monofilament SAS, first dorsally in the adventitia of the spongiosum, then in the epithelium circumferentially to obtain a watertight closure and prevent formation of a hematoma. Complete the closure of the adventitia. Finally, tack the urethra to the corpora cavernosa and triangular ligaments. Insert a silicone catheter after the deep sutures are placed. Place enough additional sutures to close the bulb hemostatically.

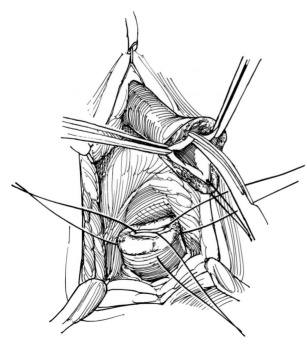

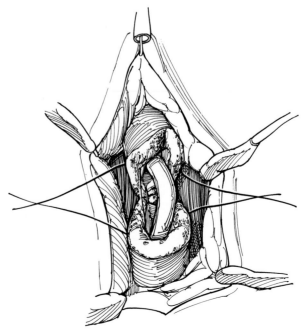

8 Approximate the bulbocavernosus muscle with interrupted sutures. Place a small suction drain. Close the dartos fascia, and approximate the skin with a running subcuticular SAS. Leave the catheter in place for 10 days or more. After the catheter has been out for a week, have the patient catheterize himself daily for the following month to prevent restricturing.

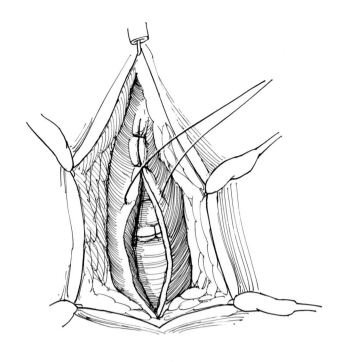

PATCH GRAFT

Patch grafts are suitable for repair of defects surrounded by relatively healthy tissue.

Position: Lithotomy. Inject dilute methylene blue intraurethrally, but realize that the stain from the dye demarcates only the epithelial deficiency, not the extent of the spongiofibrosis that must be removed.

Incision: Use a longitudinal incision for penile and midbulbar strictures; for those more proximal, an inverted-Y extension is needed, except in children. Expose the bulbocavernosus muscle. Place a ring retractor.

9 Incise down the midline raphe of the bulbocavernosus muscle, and expose the urethral and/or bulbar urethra. Insert a large curved sound in the urethra to the level of the stricture. Place two stay sutures at that level (not shown). With a #12 blade or electrocautery, cut through the penile urethra or bulb on top of the sound into the lumen distal to the stricture. Incise the urethra sharply through the entire length of the stricture, cutting at least 1 cm into normal tissue. Use a knife or Potts' scissors. Cutting on a grooved sound may help in making the incision.

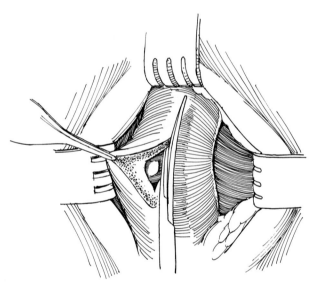

10 Catch the full thickness of the edges in stay sutures looped over the retractor for hemostasis and exposure. Insert fine running sutures as needed to control a bleeding area. Calibrate the urethra proximally with a bougie à boule to make sure that the entire strictured segment has been opened. Insert a catheter from the meatus to the bladder, choosing a size suitable for the caliber of the urethra because this determines the width of the patch when it is inserted. Measure the length and width of the defect.

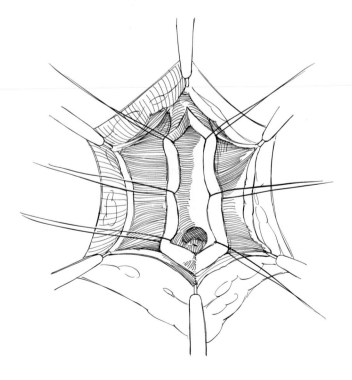

11 Outline a rectangular flap on the skin of the penis near the coronal sulcus. This may be dorsal, ventral, or preputial. Generally plenty of loose skin is available, even if the patient has been circumcised. Excise a full-thickness free graft commensurate with the defect, and close the skin with fine CCG. Alternatively, rather than taking a graft, raise a preputial flap on the dartos fascia and tunnel it into place over the defect (see pages 289 to 290). Place the graft upside down over the finger. In children, because of the small size, it is necessary to secure it on a board, using 25-gauge needles inserted in a silicone block or double-faced dermatome tape stuck on the bottom of a sterile pan. Wearing a loupe, lift up the adventitial tissue with fine forceps and trim it off with fine scissors. Leave the dermis, but take off all the tissue that is pink. Trim one end of the graft to fit (avoid overtrimming; the graft can be adjusted in situ). Alternatively, cut a template from a suture packet to fit the defect. Avoid making the patch too large, which leads to subsequent sacculation. Lay the graft in place over the catheter with the epithelial side down.

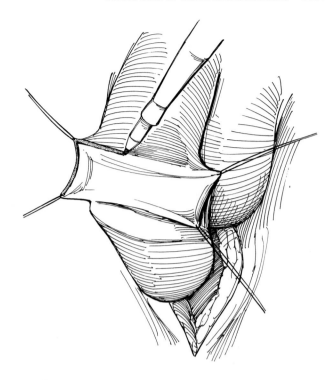

12 **A,** Place two interrupted 5-0 CCG sutures at the apex of the defect. Insert the suture from the epithelial side of the graft, then pass it through the urethral epithelium and tie the knots inside the urethral lumen (not shown). Place interrupted sutures successively down each side. Trim the graft for the final sutures. A second layer of running locked 6-0 SAS is placed to secure the urethral subepithelium and inner layer of the corpus spongiosum to the dermis of the graft. **B,** Alternatively, place four 5-0 SAS through the quadrants of the graft to hold the defect open. Start running a suture on either side from the apex, continuing alternately down one side and then the other. Trim the graft as the suturing progresses, and tie the continuous sutures to the quadrant sutures. This method provides a more watertight fit but may leave a graft that is too wide. Free the spongy tissue laterally, and suture it over the graft. When severe fibrosis is present in the spongy tissue, this cannot be done and one must depend on the bulbospongiosus muscle layer to vascularize the graft. Replace the catheter with a smaller silicone catheter (16 F). Close the bulbocavernosus muscle with suitable SAS, followed by approximation of Colles' fascia. Close the skin with a running subcuticular stitch of 4-0 or 5-0 SAS. Leave no drain, or at most place a 16-gauge minivacuum system.

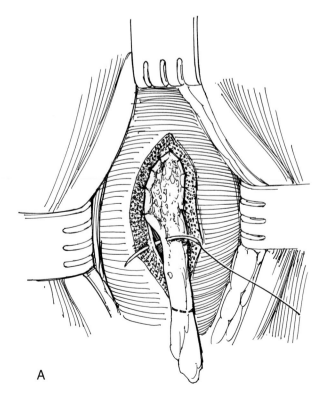

A

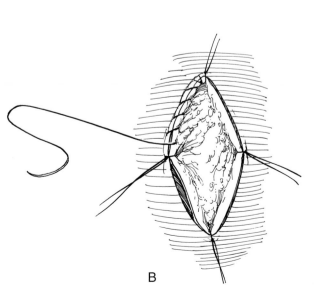

B

TUBED GRAFT

Excision and tubed graft placement may be used for longer, dense strictures, but a vascular flap is preferable.

13 Proceed as described previously, but excise the entire defect, including all surrounding scar tissue and fistulous tracts.

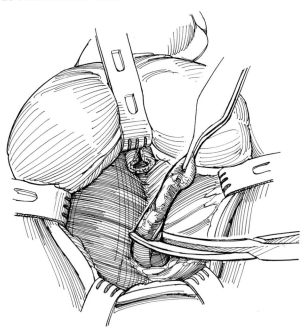

14 Anastomose the graft, usually obtained from the prepuce (Step 11), at each end with interrupted fine SAS, and close it ventrally with a continuous suture.

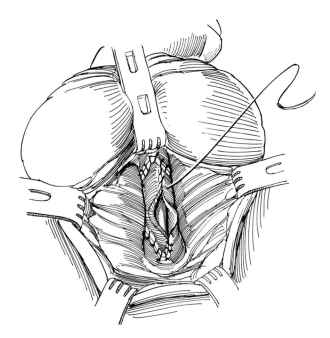

LONGITUDINAL / TRANSVERSE PREPUTIAL ISLAND FLAP (Quartey)

The Quartey flap combines the Orandi procedure with that of McAninch. Although it is an older procedure, because it provides a large island it is useful for extensive defects in the perineal portion of the urethra.

15 **A,** Make parallel incisions on the ventrum and extend them around the coronal sulcus. **B,** Raise a long flap on the blood supply from the dartos and Buck's fascia. Dissect along the corpus spongiosum and bluntly form a tunnel under the bridge of scrotum. Pass the flap into the perineum (*arrow*), and suture it onto the defect with running subepithelial sutures (Step 12).

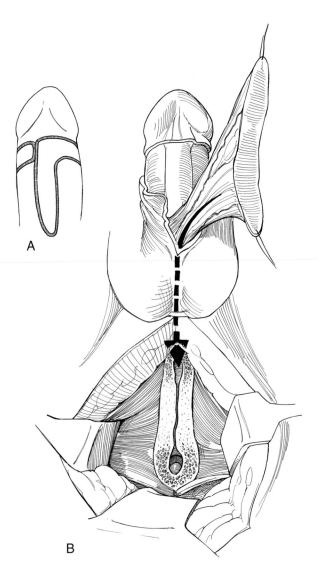

A

B

PREPUTIAL ISLAND
FASCIOCUTANEOUS FLAP
(McAninch)

Place the patient in the lithotomy position, extreme if the stricture is proximal. Protect the legs from pressure points and avoid stretching the sciatic nerve. Make a midline incision and reflect the bulbospongiosus muscle. Expose the entire stricture through an incision in the corpus spongiosum, and incise the normal urethra for at least 1 cm. Pass a 30 F bougie to check the adequacy of the channel.

16 Operative view. The cross-sectional view on the right shows the depth of incisions. Mark two parallel incisions around the shaft, one at the coronal sulcus or circumcision line and the other 2 cm proximal to it for onlay procedures or 2.5 cm for urethral replacement. Incise the distal incision through the dartos layer and Buck's fascia, avoiding the deeper layer containing the neurovascular bundle. Mobilize the penile skin back to the base. Replace the skin over the penis and incise the proximal incision along the marked line, but cut through only the dartos fascia to preserve a pedicle based on Buck's fascia. Again mobilize the shaft skin back to the base of the penis, but dissect superficial to Buck's fascia, preserving the dartos fascia and the subdermal plexus on the penile skin. Split the ring of skin in the midline ventrally, and divide Buck's fascia to the base of the penis.

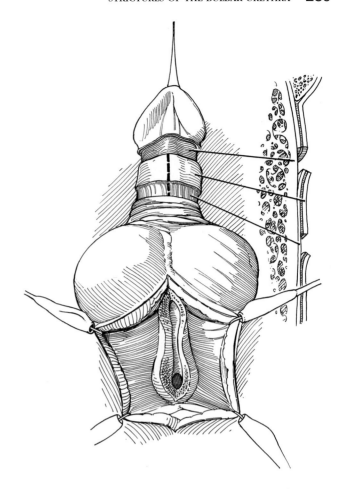

17 Raise the flap on a broad pedicle of Buck's fascia.

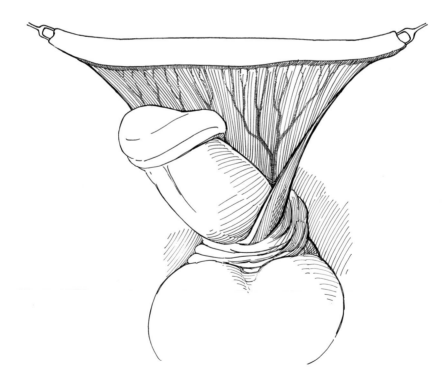

18 Create a subcutaneous tunnel into the perineal wound. Rotate the flap, and pass one end through the tunnel. If necessary, narrow the base of the pedicle to allow placement of the flap skin side down and free of tension, taking care not to impair the blood supply. With optical magnification, begin suturing proximally with a 6-0 continuous monofilament PDS, at first working on the one side from inside the flap and urethra. If the flap proves to be too short, interpose a free graft proximally. Insert a stenting catheter, and complete the closure of the other side from outside the lumen. Close the perineal wound.

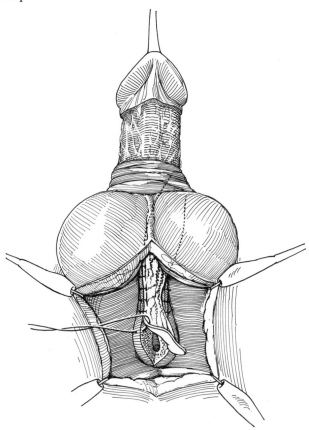

SCROTAL SKIN ISLAND FLAP
(Blandy)

Because the scrotum is easy to manipulate and lies close to the recipient site, it can be used for an island flap if a portion of it can be found to be (relatively) free of hair, usually an area in midperineum. Although the flap usually contains hairs, depilation is futile. Make a transverse incision; this allows for adequate exposure and leaves less scar. Care must be taken not to take too large a flap because the presence of the dartos muscle makes it appear smaller than it actually will be when it is secured in place. Base the flap on a lateral pedicle of the normal scrotal blood supply.

Problems are hair growth, which can lead to the formation of stones, especially with distal stenosis, and pouching of the skin with consequent dribbling.

A *dartos flap* can be raised from the scrotum, leaving the skin in place. The vascularized flap may then be rotated to cover a urethral repair (Motiwala).

FLAP ROOF-STRIP URETHROPLASTY
(Turner-Warwick)

Reserve the use of roof-strip flaps for those cases in which reanastomosis is not possible.

Position: Exaggerated lithotomy. Inject diluted methylene blue into the urethra.

Incision: Make a vertical or inverted-Y incision. Dissect the bulbospongiosus muscle laterally, and locate the stricture by placing a van Buren sound into the anterior urethra and a semicircular sound into the posterior urethra via the cystostomy tract.

Incise the urethra over the tip of the anterior urethral sound, and identify normal urethra. Open the urethra posteriorly over the transvesical sound to or into the membranous portion until a sound of the proper size passes easily into the bladder.

Excise the diseased segment and surrounding scar tissue by dividing the membranous urethra obliquely in two places. Mobilize the distal urethra and measure the length of the defect; if it is less than 2 cm in an adult or 1 cm in a child, proceed with direct anastomosis. If reanastomosis is impossible, form a roof strip by suturing the dorsal margins, and hold the distal urethra in place with fixation sutures.

To form the floor, raise an island flap from the ventral shaft skin on a dartos pedicle (or obtain it from the prepuce; see page 289). Pass the flap under the scrotal bridge, and suture it to form the floor of the urethral defect. Bring available muscle and connective tissue over the repair and tack it in place. Close the wound in layers without drainage. Leave the catheter in place at least 10 days, and check with retrograde urethrography prior to removal.

MESHED GRAFT TWO-STAGE PROCEDURE
(Schreiter and Noll)

An alternative for long strictures with considerable fibrous reaction is to remove the diseased urethra entirely because it is useless for formation of a neourethra. Cover the defect with a split-thickness graft. Subsequently, excise the graft, leaving a hairless, healthy bed for a new graft or flap.

19 **A,** *First stage:* Remove the diseased skin from the ventral surface of the penis. Mobilize the dartos fascia lateral to the urethral bed from under the penile skin for a short distance on each side, and bring the two flaps together in the midline with a running 4-0 CCG suture to provide a bed for the graft. Cut a 0.015-inch-thick split-thickness skin graft from the thigh and place it in a meshing dermatome (see page 218). **B,** Lay the graft in the defect on the ventrum of the penis. Do not expand it because the principal purpose of meshing is to provide drainage and encourage angiogenesis. Suture it in place with 4-0 CCG sutures, leaving the sutures long. Cover it with medicated gauze carefully padded with Dacron wool, and tie the long sutures over it for fixation. The defect may be reduced in size by closing the scrotum transversely on either side in the first stage and later releasing it to help cover the new graft. Insert a 14 F silicone catheter in the proximal urethrostomy, and consider inserting a suprapubic tube. Place the patient at bed rest and maintain antibiotic coverage for 5 to 6 days,

at which time the dressing can be removed. Remove the urethral catheter at this time, and remove the suprapubic catheter 1 week later.

Second stage: Allow healing for 6 months or more. If the new skin is not of satisfactory quality, remove it to provide a fresh base for a new flap secured from the skin of the prepuce or shaft. If the skin from the graft appears healthy, make longitudinal incisions 3 cm apart through the skin, sparing the dartos fascia. Raise two parallel flaps (Thiersch-Duplay, see page 140) by dissecting laterally and taking care not to undermine the new skin during mobilization of the flaps. Trim the flaps exactly to size (30 F), especially in the scrotal area, to avoid sacculation. Approximate the edges of the flaps over a 14 F catheter with several interrupted 6-0 CCG sutures to form a tube. Place a running layer of 5-0 SAS subepithelially. Cover the neourethra by approximating the lateral skin edges with interrupted 6-0 SAS or a running subcuticular suture. Apply a Bioclusive dressing.

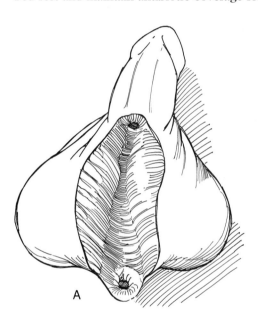

A

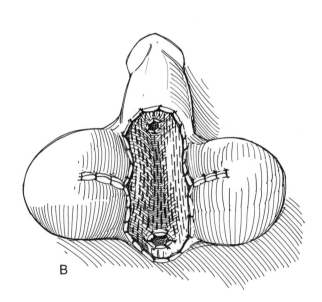

B

Commentary by Jack W. McAninch

The flap is taken from the distal penile skin; this can be done safely even in previously circumcised patients. Sufficient penile skin remains without interference with erectile function or cosmetic appearance. This flap is taken in a circular configuration and split ventrally to maximize the rich dorsal vasculature that runs along Buck's fascia. The deep dorsal penile vessels and nerves are not disturbed. When this is used as an onlay flap, approximately 13 to 15 cm of skin can be obtained in an adult. A complete tubularized urethral replacement of 8 to 10 cm can be done with this flap. The pedicle is quite substantial and well vascularized. The skin of the distal penile shaft is free of hair, which provides a great advantage in urethral reconstruction over other areas of genital skin. The flap is made adaptable to any anterior urethral stricture distal to the verumontanum by freeing the base of the pedicle back to the level of the pubic bone before rotation into the perineum. Lateral release of the

pedicle base provides tension-free flap rotation through the scrotum to the proximal anterior urethra. Long strictures that exceed the length of the flap can be reconstructed by combining free graft tissue taken from buccal mucosa, bladder epithelium, or additional penile shaft skin. Combining these tissue-transfer techniques has allowed us to reconstruct strictures up to 24 cm in length in a single stage.

A stenting 16 F urethral catheter is left in place for 2 to 3 weeks. The patients are followed carefully with urinary flow rates and urethrography at 3 and 12 months postoperatively. No dilation or instrumentation is done. The success rate is approximately 90 percent. Failures have been more common with the tubularized flap at both the proximal and distal ends. These have been managed successfully by excision of the localized segment and end-to-end anastomosis to the native stricture-free urethra.

Bulbomembranous Urethral Strictures

Fracture of the pelvis frequently results in a bulbomembranous urethral distraction defect, one that poses difficult problems for the urologist. Repair of the resulting stricture is best undertaken by those with continuous experience. An open repair is usually required if endoscopic incision fails. A less satisfactory alternative is the insertion of an expandable intraluminal stent.

IMMEDIATE MANAGEMENT

Because effective techniques are now available for delayed repair of prostatomembranous strictures, current practice is the immediate insertion of a suprapubic tube without attempting to correct the distraction defect unless the injury is a major one.

Partial Tears. Suprapubic drainage is all that is necessary. Urethral catheterization may expand the defect. Follow the healing process with serial urethrography. When extravasation has ceased, have the patient void before removing the tube. If a stricture forms, it is usually soft and amenable to dilation.

Complete Tears. Place a suprapubic tube (Johanson). This does not have to be done by an expert and can be done with local anesthesia if the patient's condition is unstable. Wait 3 or more months before proceeding with a definitive one-stage repair. In contrast to immediate repair, including traction with a balloon catheter or suture repair, delayed repair results in more successful outcomes with less adverse effect on potency and continence, less chance for infection of the hematoma, and less overall risk to the injured patient.

Severe Injuries. For major distraction of the prostatomembranous urethra, where it is (1) surrounded by a massive pelvic hematoma, (2) associated with injury to the bladder neck, or (3) associated with injury to the rectum, immediate repair is advisable. Achieve stabilization by placing the pelvis in a C-arm frame. This can decrease bleeding enough to allow primary repair of the urethra and vesical neck if that is thought to be advisable (see pages 264 to 265). Make a lower midline incision, evacuate the hematoma, and manipulate a 16 F or 18 F catheter retrogradely. Insert a similar catheter via a cystotomy through the bladder neck and prostatic urethra, and place a stitch to hold the tips of the two catheters together. Maneuver the prostate into place without excessive mobilization or division of fascial attachments. *Vest suture* (see page 462): Insert a monofilament suture through the anterior surface of the prostate, and place both ends in a long straight needle. Pass the needle into the perineum through the urogenital diaphragm at the appropriate site to prevent angulation and misalignment. Tie the suture over a rubber bolster, applying enough traction to bring the prostate to the urogenital diaphragm. Remove the suture in 7 to 10 days, the stenting catheter after a urethrogram shows no extravasation, and the suprapubic tube after voiding has begun.

EVALUATION

Synchronous cystography and urethrography are essential to detect fistulous tracts and false passages. Failure to demonstrate the prostatic urethra by antegrade filling is reassuring evidence of bladder neck competence (unless it has become stenotic after the injury). A patulous bladder neck is intrinsically damaged or is tethered by extensive retropubic fibrosis left by the resolving hematoma. The difference can be evaluated by cystourethroscopy: If the bladder neck appears normal, it probably is competent and the stricture may be repaired directly. If it appears distorted, a combined abdominoperineal approach is required. The length of the actual defect may be gauged by cystourethrography or even better by magnetic resonance imaging. The extent of the local fibrosis can be estimated by ultrasonography but observed at operation. Extrapolation from the radiographs is potentially misleading. For this reason, the surgeon must make contingency plans for a more extended procedure.

OPTIONS FOR TREATMENT

Several options are available. Simple dilation, especially if done early, may create a false passage. Internal urethrotomy is worth trying but should be reserved for strictures distal to the membranous urethra. Endoscopic incision through a completely obliterated posterior urethra, guided by an intravesical light or a guide wire, may cause further damage to the remaining sphincteric function but has been effective in selected cases. Anastomotic techniques are preferable to any other method, provided that the prostatic urethra is not involved. Substitution procedures with free patches or pedicle flaps are more adaptable but carry a greater risk of failure.

PRINCIPLES OF TREATMENT

Certain principles must be followed: Meticulously excise all the periurethral and retropubic fibrosis with accompanying infected pockets, and mobilize the bulbar urethra to allow an anastomosis free of tension on its healthy spatulated end that joins the prostate. Perform the anastomosis with perfect technique, and fill with omentum any residual dead space left after removing the fibrous tissue. Remember that once the urethra is divided, the distal portion is without proximal blood supply from the bulbar arteries and depends on a more tenuous distal supply. Both the retropubic and perineal routes are available for repair. A combined approach allows mobilization of the omentum.

TIMING

The timing of the repair depends on the size of the pelvic hematoma. For small collections, 3 months may be sufficient. For a large hematoma, a year may be necessary for resolution, even if the injury was initially treated only by suprapubic urinary drainage.

APPROACHES

Several operative approaches can be used: perineal, transpubic, or a combination of the two. Use the abdominoperineal position to provide abdominal access if the retropubic fibrosis is found to be excessive during dissection from the perineum.

For complex strictures, the procedure must combine exploration and excision with repair. Both Turner-Warwick and Webster have devised approaches in which the findings and accomplishments at each step lead to the next one. The elements are as follows: (1) placing the patient in the abdominoperineal position for access to both areas; (2) mobilizing the bulbar urethra and excising the scar tissue around the distal stricture perineally; (3) resecting the retropubic fibrosis suprapubically if necessary, even removing retropubic fibrosis by partial pubic resection; (4) examining the bladder neck directly by cystoscopy; (5) repairing the urethra with a spatulated bulboprostatic anastomosis; (6) rerouting the urethra to achieve a tension-free anastomosis; (7) diverting and stenting by suprapubic catheter and fenestrated urethral catheter; (8) placing an omental wrap if a large dead space remains; and (9) performing additional procedures, such as excising rectal fistulas and freeing the bladder neck for sphincteroplasty.

ANATOMIC RELATIONS IN THE SUPERFICIAL PERINEAL SPACE

1 The superficial urogenital muscles, the bulbospongiosus muscle, and both ischiocavernosus muscles are within the superficial perineal space. This space also contains the paired superficial transverse perineal muscles that run across from the anterior and medial parts of the ischial tuberosities. They join the perineal body in the midline in conjunction with muscle fibers from the superficial part of the external anal sphincter and the bulbospongiosus muscle.

The superficial perineal space also contains the transverse perineal artery, a branch of the internal pudendal artery that runs beneath the superficial transverse peri-

neal muscle along with a branch of the perineal nerve. The perineal branches of the posterior femoral cutaneous nerves and the scrotal arteries, veins, and nerves pass forward alongside the bulbospongiosus.

The perineal body, composed of fibromuscular tissue, is an important landmark. It lies superficial to the pelvic floor in a central position between the anal and urogenital portions of the perineum. It marks the separation of the two parts of the perineum and provides a central point of fixation for the perineal musculature. The more superficial attachments of the perineal body come from the bulbospongiosus, the superficial transverse perineal muscles, and the more superficial part of the external anal sphincter. The deeper connections are with the deep part of the external anal sphincter, the prostatic levators, and the deep transverse perineal muscles.

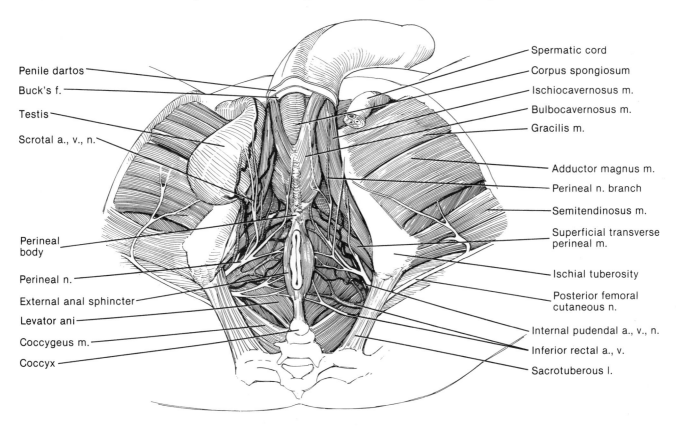

Penile dartos — Buck's f. — Testis — Scrotal a., v., n. — Perineal body — Perineal n. — External anal sphincter — Levator ani — Coccygeus m. — Coccyx

Spermatic cord — Corpus spongiosum — Ischiocavernosus m. — Bulbocavernosus m. — Gracilis m. — Adductor magnus m. — Perineal n. branch — Semitendinosus m. — Superficial transverse perineal m. — Ischial tuberosity — Posterior femoral cutaneous n. — Internal pudendal a., v., n. — Inferior rectal a., v. — Sacrotuberous l.

PATCH GRAFT URETHROPLASTY

Compared with flaps, grafts have a greater chance of stricturing.

2 *Position:* Exaggerated lithotomy. Inject methylene blue into the urethra.

Incision: Make a vertical, or better, an inverted-Y incision. Incise the bulbospongiosus muscle and displace it laterally. Locate the stricture by placing a van Buren sound into the anterior urethra and a semicircular sound into the posterior urethra via the cystostomy tract.

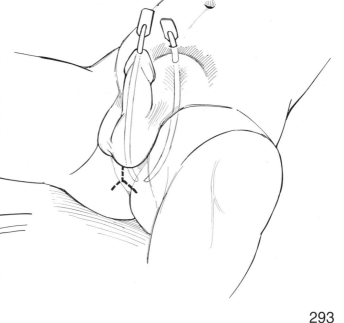

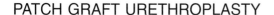

3 Incise the urethra over the tip of the anterior urethral sound and identify normal urethra. Open the urethra posteriorly over the transvesical sound to or into the membranous portion until a 30 F sound can be easily passed into the bladder. Excise the diseased segment and surrounding scar tissue. Spatulate the membranous urethra. Measure the defect. If it is less than 2 cm long, proceed with direct anastomosis (see page 272). Insert a 22 F silicone balloon catheter into the bladder through the proximal defect, inflate it, and mark the distance from the bladder neck.

4 Obtain a full-thickness graft from the penis. If this skin is not available, obtain a thick graft (0.020-inch) with a dermatome from the inner aspect of the upper arm or the medial aspect of the upper leg (see page 211). Pin out the graft, defat it, and suture it around the marked 22 F silicone balloon catheter. Use a running 4-0 SAS for most of its length, and use interrupted sutures at the end to allow for trimming after placement.

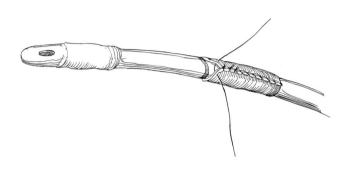

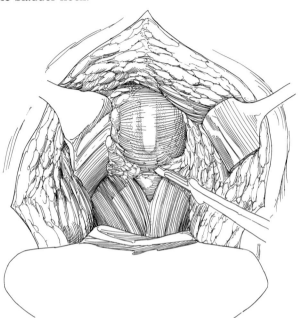

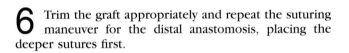

5 Insert the balloon catheter through the entire urethra and inflate the balloon. Elevate the catheter partially out of the wound, and rotate it so that the suture line in the graft lies against the deep tissue. Place three or four interrupted 3-0 SAS, approximating the edge of the graft to the membranous urethra. Continue suturing around the circumference.

6 Trim the graft appropriately and repeat the suturing maneuver for the distal anastomosis, placing the deeper sutures first.

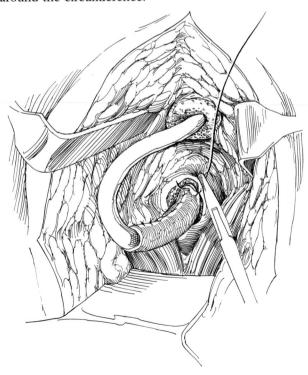

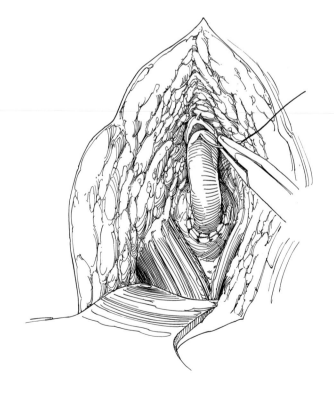

7 Bring available local tissue over the repair and tack it in place. Close the wound in layers without drainage. Leave the catheter in place 10 days.

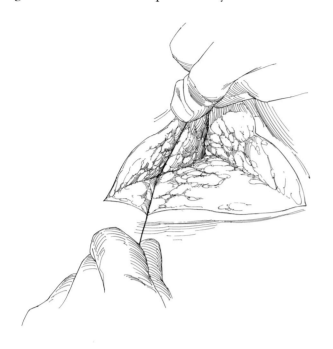

PERINEAL REPAIR
(Webster)

Defer operation until local tissue reaction has subsided (at least 3 months and as long as 1 year). Estimate the apparent extent of the stricture by simultaneous voiding cystography and retrograde urethrography. Ultrasonography may help, but accurate evaluation must wait for exposure and inspection of the quality of the periurethral tissue.

A one-stage procedure for deep obliterative defects can be divided into successive steps designed to facilitate the anastomosis, with the surgeon proceeding to the next step as the dissection develops. The operation starts with urethral mobilization. To gain more urethral length, separate the corporal bodies. Then resect a wedge from the inferior pubic ramus. For still greater length, route the urethra around one of the crura. An abdominoperineal approach is rarely needed. For patients with anterior stricture disease or prior hypospadias repair, the operation is not applicable.

Mobilizing the urethra after pelvic trauma may risk urethral devascularization if the circulation from the pudendal artery, and especially that from the proximal common penile arteries or dorsal artery of the penis, has been compromised by the injury.

Instruments: Include a ring or Scott retractor, a flexible nephroscope, and a semicircular sound. In addition, a nerve hook and an ENT (ear-nose-throat) ligature carrier can be useful for deep suturing, as can the special Turner-Warwick instruments.

8 **A** and **B,** *Position:* For deep strictures, as for perineal prostatectomy (see page 453), place the patient on a vacuum pad with his sacrum on a large sandbag or wedge and his feet in stirrups. Pull him well down to the end of the table. Angle the stirrups toward the head of the table until the perineum is parallel with the floor. Be cognizant of the potential for nerve injury and muscle injury to the legs, producing rhabdomyolysis (see page 464). Tape the sandbag in place; fold the vacuum pad over the shoulders (beware of brachial plexus injury) and evacuate it. Tilt the head of the table down slightly. For potentially complicated cases that may require a simultaneous abdominal approach, place the patient in the low lithotomy position, draped to allow simultaneous access to the lower abdomen and perineum. Place a suprapubic cystostomy. Instill dilute methylene blue solution in the urethra.

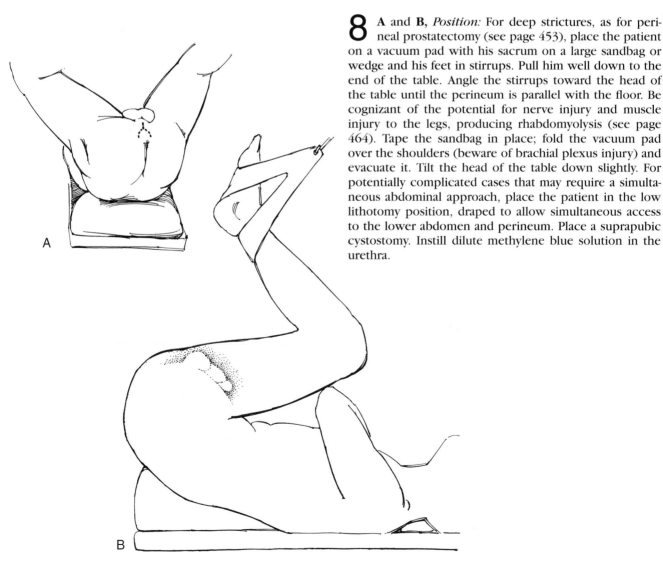

9 **A,** *Incision:* Make a midline incision in the perineum. Extended it to form an inverted-U incision
(or hemi-U) inside the ischial tuberosities. **B,** Incise
Colles' fascia in the midline, and expose the bulbocavernosus muscle. Insert sounds to the level of the stricture
from below and above. Incise the proximal end of the
bulbocavernosus muscle; split it open in the midline
without entering the erectile tissue and reflect it to expose the urethral bulb, in which the sound can be palpated. Tag the edges of the muscle for identification
during closure.

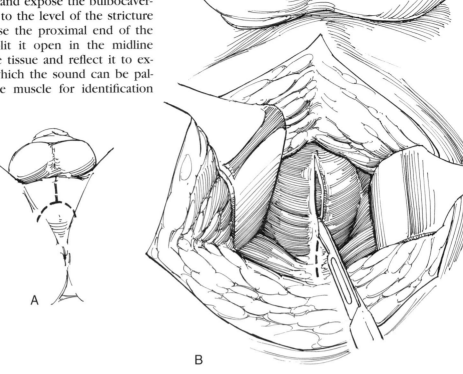

A

B

10 *Mobilization of the bulbar urethra:* Sharply and
bluntly free the bulb inside its muscular coat
both proximally to the membranous urethra and distally
to the suspensory ligament to allow for a tension-free
reapproximation. Do not dissect beyond this point to
avoid chordee. Continue the division of the bulbocavernosus muscle through the junction of the transversus
perinei muscles adjacent to the perineal body. Retract
these muscles posterolaterally to allow dissection to the
urogenital diaphragm, and develop the intercrural space.
Do not mobilize the prostate itself. Dissect and suture-
ligate the bulbourethral arteries. Place a ring or Scott
retractor with deep blades.

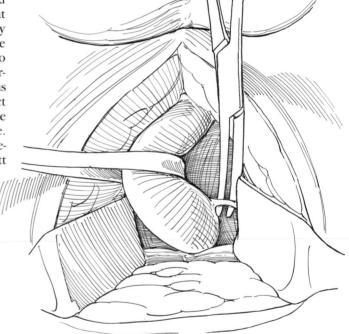

11 *Dissection to the suspensory ligament:* After transecting the urethra distal to the diseased segment, circumferentially dissect it to, but not beyond, the level of the suspensory ligament. Retain the spongy tissue, realizing that the urethra must now obtain its blood supply peripherally.

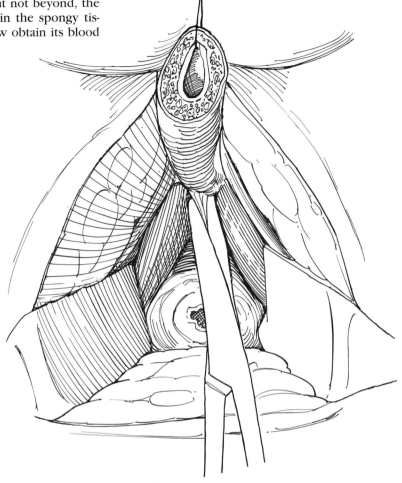

12 *Separation of the corporal bodies:* For further urethral lengthening, separate the corporal bodies from each other for 4 to 5 cm from the crus. Stay in the midline, and take care not to interfere with the dorsal-lying neurovascular bundles.

13 *Inferior pubectomy:* If further length is required, divide the periosteum over the pubis in the midline and mobilize it laterally with a periosteal elevator to preserve the vessels. Resect a wedge of pubis from the bony surface with an osteotome and rongeurs.

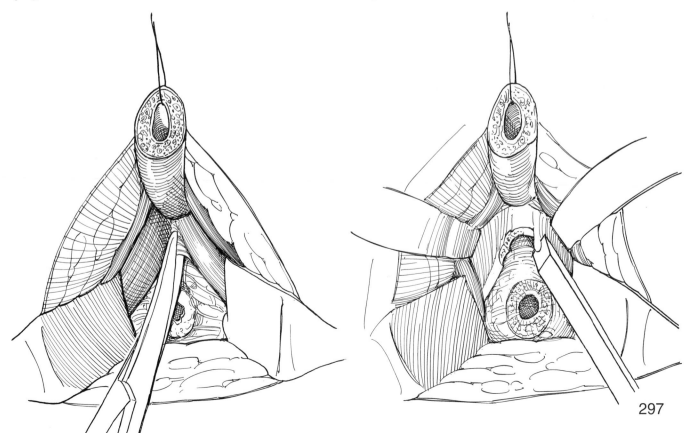

14   **A,** *Urethrourethral anastomosis:* Spatulate the prostatomembranous urethra on the dorsal aspect as high as the verumontanum, and incise the bulbar urethra similarly on the ventrum. Make the openings large enough to provide passage for a 40 F sound. Do the spatulation before rerouting; this allows a better estimate of the additional length needed. Join the urethral ends epithelium to epithelium by inserting a series of 4-0 PDS swaged on curved needles straightened into a J shape (or swaged on Turner-Warwick needles). For exposure, use a nasal or Turner-Warwick speculum. **B,** Hold the shaft of the needle vertically in the needle holder. Insert the needle from outside to inside. **C,** Grasp the protruding curve of the needle with the needle holder and advance the needle into the prostatic urethra to complete the stitch. Place the sutures first dorsally at the 12-o'clock position; then place 6 to 10 sutures, proceeding in a clockwise direction. Work for an epithelial-epithelial connection. Tie the sutures in the same sequence as they are placed. Add additional sutures in the adventitia to relieve tension on the anastomosis. Fill the dead space with the bulbocavernosus muscle (it is rarely necessary to go abdominally and mobilize the omentum). Insert a 16 F proximally fenestrated catheter. Replace the suprapubic catheter, and insert perineal suction drains.

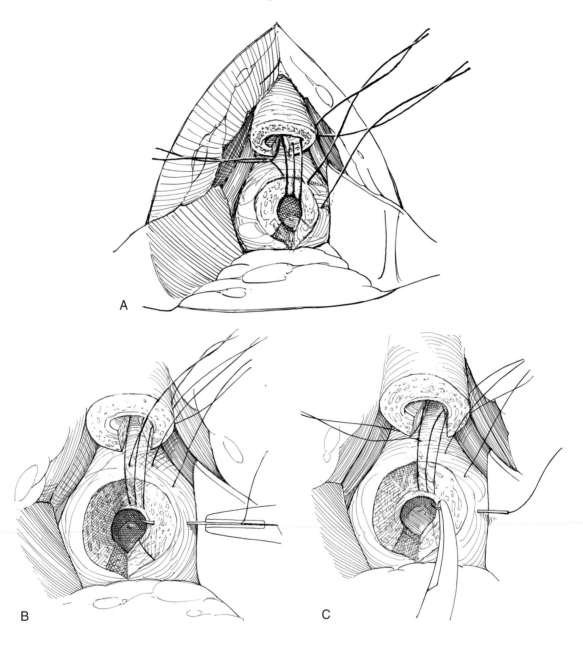

15 *Supracrural routing:* If the urethra is still too short, dissect in the soft tissue surrounding but not immediately attached to one corporal body, staying away from it because of the risk of damaging the neurovascular bundle. Gouge a channel in the symphysis to allow passage of the urethra without compression. Pass the urethra laterally and under the corporal body. Some penile torsion may be anticipated from this maneuver. Graft or flaps may be interposed if end-to-end anastomosis is not possible, although the incidence of stricture is greater than after direct anastomosis. A tubed preputial graft is an alternative, as is a tubed flap formed from overlying scrotum (Cukier).

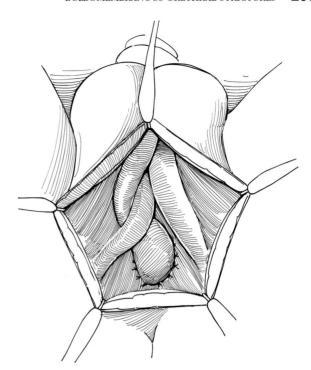

Postoperative Care

Continue antibiotics. Leave the stenting catheter in place for 2 or 3 weeks. Do retrograde urethrography around the stent; if it shows no extravasation, remove the stent. A period of trial voiding is completed before removal of the suprapubic tube.

Commentary by George D. Webster

Injuries to the posterior urethra at the time of pelvic fracture may be partial or complete. The former may heal with relatively minor stricturing that may respond to dilation or urethrotomy. However, complete disruption generally results in a distraction defect of varying length. Initial management of such injuries generally is suprapubic catheter drainage, elective delayed repair being performed 3 or more months later. Although in adults and postpubertal boys the site of injury is invariably at the bulbomembranous or prostatomembranous urethra, in prepubertal boys the injury may occur in the prostatic urethra or even at the bladder neck.

I have found a perineal anastomotic repair to be appropriate for the vast majority of such posterior urethral distraction defects, regardless of length. The absolute prerequisite for such repair is a healthy anterior urethra because the mobilized urethra must survive as a distally based flap once it has been circumferentially dissected as far as the suspensory ligament of the penis. The four steps described previously to facilitate a tension-free bulboprostatic anastomosis are performed sequentially, if necessary. It is my experience that in peripubertal boys requiring such repairs all steps are likely to be required to accomplish anastomosis. This probably is because in this age group the bulbar urethra, the most elastic portion of the urethra, is still poorly developed. Exquisite care must be taken in dissecting the small urethra circumferentially to ensure its survival as a flap.

Although considerable retropubic scar excision was advised in the abdominoperineal transpubic approach to such problems, this has not proven to be necessary with this progressive perineal approach. In fact, the perineal scar is incised vertically in the midline onto the tip of the descending urethral sound, and only a very small amount of adjacent scar is excised, sufficient to allow good visibility of the patent spatulated prostatomembranous urethra. This limited dissection avoids any further injury to nerves that may be important in erection.

It is important in performing the anastomosis itself that all of the radial sutures be placed first and tied later. I commence

with placement of the dorsal 12-o'clock position suture and then place sutures sequentially around the anastomosis in a clockwise fashion. Sutures are then all tied in the order in which they are placed, and the stenting catheter is inserted thereafter.

Indications for alternative approaches: If the anterior urethra is strictured or injured, the urethra cannot be mobilized as a flap as described previously, and this is a probable indication for a substitution urethroplasty. Although one-stage substitution urethroplasty using pedicled islands of penile skin is appropriate in some cases, in the pediatric age group, sufficient penile skin is not always available and mobilization of penile islands on a pedicle to the perineum is fraught with difficulty. Hence, in these rare instances, a staged urethroplasty probably is appropriate. These cases are exceptionally uncommon, however.

In patients with bulbomembranous urethral disruption in whom there are complicating features such as communications between periurethral tissues or pelvic floor cavity and the urethra, rectourethral fistulas, bladder base fistulas, and so forth, the abdominoperineal approach is likely to be required. This allows the additional disease to be managed. It also allows for omental pedicle support of the repair. After such injuries to the posterior urethra, continence requires a functional bladder neck. In some cases, preoperative cystography may show bladder neck incompetence, suggesting that continence may be compromised after the posterior urethra has been repaired. In some cases this too is an indication for an abdominoperineal approach because it gives an opportunity for lysis of the bladder neck from dense retropubic scar, which may fix the sphincter in the open position. Additionally, sphincteroplasty may be performed. However, it has been my experience that perineal posterior urethroplasty, even in the face of some bladder neck incompetence, is not necessarily followed by postoperative incontinence. Hence, it is my practice to complete the urethroplasty and to intervene suprapubically only at a second procedure, if incontinence demands it.

TRANSPUBIC EXCISION AND ANASTOMOSIS

The transpubic excision and anastomosis approach is used for strictures of the posterior urethra longer than 2 cm. Its advantages are that the bladder neck may be freed and reconstructed in the occasional patient who requires it. In complicated cases, it allows application of the omentum. Compared with the infrapubic approach, it has a greater morbidity. Starting the operation perineally usually allows resection of enough of the pubis from below; if not, the transpubic approach can be added.

Instruments: Provide a Gigli saw, a periosteal elevator, a medium-sized right-angle clamp, a narrow Deaver retractor, curved sounds, dilute methylene blue, a 22 F Malecot catheter, 16 F to 22 F silicone balloon catheters, bone wax, and 3-0 T-5 SAS, 3-0 PDS, 2-0 silk CE-5, and size 0 PDS.

16 *Position:* Supine with legs extended to allow a combined retropubic-perineal approach. Prepare and drape the lower abdomen and penis. Investigate the urethra from above and below with a nephroscope and cystoscope. Instill slightly diluted methylene blue intraurethrally.

Incision: Incise the skin vertically from below the umbilicus to the base of the penis, then (if desired) around the base of the penis as an inverted U.

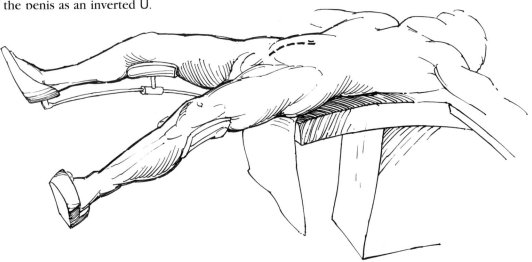

17 Separate the rectus muscles in the midline over the symphysis, and enter the prevesical space. Divide the suspensory ligament of the penis, and retract it caudally to uncover the entire anterior surface of the pubic symphysis.

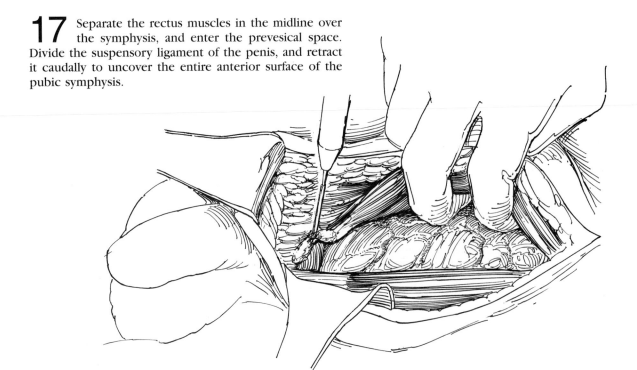

18 Open the retropubic space sharply with a knife, Mayo scissors, and periosteal elevators, and force a right-angle clamp along the undersurface of the bone. Protect the dorsal nerve plexus, artery, and vein and the prostatic plexus by keeping the instruments beneath the periosteum.

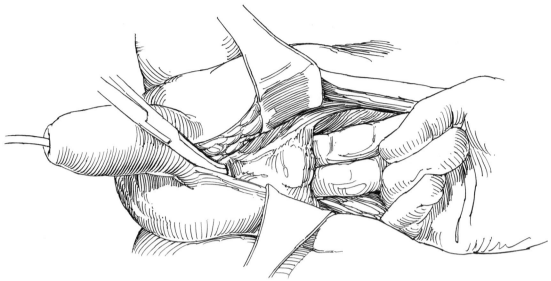

19 Separate the urogenital diaphragm from the pubic margin sharply to allow a finger to be run down the anterior wall of the membranous urethra.

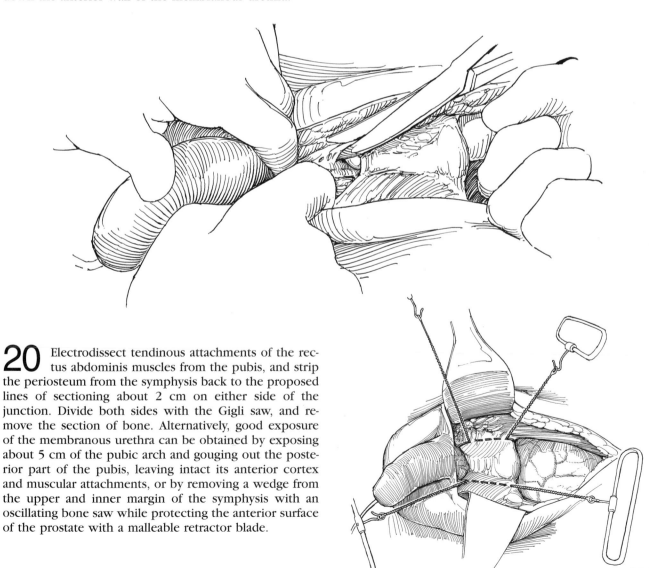

20 Electrodissect tendinous attachments of the rectus abdominis muscles from the pubis, and strip the periosteum from the symphysis back to the proposed lines of sectioning about 2 cm on either side of the junction. Divide both sides with the Gigli saw, and remove the section of bone. Alternatively, good exposure of the membranous urethra can be obtained by exposing about 5 cm of the pubic arch and gouging out the posterior part of the pubis, leaving intact its anterior cortex and muscular attachments, or by removing a wedge from the upper and inner margin of the symphysis with an oscillating bone saw while protecting the anterior surface of the prostate with a malleable retractor blade.

21 Open the bladder between stay sutures. Locate the stricture by passing a van Buren sound from below and a semicircular sound from above. Cut down on the tips of both the sounds. Excise the segment of the urethra between the tips of the sounds. Inspect the urethral lumen of both ends for deep methylene blue staining, indicating residual disease, and trim accordingly. Mobilize the urethral ends to allow them to come together without tension.

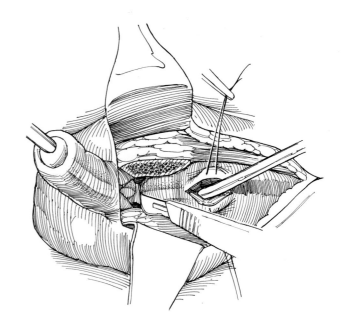

22 **A,** Place 2-0 or 3-0 SAS to approximate the posterior walls. Insert a 20 F silicone balloon catheter. **B,** Complete the anastomosis.

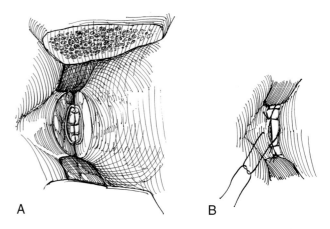

A   B

23 Draw a 24 F or 26 F Malecot catheter through the dome of the bladder and body wall and suture it to the skin with size 0 silk. Draw a Penrose drain through a stab wound at the base of the scrotum. Approximate the periosteum in the midline with two 2-0 Prolene figure-eight sutures. Close the wound in layers, taking care to simulate the suspensory ligament by suspending the penis with a row of 2-0 SAS connecting the tunica albuginea to the symphyseal periosteum.

Postoperative Problems

Incontinence is evidence that the bladder neck mechanism was compromised by the original injury. *Anastomotic stenosis* is uncommon and may respond to a single dilation or require visual urethrotomy. *Impotence* is usually already present secondary to the initial injury when the cavernous nerves lateral to the prostatomembranous urethra were disrupted. Erections can still be possible in those men who had them preoperatively if care is taken to limit dissection around the apex of the prostate to the midline. *Nerve injury* may result from compression in the groin from the extreme lithotomy position or from pressure on the peroneal nerve. *Rhabdomyolysis* can also be precipitated by this position (see page 464).

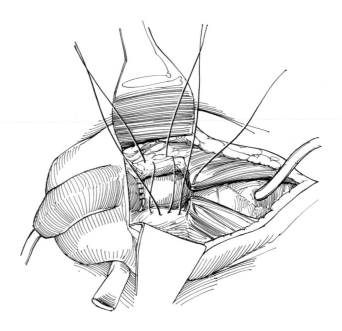

SECTION

9

Testis: Repair and Reconstruction

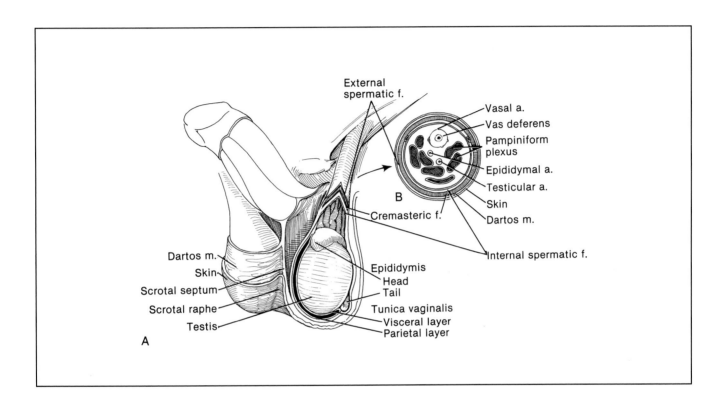

Principles of Operations on the Testis

The scrotum has two layers, a richly vascularized rugous skin and a thin nonstriated dartos muscle (dartos tunic). The three layers of fascia that form the testicular coats and covering of the cord are the external spermatic fascia, the cremasteric fascia and muscle, and the internal spermatic fascia, the last related to the transversalis fascia. The testis rests within the tunica vaginalis, the distal extension of the processus vaginalis. The spermatic cord starts at the internal inguinal ring and ends at the testis and epididymis. The external spermatic fascia is accompanied by the cremasteric nerves and vessels. The internal spermatic fascia covers the vas deferens surrounded by its vessels and lymphatics, the testicular and epididymal arteries, the pampiniform plexus, and the autonomic nerves to the testis.

The circulation approaches the testis on a stalk, permitting venous occlusion by torsion. In the parenchyma, the vessels run under the capsule both centrally and peripherally, making most of the surface unsuitable for biopsy or the placement of fixation stitches.

Related to orchiopexy, the arterial vessel to each testis arises from the anterolateral surface of the aorta just below the renal artery. As the testicular artery approaches the upper end of the testis, it divides into two tortuous main branches—an outer branch, the internal testicular artery, and an inner branch, the inferior testicular artery.

The tail of the epididymis is vascularized by a complex arrangement of vessels involving the epididymal, vasal, and testicular arteries, with supplementation from the cremasteric artery. This system provides an extensive anastomotic loop among these vessels that is important when the testicular artery must be divided to achieve scrotal placement of the testis.

The vasal artery branches to join the posterior epididymal arteries to form an epididymal-deferential loop. After ligation of the testicular artery during orchiopexy, the testis becomes dependent on the anastomosis of this loop with the terminal part or distal branches of the testicular artery, a connection that may or may not be adequate to support the testis.

Testis Biopsy

Testis biopsy can be done as an outpatient procedure. Local anesthesia is adequate for adolescents and adults if supplemented with analgesics such as midazolam or diazepam. The drawback of local infiltration is possible injury to the spermatic vessels. An alternative is to introduce a Biopty gun with a 17-mm sampling notch percutaneously to obtain one or two cores (Rajfer and Binder, 1989).

1 Because of the intragonadal distribution of the arteries in the tunica vasculosa, the biopsy should be taken from either the medial or the lateral aspect of the superior pole where the vascularity is sparse, not from the well-vascularized anterior surface (Jarow, 1990).

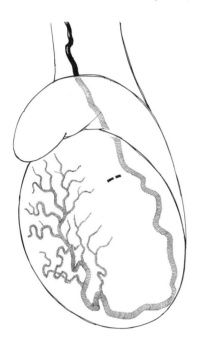

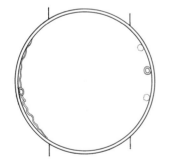

2 Stand to the left. Block the spermatic cord by pulling the testis down to relax the cremaster muscle. Grasp the cord with the left hand and place the thumb in front and the index finger behind the cord at the top of the scrotum. With the needle approaching the index finger, infiltrate both the anterolateral and anteromedial sides of the cord as it emerges from the external ring near the pubic tubercle with 1 percent lidocaine solution without epinephrine through a 2.5-inch, 25-gauge needle. Avoid injecting near the vas for fear of puncturing it. Grasp the testis in the left hand and squeeze it against the scrotal skin, being certain that the epididymis is held posteriorly out of the way. Infiltrate the skin and dartos layer with 1 percent lidocaine. Do not inject the tunica albuginea. Do not relax your grip on the testis.

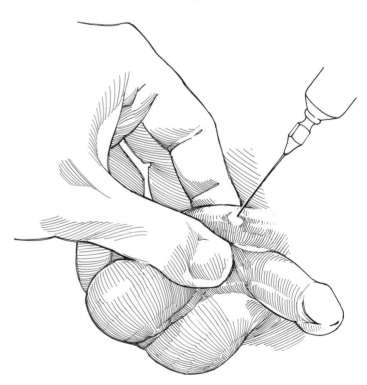

3 **A,** Incise transversely through the skin, dartos, and tunica vaginalis to follow the vasculature of the scrotum; these layers retract as the scrotum is squeezed around the testis. Place a hemostat on each side of the tunica vaginalis for exposure, but maintain a firm grip on the scrotum to hold the site in position. Manipulate the testis so that the least vascular area, either the upper medial or lateral aspect of the upper pole, is exposed. Drip 2 to 3 ml of lidocaine on the tunica albuginea and wait 30 seconds.

Alternative: Place a stay suture of 4-0 chromic catgut (CCG) in the tunica albuginea to stabilize the testis in the window; however, this causes pain and is not necessary if the testis is kept stable digitally. Incise the tunica albuginea transversely, the direction taken by the small underlying vessels. Do it sharply (and quickly, because this is the painful part of the procedure) with a #15 blade for a distance of 4 or 5 mm, to allow extrusion of a bead-sized portion of the testicular tubules. Apply pressure on the testis to promote extrusion.

B, Excise the extruded tubules with moistened small curved iris scissors, and submerge the specimen on the scissors directly in Bouin's, Zenker's, or buffered glutaraldehyde solution (not in formalin) with a no-touch technique. If desired, make a direct touch specimen on a sterile slide, have cytofixative applied to it, and have it examined for spermatozoa. Maintain your grip on the testis within the scrotum.

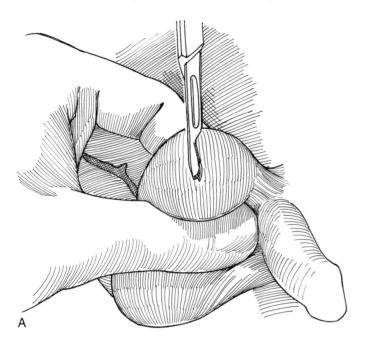

A

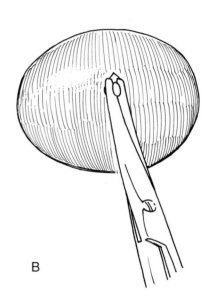

B

4 Close the tunica albuginea with one or two sutures of 4-0 CCG swaged on a needle. Observe for hemostasis, and add more sutures if necessary. Release your grasp on the testis when hemostasis is obtained. The tunica vaginalis may be closed with a mattress suture. Placing 0.25 percent bupivacaine hydrochloride (Marcaine) inside the tunic creates a Marcaine hydrocele and reduces postoperative pain.

5 Approximate the skin, together with the dartos layer, with several stitches of 4-0 plain catgut. Repeat the procedure on the other side if indicated. Apply a nonadherent dressing and a large padded scrotal suspensory.

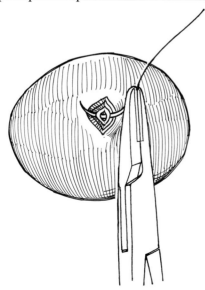

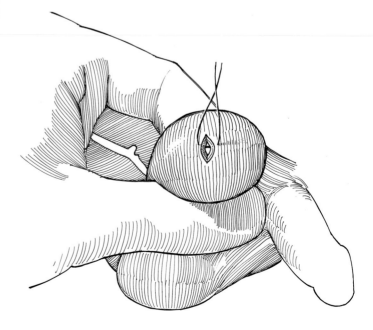

POSTOPERATIVE PROBLEMS

A *hematocele* can appear if the tunica albuginea is not closed over a subtunical vessel.

GONADAL BIOPSY FOR INTERSEXES

True hermaphrodite: Expect any combination of ovary, testis, and ovotestis, the last being most common. Look for ovotestes retroperitoneally, although half of them are found in the labioscrotal fold or the inguinal canal. Ovaries are usually in the normal retroperitoneal position.

Gonadal dysgenesis: Streak gonads of ovarian stroma lie in the normal position. With XX or Turner's type, malignancy is rare and excision is not needed. However, with the XY type the chance of future malignancy is high (30 percent); immediate gonadectomy is required.

Perform laparoscopic exploration to locate the gonad. Expose it through a labioscrotal or an inguinal incision. In hermaphroditism, take a deep biopsy of the organ because testicular tissue may exist only near the hilum, and take the sample longitudinally because the components are oriented end to end. For gonadal dysgenesis, excise the entire gonad.

Commentary by R. Dale McClure

Testicular biopsy is used primarily in the diagnostic evaluation of the azoospermic male with normal gonadotropin levels (luteinizing hormone [LH] and follicle-stimulating hormone [FSH]) to differentiate between testicular failure and post-testicular (obstructive) causes of infertility. In an azoospermic individual with low semen volume, retrograde ejaculation should be eliminated by postejaculatory urinalysis. If no sperm are found in the urine and the patient has a palpable vas, ejaculatory duct obstruction should be ruled out by rectal ultrasonography.

Biopsy is not indicated in an azoospermic individual with small testes (less than 15 cc) with a serum FSH level of twice the upper limit of normal. These individuals have primary testicular failure, for which currently there is no effective therapy.

Usually I do a unilateral biopsy, unless history or physical examination suggests asymmetric testicular pathology (e.g., unilateral testicular atrophy with contralateral ductal obstruction). In an era of intracytoplasmic sperm injection (ICSI), by which testicular sperm are obtained from a biopsy specimen, planning the biopsy sites is important, as repeated procedures may be required.

In individuals who may require future microsurgical reconstructive surgery, the testicular biopsy should be done using minimal dissection (window technique), as described previously. Vasography is not carried out at this procedure because of the potential to cause additional scarring. That radiologic procedure should be carried out at the time of definitive surgical reconstruction.

Recently percutaneous needle testicular biopsy has become available. This may be performed in the physician's office under local anesthesia. Prior to biopsy, the scrotal skin must be punctured with a scalpel. In this technique, one must stabilize the testis and secure the epididymis posteriorly. The potential disadvantage of this technique is the inadvertent and unrecognized injury to a testicular blood vessel or epididymis. Other limitations include the small sample volume and distortion of seminiferous tubule histology.

Although bleeding is the most common complication of testicular biopsy, the most serious problem is the inadvertent biopsy of the epididymis. Finally, the use of improper fixatives or crushing of the tissue may create difficulties for the pathologist reading the histology.

Inguinal Orchiopexy

After the presence of retractile testes has been ruled out by careful examination and hormonal therapy has been considered, orchiopexy is still the most effective treatment for cryptorchidism. Because many studies have shown that damage to the germ cells begins very early, at least before the end of the second year, treatment for true cryptorchidism must be done before irreversible changes occur.

Operations on infants may require magnification and special technique, especially if the testis lies high. Whether the testis is worth the effort of positioning is a matter of the surgeon's judgment. Further, the need for other than standard orchiopexy must be recognized before the testis is dissected from its bed because the option for long-loop vas orchiopexy will be lost.

The inguinal region in infants differs somewhat from that in adults, and these differences are important for surgery at this age. The superficial fascia is much thicker, resembling the aponeurosis of the external oblique, which in turn is relatively thin, with delicate medial and lateral crura. The inguinal canal runs more transversely and the cremaster is very well developed, with fibers that blend with those of the internal oblique. Before the age of 2 years, the bladder extends well into the abdomen and can be injured during medial exposure of the spermatic cord.

If the testis is not palpable, perform laparoscopy and consider proceeding with laparoscopic orchiopexy (see page 331). Or use an abdominal approach (see pages 326 to 329) or resort to a Fowler-Stephens orchiopexy (see pages 318 to 320), staged orchiopexy (see pages 321 to 322), or microvascular orchiopexy (see pages 323 to 324).

Determine serum testosterone level at 6 weeks of age. If it is low, consider early endocrine therapy. Before 2 years of age, a trial of luteinizing hormone–releasing hormone (LHRH) or human chorionic gonadotropin (hCG) may be advisable. In unilateral cases, if descent has not occurred by age 2 years, perform an orchiopexy. Perform laparoscopic exploration if the testis is not apparent to rule out anorchia. For bilateral cases, repair both sides at the same operation unless the testes are very high; repairing one side at a time is then wiser. Obtain consent from the parents for orchiectomy in case the testis proves to be not worth salvaging, and have a prosthesis of suitable size available. In boys with abnormal chromosomes or abnormal genitalia, take a testicular biopsy because of the possibility of intratubular germ cell neoplasia (Cortes et al, 1994).

Orchiopexy is usually done on an outpatient basis.

Instruments: Provide a three-power loupe (an operating microscope is probably not useful), a biopsy tray, a genitourinary (GU) fine set, a plastic set, fine Allis clamps, extra mosquito clamps, hand-held bipolar electrocautery with needle tip, two small DeBakey forceps, and a 0.25-inch vessel loop.

1 Use general anesthesia. Supplement it with either a local block (see page 76) or a caudal block to reduce the amount of inhalation anesthetic required and to diminish postoperative pain.

Position: Place the child supine with the knees bent and with the soles of the feet approximated to separate the upper legs. Prepare and drape widely in case abdominal exploration is required.

Incision: Make a 3.5- to 4.5-cm semitransverse incision in the natural skin crease, extending from the edge of the rectus muscle to a point medial to the anterior superior iliac spine. Consider making it slightly higher if the testis is not palpable. Divide and ligate the superficial circumflex iliac and superficial inferior epigastric vessels.

Pick up and divide Camper's and Scarpa's fascias with scissors to expose the external oblique fascia laterally as far as the inguinal ligament, and expose it inferiorly as well to reveal the external inguinal ring. Retract the ilioinguinal nerve medially. Place fine curved clamps on the edges of the superficial fascia to maintain exposure. Take care not to injure a testis lying in the superficial inguinal pouch, which must be freed before proceeding; these testes require minimal dissection of the cord. Push the protruding processus vaginalis down to define the external ring. Compression of the abdomen may cause the testis to extrude from the ring, simplifying the dissection.

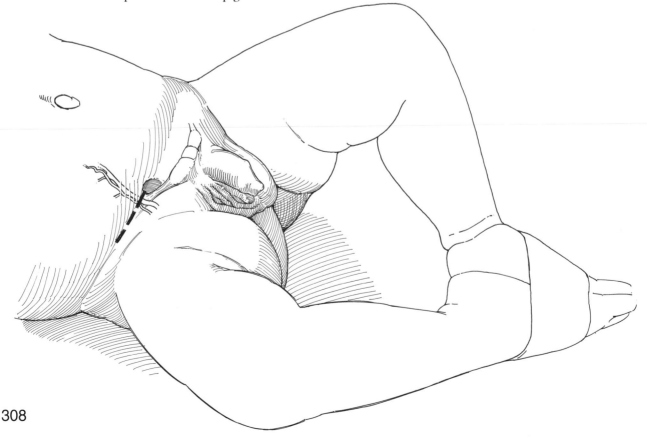

2 Sharply incise the external oblique fascia from above downward between the fibers that terminate at the external ring. Use a knife or scissors. Avoid injury to the underlying ilioinguinal nerve with its medial and lateral branches. Free the fascia from the conjoined muscle and cremasteric fibers beneath it; then look for the ilioingui- nal nerve and free it from the fascia. Divide the internal oblique muscle with the scissors or a cutting current to open the floor. Insert the index finger and move it up and down to clear the space. Mosquito clamps placed on the fascia help with exposure.

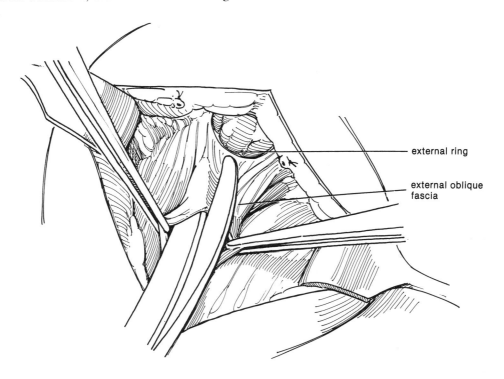

external ring

external oblique
fascia

3 Identify the testis within the tunica vaginalis. In infants, use loupes and work with inverted forceps so that hands do not obstruct vision. Open the processus vaginalis before doing any dissection of the cremaster or around the cord. Do not mobilize the tunica vaginalis until you are sure you do not need the distal collateral blood supply for a Fowler-Stephens orchiopexy. Put trac- tion on the testis, and check to be sure that the artery is long enough. If it is not, and there is a looping vas, decide at this point to do a long-loop vas orchiopexy (see pages 318 to 320). With the aid of an assistant, pick up the overlying cremasteric fibers on either side with fine smooth forceps, and sharply and bluntly peel them down and off close to the tunic to be able to locate the commu- nicating processus. It is important to completely transect the cremaster muscle fibers.

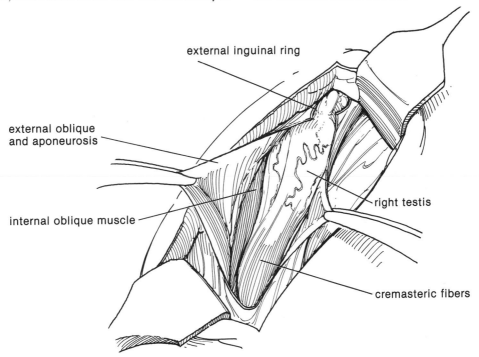

external inguinal ring

external oblique
and aponeurosis

internal oblique muscle

right testis

cremasteric fibers

4 Open the tunica vaginalis anteriorly and incise it proximally to the base of the cord. Resect the appendix testis and appendix epididymis, and superficially fulgurate the pedicles for hemostasis.

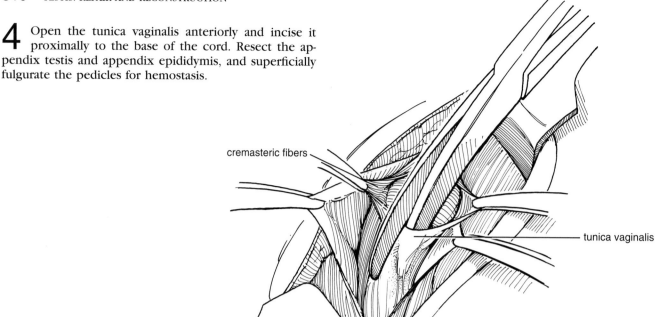

cremasteric fibers

tunica vaginalis

5 Once it is apparent that the cord will become long enough, grasp the edges of the peritoneal lining (tunica vaginalis) near the internal ring with fine forceps and insinuate fine scissors or a small straight hemostat between the lining of the hernia canal and the vessels and vas. The tunica vaginalis may appear to surround the cord. It is easiest to separate it from the vessels and vas just below the internal ring, dissecting alternately from the medial and lateral sides. Injection of saline in this plane may help the separation. Divide the delicate free edges of the sac and hold them in a series of mosquito clamps as the separation progresses. Divide the posterior and lateral connections of the internal spermatic (transversalis) fascia to the tunic.

6 Complete the division of the sac. Hold it by its edges with mosquito clamps and close the peritoneal opening with a 4-0 silk purse-string suture. With the usual small hernia sac, suture-ligation is enough. It may be preferable to postpone this step. If you do it now, the subsequent retraction needed to expose the retroperitoneal dissection frequently tears out the closure, so it may be better to close it after upward mobilization has been completed. If the peritoneum is torn, oversew the opening into the peritoneal cavity with a fine continuous absorbable suture. Be certain to get good separation of the cord structures from the peritoneum just above the internal ring during high ligation of the hernia sac.

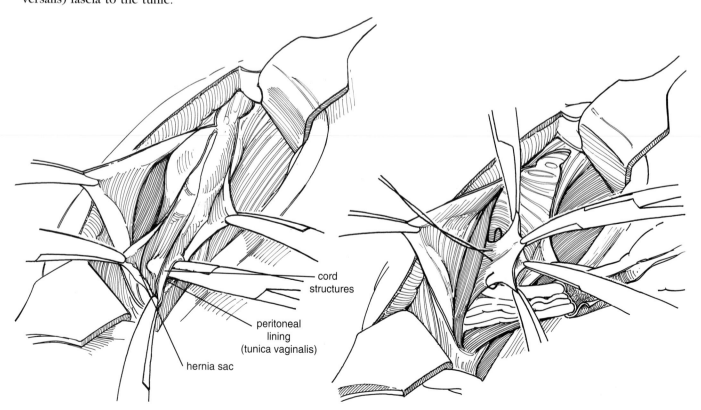

cord structures

peritoneal lining (tunica vaginalis)

hernia sac

7 Inspect the testis for size and anomalies. Gauge the length of the cord by pulling the testis over the symphysis. It is usually necessary to lengthen the cord. To do this, meticulously free the remainder of the tunica vaginalis and cremasteric fibers from the cord, working near the internal ring. Again, saline injected beneath the tunic may aid the dissection. Take care not to cut the deranged cord or splayed-out epididymis.

Caution: Avoid using the electrocautery unless the testis is well grounded; otherwise, the current runs up the relatively narrow cord and destroys the blood supply to the testis.

Place traction on the testis, and divide the cremasteric and spermatic fibers that are still attached to the cord. Continue this dissection retroperitoneally. Divide all the lateral spermatic fascia to allow the cord to be moved medially.

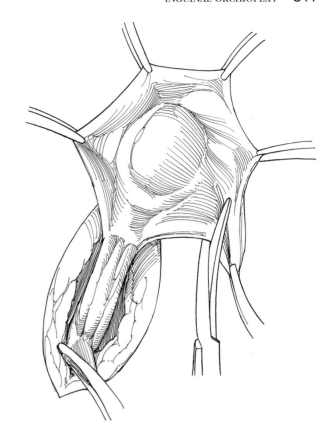

8 Locate and divide the inferior epigastric artery and vein(s) separately. Alternatively, tunnel under them. Open the associated transversalis fascial layer. Upward retraction usually provides adequate exposure of the cord after the transversalis fascia is divided, but, if necessary, open the internal ring by dividing the internal oblique muscles and more of the lateral spermatic fascia. Free the cord well retroperitoneally, using a peanut dissector to mobilize it medially, up toward the lower pole of the kidney if necessary. To avoid atrophy, dissect among the vessels, vas, and cord structures as little as possible, particularly in infants. Perform a biopsy of the testis by taking a thin wedge from the relatively avascular area on either side of the upper pole opposite the epididymis, and carry it at once on the knife without manipulation into Bouin's solution. Close the defect with one or two fine sutures. A running suture re-establishes the body-testis barrier.

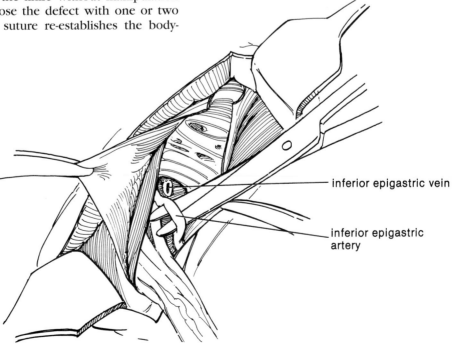

inferior epigastric vein

inferior epigastric artery

9 If the testis is at the internal ring or above, the inguinal incision can be lengthened. Elevate the skin at the upper end, and open the lateral aspect of the internal ring by dividing the lateral spermatic (transversalis) fascia with the scissors or cutting current at its point of continuity with the internal spermatic fascia. Place narrow Deaver retractors and, with a Küttner dissector, develop the retroperitoneal space. Then incise the external oblique fascia in the line of the incision, and split the internal oblique and transversalis fascias. If the testis has not been located, look for the vas or spermatic vessels adherent to the peritoneum under the subserosal fascia and trace the vas to its proximal end, either to a testis or to a blind ending. If the cord, after thorough dissection and transposition, is still too short, consider a two-stage procedure (see pages 321 to 322) or a microvascular orchiopexy (see pages 323 to 324). A long-loop vas orchiopexy is no longer an option. If orchiectomy is done because of the poor quality of the testis, consider insertion of a small prosthesis, which can be changed for a larger size at puberty. At this time, the safety of silicone prostheses has been questioned, but because no better alternatives are available, a reasonable course to follow is to advise the parents of the minimal risk and obtain informed consent. Close the neck of the scrotum behind the prosthesis.

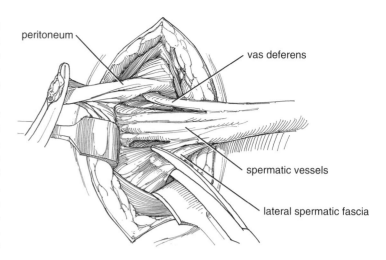

10 **A,** Pass the index finger along the usual course of descent of the testis into the scrotum until it reaches the "third inguinal ring," formed by the nondescent of the dartos fascia. Make a 2-cm incision with the scalpel through the scrotal skin, leaving the ring intact. **B,** Develop a pocket for the testis from below by bluntly freeing the skin from the dartos fascia with the back of the knife or with a mosquito clamp for a depth of 1 to 2 cm. **C,** Make a small opening in the dartos fascia tensioned over the finger, and grasp the edges with small Allis clamps or place four stay sutures.

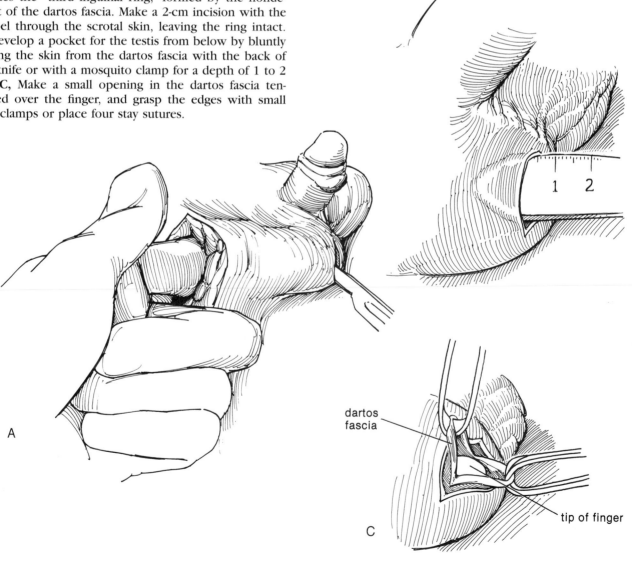

11 Pass a clamp from below. Hold the tip against the index finger as it is withdrawn upward. Grasp the cut edge of the tunica vaginalis in the clamp. Draw the testis out through the scrotal opening, taking care not to rotate the cord.

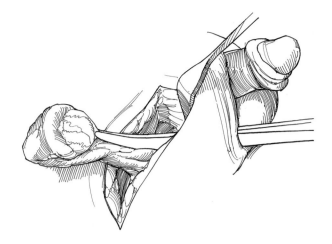

12 **A,** Close the dartos fascia behind the testis with a 4-0 synthetic absorbable suture (SAS) at each end, catching a little of the paratesticular tissue in the bite. If dartos sutures were preplaced, secure them to the paratesticular tissue. **B,** Manipulate the testis into the subcutaneous pouch. If the testis seems to retract, consider placing a fine suture in the gubernaculum or in an avascular area of the tunica albuginea near the upper pole (see page 305), bringing it through the skin and tying it over a peanut sponge, to be removed in 1 week. Close the skin with 5-0 plain catgut subcutaneous interrupted sutures and seal the wound with collodion. Any tension is an indication that the dissection should have been carried higher.

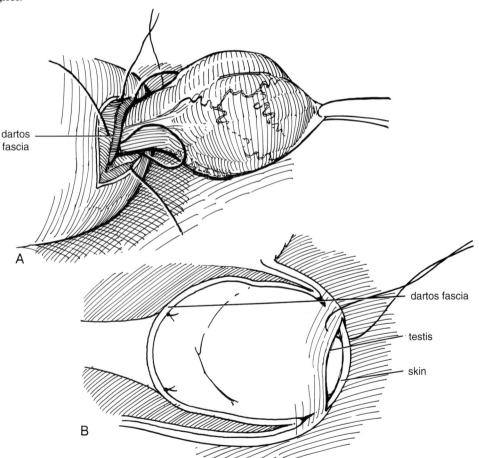

dartos fascia

dartos fascia

testis

skin

A

B

13 **A,** Reapproximate the transversalis fascia over the cord, displacing the internal ring downward. **B,** Suture the internal oblique muscle to the shelving edge of the inguinal ligament over the cord with 3-0 or 4-0 SAS.

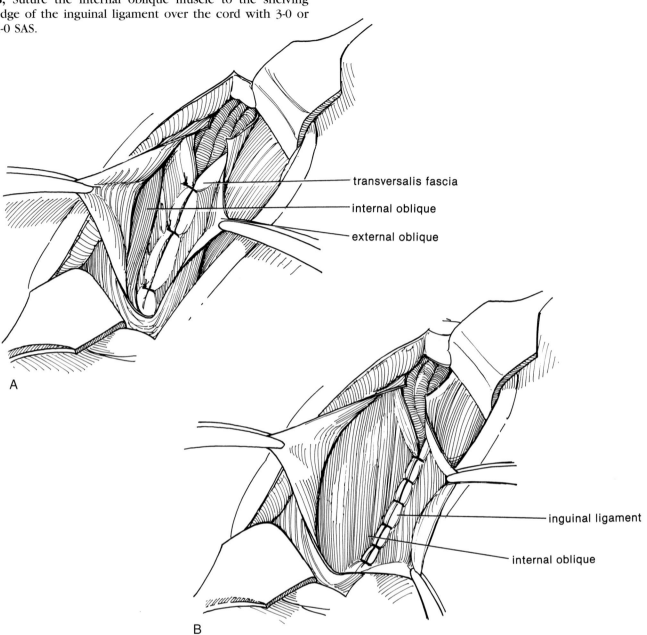

transversalis fascia

internal oblique

external oblique

A

inguinal ligament

internal oblique

B

14 **A,** Alternatively, because hernias rarely develop in children, the internal oblique muscle may simply be approximated with interrupted sutures. **B,** Close the external oblique aponeurosis with interrupted sutures from above downward to create a new external ring, but do not make the ring too tight. Loosely reapproximate Scarpa's fascia and close the skin with a running 4-0 or 5-0 SAS placed subcuticularly, sealed with flexible collodion. Instill 0.25 ml/kg of a 0.25 percent bupivacaine solution into the wound before closure to reduce pain. Perform a caudal block if it was not done at the beginning of the procedure.

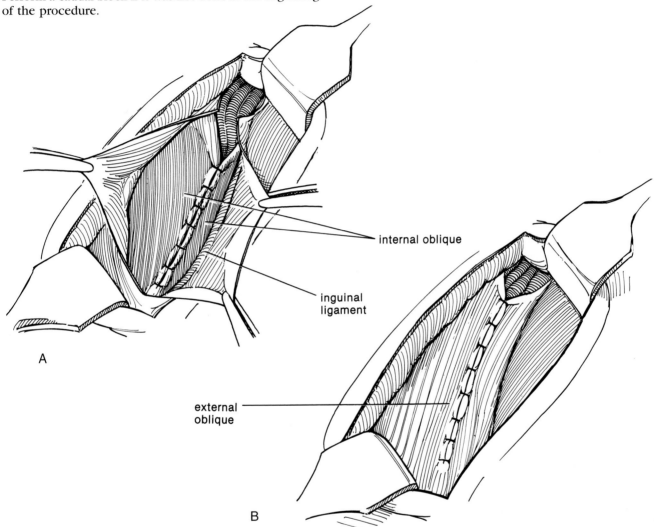

internal oblique

inguinal ligament

A

external oblique

B

POSTOPERATIVE PROBLEMS

Inadequate testis position has an incidence as high as 10 percent because of incomplete retroperitoneal dissection. It can usually be corrected in a second operation. *Retraction* of the testis after operation occurs in a small percentage of cases.

Apparent atrophy is from the preoperative size of the testis relative to age, but the most feared complication is *devascularization of the testis* during dissection of the cord, a complication that must be avoided by the use of loupes or microscope, fine instruments, and sequential dissection. *Ischemia* can be produced by a traction suture engaging a vessel in the lower pole, exacerbated by rubber band traction. Orchiectomy for an atrophic testis may be indicated at a later time for fear of cancer, at which time a prosthesis can be inserted.

Accidental division of the vas is possible. Immediate or postpubertal microvascular repair often corrects the problem.

This complication occurs more frequently in a nonpalpable case. *Epididymo-orchitis* can occur and is treated with antibiotics. *Postoperative scrotal swelling,* however, usually indicates edema rather than hematoma or infection. Progressive scrotal enlargement suggests uncontrolled bleeding and warrants exploration. Needle aspiration is seldom diagnostic and, if the swelling is due to bowel herniating through the peritoneal defect, may be harmful.

A *hydrocele* may form later from excess remnants of the tunica vaginalis. If small it can be ignored; if large it requires trans-scrotal repair (see pages 349 to 351). *Testicular extrusion* from ischemia of the scrotal skin is uncommon but may occur if the area has been electrocoagulated or if rubber band traction has been used, an unnecessary and potentially harmful practice because it can also cause testicular atrophy. *Bladder injury* has been reported from ligation of the hernia sac that includes a portion of the bladder.

Commentary by David T. Mininberg

The description provides an excellent guide to orchiopexy. We use essentially the same techniques in our practice, with a few variations. We prefer to operate on these boys close to their first birthday. All caveats concerning gentle handling of the tissues with fine instruments need to be reiterated. Magnification can be helpful, but we have not found the operating microscope useful. In the special situation of the impalpable testis, the initial step should be diagnostic laparoscopy to rule out monorchia. If an intra-abdominal testis is found, the orchiopexy should be carried out laparoscopically. If the testis is not

salvageable, a laparoscopic orchiectomy is the alternative. We have found the following two maneuvers helpful and satisfying. The empty flattened hemiscrotum is readily dilated by passing a 12 F Foley catheter with the tip cut off into the scrotum from the inguinal incision, inflating the balloon and allowing it to dilate the hemiscrotum for 5 minutes. The catheter can be grasped with a clamp to allow it to be guided easily into the inguinal canal, leading the testis down after deflation of the balloon. Where the inferior epigastric artery and/or vein impedes descent, it can be tunneled under rather than sacrificed.

REPEAT ORCHIOPEXY
(Cartwright-Snyder)

Review the previous operative report and caution the family about the possibility of orchiectomy and also about the indications for and contraindications to a prosthesis.

15 Re-enter the previous incision, extending it slightly at each end. The testis is probably found near the external inguinal ring and the pubic tubercle. Bluntly dissect the fatty subcutaneous tissue that lies over the cord structures to expose the lower pole of the testis. Place a suture in the scar tissue in the middle of the testis. With traction, dissect on both sides behind the testis with a right-angle clamp and scissors. Dissection along the floor on the transversalis fascia can be initiated bluntly; isolate and divide the medial and lateral attachments sharply. As the dissection of the cord reaches the level of the external ring, preserve a plate of external oblique fascia that adheres to the cord structures by incising the fascia on either side. Expose the fibers of the internal oblique muscle and safely transect the external oblique fascia by connecting these lateral incisions, leaving a protective strip of fascia 1 to 2 cm wide attached to the cord. At the level of the internal ring, open the internal oblique fibers and identify the vas deferens, the spermatic vessels, and the previously ligated sac. With traction on the testis, expose the anterior aspect of the

peritoneum. Open it away from the vessels and dissect, usually in fresh tissue planes, under the posterior peritoneum behind the vas deferens and spermatic vessels, as is done for an initial orchiopexy. Gather the peritoneal edges in a clamp. With the aid of Deaver retractors, dissect retroperitoneally by dividing attachments to the endopelvic fascia until enough length is obtained. Division of the lateral spermatic fascia and the inferior epigastric vessels may also be needed. Suture the peritoneal opening closed at a high level. Place the testis in a dartos pouch, or hold it with a button on the skin if scarring is excessive. Place two or three sutures from the transversalis fascia to the inguinal ligament to reconstruct the floor of the canal, thus forming a new internal ring next to the pubic tubercle, at the same time protecting the vessels and the vas. Close the internal oblique musculature with mattress sutures, and suture the external oblique muscle together. Instill 0.25 ml/kg of a 0.25 percent bupivacaine solution into the wound before closure to reduce pain. Perform a caudal block if it was not done at the beginning of the procedure.

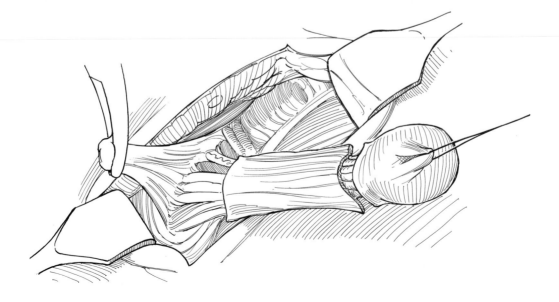

Commentary by Howard M. Snyder, III

The approach I developed is intended to avoid jeopardizing the vas and vessels, as they often lie adherent to the undersurface of the external oblique fascia. Accordingly, the dissection is carried in the subcutaneous fat distally until the testis can be elevated. Dissection is then carried back up parallel to the cord structures to the pubic tubercle. At the pubic tubercle, a strip of the fascia of the external oblique is outlined and incised medially and laterally to the adherent vas and vessels beneath. This helps to protect them. Posteriorly, the plane of dissection is usually easier on the transversalis fascia, the floor of the inguinal canal. If there is adherence posteriorly, the transversalis fascia is taken en bloc with the vas and vessels. The dissection is carried laterally with the strip of external oblique fascia until the internal oblique musculature is seen lateral to the internal ring. At that point, the incisions of the external oblique fascia are joined and the peritoneum is exposed. We try to open the peritoneum above where the processus vaginalis was tied off. This step enables the peritoneum to be separated from the vas and vessels in the retroperitoneum in a free plane where previous dissection has not taken place. At this point, the block of tissue adherent to vas and vessels is completely mobilized; if any further length of the vas and vessels is needed to achieve a good scrotal position for the testis, a retroperitoneal mobilization similar to what is done in a standard orchiopexy is carried upward until the testis can be placed adequately in the scrotum.

INSERTION OF TESTICULAR PROSTHESIS

Be certain that the parents or the patient, if he is an adult, understands the possible complications from silicone prostheses. Make a transverse inguinal or an oblique inguinoscrotal incision. If implantation is to be bilateral, place two incisions. With the index finger, stretch the scrotal sac vigorously, taking care not to tear it. Select a prosthesis a little larger than normal for the size of the child; it can be replaced with a larger size later. (Most hospitals require that a prosthesis be discarded if it has been placed into the wound because it cannot be resterilized.) Invert the scrotum into the incision, and suture the tab on the gel-filled prosthesis to the inverted scrotal wall with a 3-0 SAS. Place a purse-string suture to close the scrotal neck, taking care not to pierce the capsule of the prosthesis with the needle. It probably is not necessary either to suture the tab (just trim it off) or to place the purse-string suture.

Complications

Infection requires removal of the prosthesis. *Necrosis* of the stretched skin over the prosthesis can occur and should have been prevented by placement of a smaller prosthesis. *Scrotal hematoma* formation is rare.

Orchiopexy with Vascular Division

(Fowler-Stephens)

For the testis with a vascular cord too short to allow placement in the scrotum, this procedure uses the secondary vascular loop accompanying the congenitally long vas. The main trunk and the internal spermatic artery anastomose with the vasal artery near the lower pole of the testis and close to the hilum. From this junction a single artery bypasses the hilum, penetrates the tunica albuginea at the lower pole of the testis, and usually divides into two branches in the tunica vasculosa. In the Fowler-Stephens procedure, the internal spermatic vessels are divided and the blood supply of the testis becomes reliant on the vasal vessels and on some small branches that track across the loop to join with twigs arising from the internal spermatic vessels. It is essential to take a broad tongue of attached peritoneum along with the testis and the vas down to the scrotum. This pedicled flap furnishes essential collateral circulation to the testis.

The testis that is detected at the external ring or in the inguinal canal with a long-loop vas emerging from the external ring is ideally suited for this operation. A testis situated higher in the abdomen with the usual short vas is better suited for other orchiopexy techniques. Do not overestimate the potential value of the particular testis. Some are so poorly developed that they are best removed. A small testis found on follow-up may not be due to mismanagement of the vascular pedicle.

A first stage for vessel ligation is needed only if the testis or the loop of the vas deferens cannot be located by clinical examination. Through a short abdominal incision, the spermatic vessels and testis are identified and the vessels ligated as high as possible. Ligation may be more readily done by laparoscopic techniques (see page 333), which not only can determine the presence and location of the testis and the presence and course of the vas deferens but also allows clipping of the spermatic vessels.

1 Make an incision in the inguinal crease. Identify the special anatomic circumstances applicable to the use of this technique. Plan ahead; do not mobilize the posterior wall of the hernia sac proximal to the testis and epididymis nor disturb the floor of the inguinal canal or the epigastric vessels. Expose the processus vaginalis as for a standard orchiopexy. Dilate the internal inguinal ring or, if necessary for greater retroperitoneal exposure, incise the internal oblique muscle. Three-power loupes can be helpful. Do not dissect behind the processus or the hernia sac.

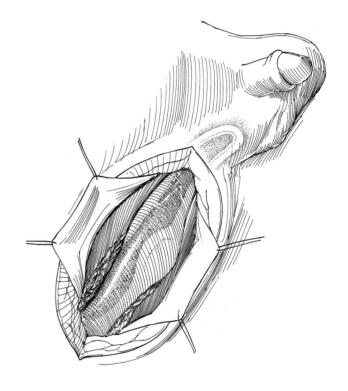

2 Open the hernia sac, identify the epididymis, and note the course of the vas with its several vascular arcades looping down the posteromedial wall of the sac below the testis. Place a traction suture superficially in the capsule of the testis; exert traction to determine if the testis has a long mesentery and can be brought into the scrotum by standard methods or a short one that requires division of the spermatic vessels. Dissect the sac well up inside the internal ring to the point where the vas turns medially, at the same time allowing the peritoneum lying more distally to remain attached medially and posteriorly to the vas. Inject saline under the peritoneum, then transect the processus (see page 310) and close it with a 4-0 purse-string nonabsorbable suture (NAS). Carefully separate the testicular vessels from the vessel to the vas and its accompanying vessels where they converge on the internal inguinal ring. If the spermatic artery was not clipped at a first stage, test the collateral circulation by placing a small bulldog clamp high on the vascular pedicle, well above the testis; then make a 3-mm longitudinal incision in the testis between the faintly visible vessels of the tunica albuginea and watch for brisk bleeding. Collateral circulation is adequate if bleeding persists for 5 minutes. In the meantime, transilluminate the cord structures. First identify the vascular anastomotic arcades between the vas and the spermatic vessels alongside the testis and epididymis. These are best seen through the back wall of the hernia sac, a view enhanced by the presence of venae comitantes. These arcades contribute to the blood supply, so divide only the arcade (or arcades) necessary to enable the loop of the vas to be straightened out and the testis to be placed in the scrotum without tension. Before dividing a major arcade, gently occlude the vessel and note whether bleeding from the tunic is impeded. Continued bleeding indicates that it is safe to divide the arcade, whereas arrest indicates a nonexpendable vessel.

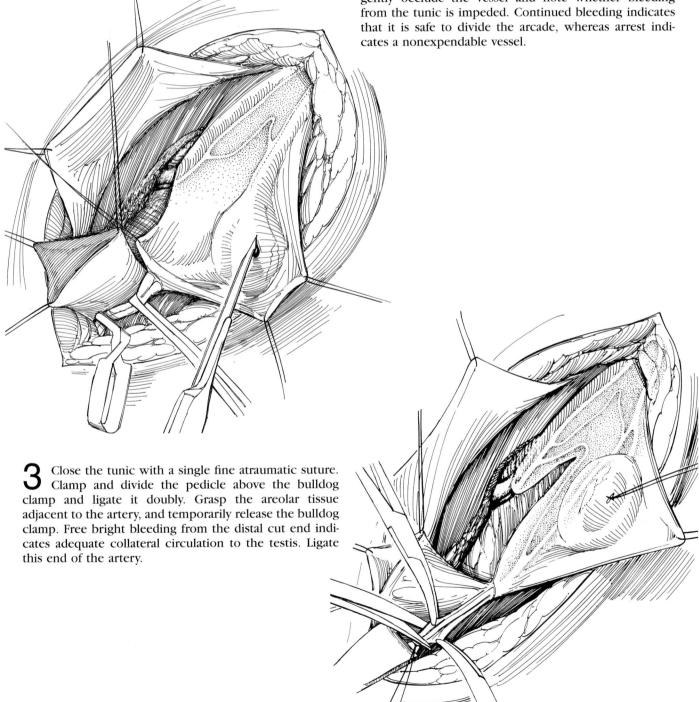

3 Close the tunic with a single fine atraumatic suture. Clamp and divide the pedicle above the bulldog clamp and ligate it doubly. Grasp the areolar tissue adjacent to the artery, and temporarily release the bulldog clamp. Free bright bleeding from the distal cut end indicates adequate collateral circulation to the testis. Ligate this end of the artery.

4 Turn the testis caudally into the scrotum. Continue as for a standard orchiopexy.

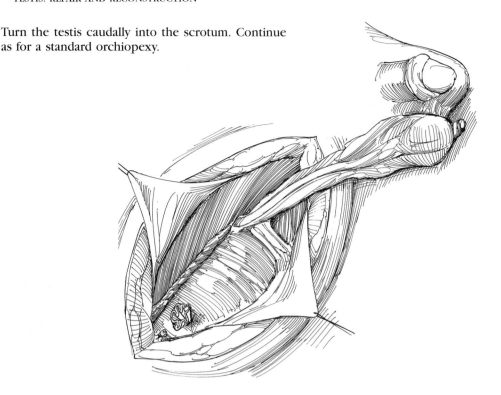

POSTOPERATIVE PROBLEMS

Testicular atrophy is the major complication. This may result from failure to incorporate an adequate strip of peritoneum medially to and accompanying the vas with loss of collaterals, from injuring the vasal artery, or from ligation of the spermatic vessels too close to the testis so that the arcades cannot function. The variable pattern of the blood supply contributes to the problem. Injury to the vas or the testis is also possible.

Commentary by F. Douglas Stephens

Division of part of the blood supply to the undescended testis can allow placement in the scrotum, but an understanding of the testicular vasculature is important. The testicular artery is the small trunk formed by the junction of the internal spermatic and vasal arteries. It arises near the hilum of the testis but does not divide and radiate from the hilum in the parenchyma in the manner of the renal vessels. Instead, it tracks under the lower pole in the tunica vasculosa beneath the tunica albuginea. It usually divides into two branches that course over the summit toward the upper pole, giving off end-artery twigs that dip into the septal compartments. Sometimes these two main branches can be identified because of the accompanying venae comitantes visible through the tunica albuginea. To avoid infarction of septal compartments during the bleeding test, incise into the vasculosa layer by a longitudinal incision of the albuginea only toward the upper pole and between the main branches, and use very fine atraumatic sutures to approximate the cut edges of the tunica albuginea, thus arresting the bleeding without incurring further infarctions.

This technique of orchiopexy is not recommended if the spermatic cord and vas deferens have been dissected or skeletonized in a failed attempt to bring the testis down into the scrotum. Hence, on recognition of the long-loop vas, conduct the operation in the stages outlined herein.

If bleeding stops almost immediately after the bleeding test incision is made, the anastomosis between the internal spermatic vessels and the artery of the vas is inadequate. Microvascular anastomoses of the inferior epigastric to the internal spermatic vessels should be considered as the means by which the viability of the testis can be maintained after division of the internal spermatic vessels.

The anatomy of the blood vessels both outside and inside the tunica albuginea governs the steps in the operation that entail the division of the internal spermatic vessels.

Blood vessels outside the tunica albuginea: The testicular artery anastomoses by one or several terminal branches with the vasal artery near the lower pole of the testis and close to the hilum. A single artery arises from the junction of these vessels, bypasses the hilum, and penetrates the tunica albuginea at the lower pole of the testis.

Blood vessels inside the tunica albuginea: Immediately beneath the tunica, the testicular artery commonly divides into two separate branches that course longitudinally toward the upper pole, giving off end-arteries that dip into and supply the tubules in the individual septa of the testis. Sometimes the vessel remains single, and sometimes the two branches at first run close together. These vessels are accompanied by veins that can be seen, if carefully scrutinized, as blue streaks under the tunic.

Precautions to preserve the blood supply to the testis: Transect the internal spermatic vascular bundle cranial to the internal ring of the inguinal canal and higher than the point of deviation of the vas deferens. In this way, the main testicular artery is divided before giving off delicate anastomosing connections to the vasal vessels. One or more of these cross-connections, which are best seen through the back wall of the hernia sac, may need to be divided under vision in order to free and turn down the testis from the descending limb of the loop of the vas and its main vessels. Venae comitantes enhance the visibility of these small channels.

The "bleeding test": Incise the tunica for the bleeding test longitudinally and toward the upper pole. Select a site for the incision between the main visible vessels in the tunica vasculosa or in an area of nonvisible vascularity. Meticulous positioning and suturing curtail the extent of infarction that follows an incision in the tunica vasculosa, which could inadvertently divide a main trunk and its septal end-arteries.

Abdominal testes: Although it is not strictly the long-loop vas problem, division of the testicular vessels and orchiopexy can be applied to abdominal testes of the triad syndrome (prune belly). In this condition, however, the vas deferens is sometimes atretic in some part of its course, and hence the bleeding test would indicate a lack of supply to the testis from the artery of the vas.

Two-Stage Orchiopexy

The need for a two-stage procedure may be revealed at the time of the initial procedure when it becomes obvious that, in spite of all cord-lengthening techniques, a standard orchiopexy will not achieve scrotal position of the testis. An unintentional two-stage orchiopexy may result when the testis recedes from the scrotum after a standard one-stage orchiopexy. The technique for an unplanned second stage is described on page 316 under "Repeat Orchiopexy."

Perform a standard orchiopexy, using all the methods described for lengthening the cord, including ligating the inferior epigastric vessels or, if not too late, using the long-loop vas technique. Resort to the two-stage procedure for the testis that has not reached the bottom of the scrotum in spite of all maneuvers.

Apply strict aseptic precautions if insertion of a silicone sheath is anticipated.

SILICONE SHEATH TECHNIQUE

First Stage

1 **A,** *Incision:* Make a skin-crease incision. **B,** Proceed with standard orchiopexy (see page 308) to find that the testis, although thoroughly mobilized, still does not reach the scrotum. Fix it to the pubic tubercle with 3-0 NAS, or, if possible, place it in a high dartos pouch. Fixation by a traction stitch is not advised because the blood supply can be jeopardized by inserting a suture on a Keith needle in the tunica albuginea and bringing it through the scrotum to attach it to rubber-band traction.

2 **A** and **B,** A silicone sheath placed around the cord (Corkery, 1975) can facilitate the second stage but causes greater capillary oozing and more fibrosis. Cut a rectangle from a sheet of 0.007-inch-thick Silastic that is long enough to reach from the internal ring to the tubercle and wide enough to encircle the testis. Cut a narrow V-shaped notch at each end. **C,** Place the notched sheath around the testis and cord and trim the sides to fit. First close the tube around the testicular fixation sutures at the pubic tubercle with a 3-0 NAS. Continue along the edges with a running 3-0 NAS. Close the external oblique fascia with similar sutures for later identification.

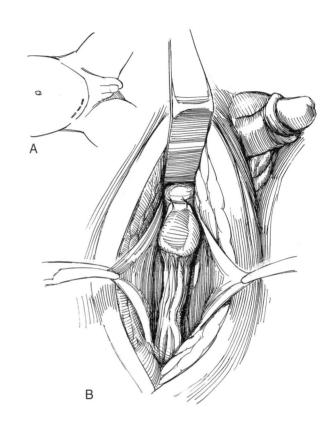

A

B

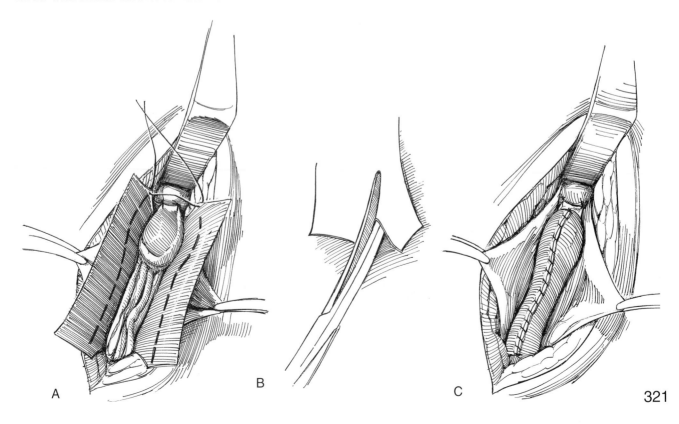

A

B

C

Second Stage

At least 1 year later (sooner in infants), open the external oblique fascia in the line identified by the NAS. Open the sheath, separate the testis from the pubic tubercle, and slip the Silastic sheet out after cutting its sutures. Dissect the testis and cord very carefully where it lies outside the sheath, using a loupe; this dissection can be tedious. Open the internal ring and free adhesions proximally.

Insert Deaver retractors and continue dissection in the retroperitoneal space, where it proceeds more easily. Adequate length is usually obtained. Scrotal placement and fixation are completed in the usual way.

POSTOPERATIVE PROBLEMS

Infection may require early removal of the sheath.

Commentary by John R. Woodard

The need for a two-stage orchiopexy may be less now than it was a few years ago. Recent experiences with laparoscopic mobilization of the spermatic cord, as well as early transabdominal orchiopexy in infants with prune-belly syndrome, have demonstrated that, with this degree of cord mobilization, an intraabdominal testis can very often be brought into scrotal position at the initial procedure.

The problem with two-stage orchiopexy is that it requires a second stage, which carries an increased risk for injury to the ilioinguinal nerve and the vas deferens. Because the optimal interval between stages is probably 1 year, the technique also results in a significant delay in achieving a scrotal environment for the testis.

I use this procedure when I have embarked upon a routine inguinal orchiopexy and have tried all of the usual maneuvers without gaining enough cord length to achieve a scrotal testis. At that point in the operation, a Fowler-Stephens procedure would likely result in atrophy, so a two-stage orchiopexy is a better option. I have not used Silastic wraps, although some find them useful and satisfactory. My reticence has been partly based on my belief that the second-stage dissection, as tedious and difficult as it sometimes is, facilitates the gain of additional length. Of course, the potential for infection of the Silastic sheath is a concern as well.

I find it useful to start the dissection for the second stage slightly lateral to the original procedure in order to allow accurate identification of tissue planes peripheral to the original scar. Beyond that, the second stage involves slow and meticulous dissection of the cord structures and testis, with mobilization to the same extent as in the first stage.

In order to avoid injury to cord structures, the group in Philadelphia (Cartwright et al, 1993) recommends that no attempt be made to dissect between the spermatic cord and overlying scarred tissues. They simply leave a strip of overlying external oblique aponeurosis attached to the cord as their dissection extends superiorly into fresh tissue planes above the site of hernia sac ligation and into the retroperitoneum (see page 316). They emphasize the importance of freeing the testis inferiorly at the start and working upward. When these maneuvers are followed, a testis that is palpable in the vicinity of the external ring following a previous procedure can almost always be placed satisfactorily in the scrotum.

Microvascular Orchiopexy

Microvascular orchiopexy is an alternative to a one- or two-stage long-loop vas orchiopexy (see page 318), with a success rate as high as 100 percent in experienced hands (Bukowski et al, 1995). For bilateral high testes, it may be reasonable to use the microvascular technique on at least one side, but at two separate operations. Infants under 2 years of age, when the procedure should be done, have well-developed genitalia and testicular vascular pedicle consequent to maternal hormonal stimulation.

Perform preliminary laparoscopy to ascertain the need for autotransplantation (see page 332).

Instruments: Provide a complete microvascular set-up with an operating room microscope, three-power loupes, and 10-0 or 11-0 nylon sutures on BV-6 or ST-7 needles. Unless you are skilled in microsurgery, consult with a microsurgeon, who usually performs the actual anastomosis.

1 *Position:* Place the boy on a heated blanket on a table that has an extension to provide space for the surgeon's knees. To keep the bladder away from the anastomosis, use suprapubic compression to manually empty it, or insert a balloon catheter.

Incision: Make a generous inguinal incision in the skin crease. Extend it well laterally as a high Gibson incision to avoid injury to the inferior epigastric vessels and to permit abdominal access (see pages 495 to 496).

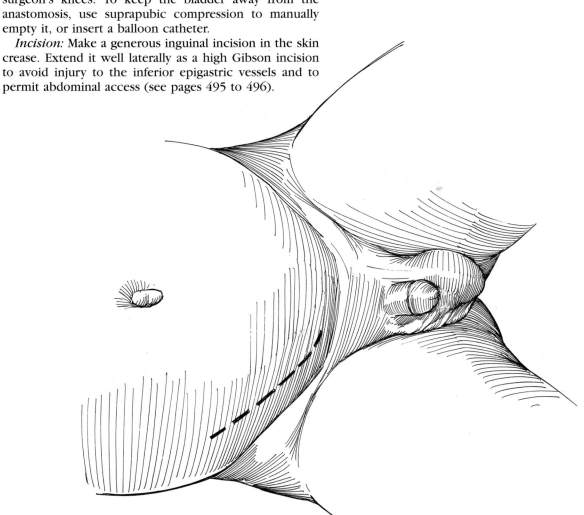

2 Open the inguinal canal and identify the gubernaculum and the processus vaginalis. Open the peritoneum at the internal ring. Locate the testis and place a traction suture in the tunica albuginea. Alternatively, expose and dissect the testis laparoscopically (see page 331). Expose the spermatic vessels. Move the testis into the retroperitoneal space and carefully dissect the peritoneum off of the vascular pedicle, obtaining as much length as possible. Close the peritoneum. Using loupes for the dissection, bluntly dissect retroperitoneally, following the spermatic vessels until they near their communication with the vena cava or renal vein and the aorta. Ensure that the dissection of the vessels extends beyond the confluence of the pampiniform plexus to form a single vein. Preserve the vasal vessels in a large patch of peritoneum as the vas is freed into the pelvis to ensure venous drainage. If the vas is too short, pass the testis under the lateral umbilical ligament (obliterated umbilical artery). Dissect through the internal oblique aponeurosis and the transversus abdominis to expose the inferior epigastric artery and (usually) two venae comitantes and hold them in a vessel loop. Ligate the arterial side branches with 5-0 silk as far from the main vessel as possible because one of them may be of suitable size for the anastomosis. Dissect the artery free. Ligate and divide both the artery and the vein high beneath the rectus muscle, placing a noncrushing microvascular clamp on the proximal end. Apply heparin solution (10 units/ml) to the cut ends. Ligate or fulgurate their muscular branches with bipolar diathermy. Prepare a dartos pouch (see page 314). Then ligate the spermatic vessels, but be sure to tag the testicular artery with a stay suture before dividing it. Divide the vessels distal to the ligature and look for back-bleeding. Place the testis in the dartos pouch before performing the anastomosis to avoid traction on the testis. Close the peritoneal defect.

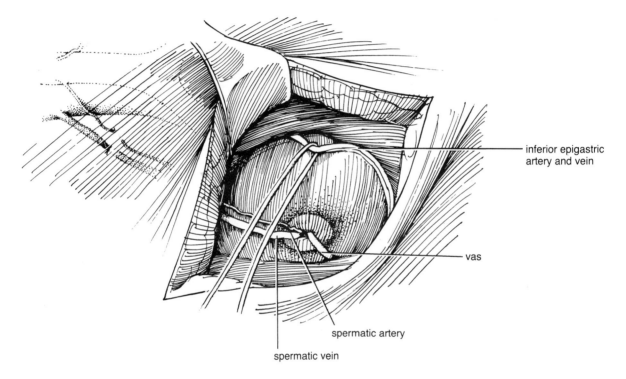

inferior epigastric artery and vein

vas

spermatic artery

spermatic vein

3 **A,** Bring the spermatic artery and accompanying veins into the microscopic field. Start by placing the veins, usually each about 1 mm in diameter, in a microvascular clamp. Depending on the urologist's proficiency, it may be wise to ask a microsurgeon to do the anastomosis. Perform the venous anastomosis first with 10-0 or 11-0 nylon. For the arteries, expect considerable disparity in size (the testicular artery usually measures 0.5 to 1 mm and the epigastric artery measures 1.0 to 1.5 mm). Cutting the testicular artery obliquely or spatulating it may compensate for the difference. A reversed venous step-down graft may be interposed. The anastomotic technique is described on pages 60 to 61. Ischemia time should be kept as short as possible. Occlusion usually occurs within 5 minutes, but observe the anastomosis for at least 20 minutes to be sure. If it does occlude, do not hesitate to resect and redo it. **B,** Before closing, incise the testis and check for fresh bleeding. Fix the testis in the scrotum, and close the inguinal wound carefully to avoid obstructing the vessels.

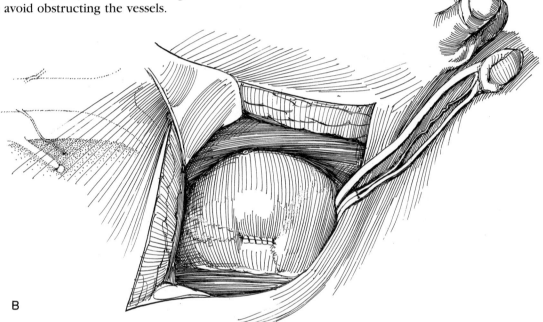

A

B

Commentary by Michael G. Packer

A number of important factors must be considered when choosing microvascular orchiopexy for the intra-abdominal testis. After a few months of age, biopsy data suggest marked reduction or absence of spermatogonia in some intra-abdominal testes. Thus, the technical challenges of this approach must be weighed carefully against the reduced fertility potential of many of these testes.

The inguinal canal should be thoroughly inspected. Once it has been determined that the testis cannot be pulled into the inguinal canal with gentle traction, the peritoneum is incised above the internal ring by the LaRoque maneuver. Spermatic vessels are carefully mobilized along with the vas with a broad pedicle of posterior peritoneum. The subdartos pouch is then created. Gentle traction on the testis can then determine whether sufficient cord length exists to bring the testis into the scrotum without cutting the spermatic vessels. This can be accomplished fairly often, avoiding the need for a microvascular approach. If the vessels are divided, it is preferable to place the testis within the dartos pouch prior to the microvascular anastomosis. This avoids further manipulation of the cord structures after the microvascular sutures are placed. Occasionally,

retraction or spasm of the spermatic or epigastric vessels makes identification more difficult. This can be prevented by placing fine tag sutures adjacent to the vessels before dividing them.

Postoperatively, the patient is kept at bed rest for 1 to 3 days, depending on the degree of postoperative swelling.

Laparoscopy now offers alternative approaches to the intra-abdominal testis. One option is to confirm the presence of an intra-abdominal testis by laparoscopy and clip (or fulgurate by laser) the spermatic vessels. One can then return in several weeks to complete the delayed Fowler-Stephens orchiopexy, either by laparoscopic or by open technique. Alternatively, the initial mobilization of the spermatic vessels, vas, and testis may be performed with the laparoscope. Depending on the length achieved for the vessels, simple orchiopexy, Fowler-Stephens technique, or microvascular approach may then be selected. The shorter operative time and reduced hospital stay with these alternative approaches may offset the advantages of the microvascular orchiopexy. With careful patient selection and safe pediatric anesthesia, the trend toward early surgery for the intra-abdominal testis should result in improved outcomes regardless of the technique.

Orchiopexy for the Nonpalpable Testis

LAPAROSCOPIC LOCALIZATION

The testis may be localized by laparoscopy in 90 percent of cases. The blind ending vas and vessels of the vanishing testis can be identified and the need for exploration eliminated. Laparoscopy can also simplify an open orchiopexy by avoiding an extensive exploratory procedure to locate the intra-abdominal or canalicular testis.

Laparoscopic inspection shows whether the vas and vessels end blindly and the testis is absent, whether the cord structures end in a closed internal inguinal ring to be attached to at most a markedly hypoplastic testis, or whether the testis is present intra-abdominally and can be corrected laparoscopically or directly through a midline abdominal incision without a preliminary groin incision. If it is seen to be hypoplastic, it may be excised by the laparoscopic technique. This approach avoids an operation for those 10 to 15 percent of boys with absent testes as proved by blind-ending vas and vessels. In bilateral cases, perform an hCG stimulation test; if there is no response, anorchia is the diagnosis and operation is not needed because the degree of response is related to the amount of testicular tissue (Davenport et al, 1995). For laparoscopic orchiopexy, see pages 331 to 337.

If the testis has not been localized laparoscopically, approach the unilaterally retained testis through a standard transverse skin-crease incision; extend the incision superiorly through the internal ring if necessary to gain added transperitoneal or retroperitoneal exposure. For bilateral cases, make bilateral skin-crease lower quadrant incisions and explore each groin. Usually extensive retroperitoneal dissection through these incisions allows the testis to be placed in the scrotum. If the testes are not found, complete the middle of the incision and open the peritoneum, essential for adequate visualization of the internal spermatic vessels and those of the cord if a long-loop orchiopexy is planned.

TRANSPERITONEAL APPROACH

1 **A,** Make a midline incision in the lower abdomen from pubis to umbilicus. **B,** Separate the rectus and underlying areolar tissue. Open the peritoneum and pack the intestines aside. The testis is often found lying intraperitoneally, usually behind the bladder and often on a short mesentery.

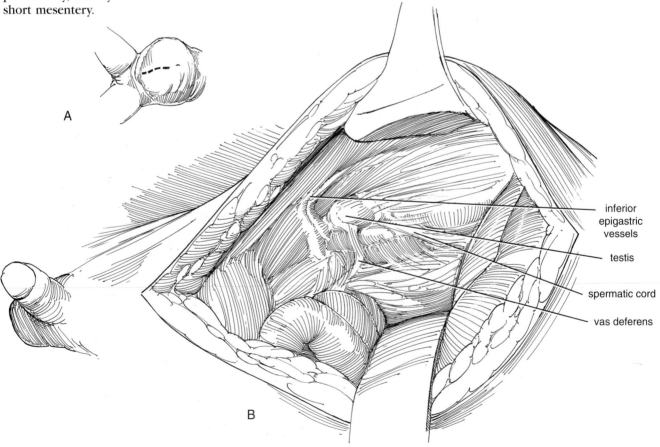

inferior epigastric vessels

testis

spermatic cord

vas deferens

2 Incise the peritoneum obliquely, and sharply free the vessels from the retroperitoneal tissue under direct vision.

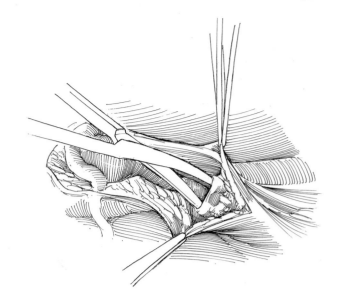

3 Sharply free the vas behind the bladder, leaving 1 cm of peritoneum on either side (not shown in the figure), until sufficient length is achieved to place the testis in the scrotum. Invert the scrotum through the external ring, as is done in palpating for a hernia, and place a curved clamp against the finger tip from above. In boys with prune-belly syndrome the ring is relatively large. Push the clamp through the transversalis fascia and the conjoined tendon as the finger is withdrawn; then dilate the canal and scrotum with the clamp and finger as necessary to form a passage for the testis. Incise the scrotum over the finger. Place a suture in the tissue adjacent to the testis, and lead the testis through the canal to the bottom of the scrotum.

Fix the testis in a dartos pouch by incising the scrotal skin and developing a pocket between the skin and dartos by blunt dissection (see page 312). Make a small nick in the dartos, and introduce a curved clamp into the inguinal canal to grasp the suture and bring the testis into the scrotum with a little traction. Anchor the testis by closing the dartos behind it with two fine NAS.

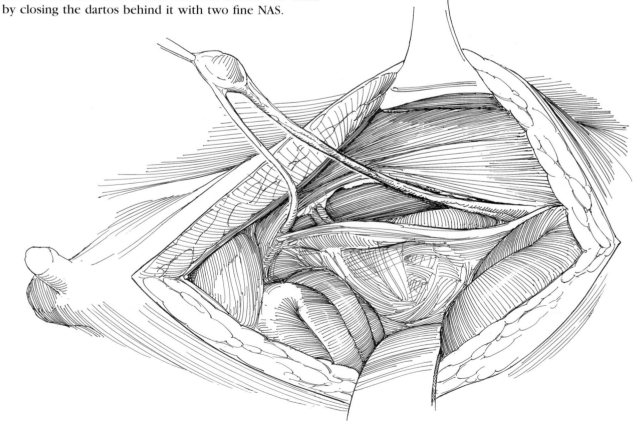

EXTRAPERITONEAL APPROACH

4 Make a lower abdominal midline incision from pubis to umbilicus (see page 487). Separate the rectus muscles and bluntly reflect the peritoneal envelope medially. Look first in the internal inguinal ring to pick up the cord structures. If found, bluntly free them along with the testis from the canal, bring them into the retroperitoneum, and divide the gubernaculum. The inferior epigastric vessels may prevent this maneuver; if they do, divide and ligate them. The internal inguinal ring may be too tight; divide it posteriorly and repair it later.

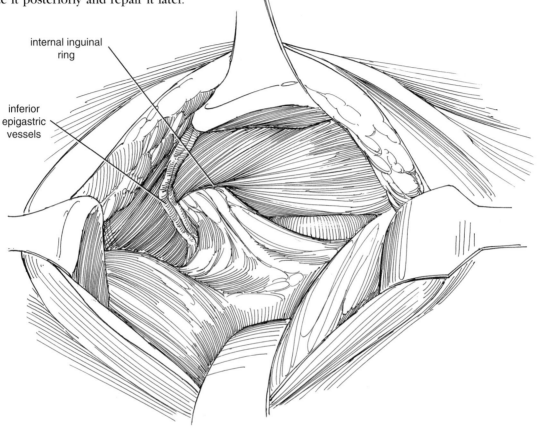

internal inguinal ring

inferior epigastric vessels

5 If the testis is not found near the internal ring, examine the posterior surface of the peritoneum within which the testis is attached. Start by locating the vas deferens behind the bladder and follow it into the canal to the testis, which is concealed because it is intraperitoneal. The blind-ending vas and epididymis may be appreciably separated from the testis.

If the vas ends blindly or in a rudimentary epididymis, identify the spermatic vessels and follow them. If they too terminate blindly, the diagnosis is an absent (vanishing) testis.

If the testis is found retroperitoneally, incise the peritoneum around it and close the peritoneal defect with a running 4-0 SAS. A pedicled flap of peritoneum, inferior to the testis, can be left attached to the testis and placed in the scrotum with it (not shown). This flap can supplement the blood supply and is necessary if a Fowler-Stephens orchiopexy is done. Encircle the testis with a small Penrose drain for traction, and bluntly and sharply free the vas down to the area of the prostate and the vascular bundle up to the level of the kidney.

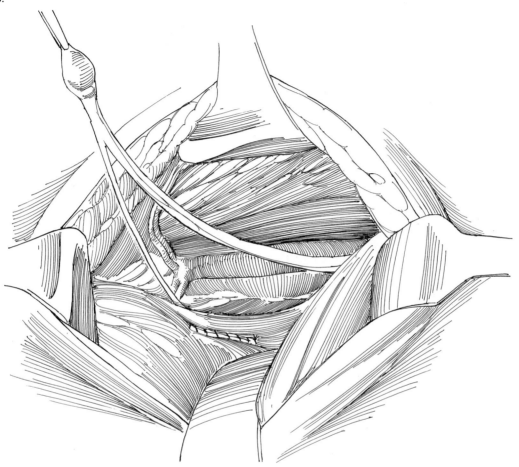

6 Make an adequate opening through the transversalis fascia and the tendinous end of the rectus muscle immediately superior to the pubis above the ipsilateral side of the scrotum. Create a scrotal pouch bluntly and install the testis in the scrotum over the dartos, as described on page 312, taking care not to twist the cord. Close the abdominal wall without drainage.

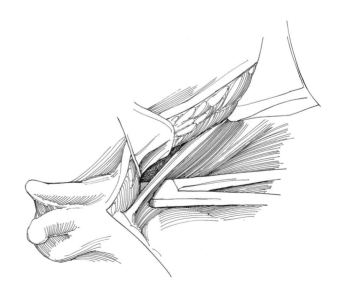

EXTENDED INGUINAL APPROACH

If the nonpalpable testis was not localized by laparoscopy, start with a standard orchiopexy incision with the expectation that the testis is located in a relatively low position, but do not extend the opening in the internal oblique muscle into the external ring. Expose the internal ring, and pull on the processus vaginalis at its point of exit to bring the intra-abdominal testis into view. Open the anterior surface of the hernia sac and look for a long, looping vas deferens or an attenuated epididymis with a testis attached. A blind-ending vas and epididymis can be found in the inguinal canal, detached from the testes and outside the hernia sac.

If the testis is not discovered, open the external oblique and retract the internal oblique muscle at the medial edge of the internal ring and open the peritoneum. Look for the vas behind the bladder near the obliterated hypogastric vessels, and trace it along with the spermatic vessels to their end, often in a nubbin that denotes anorchia. The vas should be resected for pathologic examination. If a testis is found, place a fine traction suture in the tunica albuginea at the lower pole and pull on it to assess vessel length. If it appears that enough length could be gained by high dissection of the vessels, proceed accordingly with a traditional orchiopexy. If traction shows that the vessels are too short, proceed with a long-loop vas orchiopexy (see page 318). Alternatively, if dissection has progressed and release proves inadequate, fix the testis to the pubic tubercle; perhaps cover the cord with a Silastic sheath; and return for a second-stage orchiopexy (see pages 316 and 321 to 322).

An absent testis is confirmed by the presence of blind-ending vas and spermatic vessels in the abdomen. If the vas and vessels pass through a closed internal inguinal ring, only an atrophic testis or an epididymal remnant is found. A blind-ending vas without accompanying vessels requires further abdominal exploration.

An alternative approach is through a muscle-splitting incision in a lower quadrant (see page 495). Bring the testis medial to the inguinal canal to provide a direct route for the vessels. This incision does not provide enough exposure for high intra-abdominal testes.

Commentary by Laurence S. Baskin

I approach the patient with a unilateral nonpalpable testis through a small groin incision placed in a skin crease just lateral and superior to the pubic tubercle. In the majority of cases, evidence of a testis is found during the groin dissection by identification of the spermatic vessels or the vas deferens. This fact has tempered my use of laparoscopy for the unilateral nonpalpable testis. The data suggest that antenatal torsion of a testis generally occurs after it has entered the inguinal canal. Therefore, it is unrealistic to expect laparoscopy to enable one to avoid surgical exploration in dealing with a unilateral impalpable testis. If gonadal structures are not identified, I proceed to evaluate the abdominal cavity by opening up the peritoneum. The peritoneum can be opened at the internal ring (for the peeping or emerging testis) or, in the case of the high intra-abdominal testis, through a LaRoque incision (a modification of Bevan's original groin operation for the undescended testicle), which is located 2 to 3 cm above the standard external oblique incision. In children, the rectus abdominis muscle is wider than it is in adults. The incision consequently predominantly opens the rectus fascia, with only a short extension into the external oblique. Usually, it is necessary to split the external oblique and internal oblique musculature minimally. In practice, if laparoscopy has not been performed to locate the testis prior to the incision, I proceed to open the peritoneum at the internal ring. If the testis is immediately identifiable and mobile, I proceed with the orchiopexy. If the testis is identified high in the abdomen, the incision is closed and the LaRoque maneuver performed.

Laparoscopy has confirmed the anatomic basis for the open approach to bringing down the abdominal testis. Under loop magnification, the peritoneum can be incised lateral to the spermatic vessels, all the way to the lower pole of the kidney. Still working through the relatively small inguinal skin incision with the use of Army-Navy or small Deaver retractors and a capable assistant, one can perform a high lateral dissection. Anatomically, this requires mobilization of the spermatic vessels up and out of the endopelvic or endoabdominal fascia. This retroperitoneal fascia continues down into the inguinal canal as the internal spermatic fascia around the cord structures and processus vaginalis. With this technique, we have had success in performing primary intra-abdominal orchiopexies on almost all testicles without having to resort to the Fowler-Stephens procedure. As mentioned, the key to success is optical magnification and a high lateral dissection to the lower pole of the kidney, thereby releasing the glue of the retroperitoneum.

On initial evaluation of the intra-abdominal testis, a decision must be made as to whether the testis is worth salvaging. This decision is based on testicular size, consistency, and epididymal attachment. Consideration should also be given to the normality of the contralateral testicle. To avoid persistent, excessive manipulation of the testis, I prefer to place a holding suture completely through the tunica albuginea of the testicle, avoiding the polar blood supply. The spermatic artery enters the testis near the lower pole, and placement of a clamp or suture at the lower pole, as has been historically done, does not seem wise. I find that one strategically placed holding suture allows for manipulation of the testis throughout the procedure and avoids the repeated trauma of manipulation with forceps. At the completion of the procedure, a 1- to 2-cm strip of peritoneum should remain attached laterally to the spermatic vessels. Medial to the spermatic vessels, the peritoneum or blood supply should not need to be violated.

In patients with prune-belly syndrome, make either a midline abdominal or a transverse lower abdominal incision and reconstruct the abdominal wall simultaneously with the orchiopexy. If the procedure is done in the young infant, it is possible to bring the testis down by an aggressive lateral dissection without having to resort to the Fowler-Stephens technique.

Finally, it is important to make a decision early about the need for the Fowler-Stephens procedure. Any attempt to salvage a traditional orchiopexy using the Fowler-Stephens technique is doomed to failure because a good peritoneal pedicle around the vas has not been preserved. The vasal artery provides the blood supply that maintains the testis.

Laparoscopic Techniques for Impalpable Testes

Re-examine the child under anesthesia to see if the testis can be palpated. Prepare and drape the child as for laparotomy, but leave the scrotum exposed. Insert a nasogastric tube and a urethral catheter; both stomach and bladder may become distended secondary to stress. If the child has the prune-belly syndrome, be aware of the probability of excess CO_2 absorption. For details on initiating pneumoperitoneum and techniques for inserting trocars, see pages 21 to 25. The Hasson technique is safest.

1 Schematic diagram showing sites for insertion of trocars.

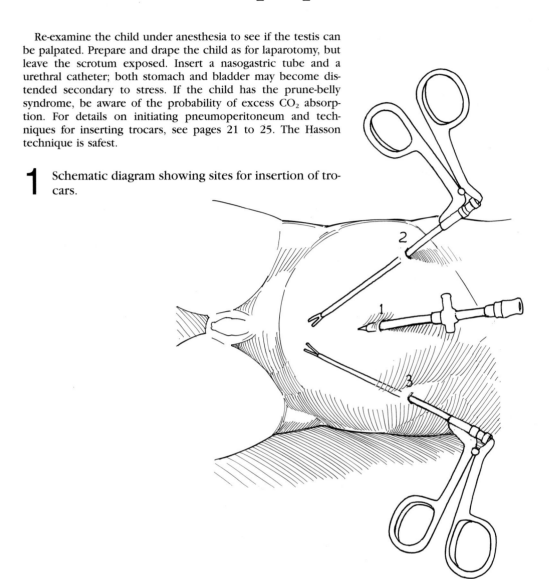

DIAGNOSTIC LAPAROSCOPY

Hasson Technique. Insert a Hasson trocar beneath the umbilicus (Step 1, site 1) by the technique described on page 25, and introduce the telescope.

Alternative for Simple Inspection (Brock, 1993). Make a short curved incision in the lower margin of the umbilicus. With operating loupes, open the fascia and hold it with two sutures. Open the peritoneum under vision and insert a 3-mm trocar without an obturator. Insufflate the abdomen, stop the filling, and insert a 0-degree lens.

2 For the impalpable testis, examine the retroperitoneal area and internal ring for the presence of the testis or related structures before proceeding with definitive surgery.

Because in children the amount of preperitoneal fat is minimal, the structures of the pelvis are readily seen. In all cases, orient yourself by locating the medial umbilical ligament (obliterated umbilical artery), which lies laterally and runs from the hypogastric artery to the umbilicus. The ureter lies medially and, like the medial umbilical ligament, is crossed by the vas deferens, the three structures making up what has been called the vasal triangle (Bloom et al, 1994). Find the median umbilical ligament (urachal remnant), which is seen running from the bladder to the umbilicus. Observe the catheter in the bladder.

Normal Side. Identify the spermatic vessels as they disappear into the internal inguinal ring. Pull on the testis in the scrotum to bring the vas and vessels into prominence. If the pelvic structures are not well visualized, check the pressure from the CO_2 insufflator; it may be too low.

Impalpable Side. Five findings are possible:

1. The processus vaginalis is patent and the spermatic cord is seen passing through the internal inguinal ring, indicating a testis or remnant in the groin area. Press on the canal externally to see if the testis can be pushed back into the abdomen. If it responds, either a standard orchiopexy or a laparoscopic orchiopexy is feasible. If standard orchiopexy is elected, proceed with laparoscopic mobilization of the spermatic vessels to the level of the kidney.

2. The testis is seen just above the internal ring, and a short but patent processus vaginalis is present. Here, too, either type of orchiopexy can be done. Laparoscopic mobilization of the spermatic vessels facilitates the orchiopexy.

3. No testis is seen, but the processus vaginalis is patent and the cord structures disappear in the canal. Use the grasper to pull on these structures to identify the position of a testicular remnant in the groin. If there is a question about this, an inguinal exploration may be indicated.

4. The testis with adnexae is seen but lies well above the patent processus vaginalis at the internal ring, and the vas is redundant. This condition is best managed by staged Fowler-Stephens orchiopexy, with preliminary laparoscopic clipping or coagulation of the spermatic vessels.

5. No testis is seen. The processus vaginalis is likely to be closed. Inspect the retroperitoneum. Look for blind-ending spermatic vessels as proof of testicular absence (vanishing testis). Even if a blind-ending vas is found at the internal ring, the entire retroperitoneum to the lower pole of the kidney must be examined, although that may require reflecting the colon by freeing its lateral attachments.

If an *atrophic* or *dysmorphic testis* is found, remove it laparoscopically (see page 379) or make a small (3- to 4-cm) muscle-splitting incision in the lower quadrant and excise it transperitoneally.

If a *movable testis* with adequate vessels is found during a diagnostic laparoscopic procedure, a determination must be made on how to proceed. Perform laparoscopic orchiopexy if the normal-appearing testis lies at or below the external iliac vessels. The alternatives are to proceed immediately with an open standard orchiopexy if the set-up is available and to reschedule for open orchiopexy at a later time. If the vessels are short, proceed with laparoscopic fulguration and/or clipping of the spermatic vessels as a first-stage Fowler-Stephens orchiopexy.

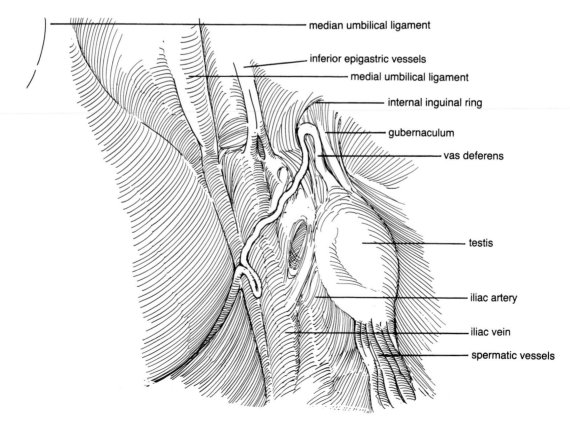

- median umbilical ligament
- inferior epigastric vessels
- medial umbilical ligament
- internal inguinal ring
- gubernaculum
- vas deferens
- testis
- iliac artery
- iliac vein
- spermatic vessels

FIRST-STAGE FOWLER-STEPHENS OPERATION: LAPAROSCOPIC VESSEL LIGATION (Bloom)

Perform the operation as an outpatient procedure. Place the child supine. For orchiopexy and other pelvic procedures, insert a rolled towel under the lower back to create lordosis, and tip the table into a 10-degree Trendelenburg position to allow the intestines to drop out of the pelvis. Shift to a 30-degree Trendelenburg position for placement of the initial port. It can be helpful after the ports are inserted to tilt the table laterally 30 degrees to raise the involved testis above the bowels.

First place two trocars, one as the telescope port and one as the access port (see Step 1, sites 1 and 2), and inspect the testis and cord. Exert traction on the testis to help decide whether to clip the spermatic vessels (the vessels are short) as a first stage or to proceed at once with laparoscopic orchiopexy (or with standard open orchiopexy). If no testis is found, use graspers to move the abdominal organs and thus reach the lower pole of the kidney to allow a search of that area. If a dysgenic testis is found, remove it. However, if an inguinal hernia is present, repair it by an open technique, preferable in adults in whom the muscular deficiency should be reconstructed.

Incise the peritoneum high over the spermatic cord, far from the testis, to preserve the collateral vessels. Dissect the vessels as high as possible, a procedure more easily done under magnification with the laparoscope than by open operation. If the testis is found close to the internal ring, enough length may usually be obtained to proceed immediately with laparoscopic orchiopexy and avoid a staged procedure.

If sufficient length of the cord cannot be obtained by dissection, insert an electrode through a 5-mm port, elevate the vessels on it, and fulgurate them using unipolar or bipolar current, or even photocoagulate them with three bursts from a laser wand passed through an 18-gauge angiographic needle.

Alternative: If a 10-mm port is in place, separate the cord into bundles, pass a loaded Hulka clip applier through the port, and clip the bundles of spermatic vessels as high as possible. Place a second set of clips so that later the cord may be divided between them. Another alternative is to place sets of vascular clips.

Remove the instrument sheath, evacuate the CO_2 to a level of 6 mm Hg, and inspect the area for venous bleeding. Remove the visualizing port. Carefully close the 10-mm port opening with 4-0 SAS to approximate both peritoneum and fascia. It is also advisable to close the 5-mm defects because the attenuated omentum of children is prone to herniate. Close the skin with subcuticular sutures and sterile tapes. Proceed with the second stage in 3 to 6 months.

SECOND-STAGE LAPAROSCOPIC FOWLER-STEPHENS ORCHIOPEXY

Wait 3 months after the first stage. As with the first stage, the procedure is done on an outpatient basis. Place the child supine. Insert a rolled towel under the lower back to create lordosis. Start with a 30-degree Trendelenburg position for inserting the initial port; then place the table in a 10-degree Trendelenburg position for the procedure. Tilt the table laterally 30 degrees to let the bowel fall away from the involved testis.

Place three trocars (see Step 1, sites 1 to 3), the larger one (#1, 11-mm Hasson trocar) subumbilically and two 5-mm trocars (#2 and 3) on either side at the same level, lateral to the rectus muscle, to avoid the inferior epigastric vessels. Place them relatively high so that the ends are not too close to the operative field. Remember that the bladder in the child lies higher than in an adult.

3 Stand on the side opposite the abnormal testis, with your assistant across from you. With an inexperienced assistant, insert the telescope through the distal trocar and the graspers and scissors through the umbilical and proximal ports to give you control. Inspect the pelvic peritoneal cavity with a 30-degree lens. Locate the median umbilical ligament (urachal remnant), the median umbilical ligament, and the sigmoid colon. Look for the internal inguinal ring with its crescentic medial margin, first on the normal side and then on the other side. The testis is attached by the gubernaculum, which is seen descending into the internal inguinal ring. The spermatic vessels as well as the site of the first-stage fulguration can be identified by having an assistant pull on the testis; the

vas deferens is seen adjacent to it. Move the colon medially for access to the spermatic vessels proximally. Formal mobilization is not needed because incision of the retroperitoneum allows its medial displacement. The incision in the peritoneum *(dashed line)* starts around the internal ring distal to the gubernaculum and bordering the testis laterally and takes a generous triangular flap of peritoneum, one that extends laterally 1 cm from the spermatic vessels, ventrally at least 1 cm from the vas deferens from the internal ring into the pelvis, and medially along the vessels from the site of fulguration toward the pelvic vas. The incision for the new canal *(dotted line)* is made between the bladder and the medial umbilical ligament, just lateral to the median umbilical ligament.

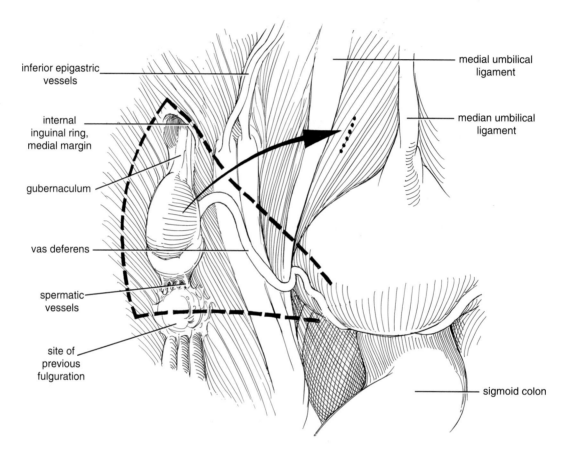

inferior epigastric vessels

internal inguinal ring, medial margin

gubernaculum

vas deferens

spermatic vessels

site of previous fulguration

medial umbilical ligament

median umbilical ligament

sigmoid colon

4 With endoscopic graspers and scissors, incise the peritoneum, starting around the internal ring distal to the gubernaculum and bordering the testis laterally. The colon falls medially once the peritoneum has been incised. Make a large triangular flap of peritoneum to provide a large peritoneal pedicle that encompasses the vas deferens and the collateral blood supply. Start dissection of the gubernaculum into the internal ring as far distally as possible to preserve all collateral vessels. Divide and fulgurate the gubernaculum, grasp it next to the processus vaginalis, and retract the testis with it. Proceed medially along the vas deferens, elevating it carefully to preserve its vessels. Bluntly mobilize the spermatic vessels to the site of the previous fulguration, and at the same time free the vas deferens. Raise the testis on the flap of peritoneum, keeping the broad isthmus of peritoneum continuous with the vas. During the dissection, watch out for the ureter, which runs over the field and lies medial to the iliac vessels. If a hernia sac is present, dissect the vessels as described, but abandon the laparoscopic approach and proceed to a standard orchiopexy and hernia repair because laparoscopic hernia repair in children not only places foreign material in the defect but also leaves staples on the peritoneal edges. Make a short incision in the peritoneum between the bladder and the medial umbilical ligament, just lateral to the median umbilical ligament, for the new inguinal canal.

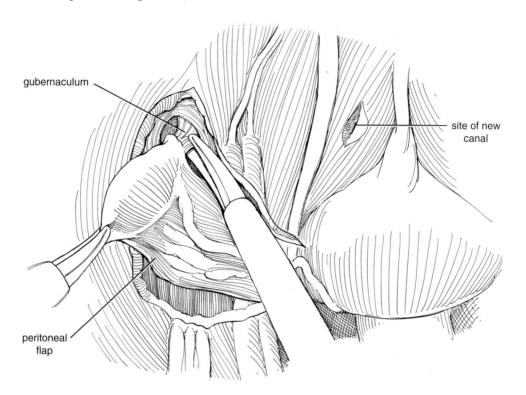

gubernaculum

site of new canal

peritoneal flap

5 **A,** Insert a curved clamp through the scrotal incision, pass it by palpation over the pubic bone alongside the pubic tubercle, and direct it through the fascia so that the tip is seen through the laparoscope lateral to the medial umbilical ligament. Insert a 10- or 11-mm trocar sheath from below along the tract, and bring the tip intra-abdominally under direct vision from above. Dilate the new canal with a Péan clamp or a Kollmann dilator and reinsert the sheath. **B,** With graspers, hold the testis against the end of the sheath and draw the testis out with the sheath. Place some traction on the testis in the scrotum, and divide any remaining retroperitoneal attachments from above. Inspect the cord to be sure that the vas is medial to the cord and that the testis has not been rotated during placement.

Alternative: Make a 2-cm incision externally on the scrotum and form a dartos pouch (see page 312). Internally, form a new inguinal canal medial to the medial umbilical ligament by passing a clamp from above through the peritoneal incision (*dotted line* in Figure 3), along the ventral surface of the symphysis, and out through the scrotal incision. Lead a clamp back from below, grasp the testis gingerly, and draw it into the scrotum. If it tends to retract, dissect further on the new cord. Fix the testis beneath the dartos with fine SAS (see page 313). Close the scrotal wound with a subcuticular SAS.

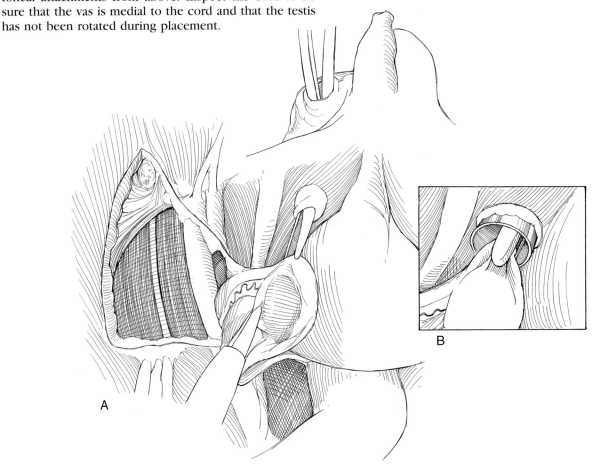

6 Reduce intra-abdominal pressure. Place the parietal peritoneum over the area of the patent processus vaginalis by clipping it in place with hernia clips. Alternatively, close the internal ring with three sutures placed between the transversalis fascia and the iliopectineal ligament; then replace the peritoneum. For a large defect associated with a hernia, insert polypropylene mesh behind the posterior wall of the inguinal canal and anchor it to the abdominal wall by its superior and lateral borders with a stapler before applying and clipping the peritoneal flaps. Inspect the vas and associated structures for torsion and the operative area for bleeding. Irrigate the peritoneal cavity and aspirate the fluid. Aspirate most of the CO_2 to reduce peritoneal irritation. Remove the instrument sheaths in order. Finally, withdraw the visualizing port after inspecting for bleeding at a pressure of 6 mm Hg. Close the 1-mm fascial opening with 4-0 SAS and the skin with subcuticular sutures and sterile tapes.

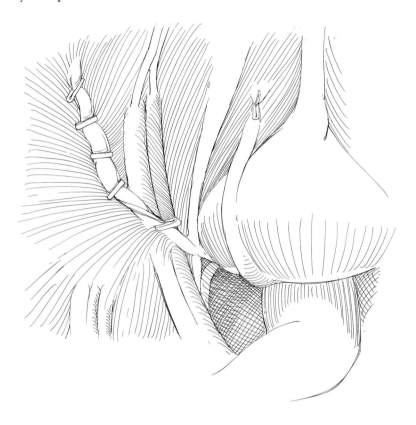

Intersex Disorders

Inspect and classify the internal sexual organs. Gonadal biopsy is the primary goal. Take a biopsy from pole to pole. Suture the incision with one or two 4-0 absorbable sutures.

Commentary by Guy A. Bogaert

The high accuracy of laparoscopy makes it the diagnostic procedure of choice for impalpable testes. Advantages are its rapidity (approximately 15 minutes) and low morbidity. Additionally, one can begin a therapeutic procedure from the diagnostic laparoscopy: One or two accessory ports are enough for all procedures. In my experience, ports larger than 5 F are almost never necessary. If I find the testicle in the groin and decide to perform a "classic" open orchiopexy, I mobilize the testicular vessels laparoscopically up to the kidney to avoid tension on them after the testis is brought into the scrotum. If the vessels still seem too short, I suggest making a new "inguinal canal" laparoscopically and bringing the testis straight into the scrotum with the Prentiss maneuver. This is much easier and faster through the laparoscope, and the length gained is impressive.

When you are ready to pull the testis into the scrotum through the new "inguinal canal" after you insert a small clamp from the scrotum, let your assistant push against the symphysis to keep the CO_2 in the abdomen. After you have pulled the testis into the subdartos pouch, little or no leakage occurs. Other methods have been described using another trocar from the scrotum or from the groin, but none has been shown to have a greater advantage than the technique described. It may not be necessary to close the peritoneal defect at the internal ring. In a few children I have coagulated the peritoneum and have observed no signs of an indirect hernia in the postoperative period. I would not recommend this in an adult patient with hernia repair, as the defect is a muscular problem.

Before ending the procedure, I make sure that no hernia is present at the internal ring. If a hernia is present, I recommend repairing it with an open procedure instead of placing foreign material in the defect and stapling the edges of peritoneum—not an attractive option in children. I have found that, in the second stage of the Fowler-Stephens orchiopexy, one can see the dilated collateral vessels around the vas deferens more clearly through the laparoscope. The magnification and the angle of dissection allow a more precise dissection around the delicate vasculature and the vas. Laparoscopy should improve the success rate of this procedure.

In a child over 10 years of age or in an adult, the intra-abdominal testis should be removed. To remove a testis laparoscopically, I recommend placing it in a sterile condom or endoscopic bag before removal to avoid spillage of cells that might become malignant. In an adult, the trocar site must be enlarged to allow removal of the testis without traction or tension.

Inguinal Hernia Repair

REPAIR OF LEFT INDIRECT HERNIA

Cooper's pectineal ligament repair is the most secure method for direct and femoral hernias, and for some large indirect hernias as well. The repair may be abbreviated in most cases of indirect hernia by attaching the conjoined tendon to the inguinal ligament, obviating dissection of Cooper's ligament and the iliopubic tract.

1 **A,** *Position:* Supine.
Incision: Make a low oblique incision that follows the skin line of the lowest skin crease. Center it over a point halfway between the anterior superior iliac spine and the pubic tubercle. **B,** Divide the skin and Scarpa's fascia, clamping branches of the superficial epigastric vessels as they are encountered medially and clamping the superficial circumflex vessels laterally. Identify the external ring and incise the external oblique fascia with a knife; then continue the incision cephalad by pushing the partially opened scissors in the direction of the fibers. Grasp the edges of the fascia with curved mosquito clamps and open the incision distally with the scissors to the external ring. Place a self-retaining retractor. Dissect the ilioinguinal nerve from beneath the external oblique fascia, move it laterally, and hold it back with a clamp on the edge of the fascia. Bluntly free the spermatic cord from the external oblique aponeurosis and from the entire inguinal ligament. Also free it from the posterior wall of the canal. Break through the thin layer of cremasteric muscle posteriorly and encircle the cord with a Penrose drain. Lift the cord. Open the transversalis fascia that forms the posterior wall of the canal *(dashed line)*. Alternatively, preserve it to strengthen the repair.

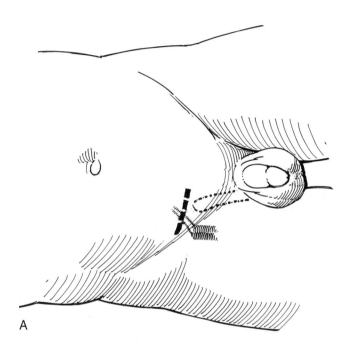

A

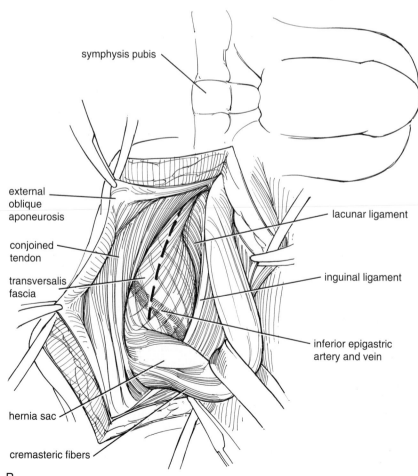

symphysis pubis

external oblique aponeurosis

conjoined tendon

transversalis fascia

lacunar ligament

inguinal ligament

inferior epigastric artery and vein

hernia sac

cremasteric fibers

B

2 The hernia sac is seen bulging within the cord. Insinuate a clamp between the cremasteric muscle and the internal spermatic fascia, and separate the cremasteric fibers at the internal inguinal ring to release the cord from the hernia sac. The external spermatic artery is exposed and may require clamping. For large hernias, expose the pectineal (Cooper's) ligament, a fibrous accretion that may be several millimeters thick and involve the periosteum of the superior ramus of the pubis along the pectineal line. Expose the iliopubic tract (the anterior femoral sheath), which appears as the thickened fibrous lower border of the transversalis fascia that runs caudal to and parallel with the inguinal ligament. Although the iliopubic tract lies very close to the inguinal ligament in its midportion, it is an entirely separate structure, part of the deep transversalis layer. Identify the conjoined tendon (transversus abdominis arch) beneath the internal oblique muscle. The hernia sac lies on the anterior aspect of the cord. Open it, place mosquito clamps on the edges, insert a finger, and dissect it free of cremasteric and internal spermatic fascias by sharp dissection. Trim it if necessary, and close it at the level of the thickened peritoneal ring with a purse-string suture to leave it flush with the peritoneum.

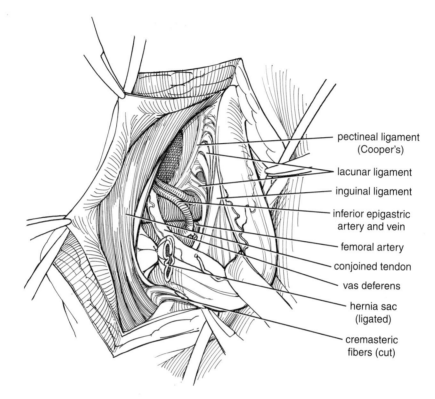

pectineal ligament (Cooper's)
lacunar ligament
inguinal ligament
inferior epigastric artery and vein
femoral artery
conjoined tendon
vas deferens
hernia sac (ligated)
cremasteric fibers (cut)

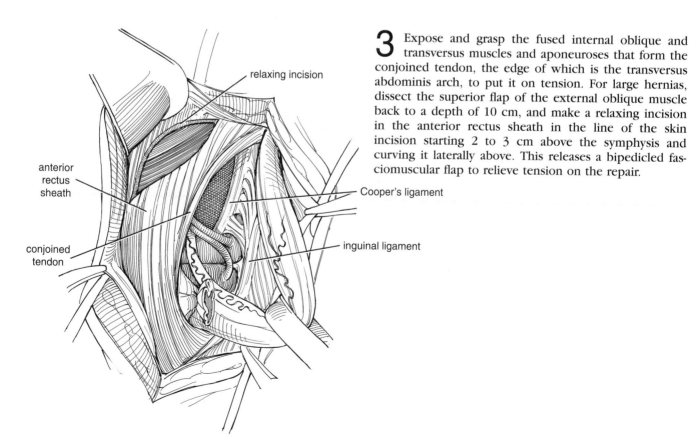

relaxing incision
anterior rectus sheath
conjoined tendon
Cooper's ligament
inguinal ligament

3 Expose and grasp the fused internal oblique and transversus muscles and aponeuroses that form the conjoined tendon, the edge of which is the transversus abdominis arch, to put it on tension. For large hernias, dissect the superior flap of the external oblique muscle back to a depth of 10 cm, and make a relaxing incision in the anterior rectus sheath in the line of the skin incision starting 2 to 3 cm above the symphysis and curving it laterally above. This releases a bipedicled fasciomuscular flap to relieve tension on the repair.

4 Grasp the edge of the conjoined tendon in an Allis clamp to manipulate it. Retract the cord inferolaterally. Starting distally, place a succession of 1-0 NAS swaged on short heavy curved needles through the edge of the conjoined tendon and then through Cooper's ligament.

Alternative: Pass the sutures through the more superficially lying iliopubic tract. In this case, take care not to penetrate the adjacent deep circumflex iliac vessels. If the iliopubic tract is poorly developed, run the suture through some of the inguinal ligament as well. Hold the sutures in a clamp.

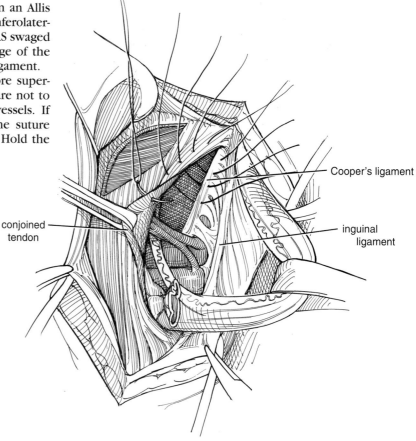

Cooper's ligament

conjoined tendon

inguinal ligament

5 Continue the closure cephalad to the end of Cooper's ligament by placing the sutures from the conjoined tendon into the anterior femoral fascia and then the inguinal ligament, leaving enough room for the cord to exit from the proximal end.

6 Tie the sutures beginning distally. Tack the edges of the relaxing incision to the internal oblique muscle with 3-0 SAS.

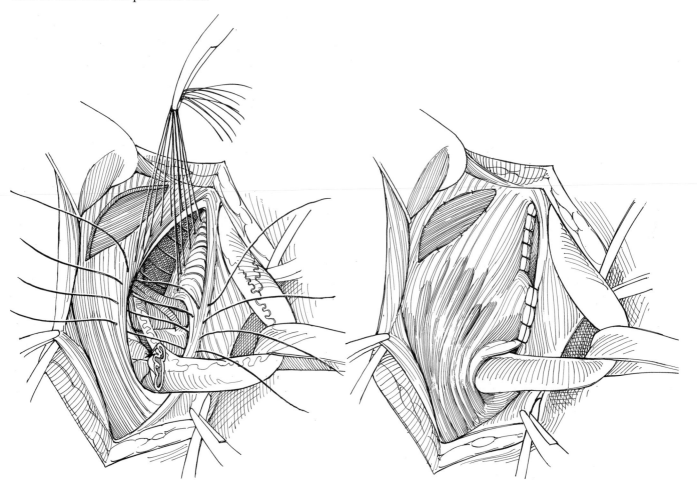

7 Close the external oblique fascia over the cord with interrupted 2-0 silk sutures, leaving a relaxed external ring. Close Scarpa's fascia with interrupted 4-0 SAS and the skin with a continuous subcuticular suture of the same material. Be certain, especially in children, to draw the testis into the proper position in the scrotum to prevent iatrogenic ascent. Inadvertent *vasal transection* should be repaired at once by microsurgical vasovasostomy (see pages 323 to 325).

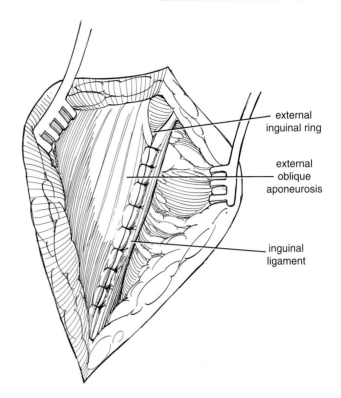

external inguinal ring

external oblique aponeurosis

inguinal ligament

Commentary by Eric W. Fonkalsrud

The purpose of the surgical repair of an indirect inguinal hernia is to anatomically correct the indirect hernia in the most efficient and effective manner while avoiding the creation of a direct inguinal hernia or injury to inguinal structures during the process. The vast majority of patients with an indirect inguinal hernia do not have a concomitant direct hernia. Thus, the essential features of indirect hernia repair should be high ligation of the indirect hernia sac while minimizing injury to the structures in the inguinal canal. It is not necessary to excise the entire hernia sac in the majority of patients. Resection of any portion of the hernia sac inferior to the pubis increases the risk of scrotal edema, hemorrhage, and pain while serving no useful purpose. Occlusion of the sac at the level of the internal ring with at least two nonabsorbable transfixion sutures is adequate for almost all patients. More extensive downward traction on the hernia sac to obtain a high ligation may result in traction on the bladder with risk of injury. Thus, a very high ligation increases the risk of injury to vital structures while providing no useful benefit in the repair.

The safest and easiest approach to the inguinal canal is incision of the external oblique aponeurosis in the direction of the fibers directly through the external inguinal ring. The mobilization of the hernia sac from the spermatic vessels and vas deferens may be performed in most patients with gentle forceps dissection. It is not necessary to mobilize the spermatic cord extensively from the inguinal canal. The cremaster muscles may be safely preserved during the dissection of the hernia sac from the cord structures because collateral blood flow to the cord accompanies these muscle fibers. In the course of repair of an indirect inguinal hernia, it is very rarely necessary to open the transversalis fascia and structures in the posterior wall of the inguinal canal.

In my experience, perhaps one of the most useful technical aspects in the repair of an indirect inguinal hernia in adults is to reef together the transversalis fascia with NAS to strengthen the posterior wall of the inguinal canal and reduce the risk of direct hernia. The tediously extensive Cooper's ligament repair is necessary only for femoral hernia that extends beneath the inguinal ligament, which is uncommon. Direct inguinal hernias are most likely to occur in the lateral aspect of the inguinal canal; thus, Cooper's ligament repair, which provides support to the narrow angle adjacent to the pubis, is rarely necessary. Furthermore, the tissues immediately beneath the medial aspect of the inguinal canal are almost always the retroperitoneal structures, usually the bladder. Bladder herniation is extremely uncommon from the medial aspect of the inguinal canal in patients with indirect inguinal hernias.

A relaxing incision in the anterior rectus sheath may be helpful for patients who have recurrent hernias, those who are obese, or those who have large direct inguinal hernias. For the vast majority of patients with an indirect inguinal hernia, however, this step is rarely necessary. Approximation of the internal oblique muscle to the shelving edge of the inguinal ligament posterior to the spermatic cord (Bassini repair) or over the spermatic cord (Ferguson repair) is adequate for the repair of the vast majority of patients with indirect inguinal hernias. More extensive repair in the medial aspect of the inguinal canal is likely to increase the amount of postoperative scrotal swelling and inguinal discomfort as well as cause the patient to ambulate in a hunched-over position, while not enhancing the surgical repair.

Preperitoneal Inguinal Herniorrhaphy

OPEN REPAIR FOR INDIRECT INGUINAL HERNIA

Perform this repair in conjunction with open prostatectomy or following pelvic lymph node dissection.

1 Consider the anatomic relationships viewed from inside the right pelvis. Removal of the transversalis fascia exposes the rectus abdominis and transversus abdominis muscles, the latter being the layer involved in both the formation and the repair of inguinal hernias. The spermatic cord and vas deferens are shown in Step 3A, next to which the indirect inguinal hernia sac is found.

The *conjoined tendon* is formed from fusion of the lowest fibers of the transversus abdominis aponeurosis, with some from the internal oblique. It begins on the lateral part of the inguinal ligament such that the tendon becomes the roof of the inguinal canal as it arches over it as the *transversus abdominis arch*, the inferior edge of the transversus abdominis muscle, to attach to the pubic crest and the pectineal line. Localization and identification of this arch are critical to successful preperitoneal hernia repair.

The *pectineal (Cooper's) ligament* lies along the pectineal line on the periosteum of the superior ramus of the pubis. The aponeurosis of the transversus abdominis and the iliopubic tract insert along the pectineal line next to the medial half of the pectineal ligament.

The *iliopubic tract* (sometimes called the anterior femoral sheath) appears as the thickened fibrous lower border of the transversalis fascia that runs caudal to and parallel with the inguinal ligament. From within the pelvis, only the iliopubic tract is visible.

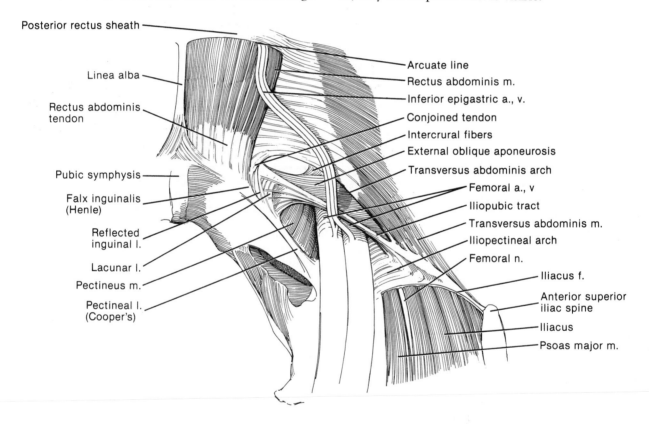

Posterior rectus sheath
Linea alba
Rectus abdominis tendon
Pubic symphysis
Falx inguinalis (Henle)
Reflected inguinal l.
Lacunar l.
Pectineus m.
Pectineal l. (Cooper's)

Arcuate line
Rectus abdominis m.
Inferior epigastric a., v.
Conjoined tendon
Intercrural fibers
External oblique aponeurosis
Transversus abdominis arch
Femoral a., v
Iliopubic tract
Transversus abdominis m.
Iliopectineal arch
Femoral n.
Iliacus f.
Anterior superior iliac spine
Iliacus
Psoas major m.

2 *Position:* Place the patient supine and slightly hyperextended over the break in the table.

Incision: The hernia repair may be a part of another operation, such as suprapubic or retropubic prostatectomy. For an independent procedure, use a shorter midline extraperitoneal or a transverse lower abdominal incision. Stand opposite the involved side. Place a flat, broad abdominal retractor on the affected side so that the assistant can elevate the rectus abdominis muscle and anterior abdominal wall. Retract the preperitoneal fat and peritoneum away from the anterior abdominal wall in the infe-

rior part of the incision to gain an interior view of the inguinal area. Expose the hernia sac as it extends from the peritoneum and through the internal inguinal ring. Insinuate a finger under the neck of the sac, including the spermatic cord. Run a Penrose drain around the neck, and use blunt dissection to pull the whole hernia sac into the preperitoneal space. In most cases, the hernia sac and preperitoneal fat can be mobilized off the spermatic cord with blunt dissection alone. In more complicated cases, an incision into the peritoneum is helpful to delineate the sac.

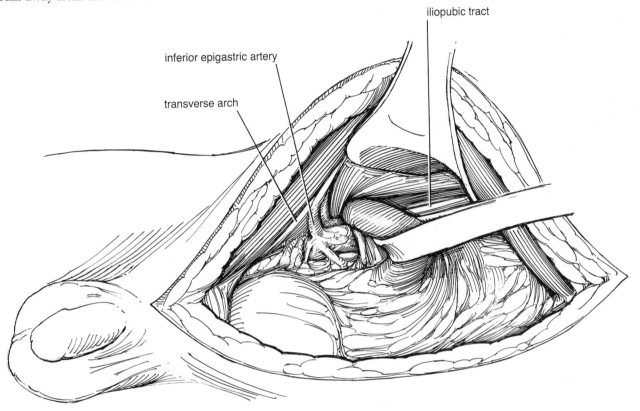

iliopubic tract

inferior epigastric artery

transverse arch

3 **A,** Separate the sac from the cord structures lying below it, and open it with scissors between clamps. **B,** Insert a finger in the opened sac to facilitate freeing it from the cord. If the sac extends distally, do not hesitate to divide it and leave that portion in place. **C,** Grasp the edges of the sac with clamps, and close the neck with a 4-0 silk purse-string suture. Trim any excess peritoneum from the sac.

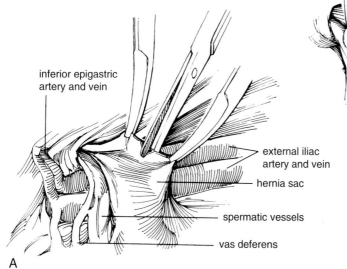

inferior epigastric artery and vein

external iliac artery and vein

hernia sac

spermatic vessels

vas deferens

A

B

C

4 Place clamps on the edges of the internal ring, and retract the cord medially. Palpate both the iliopubic tract along the inferior margin of the ring and the iliac vessels lying posteromedially. They may be exposed by displacing the overlying fat. If feasible, identify and preserve the deep inferior epigastric vessels just medial to the canal. Identify the iliopubic tract and place two or three 2-0 polypropylene sutures in it. Identify the transversus abdominis arch medial to the cord as a distinct ridge in the ring. It may help to grasp it with Allis forceps. Pass the sutures through the arch and tie them. Move the cord medially and place several similar sutures in the tract and arch lateral to the cord. Pass a curved clamp beside the cord to be certain that the vascularity of the cord is not compromised. Close the wound appropriately, or continue with prostatectomy or other operation.

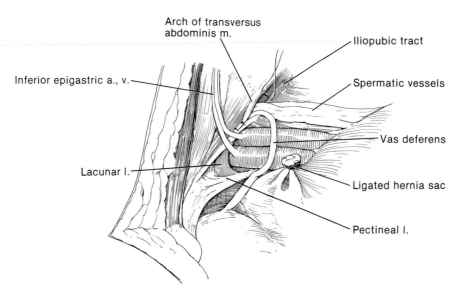

Arch of transversus abdominis m.

Iliopubic tract

Inferior epigastric a., v.

Spermatic vessels

Vas deferens

Lacunar l.

Ligated hernia sac

Pectineal l.

Commentary by Peter N. Schlegel

Preperitoneal repair of an inguinal hernia during simultaneous urologic procedures is an important addition to the surgical armamentarium of the urologist. Several considerations are important to successful repair. Both indirect and direct hernias may be repaired. However, simultaneous repair of multiple defects may cause excessive tension on the repair and/or midline abdominal incision, predisposing to incisional hernia formation or hernia recurrence. Therefore, multiple repairs should be avoided. The critical feature for repair of an indirect hernia is the accurate identification and incorporation of the transversus arch. The arch is not just the superior edge of the transversus abdominis muscle coursing over the internal ring that is covered by transversalis fascia. Therefore, the arch is typically not directly seen on internal inspection of the ring. The arch is best located by passing the index finger of the surgeon's hand corresponding to the affected inguinal ring (right index finger for an indirect right inguinal hernia) well through the ring lateral to the spermatic cord. The finger can then be hooked anteriorly toward the anterior abdominal wall. With this maneuver, the thick cord of the arch is easily palpated. I prefer to place one or two Allis clamps on the arch to facilitate suture placement. The arch, of course, is confluent with the conjoined tendon. Failure to localize the arch is likely to lead to recurrence of the hernia and is frequently associated with painful entrapment of the ilioinguinal or lateral femoral cutaneous nerves. Accurate identification of the involved structures allows rapid (two or three figure-eight sutures) and simple repair of an indirect inguinal hernia via the preperitoneal approach.

LAPAROSCOPIC REPAIR FOR INDIRECT INGUINAL HERNIA

The laparoscopic approach is essentially the same as described for the open preperitoneal hernia repair.

Required are general anesthesia, a nasogastric tube, and a urethral catheter. Prosthetic materials (prosthetic plug) are used with their attendant risk of infection. Laparoscopy also carries some risk of hemorrhage or bowel injury. It is not suitable for incarcerated or strangulated hernias, or after pelvic radiation or surgery. On the other hand, the cord structures are less likely to be injured and the patient is happy to be spared an incision. In general, open operation is preferred for initial repair, reserving the laparoscopic approach for recurrences and bilateral repairs.

Initiate pneumoperitoneum. Insert a 10-mm trocar just above the umbilicus and insert two 10- to 11-mm trocars on either side of the umbilicus at a distance of 5 cm.

5 Make a short curved incision lateral to the internal ring. Extend it medially as a transverse incision immediately below the semicircular line of Douglas. Develop a posterior peritoneal flap to expose the inferior epigastric vessels. Identify the internal inguinal ring. Dissect the sac bluntly from the underlying tissues and from the cord, and invert it by grasping its apex with a toothed grasper while pushing the surrounding tissue back with forceps along the anteromedial side to avoid the cord structures. Locate the pubic tubercle and Cooper's ligament by following the lateral border of the rectus abdominis. The iliopubic tract is seen attached to the tubercle and ligament as it continues laterally to form the medial margin of the femoral canal and the lower margin of the inguinal ring.

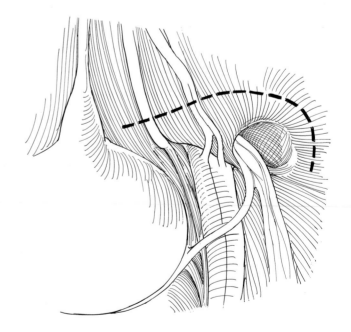

6 **A** and **B,** Cut an 8 × 10 cm patch of polypropylene mesh and roll it so that it may be drawn into a 10-mm reducing sleeve. Insert the sleeve in the ipsilateral sheath, and place the mesh in the hernia defect. Unroll it with nontoothed grasping forceps, and spread it to reach from the midline over the inferior epigastric vessels and lateral to the internal ring, as well as from below the semilunar line to below Cooper's ligament. Do not hesitate to use a second patch if the first does not cover the defect. Staple the mesh using 15 to 20 staples to Cooper's ligament and peripherally around the previously dissected area. If a staple is to be placed in the iliopubic tract, insert an instrument beneath the tract to avoid injury to the underlying femoral nerve. Hold the edges of the peritoneum together over the mesh with toothed forceps, and place staples to extraperitonealize it. Reducing intra-abdominal pressure helps bring the edges together. Evacuate the gas and remove the trocars in sequence.

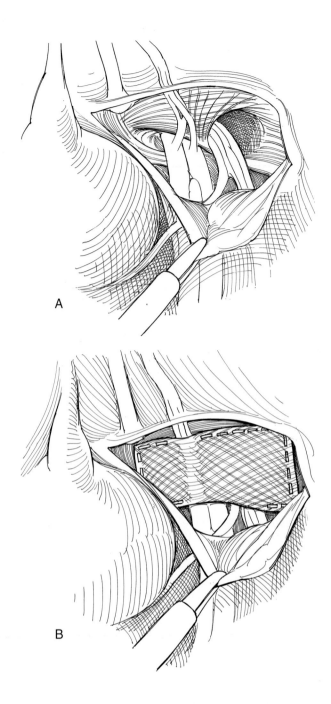

Reduction of Testis Torsion

Warn the patient and his family of possible loss of the testis. Use Doppler ultrasonography if it is available, but do not delay the surgery. In the newborn, in whom the chance for salvage is small and the risk of operation is appreciable, color Doppler imaging can rule out other potential pathologic conditions and avoid an operation at this time (Cartwright et al, 1995). Allopurinol administered at the time of detorsion may reduce reperfusion injury (Akgür et al, 1994).

Manual Detorsion. If an operating room is not immediately available, consider manual detorsion after a lidocaine cord block (see page 76). Rotate the testis from within outward. This maneuver is useful in adolescent boys, who have intravaginal torsion, but is not suitable for newborns, in whom the torsion is extravaginal.

1 *Position:* Place the patient supine. Prepare the entire genital area. Block the cord with 1 percent lidocaine where it courses over the symphysis (see page 76). In younger children, provide general anesthesia, aspirating the stomach if necessary.

Incision: Grasp the scrotum with the thumb and index finger, and press the testis forward. The scrotum may be edematous. Make a short transverse midscrotal incision. Continue the incision to the tunica vaginalis, which may appear darkened from contained bloody serum.

2 Open the tunica vaginalis, evacuate the accumulated hydrocele fluid, and extrude the testis. Observe its color after untwisting it clockwise on the right, counterclockwise on the left. Wrap it in warm saline sponges and observe it for 10 or 15 minutes (use the time to fix the contralateral testis to the scrotal wall). If the hydrocele fluid was sanguinous and the testis remains dark, consider excising it. First incise the tunica albuginea; if bleeding is not seen and if seminiferous tubules cannot be identified, remove the testis if the other one is normal to palpation and inspection. A prosthesis may replace it, but at a later time. The neonatal testis typically is infarcted and should be removed.

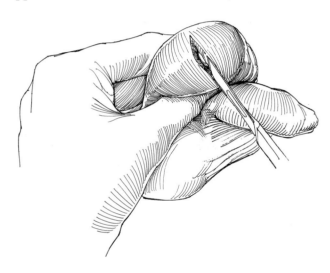

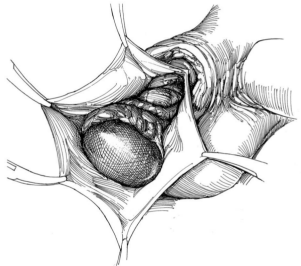

3 If the testis is to remain, trim the excess tunica vaginalis. Obtain hemostasis along the edge with thorough fulguration, keeping the testis well grounded against the scrotum.

4 Place two or three interrupted 3-0 SAS in the cut edges of the tunica vaginalis to approximate the edges behind the testis and obliterate a potential hydrocele sac.

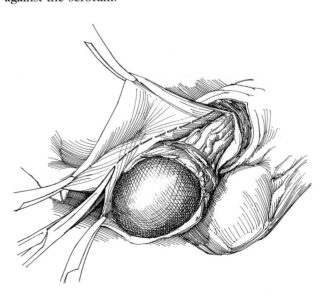

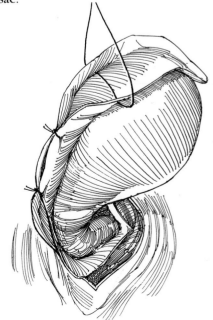

5 Invert the scrotal septum into the wound with a finger inserted from the opposite side, and fix the tunica albuginea to the septum in three places, even though this carries some risk of interfering with the intratesticular blood supply. Because of the intragonadal distribution of the arteries in the tunica vasculosa, the sutures should be placed from either the medial or the lateral aspect of the superior pole where the vascularity is sparse, not from the well-vascularized anterior surface. Use interrupted mattress 3-0 NAS and tie them after all have been inserted. Unless hemostasis is perfect, pass a clamp up through the bottom of the scrotum, incise over its tip, and draw a small Penrose drain out through the opening. Close the dartos layer with figure-eight 3-0 SAS and the skin with a 4-0 or 5-0 subcuticular SAS. Suture the drain in place. Place a dry dressing covered by a scrotal supporter.

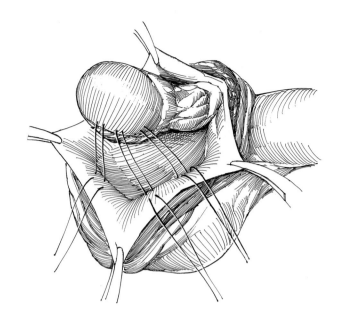

Contralateral Fixation. In all cases, anchor the contralateral testis by opening the tunica vaginalis and fixing that testis to the scrotal septum in the same way as the abnormal one. Alternatively, bring the testis into a *dartos pouch* (see page 312) for fixation (Redman and Barthold, 1995). Open the tunica vaginalis and extrude the testis. Place a few 5-0 SAS at the upper end of the cord to close the now-open tunica vaginalis along the cranial aspect of the cord. Include some of the internal spermatic fascia in the stitches. Develop a scrotal pouch by grasping the skin and dartos layer with toothed forceps, and start the dissection between the dartos and the external spermatic fascia with clamps, beginning with a mosquito clamp. If necessary, enlarge the pouch digitally. Tack the cut edge of the external spermatic fascia to the tunica vaginalis covering the cord. Insert the testis back into the pouch with the aid of U.S. Army retractors. Close the dartos with a running 5-0 SAS that catches a bite of tunic, and close the skin with a running subcuticular suture.

Alternative Approach (Peters). Incise the scrotum in the midline, and place a traction suture on either end of the septum. Open the tunica vaginalis over the involved testis first. If it is to be saved, place three NAS between the tunica albuginea and the septum. Repeat the procedure on the normal side. Close the tunica vaginalis and dartos layers vertically with a running suture. Close the skin.

POSTOPERATIVE PROBLEMS

Hematoma is rare. *Retorsion* can occur; absorbable sutures may be a factor. *Fertility* could be affected if an ischemic testis is left in place.

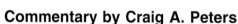

Commentary by Craig A. Peters

The most useful tool in managing the acute scrotum is a high index of suspicion; a few negative explorations are better than one missed torsion. Once a decision is made that testicular torsion is present, manual detorsion is seldom needed and may inadvertently serve to delay definitive treatment. Neonatal torsion is explored promptly at our institution as a result of experience with several synchronous and metachronous contralateral torsions.

I have found a single midline incision to be most practical in scrotal exploration for torsion. It provides access to both testes, permits effective exposure of the midline scrotal septum, and may be closed with a single suture line. I have not made a practice of resecting any tunica vaginalis. As indicated, placement of the fixation stitches is most effective with the testes out of the scrotum and the fixation stitches placed into the septum. I prefer to place three stitches in a vertical orientation. Care is taken to maintain the anatomic orientation of the testis for these sutures. During closure it is essential to perform an everting skin closure.

In the neonate, an inguinal incision is usually used in the event of a tumor unappreciated on physical examination. Although they are uncommon, we have seen two in the last 2 years.

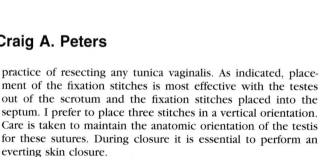

Correction of Hydrocele

The plication technique of Lord is the most effective technique for an acquired hydrocele because the dissection creates minimal interference with the surrounding loose scrotal tissues. An everting technique requires delivery of the sac from the scrotum, with appreciably more dissection of tissue planes and hence greater chance for formation of a hematoma and recurrence. In a child with a communicating hydrocele that persists longer than 24 months, plan a short transverse incision over the external ring to locate and divide the processus vaginalis, tying only the proximal end.

PLICATION TECHNIQUE
(Lord)

Instruments: Provide at least eight small Allis forceps, a Weitlaner retractor, and 4-0 SAS and 4-0 CCG sutures on half-circle needles.

Position: Place the patient supine. Prepare the lower abdomen and scrotum.

A right-handed surgeon stands on the right side of the table. Pull the testis down to relax the cremaster, and grasp the cord with the left hand, placing the thumb in front and the index finger behind the cord at the top of the scrotum. With the needle approaching the index finger, infiltrate the cord with 1 percent lidocaine solution without epinephrine through a 2.5-inch, 25-gauge needle.

1 Grasp the hydrocele in the left hand and press it anteriorly to stretch the skin firmly over the hydrocele and compress the scrotal vessels. Select a site opposite that of the contained testis and make a 4-cm transverse incision between the visible scrotal vessels. Carry it through the dartos layer down *to* the surface of the tunica vaginalis. Fulgurate any small vessels exposed in the thin dartos layer.

2 Grasp the full thickness of the incised tissue down on the tunica vaginalis, including the skin, subcutaneous tissue, and dartos, in three or four Allis forceps on each side. By keeping the scrotal tissues under tension with the left hand, each Allis forceps can be placed to evert and compress the cut edge, thus controlling any bleeding and, more importantly, preventing dissection among the layers. Release the pressure on the scrotum. At this point, digitally separate the tunica vaginalis from the dartos layer to provide a subdartos pouch large enough to hold the testis after repair.

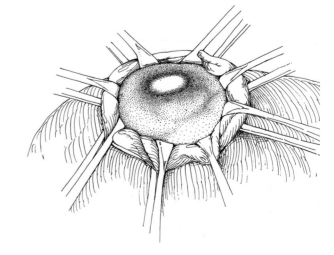

3 Holding the suction tip nearby, incise the tunica vaginalis and evacuate the hydrocele fluid. Expand the opening with scissors and squeeze the testis out. Inspect and palpate it. Lift the testis away from the scrotum to put the tunica vaginalis on stretch. Plicate the peritoneal surface of the tunica vaginalis with 4-0 SAS. Do this by picking up the free edge of the tunica with the needle and every centimeter take a small bite of the shiny surface held up by fine-toothed forceps, until the junction with the tunica albuginea of the testis is reached. Tie the suture.

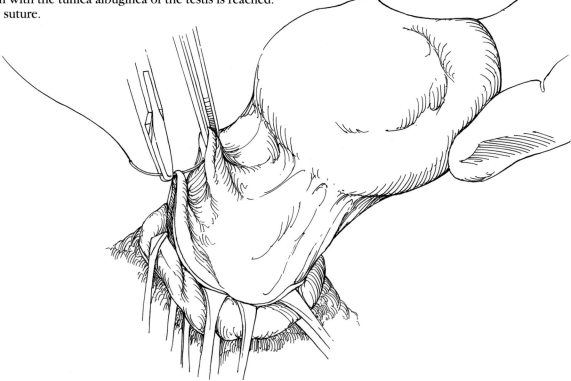

4 Repeat the suturing at intervals around the circumference of the testis, placing six to eight sutures in all. Replace the testis in the scrotum by squeezing it into the pocket beneath the dartos layer, with the aid of a flat, malleable retractor.

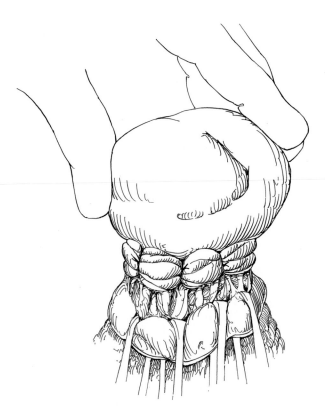

5 Place interrupted sutures of 3-0 CCG that include full-thickness skin, dartos, and all the areolar tissue as you remove each pair of Allis forceps while rotating the next pair to expose the subcutaneous tissue. Each suture obliterates the local subcutaneous space. Traction on the ends of the wound with two towel clips may help with the eversion. Place a sheet of treated gauze and several 4 × 4 inch sponges over the wound and apply an athletic supporter to provide some compression. Drainage is not necessary because only a small subcutaneous-fascial space has been opened.

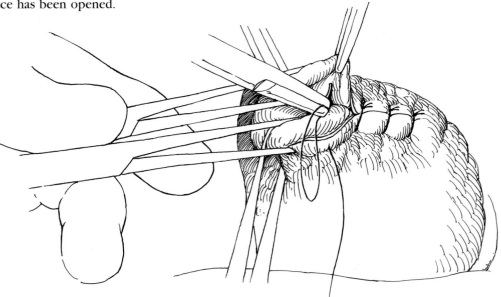

POSTOPERATIVE PROBLEMS

Hematoma formation is rare if the entire thickness of the scrotal wall is included in the Allis forceps during the incision and then in the sutures at closure. *Recurrence* of the hydrocele is likewise rare because the operation leaves no dead space for a seroma to form, around which the peritoneal lining can regenerate.

Commentary by Warren H. Chapman

For a procedure as straightforward as the repair of a hydrocele appears to be, a surprising divergence of opinion exists on how it may best be done. The Lord technique described here is probably the simplest for the smaller hydrocele because it involves less dissection and therefore less postoperative edema and hematoma. With larger and/or thicker hydroceles, the mass created by the sutures can become excessively bulky, some-times permanently so. This requires dissection of some portion of the parietal tunica vaginalis. I find that the most common complaint of patients is the amount of postoperative swelling; that is minimized by very careful placement of the suture immediately below the single layer of parietal tunic, with special care as it approaches the pampiniform plexus, shown so well in Step 4.

Varicocele Ligation

Palpate the spermatic cord while the patient is erect and doing a Valsalva maneuver. A venogram may be useful in some cases. The Doppler probe can help provide confirmation. Proceed to varicocele ligation if dilated veins are detected in a patient who is infertile without other cause.

1 The veins draining the testis, epididymis, and vas deferens connect with deep and superficial venous networks. The deep venous network has three components: the testicular vein and the pampiniform plexus (labeled A for anterior set), the funicular and deferential veins (labeled M for middle set), and the cremasteric veins (labeled P for posterior set).

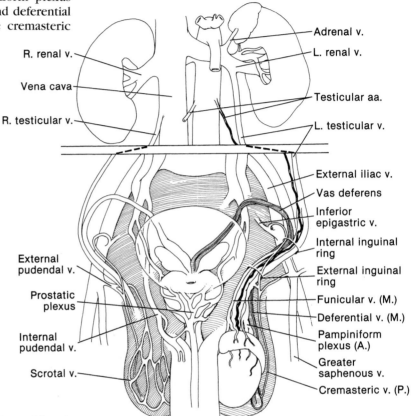

- Adrenal v.
- L. renal v.
- R. renal v.
- Vena cava
- Testicular aa.
- R. testicular v.
- L. testicular v.
- External iliac v.
- Vas deferens
- Inferior epigastric v.
- Internal inguinal ring
- External pudendal v.
- External inguinal ring
- Prostatic plexus
- Funicular v. (M.)
- Deferential v. (M.)
- Internal pudendal v.
- Pampiniform plexus (A.)
- Greater saphenous v.
- Scrotal v.
- Cremasteric v. (P.)

2 Three approaches are currently used: *A*, a subinguinal approach (Marmar); *B*, an inguinal approach (Ivanissevich), in which the spermatic artery is spared; and *C*, an abdominal approach (Palomo), in which the artery may be included in the ligation.

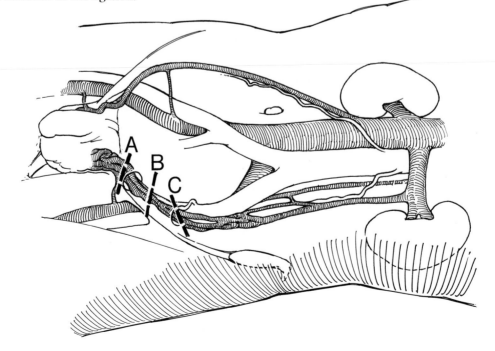

SUBINGUINAL VARICOCELECTOMY
(Marmar)

3 Under intravenous sedation with midazolam hydrochloride (1 mg/ml, up to 3 mg) and fentanyl citrate (50 μg/ml, up to 150 μg), identify the external ring digitally and infiltrate the skin over it with 1 percent lidocaine (Xylocaine) mixed with an equal amount of 0.5 percent bupivacaine (Marcaine). Make a 2- to 3-cm transverse incision directly over the external ring. Continue the incision through the subcutaneous layer and Scarpa's fascia, aided by small retractors. Identify the external inguinal ring and the spermatic cord. Inject the anesthetic agent under the cremasteric fascia with a fine needle to anesthetize the cord, and inject it also at a higher level through the canal, guided by a finger tip in the ring. Grasp the cord with a Babcock clamp, draw it slowly out of the wound, and encircle it with two Penrose drains. Keep the distal one tight to stabilize the cord, but leave the proximal one loose to maintain the superficial blood supply. Alternatively, place a tongue depressor under the cord. Clip or tie any dilated posterior cremasteric veins. Open the external spermatic fascia. With the aid of a 3.5× optical loupe or an operating microscope set at 6× to 10× magnification, identify the spermatic veins as part of the pampiniform plexus and dissect them free in groups. Displace the vas deferens and artery, but ligate the veins that accompany them if they are larger than 2 mm. Apply the operating Doppler probe to identify and avoid the spermatic artery. Preserve the lymphatics. Spray the area with 2 to 3 ml of 30 mg/ml of papaverine hydrochoride to relieve vascular spasm. Tie the veins in groups with 2-0 or 3-0 silk. Ask the patient to strain down to fill any missed veins. Close Scarpa's fascia with a single 3-0 CCG suture and the skin with a 4-0 running subcuticular SAS.

The *mini-incision microsurgical subinguinal varicocelectomy* (Goldstein) is an alternative technique that also ensures complete venous ligation. As is done for the subinguinal approach, make a 2- to 3-cm inguinal incision in the skin and the external oblique fascia over the external ring, and dissect and encircle the cord. Then draw the testis out of the wound. Identify and ligate the external spermatic and gubernacular veins, along with any other veins accompanying the gubernaculum. Return the testis to the scrotum, and dissect the veins from the cord itself. Use an operating microscope to ensure ligation of all the small veins except those accompanying the vas deferens. Spare the spermatic artery and adjacent lymphatics.

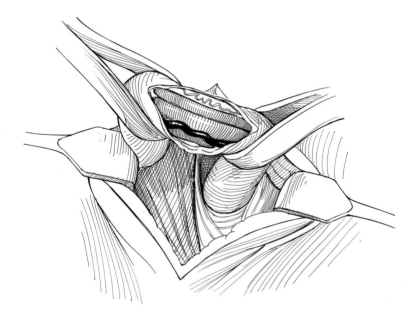

INGUINAL APPROACH
(Ivanissevich)

This approach allows management of the internal spermatic veins where they come off the cord structures at the level of the internal inguinal ring. It is easier than the abdominal approach, especially in the more obese patient, requires less assistance, and can readily be done under local anesthesia.

4 *Position*: Place the patient supine.
Incision: Make a 4- to 5-cm incision two finger-breadths above the symphysis pubis in line with the lateral aspect of the scrotum beginning above the palpable external ring and extending 3 to 4 cm obliquely along the course of the canal. Divide and ligate the superficial epigastric vessels that cross the lower end of the incision.

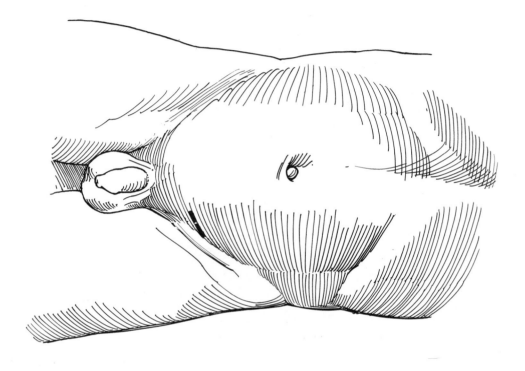

5 Divide Scarpa's fascia, and bluntly clear the connective tissue overlying the external oblique aponeurosis and external ring. Insert a self-retaining retractor. Incise the aponeurosis in the line of its fibers, beginning at the external ring and extending above the internal ring. Avoid the ilioinguinal nerve beneath. Open the external spermatic fascia. Pick up the cord between thumb and forefinger to palpate the vas and artery. Elevate the spermatic fascia with clamps to allow separation of the cord by blunt dissection.

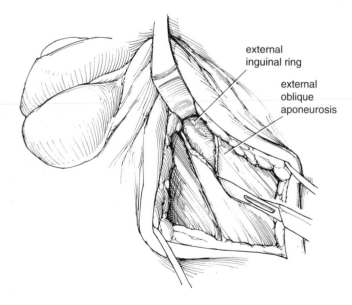

external inguinal ring

external oblique aponeurosis

6 Pass a curved clamp under the cord near the pubic tubercle and draw a Penrose drain or vessel loop through for traction to help mobilize the cord out of the wound. The incision in the internal spermatic fascia is indicated by a dashed line.

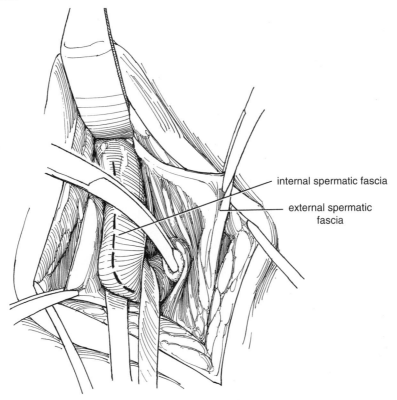

internal spermatic fascia

external spermatic fascia

7 Hold the cord in the wound by fastening the ends of the drain to the drapes on each side. Open the internal spermatic fascia. Sweep the underlying vas back out of the field. Aided by three-power loupes (an alternative is the dissecting microscope) and microvascular forceps, dissect the internal spermatic fascia from each of the (usually) three branches of the spermatic vein from each other and from the more tortuous artery and the lymphatics for 2 to 3 cm in both directions. Drip lidocaine onto the cord to help visualize the artery and the veins. A 3-mm intraoperative Doppler probe helps localize the artery, especially if it has multiple branches. Look for and ligate the cremasteric vein that runs from the spermatic cord to the pudendal vein at the external ring. In addition, the veins accompanying the vas deferens may be ligated.

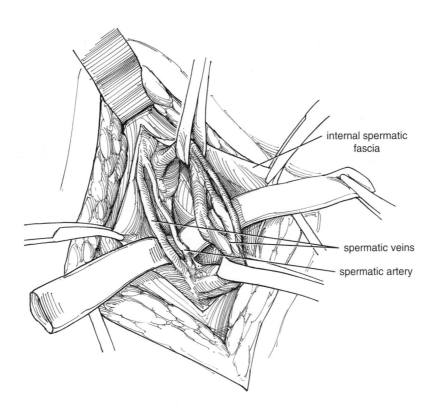

internal spermatic fascia

spermatic veins

spermatic artery

8 Doubly clamp each vein in succession, and ligate each end with a 4-0 silk tie. Tip the patient into the reverse Trendelenburg position to be sure that no veins are overlooked. Elevate the spermatic cord, and check the floor of the canal for any collateral venous branches. Remove the Penrose drain to allow the cord to return to its bed.

9 Close the external oblique fascia with interrupted or running 4-0 SAS, starting laterosuperiorly. Use the last tied suture to elevate the edge for the next stitch. At the external ring, hold the cord down with a peanut dissector while placing the last suture. Close Scarpa's fascia with a few fine sutures, and close the skin subcuticularly with a running suture. Apply a suspensory for support for the scrotum. Advise the patient to avoid activities that cause pain.

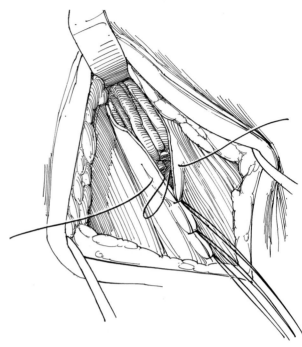

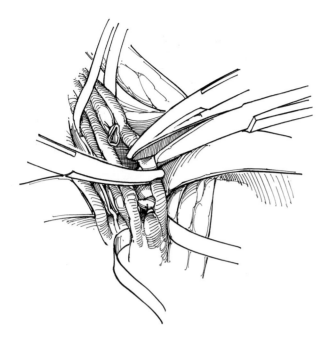

ABDOMINAL APPROACH
(Palomo)

The entire spermatic vascular pedicle can be ligated, ensuring minimal chance for failure. Because the ligation is high, adequate collateral arterial supply remains even though the artery may be included in the ligature. This method is more easily done on slender patients. Because some lymphatics are included in the ligation, hydroceles are more common postoperatively.

Instruments: Provide a basic set; a headlamp; three-power loupes; Sims, Weitlaner, and narrow Deaver retractors; vascular forceps; tenotomy scissors; and peanut dissectors.

Position: Supine, with the head elevated 10 degrees. A

foot plate allows shifting to the reverse Trendelenburg position if this is needed to fill the veins. Prepare the scrotum and lower abdomen. Local anesthesia is often adequate.

Incision: Make a short semioblique incision through the skin and subcutaneous tissue over the site of the internal inguinal ring, starting two fingerbreadths medial to the anterior superior iliac spine. Expose the external oblique aponeurosis. Insert a Weitlaner retractor.

10 Incise the external oblique aponeurosis in the direction of its fibers, taking care to avoid the adherent ilioinguinal nerve beneath it.

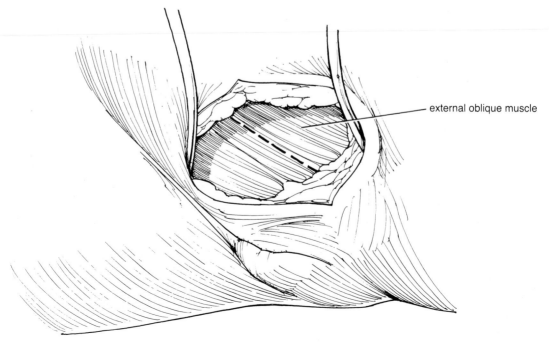

external oblique muscle

11 Separate the internal oblique muscle bluntly by inserting a curved clamp. Retract the internal oblique muscle cranially. Incise the transversus abdominis muscle.

12 Enter the retroperitoneal space 3 to 5 cm above and medial to the inguinal ligament.

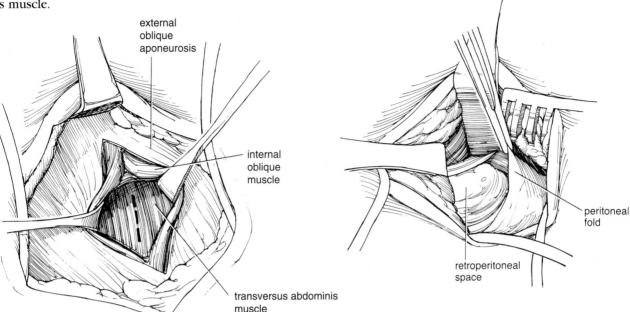

external oblique aponeurosis

internal oblique muscle

transversus abdominis muscle

peritoneal fold

retroperitoneal space

13 Push the peritoneum medially with the peanut dissector, exposing the vessels within the retroperitoneal fat as they rise to join the vas. Pulling on the testis at this point may be helpful in locating the cord structures. Deaver retractors assist in the exposure, but a retractor placed medially can hide the spermatic veins adherent to the posterior peritoneum.

14 Place a curved clamp or drain behind the vessels to elevate them into the wound. With loupe magnification, use sharp and blunt dissection to isolate all (usually two) of the flabby veins from the adjacent artery and lymphatic vessels. If the artery is not apparent, skeletonize the cord by bluntly stripping the spermatic fascia. Drip papaverine solution onto the cord to cause the artery to dilate and become visibly pulsatile. Including the artery in the ligature is rarely harmful because adequate collateral circulation comes from vasal and cremasteric vessels. Dripping papaverine solution on the spermatic artery can increase the circulation from the testis, making the veins more obvious. Placing the patient in the reverse Trendelenburg position may fill and help identify smaller veins.

Perform intraoperative venography if identification of all collaterals is in doubt, especially in children. To do this, ligate the largest vein proximally. Tent it up, make a small nick, insert the plastic cannula of an 18-gauge needle, instill contrast medium distally, and expose a film.

Ligate each vein with two silk ties and divide between them. Do not resect a segment of vein, which would require unnecessary pathologic examination. Irrigate the wound, and close each layer of the body wall. Infiltrate the subcutaneous tissue with 0.25 percent mepivacaine for prolonged regional anesthesia. Place a subcuticular 4-0 SAS to close the skin.

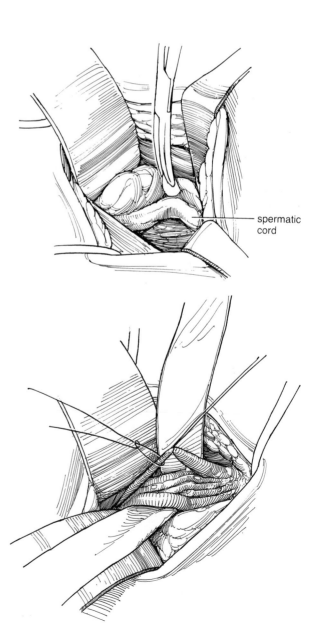

spermatic cord

POSTOPERATIVE PROBLEMS

Damage to the artery can occur with subsequent testicular atrophy. Atrophy is less likely with the retroperitoneal approach. Injury to the vas deferens should be repaired immediately. *Persistent prominence* of the veins may be expected with large varicoceles. However, if examined by color Doppler ultrasonography, usually no reflux flow of venous blood is found through these ectatic veins. *Recurrence* or persistence of the varicocele is not rare, either because a vein was missed or because the varicocele was caused by actual venous obstruction from the so-called nutcracker phenomenon.

Hydroceles presumably develop because of lymphatic obstruction. Although infrequent, they occur more often with low ligation than high ligation unless an operating microscope is used, and more often with open repair than with a laparoscopic technique. The occasional patient may note a *dull ache* in the testis on the operated side for a week or two after surgery, which usually resolves without treatment. It is most likely secondary to venous congestion within the testis from the ligation. As the venous drainage becomes rerouted, the discomfort passes.

Check semen quality in 6 months.

Commentary by Paul J. Turek

For varicocele repair, many surgeons prefer not to inject anesthetic into the spermatic cord, as this increases the risk of hematoma and arterial injury. Other options include general anesthesia and an iliac crest regional block with 0.5 percent bupivacaine. The iliac crest block of the hypogastric and ilioinguinal nerves (see page 77) is performed using a 22-gauge, 3.5-inch spinal needle and delivers excellent testis and cord anesthesia. The block involves the injection of 10 ml of anesthetic in the area of the internal ring, 2 cm medial and 2 cm caudal to the palpable anterior superior iliac spine. As the needle is pushed down through the skin and deeper tissues, a pop occurs as the external oblique layer is penetrated. After aspiration is done to ensure that the needle is not intravascular, half of the anesthetic is placed below the fascia and the other half above.

There are several ways to identify the testicular artery in these dissections. Dilute papaverine topically applied to the vessels helps visualize arterial pulsations, usually without requiring magnification. A 3-mm high-frequency (24-mHz) Doppler probe can also be used to get an audible arterial signal. Lastly, under the high magnification possible with a microscope, most arterial pulsations are visible without Doppler imaging or papaverine. Beware of arterial ligation in the inguinal and subinguinal approaches, as the testicular artery becomes an end-artery without collateralization in this region.

The subinguinal repair, unlike the other approaches, does not involve a fascial incision, as the cord is dissected below its exit from the external ring. I have found that this reduces the amount of postoperative pain that the patient experiences and thus hastens return to normal activity. With the inguinal approach, an enlarged vein is usually found on either side of the artery and another, separate enlarged vein within the cord. Two smaller veins are usually adherent to the vas deferens, but these are only infrequently enlarged to greater than 2 mm. If these vasal veins are to be ligated, consider using a microtip bipolar electrocautery to ablate them. With the abdominal approach, a muscle-splitting approach to the internal oblique and transversus abdominis muscles can be used with a curved clamp to quickly expose the retroperitoneal fat and testicular vessels. I use the abdominal approach when varicoceles recur after a lower approach or if there is evidence of prior inguinal surgery.

Laparoscopic Varicocele Ligation

The indications for laparoscopic rather than open ligation of varicoceles have not been agreed upon. General anesthesia is required, and the peritoneal cavity must be entered with the accompanying risk of vascular or visceral injury. External spermatic veins are not ligated with this approach and the lymphatics are spared, but postoperative pain is not significantly reduced and the time for convalescence is similar to that for low ligation. The patient must be well informed of risks and benefits.

Instruments: An electrocoagulating scissors (endoshears), a needle-tip grasper, a wave grasper, a dissector (endodissector), a suction-irrigation device, and a Doppler probe for identification of the testicular artery are needed. Provide papaverine or lidocaine solutions.

The details for initiating laparoscopy are described on pages 21 to 25. For varicocele ligation, use the open technique with a Hasson cannula to insufflate the peritoneal cavity and thus reduce the chance for vascular or bowel injury, complications not seen with other approaches to varicocele ligation.

Place an 11-mm video port just below the umbilicus, an 11-mm instrument port in the contralateral side slightly below the umbilical port lateral to the rectus muscle, and a 5-mm port in a similar position on the opposite side. Stand on the right and manipulate through the right and left ports. The assistant, holding the laparoscope, views a mirror image of the procedure on the monitor at the foot of the table unless a second monitor is provided. Rotate the table to elevate the affected side, and initiate a 15- to 30-degree Trendelenburg position.

1 Be familiar with the structures lying retroperitoneally. Identify the internal ring by following the vas deferens distally to the internal ring where it comes together with the spermatic cord. Move the sigmoid colon medially; freeing it may be necessary. Compress the scrotum, and observe the filling of the spermatic veins. Try to identify the spermatic artery before its manipulation results in arterial spasm. Plan a T-incision lateral to the cord *(dashed lines)*.

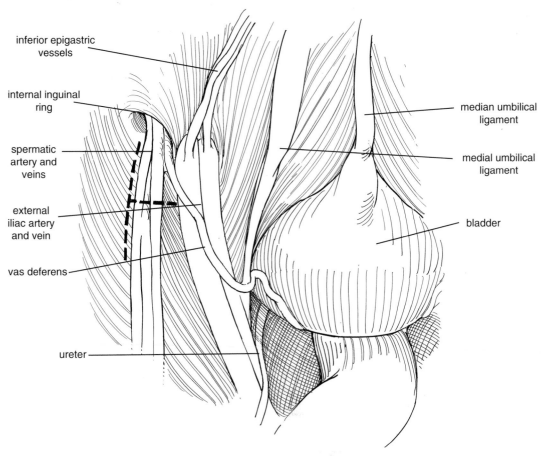

inferior epigastric vessels

internal inguinal ring

spermatic artery and veins

external iliac artery and vein

vas deferens

ureter

median umbilical ligament

medial umbilical ligament

bladder

2 Grasp the peritoneum approximately 5 cm proximal to the internal ring and slightly lateral to the spermatic vessels with grasping forceps passed through the left port. With laparoscopic scissors passed through the ipsilateral port, make a short incision first distally, then proximally to expose the vessels. Elevate the medial edge and incise a T extending to the edge of the iliac artery. Pull on the testis to identify veins adjacent to the spermatic pedicle that could allow recurrence. With a straight grasping instrument in combination with a curved dissector, free the vessels from the retroperitoneal connective tissue and the psoas muscle.

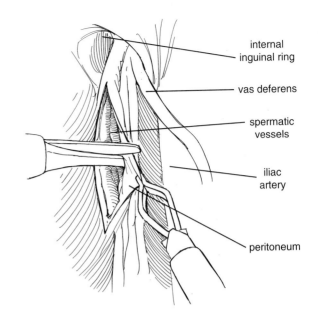

internal inguinal ring

vas deferens

spermatic vessels

iliac artery

peritoneum

3 With two graspers, bluntly dissect the three to eight veins into multiple bundles while separating the spermatic artery from them. Traction on the testis helps identify the vessels. Avoid electrocoagulation near the delicate pedicle. Elevate the venous bundles, and push the spermatic artery out of the way with a dissector. Vasospasm may make identification of the artery difficult; it can be reduced by dripping papaverine or lidocaine through an aspirator-irrigator. A Doppler probe helps identify the spermatic artery. If dissection is difficult, inject a few milliliters of saline solution through the suction-irrigation device to hydraulically separate the vessels. For the larger veins, place two 9-mm titanium vaso-occlusive endoclips proximally and two distally on each venous bundle. Cut the veins between the paired clips with endoshears. Smaller veins may still be present around the artery. Tease them away and clip them, or fulgurate them with a fine electrosurgical probe and then divide them with endoshears. A safer alternative to clip-

ping the veins may be to fulgurate them with an Nd:YAG contact laser probe, if available. The spermatic artery is easily seen and preserved. Inspect the area to be sure of hemostasis, and check the result by again compressing the scrotum. Place the patient in a reverse Trendelenburg position. Again look for dilated veins as well as for oozing; aspirate any blood or irrigant that may have collected. Remove all but the subumbilical port under direct vision. Place a single SAS in the fascia of the right 11-mm port. Remove the subumbilical port with the laparoscope in place to prevent entrapment of bowel. Tie the stay sutures that held the Hasson sheath after the abdominal cavity is deflated and the scrotum evacuated by compression. Seal the skin incisions with sterile adhesive strips covered with Tegaderm. The large varicoceles of adolescents may resolve slowly postoperatively, and the pampiniform plexus may remain palpable. Hernia repair (see page 338) may be done at the same time as varicocele ligation.

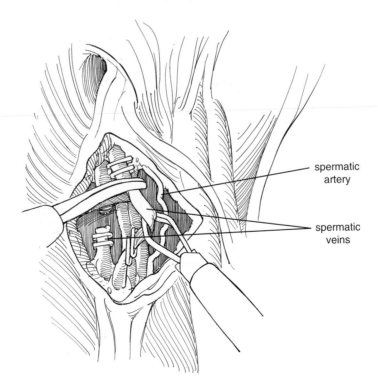

spermatic artery

spermatic veins

Commentary by Keith W. Kaye

Laparoscopic varicocelectomy is a fairly simple procedure and, with care, seems to be an excellent way of introducing surgeons to the field of laparoscopic surgery. I believe it is neither time- nor cost-effective to perform this for unilateral cases, although it may be useful for bilateral varicoceles.

Bilateral varicocele repair: The surgeon stands on the left with the assistant on the right and remains so. An 11-mm port is placed on the left side and a 5-mm port on the right. The assistant holds the camera and laparoscope in the left hand. Dissection is started on the *right varicocele,* as it is easier and has fewer adhesions. The assistant passes the needle-tip grasper through the right port and then elevates the peritoneum just *medial* to the spermatic vessels. This enables the surgeon, using a curved coagulating scissors through the left port, to have straight access for the 5-cm peritoneal incision parallel and medial to the spermatic vessels. Then, after freeing the peritoneum over the vessels, a second cut in the peritoneum from medial to lateral exposes the operative field. Rotating the scissors posteriorly, the medial and lateral borders of the spermatic vessel package are roughly defined without having to separate it completely from the underlying psoas muscle. The assistant then passes a wave grasper and applies countertraction gently on the lateral edge of the areolar tissue surrounding the vessels.

Meanwhile, the surgeon replaces the scissors with an endo-dissector and spreads the package apart. Usually at this stage one or two large veins are seen and carefully dissected. Staying close to the vein wall ensures that no attached artery or lymphatics are present. If difficulty is encountered in differentiating artery from vein, it is extremely useful to have a Doppler probe.

Once the vein is isolated on the curved grasper, the assistant uses a fallopian tube ring grasper to elevate the vein. The surgeon replaces the 5-mm reducer on the 11-mm port with a 10-mm reducer, doubly clips the vein, and transects it. Further veins are similarly dealt with, taking care to leave the artery and lymphatics intact.

For the *left varicocele ligation,* often adhesions are present from the sigmoid colon which needs to be mobilized. A short-cut, once the spermatic vessels are seen, is to stop mobilizing the colon and open the posterior peritoneum as described. The adhesions then simply fall away from the operative site. The only difference on the left side is that, with the surgeon standing on the left, the initial peritoneal incision is made *lateral* to the spermatic vessels and the second T incision passes *medially* from the first incision through the peritoneum over the spermatic vessels.

The key to the success and simplicity of this operation is having the correct instruments, dissecting close to the vein wall, and having the assistant provide good countertraction. The only real pitfall is cutting the testicular artery, which occasionally leads to testicular atrophy, and cutting all the lymphatics, which may result in a hydrocele. Keeping to the above principles, however, should avoid these problems.

Vasoligation

This procedure could be termed *vastomy* (*vas* plus Gr. *tomos*, to cut) because ligation is not essential and vasectomy implies that a section of vas is removed.

Counsel the patient concerning possible irreversibility should he later desire children, and warn him of the small chance of recanalization and the need for follow-up semen examination. Instruct him to take a shower with antibacterial soap. Provide sedation and reassure the patient as you progress with the operation. Minimal trimming of genital hair is needed. Coat the skin overlying the vas with EMLA cream (eutetic mixture of local anesthetics) 0.5 hour before surgery to anesthetize it to receive the towel clip *(scalpel technique)* or ring clamp *(no-scalpel technique)*.

SCALPEL TECHNIQUE

Instruments: Provide two towel clips, two Allis clamps, two curved mosquito clamps, a knife with a #10 blade, 1 percent lidocaine with syringe and 25-gauge needle, needle electrode, one length of 2-0 SAS with a round needle, and one length of 3-0 plain catgut suture with a cutting needle.

Prepare the area with warm solution to prevent scrotal contraction.

1 Stand on the patient's left side and retract the testis with the left hand. Palpate the vas with the right index finger against the first two fingers of the left hand. First digitally separate the vas from the other cord structures; then fix it against two left-hand fingers with the left thumb. Make a superficial skin wheal, and infiltrate the tissues proximal to the vas with 1 percent lidocaine through a 25-gauge needle. Wait 3 minutes. (Alternatively, infiltrate the cord high in the scrotum [see page 76]). Grasp the vas against the fingers of the left hand with a sharp towel clip by first slowly opening it to fit around the vas as it pushes the skin and subcutaneous tissue aside, then closing it around the now isolated vas. Tell the patient that this may be a little painful and add more lidocaine. It is possible, but not as secure, to omit inserting the towel clip, directly incise the skin and sheath transversely, and proceed with Step 3.

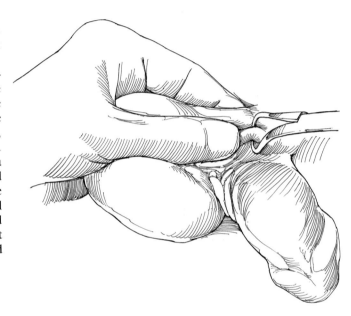

2 Elevate the clamp with the vas. Compress the scrotum on either side between the thumb and forefinger to thin the tissue overlying the vas. Inject more lidocaine under the skin and along the vas. Incise vertically through the skin and the sheath directly onto the white wall of the vas over a distance of 1.5 cm.

3 Apply an Allis clamp open just enough to push the sheath aside with its blades and close it around the vas. If needed, inject more lidocaine proximally. Raise the vas from the wound and free it from its sheath with longitudinal incisions proximally and distally. Reapply the Allis clamp as necessary, but do not remove the towel clip. Dissect beneath the vas with a mosquito clamp to free it from the sheath for a distance of 1.5 cm.

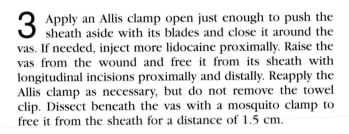

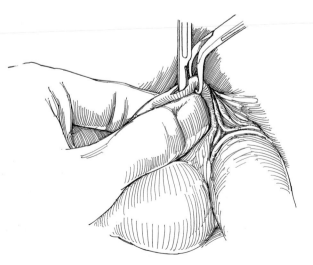

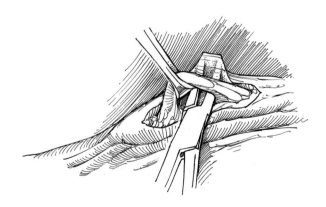

4 Clamp the distal vas with a curved mosquito clamp, and grasp the adventitia of the proximal end with another clamp. Remove the Allis clamp and divide the vas with scissors or a knife. Insert a needle electrode into the lumen of the proximal end and destroy the epithelial lining.

5 Ligate the distal vas with a 2-0 SAS swaged on a needle. Then pass the needle through the tissue deep to the vas, and tie the suture, thus partially burying that end of the vas. Clamp the ends of this suture and cut the long end. Observe for hemostasis and cauterize as needed. If hemostasis is complete, cut the other end of the suture, remove the towel clamp, and allow the ends of the vas to fall inside the scrotum, aided by traction on the testis.

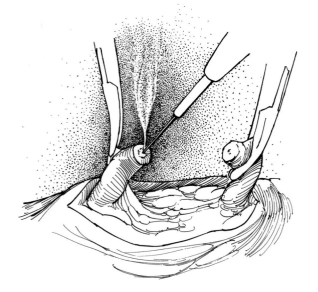

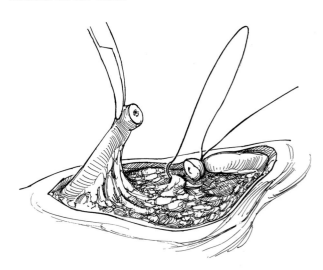

6 Close the skin and subcutaneous tissue in one layer with two 3-0 plain catgut sutures. Apply a scrotal supporter, to be worn for 1 week. After 6 weeks, check the semen on two occasions for the absence of sperm.

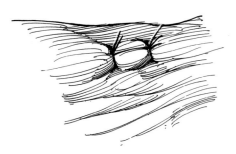

POSTOPERATIVE PROBLEMS

A *hematoma* needs to be evacuated if it is large. *Infection* is usually superficial and drains spontaneously. *Persistent fertility* is the most serious complication. In practice, tell the patient to abstain from unprotected intercourse for 6 weeks, then to bring in a semen specimen for you to look at under the microscope for motile and nonmotile sperm. If any sperm are seen, repeat the examination 2 weeks later. Persistence of sperm beyond 2 or 3 months indicates either recanalization or a technical error and requires bilateral reoperation, preferably at sites on the vasa proximal to the previous ones. A *sperm granuloma* may form if the epithelium in the proximal vas is not destroyed by fulguration. Do not intervene unless the granuloma continues to cause pain. If pain persists, evacuate the granuloma and recauterize the vas.

Commentary by Stanwood S. Schmidt

Counsel the patient about the possible irreversibility of the procedure should he later want children. Warn him of the possibility of recanalization and the need for postoperative testing. Provide the couple with all possible information, but let them make their own decision. Have the patient agree in writing to use postoperative contraception until semen testing has shown him to be sterile. The patient should take a shower with antibacterial soap.

These patients are uniformly frightened during surgery. Give sedation if the patient has someone to drive him home. Tell him when you are about to inject the anesthetic, handle the tissues gently, and add additional anesthetic as you work.

Be aware that congenital absence of the vas occurs once in 335 cases. If you cannot palpate the vas in the midscrotum or at the cauda of the epididymis or the external ring, don't search for it inside. Simply do the other side. Absence of sperm later will prove the congenital absence.

Some surgeons like to hold the vas by placing a towel clip through the skin around the vas, but this can be painful. Instead, hold the vas in the fingers of the left hand, open the skin, and then feel for the vas with a closed Allis clamp. Open it and grasp the vas. It is not necessary to clamp and ligate the distal vas; simply cauterize both ends to seal them. You may initially fail to get adequate anesthesia. If so, hold the vas gently with an Allis clamp and inject more anesthetic. Then close the clamp on the vas. Always tag the sheath of the vas with a hemostat so that you don't lose the ends of the vas.

Excising a segment of vas has no value and may complicate a future reversal. Unlike a blood vessel, the lumen of the vas stays open up to the ligature. The ligated end often falls off, leading to a spermatic granuloma and possibly to a spontaneous recanalization. Fulgurate, don't ligate! Fulguration is the best method of sealing the vas. Destroy only the mucosa and not the muscular wall. Coupled with a fascial barrier between the vas ends, I have never had the operation fail in any of the more than 6500 consecutive vasectomies I have performed.

Double-check hemostasis before closing the skin and again before applying the bandage. Ecchymosis is acceptable; hematoma is not. Be available to the patient in case of a complication, real or imagined. Ask for a semen specimen after the patient has had 15 ejaculations; no sperm should be present.

NO-SCALPEL TECHNIQUE
(Shunqiang Li)

Instruments: Special instruments are required: an extracutaneous ring clamp and a sharpened curved mosquito clamp (Chongquing Family Planning Group).

Preparation: Tape the penis onto the abdomen. Apply povidone-iodine solution to the upper scrotum.

Stand on the right side and manipulate the vas with the left hand to place it under the skin in the raphe trapped between the middle finger beneath it and the thumb and index finger over it (see Step 1). Inject 2 to 3 ml of 2 percent lidocaine through a 27-gauge, 1.5-inch needle proximally under the skin and along the vas. Repeat the procedure for the other side.

7 Manipulate one vas under the raphe. As shown for the towel clamp in Step 1, apply the ring clamp to the vas while compressing the skin on either side between the thumb and forefinger to thin the tissue overlying it. **A,** Elevate the ring clamp and puncture the skin with one blade of the sharp hemostat, held at an angle of 45 degrees. Impale the vas on the point. **B** and **C,** Insert both blades and use them to open the skin and sheath to reach the wall of the vas. Gently separate the vas from its sheath with the sharp points of the clamp. **D** and **E,** Catch the vas in one point of the clamp, rotate the clamp 180 degrees, and deliver the vas into the wound. **F,** Release the ring clamp and reapply it to the exposed loop of vas. Divide the vas and ligate or fulgurate it as described in Step 5. Bury the distal end with the suture. Repeat the procedure on the opposite side, through the same skin puncture site. Pinch the skin together for hemostasis; a suture is not needed. Apply a sterile dressing and a scrotal supporter.

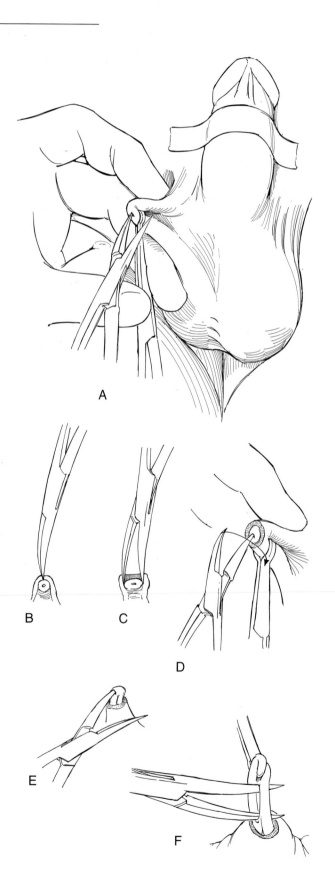

Vasovasostomy and Vasoepididymostomy

VASOVASOSTOMY

Preparation of the patient includes a pHisoHex shower the night before. Shave the scrotum in the operating room and prepare it with povidone-iodine solution.

Instruments. Include an operating room microscope with a 175- or 200-mm lens and pedals to control the zoom, focus, and position; Babcock clamps; a Medicut flexible cannula and syringe; methylene blue diluted 1:10 with saline; glass slides with cover slips; a monopolar needle-point hand-held electrode; a bipolar cautery; a vas clamp (Microspike); straight and curved jeweler's forceps; a microneedle holder; a microknife and microscissors; tenotomy scissors with blunt tips; nerve clamp; microtip marking pen; water for irrigation; microswabs; a scrotal suspensory; 2-0 monofilament thread; and 4-0 SAS. Have available 8-0 and 9-0 nylon suture on GS-16 needles and 10-0 nylon suture on LE-100 needles and a microscope nearby.

1 *Position:* Place the patient supine with the legs extended over a Bakelite (plastic) extension such as that used for operative fluoroscopy and supported on a nonrolling stool. Lower the foot of the table to provide room for your knees under the extension. Do not place pads under the patient's knees, but do pad the ankles and feet carefully. An egg-crate mattress can reduce discomfort for the patient during the long procedure.

You should be in a comfortable position with the ability to stabilize your arms. Padded armboards and a beanbag (prayer-bag) to sit on may help. Set up the operating room microscope over the scrotum, mounting a 175- or 200-mm lens, set for 10× for the anastomosis. Push the microscope aside.

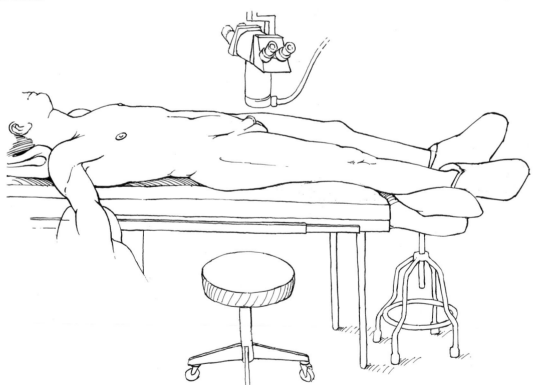

Modified One-Layer Closure

If the difference between the sizes of the distal and proximal lumina is small, a one-layer technique is satisfactory.

2 If you can feel the site of the previous vasectomy, make a 2- to 3-cm vertical incision at that site. If not, make a 2- to 3-cm vertical incision below the inguinoscrotal junction of the scrotum but at least 1 cm from the penoscrotal junction. *Note:* Orient the incision so that it may be extended into the groin in case the abdominal end of the vas retracts. Expose the extravaginal portion of the vas.

Alternative: If the site of the defect is difficult to locate, extend the incision and bring the testis out of the scrotum with the tunica vaginalis intact; it may be replaced once the vas deferens has been dissected.

Grasp the vas above and below the vasectomy defect with Babcock clamps. Replace the clamps with vessel loops to dissect the connective tissue from the vas just enough to expose its normal structure above and below the defect while preserving the sheath containing the vasal vessels. If the vas is short as a result of extensive excision at the time of the vasectomy, continue the dissection distally through the convoluted portion under magnification to allow the testis to drop upside down. The vasoepididymal complex can be dissected from the testis for additional length. Extending the scrotal incision proximally is not necessary, but digital dissection into the canal can help. The floor of the canal can be divided if necessary.

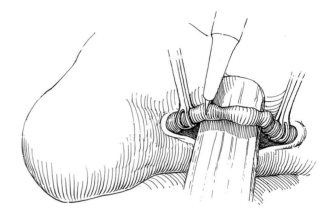

Hold the vas in a slotted neurosurgical nerve clamp, and divide it with a sharp knife above and then below the vasectomy site. Inspect the end for normal white mucosal ring and homogeneous muscularis and for bleeding. If it is abnormal, make successive cuts to expose a normal lumen. Touch the proximal end of the vas with a sterile slide or a Medicut cannula to collect fluid for examination for sperm in the operating room by the surgeon or the pathologist. Add a drop of saline to it, and cover it with a cover slip. If no sperm are seen, milk the distal epididymis and the convoluted portion of the vas.

3 Clear the loose adventitial tissue from both ends of the vas, taking care to preserve the mural vessels. Secure hemostasis with a bipolar electrode, a process that may be tedious. If tension is present, dissect the vas in both directions sufficiently to be able to bring the ends into apposition. If there is tension, place a mosquito clamp or a suture on the perivasal tissue of each end to assist with manipulation and prevent retraction. The testis, if it was removed from the scrotum, may be returned. Approximate the skin edges with a towel clamp to keep the two ends of the vas exteriorized. It may help with suturing if the ends protrude through an opening in a rubber dam.

4 Inject saline solution up the vas through a Medicut flexible cannula. If the fluid flows freely, patency is assured. Alternatively, pass a length of 2-0 monofilament suture up the vas.

Insert the two ends in a vas clamp. Place a piece of colored rubber cut from a balloon behind the vas for background. Prop up the clamp with a gauze sponge as necessary. Swing in the microscope, which provides binocular vision for you and your assistant.

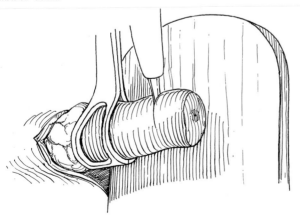

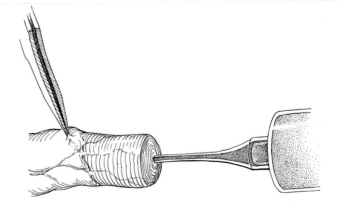

5 To maintain orientation during insertion of the sutures, first dry the ends of the vas with a small triangular sponge (microswab) and make four to six dots on each cut end of the vas with a microtip marking pen (Goldstein). To mark the starting point, place one of them more peripherally than the others. Insert curved jeweler's forceps or lacrymal probes in the proximal (smaller) lumen to stretch it and to aid the exit of the first suture. If loupes are used instead of a microscope, employ a grooved needle guide.

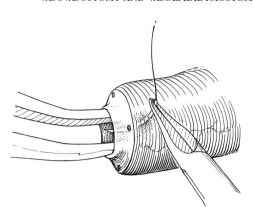

6 Place the first full-thickness suture of 9-0 nylon on a GS-16 or LE-100 needle through the entire thickness of the wall to exit between the jaws of the forceps. Run it diagonally through the wall, catching more muscularis than mucosa. Clear the field occasionally with water delivered through a cannula from the syringe. Touch the repair with microswabs to improve visibility.

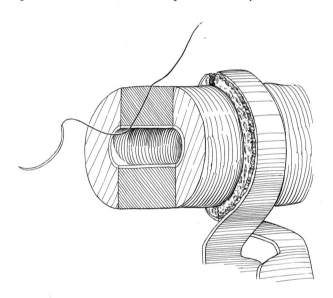

7 Continue the suture into the distal lumen, aided by an initial forceps dilation of this smaller opening; then run it out through the wall. Tie it with a square knot and cut the ends of the suture long for identification.

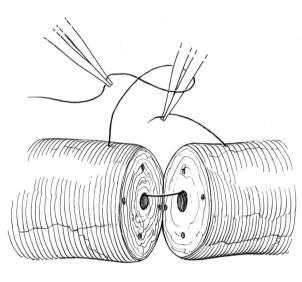

8 Place the second full-thickness suture in the same way 180 degrees from the first; tie and cut it. Place a third suture at 90 degrees from the others. Close the muscularis between these sutures with one or two 8-0 nylon sutures in each space.

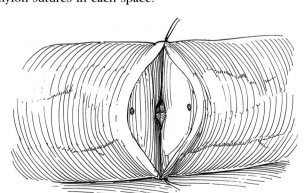

9 Invert the vas clamp. Inspect the lumen to be sure the previous deep sutures are properly placed through the mucosa. Insert a fourth deep suture between the two lateral sutures to complete the full-thickness set at the 12-, 3-, 6-, and 9-o'clock positions. *Alternatively,* place six full-thickness sutures, each spaced 60 degrees apart. Between each, place one suture in the muscularis to secure and seal the anastomosis, a total of 12 sutures.

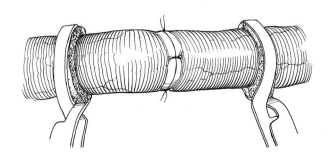

10 Close each of the remaining intervening spaces with one or two 8-0 sutures. Place these through the adventitia and half the thickness of the muscularis. Irrigate the wound with water to remove residual sperm. Support the anastomosis by approximating the adventitial tissue with 4-0 SAS.

Penrose drains are usually not needed, and if placed are removed the following morning. Close the dartos layer with a running 4-0 SAS, and place interrupted sutures for skin closure. Do the opposite side in a similar manner. Place a bulky cotton dressing inside a scrotal supporter. Discharge the patient when he is able to walk.

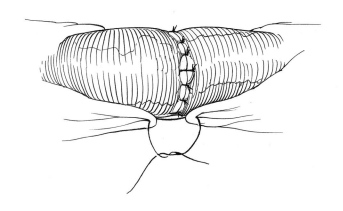

The dressing may be removed in 3 days for bathing, but the supporter should otherwise be worn for a total of 3 weeks. During this period, the patient should not be physically or sexually active. Examine the semen at 2 months and every 2 months thereafter until the count is stable.

Two-Layer Closure

When the distal end of the vas is appreciably larger than the proximal end or when the vas was ligated in the convoluted portion, a two-layer closure is advisable. It takes longer than a single-layer closure but is worth the extra effort. Proceed through preparation of the ends of the vas as described in Steps 1 to 4. Stain the mucosa with dilute methylene blue.

11 Place a 10-0 Prolene suture on an LE-100 taper-cut fishhook needle through the mucosa (opposite the microdot if one has been placed) on the far side of the larger, proximal vas, then through the mucosa of the distal vas at the matching dot. Tie the suture with five throws and cut it. Place a second 10-0 nylon suture in the mucosa approximately 70 degrees from the first. An *alternative* is to use double-armed sutures to allow inside-out placement, which reduces manipulation and avoids back-walling.

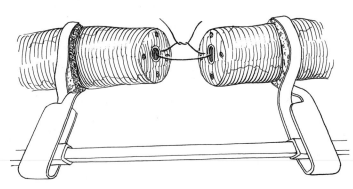

12 Rotate the vas clamp and place two or three more mucosal sutures. Before the last suture is tied, irrigate the area.

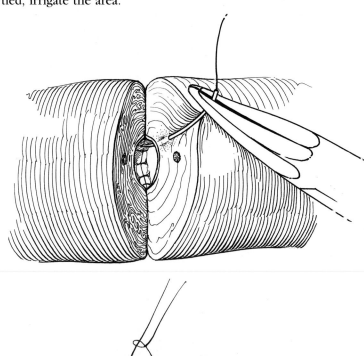

13 Close the muscularis with 8 to 12 sutures of 8-0 nylon placed on the near side between the mucosal sutures visible through the wall. If they are placed but not tied, successive sutures can be placed more accurately. Rotate the vas clamp to close the opposite side. Support the anastomosis with a few sutures in the periadventitial tissue, and close the wound as previously described.

For a *side-to-side anastomosis* without magnification (Royle and Hendry), spatulate the ends for a distance of 0.5 cm, overlap them, and perform a side-to-side anastomosis with 6-0 nonbraided synthetic NAS. The role of fibrin glue (Tisseal) and laser welding is not established.

Anastomosis of the Convoluted Vas

Anastomosis at this site is more difficult. Dissect the sheath of the convoluted portion from the epididymis, protecting its blood supply. Leave the convolutions in place; do not straighten them. Cut the vas in a plane absolutely vertical to the vasal lumen at that point; avoid an oblique cut. Insert sutures with care not to enter adjacent portions of the vas. Place multiple sutures to secure the sheath of the convoluted portion to the vasal sheath.

Postoperative Problems

A *hematoma* may form in the wound, rarely large enough to require evacuation, but enough to jeopardize the repair. Exact hemostasis is mandatory.

Anastomotic Failure

Wait 6 months for return of sperm. If sperm are present but have poor motility, look for sperm antibodies. Their presence indicates a poor prognosis and works against a second attempt at anastomosis.

Inadequate blood supply from damage to the vasal vessels at the time of vasoligation causes stenosis at the repair site and indicates that resection was inadequate at the end of the vas. The vasal vessels may also be damaged during the anastomotic procedure if too much perivasal tissue is stripped. Similarly, *diseased muscularis or mucosa* can be a factor unless the vas is adequately trimmed. *Excessive tension* on the anastomosis from inadequate initial mobilization is a cause of late failure. An obstructive *sperm granuloma* may form at the site of a leak. Finally, *technical errors,* such as back-walling with a suture or injuring the mucosa, can result in obstruction.

Repeat Vasovasostomy. Repeat operation requires more time and hence better anesthesia than the initial repair; use an epidural block. Partially divide the vas proximal to the previous repair, and examine the luminal contents for sperm. If sperm are present, resect the anastomosis and repeat the vasovasostomy. (Because of the high failure rate in a repeat operation, consider aspiration and cryopreservation of sperm.) If sperm are absent, the anastomosis may also be obstructed; test by instilling saline distally with a blunt needle. If this demonstrates that the obstruction is in the epididymis, proceed with vasoepididymostomy, using vas proximal or distal to the previous anastomosis, depending on the findings of the patency test.

VASOEPIDIDYMOSTOMY

Obtain serum FSH levels. If they are normal, perform an open biopsy of the testis using local anesthesia, or use fine-needle aspiration. If the biopsy results are normal and the ejaculate has a volume of less than 1 ml, perform transrectal sonography to rule out obstruction of the ejaculatory ducts. Operate for epididymal obstruction, using general anesthesia and an end-to-end or end-to-side technique. In general, an end-to-side anastomosis is preferred. The end-to-end technique is necessary when the anastomosis must be done high in the scrotum. Try to separate the cauda and corpus epididymis away from the adjacent testicle, leaving the efferent ducts and caput epididymis undisturbed. Turn mobilized epididymis superiorly, which adds as much as 2 to 3 cm to make up for the short vas.

End-to-End Anastomosis

Free the vas sufficiently to relieve tension, even dissecting to the external inguinal ring if needed, but preserve as much of the sheath and periadventitial tissue as possible. Make a hemivasostomy just beyond the convoluted portion. Examine the vasal fluid under the microscope to check for absence of sperm. Ascertain vasal patency by injecting saline. Dilating the vas with a 3 F Fogarty balloon catheter inflated to 0.1 ml may facilitate anastomosis (Grasso).

14 **A,** Determine the level of epididymal obstruction by serial transverse cuts made with a sharp knife, starting on the cauda epididymidis. **B,** Hold the epididymis in a slotted nerve clamp to ensure that you make clean transverse cuts. Watch for a spurt of vasal contents, and examine the cut section to locate the one specific transected tubule that is emitting sperm. Have your assistant irrigate as you examine the cut tubule using a microswab to clear the area. If two (or sometimes three) transected tubules emit sperm, it becomes impossible to know which transected tubule is the one in continuity with the testicle.

Collect fluid on a glass slide to prove the presence of sperm microscopically. Mark the specific tubule with methylene blue. Cauterize bleeding points carefully with bipolar current. Because of the high failure rate of primary vasoepididymostomy and much higher failure rate in a repeat operation, consider aspiration and cryopreservation of sperm.

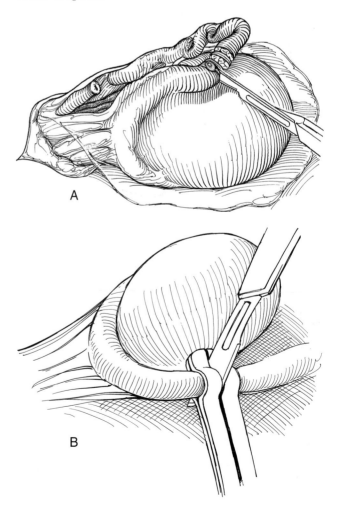

15 Place the vas and epididymis in a vas clamp. Hold the vas deferens in place with a 6-0 SAS. Place the first suture of 8-0 nylon posteriorly in the epididymal tubule to include the epididymal tunic on the back wall. Go from outside to inside. Subsequent sutures should include part of the epididymal wall to avoid tearing. Bring the vas into the field and place the sutures from inside to outside through the vasal mucosa. Tie and cut them. Alternatively, the sutures may be placed first outside-in, then inside-out to prevent back-walling of the mucosa.

16 Place two or three anterior mucosal sutures in the vas from outside to inside, and continue them in the tubule from inside to outside. Tie and cut them. Do not hesitate to place more sutures; a nonleaking anastomosis is essential.

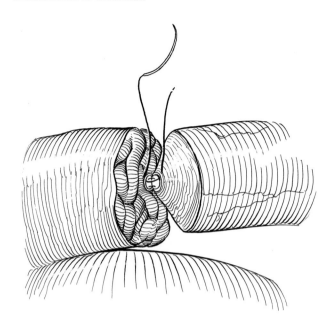

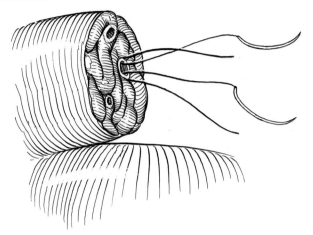

17 Suture the sheath and muscularis of the vas deferens to the epididymal tunic with at least 10 or 12 of the 8-0 nylon sutures.

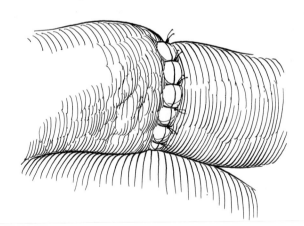

End-to-Side Anastomosis (Sharlip-Thomas)

Use in the presence of marked dilation of the epididymal tubule, although it does have a higher incidence of stenosis.

18 Open the tunica vaginalis and inspect the epididymis. Select an area with dilated tubules just proximal to the obstruction. If a site of obstruction is not seen, begin the incisions at the lower (most distal) part of the epididymis. Excise a 3-mm circular patch of the epididymal capsule on its lateral surface, enough to expose an underlying tubule.

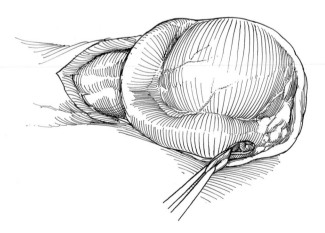

19 Mark this tubule by looping it with a 10-0 nylon suture and incise it longitudinally on its lateral wall. Make a touch preparation and have it examined microscopically for sperm. If no sperm are present, remove the stay suture and close the defect.

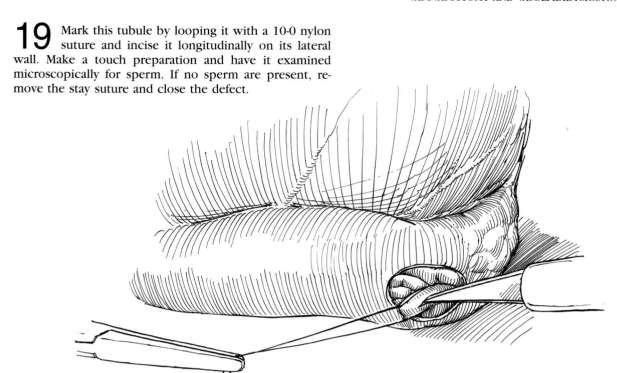

20 Repeat the procedure 0.5 to 1.0 cm more proximally. Continue up the tubule until sperm are identified.

21 When sperm are found, pass the distal end of the vas under the parietal tunica vaginalis to bring it to the site on the epididymis. Fix it there with three sutures of 6-0 Prolene between the capsule and the adventitia of the vas (not shown). Anastomose the mucosa of the vas to the edges of the opened epididymal tubule, using six sutures of 10-0 nylon on an LE-100 needle.

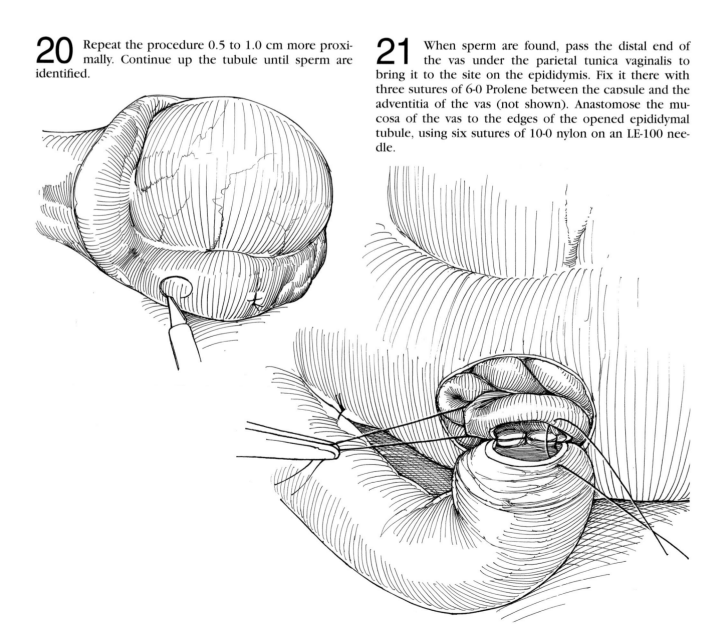

22 Suture the muscularis of the vas to the edges of the capsule with 8 to 12 sutures of 9-0 nylon, using an LE-100 needle. Return the testis and epididymis to the scrotum, and close the parietal tunica vaginalis with 3-0 SAS. Close the wound.

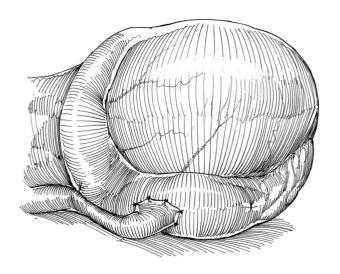

Postoperative Problems

Infection and *hematoma* are seen, in part because of prolonged exposure. A *sperm granuloma* may appear after weeks or months. It is seldom painful but may interfere with flow in the vas. *Atrophy of the testis* is rare, secondary to inadvertent interference with the testicular artery. A *hydrocele* may form. *Scrotal pain* can be a problem; its cause is unclear. Finally, *ulnar neuritis* from local pressure during anesthesia may occur. Appearance of sperm may be delayed for as long as 15 months without change in prognosis for fertility (Jarow et al, 1995).

Commentary by Stuart S. Howards

It is important to make arrangements to have your knees fit comfortably under the operating table and to have easy access with a foot to the control pedals for the microscope. I remove my shoes for better sensitivity. It is probably not necessary to drape the microscope. I do not and have had very few cases of infection.

Be certain that you cut back both ends of the vas into healthy, well-vascularized tissue. For any tension on the abdominal end of the vas, I place a perivasal suture of 3-0 CCG to prevent retraction.

Some surgeons place four mucosal sutures separated by 90 degrees; others place more sutures. I find it easy to place two mucosal sutures fairly close together with an intervening muscular suture and then to rotate the clamp. I then place another mucosal suture as far away from the initial sutures as possible and tie it. Finally, I place two more sutures, which are tied at the same time. I find this is easy and effective, the only difficult suture being the second one. I often dilate the abdominal end of the vas deferens with straight jeweler's forceps, being careful to insert and withdraw it while closed, to avoid injuring the mucosa.

For vasoepididymostomy, I find it helpful when incising the epididymal tubule to mark and elevate it with a noncutting needle, and then either incise it with a blade or cut it with microscissors. Postoperatively, I ask the patient to avoid heavy lifting and sexual activity for 2 weeks.

SECTION
10
Testis: Excision

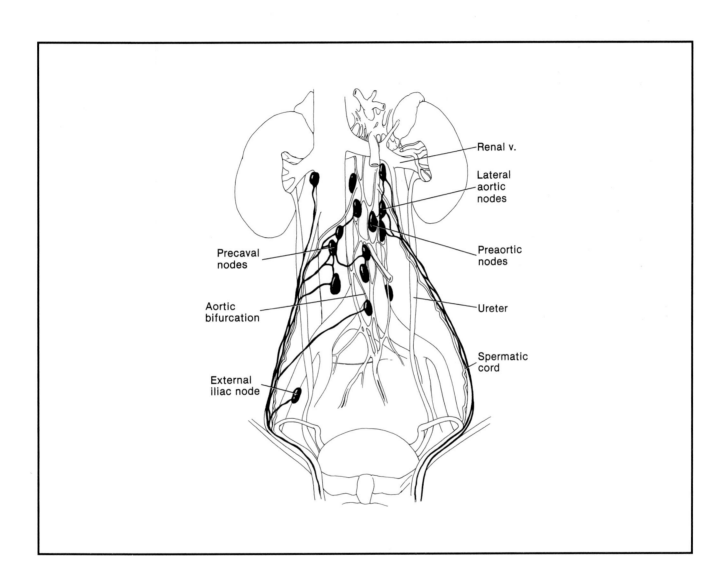

Anatomy of Testicular Excision

The testicular arteries arise from the anterolateral surface of the aorta just below the renal arteries. As the testicular artery approaches the upper end of the testis, it divides into two tortuous main branches—an outer branch, the internal testicular artery, and an inner branch, the inferior testicular artery.

LYMPHATIC DRAINAGE OF THE TESTIS

Lymphatic channels course along the upper posterior border of the testis to form a series of four to eight collector vessels that accompany the spermatic cord. At the crossing of the ureter, they separate from the blood vessels and deviate medially to terminate in the precaval nodes and the nodes around the aorta at the site of origin of the testis.

The collectors from the right testis join the aortic nodes lying between the take-off of the renal vein and the aortic bifurcation. From the left testis, two thirds of the collectors run to the lateral aortic nodes, especially those lying most cephalad, and some terminate as low as the bifurcation; the other third end in the preaortic nodes.

Although the lumbar sympathetic trunk lies posterior to the outer stratum of the retroperitoneal fascia, it may be resected with the lymph nodes, with resulting anejaculation.

Simple Orchiectomy

TRANS-SCROTAL ORCHIECTOMY

Because of the difficulty in sterilizing scrotal skin, give perioperative antibiotics.

Position: Supine.

Anesthesia: Apply a testis nerve block (see page 77). Prepare the scrotal area with iodophor solution.

1 Grasp the scrotum behind the testis with the fingers and thumb to tense the overlying skin. Make a transverse skinfold incision in the scrotum to avoid the scrotal vessels. If bilateral excision is planned, a vertical incision in the scrotal raphe is possible. Incise the dartos muscle and cremasteric layers onto the bluish tunica vaginalis. Control bleeding vessels with the electrocautery.

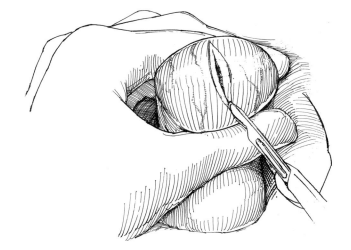

2 Push the scrotal layers away with sponge dissection, and deliver the testis within the tunica vaginalis into the wound. Alternatively, open the tunica vaginalis before delivering the testis. Draw the testis down to expose the epididymis and cord. Bluntly dissect the spermatic vessels from the vas deferens. Divide and ligate the vas with a 3-0 synthetic absorbable suture (SAS). Bluntly separate the cord into two or three parts, doubly clamp each part, and ligate them with a 3-0 SAS individually.

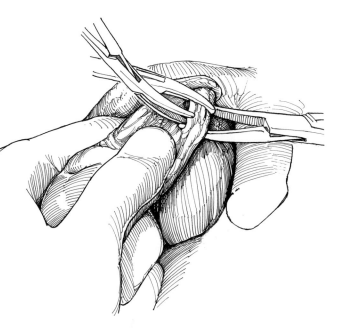

Suture-ligate the internal spermatic artery with its spermatic veins because these vessels retract after division, and loss of the ligature results in a major scrotal and inguinal hematoma. Should this occur, quickly extend the incision and reclamp the cord below the external inguinal ring. In children, individual ligation is not necessary, especially in cases of torsion. Clamp the entire cord and suture-ligate it.

Before closing, electrocoagulate any bleeders in the dartos and subcutaneous tissue to avoid a distressing scrotal hematoma. Drains are rarely necessary, but if they are placed, they should be brought out through the most dependent (posterior) portion of the scrotum with the aid of a curved clamp and fixed in place with a 2-0 suture and a safety pin. Close the dartos layer with a running SAS, and close the skin, together with the subcutaneous tissue, with interrupted 4-0 or 5-0 SAS or with a fine subcuticular monofilament running SAS. Repeat the procedure on the opposite side. Place bacitracin ointment on the wound, and add sterile fluffs held in place with a snug-fitting scrotal supporter.

Postoperative Problems

Continued oozing with formation of a *scrotal hematoma* is the most common complication and results from incomplete hemostasis, with bleeding occurring into the several loose layers of the scrotum. Placement of a drain before closure avoids the hematoma but should not be necessary if good technique is followed. Drain a hematoma only if it becomes distressingly large or infected.

INTRACAPSULAR ORCHIECTOMY

For some men, the psychological benefit of a palpable, if small, organ outweighs the remote possibility of leaving a few interstitial cells.

3 After exposure of the testis as described, incise the tunica albuginea along the entire length of the testis.

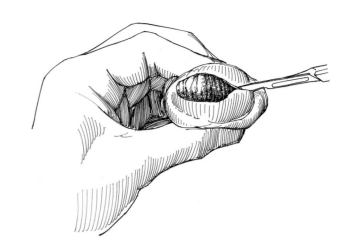

4 Grasp the edges with three clamps on each side and evert the lining. Take an opened 4 × 4 inch gauze pad over the index finger and wipe the tubules from the inner layer of the tunica albuginea, sweeping all the contents to the center. Fulgurate the vessels of the tunica albuginea as they are exposed (they tend to adhere to the electrode).

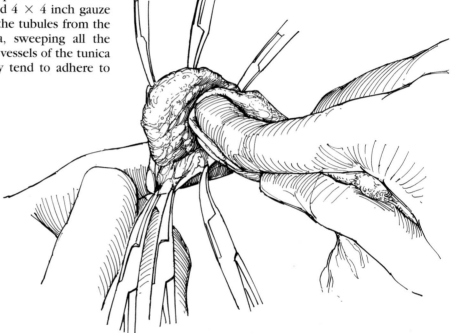

5 **A,** Ligate the hilus with a 2-0 chromic catgut (CCG) suture. Divide it with the electrosurgical knife. **B,** Fulgurate the base as well as the entire inner surface of the tunica albuginea to thoroughly destroy any residual interstitial cells.

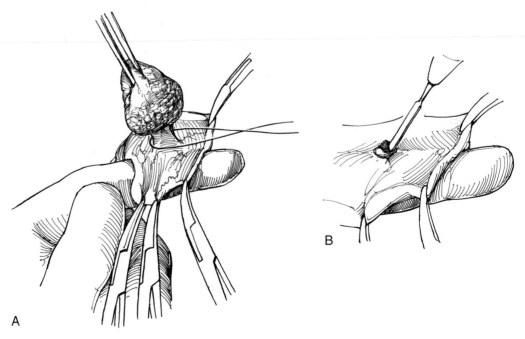

A

B

6 Close the tunica albuginea with a running 3-0 CCG suture. Control the vessels in the wound edges. Close the dartos layer with a running 4-0 SAS, placing a second layer as vertical mattress sutures. A drain is seldom necessary. Repeat the operation on the other testis. Pack with fluffs held by an athletic supporter.

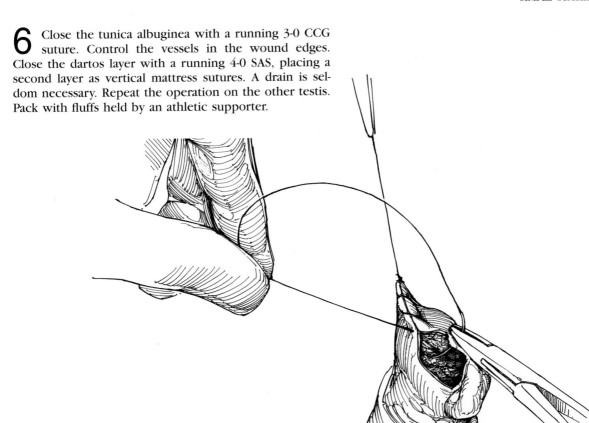

EPIDIDYMIS-SPARING ORCHIECTOMY

Like the intracapsular orchiectomy, this procedure leaves a palpable "testicular" mass.

7 Progressively clamp and ligate the numerous small vessels as they enter the hilus of the testis.

8 Suture the ends of the epididymis together with one or two figure-eight 3-0 CCG sutures to create a rounded structure that mimics a small testis. Drain the scrotum with a drain through a stab wound. Repeat the procedure on the opposite side.

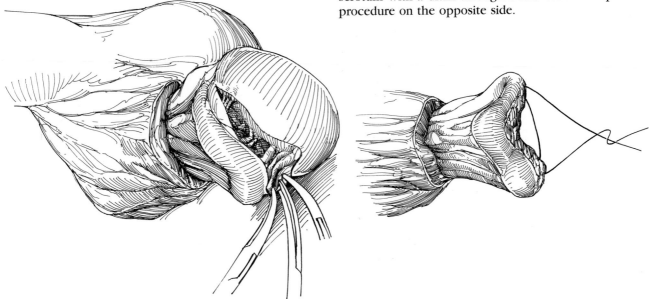

Postoperative Problems

An *enlarging hematoma* means that a spermatic vessel is incompletely ligated. Make a subinguinal incision, free the cord, draw the end into the wound, and religate it. *Retroperitoneal* *hemorrhage* can occur after inguinal orchiectomy as the inadequately secured testicular artery retracts. A scrotal hematoma on the involved side may appear, and ultrasonography helps make the diagnosis. Make an inguinal incision immediately to secure the vessel.

Commentary by Marc Goldstein

The primary complication of simple orchiectomy is bleeding. I prefer ligation of the vas, the cremasteric muscle, and the internal spermatic vessels in three separate bundles using 2-0 silk suture-ligatures. Silk is still the most secure suture material for vascular structures and does not cause problems when used below the skin and subcutaneous tissues.

Because Leydig cells are remarkably tenacious and small numbers of them are capable of producing surprising amounts of testosterone, I am not enthusiastic about subcapsular orchiectomy for prostate cancer. An epididymis-sparing procedure, on the other hand, poses no risk of residual Leydig cells. It is a bloodier operation than total epididymo-orchiectomy or intracapsular orchiectomy. Three major groups of epididymal vessels are usually encountered: superior, middle, and caudal. These should be individually ligated with 2-0 silk. I agree with drainage for the epididymis-sparing procedure.

If bleeding occurs after a scrotal orchiectomy, a 3-cm subinguinal incision within the skin lines allows the cord to be grasped with a Babcock clamp just below the external inguinal ring. This obviates opening the fascia.

INSERTION OF TESTICULAR PROSTHESIS

The patient must understand that implantation of a prosthesis is for cosmetic, psychological needs only. The risk of late complications from silicone has not been determined. Insertion after radical orchiectomy for cancer is inadvisable because the persistent mass reminds the patient of his former lesion. For adults, select a silicone gel–filled prosthesis of a size similar to that of the contralateral testis. In children, implant a somewhat larger testis to allow for growth and to delay the need for replacement. Prepare the skin well and give antibiotics.

Incision: Make an inguinoscrotal incision along the skin fold in children. An alternative is to enter through the scrotal raphe, but this practice carries a greater risk of necrosis. Stretch the scrotum vigorously with one or two fingers inside it, being careful not to tear through it, especially in children. Select the proper size because most hospitals require that a prosthesis be discarded if it has been placed in the wound. If the tab on the prosthe-sis is used for fixation, trim the sharp edges, invert the scrotum into the wound, and stitch the tab to the dartos layer with an absorbable suture. Usually the tab is unnecessary; cut it off and consider placing a purse-string suture around the neck of the scrotum, taking care not to pierce the capsule of the prosthesis with the needle. Close the wound in layers. Manually pull the prosthesis to the bottom of the scrotal sac before the patient leaves the operating room.

Postoperative Problems

Infection necessitates removal of the prosthesis. *Necrosis* of the overlying skin results from insertion of too large a prosthesis. *Hematoma* is unusual because the interior of the scrotum has few exposed vessels. *Perforation* of the prosthesis itself can occur if a needle is carelessly inserted during closure.

Replace the prosthesis in a child after growth by reopening the inguinal incision, inverting the scrotum, and shelling the prosthesis from its pseudocapsule. Stretch the scrotum, and insert a prosthesis of more appropriate size.

Laparoscopic Orchiectomy

The laparoscope provides another, simple approach for the removal of small, dysgenic testes and those associated with testicular feminization.

Place the boy in a three-quarters torque position so that he does not have to be moved. Use the Hasson technique: Through a small subumbilical incision open the peritoneum under vision, avoiding the risks associated with the Veress needle. Follow the technique and insert the trocars as described on pages 21 and 331.

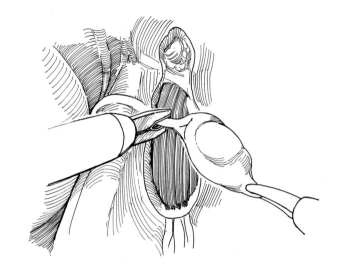

1 Locate the small testis endoscopically, and incise the peritoneum over the upper pole. Identify and fulgurate the spermatic vessels or, if the port is large enough, clip them. Dissect the testis from its bed along with a short length of vas deferens. Pull on the gubernaculum and fulgurate it. Clip the vas on the distal side. Usually the testis is small or atrophic, so it can be withdrawn through the sheath, or it can be removed after enlarging one of the accessory ports, avoiding the need for a bag.

Alternative Removal 1. Make a short inguinal incision, insert a clamp, and grasp the testis under endoscopic control. Withdraw it through the incision.

Alternative Removal 2. Place the testis and adnexae in a specimen retrieval bag (Endobag) or a sterile condom and draw the mouth of the bag to the sheath of the trocar at the anterior abdominal wall. Withdraw the sheath, clamp the bag, and draw the testis through the puncture site. This ensures that no malignant cells from a dysgenic testis are left behind. Inspect the bed.

Alternative Removal 3. Locate the testis endoscopically, make a small localized incision directly over the testis, and excise the testis with clamps, sutures, and scissors.

Commentary by David A. Bloom

Abdominal testes, once identified, should either be moved to a scrotal position or removed altogether. In instances of bilaterality, particularly in infants, relocation to the scrotum is the usual scenario. When the abdominal testis is unilateral and the contralateral testis is normal, however, removal is generally the more prudent policy. Laparoscopy offers some particular advantages in these situations. First, by means of laparoscopy, one can easily identify an abdominal testis or declare its absence if there is no gonad. Furthermore, the precise identification of the site of the abdominal testis and the size and configuration of the testis facilitate the appropriate decision and operative approach. Four laparoscopic means of orchiectomy are detailed.

None is particularly better or worse than any of the other modalities. Two ports, in addition to the optical port, are necessary for laparoscopic orchiectomy. The procedure is quite straightforward, as described. I favor clipping the spermatic vessels doubly on the retained side of the spermatic vessel leash. Perhaps even more expeditious than the complete laparoscopic orchiectomy is alternative number 3, which simply uses endoscopic inspection to locate the testis. By shining the endoscopic light through the abdominal wall at the site of the testis, one can see exactly where to make a small incision and then proceed with a so-called open orchiectomy through what is virtually a minilaparotomy incision.

Radical Orchiectomy

Obtain serum markers for alpha-fetoprotein (AFP), lactic acid dehydrogenase (LDH), and beta-human chorionic gonadotropin (beta-hCG) before orchiectomy. Stage the disease following the orchiectomy: Obtain a chest film, perform abdominal and pelvic computed tomography, and repeat the measurement of the serum markers. For patients with seminomas in Stage I or IIa or IIb and normal AFP levels, arrange for radiation therapy following orchiectomy; for patients with bulky or disseminated seminoma or other germ cell tumors, treat according to stage. Consider having the patient bank sperm, although as many as 50 percent are subfertile preoperatively.

1 *Position:* Supine. Prepare and drape the lower abdomen, including the genitalia.

Incision: Incise the skin above and parallel to the inguinal ligament, as for inguinal hernia repair (the more cosmetic transverse incision may make extraction of the testis from the scrotum more difficult). The skin incision may be shifted obliquely to the inguinal ligament to enable extension into the upper scrotum to facilitate the removal of large tumors. In children, however, follow the skinfold. Divide the subcutaneous fat, and ligate the several veins with 3-0 SAS as encountered. Incise Camper's and Scarpa's fascias.

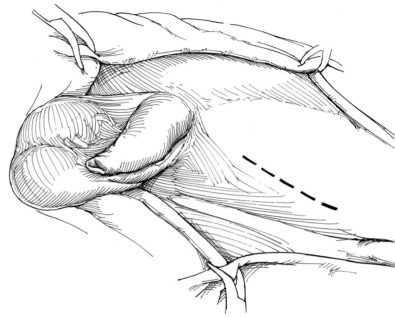

2 Identify the external ring and incise the external oblique fascia sharply, taking care not to interfere with the ilioinguinal nerve lying just beneath it.

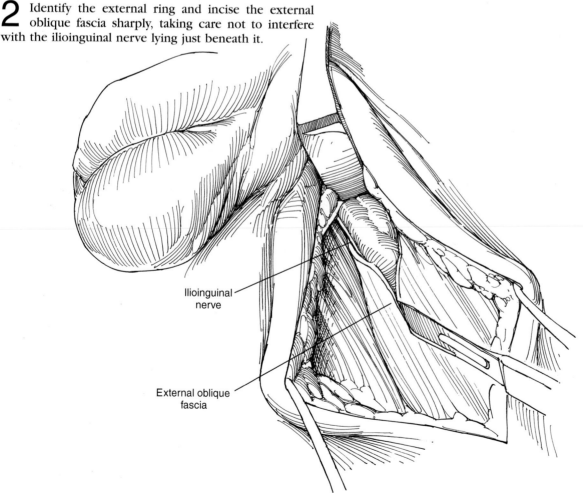

Ilioinguinal nerve

External oblique fascia

3 Grasp and elevate the lateral and medial edges of the external oblique fascia, and bluntly dissect the spermatic cord with peanut dissectors inferiorly to expose the pubic tubercle.

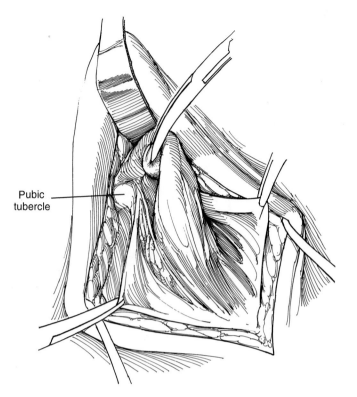

Pubic tubercle

4 Repeat the dissection medially, again to the tubercle, elevating the medial fascial edge so that all of the cord structures are exposed, including the cremaster muscle.

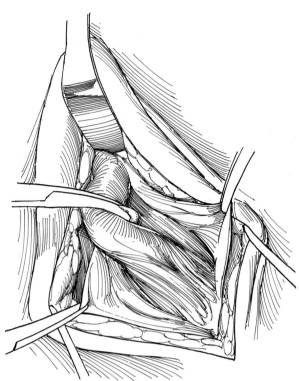

5 Surround the cord with a Penrose drain. Lift it and free the cord as far as the internal ring. Watch for a perforating cremasteric vessel that must be tied.

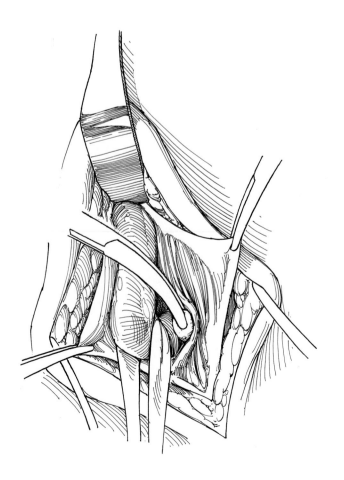

6 **A,** Pass a 14 F catheter, preferably latex, around the cord 2 cm below the internal ring to allow division of the cord at the ring without release of the constriction. Draw it up and clamp it as a tourniquet. **B,** *Alternative:* Pass a Penrose drain twice around the cord and clamp it.

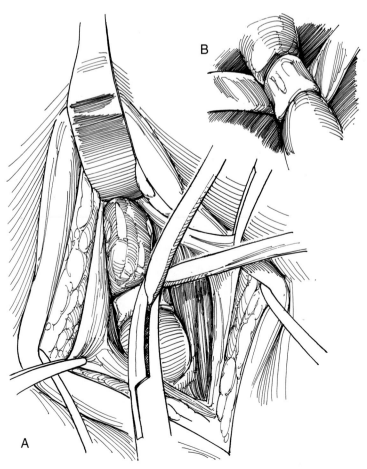

B

A

7 Stretch the neck of the scrotum from above. Push the testicle upward by pressure on the scrotum. For large tumors, Scarpa's fascia may need further division. Extend the skin incision over the anterolateral aspect of the scrotum.

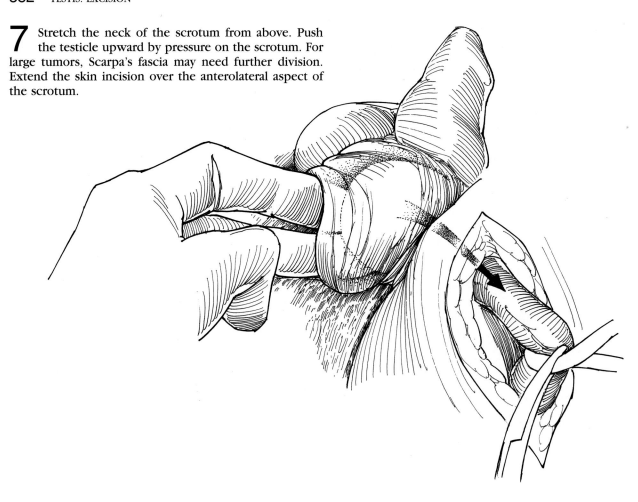

8 Clamp and divide the gubernacular attachments and ligate them. Open the internal oblique muscle at the internal ring for 2 or 3 cm, and dissect the vas and spermatic vessels as far as feasible through this incision.

9 *Inspection and biopsy:* If at this point there is any doubt about the diagnosis, place the testis on a folded sterile towel. Open the tunica vaginalis and inspect and palpate the testis. Because the tumor is usually obvious under the tunica albuginea, frozen section biopsy is rarely necessary. If there is doubt about the diagnosis, biopsy of the testis can be done without risk of spread if the testis is draped out of the field. If the report is positive for cancer, change gloves and instruments and divide the cord above the tourniquet and remove the specimen in the towel from the field (Step 10).

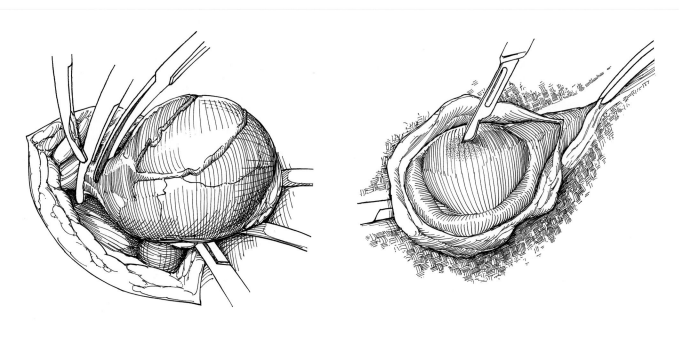

10 Doubly clamp, divide, and doubly ligate the vascular cord above the tourniquet proximal to the internal ring. Use 2-0 or 3-0 nonabsorbable sutures (NAS), preferably silk cut long for later identification at node dissection. Division above the tourniquet excludes any tumor cells that might have been driven into the cord during manipulation. Follow the vas, and clamp and divide it between nonabsorbable ligatures. The end of the cord should lie retroperitoneally so that it can be readily reached from above. Observe for hemostasis, and irrigate the wound. Should the ligatures slip and the cord retract above the canal, immediately open the external and internal oblique muscles in the line of the incision, and grasp and religate the free end of the cord.

11 **A,** Suture the conjoined tendon to the shelving edge of the inguinal ligament. **B,** Imbricate the external oblique fascia with 3-0 SAS. Close the subcutaneous tissue with fine SAS, and run a 4-0 SAS subcuticularly. Do not place drains. Use fluffs to compress the empty scrotum. Concomitant placement of a testicular prosthesis is not advisable; moreover, the patient usually prefers a scrotum free of all masses.

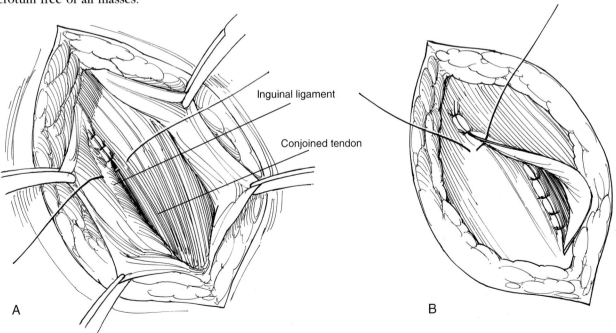

Inguinal ligament

Conjoined tendon

A

B

Benign Tumors. Opt for organ-preserving excision after ultrasonography has demonstrated a cystic or distinctive solid lesion *(epidermoid cyst)* and tumor markers are negative. Expose the testis as described in Step 9. Obstruct the cord, open the tunica vaginalis on a towel, and excise the tumor with a 2- to 3-mm margin. Make at least two biopsies of the adjacent testis to exclude an adjacent germ cell tumor. Send the specimens for frozen section diagnosis to rule out malignancy. If doubt persists, clamp the cord above the tourniquet and remove the testis.

Postoperative Problems

Hemorrhage can be a major complication, resulting from not controlling the vas and vessels separately and from improper ligation of the cord. An expanding *hematoma* or evidence of *retroperitoneal bleeding* warrants reopening and extending the inguinal incision to reach the retracted vessels.

BILATERAL TUMORS

In a patient with a neoplasm in the contralateral testis who has normal plasma testosterone levels, enucleation may be applicable if the tumor is small and confined to the organ (stage T1) and does not involve the rete testis (Heidenreich et al, 1995). After enucleating the tumor, obtain biopsies from the tumor bed and the peripheral parenchyma. Treat carcinoma in situ with 20 Gy of local irradiation. Follow the patient with serum markers and testosterone levels.

Commentary by Joseph C. Presti, Jr.

Inguinal exploration with cross-clamping of the spermatic cord vasculature and delivery of the testis into the surgical field is the procedure of choice for a possible testicular tumor. If cancer cannot be excluded by examination of the testis, then radical orchiectomy is warranted. Scrotal approaches and open testicular biopsies should be avoided, as they may result in scrotal recurrences or disruption of the normal lymphatic drainage. If scrotal violation has occurred, simple scar excision rather than hemiscrotectomy is adequate.

The incision is typically placed above and parallel to the inguinal ligament. However, in the case of large tumors, the incision should be placed obliquely so that it may be extended into the upper scrotum if necessary. Early vascular control, although no longer thought to be necessary for prevention of tumor cell spread, does facilitate a clean dissection of the cord to the level of the internal ring and at the level of the pubic tubercle. Separate division and ligation of the vas facilitate complete removal of the spermatic cord at the time of retroperitoneal lymph node dissection. Division of the spermatic cord bundles is usually accomplished between right-angle clamps. The patient's side of the cord is doubly ligated with a proximal free tie and a distal suture ligature. The ends of the suture from the patient's side are tagged to enable inspection of the stump prior to closure. Once hemostasis is established, the end of the cord is released into the retroperitoneum. The specimen side of the cord is managed with a single free tie. After removal of the specimen, inspection and palpation of the floor of the inguinal canal determine whether repair of the floor is needed. The scrotum is inverted on a finger tip into the inguinal incision for inspection for meticulous hemostasis. Patients should be instructed to limit their activity on the day of surgery to minimize swelling. Prior to the subcuticular skin closure, a local anesthetic may be infiltrated into the wound for postoperative analgesia.

Retroperitoneal Lymph Node Dissection

STAGING

Proceed with staging for nonseminomatous tumors removed at radical orchiectomy (see page 380):

1. *Abdominal and pelvic computed tomography (CT) scans:* If findings are negative or show only small involved nodes, proceed with staging retroperitoneal lymph node dissection (RPLND). For large nodes, give chemotherapy first.

2. *Whole-lung tomograms:* If findings are positive (Stage III), give chemotherapy. Subsequently do RPLND if CT scan findings show positive nodes; otherwise watch the patient carefully. If the lungs are clear, proceed with RPLND.

3. *Nodal pathologic staging:* If node findings are negative (Stage I), watch the patient. If they are positive (Stage II), either watch the patient or give chemotherapy. For markers, use alpha-fetoprotein (AFP) with a metabolic half-life of 5 days and beta-human chorionic gonadotropin (beta-hCG) with a metabolic half-life of 30 minutes.

EVALUATION

Evaluate the patient's respiratory status, especially if he has received bleomycin. Review the intravenous urogram to establish the presence or absence of ureteral obstruction or any renal malfunction on the side of the nodal mass.

PREPARATION

Explain to the patient the possibility of dry ejaculation, and have him provide sperm (even if of poor quality) for cryopreservation. In advanced cases, warn him of the possibility of removal of contiguous structures, including excision of the aorta, vena cava, and ipsilateral kidney.

Provide for monitoring with intra-arterial lines and Swan-Ganz catheters. Order adequate blood for replacement. Patients with large nodal masses need to have up to 6 units typed and cross-matched. Additional blood bank supplies should be available, as well as 1 to 2 L of 5 percent albumin. A sonogram probe may be placed in the rectum for monitoring bladder neck contraction from nerve stimulation to identify the autonomic nerves during dissection of the nodes.

Prepare the bowel. Hydrate the patient intravenously with 5 percent dextrose in half-normal saline at 150 ml/hr the night before. Intraoperatively, give mannitol prior to dissection of the renal vessels. Avoid furosemide after cisplatin or gentamicin therapy.

APPROACHES

A transabdominal approach (see page 867) is quicker and easier. It facilitates bilateral dissection in the contralateral suprahilar and iliac areas, but for muscular patients or for bulky nodes, the thoracoabdominal incision (see page 890) gives better ipsilateral exposure and less postoperative ileus.

ANATOMY AND TEMPLATES FOR NERVE SPARING

In clinical Stage I (or low-volume Stage II) disease, morbidity from loss of ejaculation may be reduced without impairing the effectiveness of the cancer operation by sparing the retroperitoneal autonomic nerves. Identify these nerves at operation. Dissect the nerves first, and then dissect the nodes for the best chance of preserving ejaculation.

1 **A,** Lymph nodes and nerve plexuses. The sympathetic trunk and ganglia lie just lateral to the vertebral bodies and contribute to the several plexuses over the aorta and vena cava. The celiac plexus, at the level of the lower margin of the 12th thoracic vertebra, joins the two celiac ganglia that are found between the adrenal gland and the take-off of the celiac artery. Each of these ganglia is connected above to the greater splanchnic nerve and is attached below, as the aortorenal ganglion, to the lesser splanchnic nerve originating from T12. This ganglion in turn supplies the renal plexus that lies at the base of the renal arteries. The superior hypogastric plexus lies below the aortic bifurcation. It is connected above with the inferior mesenteric plexus and below with the bipartite inferior hypogastric (pelvic) plexus, which contains the hypogastric ganglia. The plexiform connection between the superior hypogastric plexus and the inferior hypogastric (pelvic) plexuses is known as the hypogastric or presacral nerve. The inferior hypogastric plexus connects with the vesical plexus, the prostatic plexus, and, in the female, the uterovaginal plexus. The

hypogastric plexus as it crosses anterior to the aortic bifurcation is the most vulnerable site for injury.

B, Templates for dissection. A modified dissection done for nerve sparing is unilateral below the inferior mesenteric artery and bilateral above.

For standard lymphadenectomy, the nodal area to be resected for *right-sided tumors* stops over the aorta and includes the right iliac and right paracaval nodes. For *left-sided tumors,* resection stops medially over the vena cava and includes the interaortocaval nodes and left para-aortic nodes as well as the left iliac nodes.

With Stage I disease, a nerve-sparing technique may be applied by limiting the dissection. For *right-sided tumors,* the right para-aortic nodes (interaortocaval zone) are resected, and the right paracaval and right iliac nodes are routinely included. For *left-sided tumors,* the nodes that must be gathered for this clinical stage are from the left para-aortic and infrarenal hilar zones. Bilateral dissection above the inferior mesenteric artery is not necessary for Stage I disease, but bilateral node dissection is indicated for bulky advanced disease (Stages IIc or III).

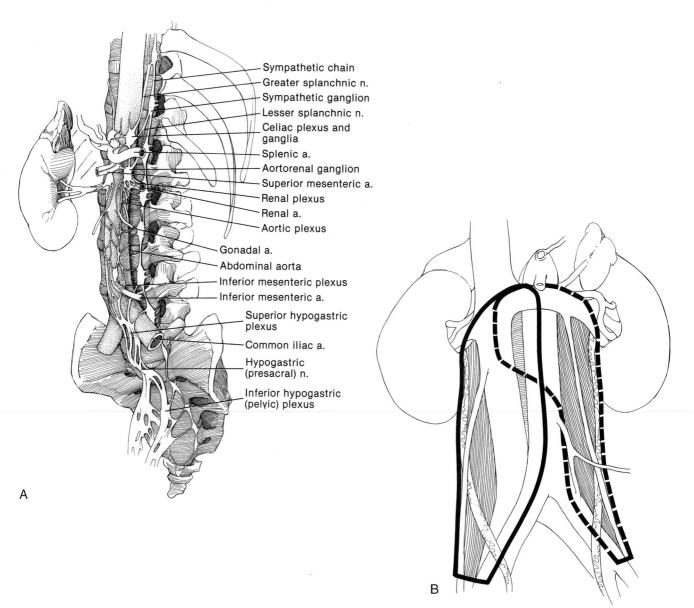

Sympathetic chain
Greater splanchnic n.
Sympathetic ganglion
Lesser splanchnic n.
Celiac plexus and ganglia
Splenic a.
Aortorenal ganglion
Superior mesenteric a.
Renal plexus
Renal a.
Aortic plexus
Gonadal a.
Abdominal aorta
Inferior mesenteric plexus
Inferior mesenteric a.
Superior hypogastric plexus
Common iliac a.
Hypogastric (presacral) n.
Inferior hypogastric (pelvic) plexus

A

B

TRANSABDOMINAL LYMPHADENECTOMY

Right-Sided Tumor

The best access to the retroperitoneum is by an anterior incision, through which both sides may be approached. It can be extended by a median sternotomy or by angling it into the 9th or 10th interspace. Also, the postoperative pain may be less than that with the thoracoabdominal approach.

2 **A,** Place a nasogastric tube. Consider hypotensive anesthesia.

Position: Place the patient supine and extended, with both arms on arm boards. If the incision is to be extended into the eighth or ninth interspace, hang the ipsilateral arm on the anesthesia screen. Prepare the skin from the chest to the upper thighs. Insert a urethral balloon catheter of suitable size and connect it to drainage.

Incision: Make a midline incision from beside the xiphoid to slightly below the pubis. Place plastic wound protectors and two self-retaining retractors.

B, Divide the falciform ligament to allow upward displacement of the liver. Palpate and inspect the liver, spleen, pancreas, bowel, and retroperitoneal lymph nodes to determine operability. Reflect the omentum, and hold the colon on the chest in a bowel bag or surrounded with warm moist packs. Pack the small bowel to the right side or exteriorize it also. Have a nasogastric tube inserted and palpate it in the stomach transabdominally.

Divide the mesentery from the cecum to the base of the foramen of Winslow by taking down the hepatic flexure. Extend it superiorly and medially over the vena cava to the duodenojejunal flexure to allow cephalad mobilization of the fourth portion of the duodenum and the pancreas (Kocher maneuver, see pages 859 and 986).

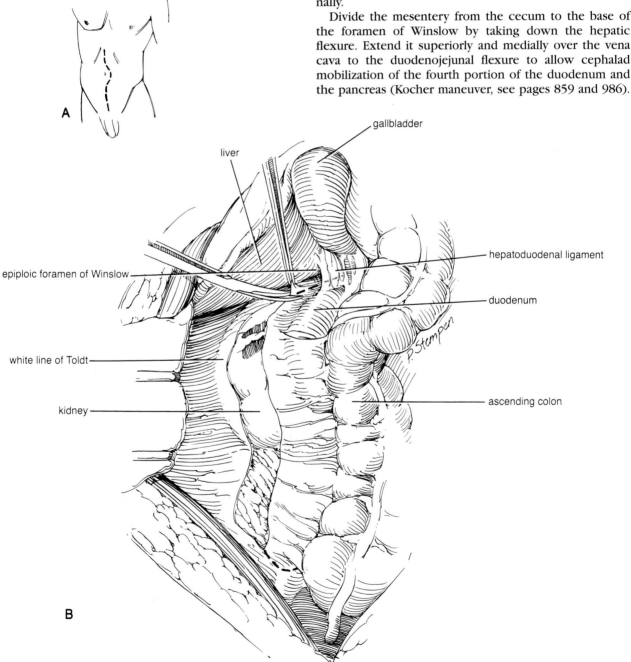

3 Continue the incision around the cecum obliquely to the left by blunt and sharp dissection of the root of the mesentery to reach the ligament of Treitz. Divide the inferior mesenteric vein, ligate it, and dissect it away from the base of the mesentery as it ascends to empty into the portal system. Clip intestinal lymphatic trunks proximally and distally as they are encountered.

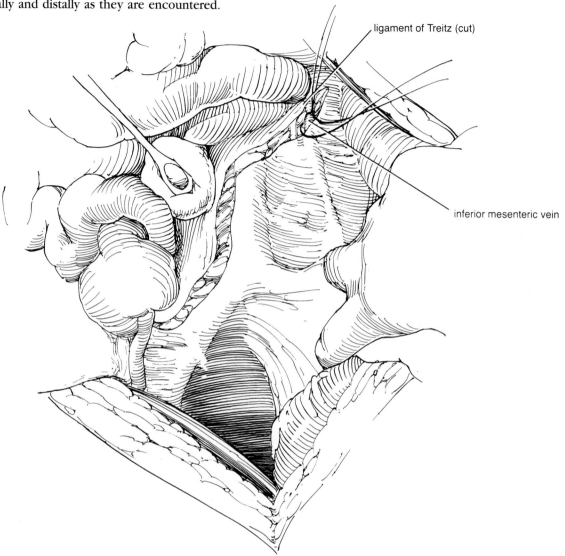

ligament of Treitz (cut)

inferior mesenteric vein

4   Separate the undersurface of the bowel bluntly from Gerota's fascia, and free the rest of the cecum, duodenum, and pancreas. Separate the pancreas bluntly from the anterior aspect of Gerota's fascia beneath it. Place the small bowel, cecum, and ascending colon in a bowel bag onto the chest, held with a broad retractor against the trunk of the superior mesenteric artery. Avoid compression of this artery. In cases that require high

dissection, divide the inferior mesenteric vein between silk ligatures and place a laparotomy pad on the head and body of the pancreas and elevate it with broad retractors, thereby improving high retroperitoneal exposure. Identify the origin of the superior mesenteric artery and preserve it with care. Locate the ureters, renal vessels, and pancreas to define the safe limits for dissection.

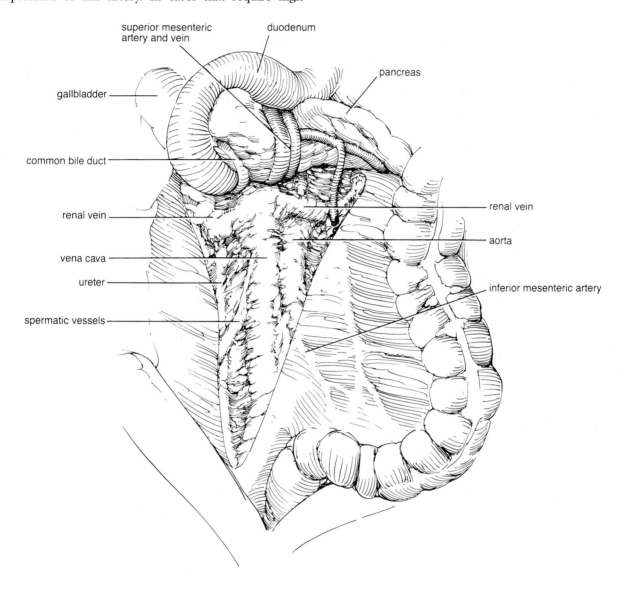

Dissection, Step 1

For a nerve-sparing operation, as the dissection progresses identify the retroperitoneal autonomic nerves before resecting the nodal tissue. Place vessel loops around the nerves as they are dissected from the lymphatic tissue posteriorly over the aorta and around the lumbar veins. If there is doubt, they may be absolutely identified by electrostimulation while observing the bladder neck by transrectal sonography (Recker and Tscholl, 1993).

5 Start dissecting on the anterior aspect of the vena cava at the level of the left renal vein. Use DeBakey or Potts forceps to grasp the adventitia and Metzenbaum scissors for dissection, keeping the tips away from the vessel. Get in the correct plane, which is right on the surface of the vessel. This step is the beginning of the "split-and-roll" technique (Donohue), in which the nodal package is split anteriorly over the inferior vena cava, aorta, and renal vessels. The three pairs of lumbar arteries are preserved, and the three left-sided and two right-sided veins are either preserved or divided as the great vessels are elevated and the underlying nodal tissue is removed. Recognize that some of these lumbar vessels may branch.

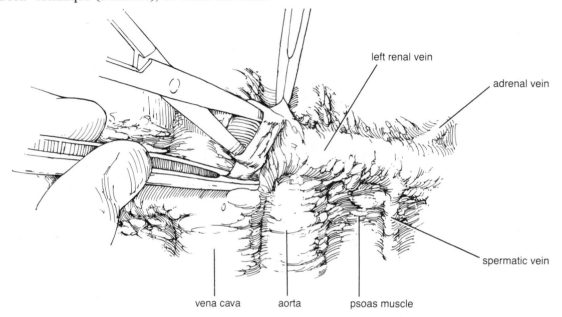

left renal vein

adrenal vein

spermatic vein

vena cava   aorta   psoas muscle

6 Dissect along the left renal vein to expose the adrenal vein. Pass sutures and doubly tie and divide the adrenal vein. (For low-stage disease, the adrenal vein need not be divided.) It is always necessary to divide the spermatic vein (Step 7). Be prepared to clip all lymph channels, even if the presence of disease is only suspected.

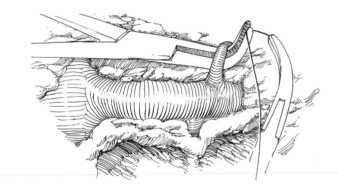

7 Mobilize the perivascular lymphatic tissue inferiorly from the left renal vein. Clip and divide the tributary (spermatic and lumbar) veins. Watch for the short lumbar vein that runs through this tissue and enters the left renal vein posterior to the left gonadal vein. Clip or ligate it close to the medial border of the psoas muscle, which then allows exposure of the left renal artery. Alternatively, the lumbar vein may enter the spermatic vein. Dissect the left renal artery free of tissue, beginning at its origin.

Enter the adventitial plane over the infrarenal aorta and clear it. Ligate and divide the spermatic arteries as soon as they are encountered. Do not place clips on the aorta or vena cava; they are easily avulsed. Lift the renal vein with a retractor and pull down on the lymphatic tissue to reach the posterior superior portion of the hilar lymphatics that lie behind the posterior layer of Gerota's fascia. Stop the dissection laterally when the pelviureteric junction comes into view.

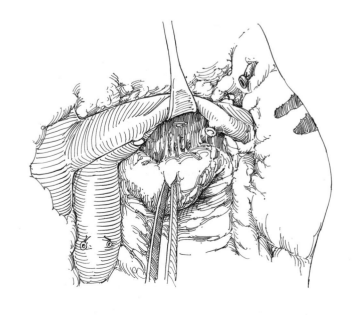

8 Dissect the hilar lymphatics from the psoas fascia toward the aorta. Incise the posterior layer of Gerota's fascia at its attachment to the spine. Mobilize the lateral retroaortic tissue.

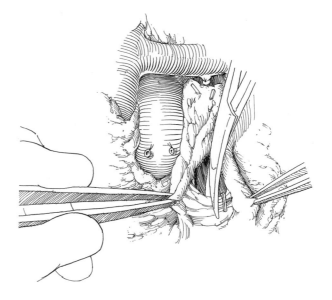

9 To visualize the lumbar vessels and lumbar sympa- thetic trunk, elevate the vena cava and clear it of nodal tissue. Dissect the first or second dorsal vein below the renal vein to its exit between the psoas muscle and the vertebral column to locate the cordlike lumbar sym- pathetic trunk. In a patient with negative findings, place vessel loops around the anterior and posterior branches of the sympathetic nerve chain and draw the nerves over the aorta. Dissect the trunk caudally in and out of the lymphatic tissue to the plexus at the base of the aorta. Usually two or three branches can be preserved as the dissection continues caudally, but sacrifice the numerous small connecting rami that enter the lymphatic mass. If the nodal findings are positive, do a block dissection, disregarding the nerves. Dissect along the anterior and lateral aspects of the aorta, watching for aberrant vessels to the lower pole of the kidney. Preserve the preaortic and para-aortic tissue below the inferior mesenteric ar- tery, which is neither dissected out nor divided.

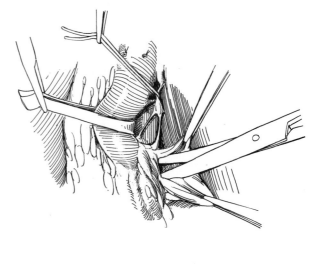

10 Continue the dissection down the aorta on the psoas fascia, ending at the bifurcation of the left external and internal iliac arteries. Watch for the iliopsoas and other muscle branches that extend from the left common iliac vessels.

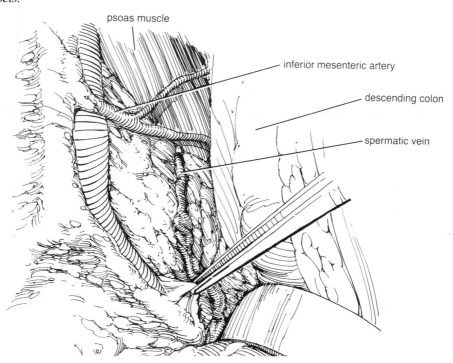

psoas muscle

inferior mesenteric artery

descending colon

spermatic vein

Dissection, Step 2

11 Pass the dissected tissue under the aorta below the renal artery *(arrow)*. Ligate and divide lumbar arteries prospectively in this area of dissection as needed, usually sacrificing the L2 and L3 branches. This provides better hemostasis, easier retraction of the aorta, and better exposure of the para-aortic nodal tissue.

12 In the more extensive dissections for gross disease, dissect caudally and ligate and divide any lumbar veins that are encountered. Pass a clamp behind the vessel, and draw a ligature around it and tie it. Apply a second ligature and divide the vessel between them. This permits a 360-degree dissection around the vena cava and aorta and allows them to be mobilized and better retracted, which in turn facilitates a full dissection (Step 11).

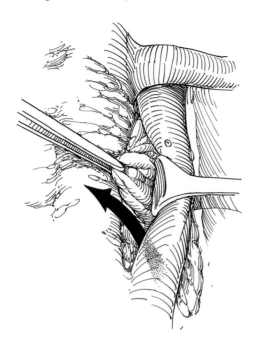

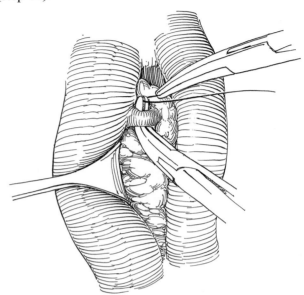

13 Dissect the tissue from the right renal vein and vena cava, beginning on the anterior surface. Ligate the right spermatic vein at the vena cava. Free the right ureter by clipping its vascular connections with the right spermatic vessels. Continue dissecting down the vena cava to the right common iliac artery and the first part of the right external iliac artery; pass the tissue to the midline. *Caution:* Lift the right common iliac artery to allow early ligation of the veins entering the left common iliac vein to avoid stubborn bleeding should they be avulsed.

Dissection, Step 3

Retract the aorta and vena cava to the left with vein retractors (not shown).

14 Isolate and clear the right renal artery behind the vena cava. Pass the dissected tissue beneath the vena cava to the midline. *Caution:* Clip *all* proximal lymphatic channels. The cisterna chyli lies just cephalad.

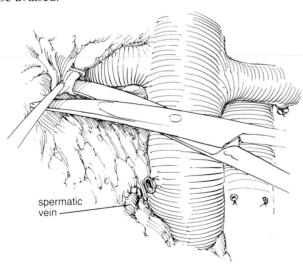

spermatic vein

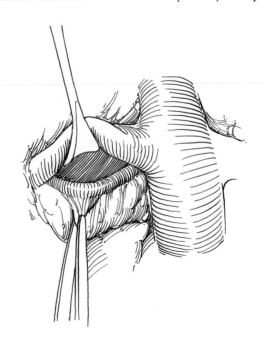

15 Dissect caudad on the anterior spinal ligament, sacrificing lumbar vessels as necessary and clearing all the interaortocaval, medial retrocaval, and retroaortic lymph tissue. A peanut dissector or a suction tip is useful here. Clip points of fixation or attachment posteriorly and divide them. It may be necessary to suture-ligate the lumbar vessels at the posterior body wall foramina, particularly when bulky masses are present. Complete the division of the tissue around the iliac artery, and remove the specimen. Follow the spermatic vessels on the side of the tumor to the external inguinal ring and remove them cleanly, including the ligated end from the previous orchiectomy along with a patch of peritoneum. Inspect the wound for bleeding and residual tissue, and irrigate it with sterile water. Attach the parietal peritoneum to the root of the mesentery as the bowel is replaced, using interrupted 3-0 silk sutures to decrease adhesions.

Elevate each renal artery with a vein retractor and inspect the suprahilar nodal areas. Drainage of lymph from the testis passes from the primary nodes that were removed as described, into the posterior mediastinum via the posterior para-aortic nodes below the right and left crura of the diaphragm. The dissection of these nodes is needed only in the event of their significant enlargement in association with gross disease below the renal hilus. Again, great care is necessary in securing the L1 lumbar vessels and proximal lymphatic trunks. Close the wound in layers without drainage.

Left-Sided Tumor

Reflect the left colon medially, and divide the splenocolic attachments and the mesocolon to allow exposure as far as the left renal and iliac vessels. Pack the bowel.

Palpate along the dorsolateral aspect of the aorta for the left sympathetic chain (Step 1). Sharply and bluntly dissect the areolar tissue to expose the fibers from the chain that divide superficial to the aortic adventitia on the anterolateral aspect. With a right-angle clamp, dissect them free and contain them in a vessel loop. Follow them medially to their respective trunks, which are in turn encircled with vessel loops. As the nodes are dissected cephalad, they are found under the chain, requiring delicate handling. Division of some of the lumbar arteries and veins may help the dissection. To retrieve all of the nodal tissue, it must be divided into segments.

Closure

Close the anterior peritoneum as a separate layer and approximate the fascia with interrupted 1-0 SAS. Close the subcutaneous tissue with interrupted plain catgut and the skin with staples. Consider placing a gastrostomy (see page 673) as an alternative to a Salem sump tube.

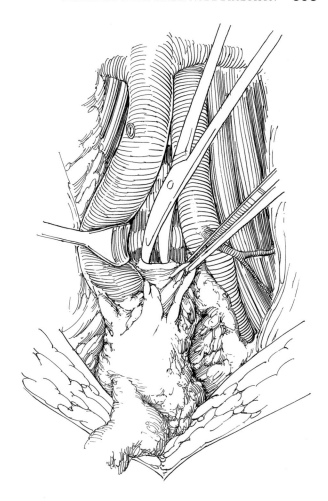

THORACOABDOMINAL LYMPHADENECTOMY

The thoracoabdominal incision (see page 890) can provide adequate exposure for removal of large retroperitoneal nodal masses detected preoperatively above the true pelvis. Although it may be used for routine lymphadenectomy, especially in heavy men, this incision particularly facilitates dissection above the renal vessels and in the posterior mediastinum. The operation is on the left or right side, depending on the location of the mass as defined by the site of the initial tumor and preoperative CT scanning. Occasionally, sequential left-sided and right-sided operations may be necessary for bulky bilateral disease, especially with retrocrural or mediastinal deposits.

Left-Sided Approach

16 Place the patient in the torque flank position, with the shoulders at a 30- to 45-degree angle and the back close to the edge of the table, held by a roll. The pelvis may lie flat on the hyperextended table, or a sandbag may be placed under the ipsilateral buttock. Flex the opposite knee, and place the left arm on an arm support. Tape the patient in place.

Incision: Usually select the ninth interspace. Start the incision near the posterior axillary line over the 10th rib and carry it straight toward the epigastrium, halfway between the xiphoid and the umbilicus. There, turn it down as a midline or paramedian incision. In a thin patient with limited disease, begin the incision at the costochondral junction.

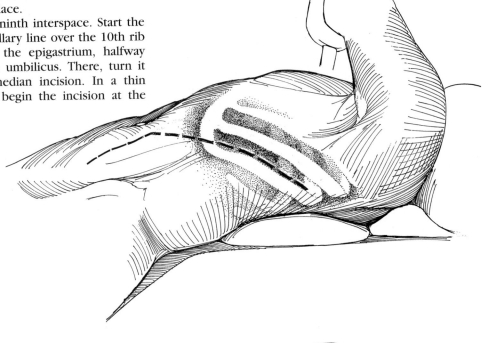

17 Divide the lateral body wall muscles, cutting directly onto the rib with electrocautery.

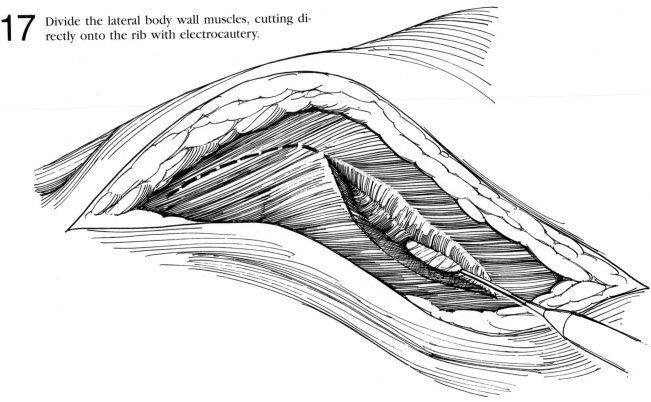

18 Cut the intercostal muscle above the 10th rib (see page 881), or resect the rib (see pages 875 to 876) and enter the pleura, taking care to avoid the lung. Palpate the lung and mediastinum for metastatic tumor.

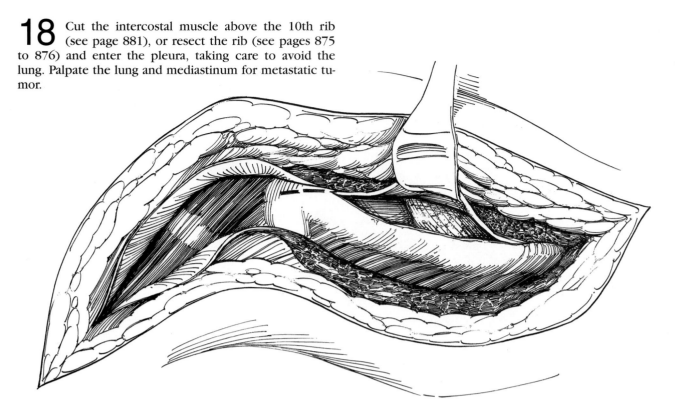

19 Divide the anterior rectus sheath, and continue the incision upward to join the pleural incision. Insert and spread Mayo scissors beneath the connecting costal cartilage; then resect it, entering the plane between the peritoneum and abdominal wall. Mobilize the rectus muscle laterally. Divide it at the upper end to reduce denervation.

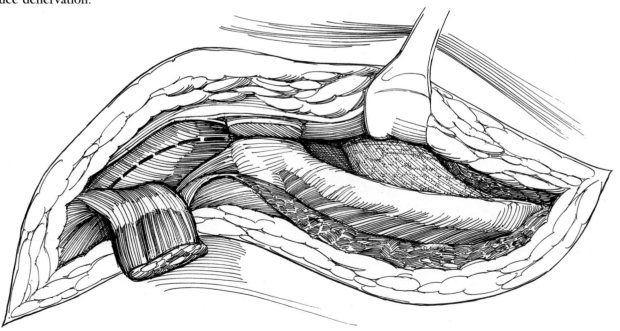

20 Dissect the peritoneum from the rectus sheath to the linea alba. Use delicate sharp dissection supplemented by digital dissection. Split the fibers of the transversus abdominis muscle, and incise the posterior rectus sheath.

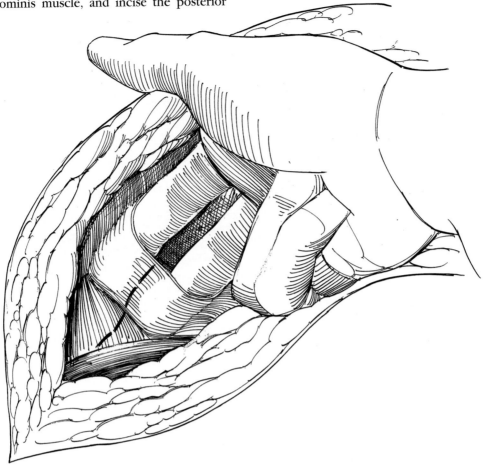

21 Dissect the peritoneum from the diaphragm as your assistant elevates the upper edge of the incision while you place countertraction on the peritoneal envelope. Avoid cutting the muscular diaphragmatic fibers and entering the peritoneum. Close any small tears in the peritoneum; large tears are best left until the wound is to be closed. Alternatively, open the peritoneum widely, especially in obese patients.

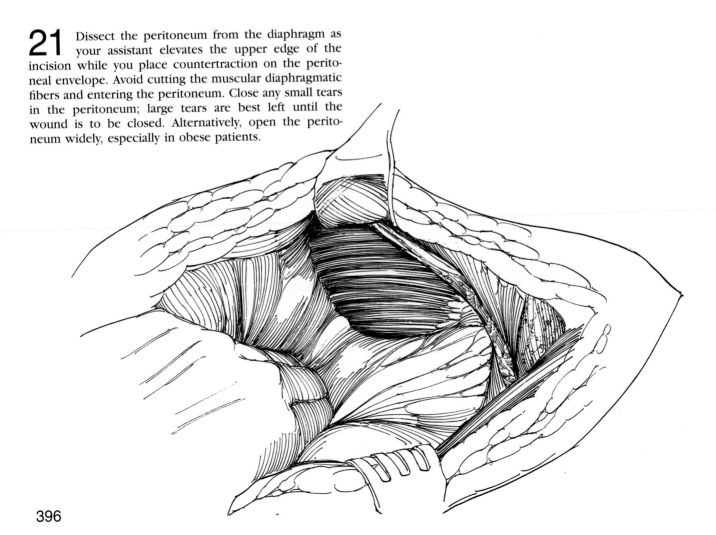

22 **A,** Divide the diaphragm by a convex incision that ends near the 12th thoracic vertebra. **B,** Continue the dissection to include the central tendon of the diaphragm.

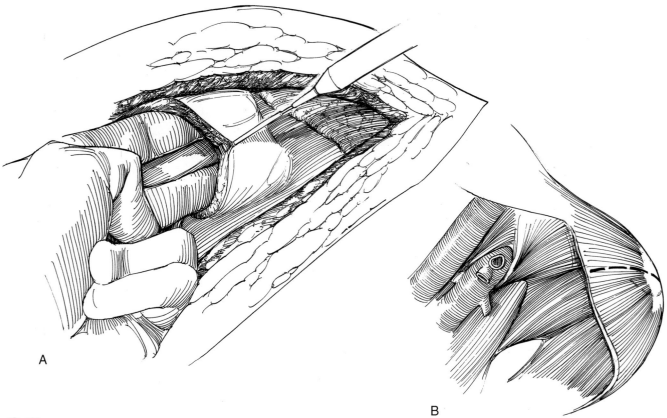

A

B

23 Mobilize Gerota's fascia from the lumbar muscles laterally to the margin of the aorta medially and to the iliac vessels and inguinal ligament inferiorly. Place a self-retaining retractor with the upper blade against the cut costal cartilage and the lower blade secured with a towel clip in the drapes to prevent it from slipping down.

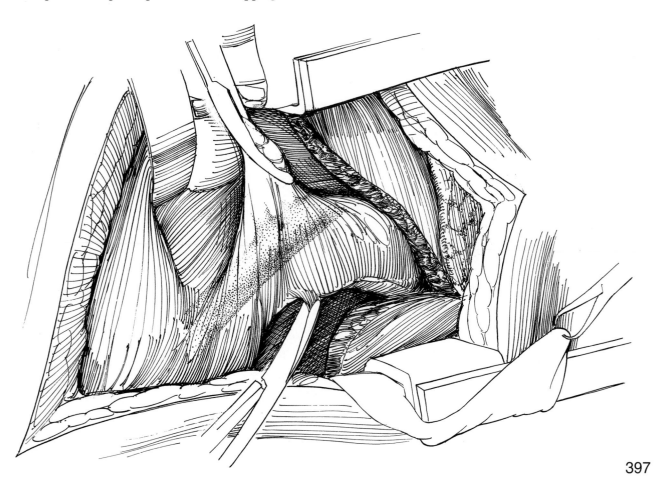

24 For posterior mediastinal dissection on the left, locate the left crus of the diaphragm. Pass the index finger underneath it parallel to the vertebral bodies. This movement pushes the aorta away and allows the crus to be opened for a distance of 3 to 5 cm. Lift the aorta and dissect the tissue in the posterior mediastinum.

For mediastinal dissection on the right, delay opening the crus until the tissues have been removed around the inferior vena cava above the right renal vein, including ligation of the adrenal vein and removal of the periadrenal tissue with or without the adrenal gland.

For massive tumors, optimal exposure is obtained by opening the peritoneal cavity, freeing the ascending colon and small bowel, and placing them in a bag on the chest, recognizing the complications of transperitoneal surgery, such as ileus, adhesions, and evisceration.

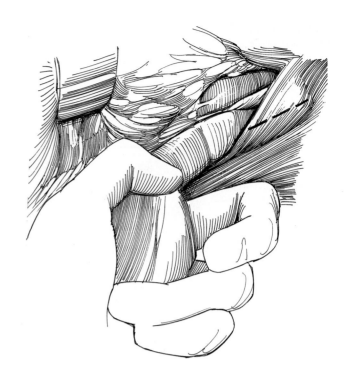

25 For an extraperitoneal approach, separate Gerota's fascia from the peritoneum, cutting the fine strands along the avascular plane to reach the left renal vein—the central anatomic landmark. For right-sided dissection, free the peritoneum from Gerota's fascia until the duodenum and head of the pancreas are exposed. A Kocher maneuver under the duodenum allows them to be mobilized medially (see pages 859 and 986).

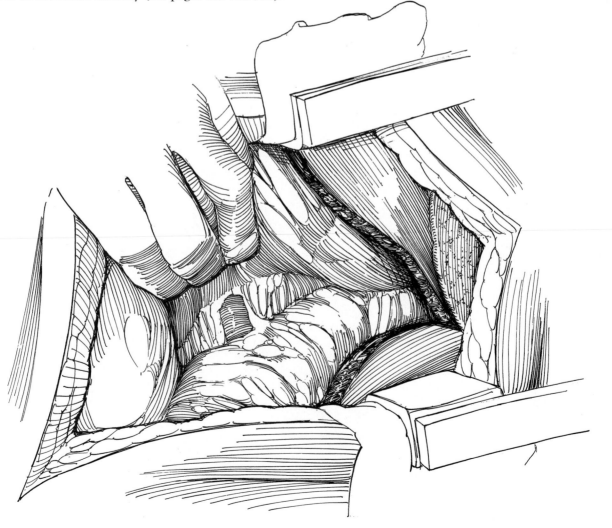

26 Identify the superior mesenteric artery cephalad and the aorta, the origins of both renal arteries, and the inferior vena cava below as you mobilize the peritoneum, pancreas, and duodenum anteriorly. For division of the superior margin, expose the adventitia of the superior mesenteric artery, and follow it to the aorta by dividing the tissue over it. Be sure to clip all lymphatics there.

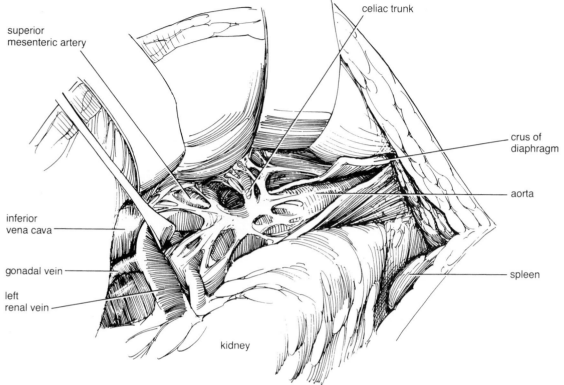

27 For exposure of the aorta and vena cava, grasp the suprahilar nodal tissue lying between the upper pole of the kidney and the diaphragm and aorta between the fingers, and successively clip and divide it. Continue that line of dissection over the vena cava.

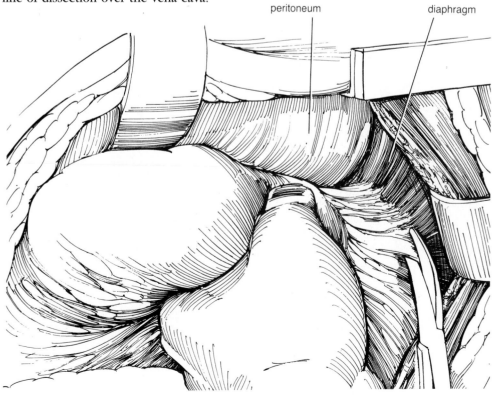

28 Divide the tissue over the renal vein to expose the left adrenal and spermatic veins, which are ligated and divided. Retract the renal vein, and clip and divide the tissue down the aorta to the inferior mesenteric artery. A finger against the aortic adventitia helps the dissection.

29 Divide the inferior mesenteric artery. Continue dissection across the vena cava at the superior margin to the base of the right renal vein. Be careful to clip all tissue; then divide the tissue down the vena cava. Dissect the tissue from the aorta. Identify each lumbar artery, ligate them with 3-0 silk ties, and divide them as the dissection progresses. Inject mannitol intravenously.

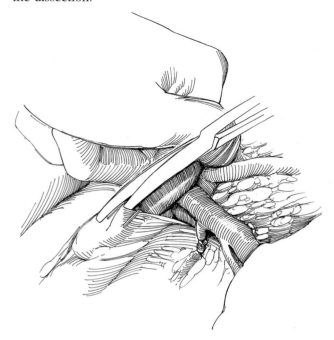

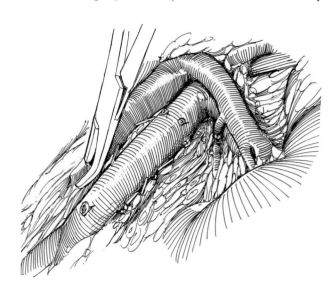

30 A, Dissect the tissue from the left renal vessels by first splitting Gerota's fascia over the lateral border of the kidney and reflecting it medially. B, Divide the resulting ring of tissue, keeping the renal pedicle in view to avoid damage to the vessels. Do not be concerned about inadvertent division of a polar vessel because hypertension is a very unlikely sequela.

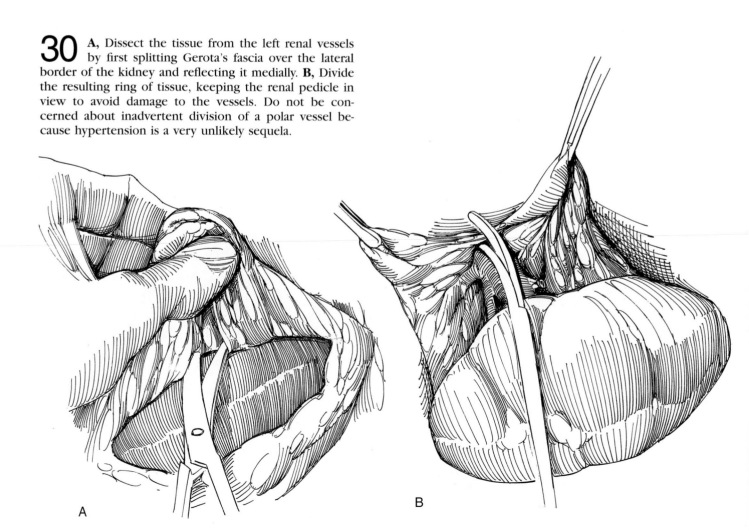

A

B

31 For dissection between aorta and vena cava, expose the right renal artery by retracting the vein. A small Penrose drain around the left renal vein may aid in dissection. Later use the same technique for the vena cava and aorta. A vasodilator (2 percent lidocaine and 1 percent papaverine) may be applied to the renal vessels during dissection to reduce spasm. Dissect the tissue above the right renal artery between the great vessels; then clip and divide it. Identify the adrenal blood supply, and ligate it as far from the renal artery as possible.

Continue dissection behind the vena cava down to the fascia of the prevertebral ligament, progressively clipping and dividing the tissue. Ligate and divide the left lumbar veins, clipping the distal ends and ligating the origins on the vena cava.

Stop the dissection inferiorly after exposure of the right common iliac artery and vein. If ejaculatory ability is to be preserved, it is vitally important to avoid the sympathetic tissue of the hypogastric plexus at the bifurcation of the vessels.

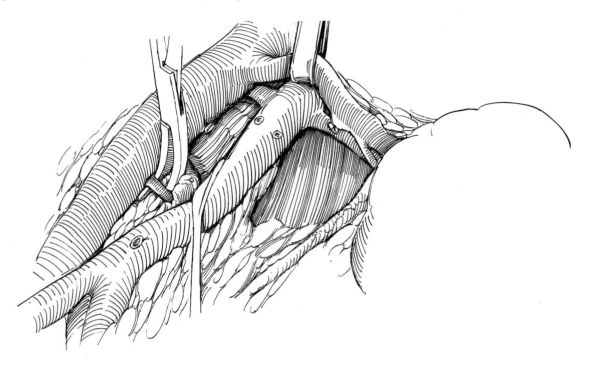

32 Divide the right lumbar arteries. Place a clip on the distal segment, and ligate the end arising from the aorta to prevent dislodgment during dissection. If a tie or clip is dislodged, grasp the vessel with an Allis clamp and oversew it with a 4-0 arterial silk suture. The spinal cord is not devascularized as long as the lumbar arteries above the renal pedicle are spared. Lift the aorta and pull the nodal tissue under it.

To complete the dissection, bluntly free the ureter from the specimen. With large masses, first identify the ureter at the pelvic brim and trace it up into the mass. Trace the left spermatic vessels to the external ring, where the marking ligature on the vessels from the radical orchiectomy is recovered. Clip the vessels behind the aorta on the left. Preserve the sympathetic chain as it is encountered.

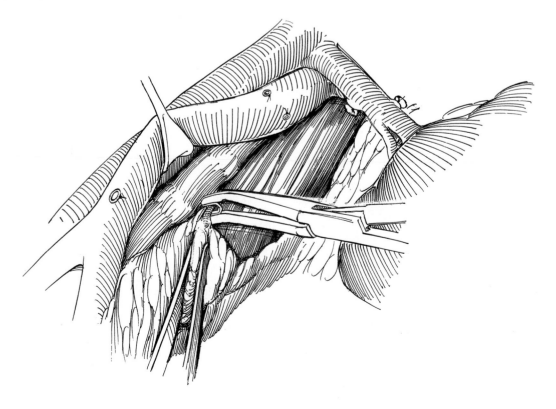

33 *Closure:* Before closing the wound, retrace the steps of the operation. Place clips on all the ligated branches of the aorta. Check the flow in the renal arteries. Look for lymphatic leaks, especially the lacteals at the base of the superior mesenteric artery. If the ureter has been extensively mobilized, wrap it in omentum. Perform a nephropexy with a 2-0 figure-eight SAS on the renal capsule over fat bolsters. Level the table. Close the diaphragm watertight in two layers with 2-0 SAS. Alternatively, place one layer of NAS in it.

Inspect all the ligated vessels, adding hemoclips where needed, and check the upper and lower limits of the dissection for gross lymphatic leakage, especially around the base of the superior mesenteric artery.

Straighten the table. Close the diaphragm in a water-tight fashion in two layers with a running suture of 2-0 synthetic absorbable material. Place a plastic thoracotomy tube (36 F) one interspace above or below the incision, to remain 2 or 3 days. Connect it to water-sealed, three-bottle suction under a negative pressure of 15 to 20 cm H_2O. Close the chest in one layer with 1-0 figure-eight interrupted SAS. Place all the sutures before tying them. Include the diaphragm in the more medial sutures to separate the pleura from the retroperitoneal space. Close the abdomen in layers with the same suture technique. Block the appropriate intercostal nerves with 5 ml of 0.75 percent bupivacaine percutaneously. Drains are probably unnecessary.

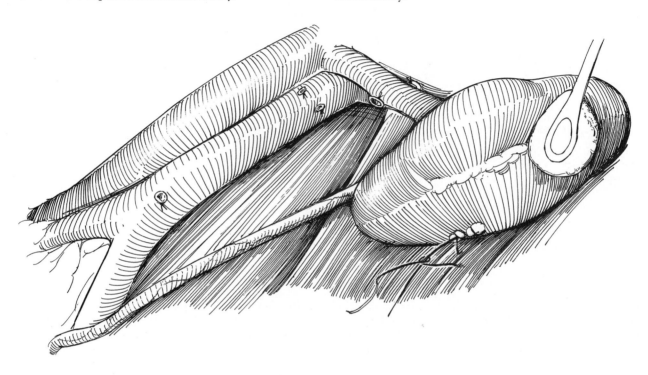

Right-Sided Approach

Start the dissection below the insertion of the lowest hepatic vein on the vena cava. Ligate the adrenal vein; then resect the adrenal gland. Free the vena cava, and clear the right crus of the diaphragm behind the vena cava. Follow the steps for left-sided dissection (Steps 16 to 33).

INTRAOPERATIVE MANAGEMENT

Monitoring: Follow volume changes throughout the operation. Continue infusion of 5 percent albumin solution (1 to 1.5 L) and 5 percent dextrose in 0.3 percent saline with 20 mEq/L of potassium chloride (3 to 4 L) during the operation and in the recovery room, continued in the patient's room for 2 to 3 days. Follow the hematocrit value and the levels of sodium and potassium in the urine as the third-space fluid is resorbed.

Vascular injuries are managed in the usual way (see page 81). With a large tumor, the segment of the vena cava below

the renal veins can be resected with the tumor. Most vessels can be repaired, although nephrectomy may become necessary. *Ureteral injuries* are uncommon and are treated by intraoperative repair with stenting (see page 68).

Appendectomy. Appendectomy is contraindicated in retroperitoneal lymphadenectomy because of the greater incidence of infection (Leibovitch et al, 1995).

POSTOPERATIVE MANAGEMENT

Check lung expansion by a chest film. Third-space loss must continue to be replaced by large infusions of saline and 5 percent albumin solution. As much as 3000 to 4000 ml of saline and 1000 to 1500 ml of 5 percent albumin are needed during the operation. Give 5 percent dextrose in saline at a rate of 150 ml/hr in the recovery room and 5 percent albumin at 50 ml/hr for the first 18 to 24 hours. Monitor hematocrit and urine output. By the third day, urine output increases significantly as the fluid in the third space is resorbed. Maintain 15 to 20 cm H_2O closed-vent suction on the chest tube until drainage falls below 100 ml/day. Then use a water seal and remove the tube the next day.

A decision must be made for or against adjuvant chemotherapy. With negative nodes, actinomycin D can be given at surgery and again for a 5-day course after 2 months. For other stages, the decision must be individualized.

Check the patient every 2 months for the first year, and closely thereafter, with examination of the supraclavicular nodes, the abdomen, and remaining testis; a chest film; and testing for beta-hCG and AFP.

POSTOPERATIVE PROBLEMS

Complications after postchemotherapy node dissection are appreciably greater than after dissection for low-stage disease.

Wound infection is seldom a serious problem, especially when wound protectors are used. Dehiscence is rare. *Respiratory complications* are serious after bleomycin therapy, which may cause pulmonary fibrosis with resulting high risk for respiratory morbidity. Be sure to evaluate pulmonary function postoperatively as well as preoperatively. Enforce pulmonary physiotherapy, and routinely give a broad-spectrum antibiotic. Complications can be lessened by a reduced level of oxygen saturation during surgery and by the avoidance of overhydration. *Atelectasis*, evidenced in the first 24 hours by increased temperature and pulse rate, is managed with early ambulation and rebreathing techniques plus aerosol inhalation. *Pneumothorax* is avoided by the placement of a chest tube. Pleural effusion may require aspiration or reinsertion of a chest tube.

Bleeding appears immediately unless a major vessel has been injured and repaired. Injuries are repaired by standard vascular techniques. *Pancreatitis* can occur after suprahilar dissection. Pancreatic injuries must be closed with NAS and drained carefully.

Ileus usually lasts 3 to 4 days; it is less common after an extraperitoneal thoracoabdominal operation than after a transabdominal one. If ileus persists, suspect a retroperitoneal problem, such as hematoma, urinary extravasation, or pancreatitis. Mechanical *bowel obstruction* is rare if the mesentery was closed accurately and the bowel was placed in a bowel bag and seldom requires operative intervention.

Chylous ascites from failure to ligate the cisterna is uncommon but may be signaled soon after operation by abdominal distention with or without pleural effusion. Identifying the major lymphatics entering the cisterna chyli and doubly ligating the cisterna itself help prevent chylous ascites. If it is clipped, include some perilymphatic tissue to prevent the clip from cutting through. Abdominal ultrasonography and paracentesis help establish the diagnosis. Treat with low-fat diet, medium-chain triglycerides, diuretics, and, if necessary, hyperalimentation, but ligation of the open vessel or peritoneovenous shunt may be required. A *lymphocele* may develop; aspirate it under CT guidance.

Loss of ejaculation, either retrograde ejaculation or anejaculation, can often be avoided by preserving the sympathetic fibers in the preaortic area between the inferior mesenteric artery and the aortic bifurcation. Loss may occur in spite of preserving the nodal tissue on the contralateral side below the superior mesenteric artery, the nerve-sparing technique. Anejaculation (no sperm in the urine), however, is common after bilateral postchemotherapy lymphadenectomy because of disruption of the thoracolumbar sympathetic outflow (T12-L3), but normal ejaculation may return months later if the dissection does not include removal of the contralateral iliac, preaortic and precaval, and interaortic nodes below the point of origin of the inferior mesenteric artery, especially the hypogastric plexus below the bifurcation of the aorta. If sperm were not banked, consider sperm aspiration from testis or epididymis.

Ureteral injury can occur where the gonadal vein crosses in front of the ureter when the vessel is elevated, angulating the ureter. Freeing the ureter prior to this dissection can prevent injury. If the ipsilateral kidney is functioning poorly, as shown on preoperative urograms, nephrectomy should be performed. If the kidney has good function, the ureter should be repaired over a suitable stent. Alternatively, resect the distal portion and reimplant it with the aid of a psoas hitch, because the ureter has been partially devascularized.

Anorexia and *weakness* may continue for as long as 6 weeks after surgery, especially if the patient received chemotherapy. Consider hyperalimentation if anorexia is severe.

SALVAGE SURGERY

After chemotherapy, suspect the presence of a mature teratoma or residual immature tumor elements if a 2-cm or greater mass persists. Excise any suspected residual tumor. If, after chemotherapy, the markers remain abnormal, repeat a course of chemotherapy. Proceed with salvage surgery if the markers do not return to normal. Wide lymph node dissection is needed only in patients with larger tumors or those with suspected viable tumor.

Commentary by John P. Donohue

The templates for left and right dissection shown in Step 1B are correct. For low-stage disease (clinical Stages I and IIa), transabdominal retroperitoneal lymph node dissection has been modified to maintain ejaculation by preserving preaortic sympathetic fibers below the inferior mesenteric artery (as shown in Step 1C). The template of dissection captures the primary nodes of spread for the respective side of the primary tumor. With right-sided primaries in low volume, dissection above the inferior mesenteric artery need not be bilateral because none of the low-volume Stage IIb disease was suprahilar and only one case was positive contralaterally. Similarly, no left-sided low-volume Stage II disease is bilateral. For bulky, advanced disease (clinical Stages IIc or III, including node dissection after chemotherapy), I do bilateral node dissections. The lateral borders of the dissection are either ureter; it may be necessary to extend the dissection cephalad into the retrocrural (suprahilar) areas, caudad into the pelvic (external iliac, hypogastric, and obturator) areas, or both in cases of clinical (CT) or gross (visual or palpable) involvement.

For both low-stage and high-stage disease, the fundamental principle of dissection involves the "split-and-roll" technique. The lymphatic and nodal package is split at 12 o'clock over the aorta and vena cava and the iliac and renal vessels and rolled laterally off the vessels. Lumbars are divided so as to complete the roll en bloc. The tissue is then removed from its attachments to the posterior body wall.

Rather than "cold cutting," which is acceptable but costly in terms of lymph and red blood cells over an extended time period, the cautery and clipping are helpful in conserving these. I use the hand-held unit with an extender for the electrode.

Laparoscopic Modified Retroperitoneal Lymph Node Dissection

(Stone, Waterhouse)

Limit the dissection superiorly by the renal hilum, laterally by the ureter, medially by the vena cava for left-sided testicular tumors and by the aorta for right-sided tumors, and inferiorly at the level of the inferior mesenteric artery. Extend it to the bifurcation of the common iliac vessels, and include the stump of the spermatic vessels.

Prepare the bowel preoperatively. Magnesium citrate is better than GoLYTELY because the bowel is not distended and is easier to retract. Consider donations of autologous blood. The potential for a serious complication is greater than for an open procedure, and the patient should be advised that open surgery may be necessary if complications occur.

Cystoscopically insert a ureteral stent on the affected side. Place a nasogastric tube. While the patient is supine, induce pneumoperitoneum and insert five trocars: one supraumbilical observation trocar, three ipsilateral trocars in the midclavicular line, and one contralaterally in the midclavicular line. Move the patient into the semilateral position.

After freeing any interfering adhesions, incise the posterior peritoneum with scissors along the white line of Toldt, including the hepatic flexure on the left and the splenic flexure on the right. Put traction on the medial peritoneal edge, and use blunt and sharp dissection to free the colon from the retroperitoneal tissues.

Right Modified Dissection

1 Start by exposing the bifurcation of the common iliac vessels (marking the *inferior margin* of the dissection). Uncover the inferior mesenteric vessels superiorly, and draw them medially and anteriorly with the colonic mesentery, exposing the medial margin of the vena cava *(medial margin)*. Identify the ureter *(lateral margin)*, and begin blunt dissection of the nodal tissue medially. Identify the spermatic vein near the internal

ring, and divide it between clips. Dissect it to the renal vein, taking care not to avulse it *(cephalad margin)*. With the spoon forceps, bluntly and sharply dissect the tissue from the psoas muscle and the spine. Divide the lymph channels with the electrocautery scissors. Clip small vessels from the aorta and vena cava. Elevate the renal vein, and retract it medially to dissect beneath it. Return the patient to the supine position, and clip the retroperitoneum together. Terminate the procedure in sequence.

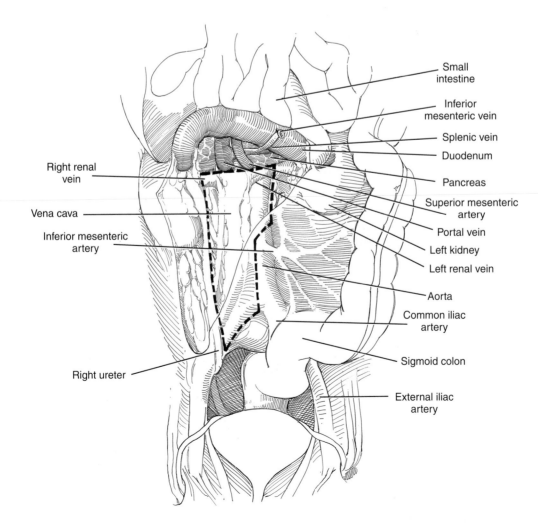

Limited Template Technique (Janetschek et al, 1994). Apply a two-step procedure. *Step 1:* Approach ventrally to free the colon and excise the spermatic vein to define the borders of the dissection. *Step 2:* Approach laterally to allow straightforward transection of the lumbar vessels.

Intraoperative and Postoperative Problems

Injury to a vessel, particularly the spermatic vein or the inferior mesenteric artery, may necessitate immediate open exposure for control. *Lymphoceles* can occur, to be drained percutaneously. *Bowel injury* is possible. With the proper template, ejaculation is maintained.

Commentary by Paramjit S. Chandhoke

Laparoscopic retroperitoneal lymph node dissection (RPLND) is a difficult procedure even for the well-trained laparoscopic surgeon. Because dissection is near major vessels, bleeding injuries can be difficult to control; this is the reason that the retrocaval and retroaortic nodes are not dissected out. Unlike laparoscopic pelvic lymphadenectomy, for which studies have documented the adequacy of the dissection, no studies have been reported in which laparoscopic RPLND was followed by an open evaluation. Therefore, this procedure should be considered experimental at present.

It is helpful to have laparoscopic fan retractors to retract bowel and laparoscopic vein retractors to gently retract vascular structures. Retraction injury of the spleen, liver, or bowel should be carefully avoided.

Because open RPLND may be a cure for Stage II testicular cancer in two thirds of the patients, the question lingers whether laparoscopic RPLND can achieve the same success. Currently, all patients undergoing laparoscopic RPLND also undergo chemotherapy if any nodes are found positive, chemotherapy that would not have been necessary if the patient had had an open procedure. If appropriate studies are not conducted, the potential for an inadequate dissection must be weighed against the lower morbidity of the laparoscopic procedure.

Spermatocelectomy

Caution the patient about a possible adverse effect on fertility.
Prepare the genitalia after limited shaving. Infiltrate the cord at the base of the scrotum with 1 percent lidocaine (see page 77).

1 Grasp the scrotum with the left hand to force the contents against the skin, and rotate the upper pole anteriorly. Incise the tissue transversely exactly to the thin surface of the spermatocele. Extrude the testis and epididymis without entering the tunica vaginalis at this stage. Place hemostatic Allis forceps on the skin and dartos layers, as done for hydrocele (not shown).

2 **A** and **B,** Cautiously dissect bluntly and sharply directly against the bluish cyst wall, trying not to puncture it (it is very tenuous). Curved arterial clamps are useful. Tie or fulgurate any small vessels. Remember that spermatoceles are usually multilocular. It may be helpful to open the tunica vaginalis at this point and dissect from inside.

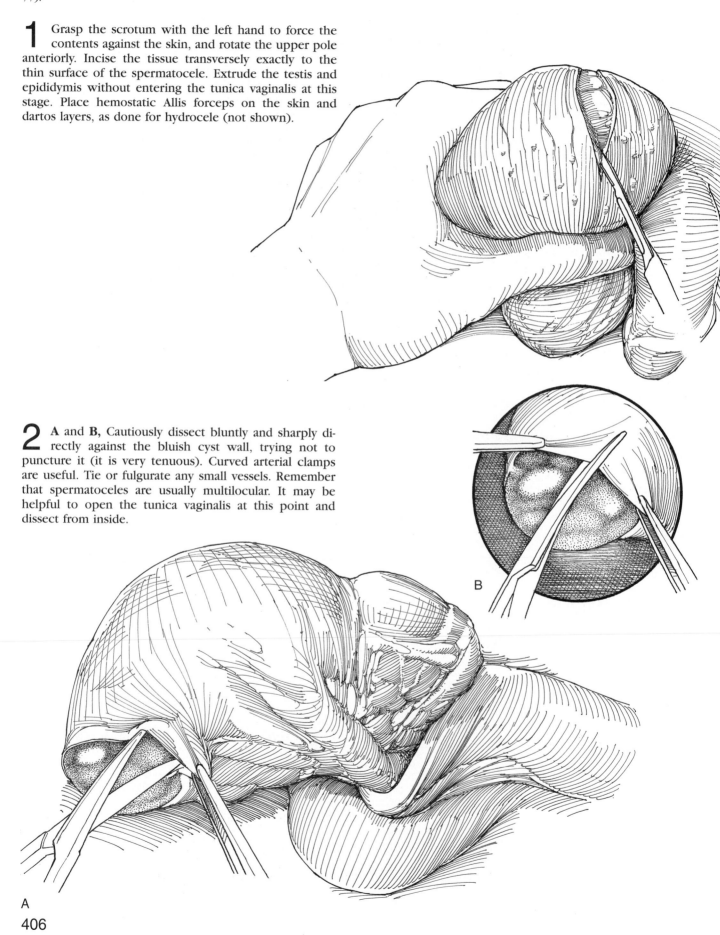

A

B

3 Continue the dissection by "shelling" out the locules to reach the thicker base where the cyst joins the epididymis. Fulgurate the small epididymal vessels. Use gauze over the index finger to push the areolar tissue aside, or elevate and dissect the spermatocele with scissors until it is exteriorized. If the spermatocele is large, it may help to open it, allow two thirds of its contents to escape, and clamp the opening closed with a mosquito clamp before proceeding with the dissection.

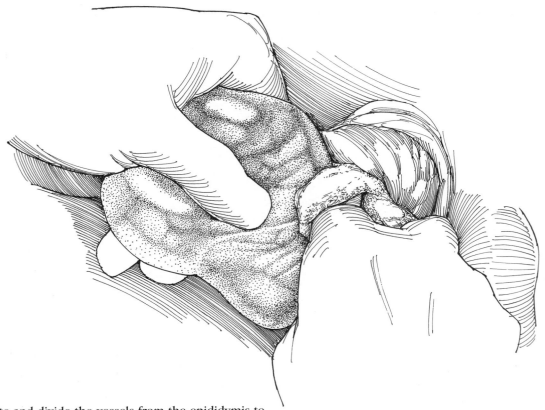

4 Ligate and divide the vessels from the epididymis to the spermatocele, and divide the remaining attachments. Secure absolute hemostasis to avoid drains. Close the dartos layer with one or two figure-eight 3-0 CCG sutures and the skin with fine subcuticular running plain catgut sutures. Apply a dry dressing in a suspensory, and send the patient home.

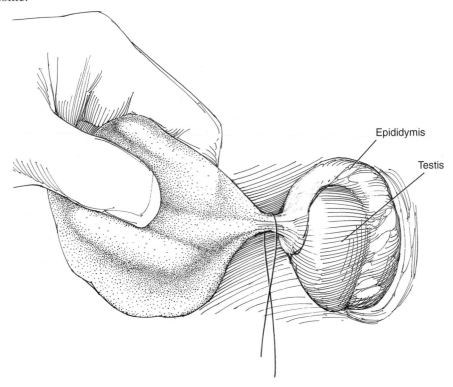

Epididymis

Testis

Commentary by Harris M. Nagler

Spermatoceles are located superior to the testicle. Although they are palpable as discrete structures, they are intravaginal in location. The removal of a spermatocele may proceed initially extravaginally, but the tunica vaginalis must be entered to excise the spermatocele. I approach spermatoceles by opening the tunica vaginalis immediately. The spermatocele can then be visualized as it arises from the epididymis. This intravaginal approach minimizes the potential for iatrogenic injury. Furthermore, the "avascular" plane of gossamer-like tissue immediately surrounding the spermatocele is more easily entered. Great care must be exercised in arriving at the right plane. As the dissection proceeds, the spermatocele looks almost like a gelatinous mass that is easily separated from the surrounding tissues. This plane is almost bloodless. Hemostasis may be achieved with fine bipolar forceps. The dissection should proceed carefully until the spermatocele narrows to a fine stalklike attachment to the caput of the epididymis. This can be ligated on both the specimen and the epididymal side. The stalk is divided, and the specimen may be removed without being entered.

Spermatocelectomy should be avoided in young men who still desire children. Epididymal obstruction may result even when the greatest care has been exercised.

Epididymectomy

Position: Supine. *Anesthesia:* Local cord infiltration (see page 76).

1 Manipulate the testis under the skin and make a transverse incision in the scrotum over it. To make closure easier, gather the successive layers with a suture placed at either end or in Allis clamps (see page 349). Open the tunica vaginalis. If epididymectomy is performed for tuberculosis, the incision should extend to the external inguinal ring to allow early ligation and subsequent removal of the distal vas and should include any sinus openings. Place a traction suture in the globus major, and begin dissection sharply at its apex. Divide and ligate the efferent tubules. Keep close to the epididymis to avoid injury of the vessels to the testis that run along the medial aspect. If they are injured, do not rush to orchiectomy because collateral vessels may supply adequate circulation. Identify and clamp the epididymal branch of the testicular artery.

Alternative: Begin the dissection at the lower pole to have more of the epididymis free before encountering the rete and vessels.

2 Free the body to the globus minor bluntly and sharply, aided by traction on the stay suture.

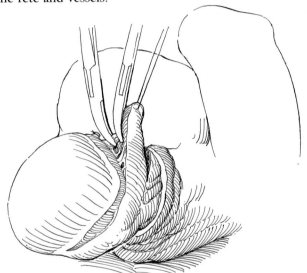

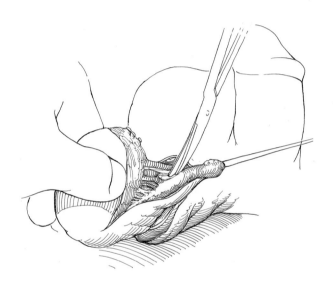

3 Elevate the specimen and clamp, divide, and ligate the vas with 3-0 CCG ties. Remove the specimen.

4 Close the defect with interrupted 3-0 CCG sutures. Replace the testis in the scrotum, and close the subcutaneous layers and the skin with 3-0 CCG sutures. A drain is usually not needed and is contraindicated with tuberculosis. Apply a scrotal support.

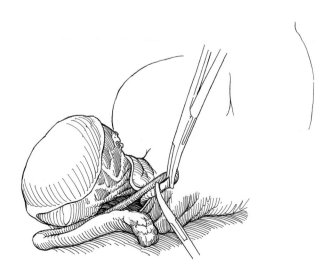

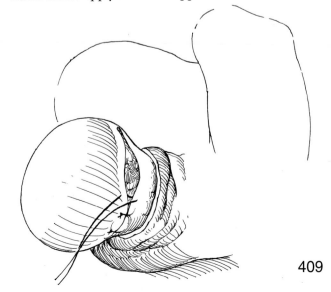

POSTOPERATIVE PROBLEMS

Persistent bleeding from scrotal surgery with formation of interstitial collections or hematomas in the loose scrotal sac is the most common complication. Although it is seldom life threatening, it does frighten the patient and delays his recovery. If infection supervenes, the problem becomes quite serious. Bleeding can be prevented by minimal dissection of planes and by meticulous fulguration of even the smallest vessels, especially on the cut edge of the tunica vaginalis. The dartos must be closed before the skin to achieve hemostasis at that level. If dissection has been extensive, insert a drain drawn out through a stab wound in the dependent portion of the scrotum; otherwise avoid drains because they act as bacterial conduits. Finally, to immobilize the area, apply either a nonelastic extra large scrotal suspensory that is well padded with gauze or an athletic supporter with a hole cut for the penis. Compression dressings are not feasible. If you find swelling and ecchymosis, delay intervention unless an obviously expanding hematoma is present. It is usually not possible to drain a significant accumulation because the distribution of blood is too diffuse. Of course, drainage is needed for an infected hematoma.

Commentary by Harris M. Nagler

Epididymectomy is a procedure that is seldom indicated. Draining scrotal sinuses should make the physician consider the diagnosis of tuberculosis. Appropriate antituberculous regimens must be instituted. Epididymectomy may also be done in the patient with chronic painful epididymitis. However, the surgeon must be aware of the pitfalls of operating for the relief of pain. This approach should be used only when all other approaches to pain management have been exhausted. All patients undergoing epididymectomy must be aware of the potential loss of the testicle either operatively or by subsequent atrophy.

As the author highlights, meticulous hemostasis must be achieved in scrotal surgery to avoid an unnecessarily long and uncomfortable recovery. I routinely invaginate the scrotal skin, expose the inside of the scrotal compartment (the inner surface of the dartos), and fulgurate all bleeding points.

SECTION

11

Prostate: Excision

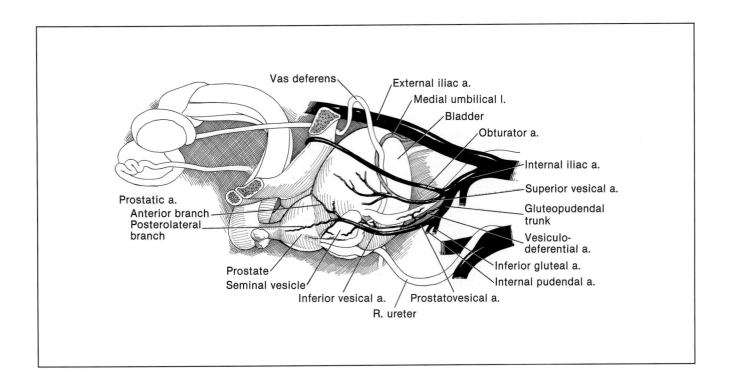

Anatomy and Principles of Excision of the Prostate

Although most benign obstructions requiring surgery are treated by transurethral techniques, open prostatectomy may still be preferable for very large glands, despite the increased stress on the patient, the need for a longer hospital stay, and a slightly increased mortality rate.

BLOOD SUPPLY

1 Control of the vessels to the prostate is important whether a simple or a total excision is done. The prostatovesical artery divides into the inferior vesical artery to supply the base of the bladder and lower part of the ureter and the prostatic artery to supply the prostate. The prostatic artery in turn divides at the base of the prostate to form a major posterolateral branch supplying most of the gland and an anterior branch supplying only the anterolateral portion. Their subsequent course depends on the level at which they enter. The penetrating or urethral branches are the proximal branches that enter through the prostatic capsule posterolaterally, just distal to the bladder neck. These run concentrically, parallel to the urethra in the preprostatic sphincter, to supply the transition zone. With the development of benign prostatic hyperplasia they become very large. The capsular branches, as posterolateral offshoots, enter the prostate more distally and peripherally than the urethral group. They supply the central and peripheral zones that make up more than two thirds of the mass of the normal prostate.

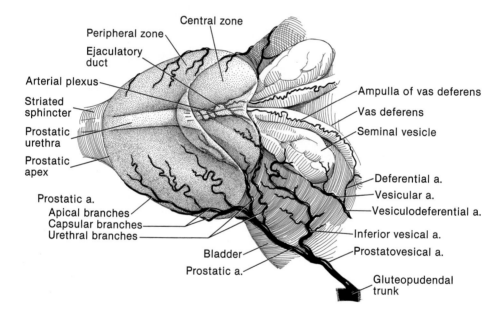

Central zone
Peripheral zone
Ejaculatory duct
Arterial plexus
Striated sphincter
Prostatic urethra
Prostatic apex
Prostatic a.
Apical branches
Capsular branches
Urethral branches
Bladder
Prostatic a.
Ampulla of vas deferens
Vas deferens
Seminal vesicle
Deferential a.
Vesicular a.
Vesiculodeferential a.
Inferior vesical a.
Prostatovesical a.
Gluteopudendal trunk

APPROACHES

For *simple prostatectomy*, the suprapubic approach is the easiest to learn but lacks the control available in retropubic enucleation. The perineal route is best for control of bleeding. In 1903, H. H. Young wrote, "Why these gentlemen prefer darkness to light and object to a technique carried out under full visual control is incomprehensible. In my opinion, the near future will see the surgery of the prostate on the same rational basis of careful technique under visual inspection as that of other parts of the body. I may also add that the instrument which I have called my 'prostatic tractor' has transformed, for me, the operation of prostatectomy. Where before it was (with me—perhaps not with others) an operation done somewhat haphazardly, depending largely on the sense of touch, and in the dark; now the entire operation is performed in a shallow wound, accurately under visual control, proper regard being paid to the urethra and to the ejaculatory ducts, so that they are preserved to continue their pleasant duties." This approach, however, although less familiar to urologists, is being used more often, in conjunction with laparoscopic pelvic lymph node dissection, for total prostatectomy. A retropubic plastic procedure is useful for fibrous prostatic obstruction.

For total *prostatectomy* for carcinoma limited to the prostate, the retropubic route has the advantage of familiarity, and it also allows nodal sampling through the same incision. Total perineal prostatectomy, more difficult to learn but quicker and more precise when the urologist becomes skilled with it, does require either an abdominal incision or, preferably, a laparoscopic procedure if node dissection is necessary. Now that it can be performed with a nerve-sparing technique, it may regain some of its former popularity.

POSITION

The low lithotomy (frog-leg) position may make the prostate slightly more accessible retropubically. The exaggerated lithotomy position with the perineum parallel to the floor provides the best access to the prostate from below. Either position requires careful padding to avoid nerve injury. Injuries from the lithotomy position include the compartmental syndrome, deep venous thrombosis, and peroneal nerve palsy.

PREOPERATIVE MANAGEMENT

Because these patients are usually elderly, often with chronic obstructive pulmonary disease or hypertension, evaluate the patient carefully, remembering that this is usually an elective procedure. Check renal function by a creatinine determination. For routine cases, an intravenous urogram or urodynamic studies are probably not cost effective; a plain film of the abdomen and a renal sonogram are alternatives.

Antibiotic coverage: Culture the urine and treat infection. Provide perioperative antibiotic coverage, usually with ampicillin or cefazolin sodium (Kefzol) limited to three doses. Start coverage again when the catheter is removed, usually with trimethoprim-sulfamethoxazole (Septra) or ciprofloxacin (Cipro).

Suprapubic Prostatectomy

This is a standardized safe procedure for larger adenomas, as an alternative to a retropubic approach or an operation for those less skilled in transurethral resection.

Provide preliminary catheter drainage if azotemia is detected. Correct fluid and electrolyte imbalance, especially dehydration and hypokalemia. Have the patient thoroughly evaluated for cardiovascular and pulmonary problems. Epidural is preferable to general anesthesia. Provide perioperative antibiotics.

Have blood available. Vasoligation is not necessary.

Instruments: Provide a prostatectomy set with lobe forceps, Allis clamps, three Deaver retractors, a Balfour retractor equipped with a flexible blade or a three-bladed bladder retractor (Jacobson), 2-inch vaginal packing, and a cystoscopy set.

Perform cystoscopy, if not previously done.

1 *Position:* Place the patient supine with the pelvis somewhat elevated on a sandbag or folded sheet. Break the table slightly. If you plan to digitally elevate the prostate from the rectum during enucleation, leave the left leg free. A right-handed surgeon stands on the patient's left side. Insert a Robinson catheter, and fill the bladder by gravity with 300 ml of sterile water. Remove the catheter before preparing the operative area, penis, and scrotum. Drape the penis in the field; after the drapes are in place, cover it with a folded towel. Make a midline extraperitoneal incision (see page 487) extending from the anterior surface of the symphysis to the left side of the umbilicus. Make a longer incision in obese patients.

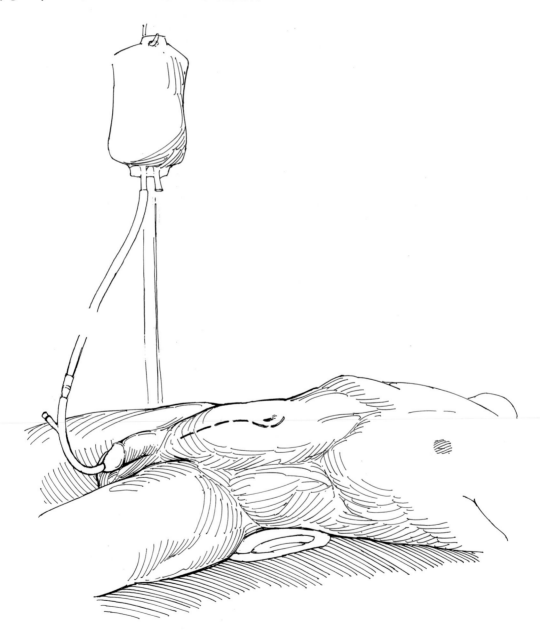

2 Split the linea alba in the midline and retract the rectus muscles. Incise their investing fascia to one side of the midline to expose the underlying retroperitoneal connective tissue, the transversalis fascia. Place a padded Balfour retractor.

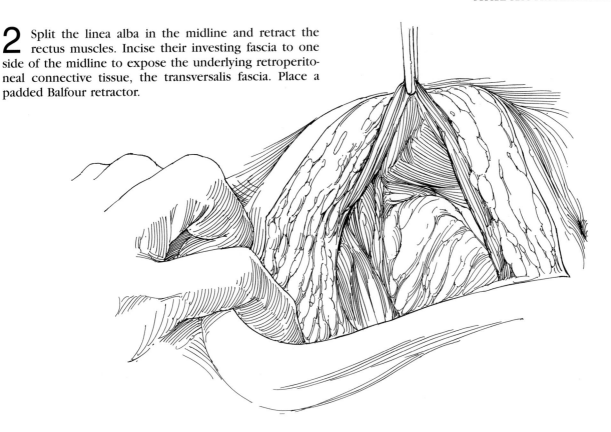

3 Expose the bladder in the space of Retzius by bluntly pushing the peritoneal reflection upward and the perivesical tissue laterally and downward. Avoid injuring the inferior epigastric vessels. Dissection is unnecessary over the vesical neck, although it must be identified.

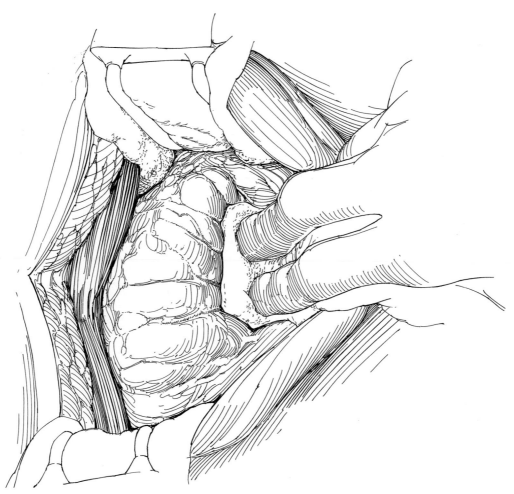

4 Place stay sutures above and below the site of the intended incision above the bladder neck. Avoid placing them too low because of the possibility of tearing into the prostatic capsule. Open the bladder with a knife or cutting current between the stays, and aspirate the bladder contents. Insert a Mayo clamp to enlarge the incision; then stretch it open with two index fingers, a technique preferable to enlarging it sharply because fewer vessels are entered. Insert a three-bladed bladder retractor if available. Or elevate the dome of the bladder by packing it with a laparotomy tape held by a Deaver retractor and place two narrow Deaver retractors on either side, held by an assistant. Visualize and palpate the vesical neck. Inspect the interior of the bladder and remove any vesical calculi. Identify the trigone and ureteral orifices.

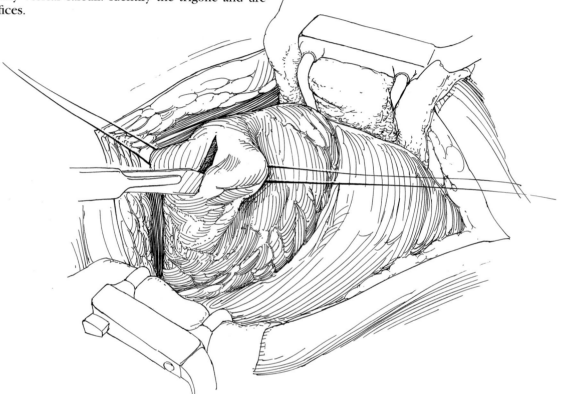

5 Incise the vesical epithelium circumferentially around the protruding adenoma with the electrosurgical knife. Separate the epithelium from the adenoma with curved scissors. Remove the retractor. Shift the patient to the Trendelenburg position. Use sponge sticks to push the intravesical portions aside. Have a moistened 2-inch vaginal pack ready on the instrument table.

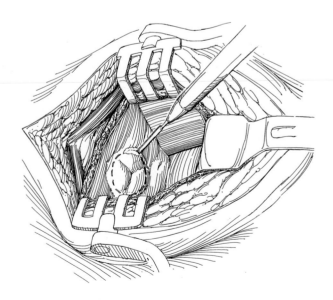

6 **A,** Insert the index finger into the distal third of the prostatic urethra along the roof between the lobes of the adenoma. **B,** Force the tip of the finger through the urothelium in the midline anteriorly, using the fingernail as a wedge.

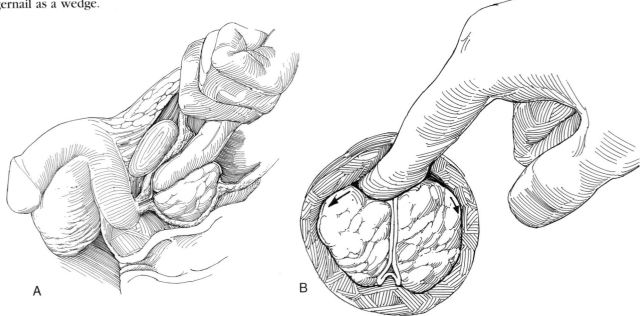

7 Sweep and roll the tip of the finger laterally, alternating from side to side. Be sure to start the enucleation of both lobes before proceeding to free either one completely. In obese patients, insert a finger of the left hand in the rectum to elevate the prostate to help with a difficult enucleation. Do not hook into the capsule with the sharp finger tip; keep close to the adenoma. Free each lobe laterally; then continue posteriorly across the midline and behind the middle lobe.

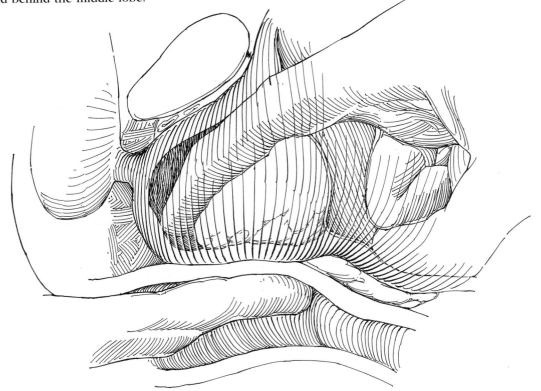

8 Push the urethral epithelium distally with the fingernail at the apex to sever the urethra. Pinching it off between thumb nail and finger helps, but try not to put traction on this section for fear of injuring the external sphincter.

If adhesions are met during enucleation, try angling the elbow or standing with your back to the table. Use either hand. Do not persist if one area is stuck; withdraw the finger from that groove and approach the dissection from another angle, leaving the adherent area until last. Finally, pinch off the adenoma from the vesical epithelium.

9 Grasp the adenoma with sponge or lobe forceps, and remove it while trimming any adherent vesical epithelium with scissors. Palpate the fossa gently for residual lobes, but do not waste time performing hemostatic maneuvers.

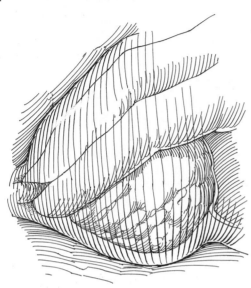

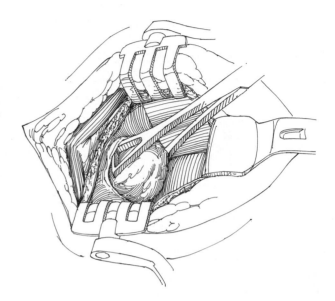

10 Quickly pack the fossa with a warm, moist 2-inch vaginal pack, using long forceps. Hold the pack down with a Deaver retractor for 5 minutes to allow the fossa to contract to aid in hemostasis.

Manipulate the retractor and suction tip to bring the posterior lip of the vesical neck into view. Grasp it with two Kocher clamps. Place figure-eight sutures of 2-0 chromic catgut (CCG) at the 4- and 8-o'clock positions, avoiding the ureteral orifices. These sutures should include a little bladder epithelium and should catch a deep bite of the prostatic capsule, extending 1 cm deep and 1 cm caudad so as to include the main prostatic arteries that enter at these sites (see Step 11). After placing one bite, the suture can be used to elevate the neck, facilitating placement of a second, deeper stitch. Place two more sutures at the 11- and 1-o'clock positions to catch the anterior arterial branches. Leave the sutures uncut; they help during inspection of the fossa for hemostasis. Place further sutures of 3-0 CCG swaged on small round needles as needed. If the neck is small or fibrous, excise a wedge from the posterior lip (see page 425). Tack the vesical epithelium over the rim of the fossa with fine plain catgut (PCG) sutures to prevent vesical neck contracture. Remove the pack slowly. Pull down on the four sutures and fulgurate any small bleeders. Inspect the fossa for residual lobes.

Insert a 24 F 30-ml silicone balloon catheter, and grasp the tip with a long curved clamp. If bleeding seems to be a problem, place a three-way catheter to allow postoperative irrigation. Control venous ooze by drawing the catheter, inflated to as much as 45 ml, down to the neck, but do not inflate it in the fossa. A square of absorbable hemostatic gauze in the neck under the balloon may help.

If hemostasis is less than adequate, consider placing purse-string sutures (Step 12) or plicating the neck (Step 13). If either of these maneuvers is done, insert a cystostomy tube to allow through-and-through irrigation. To do this, make a stab wound in the skin lateral to the incision and insinuate a Mayo clamp through the body wall and the wall of the bladder. Cut the end obliquely from a 30 F Malecot catheter, and draw it out through the tract. Hold it against the bladder wall away from the trigone with a purse-string suture of *plain* catgut at the site of exit from the bladder. Suture the catheter to the skin with heavy silk and secure it with tape.

Close the bladder with a running subepithelial stitch of 3-0 PCG swaged on a fine needle. Place a second layer of interrupted 2-0 CCG or synthetic absorbable sutures (SAS) in the muscle, but do not penetrate the epithelium.

Drain the area with a large Penrose drain placed near the suture line and exiting through the incision. Irrigate the catheter(s) to test for watertightness and bleeding. Approximate the recti loosely, and close the rectus fascia with interrupted 3-0 CCG sutures. Complete wound closure. Apply Montgomery straps and abdominal pads to allow for dressing changes, and tape the suprapubic tube firmly to the abdomen and the urethral catheter to the penis (see page 13) with the aid of tincture of benzoin. Connect the catheter(s) to sterile drainage; traction is not necessary if the purse-string suture is in place. Irrigate if clots form; if clotting cannot be controlled, return the patient to the operating room for clot evacuation through a resectoscope and placement of a suprapubic tube for continuous irrigation.

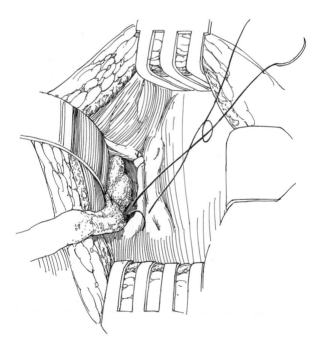

INTRAOPERATIVE HEMOSTATIC PROCEDURES

11 The blood supply to the adenoma comes from the urethral branches of the prostatic arteries that enter near the vesical neck at the 5- and 7-o'clock positions. *Excessive bleeding*, if bright red, probably comes from the urethral branch of the prostatic artery that enters at the 5- or 7-o'clock position distal to the vesical neck and constitutes the blood supply to the adenoma. Dark blood suggests venous bleeding from the posterior capsule, which has not contracted adequately owing to clot or interference from a catheter. Endoscopic fulguration fails to control bleeding here. If the capsule is torn, first suture-ligate the vessels near the neck; then convert the transvesical approach into a transcapsular one by a vertical incision in the capsule toward the apex, and insert a mastoid retractor (see page 427). Another source of bleeding is the deep dorsal vein of the penis.

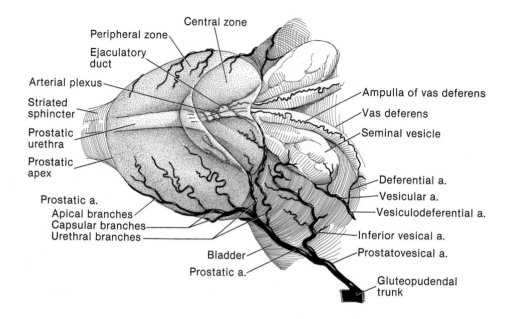

Purse-String Partition Closure (Malament)

12 **A** and **B,** Insert a purse-string double-swaged suture of 1-0 nylon or polypropylene at the posterior margin of the vesical neck through the mucosa and into the muscle. Carry it around in both directions to cross in the midline anteriorly and exit through the entire thickness of the anterior bladder wall. Be careful not to cross the stitches or the suture will be difficult to remove. Insert a 24 F or 26 F 30-ml silicone balloon catheter, inflate the balloon, and draw the purse-string suture around the catheter to close the neck. Partially close the bladder, taking care that the closure stitches do not catch the purse-string suture (or the balloon of the catheter). Cut the needle from each end of the nylon suture, and thread both ends on a large curved cutting needle. Pass the sutures through the body wall above the symphysis, and put them under enough tension to close the bladder neck around the catheter to partition the fossa from the bladder. Tie them together over a button or gauze pledget. Insert a Malecot cystostomy tube. Complete closure of the bladder. Insert a Penrose drain retropubically and close the wound. Withdraw the purse-string suture the following day, taking care to cut only one end. Remove the balloon catheter on the second postoperative day and the suprapubic tube on the fifth day.

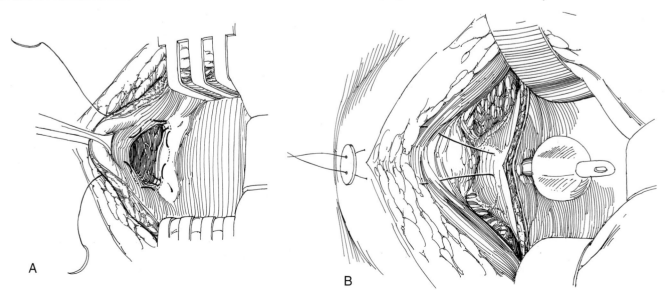

A   B

Capsular Plication
(O'Conor)

13 For persistent bleeding without an obvious source, plicate the capsule. Place a 1-0 CCG on five-eighth curved needles in the posterior capsule, one near the neck and the other more distally, running from one side of the fossa to the other to bring the capsule together and mimic physiologic contraction.

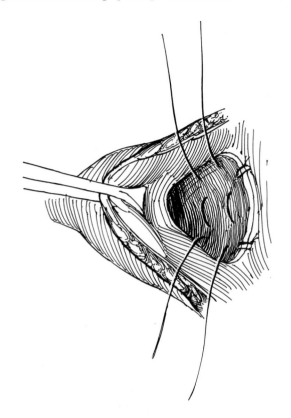

POSTOPERATIVE CARE

Postoperatively, supply adequate hydration. Oral intake can begin as soon as the anesthetic has worn off. Encourage the patient to breathe deeply, move his legs, and get out of bed. Remove the purse-string suture the day after surgery. Partially deflate the balloon catheter as hemostasis is secured, unless a purse-string suture was used and the balloon was not responsible for hemostasis, and remove it as early as the second day. Remove the suprapubic tube on the fifth day. If suprapubic drainage persists or if voiding is unsatisfactory, insert a 22 F 30-ml balloon catheter on a straight stilet for a few days. Remove the Penrose drain last, and discharge the patient.

POSTOPERATIVE PROBLEMS

Bleeding may persist and require endoscopic fulguration if tamponade fails because tamponade itself prevents capsular retrac-

Table 1. Diagnosis of Postoperative Bleeding Disorders

	Dilutional Coagulopathy	Disseminated Intravascular Coagulation	Primary Fibrinolysis
Prothrombin time	+	+	+
Thrombin time	+	+	+
Fibrinogen level	−	− −	−
Platelet count	− −	− − −	
Activated partial thromboplastin time	+	+	+
Plasma protamine paracoagulation test		+	
Factor VIII	N	− −	
Fibrin split products		+	
Schizocytes		+	

+ indicates increased; −, decreased, slight; − −, decreased, moderate; − − −, decreased, major.
Adapted from Peterson NE: Management of operative prostatic hemorrhage. Monogr Urol 5:66, 1984.

tion. Look for clotting disorders. The patient will have had a hematocrit and an estimate of platelets on the blood smear. Order a thrombin time to evaluate fibrinogen and antithrombins. Test for plasma protamine paracoagulation to measure fibrin monomers and fibrin split products for estimating clot digestion. Get a fibrinogen level (for clot substrate), another prothrombin time, and an activated partial thromboplastin time. Table 1 summarizes the tests for differentiating clotting disorders.

Wound infection is not common, and even more rare is *epididymo-orchitis. Incontinence* seldom occurs. *Contracture of the bladder neck,* from inadequate coverage of the vesical neck with vesical epithelium, is seen in a few patients. In contrast to that after transurethral resection of the prostate, it responds readily to dilation.

Prolonged suprapubic leakage postoperatively usually stops with urethral catheter drainage. Try inserting a silver nitrate stick, or thread a (new) wood screw into the fistula and pull it out to denude the tract. If leakage does not stop, perform cystography and also look into the urethra and bladder with a cystoscope for an obstructive cause.

After release of chronic obstruction, watch for *postobstructive diuresis.* Urinary output can be excessive, with resulting loss of salt and water. Patients fit into one of three categories: moderate, high, and very high output. *Moderate output:* If the diuresis is 100 ml/hr or less, treat the patient with oral fluids and salt. *High output:* If it is between 100 and 200 ml/hr, replace the urine volume with 0.075 M NaCl in 5 percent dextrose. Follow the body weight. If it is stable the next day, cut the infusion rate in half, making further cuts as the weight declines. If the urine output is more than 200 ml/hr, measure the urinary sodium concentration and use a proportionately more concentrated NaCl solution for 2 days, then progressively decrease it as the urine flow falls and the blood pressure remains stable. If this does not occur, go back to the earlier rate of infusion for 2 more days. *Very high output:* For rates of diuresis over 300 ml/hour, proceed as above for 4 days; then reduce the infusion rate no more than 25 percent while monitoring blood pressure and pulse as well as urinary potassium and serum electrolytes.

Commentary by Ray E. Stutzman

The management of benign prostatic hyperplasia has significantly changed over the past several years with the emphasis on pharmacologic treatment and minimally invasive procedures. Definite indications for suprapubic prostatectomy still exist. With a low transvesical incision, the prostatic fossa is very easily visualized following enucleation of the adenoma. Placement of hemostatic sutures posteriorly at the 5- and 7-o'clock posi-

tions adjacent to the bladder neck provides good hemostasis. Such exposure offers the advantages of the transvesical approach as well as visualization and hemostasis obtained during the retropubic approach. The techniques described in this chapter are easily learned and are still very applicable in patients with large prostates and other indications for transvesical exposure.

Retropubic Prostatectomy

Clear urinary infection and start the patient on prophylactic antibiotics just before the operation. Be certain that the patient has evacuated his bowel. Apply veno-occlusive stockings. Epidural anesthesia is best.

Instruments: Provide a basic set; prostatectomy instruments; Millin, Balfour, and Deaver retractors; a curette; a bladder neck spreader; a T clamp; lobe forceps (large, medium, and small—two each); curved sponge sticks; 9-inch Mayo scissors; curved and straight Metzenbaum scissors; a joker; bipolar coagulating forceps if available; and a cystoscopy set.

1 Review the vascular supply of the prostate before starting the operation. The prostatovesical artery provides the major portion of the blood supply to the prostate. Most commonly it arises from the gluteopudendal trunk of the internal iliac artery, although it may come from the superior vesical artery, from a common trunk in company with the vesiculodeferential artery, or even from the internal pudendal or obturator arteries. It runs medially on the surface of the levator ani to the bladder base. There the prostatovesical artery divides into (1) the inferior vesical artery to supply the base of the bladder and lower part of the ureter and (2) the prostatic artery to supply the prostate. The prostatic artery in turn divides at the base of the prostate to form a major posterolateral branch supplying most of the gland and an anterior branch supplying only the anterolateral portion.

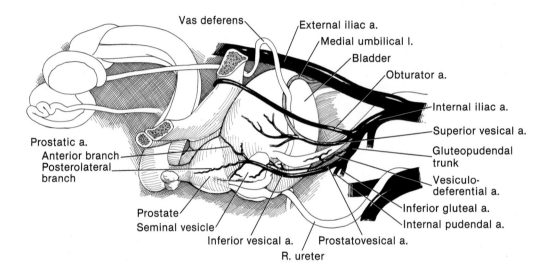

2 *Position:* Place the patient supine on the table. It may be helpful to slightly flex the table to elevate the pelvis, but that puts tension on the rectus muscles if a midline incision is used. Tilt the table to a 20-degree Trendelenburg position to displace the peritoneal contents. Prepare the abdomen and genitalia. Perform preliminary cystoscopy.

Incision: If you are right handed, stand on the left side of the table. Make a midline extraperitoneal incision, extending well down over the pubis (see page 487). (A good alternative is the Pfannenstiel incision [see page 490], especially if a hernia is to be repaired [see page 342]. Exposure is excellent, and weakness of the wound with herniation is rare.)

Retract the rectus muscles laterally, and open their investing fascia 2 to 3 cm from the midline to reach the retroperitoneal connective tissue, the transversalis fascia. Continue in this plane inferiorly into the space of Retzius, retracting the peritoneum and bladder cephalad with the left hand. Alternatively, spread a wet laparotomy tape on the bladder and retract it with a broad Deaver retractor. Dissecting laterally, the vasa deferentia may be divided and ligated to prevent epididymitis. The blood supply to the prostatic capsule can be reduced by initially ligating the lateral prostatic pedicles (Gregoir, 1978).

Expose the anterior surface of the prostate by very gently sweeping the fat superolaterally in the direction of the vessels with cherry sponges. Tease the fat with closed scissors or a hemostat, taking care not to tear the veins on either side of the prostate. Lateral packs are seldom helpful. Insert a Millin or Balfour retractor, padded over the wound edges, and adjust the blade to hold the bladder back. Have the assistant retract the tissue lateral to the vesical neck with two sponge sticks.

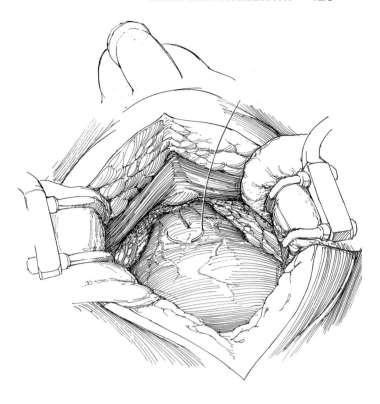

TRANSVERSE CAPSULAR TECHNIQUE (Millin)

3 Locate the vesical neck by palpation of the balloon and by a difference in texture of the tissue, the distal prostatic tissue being firmer to palpation. Place a suture deeply in the capsule of the prostate just below the vesical neck and a second suture distal to that. Use size 1-0 CCG sutures on a five-eighths curved needle. Tie them and tag the ends with clamps. An entire double row of 2-0 CCG sutures can be placed across the prostate as shown. They are traditional but probably not necessary for hemostasis. Remove the urethral catheter.

Make a transverse incision progressively through the capsule into the adenoma with a scalpel or with the more traumatic cutting current, extending across the entire anterior surface. The larger the adenoma, the longer the capsular incision. Hold the suction in the left hand and cut with the right, as the assistant retracts the bladder cephalad with the left hand over a sponge. Place pressure on the upper lip of the capsule, and put it under tension to compress the vessels. Catch and fulgurate them in the cut surface.

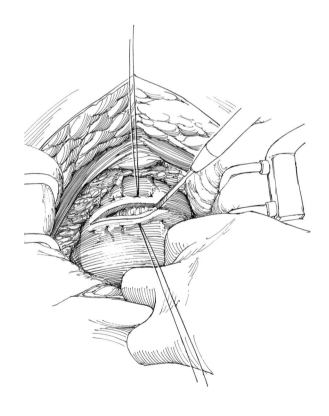

4 Identify the plane between adenoma and capsule by teasing with the joker. Be sure to get in the right plane. Begin separation with curved Metzenbaum scissors; then insert the index finger and start the enucleation. Progress from the easiest areas to those where the adenoma is more adherent. In the unlikely event of a tear into the rectum, close the defect in two layers. In that case, it may be advisable to apply an omental flap and place a cystostomy tube. A transverse colostomy is seldom needed.

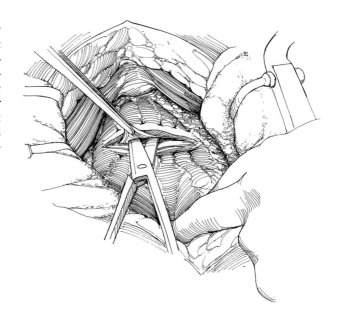

5 Approach the apex with care. Try to divide the junction of the prostatic urethra with the membranous urethra with scissors under vision to avoid damage to the sphincters. A stay suture in the adenoma instead of lobe forceps for traction may help. Enucleate the remainder of the lateral lobes (and median lobe, if present). The attachment to the vesical neck may be divided under vision. Pack the fossa with warm, moist roller gauze for 5 minutes.

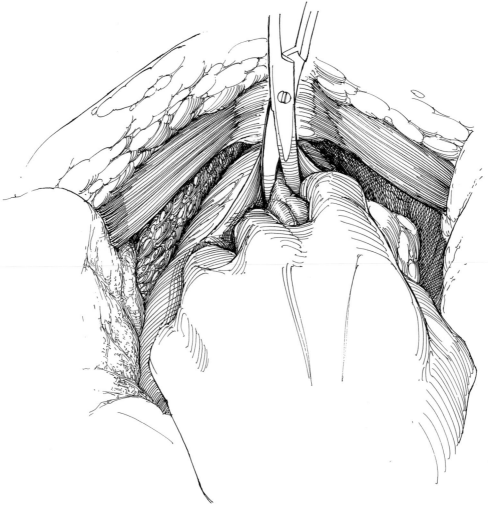

6 Place figure-eight 2-0 CCG sutures at the 5- and 7-o'clock positions through the vesical neck and proximal capsule for control of the prostatic arteries, which can usually be seen spurting. Suture-ligate any visible bleeding vessels in the fossa. Identify the ureteral orifices. (Ask the anesthetist to give indigo carmine intravenously if you have any doubt.) Remove any vesical calculi. Identify the ureteral orifices; consider inserting ureteral catheters.

7 Resect a generous wedge from the posterior lip of the vesical neck, and suture the edge, including the superficial trigone, down over the defect to the inner surface of the capsule posteriorly as low as possible with a running suture of 2-0 CCG to prevent vesical neck contracture. Insert a straight catheter with multiple holes held with a skin bolster (see Step 16). Alternatively, insert a 22 F 30-ml three-way irrigating balloon catheter into the fossa and grasp it with a long clamp, steering the tip into the bladder. Support it with a suture through a skin bolster so that it may be deflated and kept in place. After filling the balloon, tie the filling tube with heavy silk to prevent loss of water.

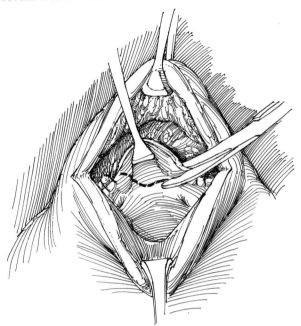

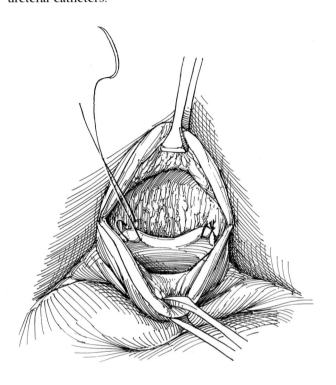

8 Close the capsule from both ends with two continuous 2-0 CCG sutures, placing the stitches close together. The balloon catheter may then be pulled down to tamponade the prostatic fossa and, if necessary, may be left on traction for a while. A cystostomy tube may be inserted but is rarely needed unless bleeding is a problem. Place a Penrose drain in the space of Retzius to remain 2 days or a tube drain to remain until drainage stops. Irrigate and close the wound. A purse-string closure of the vesical neck (see page 420) may stop uncontrollable bleeding.

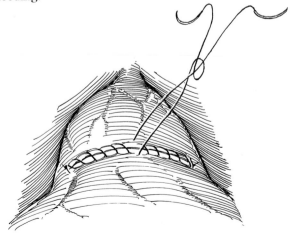

VESICOCAPSULAR TECHNIQUE

This technique is easier to perform than the transcapsular approach but somewhat more likely to leak, and it may be associated with a capsular tear or downward extension into the sphincter.

Additional instrument: Mastoid retractor. Place an 18 F balloon catheter with the connector draped within the operating field. Leave the bladder partially filled.

9 Approach the space of Retzius, and depress the prostate and bladder neck. Place a 2-0 CCG five-eighths curved genitourinary (GU) suture as low as possible into the prostatic capsule in the midline. Tie the suture and hold the ends in a clamp. Bending the needle to reduce the radius helps rotation in the depth of the wound.

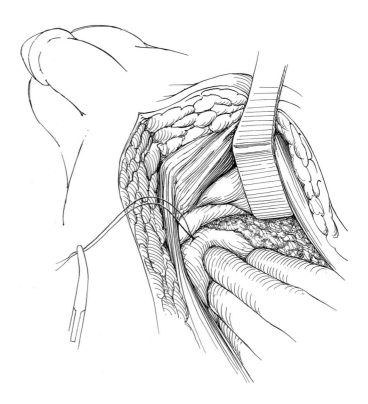

10 Place two stay sutures of 2-0 CCG on each side at the vesical neck. Incise vertically through the bladder wall just above the prostate with the electrocautery in one hand and the suction in the other. Aspirate the bladder contents.

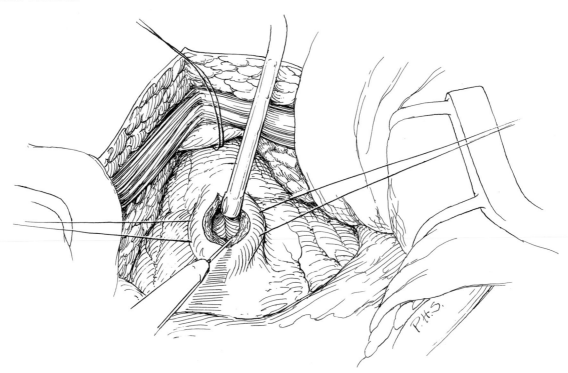

11 Enucleate the adenoma as described for suprapubic prostatectomy. Insert the right index finger into the bladder and then into the prostatic urethra between the prostatic lobes. Break through the urethra anteriorly, begin enucleation laterally, and then move posteriorly, finally freeing the vesical neck, as described on pages 417 to 418. Leave the apex intact at this time.

12 Split the capsule with curved Mayo scissors down to the previously placed stitch.

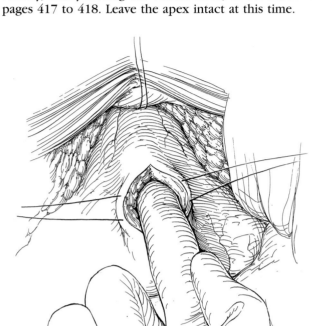

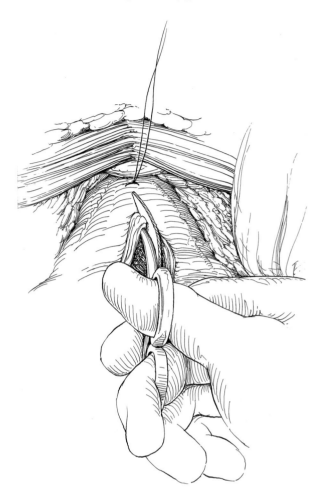

13 Place a mastoid retractor. Divide the urethra at the apex of the prostate with scissors under vision. Remove the adenoma. Locate the ureteral orifices to avoid them during hemostasis.

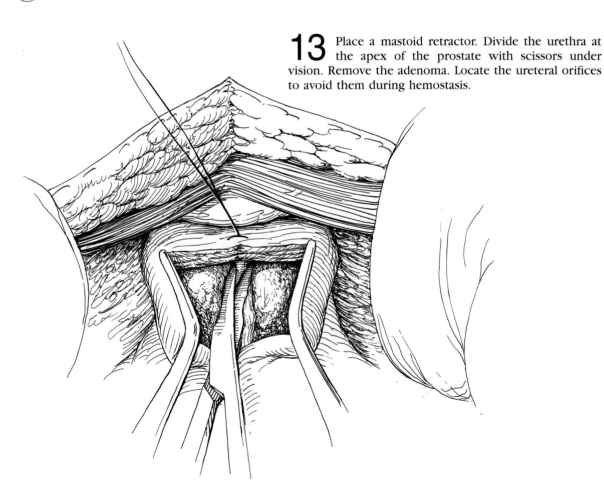

14 Place figure-eight sutures of 2-0 CCG from the bladder neck deep into the capsule at the 4- and 8-o'clock positions at the sites of the urethral branches of the prostatic arteries. Use additional sutures and electrocoagulation as needed to control bleeding. Remove a wedge of vesical neck posteriorly if it appears obstructive, or form a triangular lip of bladder mucosa to suture to the floor of the prostatic urethra. At the least, tack the vesical mucosa at the neck into the fossa with 3-0 PCG sutures to cover the exposed muscles of the vesical neck and thus prevent contracture. Insert a 24 F 30-ml balloon catheter, but do not inflate it.

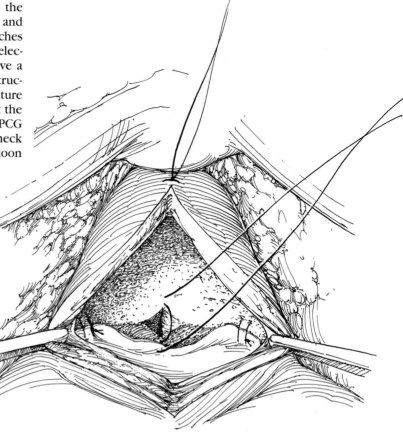

15 Place a running 3-0 PCG suture submucosally around the cystostomy incision and part of the bladder neck as a purse-string suture. Start the suture at the 8-o'clock position at the vesical neck and end it at the 4-o'clock position. Tie it, thus closing the original opening into the bladder.

16 Close the capsule with interrupted 2-0 SAS, beginning at the distal stitch that was placed initially and continuing the sutures cephalad to approximate the prostatic capsule; then close the bladder muscle and adventitia. Inflate the balloon catheter and irrigate the bladder, leaving some fluid behind to reduce clotting. Place a Penrose drain in the space of Retzius and close the wound.

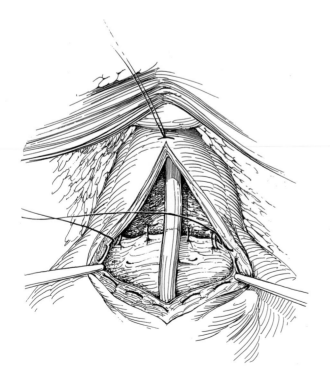

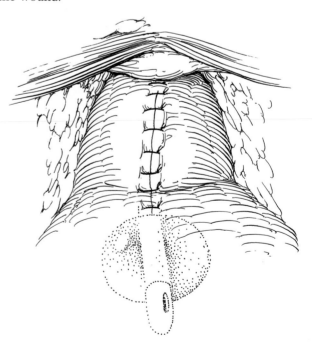

Remove the Penrose drain on the second postoperative day, early enough to give the retropubic space time to seal before the catheter is taken out on the fifth day.

Alternative Catheter Technique

17 Cut extra holes in a 24 F Robinson catheter. Pass a 2-0 CCG suture through an eye and out the tip. Put both ends of the suture in a large curved cutting needle and pass them through the upper wall of the bladder, then through the body wall, and tie them over a bolster to hold the catheter in the proper position.

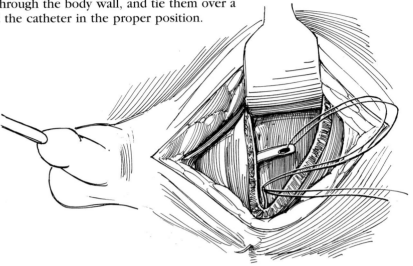
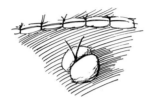

YV-PLASTY FOR SMALL FIBROUS PROSTATE OR CONTRACTURE OF THE VESICAL NECK
(Bonin)

18 **A** and **B,** If transurethral resection was inadequate, apply the Y-V principle. Excise a triangular wedge from the anterior vesical neck. At the same time, take a posterior wedge of prostate, and enucleate prostatic lobes if present.

19 Close the defect in the anterior capsule by advancing the bladder wall into it.

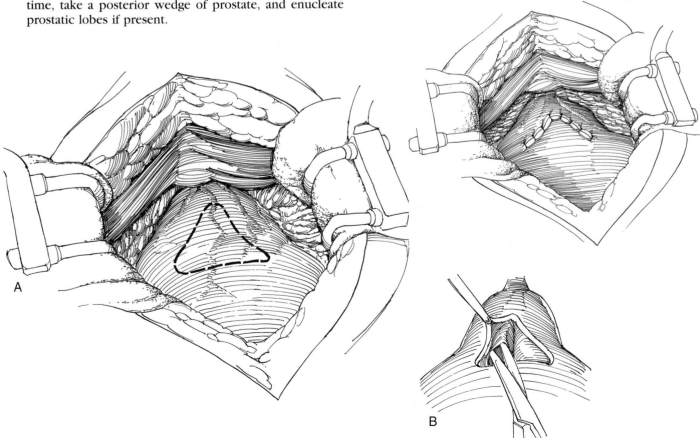

Postoperative Problems

For *inadvertent loss of the catheter,* very carefully manipulate an 18 F straight sound through the fossa (through the anastomosis if a radical operation has been done) into the bladder. Replace it successively with 20 F and 22 F straight sounds, then with an 18 F balloon catheter on a straight stilet. A curved sound or a catheter on a curved stilet cannot be as accurately guided because of the spatial relation of the curve. For primary or secondary *bleeding,* apply traction on a balloon catheter. Bleeding may be copious enough to require taking the patient to the cystoscopy suite, inserting a resectoscope under anesthesia, and evacuating the clots. Often no bleeding site is seen, but suspicious areas should be fulgurated. If severe bleeding continues, reopen the wound, pack the fossa with 2-inch gauze, and again apply traction on the balloon. *Deep venous thrombosis* with subsequent pulmonary emboli is a concern.

A *suprapubic fistula* requires replacement of the catheter. Consider the need for later resection of residual obstructing tissue. *Ureteral obstruction* may result from placing the hemostatic sutures too high at the bladder neck. If there is doubt during the operation, check for efflux with indigo carmine. Flank pain postoperatively is an indication for intravenous urography, followed by percutaneous nephrostomy if ureteral obstruction is the cause.

Bladder neck contracture secondary to delayed epithelialization of the aglandular vesical neck can be prevented by incising a wedge at the neck and tacking the vesical epithelium over it. Once contracture develops, dilation with a Kollmann dilator (if it will pass) or transurethral incision usually corrects it. If not, a YV-plasty (see page 429) is necessary. *Urethral strictures* are rare but respond to dilation or endoscopic incision.

Urinary incontinence is the result of tearing the apex of the prostate from its bed along with the passive sphincter mechanism lying just distal to it. If the injury is mild, continence may return in time when aided by perineal exercises and anticholinergic drugs. If it persists, implantation of an artificial sphincter (see page 580) or reconstruction of the vesical neck (see page 573) may be necessary. *Inability to void* postoperatively is usually the result of local spasm and a relaxed detrusor. Replace the catheter (mount it on a straight stilet to be able to steer it into the bladder) and wait a couple of days. If retention persists, the patient should undergo cystoscopy looking for residual lobes or tissue flaps.

Impotence may result from anxiety or natural disinclination; rarely is the nerve supply disrupted in suprapubic or simple retropubic prostatectomy. Retrograde ejaculation is more common and results from incompetence of the bladder neck. Techniques to prevent it lead to vesical neck contractures, so the patient must be forewarned.

Commentary by Ross O'Neil Witherow

This operation is generally reserved for the large prostate, an impression gained from digital rectal examination and confirmed by transrectal ultrasonography. The latter has the advantage of identifying foci of carcinoma in a large gland, which can undergo biopsy and should avoid the unpleasant experience of attempting to enucleate a malignant gland, which led to many of the complications in the past. Prostates with a measured volume of 80 ml or more are best enucleated retropubically, but a less experienced resectionist may wish to perform a retropubic prostatectomy for a smaller benign gland. If at preliminary cystoscopy the gland appears to be much larger than expected, it may well be safer to perform a retropubic prostatectomy rather than try to resect a very large gland. Small fibrous or neoplastic glands are not suitable for retropubic enucleation, as the risk of rectal injury is significant; they are better resected.

In addition to the instruments outlined, I like to use a small Turner-Warwick ring retractor with four curved blades to hold the wound open, and in this respect a Pfannenstiel incision always appears perfectly adequate for access. If one sutures the inferior skin margin together with the inferior border of the rectus sheath to the upper edge of the pubic symphysis, access is improved further.

If access is still difficult, the recti can be divided 1 inch above their insertion into the symphysis pubis and resutured at the end of the procedure (see page 493). The vasa need not be divided, as epididymitis is very unusual with the use of prophylactic antibiotics.

I prefer the transverse capsular technique to avoid dividing the bladder neck musculature anteriorly. After making the transverse incision through the capsule and adenoma, I continue this until it enters the urethra. One can then split the prostatic lobes anteriorly, remove the urethral catheter, and identify the veru in the floor of the prostate, either under vision or by feeling it with the forefinger. Immediately lateral to the veru, the elastic tissue of the prostatic apex can be felt, and one can then dissect the left lateral lobe of the prostate accurately at

the apex in the posterolateral groove, initially using the index finger. This lateral split can be developed proximally with the intention of leaving a posterior strip of urethral mucosa. Enucleation can then proceed from the apex proximally and anteriorly toward the bladder neck. Damage to the distal sphincter is much less likely with this method than with the described method of pulling the enucleated gland toward one to divide the urethra with scissors. The same technique is applied to the other lobe, preserving the posterior urethral strip.

For the right hander, it is often helpful to turn away from the table and perform the enucleation behind one's back, as it were. If no middle lobe is present and the bladder neck is not unduly occlusive, the presence of the posterior urethral strip of mucosa makes resection of the bladder neck unnecessary. Any small pieces of epithelium missed on the lateral walls can be grasped with forceps and dissected off with scissors.

Hemostasis can usually be achieved by deep sutures placed into the capsule at either end of the incision, passing the needle right through the wall of the capsule from outside to inside and out again. Once tied, these usually control the prostatic arteries, avoiding the figure-eight sutures into the vesical neck and proximal capsule, which carry the risk of catching the ureteric orifices. If bleeding is not excessive, one can avoid packing the cavity for a few minutes and proceed with closure of the capsule as described.

I like to place a 22 F irrigating catheter in the bladder before the capsule is finally closed. When the capsule is closed, it is worth irrigating the bladder to make sure that no leakage occurs through the suture line which may require an extra interrupted suture. One can then irrigate the bladder with saline with confidence, avoiding the need for washouts. A 20 F tube drain is preferable to suction drainage, which may cause a fistula.

Acute dilation of the stomach was a complication of this procedure in the past, and a nasogastric tube should be placed postoperatively for 24 hours if the patient has hiccups or vomiting, but it need not be placed routinely. Incontinence is extremely unusual with this technique.

Total Retropubic Prostatectomy

Determine prostatic-specific antigen (PSA) for a baseline (less than 15 ng/ml). Obtain a transrectal needle biopsy (positive). Perform seminal vesicle needle biopsies if the sonogram suggests involvement. Vesicle involvement is more likely if the Gleason score is 4 or more, if the PSA level is greater than 10 ng/ml, or if the clinical stage is TIIb or more (Stone et al, 1995). If the PSA level is 15 ng/ml or greater or the Gleason score is 7 or greater, perform pelvic lymph node dissection (see page 465) preliminary to prostatectomy. If the nodes are negative, proceed with total prostatectomy.

Have available adequate blood replacement (the average blood loss is 1000 ml) by asking the patient to donate 3 autologous units preoperatively. Sequential compression devices reduce venous complications; it has not been determined if they reduce blood loss. Minidose heparin may induce lymphoceles. Consider preparing the bowel.

Instruments: Include a Basic set, GU long and GU vascular sets, prostatectomy specials, a cystoscopy set, medium and large clip appliers, long vascular forceps, Russian forceps, Satinsky-Cranford forceps, toothed Cushing forceps, extra-long Allis clamps, a fiberoptic suction tip, a hand-controlled electrosurgery unit, two head lamps, 22 F and 24 F 5-ml and 30-ml silicone balloon catheters, a 24 F Robinson catheter, lubricant, two 0.75-inch Penrose drains, 5 F and 8 F infant feeding tubes, a 6-mm Jackson-Pratt drain, and Montgomery straps. A Buchwalter retractor may be useful.

Position: Place the patient in the supine position with the legs moderately spread and supported on airplane splints, or insert bed rolls under the knees. Place the perineum at the edge of the table to allow an assistant access for applying compression during urethral anastomosis. Elevate the pelvis by breaking the table and tilting it to a 20-degree Trendelenburg position. Prepare the abdomen and perineum. Empty the bladder with a 22 F 30-ml balloon catheter, and leave it in place for later manipulation of the prostatic apex. Place a rectal tube if desired.

1 *Incision:* Make a vertical midline incision extending from the symphysis to the umbilicus; transverse incisions are less satisfactory for reaching the deep pelvis. Split the rectus muscles in the midline. Lift the semilunar line, and dissect the peritoneum and fascia off the posterior abdominal wall. Be sure to carry the dissection beneath the transversalis fascia to avoid injury to the inferior epigastric vessels. Free the peritoneum from the internal inguinal rings. Insert a retractor with a malleable blade to hold the bladder superiorly.

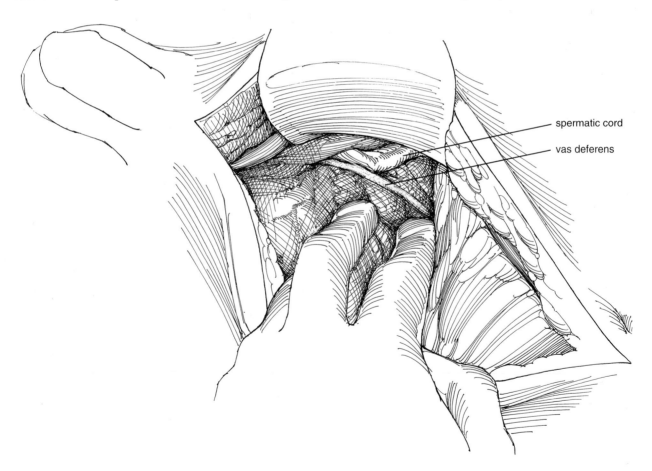

spermatic cord

vas deferens

2 Ligate the vasa deferentia. Identify and elevate the obliterated hypogastric artery.

If the tumor has not extended locally, proceed with modified pelvic lymph node dissection (see page 465), and send the nodes for frozen section pathologic examination. Gently tease the retropubic fat from the anterior prostatic surface, moving it laterally and proximally.

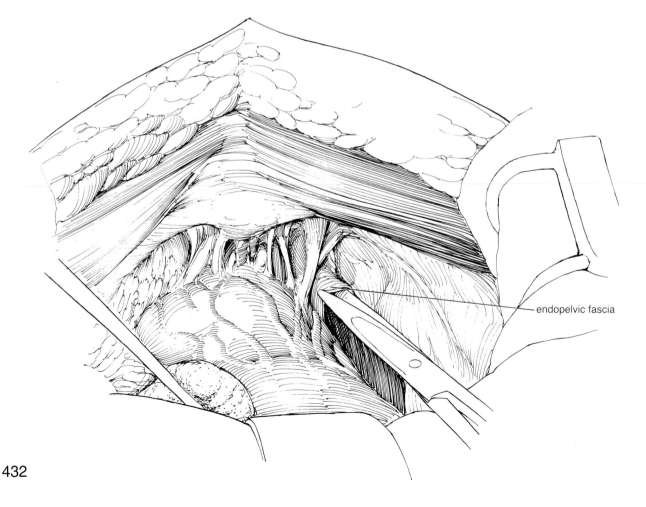

obturator nerve

obliterated hypogastric artery

internal iliac artery, anterior trunk

NERVE-SPARING TECHNIQUE
(Walsh)

3 Enter the endopelvic fascia near the pelvic side wall on both sides of the prostate with scissors. Keep away from the fascial attachment to the prostate and bladder, under which run large veins. Open the space close to the bellies of the levator ani muscles and well lateral to the apex of the prostate by blunt finger dissection. Place vessel loops around the hypogastric arteries that were exposed by the node dissection, and occlude both arteries above the take-off of the obliterated hypogastric (umbilical) artery with rubber-shod bulldog clamps.

endopelvic fascia

432

4 Place a malleable retractor blade so that it elevates the bladder by impinging on the catheter balloon in the bladder. Clear away the areolar tissue from the two puboprostatic ligaments, and fulgurate or ligate and divide them. Reduce blood loss by preliminary fulguration or suture-ligation of the superficial preprostatic vein(s) on the anterior and lateral surfaces of the bladder neck and prostate (Narayan, 1991) that enters the deep dorsal vein (Myers, 1989).

Insert the scissors behind one ligament to separate it from the anterior prostatic fascia that encloses the dorsal vein complex, and divide it midway from the pubis. Leave the ligamentous urethral attachments intact to assist in maintaining continence (Steiner, 1994). The puboprostatic ligaments do not need to be ligated. Push them off the pubis with the index finger, being careful not to injure the dorsal vein.

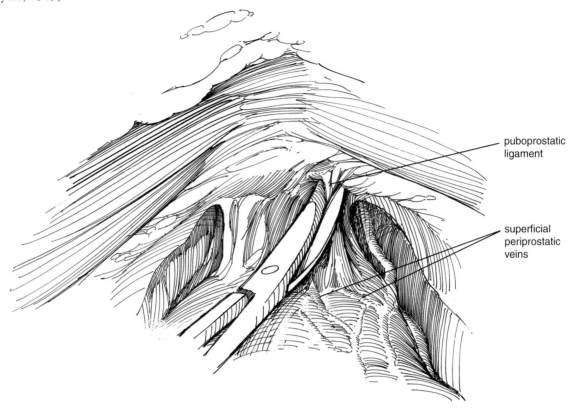

puboprostatic ligament

superficial periprostatic veins

5 Pass a right-angle clamp through the lateral pelvic fascia (endopelvic fascia) beneath the tissue containing the deep dorsal vein and over the urethra containing a catheter that is palpable. Gathering the veins and underlying fascia proximally in an Allis, Babcock, or curved Kocher clamp (Miller, 1994) aids in exposure and ligation.

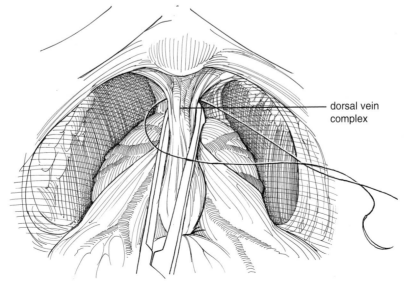

dorsal vein complex

6 Avoid the posterolateral tissue containing the neuro-vascular bundle.

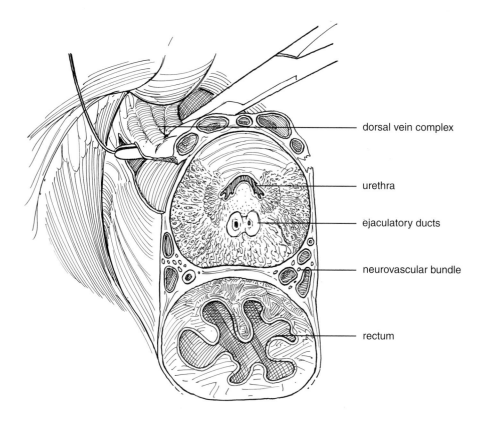

dorsal vein complex

urethra

ejaculatory ducts

neurovascular bundle

rectum

7 Pass a 1-0 SAS on the clamp under the tissue con-taining the deep dorsal vein, and doubly ligate it. Alternatively, gather the vein complex in an Allis clamp to consolidate it before ligation. Divide the dorsal vein tissue on the bladder side of the ligatures. Temporarily pack small laparotomy tape sponges toward each obtura-tor fossa to arrest any ooze. If bleeding continues from the dorsal vein, religate it with a 2-0 CCG suture swaged on a five-eighths curved needle, using a figure-eight stitch against the pubis, or oversew it with the suture. Pulling down on the balloon catheter intermittently compresses the vein against the pubis and facilitates ligation. Do not proceed until hemostasis has been secured.

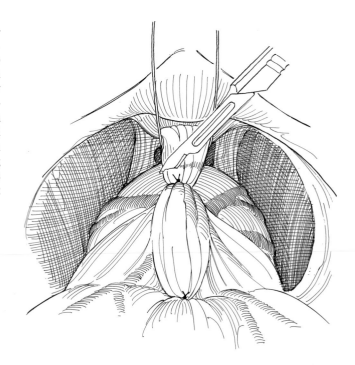

8 Separate the neurovascular bundles, located posterolaterally, from the urethra and prostatic apex. Use
scissors, then a right-angle clamp, to push them off the
surface of the prostate. Do not hesitate to include one
nerve with the specimen if local involvement is suspected. If in doubt, mark the area of the prostate that
abuts the nerve with India ink and excise it for a frozen
section. If it is positive, resect the nerve and adjacent tissue.

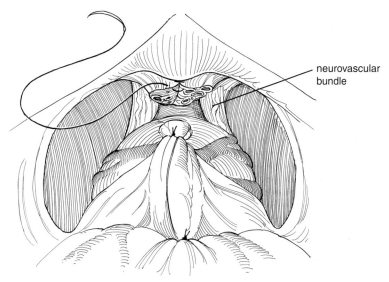

neurovascular
bundle

9 Dissect closely around the urethra just below the
apex of the prostate. Pass a right-angle clamp from
medially to laterally to avoid rectal injury, and pass a tape
beneath the urethra.

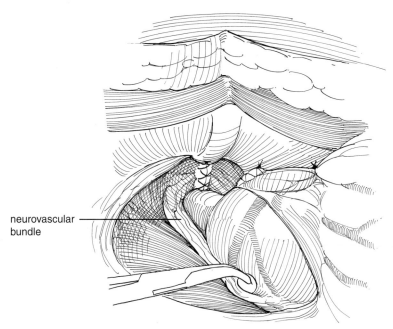

neurovascular
bundle

10 Partially divide the urethra anteriorly at its junction with the prostate. Cut it obliquely because the apex of the prostate extends more distally on the lateral and posterior aspects of the urethra. Place traction sutures at the 2- and 10-o'clock positions.

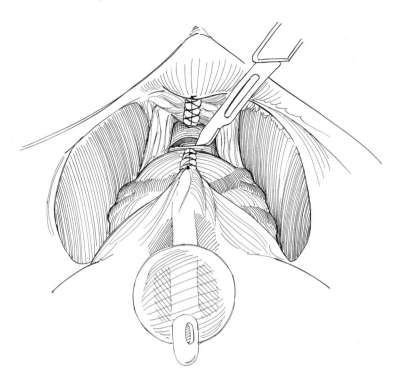

11 Cut the catheter and use it for traction to assist with accurate division of the posterior portion. Sharply divide the posterior half of the urethra to expose the posterior leaf of Denonvilliers' fascia and the recto-urethralis muscle. Elevate the fascia with a right-angle clamp, and sharply divide it at a right angle so that it may be incorporated into the anastomosis. Cut the catheter and draw the now-distal end into the wound. At this time it may be advantageous to place six, or preferably eight, sutures of 2-0 monofilament SAS in the distal stump and hold them in rubber-shod clamps.

Complete the division of the urethra, and send the specimen of the prostatic apex for frozen section to be sure that the anastomotic line is clear of tumor. If tumor is present, either resect more of the tissue on the distal urethra or resort to postoperative radiation.

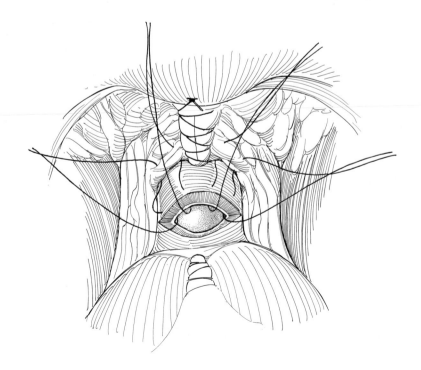

12 **A,** Retract the apex by traction on the cut urethral catheter. **B,** Divide the remainder of the rectourethralis muscle and Denonvilliers' fascia with scissors in the midline to avoid the neurovascular bundles.

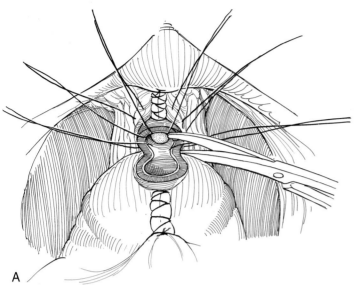

A

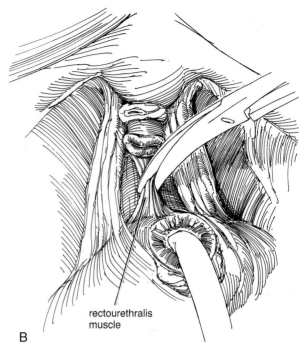

rectourethralis
muscle

B

13 Use finger dissection and scissors to separate the posterior layer of Denonvilliers' fascia from the anterior wall of the rectum. Divide the lateral pelvic fascia, and clip the small branches going to the prostate from the neurovascular bundle.

14 Release the rectum and expose the vasa and seminal vesicles. Inadvertent dissection within the trigonal layers may damage the ureter; in that case, reimplant it.

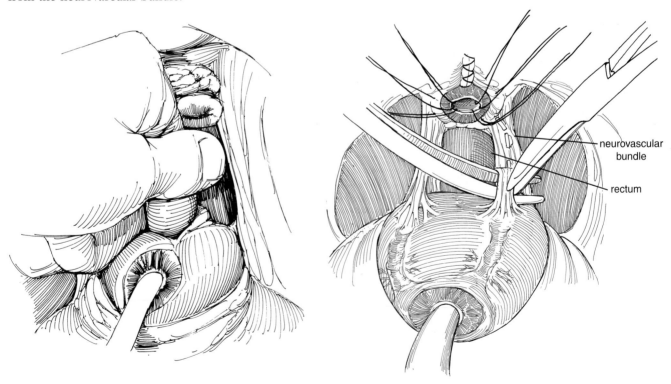

neurovascular
bundle

rectum

15 Dissect laterally to free the prostatic fascia and neurovascular bundle from the prostate up to the lateral pedicle. Ligate and divide the vessels on the lateral surface of the seminal vesicles near the prostate.

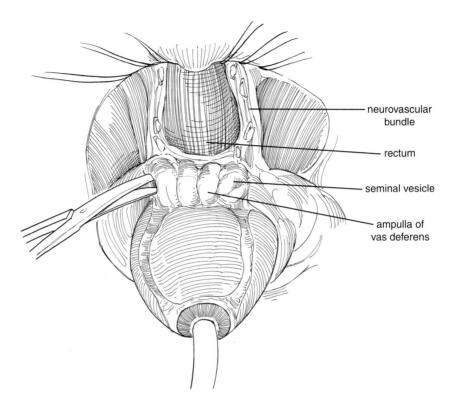

neurovascular bundle

rectum

seminal vesicle

ampulla of vas deferens

16 Pull on the prostate by traction on the balloon catheter to extrude the vesical neck. Make a short incision in the groove between the prostate and the vesical neck, and transect it distal to the circular fibers. Inject 1 ml of indigo carmine intravenously; if it fails to flow from the orifices, pass ureteral catheters.

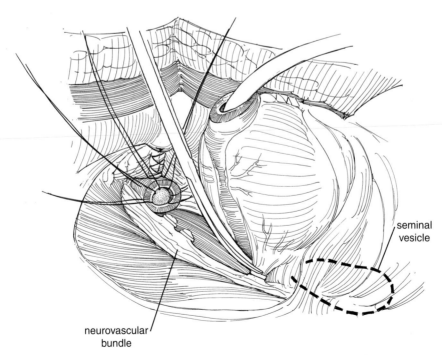

seminal vesicle

neurovascular bundle

17 Divide the posterior portion of the vesical neck. Take care to preserve the circular fibers and to avoid tearing the bladder neck after the trigone has retracted.

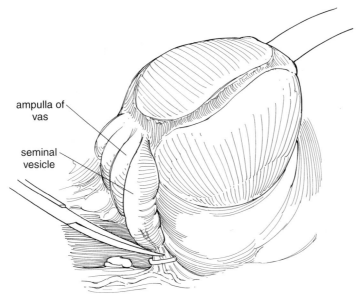

ampulla of vas

seminal vesicle

18 Push the bladder cephalad and free the prostate from the rectum from above downward. Pass a right-angle clamp under the terminal plate of Denonvilliers' fascia and the fibers of the rectourethralis under direct vision. This reduces the chance for rectal injury during dissection of the apex in the plane between the rectum and Denonvilliers' fascia. If the rectum is entered, close it in two layers. Have the assistant dilate the anus widely. If possible, draw the omentum through the cul-de-sac and place it between rectum and urethral anastomosis.

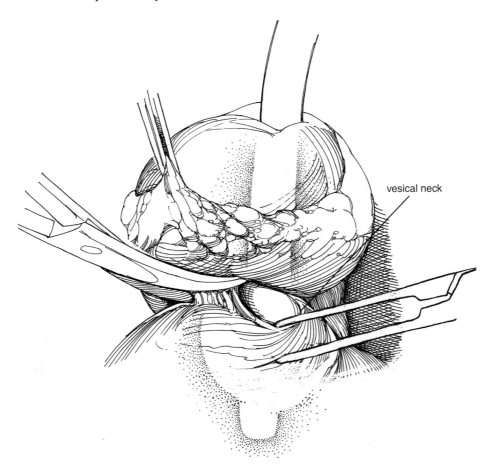

vesical neck

19 Identify and dissect the vasa deferentia directly behind the bladder neck in the midline. Clip and divide them (they are friable).

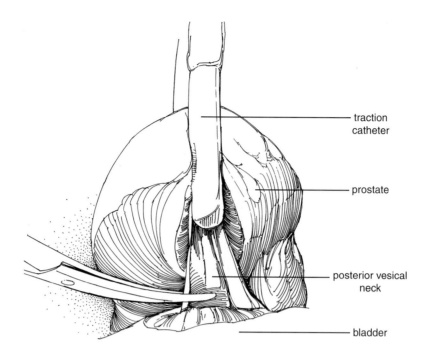

traction catheter

prostate

posterior vesical neck

bladder

20 Clip the vessels at the tips of the seminal vesicles. Remove the specimen. If the bladder neck has been spared, obtain quadrant biopsies for residual prostatic tumor. The specimen may be coated with artist's pigments, blue for the left side or green for the right side (Noldus and Huland, 1995), to aid the pathologist in identifying involved margins.

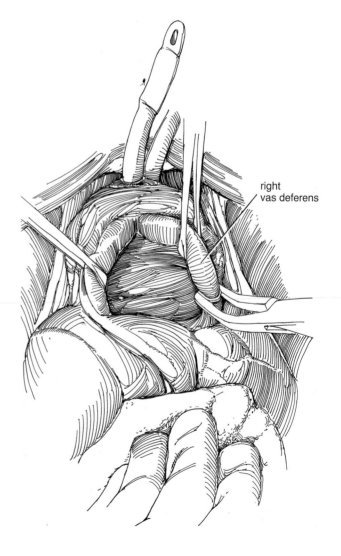

right vas deferens

POSTERIOR CLOSURE TECHNIQUES

Standard Closure

21 Begin inserting interrupted 2-0 CCG sutures from the posterior margin of the bladder neck that include the full thickness of bladder wall. Continue anteriorly until the opening is approximately 1 cm in diameter, such that it admits the tip of the index finger. Hold the sutures in rubber-shod clamps. Stomatize the opening by everting the vesical epithelium with fine sutures. Pass a 20 F 5-ml silicone balloon catheter through the urethra into the bladder and inflate it. Have the assistant double the filling tube on itself, and place a silk tie around it to prevent inadvertent loss of fluid.

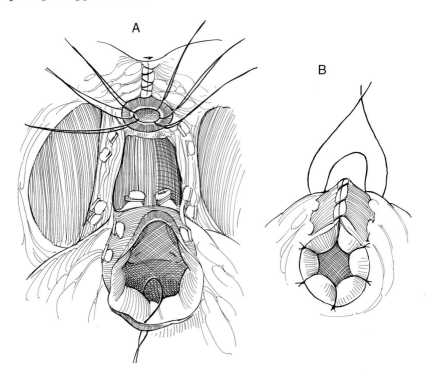

22 If sutures were placed at the time of urethral division (optional Step 11), pick up the proximal ends of the urethral sutures and pass them through the edges of the new vesical neck. Tie the sutures successively, using traction on the catheter to aid apposition. If they were not placed initially, pressure on the perineum by the assistant elevates the distal end of the urethra and makes insertion of the sutures easier.

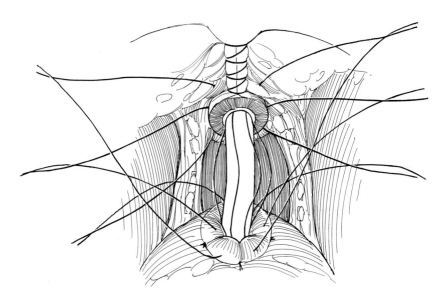

23 *Alternative urethral suture method:* Wait until the vesical defect is partially closed before placing urethral sutures. Insert a 20 F 30-ml balloon catheter into the urethra through the penis to a point at which the tip is just visible emerging from the cut end. Inflate the balloon now lying in the urethral bulb with 1 to 3 ml of water. Catch the tip of the catheter with a long clamp, and pull the urethral stump into view. Or insert a stilet in the balloon catheter to lever the balloon and urethra into position (Bell, 1993). Place six 2-0 SAS into the urethral stump and into the margin of the bladder neck, starting posteriorly, and hold them in rubber-shod clamps. Deflate the balloon and remove the catheter. Insert a new 22 F 5-ml silicone balloon catheter into the bladder and inflate the balloon.

24 Push the bladder down while pulling on the catheter and tie the sutures, beginning posteriorly. Place a suction drain (Jackson-Pratt type) to the area of anastomosis. A suprapubic tube is rarely necessary. Close the wound with 1-0 SAS for the rectus fascia and 2-0 PCG sutures subcutaneously. Suture the drains (and suprapubic catheter if placed) to the skin. Tape the urethral catheter to the penis. Remove the urethral (or suprapubic) catheter in 8 days and the drains in 9 days.

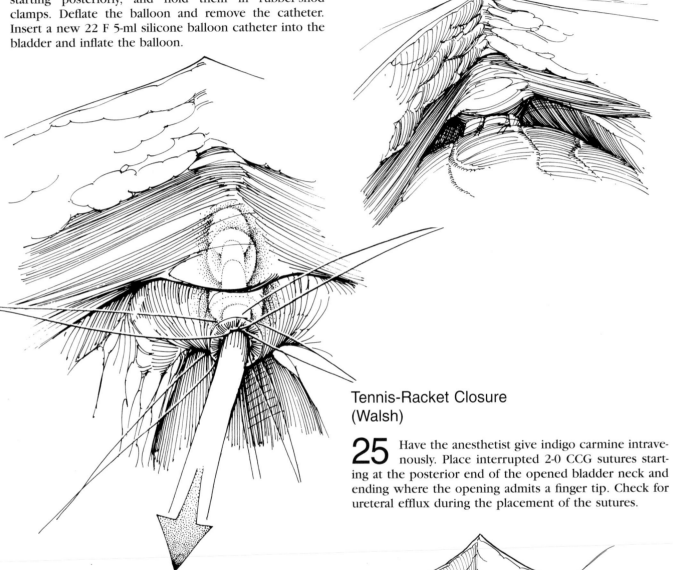

Tennis-Racket Closure (Walsh)

25 Have the anesthetist give indigo carmine intravenously. Place interrupted 2-0 CCG sutures starting at the posterior end of the opened bladder neck and ending where the opening admits a finger tip. Check for ureteral efflux during the placement of the sutures.

26 Insert 4-0 CCG sutures to evert the vesical epithelium and tack it to the vesical muscularis. Narrow the opening further to fit it around a 20 F balloon catheter. Insert traction sutures in the striated sphincter at the 5- and 7-o'clock positions to keep it away from the neurovascular bundles during closure. Place a silk suture through the eye of the balloon catheter so that the epithelial lining can be identified and everted as the catheter is drawn in and out through the sphincter area.

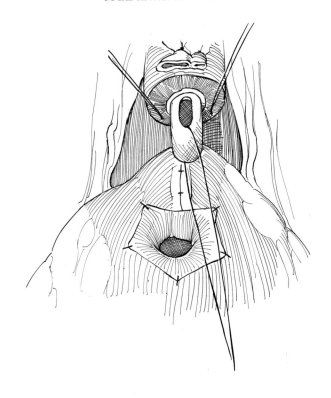

27 Place a 4-0 SAS at 6 o'clock through the edge of the striated sphincter and then into the urethral lumen. Insert similar sutures at the 3- and 9-o'clock positions. Pass a 4-0 SAS at the 12-o'clock position through the dorsal vein complex, the striated sphincter, and the urethral lumen.

Insert the four urethral sutures in the quadrants of the vesical opening. Test the balloon, deflate it, and advance the catheter into the bladder. To prevent the catheter from inadvertently falling out postoperatively, consider placing a heavy silk suture on a large curved Keith needle through the eye of the catheter and then through the bladder and body wall, to be tied over a bolster (see page 429).

Tie the urethrovesical sutures starting with the anterior one, then the right lateral, posterior, and left lateral in that order. Inflate the balloon to 15 ml, or hold it in place with the previously inserted heavy silk suture. Place small suction drains and irrigate the wound. Close the wound with 1-0 SAS for the rectus fascia and 2-0 PCG subcutaneously. Suture the drains (and suprapubic catheter if placed) to the skin. Tape the urethral catheter to the penis and the leg.

Perform retrograde cystography at 8 days and remove the urethral (or suprapubic) catheter if no extravasation is seen. The drains may be removed the next day. If extravasation is detected, leave the catheter for another week, and repeat the cystography.

Alternative Technique for Suture Placement (Fourcade, 1994). Insert a resectoscope sheath with a 70-degree lens. The light and irrigation allow placement of the sutures under direct vision, and a video attached to the lens allows an internal view. A suture guide (Greenwald) may help grip the urethra for insertion of sutures.

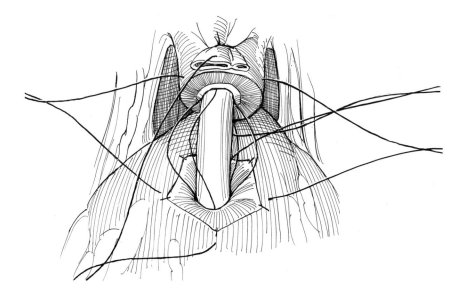

Tubularized Neourethra
(Steiner)

28 After placement of sutures to partially close the vesical neck, leave the last one long for traction (Step 21). Insert two stay sutures at the 10- and 2-o'clock positions. **A** and **B,** Incise the neck obliquely on either side distal to the stay sutures for a distance of 1.5 to 2 cm. Insert a 20 F balloon catheter through the urethra into the bladder and inflate it. Bring the stay sutures together to start formation of a tube. **C,** Close the tube with 2-0 CCG sutures. Anastomose the new orifice to the urethra, everting the mucosa (Steps 21 to 24).

Vest Sutures. Long sutures placed in the prostatic capsule and brought out through the perineum can bring the cut ends of the urethra together without direct anastomosis, but they do not ensure epithelium-to-epithelium apposition and so are less effective than direct anastomosis in reducing vesical neck stricture (Levy et al, 1994). They may, however, be associated with better continence (Novicki et al, 1995).

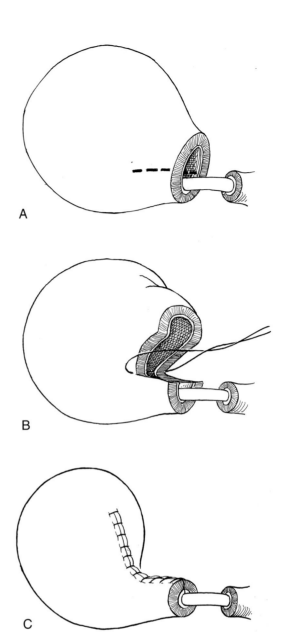

A

B

C

POSTOPERATIVE CARE

Maintain intermittent leg compression for 2 or 3 days. Remove the suction drains after 5 days or when drainage is minimal. Remove the catheter in the office at 2 weeks. Obtain a cystogram if drainage is excessive or if the catheter is to be removed earlier. Instruct the patient in securing incontinence pads and in performing Kegel exercises four times a day.

POSTOPERATIVE PROBLEMS

Immediate Problems

Catheter replacement in the early postoperative period is necessary but hazardous. One method is to manipulate an 18 F straight sound very gingerly into the bladder, then a 20 F and 22 F straight sound, followed by a 20 F balloon catheter on a straight stilet. Do not persist. Another approach is to cystoscopically place a guide wire, over which an 18 F Councill-tip catheter is passed.

Postoperative hemorrhage, evidenced by significant hypotension even though 2 or 3 units of blood have been given during surgery, requires blood replacement and early reoperation to stop the bleeding. (Open vessels are usually not found; the bleeding is more often due to factors in the blood.) More importantly, for prevention of a bladder neck contracture and incontinence, reoperate to evacuate a *pelvic hematoma* and to repair a *disrupted anastomosis.*

Persistent *drainage,* continuing after the third or fourth day, is either lymph or urine. Test the creatinine concentration or give indigo carmine. If it is lymph, stop suction and slowly advance the drains. If it is urine, it probably comes from the urethrovesical anastomosis. Check the site with cystography. Stop suction and move the drain away from the anastomosis. Spontaneous closure may take 3 to 4 weeks.

Urinary extravasation and *wound infection* occur in a small percentage of patients. *Ureteral obstruction* occurs from edema of the floor of the bladder. It is rarely possible to catheterize the orifices, so a percutaneous nephrostomy must be placed. In difficult cases in which the vesical neck repair was close to the orifices, a ureteral stent should be left in place.

Thrombophlebitis and *pulmonary embolism* result from venous stasis. Maintaining the head-down position and intermittent compression stockings during surgery and for a day after help in prevention, as do early ambulation and avoidance of sitting in a chair without elevation of the legs. The necessity for postoperative anticoagulation has not been demonstrated. Prolonged compression of the rectus muscle by a self-retaining retractor may result in *muscle necrosis.*

Ureteral injury may occur during node dissection if the bladder is incompletely freed from the pelvic wall. The presence of a large medial prostatic lobe may cause the ureter to pursue a J course, where it could be involved during transection of the posterior aspect of the bladder neck. The injury must be recognized intraoperatively, aided by the intravenous injection of indigo carmine as the bladder neck is transected.

Rectal injury is infrequent and may be closed primarily if the bowel has been prepared. It requires a meticulous closure (see page 87). Débride any nonviable edges. Close the defect transversely with interrupted 3-0 SAS supplemented by omental interposition. Overdilate the anal sphincters digitally. Irrigate the pelvis copiously, and place drains to the area. A diverting colostomy should be considered if the repair is tenuous, if the bowel was not prepared, if gross fecal contamination is present, or if the injury is related to prior irradiation.

Late Problems

Lymphoceles can be diagnosed by ultrasonography and treated most often by aspiration with a needle and syringe, either percutaneously or laparoscopically. For large collections, a window into the peritoneal cavity can be created through the laparoscope.

Severe to total *urinary incontinence* occurs in some 5 percent of patients and moderate incontinence in 20 percent as a result of interference with the passive continence mechanism. It usually decreases with time, during which the patient should follow a program of perineal exercises. Anticholinergic or sympathomimetic drugs may help. Evaluate the problem urodynamically to differentiate it from bladder instability. Management is by a penile clamp, a condom catheter, or implantation of an artificial sphincter. Injection of bulking agents may be helpful. It is advisable to delay radiation therapy until incontinence has resolved. *Impotence,* if the patient was potent preoperatively, is now less common. Wait 6 to 12 months for return. Postoperative radiation further impairs weak erections. Rarely, impotence results from ligation of the occasional accessory internal pudendal arteries that either were not recognized during the operation or were not dissected free because of concern over excessive bleeding from the dorsal vein complex (Polascik and Walsh, 1995). The patient must be warned of the possibility and have the alternative of a prosthesis explained. If potency does not return in 12 months, consider intracorporal vasodilators, vacuum erection devices, or implantation of a penile prosthesis.

Fecal fistulas may appear immediately or after a week or more; they are due either to direct rectal injury at the time of operation or to ischemia and subsequent necrosis of the rectal wall. They are unlikely to close spontaneously and require formal closure (see page 476).

Contracture at the vesicourethral anastomosis has an incidence of 3 to 12 percent. It is secondary to inadequate apposition of the epithelial edges during the anastomosis associated with prolonged urinary leakage or with prior prostatic resection. Another cause may be disruption of the anastomosis in the postoperative period. Treat the stricture first with gentle filiform-guided dilation. Try fluoroscopically guided balloon dilation followed by a period with an indwelling catheter. If the stream narrows, instruct the patient to intermittently catheterize himself. If these measures fail, incise the vesical neck transurethrally either anteriorly or at 4- and 8-o'clock positions with a cold knife. Extend the incision to—but not into—the normal sphincteric fibers because incontinence may result. Obtain hemostasis with a small electrode, and leave a catheter in place for 3 days.

A vesical neck stricture may be repaired by an abdominoperineal approach (Schlossberg et al, 1995). Dissect by an anterior approach to the area of the stricture; then expose it perineally, as done for radical perineal prostatectomy. Open the cul-de-sac from above to join the perineal dissection. Divide the area of obstruction over a sound. Excise the scarred area. Bring in an omental flap. Construct a new vesical neck situated more anteriorly, using six 2-0 SAS. Leave a urethral catheter and a suprapubic tube for 4 weeks.

If the patient is already incontinent, proceed directly to incision/resection of the stricture with the electrosurgical unit and implant an artificial sphincter.

Perineal Prostatectomy

Clear infection and begin antibiotic prophylaxis. Preparation of the bowel because of the possibility of rectal injury is especially indicated in patients after previous perineal surgery. Ascertain that the patient has enough cardiopulmonary reserve and suffi-cient mobility in knee and hip joints to withstand the extreme lithotomy position. Shave only the perineum.

Instruments and *position* are those for total perineal prosta-tectomy (see page 451).

1 Proceed as for total perineal prostatectomy, Steps 1 to 10 (see pages 451 to 457). Make the original incision vertically in the rectal fascia (posterior lamella of Denonvilliers' fascia) (Step 10).

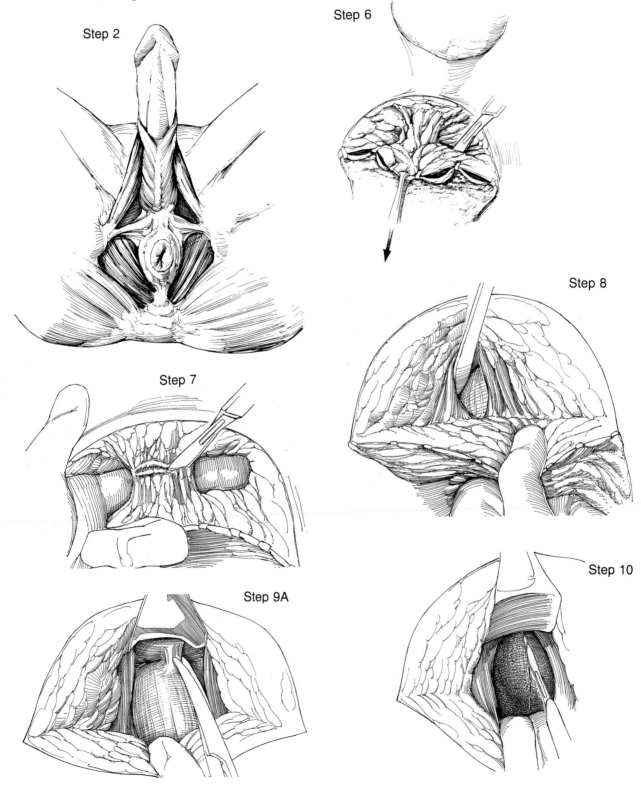

Step 2

Step 6

Step 7

Step 8

Step 9A

Step 10

2 **A** and **B**, Make the original incision in the rectal fascia (posterior leaf of Denonvilliers' fascia) vertically. Dissect the rectal fascia laterally from the body of the prostate to preserve the neurovascular bundles containing the cavernous nerves.

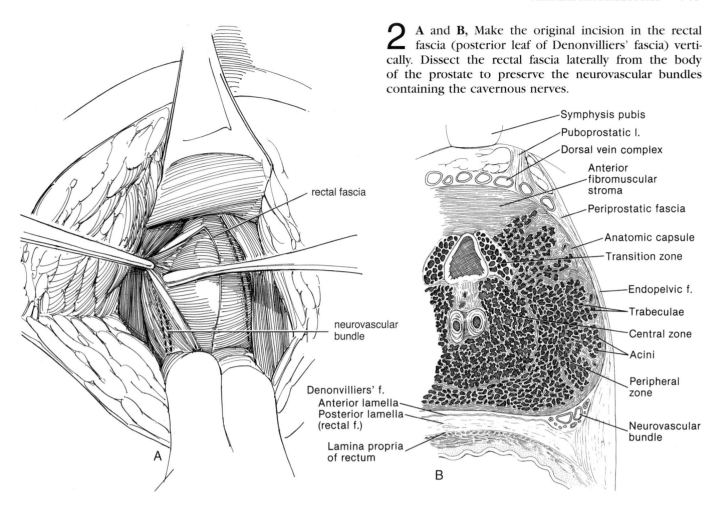

A

rectal fascia

neurovascular bundle

Denonvilliers' f.
Anterior lamella
Posterior lamella (rectal f.)

Lamina propria of rectum

B

Symphysis pubis
Puboprostatic l.
Dorsal vein complex
Anterior fibromuscular stroma
Periprostatic fascia
Anatomic capsule
Transition zone
Endopelvic f.
Trabeculae
Central zone
Acini
Peripheral zone
Neurovascular bundle

3 Hold the rectum back with the padded posterior retractor. Make an inverted U-shaped incision in the surgical capsule of the prostate with its apex slightly proximal to the verumontanum, which may be felt as a soft spot in the capsule. Incise through the capsule deep enough to expose the cleavage plane between the capsule and the adenoma.

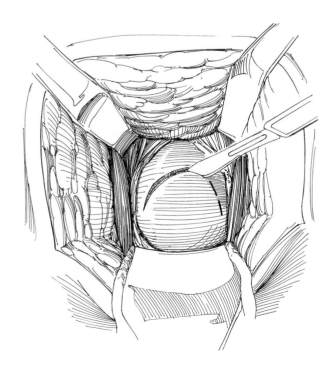

4 Turn the U flap outward with an Allis clamp, freeing that portion of the capsule bluntly from the underlying adenoma.

Start dissecting the adenoma laterally with a joker. Be certain to get in the proper plane initially. Continue the dissection digitally, taking care around the apex of the adenoma to outline the urethra. During the enucleation, remove the long tractor and the lateral and posterior retractors from the wound to avoid injury and tearing.

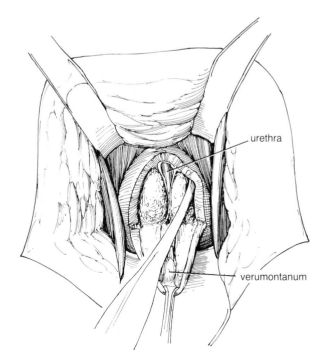

urethra

verumontanum

5 Divide the dorsal wall of the urethra to free the apex of the adenoma; then sharply divide the remainder of the urethra at the apex to avoid tension on the sphincters. Insert the index finger into the cleavage plane and complete the enucleation, leaving the adenoma attached at the vesical neck.

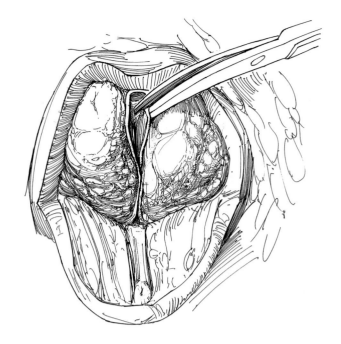

6 Place prostatic lobe forceps or thyroid forceps on the adenoma, and complete freeing it by pushing back the circular fibers of the vesical neck. With scissors, enter the cone of epithelium thus formed transversely, and grasp the bladder wall with an Allis clamp to hold the bladder in the wound. Complete the transection, preserving as much epithelium as possible. Be sure to remove all subtrigonal and subcervical lobes. A large median lobe may have to be "popped" out of the bladder by digitally dilating the bladder neck. Fulgurate or suture-ligate vessels entering the adenoma at the vesical neck as they are encountered. Inspect the fossa for residual tissue. Because visualization is excellent, bleeding points can be fulgurated or oversewn.

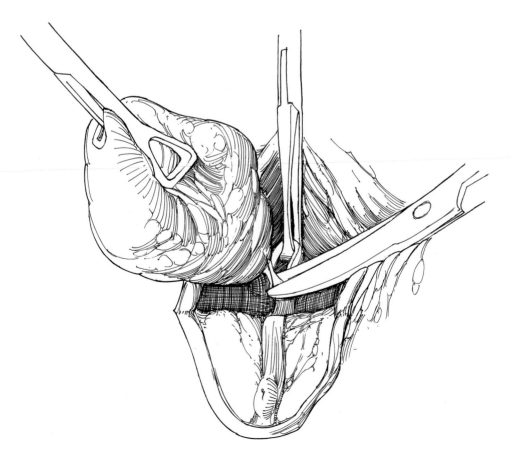

7 Place another Allis clamp on the vesical neck and draw it into view. Deep lateral retractors help with exposure. Insert a figure-eight 3-0 CCG suture in the mucosa and muscle of the neck at the 5- and 7-o'clock positions to control the urethral branches of the prostatic artery that usually can be seen spurting. Leave these sutures long. Draw the posterior vesical neck into the fossa, and suture it circumferentially to the posterior capsular flap with interrupted 3-0 PCG sutures.

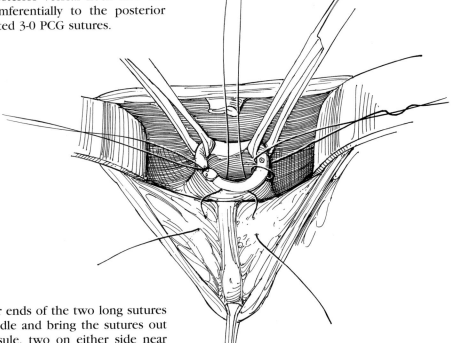

8 Place each of the four ends of the two long sutures in a large curved needle and bring the sutures out through the prostatic capsule, two on either side near the incision. Tie them in pairs. This collapses the space previously occupied by the adenoma and provides hemostasis. Avoid placing sutures laterally that could involve the neurovascular bundle. Insert a 24 F 30-ml balloon catheter through the urethra into the wound, and lead it into the bladder on a curved clamp. Inflate the balloon and suture the catheter to the frenulum with a size 1-0 silk suture. Irrigate the catheter to free the bladder of clots, which can accumulate in the sump, and to be very certain that the balloon lies within the bladder.

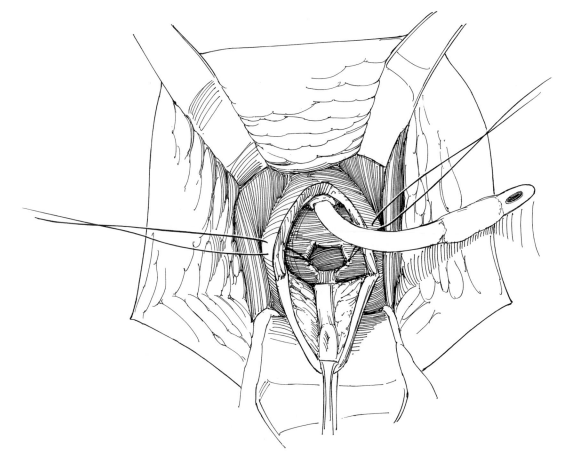

9 Suture the U-shaped flap into the defect in the capsule with a running 2-0 CCG suture, keeping the stitches close to the edges. Insert a Penrose drain and approximate the levators. Close the wound with subcutaneous sutures and a running, preferably subcuticular, 3-0 SAS. Tape the catheter to the penis (see page 13) and to the leg. Place a fluffed-gauze dressing held by a perineal binder. Remove the drain in 3 or 4 days and the catheter in 7 days.

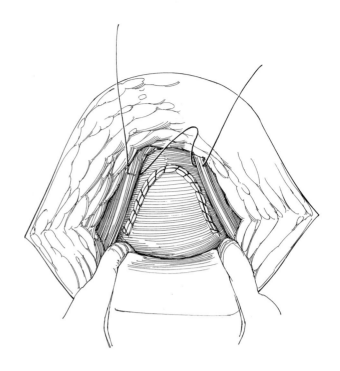

POSTOPERATIVE PROBLEMS

For *premature removal of the catheter,* gently insert a straight 28 F sound into the bladder. Remove it and follow it immediately with a balloon catheter on a straight stilet. This allows tactile guidance of the tip of the catheter. *Rectal perforation* should be detected intraoperatively. Because it usually occurs on the approach, one may decide to terminate the procedure before the urethra is broached. If perforation is detected during closure, close it in two layers with fine absorbable sutures, overdistend the anal sphincters, prolong the period of catheter drainage, and provide antibiotic coverage. If a *fecal fistula* develops, make a diverting colostomy and wait. If the fistula does not close spontaneously, a formal closure is required (see page 476).

Commentary by C. Eugene Carlton, Jr.

The great advantage of perineal prostatectomy, both simple and radical, is the precise anatomic dissection that can be carried out. This leads to doing the operation under direct vision, which in turn allows for precise capsular reapproximation in the simple operation and precise vesicourethral anastomosis in radical perineal prostatectomy. Another great advantage is the ability to visualize the neurovascular bundle directly early in the procedure, allowing for its retraction and protection. The patient's tolerance of this operation is so much better than with the abdominal approach for either the radical or simple retropubic prostatectomy: The patient can have a normal diet on the evening of surgery, can be ambulatory on the afternoon of surgery, can be dismissed home on the second postoperative day, and experiences little if any discomfort after the operation. Blood loss is significantly less than with the abdominal approaches.

Perhaps the secret to this operation is the development of the proper plane between the bulbocavernosus muscle and the anterior wall of the rectum early in the dissection. In order to do this, after dividing the central tendon, one must look carefully for the fibers of the bulbocavernosus and median raphe forming an inverted triangle, with the apex posteriorly meeting the levator fibers coming off the anterior wall of the rectal sphincter, again in a triangular fashion. Where these two triangular tips meet is the deep perineal body. Identification and dissection of this body and establishment of the plane between these two structures early in the procedure allow one to stay out of both the rectum and, more importantly, the bulbocavernosus muscle. Proper retraction then allows easy identification and dissection of the prostate.

I find that a self-retaining perineal retractor adds greatly to the ease with which this procedure can be carried out.

Total Perineal Prostatectomy

The two standard approaches are the extrasphincteric approach of Young and the Belt subsphincteric technique. Either may be combined with a nerve-sparing technique (Weldon and Tavel, 1988). A perineal operation is difficult for prostates weighing more than 100 g. Perform pelvic lymph node dissection by an open approach (see page 465) or, better, by a laparoscopic approach (see page 469) if the PSA level is 15 ng/ml or greater or the Gleason score is 7 or greater. If the laparoscopic approach is used and the nodes prove to be negative for cancer, proceed laparoscopically to mobilize the seminal vesicles up to their entry into the ejaculatory ducts; this makes subsequent prostatectomy easier.

Correct blood volume. Have two units of blood or packed cells available (these units can be released at the end of the operation if not used because postoperative blood loss is seldom significant). Prepare the bowel with clear liquid diet, Go-LYTELY, and gentamicin, in case the rectum is entered. Start intravenous fluids to provide diuresis during surgery (which also have the benefit of increasing the rate of excretion of indigo carmine if it is given to identify the ureteral orifices). Consider minidose heparinization (5000 units twice a day for 2 days) unless simultaneous pelvic lymphadenectomy is performed, with its increased risk of lymphocele. Consider applying compression stockings.

1 *Instruments:* It is important to have perineal prostatectomy specials as illustrated. Provide GU long and GU fine sets, male sounds with lubricating jelly, long Allis clamps, an irrigating syringe, a 16 F 5-ml silicone balloon catheter, and 0.5-inch and 1-inch Penrose drains.

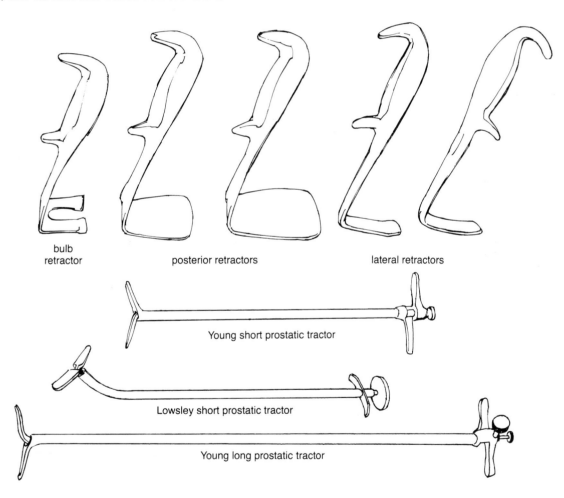

bulb retractor

posterior retractors

lateral retractors

Young short prostatic tractor

Lowsley short prostatic tractor

Young long prostatic tractor

2 The *Young approach (open dashes)* enters anterior to the subcutaneous, superficial, and deep portions of the external anal sphincter, passing through the ischiorectal fossa to the perineal body. The *Belt approach (closed dashes)* enters over the subcutaneous portion of the external anal sphincter and under its combined superficial and deep portions to drop immediately onto the lamina propria of the rectum. The dissection then follows the lamina propria to the perineal body and the attachment of the rectourethralis muscle. This feature makes it easier to learn and perform this approach.

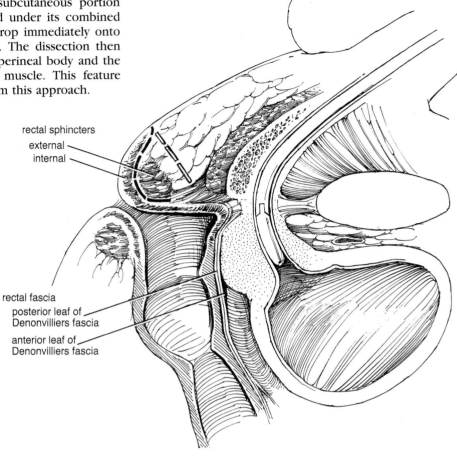

rectal sphincters
external
internal

rectal fascia
posterior leaf of Denonvilliers fascia
anterior leaf of Denonvilliers fascia

BELT APPROACH

3 The external anal sphincter has three parts, two of which are elevated. Depression of the anal verge and subcutaneous part of the rectal sphincter exposes the lamina propria of the rectum. Dissection is done posterior to the transverse perineal muscles; entering the bulb must be avoided.

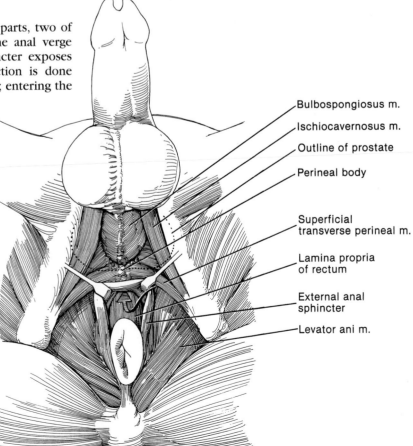

Bulbospongiosus m.

Ischiocavernosus m.

Outline of prostate

Perineal body

Superficial transverse perineal m.

Lamina propria of rectum

External anal sphincter

Levator ani m.

4 **A,** Provide spinal anesthesia or use general anesthesia with intubation (the patient's vital capacity may be reduced by the exaggerated perineal position, although splinting the diaphragm by the increased intra-abdominal pressure may aid some patients in respiratory exchange).

Position: Place the patient on a vacuum bag if available. Proper positioning of the patient in the extreme lithotomy position is most important. Unless the perineum is in the same plane as the floor, the operation is difficult to perform. Place the patient's feet in padded stirrups. Lower the end of the table. Brace your knee against the table, grasp the thighs, and pull the patient down until the buttocks extend well over the end of the table. Rock the legs back with the leg supports. Carefully pad the proximal end of the fibula to protect the peroneal nerve. Insert a large wedge or sandbag deep under the sacrum. Place well-padded shoulder braces laterally against the acromial processes, away from the brachial plexuses. Do not abduct the arms. Evacuate the vacuum bag under the patient to cradle the shoulders and hold the patient in position. Flex the thighs further until the perineum is absolutely parallel with the floor. One can tilt the head of the table down slightly to improve the position.

Recheck the padding at all points of contact. Adjust the height of the table to allow operating while standing.

The first assistant stands to the left of the right-handed surgeon so that he or she may assist with the right hand, and the second assistant stands to the right. Prepare the suprapubic region and perineum. Drape the area with towels, leg drapes, and an inverted laparotomy sheet. An adhesive drape with integral finger cot may be applied if available. Drape the penis and scrotum in a separate field. Insert a rectal tube to evacuate the rectum of the fluid from the bowel preparation.

Inject a copious amount of lubricant into the urethra. Insert a long Young or Lowsley prostatic tractor into the bladder to be certain that it can be passed later. A curved 28 F sound with a clamp-on handle or even a balloon catheter can be substituted, but they are much less satisfactory. Partially withdraw the closed tractor so that its angle lies in the bulb, allowing palpation of the site of the prostatic apex. Have the second assistant support the tractor with the right hand.

B, Palpate the ischial tuberosities and make a U-shaped skin incision from the middle of the perineum running just within them (so that the patient will not have to sit on the incision). Carry the incision well posterior to the anus on both sides to enable the rectum to be dropped back for greater exposure. Preserve the subcutaneous fat on the flap.

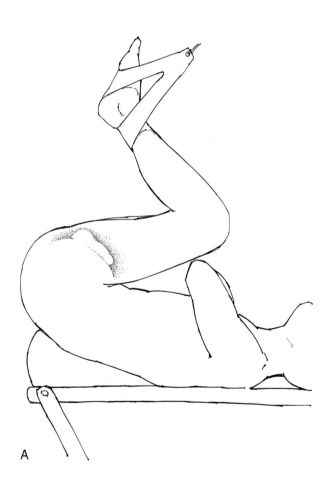

A

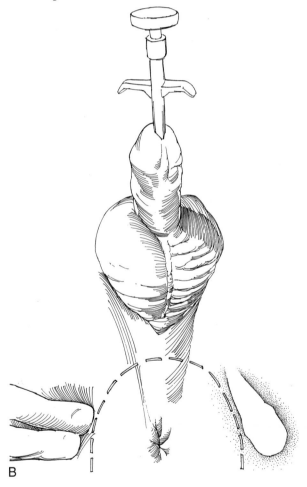

B

5 Clip a folded 4 × 4 inch sponge saturated with iodophor solution to the skin edge to mask the anus, and grasp the apex of the skin flap together with the apex of the sponge with an Allis clamp. Using the cutting current, divide the exposed superficial fascia in the line of the incision. Palpate the angle of the tractor in the bulb for orientation. Use a #10 scalpel to penetrate upward and laterally through the superficial perineal fascia into the ischiorectal fossa on each side near the lateral angles of the wound for a depth of 3 or 4 cm.

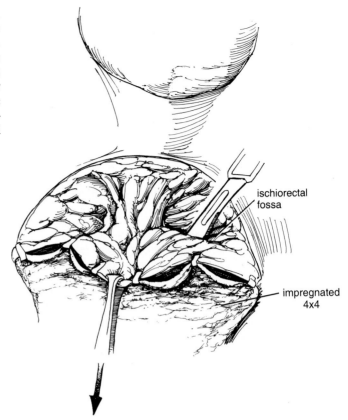

6 Insert an index finger on each side, directing it forward and cephalad along each side of the rectum under the external striated rectal sphincters. Work the fingers over the rectal wall until a finger can be passed from one side to the other around the central tendon. If the fingers do not penetrate the tissue easily, move them more posteriorly. Stay well behind the transversus muscles and the bulbar urethra. Divide the central tendon of the perineum progressively with knife or cutting current.

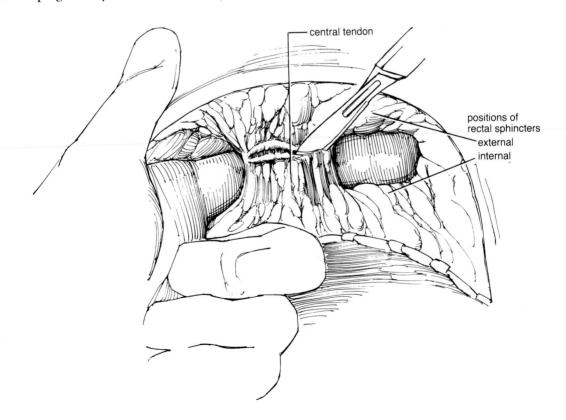

7 Continue the division of the tendon directly down to the rectal wall. The surface of the rectum is easily recognized by the whitish longitudinal fibers in the lamina propria. Use these fibers as a landmark as the dissection progresses proximally. Put an extra glove on your left hand and place the index finger in the rectum; this helps you follow this important surface with less fear of penetration. Place a moist opened 4 × 4 inch gauze under the left thumb to draw the rectal wall taut. With the knife handle, progressively lift the external rectal sphincter away from the rectal lamina propria, supporting it with lateral retractors.

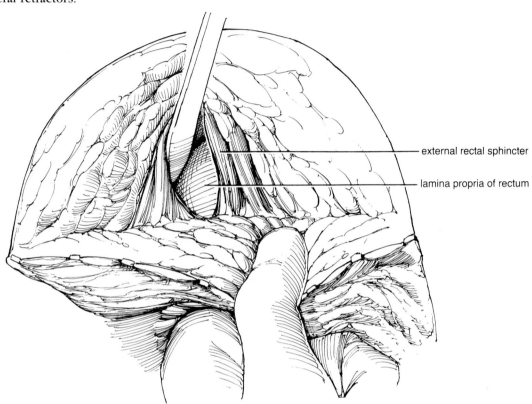

external rectal sphincter

lamina propria of rectum

8 **A** and **B,** Follow the rectal wall along its longitudinal striations as you push the levator ani muscles aside and upward. No other structures are encountered until a condensation of muscular tissue, the so-called rectourethralis muscle, is exposed in the midline. Advance the prostatic tractor well into the bladder, and open and lock the blades after making sure they are inside the cavity. Have your assistant use the tractor as a lever over the symphysis to elevate the prostate into the wound. Identify the apex of the prostate. Burrow with the knife handle and finger tip on either side close to the rectum. Minimally displace the rectum backward, because the pelvic nerve plexus and cavernous nerves course in the lateral rectal and lateral pelvic fascias close to it. Insertion of a self-retaining retractor anchored to the table may help with exposure, especially if only one assistant is available. Grasp the rectourethralis muscle with forceps and continue spreading the decussation of the levator ani muscles, which often reveal the white surface of

Denonvilliers' fascia covering the prostate on either side near the apex. Remember, the rectum is tented up by the rectourethralis muscle at this point and is easily entered. Divide the rectourethralis muscle sharply with Lahey scissors at its junction with the rectal wall. It must not be divided too far anteriorly, where the bulb could be entered, nor too far posteriorly, risking entry into the rectum.

Alternative: Divide the rectourethralis muscle vertically, as is done for Denonvilliers' fascia (Step 9). Position the padded posterior retractor yourself, making certain that the assistant holding it does not relax and tip the blade posteriorly, thus compromising the rectal blood supply. A weighted retractor may be a good substitute. Look for evidence of malignancy in the periprostatic tissues, and make a decision about sacrificing the neurovascular bundle(s) and whether a wide-field technique should be followed.

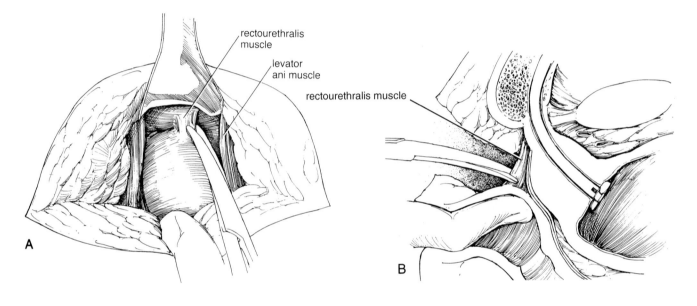

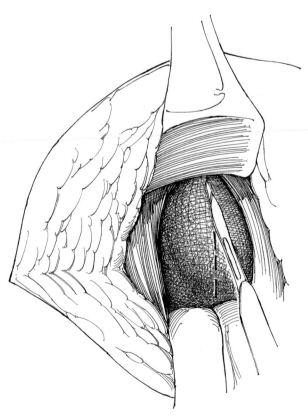

9 Have the second assistant raise and tilt the Lowsley tractor to move the prostate into the wound (the symphysis acts as a fulcrum). Bluntly expose the apical portion of the ventral rectal fascia (the posterior lamella of Denonvilliers' fascia) with the knife handle. These are the "pearly gates" of Young that admit you to the prostate itself. Make a vertical cut just through the posterior lamella starting at the apex, which is readily palpable against the tractor. A vertical incision, in contrast to the traditional transverse one, protects the cavernous nerves located laterally.

10 Use the joker dissector and knife handle to separate the posterior lamella containing the nerves from the anterior lamella of Denonvilliers' fascia on the prostate gland. The two layers are adherent near the prostatic apex. Divide the adhesions sharply against Denonvilliers' fascia to protect the nerves on the reflected ventral (rectal) fascia. Continue dissection laterally and posteriorly all the way to the base of the seminal vesicles, where Denonvilliers' fascia must be incised transversely to allow access to the vesicles and ampullae. Some surgeons identify and ligate the lateral vascular pedicles at this point. Bluntly free the prostate laterally inside the fascia and on either side of the apex, but avoid strong lateral retraction that could injure the nerves.

Pad the exposed surface of the rectum with moist gauze, and again place the angled posterior retractor. Never allow assistants to place retractors because they have an incomplete view of the field. Position them yourself, and see that they are maintained in that position. Have the second assistant hold the rectum back with the retractor to create tension. To avoid ischemic injury to the rectum, the assistant must not tilt the tip of the blade too deeply into the wound. If the prostate is large, additional room may be obtained by dividing some of the fibers of the levator ani muscles transversely.

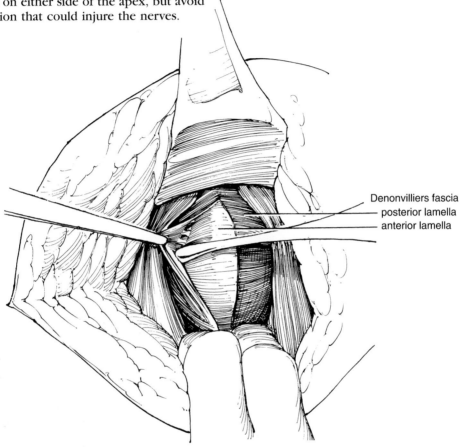

Denonvilliers fascia
posterior lamella
anterior lamella

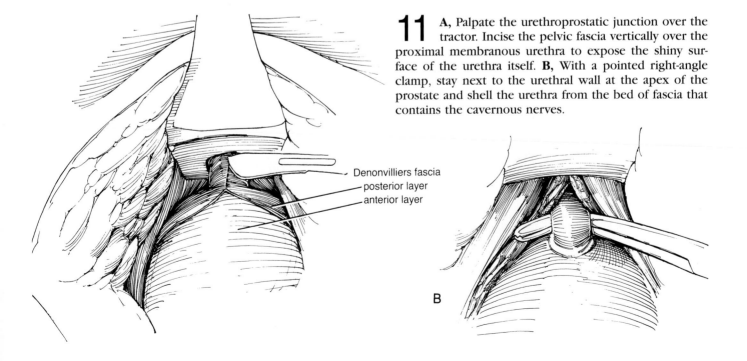

Denonvilliers fascia
posterior layer
anterior layer

B

11 **A,** Palpate the urethroprostatic junction over the tractor. Incise the pelvic fascia vertically over the proximal membranous urethra to expose the shiny surface of the urethra itself. **B,** With a pointed right-angle clamp, stay next to the urethral wall at the apex of the prostate and shell the urethra from the bed of fascia that contains the cavernous nerves.

12 Cut down onto the clamp at the urethroprostatic junction. Remove the long tractor, and replace it with a short one passed through the new opening in the cut urethra. Divide the remainder of the urethra under direct vision against the clamp with the scissors angled obliquely downward. Because the dissection stays close to the surface of the urethra and prostate, the dorsal veins are avoided. If Santorini's plexus anterior to the prostate bleeds, pass a large Mayo needle blunt end first to ligate the whole venous complex, although at the same time jeopardizing the prospects for potency. The puboprostatic ligaments, if encountered holding the prostate near the bladder neck, can be divided sharply without risk of bleeding.

13 Pull down on the short tractor to allow blunt dissection of the anterior surface of the prostate. Keep close to the prostate itself (the surgical capsule) to avoid the dorsal vein system and the need to divide the puboprostatic ligaments. Continue the dissection until the vesical neck is reached (identified readily by palpation on the tractor blades). Use the fingernail or scalpel handle to create a groove between the prostate and vesical neck anteriorly down to the vesical epithelium.

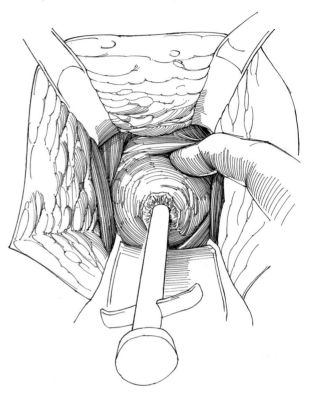

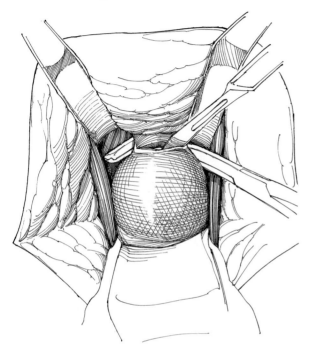

14 Remove the short tractor. Insert a right-angle clamp into the urethra; pass it to the vesical neck and cut through the remaining tissue at the bladder neck against the point of the clamp. Use the clamp to grasp the tip of a 20 F Robinson catheter or the end of a length of umbilical tape, and draw it out the urethra. Clamp the ends and use the loop for traction.

15 Divide the anterior wall of the bladder at its junction with the prostate. Clamp and ligate or cauterize vessels as they are encountered (use small right-angle clamps). For a more hemostatic alternative, place a row of 3-0 CCG sutures along the exposed vesicoprostatic junction, and divide the bladder distal to them. Ask the anesthetist to give a bolus of 5 ml of indigo carmine intravenously, which in the presence of the existing diuresis soon allows visualization of the ureteral orifices. Ureteral catheters are not needed.

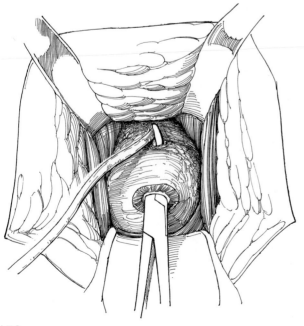

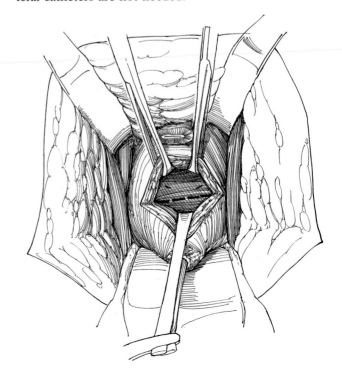

16 Continue division of the vesical neck posteriorly. This exposes the base of the seminal vesicles and ejaculatory ducts. Watch for the ureteral orifices with their blue-green efflux. The prostate is held laterally by vessels that arise from the prostatic branches of the inferior vesical artery. Isolate these adjacent to the prostate with Mixter or right-angle clamps. Clamp them proximally, divide them, and ligate or clip the proximal ends. Avoid mass ligation. The neurovascular bundle containing the erector nerves lies laterally and is not exposed in this dissection, but the nerves may be injured by vigorous lateral traction. (For a more radical operation, excise the adjacent rectal and lateral pelvic fascia and sacrifice the neurovascular bundles.) As the last few fibers of the detrusor are divided, pull down on the specimen and elevate the posterior lip of the bladder with an Allis clamp to expose the anterior leaf of Denonvilliers' fascia that covers the seminal vesicles.

prostatic branch of inferior vesical artery

ampulla of vas deferens

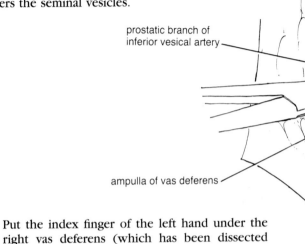

17 Put the index finger of the left hand under the right vas deferens (which has been dissected previously from behind), grasp it with two clamps, and divide and ligate it. Repeat this procedure for the left vas.

ampulla of vas deferens

18 This frees the specimen so that a little traction on it allows blunt dissection of the seminal vesicles to their proximal ends.

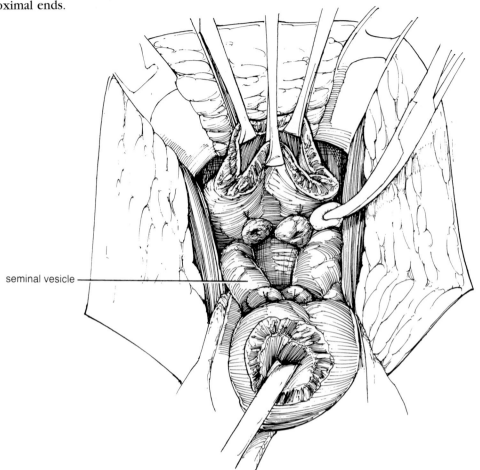

seminal vesicle

19 Elevate the specimen and clip the vesicular arteries at the tip of the seminal vesicles. Clamp and divide the last remaining muscle fibers enclosing the arteries. Remove the specimen and place ties of 3-0 CCG or clips above the clamps.

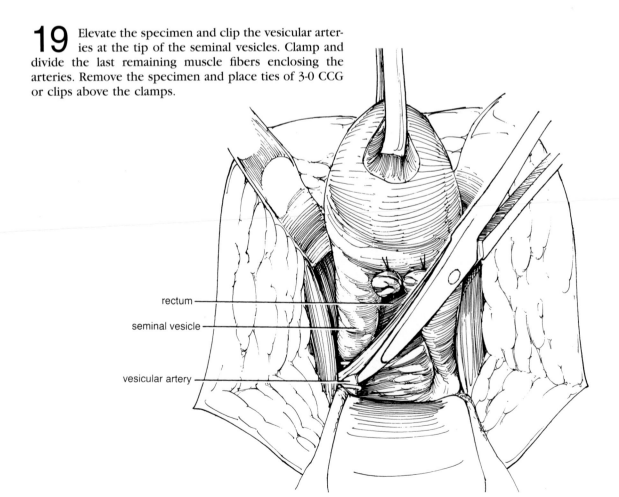

rectum

seminal vesicle

vesicular artery

20 Insert a 22 F silicone Robinson or balloon catheter through the urethral meatus. Grasp it as it exits at the site of urethral transection and clamp the ends together. Elevate the urethra with the looped catheter to expose the ventral rim of the transected membranous urethra. Insert one 3-0 CCG suture through the remnant of the prostatic apex from the outside in; then pass it through the wall of the bladder, being certain that the suture is placed to evert the epithelial surfaces. Insert a second suture close by, and tie them both. Do not place sutures in the so-called urogenital diaphragm or in the periurethral fascia, thus avoiding the cavernous nerves within. Take care not to tear the tissue while inserting the sutures.

21 Place two more sutures on each side and tie them. Insert the tip of the catheter into the bladder. Continue suturing the circumference of the urethra with two or three more sutures. Because the opening in the bladder is larger than the urethral diameter, complete the closure of the bladder defect vertically (racket handle) with similar sutures. Test for watertightness by filling the bladder, and add sutures if needed. Irrigate the wound and fulgurate any bleeding points. Check the surface of the rectum for injury. Place a ⅝-inch Penrose drain, to exit at a corner of the wound. Loosely connect the edges of the levators in the midline with 2-0 SAS. Reapproximate the central tendon and Scarpa's fascia. Place a few interrupted subcutaneous sutures, and close the skin with a running 2-0 SAS. Place a gauze dressing held in place by a net stocking or mesh pants. Ambulate and feed the patient on the day of surgery. Remove the drain on the second day and stop prophylactic antibiotics. Discharge the patient and have him return in 2 weeks for removal of the catheter. At that time give instructions for traffic exercises (stop and go during urination) and for exercises to strengthen the perineum.

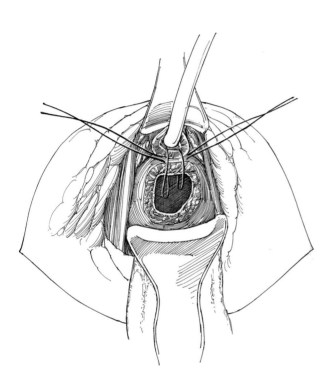

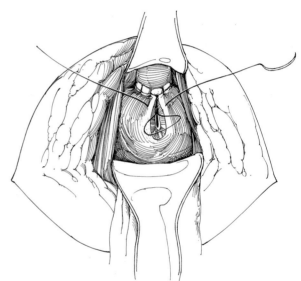

ALTERNATIVE METHODS OF CLOSURE

22 *Closure I (posterior insertion):* Beginning ventrally, first partially close the bladder defect, leaving an opening of the same size as the urethra. Anastomosis is done as described above.

23 *Closure II (bladder flap, Flocks):* When continence is a concern, form an anterior bladder flap into a tube (see page 573) and suture the tube to the urethra.

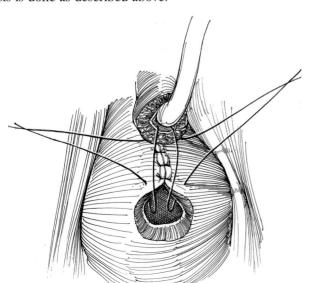

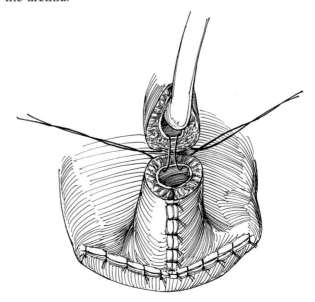

24 *Closure III (Vest):* To support any type of anastomosis, place one suture of 2-0 CCG into the bladder on either side of it. Bring the ends onto the perineum on long needles, and tie them over bolsters (Vest sutures) to put traction on the bladder neck and hold it against the membranous urethra.

25 *Closure IV (Hodges):* After placing an anterior and two lateral sutures, place a mattress suture at the apex, bring it subcutaneously, and tie it. Close the vesical defect vertically.

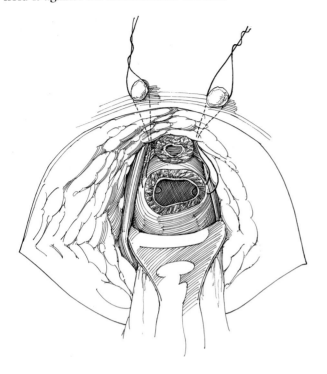

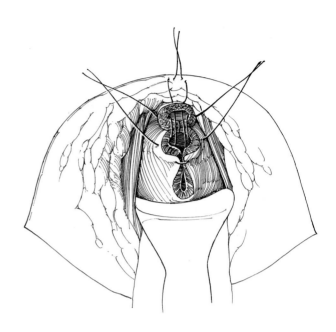

26 Approximate the levators loosely in the midline with interrupted 3-0 CCG sutures, taking care not to include the lateral bundles, especially anteriorly, or the rectum. Place several 3-0 PCG sutures to close the subcutaneous space around a medium-sized Penrose drain placed in either angle of the perineal wound (or brought out through a stab wound).

27 Close the wound with a 4-0 SAS placed subcuticularly. Alternatively, place interrupted absorbable sutures percutaneously, leaving the ends long so that they cannot cause perineal discomfort. Tape the catheter to the penis, using tincture of benzoin on the skin (see page 13). Apply a nonstick dressing generously covered with fluffs. Perineal compression with a sandbag may reduce oozing.

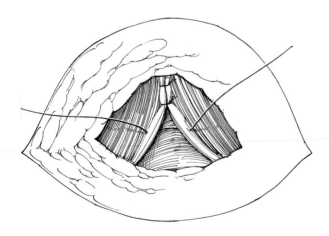

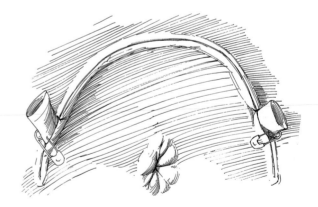

WIDE-FIELD TOTAL PROSTATECTOMY (Paulson)

Wide-Field Radical Perineal Prostatectomy. If palpation or ultrasonography indicates involvement of the periprostatic tissue, total prostatectomy may not be curative. A so-called wide-field radical perineal prostatectomy has been advocated in which the periprostatic fascia and the neurovascular bundle are resected (Paulson, 1986).

Proceed through Step 13. In dividing the urethra, cut the endopelvic (lateral pelvic) fascia widely where it reflects onto the bladder. Control the bleeding with clips. This divides the neurovascular bundle(s). Divide Denonvilliers' fascia posteriorly over the seminal vesicles, and clamp and divide the fibrovascular pedicles. Continue freeing the seminal vesicles and removing the prostate.

POSTOPERATIVE CARE

Ambulate the patient as soon as possible. Postoperative pain may be managed by administering ketorolac tromethamine (Toradol), 30 to 60 mg IM in the operating room, followed by 30 mg intramuscularly every 8 hours for three doses. Morphine may be given by percutaneous pump (expensive), followed by oxycodone hydrochloride and acetaminophen (Percocet) given after 2 days. Provide stool softeners (Dulcolax suppositories) to avoid constipation. An alternative is to give a 30-ml dose of mineral oil orally twice daily until the patient objects. Give no enemas! Give sips of water on the day of surgery, full liquids on postoperative day 1, and select diet on postoperative day 2. Remove the drain in 2 or 3 days, and discharge the patient from the hospital. Remove the catheter in 4 to 7 days. Warn the patient about temporary impairment of control.

INTRAOPERATIVE COMPLICATIONS

Inability to Introduce a Long Tractor (Young or Lowsley). Try guiding the tip through the sphincter and over the prostate with the fingers behind the scrotum or a finger in the rectum. If that fails, use a 20 F straight sound to map the posterior urethra, and then try again with the tractor. If all attempts fail, pass a 24 F balloon catheter and use it for traction.

Dissecting Too Far Anteriorly. Watch out for the transverse perineal muscles. If they or the bulbar urethra is encountered, the dissection has gone too far forward. Back out. Begin again nearer the rectum; otherwise severe bleeding comes from the bulb and the urogenital diaphragm is placed in jeopardy.

Ureteral Injury. Damage may occur if dissection extends behind the trigone in an attempt to find a plane of cleavage between the bladder and seminal vesicles. Injury can also follow division of the posterior bladder neck at too high a level. Intravenously injected indigo carmine identifies the orifices. During closure, the ureters could become obstructed with a stitch; if doubt exists at that time, place stents to exit through the perineal incision.

Rectal Injury

Rectal injury is more common after perineal prostatectomy than after retropubic excision because of the tenting of the rectum by the rectourethral muscle.

28 Routinely prepare the bowel to reduce the complications from injury to the rectum. If the bowel has not been prepared, provide a diverting colostomy (see page 669). Consider fecal diversion if the repair is tenuous, if gross fecal contamination is present, or if the injury is related to prior irradiation.

A, Be aware of the possibility of rectal injury and look for perforation at the time of posterior rectourethral dissection. The real danger is in overlooking the significance of bleeding from the submucosal vessels or bulging of the rectal mucosa. If the rectum is entered, wait until the end of the operation before repairing the injury. An alternative for a large defect is to repair it, close the perineal incision, and proceed to remove the prostate by the retropubic approach.

B, For intraoperative repair, place a running 4-0 CCG suture transversely to invert the submucosal and mucosal edge, with the knots in the rectal lumen.

C, Close the muscularis and lamina propria longitudinally with interrupted 4-0 CCG sutures. If possible, suture the deep external rectal sphincter to the levator ani muscles, placing it proximal to the site of repair. Alternatively, suture all layers with interrupted 4-0 CCG sutures and infold this suture line with a second (and even third) layer of muscularis. Suture the external anal sphincter to the rectal lamina propria above the site of the injury to ensure that any leakage does not pool (Resnick, 1995). Irrigate the incision copiously with iodophor solution, dilate the anus widely, and drain the area well with two Penrose drains. Start the patient on a low-residue diet postoperatively and provide stool softeners. Place a punch cystostomy to help divert the urine. Repair of rectourethral fistulas is described on page 476.

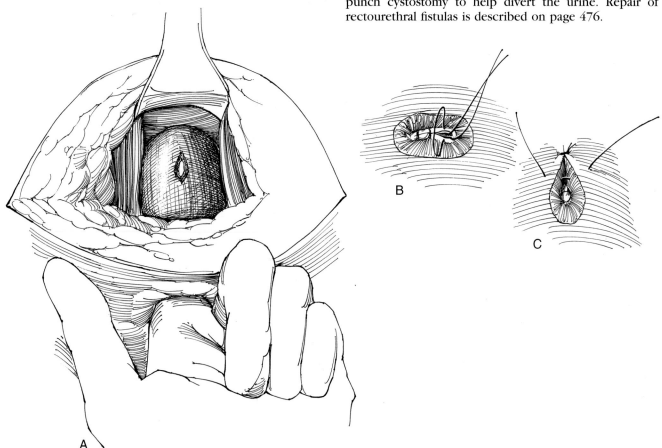

POSTOPERATIVE PROBLEMS
Immediate Problems

Replacement of the urethral catheter may not be necessary if the anastomosis is solid. If the catheter falls out or if the patient is unable to void when the catheter is removed on the 10th or 12th postoperative day, give the patient intravenous valium. Place a 24 F Robinson or balloon catheter on a straight stilet. Overfill the urethra with lubricant. With a finger in the rectum, gently guide the catheter into the bladder. Alternatively, first insert a smaller straight sound to map the route before inserting the catheter on a straight stilet. Flexible cystoscopy may be used. Endoscopic introduction of a guide under anesthesia is a possibility, but a better immediate solution is insertion of a disposable punch cystostomy device.

Constipation can be avoided by stool softeners. Enemas must not be given; a tube could injure the rectum where it was weakened by the dissection.

A *urethrorectal fistula* can follow unrecognized rectal injury. First replace the urethral catheter, provide an elemental diet, and reduce bowel activity for a few days' trial. If the fistula is discovered within the first 2 weeks, it can be corrected transrectally. Dilate the sphincter, locate the tear, and close it under direct vision with fine SAS. Leave a perineal drain in the wound to prevent an abscess. If this maneuver fails, wait 3 or 4 months and close the fistula by one of the techniques described in the text (see page 476). The safest way is to divert the fecal stream with a colostomy (see page 669) and the urine with a cystostomy (see page 625) before proceeding. However, a colostomy may not be necessary if repair is done meticulously.

Ureteral occlusion can result in anuria or flank pain. This complication is rare with the use of diuretics and indigo carmine. If one or both ureters become obstructed by sutures placed for hemostasis or during vesicourethral anastomosis, wait a few days for the sutures to absorb. It is rarely feasible to pass a small resectoscope and try to cut the sutures. Temporary percutaneous nephrostomies give more time for the suture to become absorbed.

Hemorrhage via the catheter is rarely a problem as it is with a radical retropubic prostatectomy because the vesical neck is brought down and anastomosed for good vascular control. However, perineal bleeding from the prostatic pedicles and adjacent structures may be more difficult to control during the operation and may continue to ooze. A Penrose drain prevents a hematoma, and a sandbag pressed into the perineum reduces the ooze. Reopen the operative site as a last resort, because considerable and potentially disturbing exposure is required to find the bleeding points that were missed.

Catheter obstruction from clots may require movement of the catheter to achieve irrigation; be sure the catheter is taped to the penis when the balloon is deflated. If it cannot be cleared and must be replaced, reinsert the new catheter without delay. Placing a cystostomy may be the better choice.

Perineal urinary leakage that lasts longer than 2 weeks with catheter drainage should be investigated by panendoscopy under anesthesia, fistulography, and voiding cystography. However, most perineal fistulas close spontaneously.

The extreme lithotomy position may result in *nerve injury,* either by pressure in the groin or pressure on the peroneal nerve. *Rhabdomyolysis* with renal failure may follow prolonged angulation in this position. Look for smoky urine and obtain a creatine phosphokinase determination; if it is greater than 20,000, myolysis has occurred. Correct electrolytes, keep the patient hydrated, and alkalinize the urine. *Hypotension* may follow taking the patient out of the extreme lithotomy position.

Late Problems

Urinary incontinence is not common if the urethra is carefully dissected at the apex. When present, it is usually temporary. Wait at least 6 months before considering an operation for it. Possible remedies are injection of bulking agents, formation of a bladder tube (see page 573), and implantation of an artificial sphincter (see page 580). *Impotence* after the perineal approach was the rule in the past, but techniques that respect the neurovascular bundles have reduced the incidence. A *stricture* at the urethrovesical anastomosis may appear after 4 to 6 months owing to failure to evert the vesical and urethral epithelial surfaces during anastomosis (Step 20). Treat the stricture with filiform-and-follower dilation to 18 or 20 F. If this fails, resort to direct-vision urethrotomy.

Persistence of carcinoma is signaled by PSA levels greater than 0. A stricture appearing after several years suggests recurrence of the carcinoma.

Commentary by Martin I. Resnick

Radical perineal prostatectomy is a valuable procedure used in the management of patients with localized carcinoma of the prostate. Although the approach does not permit access to the regional lymph nodes, it does allow for excellent exposure and removal of the prostate with reduced blood loss and an easily performed vesicourethral anastomosis. As with all techniques, most surgeons develop minor modifications that work well in their hands so that the procedure can be performed safely and effectively. As with all procedures, one must consider preoperative preparations and positioning, intraoperative techniques, and postoperative care. Blood loss with radical perineal prostatectomy is low, and it has not been found necessary to type and cross-match patients for either autologous or banked blood. All patients are typed and screened; if blood loss is greater than expected, cross-matching and transfusion are carried out either intraoperatively or postoperatively.

The exaggerated lithotomy position is routinely used, but care must be taken not to "overflex" the thigh, as this may result in injury to the femoral nerves. Stirrups that support the lower leg and take tension off the thigh are valuable in avoiding this potential complication. Additionally, shoulder braces are not routinely used, thus avoiding the potential of injury to the brachial plexus.

The Belt approach is used most commonly, and many believe that it provides more ready access to the apex of the prostate with reduced blood loss. The use of a self-retaining retractor is also very helpful and provides continuous and adequate exposure throughout the procedure. A direct vesicourethral anastomosis can be obtained without bladder neck reconstruction in most instances, and usually six to eight 3-0 polyglycolic acid sutures are used. If bladder neck reconstruction is required, it is done in a tennis-racket fashion (see Fig. 21).

Postoperatively patients are often able to begin eating after the effects of anesthesia have dissipated. Non-narcotic agents are often satisfactory in controlling pain (e.g., ketorolac tromethamine). Epidural anesthesia is not routinely used. More than 50 percent of patients are able to be discharged within 48 hours. Catheter drainage is maintained for 14 days.

The radical perineal prostatectomy had its origins in the early days of urology, and such eminent names as Hugh Hampton Young and Elmer Belt are closely associated with the procedure. It continues to be an important procedure that is useful in the management of patients with localized carcinoma of the prostate. Because of the development of laparoscopic techniques for assessing lymph and the greater realization (based on tumor grade and serum PSA) that not all patients require lymphadenectomy, its application in modern-day urology is greater than ever.

Modified Pelvic Lymph Node Dissection

Pelvic node dissection is done before total prostatectomy if the Gleason score is 7 or greater and if the PSA level is 15 ng/ml or greater. Evaluate the venous system of the lower extremities for deep vein occlusion, phlebitis, and edema. If a symptomatic inguinal hernia is present, it is possible to repair it from inside the pelvis (see page 342). If interstitial radioactive implantation is contemplated, obtain blood studies (bleeding time, prothrombin time [PT], partial thromboplastin time [PTT], and platelet count). Obtain urine cultures. Place the patient on a low-residue diet, and prepare the bowel in case the rectum must be entered.

Begin prophylactic antibiotics. Consider installing a central venous line preoperatively.

Incision: Lower midline extraperitoneal incision (see page 487). If node dissection is performed prior to total perineal prostatectomy, a lower abdominal transverse incision is suitable, done without mobilizing the rectus sheath and muscle (see page 490). The transverse incision may also be used for total retropubic prostatectomy if the rectus muscles are divided at their junction with the pubis (Cherney incision, see page 493).

1 Enter the prevesical space. Open a space between the bladder and iliac vessels with the forefinger. Sharply dissect the peritoneum from the anterior abdominal wall, from the iliopsoas region, and from the internal ring. Free the spermatic cord and loop it out of the way with a Penrose drain.

2 Place retractors to hold the bladder medially and the colon and peritoneal envelope superiorly. Elevate the abdominal wall laterally with a rake retractor. Divide the fibrofatty tissue over the iliac vein. Carry the dissection distally far enough to reach and resect the large medial retrocrural lymph node of Cloquet near the inguinal canal, to clear all the fibrofatty tissue from the bony surface of the pelvis and over Cooper's ligament. Stop at the circumflex iliac vein.

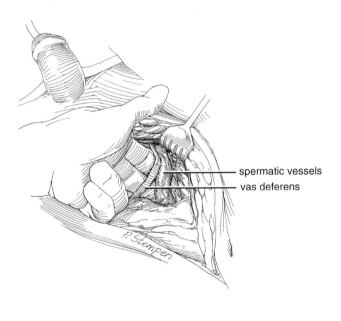

spermatic vessels
vas deferens

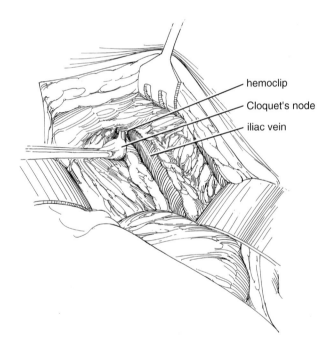

hemoclip
Cloquet's node
iliac vein

465

3 Separate the tissue between the iliac artery and vein. The artery is thus exposed along its medial and anterior surfaces. The lateral tissue is left intact.

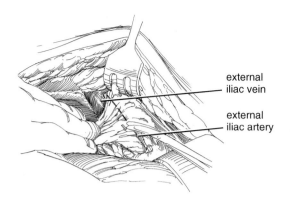

external iliac vein

external iliac artery

4 Pass the tissue under the iliac vein.

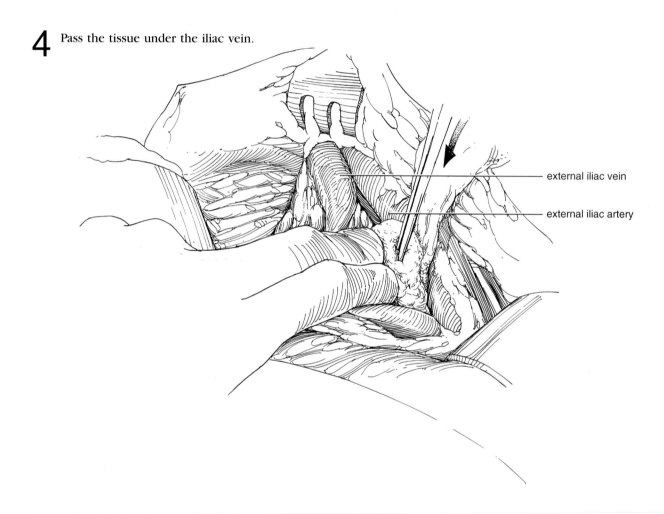

external iliac vein

external iliac artery

5 Free this mass of tissue at its superior margin to expose the obturator nerve. Pick up the obturator nodal tissue and dissect it to the obturator canal along with the rest of the tissue.

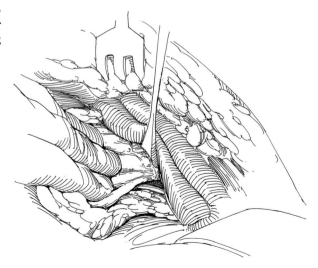

6 Clip the obturator artery and vein. (If the vein is torn flush, pack the canal with synthetic foam.) Be sure to clip all the lymphatics coming from the leg. Watch out for an accessory obturator vein arising from the medial aspect of the external iliac vein. If it is present, ligate it rather than clip it to prevent troublesome bleeding later on. Bluntly clear the tissue dorsal to the obturator nerve, where few nodes are encountered. Remove the resected tissue.

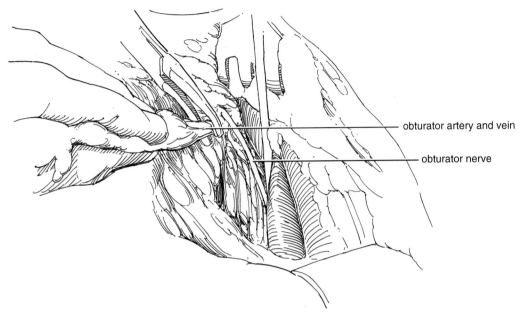

obturator artery and vein

obturator nerve

7 Resect the fibrofatty tissue around the internal iliac artery and its branches to the pelvis. If the obliterated hypogastric artery is in the way, ligate and divide it. Avoid dissection behind the internal iliac artery, but place a large clip in it to aid in hemostasis during removal of the prostate. Repeat the procedure on the opposite side. Proceed with radical prostatectomy.

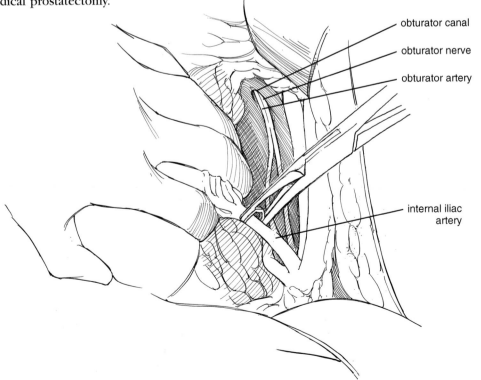

obturator canal

obturator nerve

obturator artery

internal iliac artery

POSTOPERATIVE PROBLEMS

A *lymphocele,* presenting as pelvic pain and swelling of the leg, is the result of not clipping all the afferent lymphatics. With the modified operation, lymphoceles are less frequent and smaller, resolving spontaneously after a time. It is advisable to place a drain to the operative area if lymphadenectomy is done as an isolated procedure. Confirm the diagnosis by pelvic computed tomographic scan or ultrasonography. Treat the lymphocele with radiographically guided aspiration and tube drainage, withdrawing the tube over a 1- to 2-week period. Alternatively, use a three-port *laparoscopic approach* (Gill et al, 1995), locating the lymphocele by real-time intraoperative ultrasonography. Confirm the location of the lymphocele by needle aspiration, and distinguish it from the bladder by vesical distention through a catheter. Incise a 3- to 4-cm window in the thinnest portion, advance the laparoscope, and disrupt any septa. Repeat ultrasonography to determine that evacuation is complete. A lymphocele may also be treated by open marsupialization, making a window and suturing the edges. Another alternative is ethanol sclerosis. *Thrombosis* of the pelvic veins may lead to pulmonary emboli. *Lymphedema* of the genitalia and legs is not common unless the patient has received external beam radiation.

Commentary by Lance J. Coetzee and David F. Paulson

Staging pelvic lymphadenectomy has traditionally been considered an integral part of the radical surgery for control of prostatic adenocarcinoma clinically confined to the prostate. Since the popularization of PSA as an aid in the management of prostate cancer, the profile of the disease has changed somewhat. The preoccupation of the urologic and, of late, the lay press with PSA has focused a great deal of attention on prostate cancer. This greater awareness has led to a greater index of suspicion, more widespread screening for prostate cancer, more aggressive intervention to establish the diagnosis, and earlier detection of prostate cancer. This earlier detection of prostate cancer has impacted on the incidence of lymph node metastases at the time of diagnosis and has resulted in a marked reduction in findings of positive pelvic nodes at the time of surgery compared with those of the pre-PSA era, when most patients with prostate cancer were diagnosed and staged clinically and therefore tended to be picked up at a more advanced stage of the disease. This finding of a reduced incidence of positive pelvic lymph nodes in cases of clinically confined prostate cancer has led to a re-evaluation of the role of pelvic lymphadenectomy, especially when a perineal prostatectomy or laparoscopic pelvic lymphadenectomy is planned and would mean an additional procedure for the patient. A number of centers have attempted to establish a risk profile for each patient to predict what that patient's chances of having positive lymph nodes might be. Using preoperative PSA and a Gleason grade of 7, a few retrospective studies have reported positive predictive values for negative lymph nodes of more than 95 percent in clinically confined prostate cancer. By employing the above variables and if one can accept a false-negative incidence for positive lymph nodes of 3 to 5 percent, a number of patients with well-differentiated and moderately differentiated cancers can be spared the morbidity of a pelvic lymphadenectomy. Having said this, it should be realized that failure to identify positive lymph nodes puts these few patients at a significant disadvantage in that they are undergoing an operative procedure designed for control of localized disease when in fact they already have systemic disease.

In patients in whom a modified pelvic lymphadenectomy is performed, the area of dissection includes primary, secondary, and tertiary levels of drainage. This has been shown to have predictive impact equivalent to that of more extended traditional dissection. In our dissection technique, the area is restricted even further than described. After exposure of the perivesical space, the vessels are identified. The fibrofatty tissue overlying the external iliac vein is split from the level of the bifurcation of the common iliac vein down to the take-off of the circumflex iliac vein. Dissection then is carried medial to the vessel, and tissue superior and lateral to the vessel is left undisturbed. No tissue is passed around the vessel to be incorporated with the specimen. Instead, the dissection is carried distally to the pelvic floor and then is carried down to the level of exit of the iliac vasculature from the pelvis. The dissection is then dropped posteriorly along the bony and musculopelvic floor to the site of exit of the obturator nerve and vessel. The nodal channels that are transected are first controlled with surgical clips. At this point the node package is not fixed and, being grasped with ring forceps, can be bluntly dissected from beneath the external iliac vein and elevated from the obturator nerve and vessels. The obturator vessels may be incorporated with the node package or may be left behind. The vessels frequently lie beneath the obturator nerve and may be left undisturbed. As the node package is freed moving from caudad to cephalad, the package becomes progressively narrower as the bifurcation of the external and internal iliac vein is approached. At this level, the node package may be controlled with a surgical clip on the distal side and the specimen removed. A true dissection may not be carried out medial to the obturator nerve and around the hypogastric vasculature because the posterior and medial branching vessels of the hypogastric prevent a clean dissection. The tissue medial to the obturator nerve and superior to the hypogastric vasculature is best removed piecemeal. Following completion of the bilateral dissection, a Penrose drain is split and one arm is led down into either perivesical space. This drain is usually left in place approximately 24 hours before removal because careful attention to detail during the dissection prevents damage to the pelvic vasculature and ureter.

Laparoscopic and Minilaparotomy Pelvic Lymph Node Dissection

LAPAROSCOPIC NODE DISSECTION, TRANSPERITONEAL APPROACH

A node dissection by the laparoscopic route may be performed immediately preceding total perineal prostatectomy.

An extraperitoneal approach is an alternative to a transperitoneal one. It is preferable in obese men or patients who have undergone significant intraperitoneal surgery previously. Because either of these approaches may be time-consuming and require a significant learning period, consider a minilaparoscopy procedure through a 6-cm incision (Step 5). One disadvantage of the laparoscopic approach is that it may be accompanied by herniation of the bowel into the retroperitoneal space, placing the bowel more at risk during radiation therapy. Another is that severe ileus may occur, placing the incision for retropubic prostatectomy at risk for dehiscence.

Inform the patient of the possibility of conversion to an open procedure if a complication occurs or the operation cannot be completed laparoscopically. Screen for blood type and antibodies. Prepare the bowel in patients with previous surgery and in those who, if the nodes are negative, will undergo prostatectomy. Otherwise, give an enema the night before to decompress the rectum and sigmoid. Consider giving a broad-spectrum antibiotic 1 hour before the procedure and twice postoperatively.

Instruments: Laparoscopic instruments include a pair of 5-mm cutting-coagulating scissors, two 5-mm coagulating-dissecting graspers, a needle driver, ligators, hemostats, stapling devices, a fan-type bowel retractor, a 10-mm spoon-shaped grasper, an ultrasonic attachment, baskets or netting devices, and a suction-irrigation instrument. In addition, include a robotic arm to hold instrumentation, an aquadissection system, a bipolar or unipolar cautery, an argon beam coagulator, and laser systems. A robot arm also allows the surgeon to direct the camera.

Provide general anesthesia. Insert a catheter in the bladder and a tube in the stomach. Prepare the entire abdomen. Place a sacral roll, and pad all pressure points. Secure the patient to the table with the arms at the side prepared for Trendelenburg tilting. Start with a 15-degree Trendelenburg position. Drape the patient so that the genitalia are exposed in case traction on the testis is desired for orientation or orchiectomy is to be done for positive nodes. Insert a balloon catheter and drain the bladder.

Insufflation: Follow the steps given on page 21. If retropubic prostatectomy is anticipated, make a short vertical incision in the inferior umbilical crease instead of a transverse one. Insert the Veress needle and insufflate the peritoneal cavity to a pressure slightly higher than working pressure to aid in trocar insertion (15 to 20 mm Hg).

1 Insert the 10- or 11-mm trocar unit at the umbilicus and attach the full-beam camera. Check for intraperitoneal injury and systematically inspect the contents of the abdominal cavity. Proceed with insertion of the *three working ports* in a diamond configuration under direct laparoscopic visualization: Transilluminate the body wall to visualize any vessels in the abdominal wall and place a 10- or 11-mm trocar in the midline 3 to 5 cm above the pubic symphysis. Insert a 5-mm (or 10-mm) trocar on each side one third to one half of the distance from the anterior superior iliac spine to the umbilicus. Place them beside the rectus muscle, not through it. For better maneuverability, especially in obese patients, use *four working ports:* Instead of a single suprapubic trocar, insert a pair of 5-mm ports two thirds of the distance from the spine to the pubis. The superior ports should then both be 10 or 11 mm in size. Secure the ports to the abdominal wall with sutures. Increase the Trendelenburg tilt to 30 degrees, and rotate the patient laterally 15 to 30 degrees to elevate the side of dissection.

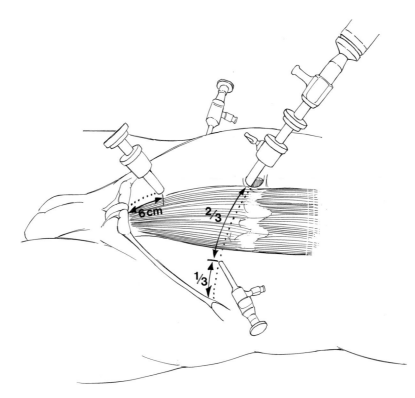

2 Orient the camera for anatomically correct visualization. Identify the medial umbilical ligament (obliterated umbilical artery) as it passes beside the bladder toward the umbilicus; the lateral umbilical fold (inferior epigastric); the median umbilical ligament (urachus) rising from the dome of the bladder; the vas deferens and spermatic vessels traversing through the internal inguinal ring (identified clearly by traction on the testis); the inferior epigastric vessels passing vertically up the anterior abdominal wall immediately lateral to the medial umbilical ligament and anterior and medial to the internal inguinal ring; the ureter; and the pulsating common and

external iliac arteries. Lyse any adhesions and, if necessary to reach the obturator nodes on the left, release the sigmoid colon and, on the right, free the appendix and cecum.

Start the first incision in the posterior peritoneum anteriorly high over the pubic bone immediately *lateral* to the medial umbilical ligament. Extend it posteriorly, staying medial to the external iliac artery and ending near its junction with the common iliac artery. A second peritoneal incision 2 or 3 cm lateral to the first may provide better exposure by allowing laying back of a triangle of posterior peritoneum.

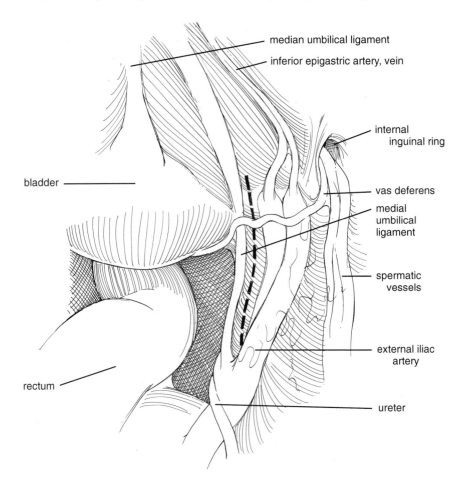

3 As the vas deferens is crossed, clip or coagulate and divide it, allowing improved access to the iliac-obturator region.

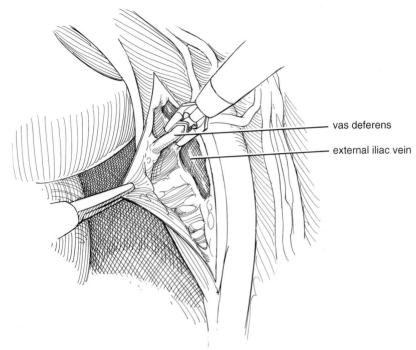

vas deferens

external iliac vein

4 Identify the pubic bone by contact. Expose the medial border of the external iliac vein and first clear its anterior surface, which has no tributaries. Continue along its medial surface to the pubic bone, thus defining the *lateral inferior margin* of the dissection. Be alert for the circumflex vein and for an aberrant obturator vein where the external iliac vein passes over the pubic bone.

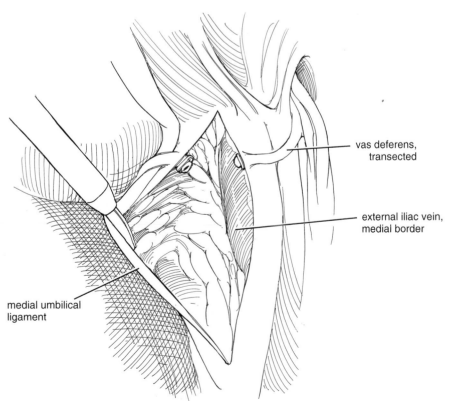

vas deferens, transected

external iliac vein, medial border

medial umbilical ligament

5 Retract the medial umbilical ligament medially, and enter a plane immediately lateral to it to define the *medial margin* of the dissection. Free the nodal tissue directly below the pubic bone, coagulating any small vessels.

Locate the pubic bone and the anterior surface of the obturator nerve and its vessels, marking the *distal margin* of the nodal packet.

Tease the tissue from the obturator fossa and strip it back toward the iliac bifurcation. Bleeding is easily controlled with coagulation. Have your assistant retract the external iliac vein laterally to expose the deeper area. Continue the dissection over the connective tissue layer overlying the internal iliac vein to reach the bifurcation of the common iliac artery, constituting the *cephalic margin*. Be aware of the ureter here; it crosses the vessels at a point lower than that shown in Figure 5.

To *retrieve the specimen,* hold the flap-valve on the sheath open so that it does not catch the specimen. Grasp the tissue with spoon-shaped graspers, and extract it through the 10- or 11-mm suprapubic port under observation to detect detached tissue. Send the specimen for frozen section. Proceed with dissection of the left side after incision of sigmoid adhesions.

Inspect the pelvic and peritoneal contents. Remove the trocars one by one under direct vision. Close the larger sites with fascial and subcutaneous sutures and adhesive strips. Remove the nasogastric tube, but it may be worthwhile to keep the balloon catheter in place to monitor urine output. Start oral fluid the evening of the procedure and discharge the patient the following day with instructions to report abdominal pain or distention, fever, edema of the legs, shortness of breath, and inflammation at the trocar sites.

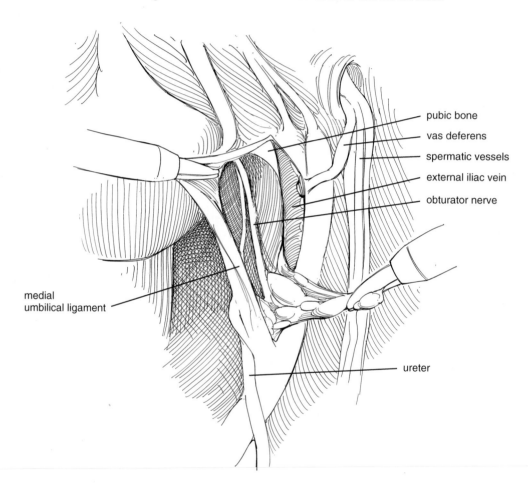

pubic bone
vas deferens
spermatic vessels
external iliac vein
obturator nerve

medial umbilical ligament

ureter

Mobilization of the Seminal Vesicles Before Perineal Prostatectomy. If the nodes are negative and total perineal prostatectomy is planned, proceed with release of the seminal vesicles (Teichman et al, 1995). Retract the rectum posteriorly with a fan retractor, and hold the bladder up with the suction-aspirator to expose the retrovesical pouch. Grasp the vas deferens that had been cut during the node dissection, and dissect along it in the retrovesical space to reach the medial surface of the seminal vesicle. Grasp the tip of the vesicle and dissect it from

its bed with endoshears, cautery, and a 5-mm argon beam coagulator probe. Continue the dissection to the insertion of the vas into the ejaculatory duct.

Check for hemostasis and visceral injury, and inspect the sites of entry. Irrigate and aspirate the wound. Remove the sheaths under vision and evacuate the gas. Close all 10- or 11-mm sites with fascial sutures, and apply sterile adhesive strips. Proceed with total perineal prostatectomy (see page 451).

INTRAOPERATIVE EMERGENCIES

Vascular injury to large vessels may require stopping the laparoscopic approach and converting to an open operation. Grasp the vessel above and below the site of injury, and maintain the pneumoperitoneum to control the bleeding until the vessel can be secured and repaired by an open approach. Transection of the proximal aspect of the medial umbilical ligament may result in significant hemorrhage. *Intraperitoneal bladder injury* may be repaired laparoscopically or, if not recognized, may require later operation. *Ureteral injury,* whether detected early or late, usually necessitates open repair, as does *bowel injury.* These complications are correlated with each surgeon's learning curve. *Body habitus* or *technical difficulties* may demand abandonment of the procedure.

POSTOPERATIVE PROBLEMS

Postoperative hemorrhage may require emergency laparotomy. *Lymphoceles* may occur after partial reperitonealization. They may be marsupialized laparoscopically. *Small bowel obstruction* is uncommon. *Ureteral injury* is recognized late as the patient complains of pain and nausea. A urinoma is found. Treatment may require resection of the damaged ureter. *Visceral injuries* are rare but require open intervention. Hernias have been reported in trocar sites. *Deep venous thrombosis* is not peculiar to laparoscopic surgery, but prevention involves the use of venous compression devices.

LAPAROSCOPIC SEMINAL VESICULECTOMY
(Kavoussi)

The seminal vesicles may be removed from above following laparoscopic node dissection prior to total perineal prostatectomy (see page 451). Start while waiting for the report on the frozen sections.

Using the four or five ports already placed for the laparoscopic pelvic lymph node dissection, incise the anterior peritoneum in the rectovesical pouch, using the medial aspect of the vas deferens as a guide. Have the assistant hold the anterior leaf and the bladder anteriorly as you push the rectum and posterior peritoneum back. As the peritoneum is teased away, identify, isolate, and clip the ampulla of the vas deferens bilaterally. Put traction on the tips to reveal the seminal vesicles. Bluntly dissect them starting medially, keeping in mind that the ureter lies lateral and posterior to the vas deferens. Isolate and clip the seminal vesicular artery. Draw the vesicle medially to free it laterally from the neurovascular bundle. Avoid electrocauterization near the nerves. Pull the ampullae anteriorly and push the rectum off the posterior surface of the prostate. The chance of rectal injury is reduced, and the dissection is facilitated by having an assistant place a finger in the rectum.

Irrigate the area with heparin-saline, and reduce intra-abdominal pressure to check for bleeding. Tuck the vesicles behind the prostate and close the peritoneum with the hernia stapler.

Remove the trocars and place the patient in the extreme lithotomy position for total perineal prostatectomy (see page 451).

EXTRAPERITONEAL APPROACH TO LAPAROSCOPIC NODE DISSECTION
(Das and Tashima)

The extraperitoneal approach can be more difficult because the vas and medial umbilical ligament, which are elevated with the peritoneum, cannot be used as landmarks. The surgeon must rely on the iliac vessels and an obturator nerve as guides to the limits of dissection. More CO_2 is absorbed. However, it may be preferable for obese patients, those with previous operations, and those who elect external radiation therapy.

Place the patient supine in a 15-degree Trendelenburg position, and make a 3-cm midline incision either in the inferior umbilical crease or 2 cm below the umbilicus. Incise the subcutaneous tissue and linea alba. Place stay sutures on the rectus fascia. Digitally develop a space in the retroperitoneum laterally behind the rectus abdominis, inserting the index finger toward the pubis. When the pubis is felt, swing the finger laterally to develop the space of Retzius. Insert a distending balloon (Gaur; see page 994). Inject 800 to 1200 ml of normal saline, wait 5 minutes for vascular tamponade, then drain and remove the balloon. Insert a Hasson cannula and fix it with stay sutures. Start CO_2 insufflation to maintain a pressure between 10 and 15 mm Hg. Manipulate the laparoscope in a circular fashion if necessary to create space for the other ports. Insert a second 10-mm trocar 3 cm above the symphysis pubis in the midline, and develop the lateral aspects of the space of Retzius. Then place two 5-mm working ports lateral to the rectus midway between the umbilicus and symphysis. Take care not to traverse the peritoneal membrane because the pneumoretroperitoneum will be lost and the operation converted to a transperitoneal one. (This is a real possibility in a patient who has had previous lower abdominal surgery.) Stand together with the assistant on the contralateral side. Insert the camera through the lateral port to look across the pelvis into the obturator fossa. The traditional landmarks are not present. Look for the pubic ramus and dissect laterally from it.

Clear the node of Cloquet from the femoral canal; then work laterally over the external iliac vein. Retract the vein laterally to reach to the pelvic side wall. Retract the bladder and perivesical fat to allow dissection of the obturator nerve, which marks the most posterior extent of the dissection. Free the obturator packet back toward the iliac bifurcation. Seal the lymphatic channels with cautery or clips (so that lymphatic leakage does not have access to the peritoneal cavity). Move to the opposite side of the table, and repeat the procedure on the other side. Lower the gas pressure and check for bleeding. Remove the trocars appropriately and follow with prostatectomy if the nodes prove to be negative for tumor. (Delayed retropubic prostatectomy may be more difficult after extraperitoneal laparoscopic node dissection.)

The complication rate is lower because the peritoneal cavity is not entered, but the rate of formation of lymphoceles may be higher.

Commentary by Howard N. Winfield

The minimally invasive nature of a staging laparoscopic pelvic lymph node dissection (LPLND) may be realized by careful selection of patients and by experience of the surgeon. The formation of a laparoscopic surgical team, full working knowledge of the laparoscopic videocamera equipment, insufflators, and hand instruments, and critical attention to technical detail diminish the risk of complications.

Creation of the CO_2 pneumoperitoneum is crucial to the success of the intraperitoneal approach. If insertion of the Veress needle fails from the inferior crease of the umbilicus, I try from the superior crease aiming toward the sacral promontory. This should drop the needle into the peritoneal cavity directly below the umbilicus, where all abdominal wall fascial layers fuse. Failing this, I do not hesitate to employ the Hasson cannula "open laparoscopy" technique. In fact, some surgeons use only the Hasson approach so as essentially to eliminate the risk of visceral or vascular injury from blind Veress needle and trocar punctures.

The extraperitoneal approach is helpful in obese patients, in whom a large working space may be created by using one of the balloon inflation devices. With the peritoneal membrane intact, loops of fat-laden bowel and mesentery are retracted naturally out of the surgical field. Care must be taken to mobilize the peritoneal membrane cephalad prior to inserting lateral ports. Penetration of the peritoneal membrane results in leakage of CO_2 into the intraperitoneal space, leading to compression and eventual collapse of the space of Retzius. The experienced laparoscopic surgeon is then able to convert to an intraperitoneal approach. Beware of increased subcutaneous emphysema and CO_2 absorption with the extraperitoneal route, perhaps a relative contraindication for patients with compromised pulmonary function. Furthermore, the extraperitoneal approach is associated with a higher rate of lymphocele formation. For average-sized patients, my preference is still the intraperitoneal route.

Obturator lymph nodes are the first echelon of metastatic spread from prostate cancer in more than 85 percent of cases. Therefore, an obturator LPLND should detect metastatic disease, if present, while resulting in minimal morbidity. My approach is first to locate the medial border of the external iliac vein and then to follow it distally toward the pubic bone. In this way the accessory obturator vein is encountered safely and dealt with if it needs to be freed from the obturator packet. Using the anterior surface of the obturator nerve as a plane of dissection, injury to the obturator vessels that lie posteromedial should be avoided. I do not hesitate to transect these vessels if they are entangled within the lymph node packet. Extended LPLND may be indicated in select patients who have suspicious adenopathy overlying the external or common iliac arteries and in patients harboring malignancies of the bladder, penis, or urethra. Surgical morbidity directly correlates, however, with the extent of the dissection.

Owing to the technology-intensive aspects of laparoscopic surgery, these procedures are best performed by urologists who regularly undertake this form of minimally invasive intervention. In this way success is high, morbidity is low, and financial costs are competitive with the more invasive open surgery or minilaparotomy.

MINILAPAROTOMY PELVIC NODE DISSECTION
(Steiner and Marshall)

Diagnostic node dissection can be done through a limited incision without extensive training or special equipment and in a shorter time than that required for the laparoscopic technique. If the nodes are negative, the minimal incision can be extended to allow retropubic prostatectomy, or the patient can be repositioned for a perineal approach.

Instruments: The exposure is facilitated by special retractors (Mohler, 1995), including a narrow vein retractor at the end of a flat retractor to retract the iliac vein and a narrow and deep (10 cm) tapered malleable retractor to retract the inferior and superior aspects of the wound.

Position: Supine, with table slightly hyperextended. Insert a catheter with a 30-ml balloon inflated to 50 ml.

Incision: Make a vertical midline incision 6 cm long beginning 2 cm above the symphysis. Extend it through the linea alba and transversalis fascia. With a Richardson retractor, pull the entire incision to the right. Mobilize the peritoneum and enter the space of Retzius. Rotate the table 20 degrees to the left for a direct view of the obturator fossa.

6 Free the peritoneum from the external iliac vessels as high as the bifurcation while displacing the vas deferens and peritoneum upward. Insert a medium Richardson retractor to draw the incision laterally; insert a broad blade retractor to hold back the bladder and a Deaver retractor superiorly to retain the vas deferens and peritoneum. Alternatively, insert a small Balfour retractor. Or use an Omni retractor (Minnesota Scientific) if available, as shown. Proceed with right pelvic lymphadenectomy (see page 465). Begin by incising the sheath over the medial aspect of the external iliac artery in the angle between the external iliac vein and the internal iliac artery, and end by removing the collection from the obturator nerve. Repeat the procedure on the left after rotating the patient to the right. Send the nodes for frozen section examination. If they are negative, proceed with total prostatectomy; if they are positive, close the wound in layers.

Alternative, Outpatient Procedure (Mohler, 1995)
Start on the more suspicious side by making an oblique 3-cm incision one fingerbreadth above a point located two thirds of the way along a line connecting the pubic tubercle and the anterior superior iliac spine. Expose the external oblique muscle and the rectus fascia. Make a 4-cm incision at this junction, extending medially over the sheath. Retract the rectus muscle medially. Place a fixed retractor ring, and retract the superior and inferior margins with special malleable, deep retractors. Have the assistant retract the medial aspect of the wound with a folded 4 × 4 inch gauze pad on a 60-degree angled Fogarty clamp. With a headlight, proceed with lymphadenectomy. Send the specimen for frozen section examination. Repeat the procedure on the opposite side.

If the nodes are reported negative for cancer, extend the incision and proceed with total retropubic prostatec-

tomy. If the nodes are positive or if a total perineal prostatectomy is elected, close the fascial incision with a running 1-0 synthetic monofilament suture without drainage, and close the skin with a subcuticular SAS. Reposition the patient.

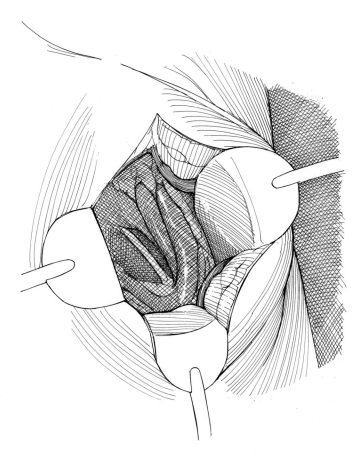

Commentary by Mitchell S. Steiner

A minilaparotomy staging pelvic lymphadenectomy (minilap) is an excellent alternative to standard or laparoscopic pelvic lymphadenectomy. This procedure uses a smaller incision, which is more than adequate to perform a full pelvic lymph node dissection under direct vision. The minilaparotomy does not require any additional technical training or expensive equipment, as standard retractors may be used. Moreover, the option to proceed to a radical retropubic prostatectomy or perineal prostatectomy is available if the lymph nodes are negative for cancer without subjecting the patient to an additional anesthetic. Postoperatively, as with the laparoscopic pelvic lymphadenectomy, patients require minimal pain medication, have a shorter hospitalization (24 to 48 hours), and may return to work sooner than is possible with a standard pelvic lymphadenectomy.

After making the midline vertical abdominal incision, it is very important to develop the space of Retzius completely and, if necessary, to extend the fascial portion of the incision an additional 1 or 2 cm to increase visibility. The vertical incision can be easily moved laterally to the side of the node dissection using a Richardson retractor, obviating a second incision. In addition, to provide ideal surgical exposure, the bladder can be retracted medially using a broad retractor, like a sweetheart retractor, and the vas deferens and peritoneum can be mobilized and retracted superolaterally with a deep Deaver retractor. Tilting the surgical table approximately 15 to 30 degrees also helps to bring the obturator fossa into full view.

During the pelvic lymph node dissection, special care must be taken to avoid lacerating the accessory obturator vein, which

courses from the obturator foramen to the external iliac vein. Bleeding there may be difficult to control, and consequently, it is probably best to end the distal portion of the pelvic lymph node dissection at the accessory obturator vein. This vein is present more often than has been appreciated previously in the literature; we found it to be present in 80 percent of patients (bilateral in 96 percent of these cases). When the ipsilateral pelvic lymphadenectomy is completed, the incision may be pulled to the contralateral side to perform the pelvic lymph node dissection in a similar fashion.

The minilaparotomy had an average intraoperative time (excluding the time necessary for a pathologist to process frozen sections for suspicious lymph nodes) of 32 minutes (range 27 to 45 minutes), and the intraoperative estimated blood loss was less than 20 ml. The mean number of pelvic lymph nodes removed was similar to that for standard pelvic lymphadenectomy.

The minilaparotomy shares the advantages of both the standard and the laparoscopic pelvic lymphadenectomy. Like the standard pelvic lymphadenectomy, the minilaparotomy allows for complete pelvic lymph node dissection under direct vision and full control. Furthermore, if the pelvic lymph nodes are clinically negative for prostate cancer, a radical prostatectomy may be performed using a single anesthetic. Similar to the laparoscopic pelvic lymphadenectomy, the minilaparotomy has low morbidity, shorter hospitalization, and a cosmetic incision. For these reasons, the minilaparotomy is an attractive alternative for patients at high risk for metastatic prostate cancer who require a staging pelvic lymphadenectomy.

Closure of Rectourethral Fistula

PERINEAL APPROACH
(Weyrauch)

Prepare the bowel; a colostomy is probably not needed, but a cystostomy may be protective. Examine the urethra with a panendoscope. Consider ureteral catheterization if the dissection may be extensive.

1 Place the patient in the extreme lithotomy position and proceed to obtain wide exposure as for total perineal prostatectomy (see page 451). If a subsphincteric route was used before, approach by the classic Young operation (see page 452); if the previous operation was by the Young approach, dissect beneath the sphincter. Use the Young or Lowsley long tractor to bring the fistula into the wound, and insert a finger into the rectum as a guide. Divide the fistula and excise all surrounding scar tissue. Remove asymmetric ellipses of tissue around both the rectal and urethral openings.

2 Replace the tractor with a 20 F 30-ml balloon catheter and fill the balloon. Have your assistant draw up on the catheter. Continue blunt and sharp dissection between the rectum and prostate well above the fistula to reach normal tissue. Close the rectal fistula first while the catheter traction holds the prostate up out of the way. Place two layers of 4-0 SAS, one continuous layer in the mucosa and submucosa and the other at right angles as interrupted sutures in the muscularis.

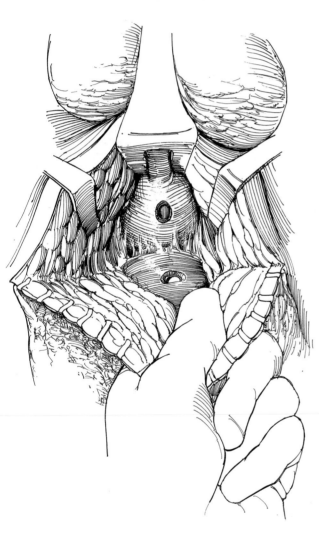

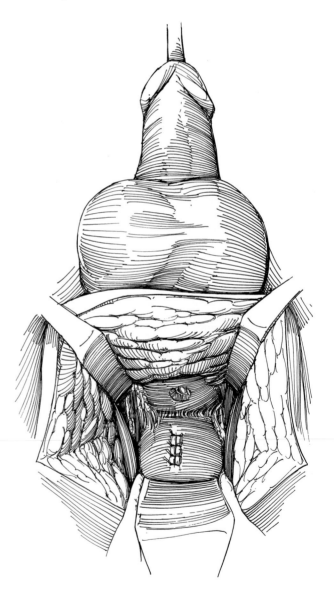

3 Close the urethral defect in two layers with 4-0 SAS. Pull the rectum down so that the suture lines are not juxtaposed. Bring any available soft tissue across and suture it in the midline. If none is available and the closure is tenuous, mobilize the *gracilis muscle* and interpose it between the rectum and urethra, as described for vesicovaginal fistulas (see pages 590 to 592). If scarring does not prevent it, mobilize and tack the levator ani muscles together, but avoid deep bites and tension.

Irrigate the wound thoroughly with bacitracin-neomycin solution. Approximate the subcutaneous tissues and place a Penrose drain. Close the skin with interrupted nonabsorbable sutures or with a subcuticular SAS. Deflate the balloon to 5 ml and tape it to the penis. Continue antibiotic administration and a low-residue diet postoperatively. Shorten the drain in 3 days and remove it the next day. Remove the catheter or cystostomy no sooner than the eighth day.

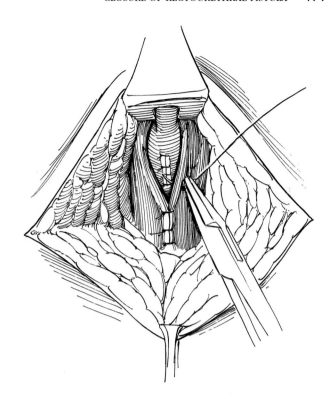

Commentary by Sam D. Graham

The perineal approach is an excellent one for a rectourethral fistula. The view provided is completely unobstructed by other anatomic structures such as the symphysis pubis. The Lowsley retractor is ideal for bringing the fistula closer to the skin incision, and it also provides a landmark for dissection if there is intense fibrous reaction from the fistula. Also, a finger inserted into the rectum serves as a guide to protect the rectum. Generally, if possible, dissection directly onto the white fascia of the rectum as soon as feasible allows one both to identify the rectum and to go straight to the fistula without injuring the bulb or more distal urethra.

For small fistulas, the Weyrauch approach with simple closure is an excellent option, with interposition of other soft tissues between the closures. However, it is generally limited in that an omentum is not available through the perineal approach, and the only significant soft tissue may be the gracilis muscle.

For larger fistulas, the Young-Stone operation is probably a better procedure. However, it does involve a distal anal pull-through, and care should be taken not to injure the rectal sphincter.

Both approaches require copious drainage and intense use of antibiotics and generally are preceded by a temporary diverting colostomy.

TRANSRECTAL TRANS-SPHINCTERIC REPAIR
(York-Mason)

After general anesthesia is induced, place the patient prone in the jack-knife position. Tape the buttocks apart.

4 Make an incision from the tip of the coccyx through the rectal wall and anal sphincters. For more exposure, either excise a portion of the coccyx or extend the incision beside it. When dividing the anal sphincter, be certain to tag both the mucocutaneous junction and each segment of the sphincter (external, internal, and deep) to allow them to be accurately reapproximated later. Retract the rectal walls, and visualize and excise the fistula with an oval incision. Close the defect in the prostate with interrupted 3-0 absorbable sutures to the mucosa. With fine running absorbable sutures, approximate the muscularis of the anterior rectal wall; then close the rectal mucosa. Close the posterior rectal wall with interrupted absorbable sutures. Tie the tagged sutures in the anal sphincter together; extra sutures may be added between them. Close the skin with interrupted sutures.

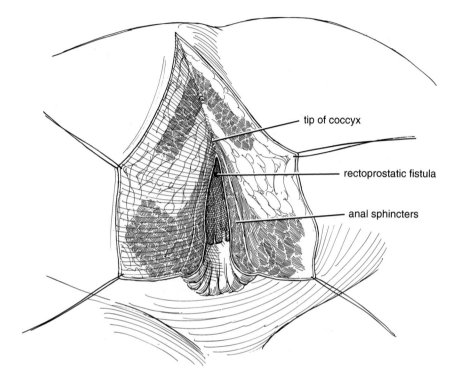

tip of coccyx

rectoprostatic fistula

anal sphincters

TRANSANORECTAL REPAIR
(Gecelter)

This procedure is similar to the York-Mason operation but provides more exposure. If the fistula is small and below the peritoneal reflection, as it usually is, a colostomy is not necessary, but if the case is complicated, fecal diversion should be done weeks before the operation (see page 669). Provide bowel preparation and antibiotic coverage.

5 **A,** Place the patient in the exaggerated lithotomy position. Insert a suprapubic cystostomy tube (see page 625). Make a vertical incision anterior to the anus, starting from the anal verge and carried as far forward as needed. Make lateral incisions from its anterior end to expand the exposure, but avoid crossing over the ischial tuberosities.

B, Divide both rectal sphincters exactly in the midline to avoid injury to nervous or vascular structures, and continue to open the rectum itself longitudinally. Pack the rectum with roller gauze so that blood and irrigant do not pool there. Continue the incision in the rectum until the fistula is reached. Transect the fistula and excise the scar tissue from both the rectal and the urethral walls.

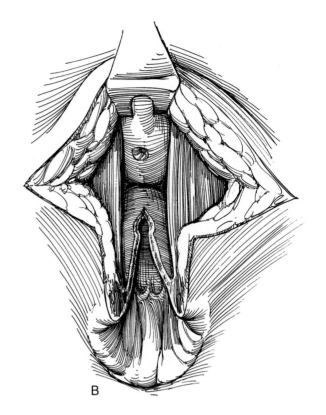

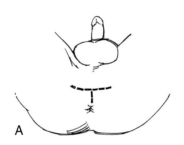

A   B

6 Close the urethral opening with a 4-0 continuous SAS, and add a second layer with interrupted sutures. If approximation is not possible without tension, insert a dermal graft. Approximate the mucosa-submucosa of the rectum and anal canal with a running 4-0 SAS.

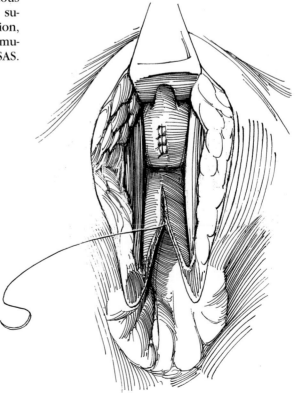

7 **A,** Place interrupted sutures to approximate the muscularis of the rectum. **B,** Interpose any available soft tissue, and mobilize the levator ani muscles to approximate them in the midline. Place a Penrose drain, to be removed in 3 days. Continue suprapubic drainage for at least 14 days, longer if the tissues appear compromised. Obtain a voiding cystourethrogram before removing the catheter.

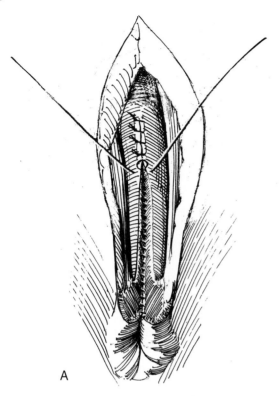

A

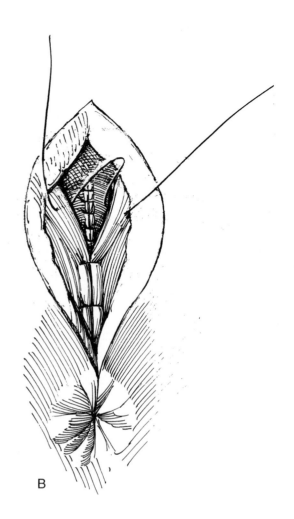

B

Commentary by Louis G. Gecelter

Anterior transanorectal repair of a urethrorectal or prostatorectal fistula is the most direct approach to the problem. Surgeons have a natural aversion to incising the anorectal canal to gain exposure to the lower genitourinary tract. But with modern aseptic and antiseptic techniques, this procedure should have no serious contraindications. Function of the anorectal canal is in no way compromised by this incision, and anal tone and function are rapidly regained after surgery.

The incision must remain strictly in the midline without any lateral skin or deep muscle extensions. The vascular and nerve supply does not cross the midline. The perineal and pudendal structures are out of the field, eliminating the possibility of impotence. It is not always necessary to incise the anorectal mucosa and submucosa, and an attempt should be made to strip this layer off the deeper incised muscles.

TRANSANAL ENDOSCOPIC REPAIR (Wilbert)

Insert a large-bore operating rectoscope with a binocular endoscope and videocamera to the level of the fistula. Consider obtaining guidance from an experienced rectal surgeon. Excise the fistula with a monopolar electrode. Mobilize the rectal wall with scissors, and close the muscular defect and then the mucosa with continuous 3-0 SAS, secured by clips on the ends. Drain the bladder for 2 weeks.

POSTOPERATIVE PROBLEMS

If the fistula is not closed initially, *contamination* of the urinary tract is to be expected, with greater risk in infants, in whom reflux is common. Also look for *hyperchloremic acidosis* from colonic filling. Treat it with oral bicarbonates, at the same time looking for urethral obstruction. Recurrent *epididymitis* is not rare, but it is less frequent with prophylactic antibacterial therapy.

Seminal Vesiculectomy

TRANSPERITONEAL APPROACH

1 *Incision:* Midline (see page 487) or Pfannenstiel (see page 490). Open the peritoneum.

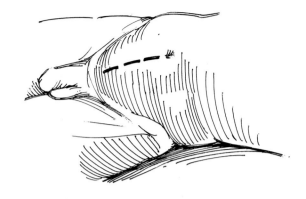

2 Make a transverse incision through the retroperitoneum where it joins the bladder wall in the cul-de-sac, and develop a cleavage plane between the bladder and rectum.

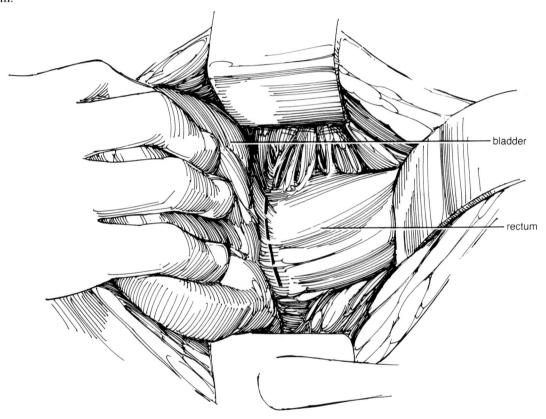

bladder

rectum

3 Identify the seminal vesicles adherent to the back of the bladder. Find the vas deferens and trace it down until its wall thins and dilates. Watch for the ureter, which passes beneath the vas. It may help exposure to divide the superior and middle vesical pedicles. Dissect the vesicle and vas from the rectum posteriorly and the bladder and prostate anteriorly. Do not dissect lateral to the vesicle; avoid the neurovascular bundle.

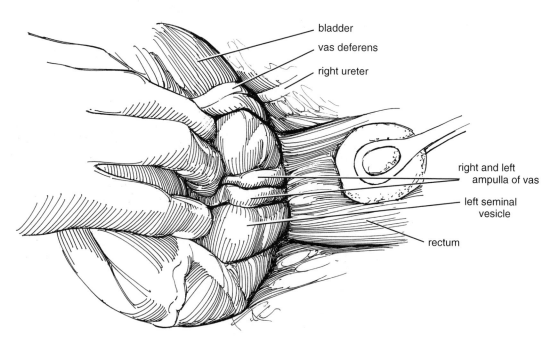

bladder
vas deferens
right ureter
right and left ampulla of vas
left seminal vesicle
rectum

4 Divide the vesicular duct where it joins the vas, ligate the distal end, and remove the specimen.

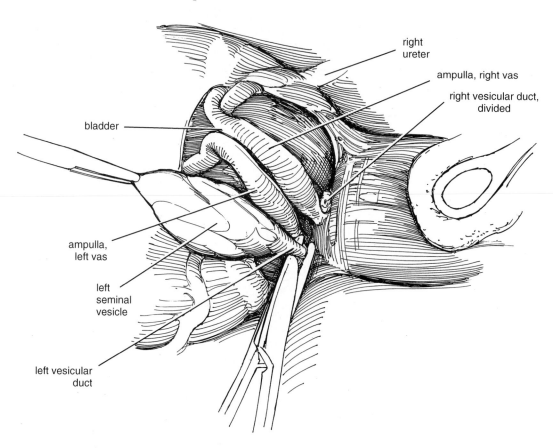

right ureter
ampulla, right vas
right vesicular duct, divided
bladder
ampulla, left vas
left seminal vesicle
left vesicular duct

PERINEAL APPROACH

5 Approach the vesicles as for perineal prostatectomy (see page 452). Open Denonvilliers' fascia vertically, and use it to free the vesicles from the rectum. Elevate the prostate with the prostatic tractor, and continue the dissection behind the prostate. Keep as close to the midline as possible to avoid the neurovascular bundles. Clamp the tip of each vesicle with a right-angle clamp; then divide and ligate. Clamp, divide, and ligate the vesicular ducts bilaterally and remove the specimen.

TRANSVESICAL TRANSTRIGONAL APPROACH

6 This is probably the most direct route to the vesicles and utricle (see page 228 for excision of utricular cyst). Place ureteral catheters; later, at closure, bring them out through the bladder and abdominal wall as stents. Make a longitudinal incision in the trigone above the bladder neck.

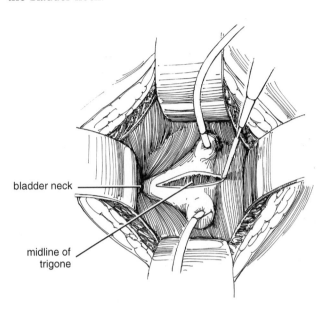

bladder neck

midline of trigone

7 Hold the bladder wall with stay sutures, and dissect down the posterior surface of the vasal ampulla and seminal vesicle with Lahey scissors under direct vision while pushing the peritoneal fold cephalad. Avoid the urethral wall and sphincters by identifying their location with the aid of a catheter. Free the seminal vesicle and divide it where it joins the vas deferens or remove it with the ampulla of the vas, as shown. Approximate the deep trigone with interrupted 3-0 SAS and the vesical epithelium with a running 4-0 SAS placed subepithelially.

ampulla, left vas

left seminal vesicle

ampulla, right vas

right seminal vesicle

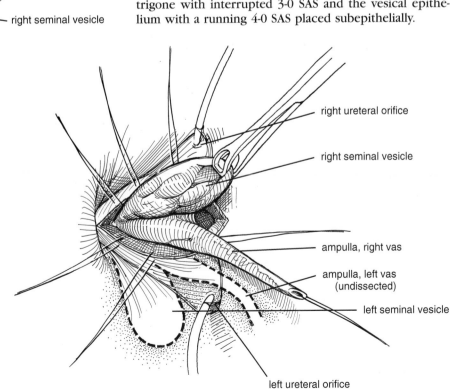

right ureteral orifice

right seminal vesicle

ampulla, right vas

ampulla, left vas (undissected)

left seminal vesicle

left ureteral orifice

8 *Excision of the prostatic utricle:* If the utricle is large and symptomatic, expose it as described but stay in the midline between the vasa. Excise the sac as low as possible. Close the stump with a running 4-0 SAS.

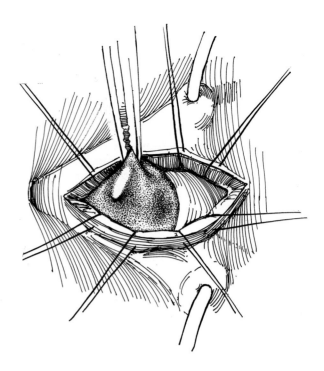

Commentary by Robert C. Flanigan

In modern practice, isolated removal of the seminal vesicles has few indications. The operative approaches are not difficult, however, if the basic principles used in the more common urologic procedures such as cystectomy and perineal prostatectomy are applied.

Three routes are available for excision or drainage (marsupialization) of the seminal vesicles. The transabdominal route is the longest, the perineal route is the most direct but involves a significant amount of dissection, and the transvesical route traverses the least amount of tissue.

For the transvesical route, use electrocautery to divide the trigone, either vertically or transversely. After the ampullae of the vasa and the seminal vesicles have been identified, I use a Küttner dissector for blunt dissection and small hemoclips to control any vessels that are encountered. Ligate the vas with large Ligaclips; these are better than sutures, which may cut through the wall when tied. Continue traction to allow dissection to the ejaculatory duct, which is clamped, divided, and suture-ligated. If drainage is necessary, tunnel laterally under the trigone into the retrovesical space and draw a drain through, to be brought out through a stab wound. Remove the stents in 3 to 4 days. It may be wise to remove them sequentially to avoid an episode of anuria from edema.

A laparoscopic approach is practical following laparoscopic node dissection before total perineal prostatectomy.

Bladder: Approaches

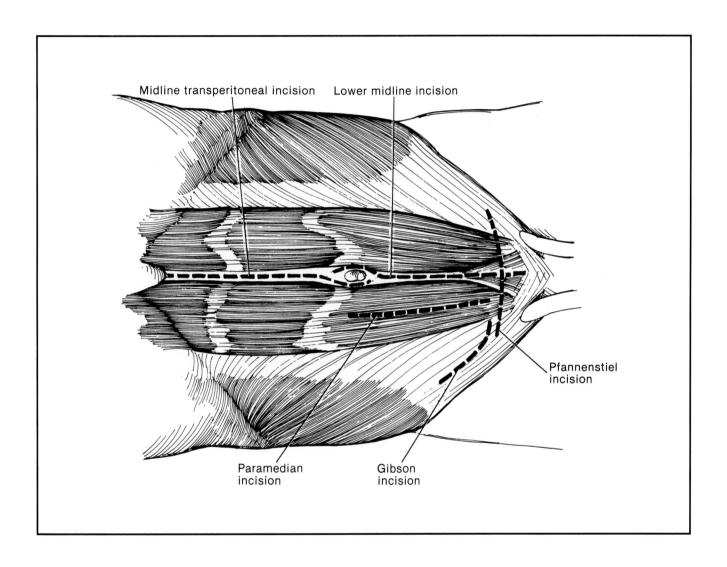

Midline transperitoneal incision   Lower midline incision

Pfannenstiel
incision

Paramedian
incision

Gibson
incision

Principles for Bladder Incisions

The bladder is usually approached through a lower abdominal midline (see page 487) or transverse incision (see page 490). Either requires incision of the anterior rectus sheath that is formed from combined aponeuroses of the anterior abdominal wall muscles.

The anterior rectus sheath covers the muscle for its full length and is firmly attached to it at the tendinous intersections. Below the arcuate line, the aponeurosis of the transversus abdominis contributes a deep part to the anterior sheath, where the posterior rectus sheath is missing. This leaves the investing fascia of the lower third of the muscle in contact with the intermediate stratum of the retroperitoneal connective tissue.

Under the muscle inside the sheath are the superior and inferior epigastric vessels and the ends of the lower six intercostal nerves that supply the muscle and the overlying skin. About half way between symphysis and umbilicus, perforating vessels

from the inferior epigastric arteries run into the rectus muscle, vessels that can form the pedicle for rectus flaps.

LINEA ALBA

The linea alba lies between the rectus muscles and extends from the xiphoid to the symphysis. It is composed of interlacing fibers from the aponeuroses of the three major abdominal muscles. The structure is narrower below the umbilicus than above because the rectus muscles diverge in the epigastrium to leave a relatively weak area where the generation of midline hernias commonly occurs. Its superficial fibers attach to the symphysis anteriorly; its deeper fibers form a triangular layer that adheres to the posterior surface of the pubic crest. The linea alba is especially dense where it is penetrated by the umbilicus.

BLOOD SUPPLY TO THE ANTERIOR ABDOMINAL WALL

1 The inferior epigastric artery arises from the external iliac artery just above the inguinal ligament in the subperitoneal connective tissue and takes a course medial to the deep inguinal ring. There it lies deep to the spermatic cord, with transversalis fascia intervening. It then passes through the fascia behind the rectus abdominis to enter the space between the muscle and the posterior rectus sheath at the arcuate line. In addition, intercostal arteries from the lower two or three intercostal spaces come forward in the neurovascular plane over the transversus abdominis to provide important blood

supply to the rectus. The veins run with the respective arteries.

The superior epigastric artery supplying the upper portion of the rectus abdominis originates from the inferior mammary artery (internal thoracic artery) that runs anterior to the upper margin of the transversus abdominis to pass through the rectus sheath behind the rectus abdominis near its lateral border. As it runs caudad on the anterior surface of the posterior rectus sheath, it penetrates the muscle to supply it and then passes through the anterior rectus sheath to supply the overlying skin. The falciform ligament supporting the liver contains vessels from a branch of the superior epigastric artery that are destined to enter the hepatic artery and thus requires ligation after division.

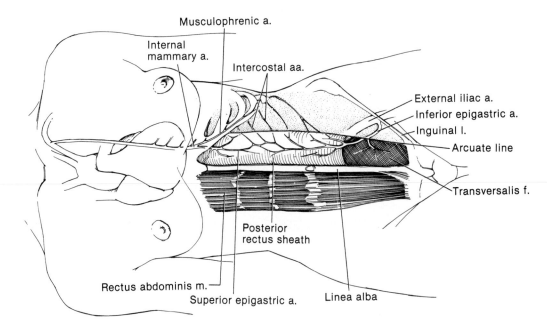

Musculophrenic a.
Internal mammary a.
Intercostal aa.
External iliac a.
Inferior epigastric a.
Inguinal l.
Arcuate line
Transversalis f.
Posterior rectus sheath
Rectus abdominis m.
Superior epigastric a.
Linea alba

Midline Lower Abdominal Extraperitoneal Incision

This incision provides exposure of the lower ureter and bladder. For extensive pelvic surgery, use the midline transperitoneal incision (see page 867).

1 *Position:* Place the patient supine with the buttocks over the kidney rest. Elevating the pelvis may help in exposure even though it tenses the rectus muscles, as does tipping the patient slightly head down in about a 15-degree Trendelenburg position.

Incision: Make a midline paraumbilical skin incision to the left of the umbilicus, extending over the symphysis pubis, and extend it to the fascial layer with the cutting current. In making the incision, place tissue forceps on the umbilicus and have the assistant lift in a cephalad direction. This places the upper portion of the incision on tension while the umbilicus is skirted. The upper part of the incision can then be made in a controlled fashion approximately 1.5 cm around the umbilicus; if the umbilicus is not held tense, irregularity of that part of the incision can result. The width of the exposure can be increased by separating the rectus tendons from each other and from the underlying pubic periosteum well down over the symphysis. Use the cutting current or a scalpel; this is a relatively bloodless field.

In overweight patients, mobilize the superficial fat for a distance of approximately 1 cm on either side of the midline to help identify the linea alba. The linea alba itself can be picked up most easily just below the umbilicus by identifying crossing fibers in the midline. Then extend the incision up and down throughout the length of the skin incision. Separate the rectus tendons.

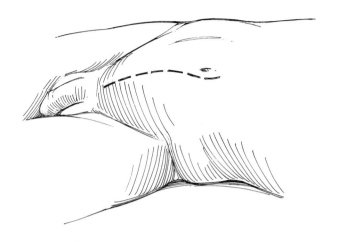

2 Incise the linea alba of the rectus fascia for a short distance with the electrocautery. To be certain of the location of the midline, look for the edge of the rectus muscle on one side or the other of the cut. Continue the incision over the symphysis pubis to the level of the insertion of the fascia to allow it to open to the fullest extent at the lower hinge. Extend the incision with curved scissors for the entire length of the wound to the depth of the insertion of the anterior sheath.

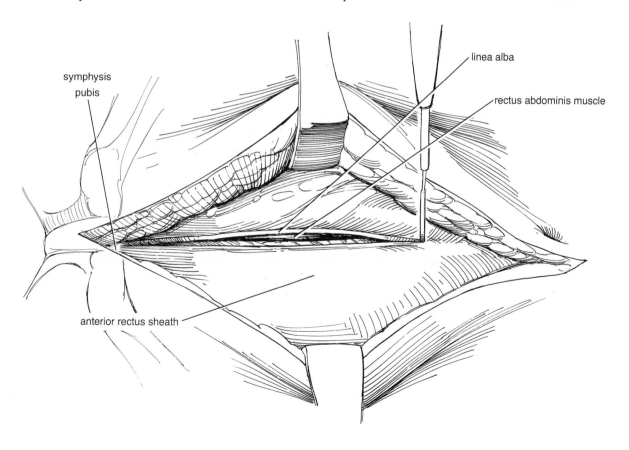

symphysis pubis

linea alba

rectus abdominis muscle

anterior rectus sheath

3 Retract the rectus muscles laterally and incise their investing fascia. Sharply open the contiguous thinned transversalis fascia laterally where it lies beneath the rectus muscle to expose the retroperitoneal connective tissue. Pick up the blood vessels as they are seen and coagulate them successively, particularly in the lower portion of the wound. Before mobilizing the peritoneum medially, gently incise the fascia on the lateral side of the ascending colon. Open this plane with blunt dissection, mobilizing the peritoneum medially and keeping the inferior epigastric vessels in the anterior plane.

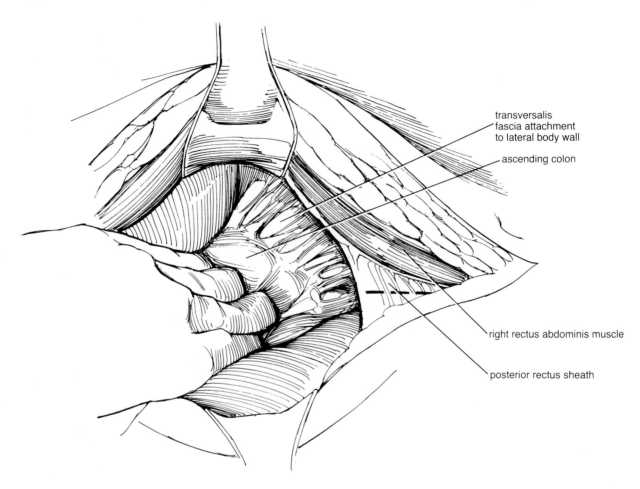

transversalis
fascia attachment
to lateral body wall

ascending colon

right rectus abdominis muscle

posterior rectus sheath

4 Dissect anterior to the retroperitoneal connective tissue inferiorly and laterally with a stick sponge, thus mobilizing the peritoneum medially but staying deep to the inferior epigastric vessels. It is at this point that the peritoneum can be inadvertently opened, as it tends to be tethered at the level of the internal inguinal ring and, in the female, in the region of the infundibulopelvic ligament. Formally close any small window made in the peritoneum at this stage with a fine continuous catgut suture to contain the intraperitoneal organs.

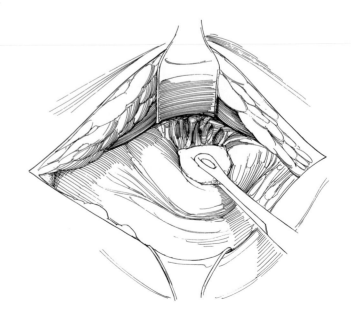

5 Follow the obliterated hypogastric (umbilical) artery to the superior vesical pedicle, if indicated, and follow the vas (or round ligament) to the internal inguinal ring.

Closure

Before closing the wound after the urinary tract has been opened, bring a Penrose or suction drain through a stab wound. Close the rectus fascia with a running absorbable or nonabsorbable suture (NAS) or with interrupted sutures, and close the subcutaneous tissue with interrupted plain catgut sutures and the skin with a subcuticular 4-0 or 5-0 synthetic absorbable suture (SAS).

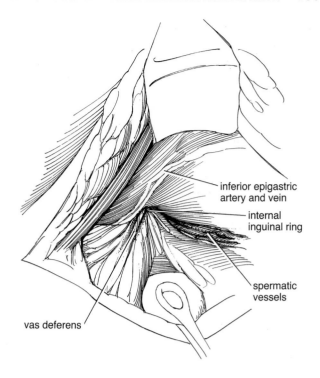

inferior epigastric artery and vein

internal inguinal ring

spermatic vessels

vas deferens

Commentary by R. Wyndham Lloyd-Davies

The lower vertical midline incision is an excellent approach, particularly when both ureters are being explored. When this is carried out on only one side, I personally prefer an oblique muscle-cutting Rutherford-Morrison incision, which places the wound directly above the ureter and requires less medial traction upon the peritoneum and the intraperitoneal structures and demonstrates the ureter very satisfactorily for the whole of its lower course. Where both ureters need to be explored, the midline incision is the incision of choice, as it is for vesical diverticulectomy.

TRANSPUBIC APPROACH

For additional exposure of structures behind the pubis, perform a *partial pubectomy.* Extend the abdominal incision over the symphysis to a point 2 cm above the penile root and laterally on either side along the pubic arch. Detach the tendons of the rectus abdominis and pyramidalis muscles (see page 301). Divide the suspensory ligament. Ligate the dorsal vein of the penis if necessary. Clear the tissue from the posterior surface of the symphysis and open into the space of Retzius. Drill two holes approximately 5 cm apart midway up the symphysis. Insert a Gigli saw (see page 493) in one, and cut the inferior border of the symphysis at an angle on one side to meet the hole. Repeat the procedure through the other hole. Re-insert the saw through the drilled holes to run transversely, and resect the central section. Enlarge the defect with rongeurs if necessary.

Transverse Lower Abdominal Incision

(Pfannenstiel)

The Pfannenstiel incision is useful for operations on the bladder and urethra as well as for other pelvic operations. The lower ureter can also be exposed transperitoneally. In selected cases it may be used for procedures involving bowel, such as ileocystoplasty.

1 **A,** The aponeuroses of the anterior abdominal muscles combine to form the anterior rectus sheath. The posterior rectus sheath, composed of the aponeuroses of the transversus abdominis and part of the aponeuroses of the internal oblique, ends below the arcuate line, leaving only transversalis fascia separating the rectus muscle from the peritoneum.

B, *Incision:* Make a symmetric, semilunar incision through a point two fingerbreadths above the symphysis pubis. With the electrocautery, carry it down to the rectus sheath. Before incising the sheath, check the distance above the symphysis by palpation.

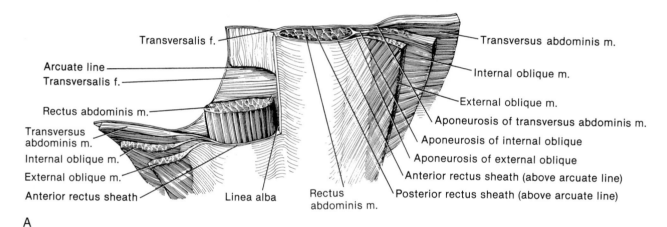

Transversalis f.
Arcuate line
Transversalis f.
Rectus abdominis m.
Transversus abdominis m.
Internal oblique m.
External oblique m.
Anterior rectus sheath
Linea alba
Rectus abdominis m.
Transversus abdominis m.
Internal oblique m.
External oblique m.
Aponeurosis of transversus abdominis m.
Aponeurosis of internal oblique
Aponeurosis of external oblique
Anterior rectus sheath (above arcuate line)
Posterior rectus sheath (above arcuate line)

A

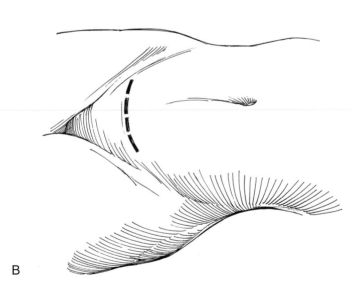

B

CHERNE

For greater
muscles at th
that the subs

7 Free th
Pfanne
tions of the
attachment
intraperiton

2 Incise the rectus sheath with a needle electrode in an arc to avoid the inguinal canals. Continue the incision laterally to divide the external and then the internal oblique aponeuroses. Split the transversus abdominis muscles at each extremity and incise the transversalis fascia.

If this incision is used for *pelvic node dissection* prior to total perineal prostatectomy, it is not necessary to mobilize the rectus sheath and muscle. Mobilize the peritoneum medially and superiorly with a large retractor. Expose the retroperitoneal space with the bifurcation of the iliac vessels, the internal and external iliac vessels, the ureter, and the genitofemoral nerve lying on the psoas muscle. Proceed with node dissection.

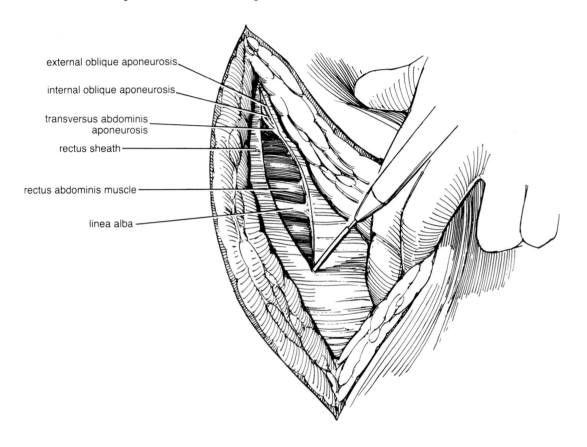

3 Grasp the upper edge of the rectus sheath with Kocher clamps, elevate it, and divide its midline attachment, the linea alba, with the cutting current for at least 10 cm. Push down on the muscle with stick sponges to free it from the sheath. Either take care to avoid the two symmetric perforating branches of the inferior epigastric vessels, or coagulate and divide them.

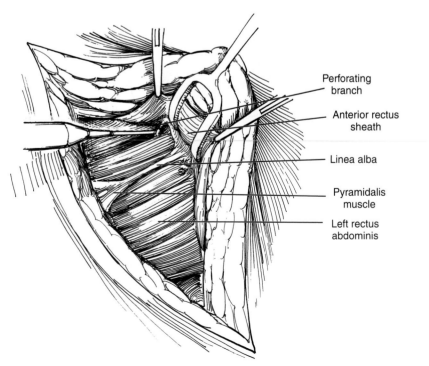

4 Free the
  ment to
tion on either
they are well
rectus sheath.

Symphysis
pubis

6 Incise a
  cia in th
the bladder a

Closure

Begin by tac
Loosely app
external obl
sion. Close t
0 SAS, the su
skin with a

Commentary by John F. Redman

In an age when discerning patients favor cosmesis, the prospect of a low transverse incision for pelvic surgery may make an operation more acceptable. I have been increasingly impressed by the degree of exposure that can be achieved with this incision when it is properly developed and then held open by the versatile blades of a fixed ring retractor such as the Buchwalter. In addition to spreading the wound, it provides upward and outward retraction, which opens tissue planes in a vertical direction as well. The smaller rings and blades that are now available allow this retractor to be used even in infants. In most cases there is no need to extend the lateral limits of the incision past the lateral edge of the rectus muscle itself. If more exposure is needed—for instance, to bridge a long Boari flap to the ipsilateral midureter, the incision may be modified into a Gibson incision with or without cutting the ipsilateral rectus muscle.

Although the Pfannenstiel incision is a transverse incision through the anterior rectus sheath, it is actually a midline incision with regard to the rectus muscles. It is therefore imperative, for the greatest exposure, to elevate the anterior sheath from the recti cranially to just caudal to the umbilicus and caudally to the pubis. To elevate the sheath, I use the cautery to incise the attaching fibroareolar tissue and any vessels encountered. When the pyramidalis is prominent, I leave it attached to the caudal leaf of the rectus sheath as I elevate it and therefore need only separate the recti to visualize the transversalis fascia.

Once the recti have been separated, the prostate or vesical neck and even the bladder can be quickly exposed by breaking through the thin transversalis fascia that covers the dorsal surfaces of the recti just cranial to the pubis. A transperitoneal incision requires little more than an opening of the transversalis fascia and the closely associated peritoneum. However, full retroperitoneal exposure of the pelvic sidewalls and the retroperitoneum craniolateral to the bifurcation of the iliac vessels requires a more formal dissection of the tissue dorsal to the rectus abdominis muscles. Following separation of the recti, the underlying layer is the transversalis fascia, which is thickened by slips of the medial aponeurosis of the transversus abdominis muscle. From the pubis to just caudal to the umbilicus, where the arcuate line of Douglas marks the caudal margin of the posterior rectus sheath, the thickening gradually becomes greater. The fascia may be thin, however, and easily confused with the underlying peritoneum. Lifting up this layer and incising it just lateral to the midline cause the underlying fat-laden intermediate stratum and peritoneum to drop away. Incising the fascia cranially and caudally, paralleling the midline, produces an edge that may be grasped with Allis clamps and then separated away from the underlying fat-laden connective tissue using broad-based traction to develop the incision to its full extent.

As the dissection reaches the lateral border of the rectus, the inferior epigastric vessels are noted as they penetrate the transversalis fascia; therefore, the plane of dissection passes dorsal to them. At the level of the internal ring, either the spermatic cord or round ligament is encountered. The round ligament may be transected with a cautery. Freeing the peritoneum from the spermatic cord requires first an incision of the intermediate stratum surrounding the cord and then a purposeful dissection of the internal spermatic vessels cranially and the vas medially.

The peritoneal envelope can then be lifted far cranially in the pelvis, giving a striking exposure of the retroperitoneum, extending as high as the iliac crest in some cases. I have a series of patients in whom over the past 4 years I have successfully performed ileocystoplasties with concomitant ureteral reimplantation utilizing standard Pfannenstiel incisions.

Gibson Incision

Access to the lower third of the ureter can be obtained by a variety of incisions. Because the ureter terminates near the midline, a direct approach can be made equally well through an oblique muscle-splitting incision in a lower quadrant—the Gibson incision—or through a midline or transverse incision. In the female, a transverse incision is more acceptable cosmetically.

1 **A,** *Position:* Place the patient supine in a partial Trendelenburg position. *Incision:* Make a hockey-stick incision extending from 2 cm medial to the anterior superior iliac spine, running 0.5 cm above the inguinal fold, and ending at the border of the rectus muscle.

B, Divide the external oblique aponeurosis in the direction of its fibers.

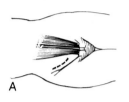

A

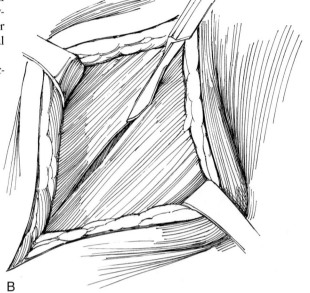

B

2 Incise the perimesium to allow separation of the internal oblique muscle in the direction of its fibers. Open the transversus abdominis muscle layer. If greater exposure is required, divide the muscle.

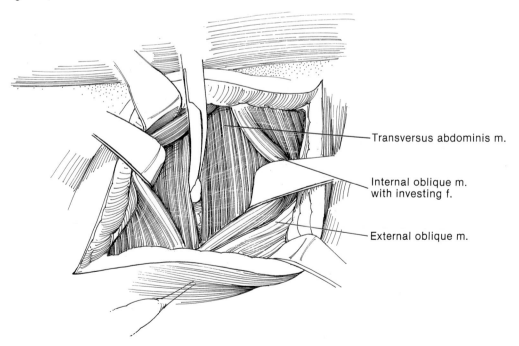

Transversus abdominis m.

Internal oblique m. with investing f.

External oblique m.

3 Draw the transversalis fascia medially (at this level it is a thin structure), carrying the peritoneum off the vessels and the lateral body wall. Divide the residuum of the processus vaginalis at the internal ring (or divide the round ligament in females) so that the peritoneum can be completely mobilized medially. This opens the lateral subperitoneal spaces and exposes the iliac vessels. In the male, mobilize the vas deferens inferiorly. Divide the inferior epigastric vessels for further exposure.

4 Identify the ureter against the peritoneum as it crosses the iliac vessels. Grasp it in a Babcock clamp, or encircle it with a Penrose drain, for further dissection.

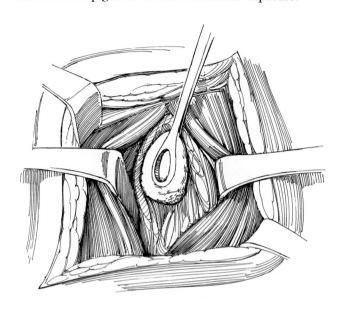 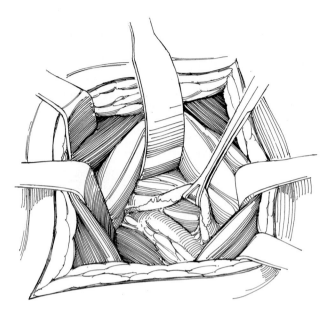

Commentary by Yoshio Aso

To an old-time urologist, a Gibson-type incision is a nostalgic approach to the treatment of the lower third of the ureter. As you know, the ureter is divided into upper, middle, and lower portions, with the upper margin of the fifth lumbar vertebra and the lower margin of the sacroiliac joint serving as anatomic landmarks.

Once the transversus abdominis muscle is divided, it is easier to separate it from the peritoneum starting at the lateral portion because the medial side is in close proximity to the peritoneum and more fatty tissue is present in the lateral part.

When a ureter is not located where you expect it to be, always look for it over the external iliac artery where it joins the internal iliac artery. Otherwise, it takes an unexpectedly longer time to find a ureter.

If an incision is made a little higher, a stone in the midureter can be removed through a Gibson incision. If we make this type of incision longer, lowering the median portion to just above the symphysis, and incise the muscular layers—including the rectus muscle—along the skin incision, the iliac fossa is fully exposed, enabling us to perform renal transplantation and ureteropelvic junction repair.

Currently a ureteral stone is usually treated with extracorporeal shock wave lithotripsy or endoscopy. Therefore, there are only a limited number of indications for this incision, including idiopathic retroperitoneal fibrosis, congenital ureteral anomalies, inflammatory conditions, benign ureteral tumors, ureteral malignancies of patients at high risk, and renal transplantation.

Suprapubic V-Incision

(Turner-Warwick)

As an alternative to the Pfannenstiel incision, the suprapubic V-incision provides better access to the pelvis and avoids approaching the inguinal canal. It is suitable for repair of an inguinal hernia at the time of retropubic prostatectomy (see page 342) or for simple vesicovaginal fistulas.

1 **A,** *Incision:* Make a transverse lower abdominal incision as for a Pfannenstiel procedure, and expose the rectus sheath.

B, Beginning just *below* the upper border of the pubis, make a 4-cm horizontal incision in the rectus sheath. Extend each end of the incision obliquely upward at an angle of about 45 degrees, staying over the rectus muscle.

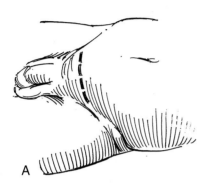

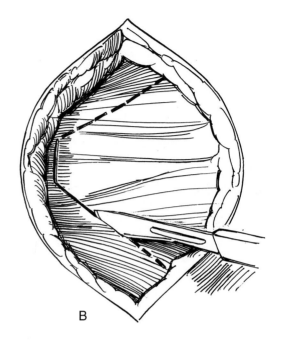

2 Tack the lower skin edge to the fascia with 2-0 SAS to expose the upper border of the pubis. Elevate the rectus sheath flap, and control the perforating vessels. Separate the rectus muscles vertically in the midline well down over the anterior surface of the pubis.

3 Increase retropubic access by lifting the caudal extension of the rectus aponeurosis off the front of the pubis by sharp dissection to expose 3 to 4 cm of its upper surface.

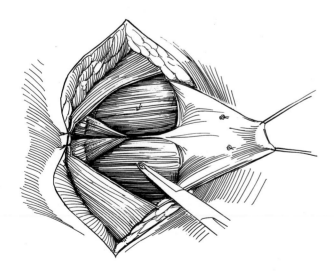

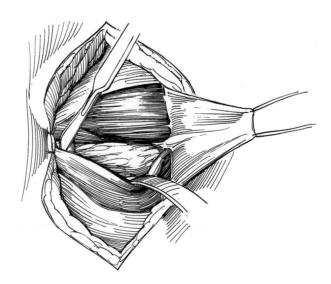

497

4 Insert a ring retractor to achieve the maximum exposure. Mobilize the peritoneum to expose the bladder.

5 For exposure of the ureter as far as the lower pole of the kidney, retract the belly of the ipsilateral rectus muscle medially and incise the lateral abdominal wall muscles toward the tip of the 12th rib. The incision can be extended even farther as a supracostal incision (see page 879) to expose the kidney.

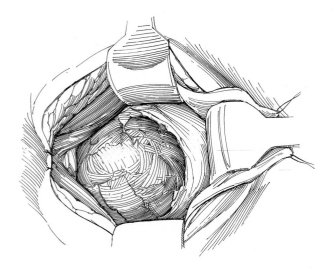

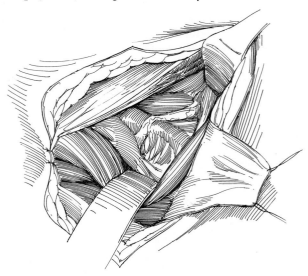

Closure

Begin by loosely approximating the rectus muscles. If a drain is needed, bring it through a stab wound. Close the fascia with continuous or interrupted 2-0 SAS.

Commentary by Richard Turner-Warwick

The classic Pfannenstiel incision can be modified to improve the exposure of both the retropubic space and the lower abdomen, and at the same time avoid the inguinal canal. Repair of a coincidental inguinal hernia can be done through it.

By extending the incision upward and laterally without dividing the rectus muscle, good exposure can be provided for a synchronous nephroureterocystectomy. However, it is not advocated for the closure of a complex vesicovaginal fistula because exposure of the greater curvature of the stomach is insufficient for the proper mobilization of the gastroepiploic pedicle of the omentum, when this is required to ensure the success of an unexpectedly complex fistula.

SECTION

13

Bladder: Excision

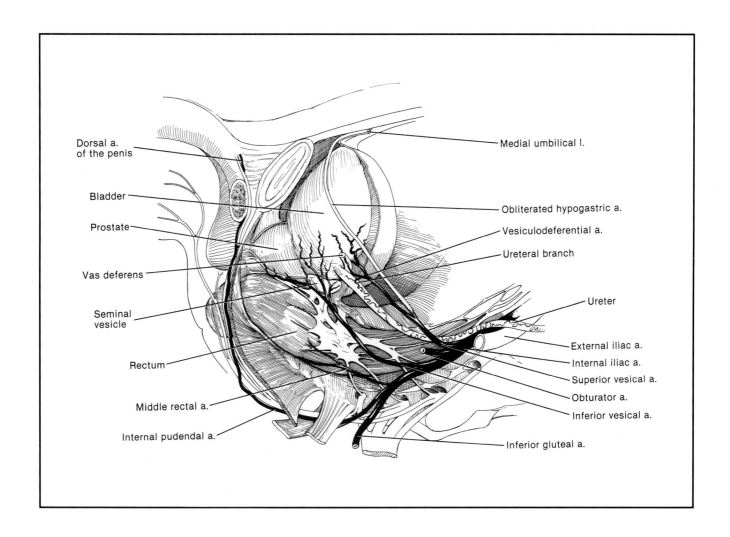

Dorsal a.
of the penis

Bladder

Prostate

Vas deferens

Seminal
vesicle

Rectum

Middle rectal a.

Internal pudendal a.

Medial umbilical l.

Obliterated hypogastric a.

Vesiculodeferential a.

Ureteral branch

Ureter

External iliac a.

Internal iliac a.

Superior vesical a.

Obturator a.

Inferior vesical a.

Inferior gluteal a.

Anatomy and Principles for Excision of the Bladder

Partial cystectomy is best restricted to primary solitary lesions unsuitable for removal by transurethral resection and to residual tumor at repeat resection 2 months later. The tumor must also lie at a site that allows 2 cm of normal tissue around it to be removed. Finally, the bladder must have adequate capacity and compliance to be functional after removal of part of its wall.

Radical cystectomy is designed to remove not only the bladder but the pelvic peritoneum, prostate, and seminal vesicles in men and the urethra, uterus, broad ligaments, and anterior third of the vaginal wall in women. In both sexes, pelvic lymphadenectomy is an integral part of the operation. In each case, some form of urinary diversion must be created.

1 Of importance surgically is the dual blood supply to the bladder by way of the superior vesical pedicle, which carries the superior vesical artery, and the inferior vesical pedicle, which contains the inferior vesical artery. The inferior vesical artery supplies the bladder base, the proximal urethra, and the prostate.

The nerves from the vesical plexus run with the arteries to the bladder at its base. The anterior part of each inferior hypogastric plexus constitutes the vesical plexus. The parasympathetic nerves from the prostatic plexus may provide some supply to the external urethral sphincter.

The lymph collectors from the bladder drain into the external iliac nodes. Some lymph from the base may pass directly to internal iliac and common iliac nodes, and some from the neck may go directly to the sacral nodes. Lymphatics from the posterior wall reach the internal iliac nodes. Those from the anterior wall meet sets of collectors from the prostate and adjacent organs and end in the middle chain of the external iliac group.

Clinically, metastases from bladder carcinoma have been found to spread principally to the obturator and the external iliac nodes, although the sacral nodes are involved in more than one fifth of cases.

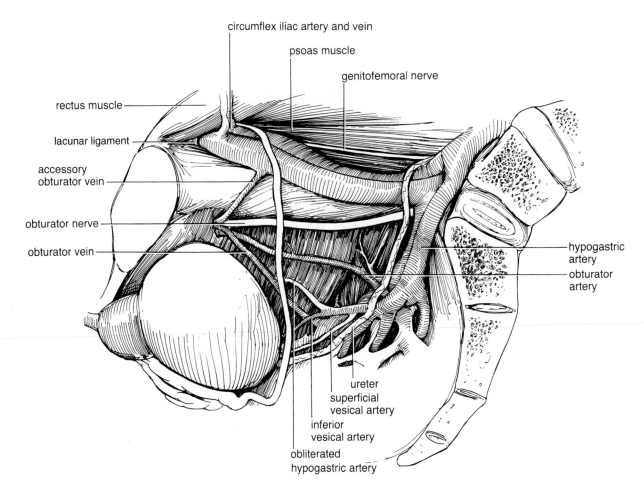

circumflex iliac artery and vein
psoas muscle
genitofemoral nerve
rectus muscle
lacunar ligament
accessory obturator vein
obturator nerve
obturator vein
hypogastric artery
obturator artery
ureter
superficial vesical artery
inferior vesical artery
obliterated hypogastric artery

Partial Cystectomy

Partial cystectomy is suitable for single tumors of moderate grade, not deeply infiltrating by CT scan, and situated away from the bladder base. It is an alternative to transurethral resection repeated at 2 months or to total cystectomy. Exclude high-grade tumors and carcinoma in situ.

Preoperatively, the lesion should be examined cystoscopically and samples for biopsy taken from the lesion and randomly from the adjacent mucosa.

Either a transperitoneal or an extraperitoneal approach may be used. The transperitoneal approach is suitable for more posteriorly situated tumors. The same surgical principles apply to both. Consider continuous epidural block for anesthesia.

Position: Place the patient supine, in a slight Trendelenburg position. Perform bimanual palpation with the patient under anesthesia. Drape the genitalia into the field, and insert a balloon catheter. Flush the bladder several times with sterile water through a catheter, then partially drain the bladder, clamp the catheter, and immediately attach the catheter to a sterile drainage bag to avoid spillage. If localization may be a problem, insert a flexible cystoscope and fulgurate around the tumor, or inject methylene blue around it through a 25-cm, 21-gauge needle to stain the serosal surface (Nargund and Hamilton-Stewart, 1994).

TRANSPERITONEAL APPROACH

1 **A,** *Incision:* Make a midline transperitoneal incision (see page 867) that extends from just above the umbilicus to well over the pubis.
B, Open the peritoneum in the midline. A peritoneal flap is not necessary.

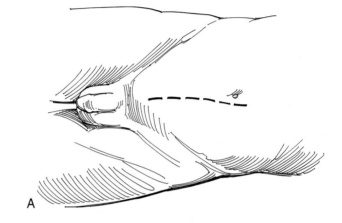

A

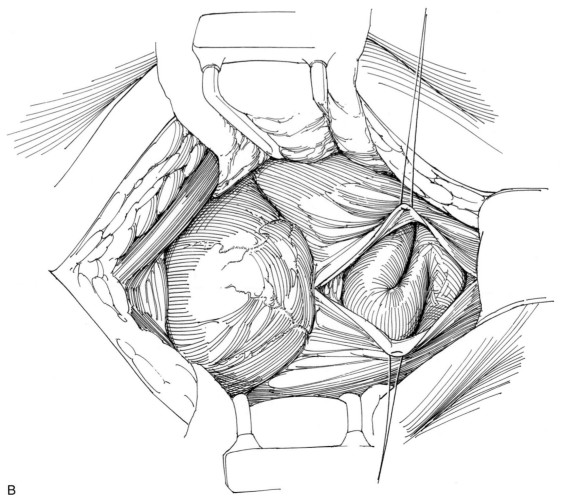

B

2 Incise the peritoneum over the iliac vessels and the nodes. Unilateral lymph node dissection may be of value for staging (see page 465). With positive nodes, partial cystectomy may still be a reasonable procedure for local control; total cystectomy does not improve the outcome.

3 Follow the obliterated hypogastric artery to the take-off of the superior vesical artery. Divide and use the vas as a guide. It is important to mobilize the bladder for tumors near the base by dividing most of the lateral leash of vessels emerging from the hypogastric artery and vein, best seen before dividing the superior vesical artery. Clip and divide them to the entrance of the ureter into the bladder. Clamp, divide, and ligate the superior vesical artery. Bluntly and sharply free the bladder farther posteriorly as needed, leaving the peritoneum attached. Incise the peritoneal reflection behind the bladder and displace the rectum posteriorly. Pack the wound edges and hold them away from the bladder with the blades of a retractor. Isolate the bladder with plastic drapes to reduce the risk of tumor implantation.

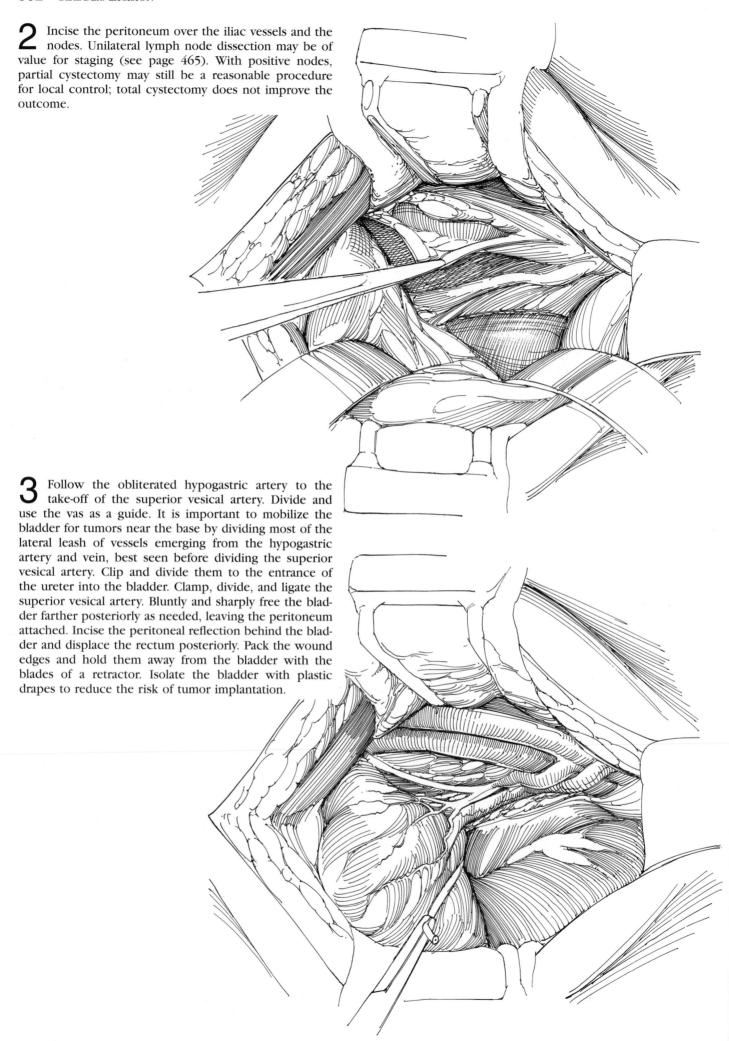

4 Protect the rectum with a moist gauze pack in the cul-de-sac. Drain the bladder and open it between stay sutures at a site known from cystoscopic examination to be distant from the tumor. Mark the wall 2 cm from the tumor by coagulation while the bladder is mildly stretched. Circumscribe the entire lesion with the electro-surgical knife, and remove it en bloc with the perivesical fat and with overlying peritoneum if necessary. Place Allis clamps both for exposure and for control of the brisk bleeding while the bladder wall is divided with the cutting current. Release the Allis clamps successively, and fulgurate or clamp and ligate the bleeding vessels in the bladder wall. Send multiple biopsy samples of the margin for frozen-section examination; if they are positive, resect more of the bladder wall.

If a 2-cm margin from the ureteral orifice is not possible, proceed with total cystectomy rather than resect the orifice and reimplant the ureter.

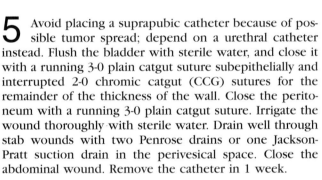

5 Avoid placing a suprapubic catheter because of possible tumor spread; depend on a urethral catheter instead. Flush the bladder with sterile water, and close it with a running 3-0 plain catgut suture subepithelially and interrupted 2-0 chromic catgut (CCG) sutures for the remainder of the thickness of the wall. Close the peritoneum with a running 3-0 plain catgut suture. Irrigate the wound thoroughly with sterile water. Drain well through stab wounds with two Penrose drains or one Jackson-Pratt suction drain in the perivesical space. Close the abdominal wound. Remove the catheter in 1 week.

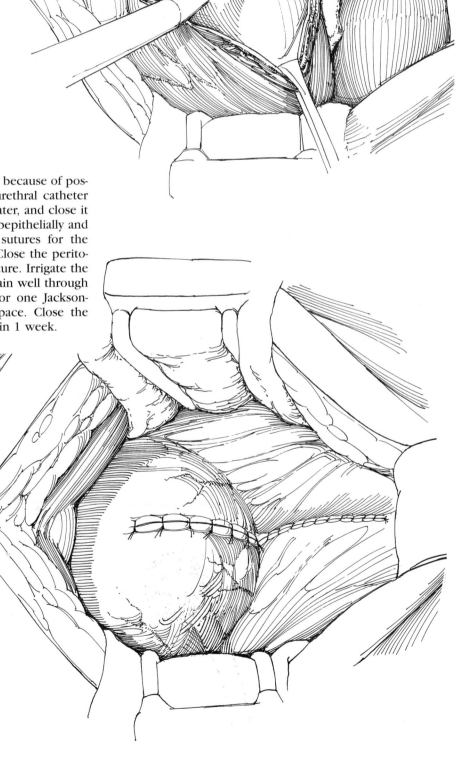

EXTRAPERITONEAL APPROACH

For the extraperitoneal approach, expose the anterior surface of the bladder and mobilize the peritoneum where it is readily separated from the bladder. Over the dome it is usually necessary to circumcise a patch of peritoneum, leaving it attached to the bladder. Free the bladder laterally and posteriorly, well beyond the site of the tumor. If necessary, expose and divide the superior vesical pedicle (see page 507). Leave the perivesical fat attached to the bladder over the area of the tumor. Proceed as for transvesical excision.

POSTOPERATIVE PROBLEMS

Leakage from the suture line usually stops in time if drainage is maintained. Avoid removing the drain until the wound has been dry for a day or two. If leakage continues, perform cystoscopy. *Bleeding* is uncommon with a two-layer closure, but clot retention can be a problem. *Prevesical infection* with formation of an abscess may require probing the wound and inserting a cut-off Robinson catheter.

Ureteral obstruction should be suspected if the patient has flank pain; sonography or intravenous urography can make the diagnosis. Endoscopic intubation will probably fail, but a percutaneous nephrostomy can divert the urine in the hope that the obstruction is temporary. If a stent had been left in place during the operation and then removed, edema may close the orifice, but only for a short time. *Incontinence* from poor detrusor compliance and uninhibitable contractions improves with time and anticholinergic medication.

Implantation of tumor cells is a real concern. Flushing the bladder with water preoperatively, protecting the wound edges, using care in manipulation of the tumor, and copiously irrigating the wound with water before closure are measures that reduce the risk.

Commentary by Mark S. Soloway

A partial cystectomy is an excellent operation for the treatment of bladder cancer, provided that the patient fits the criteria so well established in the urologic literature. These criteria are designed to minimize the chance that the patient will later require total cystectomy. The strict criteria include all of the following: (1) no prior history of bladder cancer; (2) no malignancy such as carcinoma in situ (CIS) or papillary tumor distant from the obvious tumor; and (3) a solitary muscle-invasive tumor located well away from the ureteral orifices and amenable to a partial cystectomy, which includes 1.5 to 2 cm of normal bladder around the lesion. High-grade tumors should not be excluded if the above criteria are met. Tumors confined to the urothelium (Ta or CIS) or tumors involving the lamina propria (T1) can usually be managed, at least initially, by transurethral resection with or without intravesical therapy.

The most common lesions amenable to partial cystectomy are Grade II or Grade III transitional cell carcinomas or adenocarcinomas located on the posterior wall or dome. The presence of CIS is usually a contraindication, primarily because CIS is usually multifocal. I do not think that the increasing use and success of continent diversions or neobladders make partial cystectomy a less valuable operation, provided that the indications are strict. A native bladder is far superior, in my view, to a neobladder. I have not found that instilling methylene blue or any other method to mark the tumor has been helpful or, for that matter, necessary. If there is any doubt about the location of the tumor, transurethral fulguration of the tumor or flexible cystoscopy prior to beginning a partial cystectomy helps identify the area to be removed. Usually, these tumors are palpable from the outside of the bladder. Even if the initial opening in the bladder is away from the obvious solitary tumor, this usually does not present a problem because a wide excision is necessary.

Preoperative low-dose radiation has been suggested, but more recent information suggests that it is not necessary. If the tumor is Grade III, cT2b-T3b, I suggest 2 to 3 months of systemic chemotherapy prior to the partial cystectomy. The main risk for such patients is micrometastasis, and it may be preferable to treat these prior to surgery. Obviously, successful treatment limits the risk of tumor implantation. The list of instruments used is much more extensive than is usually necessary. Because I would not perform the procedure if the tumor is close to the ureteral orifices, I would not use stents. If the ureter would have to be reimplanted, a total cystectomy is my procedure of choice. The concern, of course, is that an adequate margin would not be obtained.

I initiate the procedure with a modified bilateral pelvic lymph node dissection. This lymph node dissection is similar to the one we use for radical prostatectomy. The lymphatic tissue surrounding the external iliac vein and obturator nerve is removed, along with any lymph nodes around the internal iliac artery. If nodal involvement is limited, I probably would still proceed with removal of the primary tumor if this could be done with a partial cystectomy as planned. Thus, as a rule, I would not submit the nodal tissue to frozen section because the findings are not likely to alter my approach.

Because I am concerned about a positive margin, I would rather remove more than less of the bladder. Thus, I always divide both obliterated umbilical vessels and, on the side of the lesion (assuming it is not directly in the midline), I ligate and divide the superior vesical vessels.

I find it important to mobilize a sufficient portion of the bladder prior to opening the bladder. I believe this mobilization is best carried out with the bladder moderately filled with sterile saline or water. This fluid in the bladder is then emptied through the urethral catheter prior to opening the bladder. I emphasize the importance of frozen sections following the partial cystectomy and prior to closure of the bladder. This can be done either from the removed tissue or by taking extra sections once the partial cystectomy has been completed. The objective, of course, is to achieve a negative margin.

There are many ways to close the bladder. My preference is to use a running 2-0 CCG to the mucosa with incorporation of some of the muscle. I then close the rest of the muscle and serosa with a horizontal mattress 1-0 CCG suture, which inverts the first layer. It is important to avoid a suprapubic catheter. Assuming excellent hemostasis, there should be no reason for it. A 20 F or 22 F urethral catheter should work well because bleeding should be minimal once the bladder has been closed. I currently prefer using a closed drainage system such as a Jackson-Pratt drain.

Radical Cystectomy

Pulmonary evaluation and preparation take priority. Breathing exercises, cessation of smoking, correction of dental disease, and culturing the sputum are important. Anemia and hypoalbuminuria must be corrected. Nutrition cannot be substandard; perioperative hyperalimentation may be needed. Have the patient talk with someone who has had the procedure and meet with an enterostomal therapist, even if internal reconstruction is planned, to become familiar with urinary diversion and appliances. Preoperatively, select two alternative sites for a stoma with the patient in sitting and standing positions, and mark them with a needle scratch (see page 647). Perform intravenous urography. Consider preoperative radiation therapy, limited to 5000 rads. Apply elastic stockings or pneumatic compression boots the night before surgery, to remain until the patient is fully ambulatory.

For mechanical bowel preparation, give polyethylene glycol electrolyte solution (GoLYTELY). Give oral neomycin sulfate and erythromycin base in three doses of 1 g the day before surgery and a parenteral antibiotic the morning of surgery. Prepare the bowel. Begin intravenous hydration with lactated Ringer's solution or 5 percent dextrose in 0.5 percent normal saline solution the afternoon before surgery.

Consider hypotensive anesthesia with continuous epidural block. Place a central venous line. Shave the patient from the nipples to the upper thighs.

Instruments and Sutures. Provide a basic set; a GU long set; a GU extra-long set; a GU fine set; a Major retractor set; a Buchwalter retractor; a large Deaver retractor; GI specials; a suction tip; smooth and toothed Cushing forceps; 9-inch vascular forceps; 11-inch Mayo scissors; smooth Adson forceps; Stevens, iris, tenotomy, and Lahey scissors; 5 F and 8 F infant feeding tubes; single-J or figure-four diversion stents with mineral oil; 4-0 polyglycolic (PR4) sutures (ureter); 4-0 silk detachable sutures; 3-0 polyglycolic sutures (stoma); a urostomy set; a Smith ring retractor; large, medium, and small hemoclips with long and medium clip appliers; a right-angle clip applier for large clips; straight rubber-shod Doyen clamps; curved Jones clamps; a square pan with towel in field; and a Jackson-Pratt drain with medium Hemovac needle.

CYSTECTOMY IN THE MALE

1 *Position:* Supine. Fix the legs abducted and very slightly flexed at knees and hips, held by foot stirrups or airplane splints. This position and support allow the legs to be adjusted for urethrectomy. If urethrectomy is not contemplated, place the patient with the umbilicus over the break in the table in a hyperextended position. Apply a 20-degree Trendelenburg tilt until the legs are parallel to the floor. For urethrectomy, subsequently elevate the legs and braces together.

Preparation: Prepare the abdomen and perineum, including the vagina, and drape these areas. Insert a preconnected 24 F urethral catheter with a 30-ml balloon filled to 50 ml, and drain the bladder. Clip the gravity drainage to the drapes under the leg for accessibility. Drape out the perineum with a folded towel. Stand on the left side of the table.

Incision: Make a lower midline abdominal incision from the symphysis pubis to 4 cm above and to the left of the umbilicus (see page 867). Incise the anterior rectus fascia, and bluntly separate the rectus muscles in the midline.

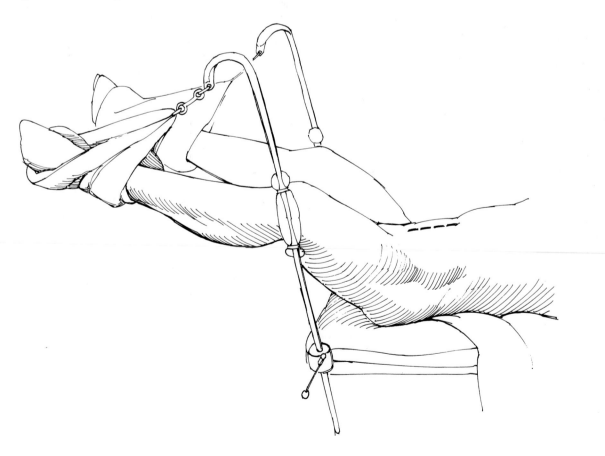

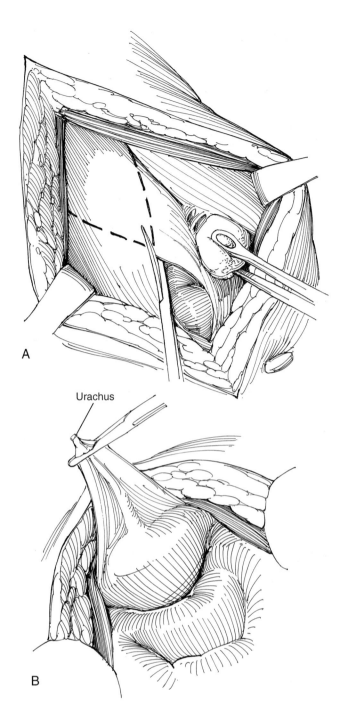

2 **A** and **B,** Incise the transversalis fascia, and bluntly open into the space of Retzius. Incise the peritoneum in the line of the abdominal incision in the upper half, but for the lower portion, after dividing the urachus, cut the peritoneum in a V shape. *Note:* If node dissection is to precede cystectomy, do not open the peritoneum but bluntly mobilize it from the pelvic sidewall. Open the V to the level of the internal iliac vessels to provide a peritoneal cuff on the bladder. A Kocher clamp on the urachus is useful for traction. Divide the vasa deferentia and ligate them, leaving the suture long to facilitate dissection of the seminal vesicles.

Check the mobility of the tumor with a thumb in the preprostatic space and the fingers in the cul-de-sac. Explore the abdomen, palpating especially the liver and preaortic and pelvic nodes. Send any suspicious nodes for pathologic examination by frozen section. Release intra-abdominal adhesions at this time. If the lesion appears operable, instill 30 to 60 ml of 10 percent formalin into the bladder, let it stand 10 for minutes, and drain it.

A

Urachus

B

3 *Triangulation technique* (Skinner): On the *right* side of the retroperitoneum, open the parietal peritoneum in the shape of a triangle, with the ileocecal region forming the apex by cutting along the length of the white line of Toldt to mobilize the cecum and ascending colon (the right side of the triangle). Incise along the medial border of the left colonic mesentery (the left side of the triangle). The duodenum forms the base of this peritoneal triangle. Pack the right colon and small bowel into the upper abdomen using several laparotomy tapes and successive packing maneuvers (see page 11). Hold them in place with a rolled towel, using a large Deaver retractor over the towel for greater exposure. Alternatively (usually not necessary), place the intestines in a bowel bag on the chest.

On the *left* side, incise along the entire white line of Toldt *(dashed line)* as high as the kidney and well over the sacrum. This allows elevation of the sigmoid colon and facilitates the passage of the left ureter under it. Place a large self-retaining retractor.

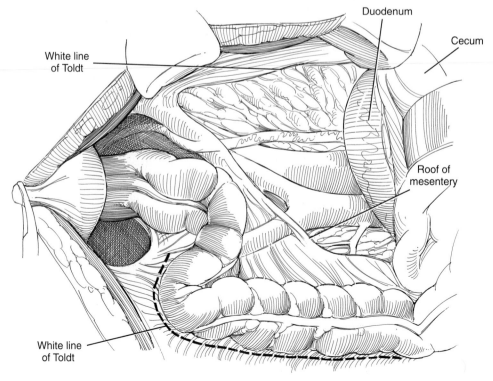

Duodenum

Cecum

White line of Toldt

Roof of mesentery

White line of Toldt

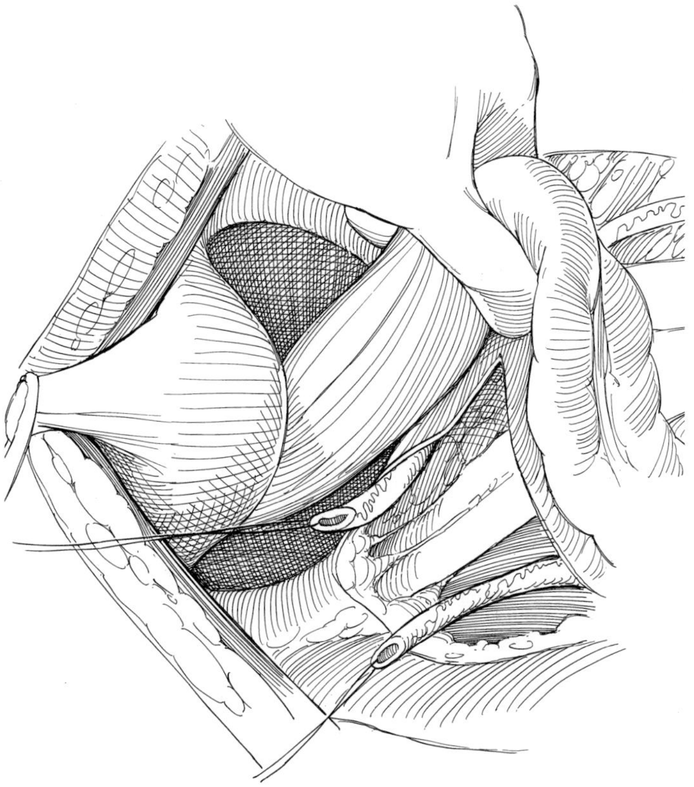

4 Free the right ureter with its adventitia, clamp it with a right-angle clamp, insert a stay suture proximally, and divide it distal to the suture.

Ureteral biopsy: If the patient is at risk for carcinoma in situ (CIS), take biopsy samples of the terminal ureters and send the specimens for frozen section. If the margin is positive, resect a segment of ureter and repeat the frozen-section examination. Free the left ureter higher than on the right and transect it similarly. Burrow with the fingers from one retroperitoneal opening to the other under the sigmoid colon, making a generous passage; insert a curved clamp; and draw the right ureter through by traction on the suture (as shown). Alternatively, draw the left ureter under the sigmoid for anastomosis to the urinary diversion. Be sure that the ureter is not twisted and that it runs in a smooth curve.

Proceed with *pelvic lymphadenectomy* (see page 517), exposing the iliac and internal iliac arteries. (For salvage cystectomy, this step is generally not feasible because of irradiation fibrosis.) Place long silk sutures on the distal ureters as an aid in their dissection.

DIVISION OF LATERAL PEDICLE

5 **A** and **B,** Insert the index finger of the left hand behind the internal iliac (hypogastric) artery while the rest of the fingers retract the bladder. Sweep the finger parallel to the sacrum down to the endopelvic fascia to separate the pedicle to the bladder from that to the rectum.

Clear the internal iliac artery and identify its first branch, the superior gluteal. Dissect distal to the gluteal branch. Pass a right-angle clamp gingerly behind the internal iliac artery, draw a 2-0 silk suture through, and ligate the artery. Clip the remainder of the vesical pedicle down to the endopelvic fascia with large clips on right-angle appliers, using the index finger to develop the plane and protect the rectum. Be sure enough tissue (0.5 to 1.0 cm) projects beyond each proximal clip to avoid dislodgment. Do not ligate the internal iliac artery, but if it becomes necessary to control it because of bleeding, put a bulldog clamp on it.

Avoid the autonomic nerves from the superior internal iliac, pelvic, and vesical plexuses when dividing the superior and inferior vesical pedicles. These innervate the sphincteric mechanisms and maintain continence after bladder substitution.

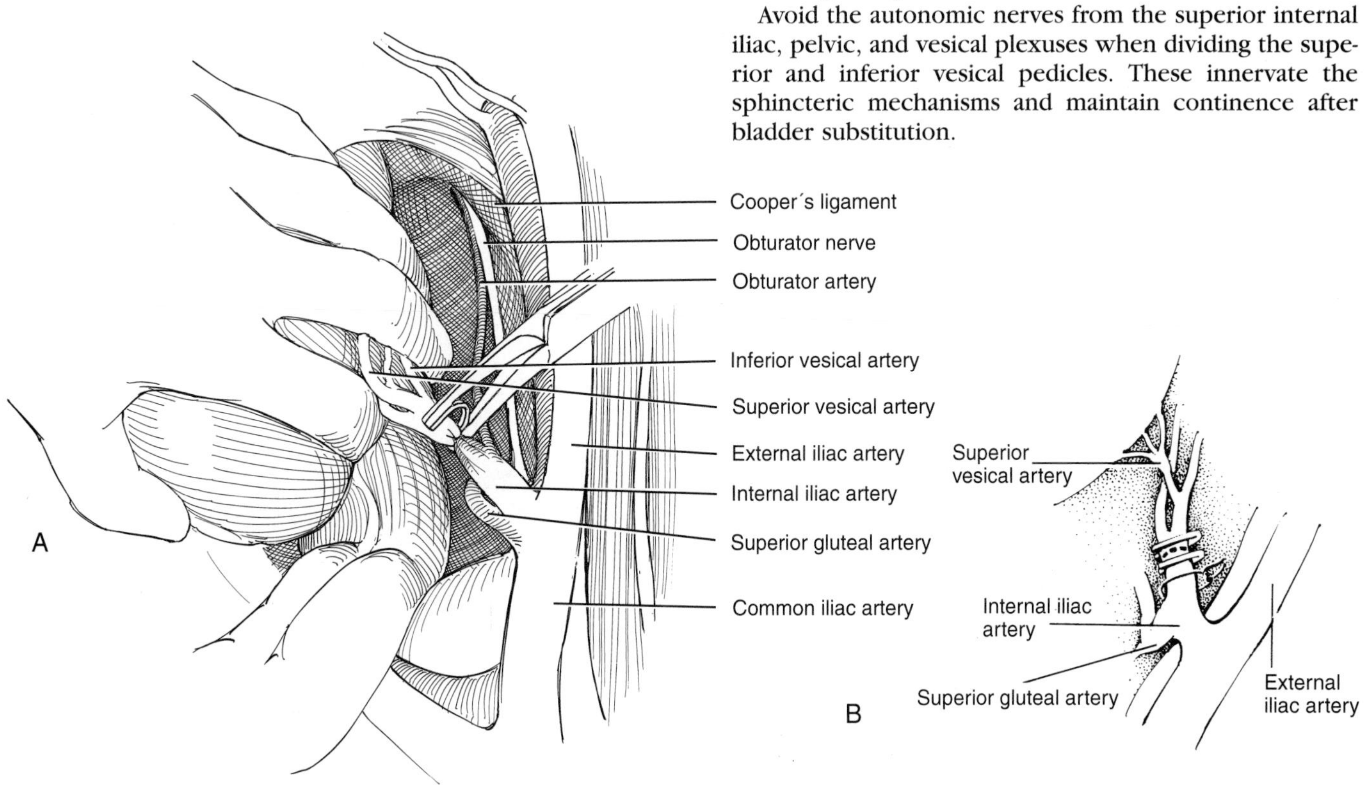

DIVISION OF POSTERIOR PEDICLE

6 **A,** Draw the bladder (uterus) up to be able to view the cul-de-sac. Incise the peritoneum and only the peritoneum, beginning on either side of the rectum, and join the incisions in the cul-de-sac exactly at its junction with the anterior rectal wall. Develop a plane behind the bladder by sharp dissection, and continue it bluntly with the palm up, sweeping the rectum from the bladder.

B, Dissect on the rectal wall, leaving the doubled fascial fold composed of the anterior and posterior lamellae of Denonvilliers' fascia (rectal fascia) anteriorly. Continue the dissection until the seminal vesicles are exposed.

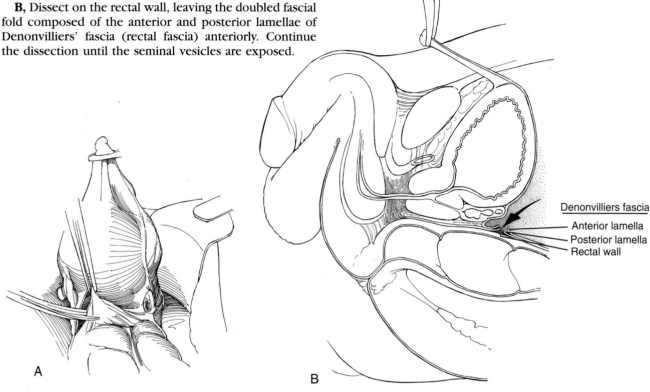

Denonvilliers fascia
— Anterior lamella
— Posterior lamella
— Rectal wall

A   B

7 **A,** Enter the plane under Denonvilliers' fascia, and bluntly sweep the rectum back from the bladder, seminal vesicles, and prostate (or posterior vaginal wall) to develop the posterior pedicles on either side. *Note:* If this plane has been obliterated by previous radiation therapy or by carcinoma, begin the operation by the perineal route (see page 451).

B, Dissect the pedicles lateral to the seminal vesicles to avoid the neurovascular bundles. The bundles are seen on the ventrolateral surface of the rectum. Clip and divide the pedicles along the anterolateral border of the seminal vesicle until the endopelvic fascia is reached. If extravesical extension of the tumor is encountered, widely excise the neurovascular bundle on that side, including the pelvic plexus, and divide the pedicle close to the pelvic wall.

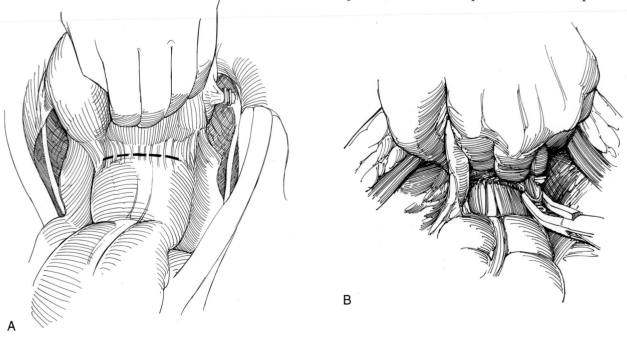

A   B

URETHRAL DIVISION

8 Return anteriorly to proceed as for total retropubic prostatectomy (see page 431). Dissect the prostate from the pubis. *Note:* If the prostate is densely adherent, open the periosteum with the cutting current and develop a subperiosteal plane to the level of the urethra. Clip the puboprostatic ligaments close to the pubis using a large right-angle clip carrier, and divide them with scissors.

9 Lift up the dorsal vein of the penis with a right-angle clamp. Clip and divide it.

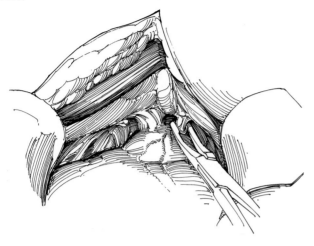

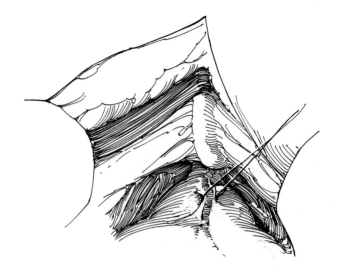

10 Pass a right-angle clamp under the urethra, avoiding the neurovascular bundles that lie posterolaterally. Draw an umbilical tape through and stretch the urethra. Place a silk ligature around the urethra to prevent contamination at the time of division. With traction on the tape, the urethra can be mobilized from the urogenital diaphragm preparatory to perineal urethrectomy (see page 513). Clamp the urethra near the prostate using a large, curved pedicle clamp placed carefully to avoid injuring the rectum, especially in radiated cases. (If the rectum is injured, close the defect in two layers and partially fill it with organic iodine solution. Subsequently dilate the anus. Consider proximal colostomy.) Pass the left index finger behind the urethra, and divide the space along the indwelling catheter. Elevate the rectourethralis muscle with a clamp, and sharply divide it under vision, again avoiding the neurovascular bundles that lie immediately adjacent in the posterolateral quadrants.

11 Divide the remaining lateral connections of the endopelvic fascia to allow the neurovascular bundles (which lie quite close to the urethra) to fall posteriorly. Try to preserve at least one of them. Mobilize and clip the small vessels at the apex of the prostate. Place 2-0 CCG sutures in the distal urethra preparatory to anastomosis of a substitute bladder, if that is planned. Remove the specimen. Before closing, place a figure-eight 1-0 synthetic absorbable suture (SAS) through both levators anteriorly just behind the pubis. Check for bleeding elsewhere.

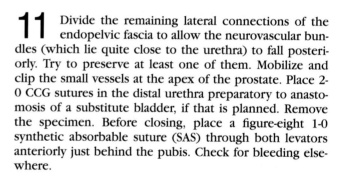

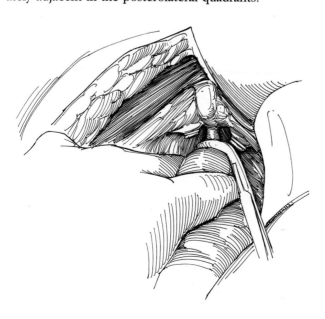

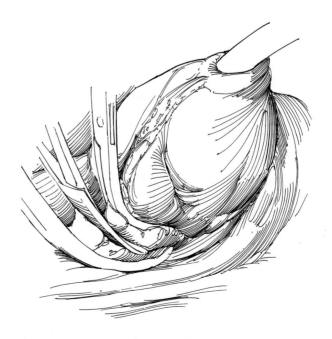

Urethrectomy

If the tumor is at the bladder neck or in the prostatic stroma or prostatic urethra, or if CIS was found on random biopsy, perform urethrectomy (see page 513). A two-team approach saves time and allows removal of the urethra in continuity. If an ileal neobladder is formed, the risk of urethral recurrence is reduced (Freeman et al, 1996).

Pack the pelvic space, and proceed with urinary diversion or with substitution if indicated. In patients who have undergone pelvic irradiation, place a Dexon mesh barrier across the abdominal cavity above the radiated area to keep the intestine off the raw surface. It does not dissolve until the peritoneum has had an opportunity to grow over it. If there is question of rectal injury, fill the pelvic cavity with water and instill air through a catheter placed in the rectum to detect a leak (Pisters and Wajsman, 1992).

Replace the bowel carefully, and pull the omentum down to cover the anastomoses. Suction drainage is usually needed for protection of the diversion. If a bladder substitute is not constructed, a balloon catheter placed through the urethra helps drain the pelvic cavity for the first few days postoperatively. Close the wound appropriately.

Give coumarin in the recovery room to keep the prothrombin time 1.5 to 2 times normal. Subsequently maintain serum protein at normal levels.

CYSTECTOMY IN THE FEMALE

Clip and divide the right posterior pedicles along with the cardinal ligaments 4 to 5 cm beyond the cervix. *Note:* The dissection on the left side is easier if the surgeon stands on the right side of the table and returns to the left to clip and divide this pedicle. Proceed with total hysterectomy (see page 254) if indicated. Perform minimum dissection where the internal iliac artery crosses the common iliac artery.

Open the vagina posteriorly just below the cervix, and divide it circumferentially. Save the urethropelvic ligament and the paraurethral vascular and nerve plexus, and dissect the urethrovesical junction from the anterior vaginal wall. Clip and divide the distal pedicles so formed. In older women, cut the vagina longitudinally down either side, leaving as much vagina behind as possible while a strip of vaginal wall is removed with the bladder specimen (Stenzl et al, 1995). Use the same sutures to tack the previously closed vagina to Cooper's ligament to prevent its descent. Approximate the levators for hemostasis. Place a figure-eight 1-0 SAS through both levators anteriorly just behind the pubis. Check for bleeding elsewhere.

Close the free edges of the introitus and vaginal wall with a running lock stitch of 2-0 SAS for hemostasis. For younger women, close the vaginal defect with a small patch of ileum.

If the tumor is at the bladder neck or if CIS was found on random biopsy, perform urethrectomy (see page 513). A two-team approach allows removal in continuity. If the bladder neck is clear by frozen-section biopsy and no evidence of vaginal extension is seen, perform orthotopic continent diversion (Stein et al, 1995). Otherwise, pack the pelvic space and proceed with urinary diversion or with substitution if indicated. Insert suction drainage to protect the diversion, and close the wound appropriately.

Consider anticoagulation with coumarin or dose-adjusted heparin postoperatively.

PROBLEMS INTRAOPERATIVELY

Coagulopathy. After 10 units of blood replacement, coagulopathy becomes a problem, mainly because of hemodilution. Replace the blood lost, but if abnormal bleeding appears, obtain a "clotting screen" and give a platelet pack. If clotting factors are found to be significantly deficient, give at least 3000 ml of fresh frozen plasma.

Vascular Injury. Repair injured vessels without compromising the lumen (see page 81). Do not hesitate to ask for the assistance of a vascular surgeon. Be aware that ligation of the internal iliac artery to control bleeding may result in ischemia of the limb if significant obstruction is present in the external iliac or femoral arteries.

Injury to the Bowel. Rectal injury is more likely after radiation therapy. Take care when bluntly dissecting the prostate from the anterior rectal surface. Close the defect in two layers. Unless the defect is large or the patient has had radiation therapy, a diverting colostomy is not required. A pelvic abscess or rectocutaneous fistula results if the injury is not recognized.

POSTOPERATIVE CARE

Continue intravenous antibiotics (a third-generation cephalosporin) for 2 days. Maintain compression boots until the patient is ambulatory, usually the next day. Keep the nasogastric tube in place for several days until flatus is passed. A gastrostomy (see page 673) occasionally may be needed. Start intravenous hyperalimentation, and continue until the patient can tolerate a regular diet. Remove the stents after 7 to 10 days, and, if an intravenous urogram shows no leakage, remove the drains.

EN BLOC EXCISION WITH PUBECTOMY

Extend the abdominal incision down onto the periosteum of the pubis. Divide the insertions of the rectus abdominis muscles. With the periosteal elevator, free the periosteum as far as the medial edge of the obturator foramen. Divide and ligate the suspensory ligament and dorsal vein of the penis. Pass a large right-angle clamp beneath the pubic arch, draw back one end of a Gigli saw, and cut a wedge-shaped segment of pubis. Divide the puboprostatic ligaments and remove the segment.

Divide the urogenital diaphragm, and free up the membranous urethra. Reach the plane against the bulbar urethra, and dissect the urethra all the way to the corona. Excise a wedge including the glanular urethra, and suture the meatus closed. Cut the wedge transversely at the corona, and free it subcutaneously back to the previously dissected corpus spongiosum. Proceed with dissection of the prostate. Drain and close the wound appropriately, and provide for anticoagulation postoperatively with coumarin or dose-adjusted heparin.

PERINEAL CYSTOPROSTATECTOMY FOR SALVAGE
(Schmidt-Ortiz)

This approach is a minimally invasive technique suitable for minimally invasive bladder cancer in male patients suspected of having rectal adherence.

Instruments: A perineal prostatectomy set, a thoracic set (long instruments), and straight and angled clip appliers are needed.

Be certain that the patient is in optimal health. Consider staging the procedure, diverting the urine for 6 weeks before cystectomy. If the urine is not diverted, perform cystoscopy on the patient and insert ureteral catheters. Start the operation with a perineal incision, as described for total perineal prostatectomy (see page 451) because it may be impossible to separate the layers of Denonvilliers' fascia. Take care in freeing the prostate from the rectum. If the rectum is injured, close it in two layers, instill iodine solution in the rectum, and dilate the anus at the end of the operation. A proximal colostomy probably is not necessary.

After mobilizing the prostate, secure the lateral pedicles with clips and divide them. Mobilize the lateral and posterior aspects of the bladder bluntly and sharply until it is attached by peritoneum and urachus. Bluntly dissect the peritoneum free, and divide the medial umbilical ligament (urachus). If the peritoneum is adherent, enter the cul-de-sac and leave a patch of peritoneum on the bladder. Remove the specimen, approximate the levators, and close the wound. In females, an anterior exenteration is an option (see page 525).

POSTOPERATIVE PROBLEMS

Problems from the Cystectomy

Bleeding can come from one of several sources and should be controlled intraoperatively. During the node dissection, especially after irradiation, smaller veins may be torn. They can be controlled temporarily with a pack, but the pack cannot be expected to stop the bleeding. Suture-ligatures or clips are needed.

Pulmonary problems can be reduced with aggressive physiotherapy and early ambulation with adequate pain medication. If atelectasis intervenes, treat it aggressively, even resorting to bronchoscopy. Treat pneumonia with specific antibiotic therapy.

Cardiac problems are usually the result of fluid overload; give 10 to 20 mg of furosemide. Monitoring central venous pressure helps keep a balance between continuous loss of serum in the abdomen that requires correction with crystalloid and colloid solutions and excessive volume expansion with the consequent strain on the heart and lungs.

Deep vein thrombosis can be reduced by use of intermittent pressure stockings and early ambulation. Low-dose anticoagulation may be used, but it may increase bleeding and also increase lymphatic flow, leading to lymphocele formation. Routine radiographic or nuclear imaging studies are not cost effective.

Wound infection and dehiscence may be a problem (see page 18). *Adhesions* may cause intestinal obstruction, which usually resolves spontaneously with gastric decompression and total parenteral nutrition. Internal hernias, the result of mesenteric defects, may require reoperation. *Ileus* is reduced if nasogastric suction is maintained for 4 or 5 days. A gastrostomy (see page 673) is more comfortable for the patient but has disadvantages: It takes more operating time and in some cases allows intraperitoneal leakage or cutaneous leakage of gastrointestinal contents.

Diarrhea may occur from bacterial overgrowth from the bowel preparation. Superinfection with *Clostridium difficile* is secondary to antibacterial suppression of normal flora, fostered by bowel stasis and transmitted through spores from colonized patients or the hands of attending personnel. Symptoms begin postoperatively with fever and diarrhea. Pseudomembranous colitis can result. Look for polymorphonuclear leukocytes in the stool, obtain a latex agglutination immunoassay to detect the cytopathic toxin in the stool, and obtain a *C. difficile* blood titer. Stop the antibiotics and give oral metronidazole (Flagyl) first. If the infection persists, give vancomycin orally.

Gastric ulcers can be prevented by starting H$_2$-blocking agents postoperatively.

Nutrition is deficient if the patient cannot begin eating by the fifth to seventh day. If complications intervene, start total parenteral nutrition at once.

Lymphatic problems may take several forms. Lymph drainage from the wound may persist, a lymphocele may form (although because the operation is intraperitoneal, this is an uncommon complication), or lymphedema may appear in the genitalia or lower extremities, especially after radiation therapy.

Femoral neuropathy, causing weakness of the thigh and paresthesias, may occur secondary to prolonged compression of the femoral nerve by a deep-bladed self-retaining retractor.

The chance of *urethral carcinoma*, if urethrectomy was not done, warrants testing of urethral washings every 6 months.

A *fecal fistula* or *pelvic abscess* may develop especially after rectal injury, requiring diversion of the fecal stream with a colostomy or loop ileostomy (see page 669), drainage of the abscess, and provision of parenteral nutrition. The fistula will probably close spontaneously. However, if it is associated with an orthotopic neobladder as a rectourethral fistula, spontaneous closure is not to be expected; remove the neobladder, provide an ileal conduit, and close the rectal defect. If the defect is in the small intestine, resect a segment of bowel.

Sexual function may be preserved by a nerve-sparing procedure in a small proportion of highly motivated patients with cancers not involving the perivesical nodes and adjacent tissues.

Problems from the Diversion

Leakage may be managed conservatively if the area has been adequately drained. A percutaneous nephrostomy may divert enough urine to allow healing of the defect. Decompress the conduit or reservoir with a catheter even if stents are in place because they do not divert all the urine. Be certain that mucus is not blocking the outlet. Suction drainage (Jackson-Pratt) is better than Penrose drainage because it allows measurement of output, is associated with less contamination, and keeps the patient dry. Suction drainage itself may prolong leakage, as it diverts the urine from its intended course or, by contact of the tip of the drain with the anastomotic site, prevents closure of the leak. Silastic single-J stents placed intraoperatively reduce the incidence of leakage. Should *dehiscence of the ureteral anastomosis* occur, caused by inadequate mobilization of the ureter (tension), too much mobilization (ischemia and kinking), or failure to construct a watertight uroepithelium-to-uroepithelium anastomosis, conservative management usually fails and reoperation is needed. *Obstruction* of the ureteral anastomosis detected soon after operation in the absence of a stent may be due to edema or possibly to angulation at the site; a hematoma may compress the ureter. Percutaneous nephrostomy is necessary. Late obstruction is more common, increasing with time. It is usually due to local fibrosis from an early leak, although it may be caused by persistent cancer inside or outside the ureter at the anastomotic site or by a stone. Try endoscopic dilation; if necessary, excise the stricture and reanastomose the ureter. Because late strictures are not uncommon, long-term follow-up is mandatory.

Leakage at the intestinal reanastomosis is infrequent, especially with the staple technique. A *pelvic abscess* may be evidence of failure of the perioperative antibiotics but usually occurs in association with a pelvic hematoma or a urinary or fecal leak. Most can be drained percutaneously if drainage is necessary. *Pyelonephritis* is not uncommon, but an obstructive cause must be ruled out. Its onset may be delayed because of the persistent effects of perioperative antibiotics. These agents may also allow fungal overgrowth.

Late problems include *diarrhea,* especially in radiated patients. The *short bowel syndrome* appears as diarrhea, malabsorption of bile salts, and vitamin B_{12} deficiency. Treat bile salt deficiency with cholestyramine. *Vitamin B_{12} deficiency* may also appear as anemia, mental changes, or neurologic defects after the terminal ileum is harvested. Detect the disorder by obtaining vitamin B_{12} or methylmalonic acid levels at regular intervals; life-long parenteral supplementation may be needed. Carotene and folate levels also may be reduced and require supplementation. *Magnesium deficiency* may become evident with the onset of neuromuscular dysfunction and personality disorders. In contrast to the consequences of ureterosigmoidostomy, patients who have lost a large segment of colon may have a chronic mild acidosis and hypovolemia from fluid loss. *Renal failure* occurs in as many as one fifth of patients owing to pyelonephritis, stenosis at the ureteral anastomosis, electrolyte

imbalance, and reflux. *Renal calculi* are associated with chronic upper tract infection, and those in the reservoir or conduit are associated with foreign bodies, usually metal staples. Treat them endoscopically, with removal of the staple. Finally, *carcinoma* may develop, although less frequently than after ureterosigmoidostomy.

For *stomal problems,* revision may be necessary. A good enterotherapist and a supportive ileostomy association are invaluable to prevent development of such problems.

In females with bladder substitution in whom the urethra has been retained and supported, *incontinence* is rare. Whether it is desirable to spare the sympathetic innervation along the later vaginal wall has not been determined. In contrast, *hypercontinence* is more common, usually occurring late and requiring intermittent catheterization (Hautmann et al, 1996).

Commentary by Joseph D. Schmidt

Radical cystectomy and its accompanying pelvic lymph node dissection and removal of other anterior pelvic structures are formidable procedures, often performed in patients well over the age of 70. With all the improvements in surgery and anesthesia as well as perioperative support, the current mortality should be approximately 1 percent. I personally do not use anticoagulation postoperatively. The use of compression stockings as well as early ambulation generally is sufficient to prevent thromboembolism. Similarly, in my practice the indications for nerve-sparing radical cystectomy are indeed few and far between. Certainly the occasional younger male patient, particularly one with extensive CIS, may benefit from such modification.

I should like to comment on a few variations of the technique of radical cystectomy. First, rather than use formalin in the bladder, I prefer a solution of the alkylating agent thiotepa at a 1 mg/ml concentration. I am concerned with the use of formalin because any inadvertent entry into the lower urinary tract might cause serious damage to adjacent pelvic structures.

Second, the associated pelvic lymphadenectomy can be performed either extraperitoneally or intraperitoneally. For patients at high risk for lymph node metastases, open extraperitoneal lymphadenectomy can be accomplished much like that done with radical prostatectomy. Also an alternative would be laparoscopic lymph node dissection to avoid a major invasive procedure with all of its attendant risks. On the other hand, in the standard cystectomy, I extend the posterior peritoneal incisions over the iliac vessels to the inguinal ligaments and perform the en bloc lymphadenectomy in a combined intraperitoneal and extraperitoneal fashion along with removal of the bladder.

Third, in regard to the ureteral-intestinal anastomoses, I prefer to bring the bowel segment to the left ureter rather than the left ureter to the bowel segment. Most instances of ischemic stenosis of the ureteral-intestinal anastomosis occur on the left side because of excessive ureteral mobilization and ischemic scarring of that structure. Depending on the length and mobility

of the mesosigmoid colon, the bowel segment used for the conduit can be brought either through or under the mesosigmoid so that the left ureteral-intestinal anastomosis is actually made lateral to the sigmoid colon.

Fourth, as an alternative to the wide mobilization of the colon, as indicated in the text, I recommend starting with rather small posterior peritoneotomies to isolate the ureters and request frozen sections for the proximal margins of the distal ureters. These peritoneotomies can then be extended in either direction to accomplish the lymphadenectomy and cystectomy.

Fifth, with the use of urinary diversion stents that are either single J's or figure-fours, the suction and pelvic drains can be removed within the first several days, with the stents removed some 7 to 10 days postoperatively after some type of transport study has been accomplished to show that no leaks are present at the anastomoses and that good urinary transport is possible.

I would like to add some fine points to avoid the common problems of radical cystectomy. During dissection of the lateral and posterior pedicles on the first side of the cystectomy, I recommend double, if not triple, clipping of the vasculature to minimize back-bleeding. This, of course, is not required when the remaining side is controlled. For male patients who are undergoing a salvage cystectomy because of failure of prior radiation therapy, I believe that a perineal exposure of the prostate and rectum is mandatory in an attempt to minimize rectal injury. If radical cystectomy is not possible because of more extensive disease than initially determined, the perineal wound can easily be closed, with Penrose drainage for a day or two.

Lastly, a reminder on the technique for closing any inadvertent rectal injury at the time of radical cystectomy: I recommend an initial continuous suture of absorbable material for the mucosa and submucosa followed by interrupted Lembert nonabsorbable sutures (NAS) in the rectal muscularis. I certainly do agree with the testing of the rectotomy closure, as indicated in the text along with anal sphincter dilation.

Urethrectomy

URETHRECTOMY IN THE MALE

Consider urethrectomy, especially if bladder tumors are multiple or involve the bladder neck or posterior urethra or if carcinoma in situ (CIS) is present in the bladder or prostatic urethra. Urethrectomy may not be indicated for the elderly or poor-risk patient or for those with advanced disease, but these patients must be followed diligently with urethral washings. With positive findings, urethrectomy is necessary. Potency is less easily preserved than after radical cystectomy alone because the erec-

tor nerves accompany the urethra closely through the urogenital diaphragm.

At the completion of the cystectomy up to division of the puboprostatic ligaments (see page 510), clamp the balloon catheter just outside the urethral meatus and divide it.

Position: Place the patient in an exaggerated lithotomy position by raising the leg braces until the hips are flexed 60 degrees.

1 *Incision:* Incise the midline of the perineum from the base of the scrotum to within 3 cm of the anus, ending over the palpable urethral bulb. For greater exposure, the alternatives are a U-shaped incision as for perineal prostatectomy *(shaded dashes)* or a midline incision with two lateral extensions placed at 120-degree angles (Mercedes-Benz incision) *(black dashed lines)*.

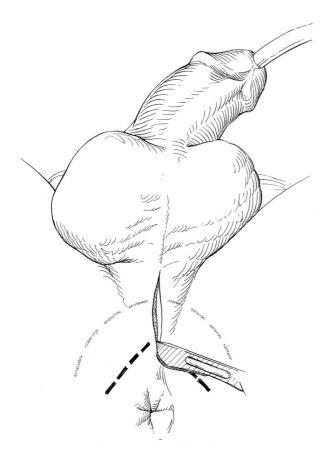

2 Divide the subcutaneous tissues to expose the bulbocavernosus muscle. Insert a ring retractor. Sharply incise the fibers of the bulbospongiosus and superficial transverse perineal muscles in the midline, and retract them to expose the corpus spongiosum. Pass a small Penrose drain around the exposed corpus. Identify and ligate the arteries to the bulb. The argon coagulator helps in attaining hemostasis on raw surfaces.

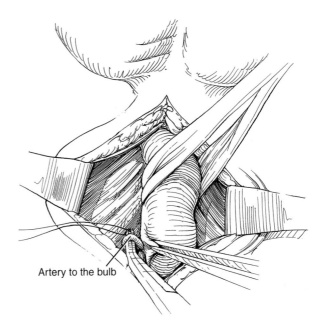
Artery to the bulb

3 Separate the distal portion of the corpus spongiosum and urethra from the undersurface of the corpora cavernosa, progressively invaginating the penis into the penile skin up to the base of the glans (Whitmore and Mount, 1970). Close an opening into the body of the corpora cavernosa with a figure-eight stitch. Expect corporal tumescence, which subsides after evagination of the penis.

4 Place a Penrose drain around the urethra and complete the dissection. Divide the urethra under vision where it enters the proximal part of the glans *(dashed line)*. Let the penis return to its normal position.

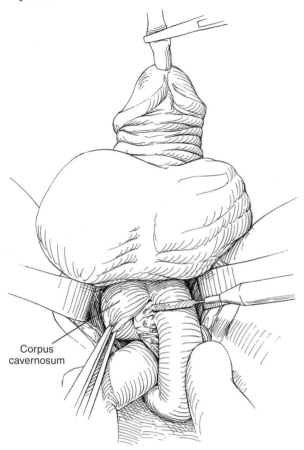

Corpus
cavernosum

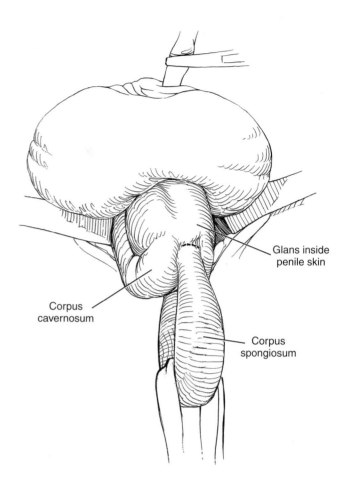

Glans inside
penile skin

Corpus
cavernosum

Corpus
spongiosum

5 Excise the distal urethra, including the fossa navicularis, by a wedge resection. Close the wound in the glans; be alert for oozing.

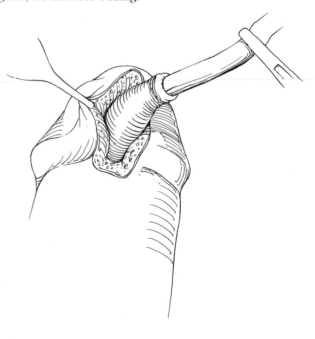

6 Dissect proximally with the scissors and electrocautery, incising the bulbocavernosus muscle to the urogenital diaphragm. Avoid too much traction, which might tear the urethra away at the triangular ligament. Keep close to the urethra as the urogenital diaphragm is approached to preserve the erector nerves. Enlarge the urethral hiatus through the diaphragm. Palpate and isolate the large bulbourethral branches of the internal pudendal arteries. Clip and divide them where they enter the bulb at the 4- and 8-o'clock positions. Avoid fulguration there. Divide the puboprostatic ligaments from above (see page 509), and sharply dissect the remaining attachments from above and below in order to withdraw the specimen from the abdominal wound.

Female Urethrectomy

7 If the urethra has not already been resected from above, make a horseshoe incision around the urethra and connect its limbs to the vaginal incisions made from above. Remove the urethra with the anterior wall of the vagina. Either retubularize the vagina with absorbable sutures, or close the vagina by bringing the posterior inferior vaginal edge to the subclitoral edge. Reinforcement of the perineum may be required. If so, use a myocutaneous gracilis flap, which facilitates subsequent vaginal construction (see pages 50 to 53).

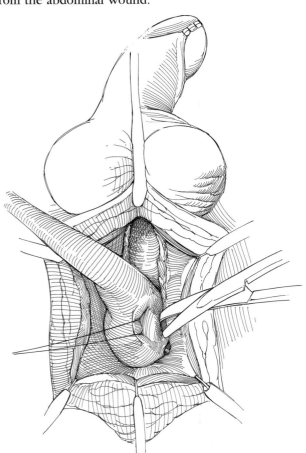

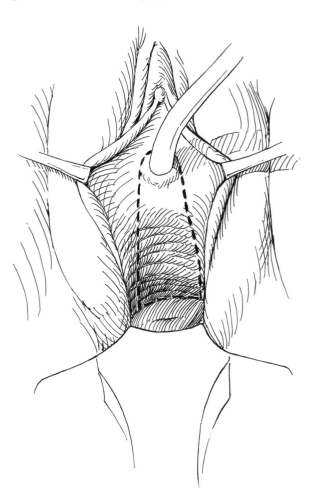

Male Urethrectomy as a Separate Procedure

Place the patient in the exaggerated lithotomy position, and insert a sound in the urethra to facilitate the dissection. Care must be used in excising the proximal urethral end because small bowel is often lurking just above the urogenital diaphragm.

Enlarge the urethral hiatus through the urogenital diaphragm. Dissect the proximal portion cautiously to avoid avulsion. Very carefully divide the urethra at its junction with the pelvic contents; it may be adherent to the bowel. Remove the specimen.

Close the bulbospongiosus muscle, subcutaneous tissue, and skin after placing a small Penrose drain in the tract to exit through a small incision near the frenulum. A bulky dressing held in place by elastic adhesive tape can reduce postoperative oozing.

For *posterior urethral carcinoma*, approach the urethra perineally, and remove the perineal soft tissue with the specimen. For extensive carcinoma, resect the inferior aspect of the pubic bone as well.

POSTOPERATIVE PROBLEMS

Bleeding is seldom of concern, although temporary *edema* and *hematoma* formation are common. *Penile ischemia* is very unlikely. *Perineal hernia* may appear if the area around the urogenital diaphragm has been involved in infection, radiation, or transurethral resection of the prostate such that dissection must be performed laterally in the levators and transverse perineal musculature. Bring the ischiocavernosus muscles together in the midline, and reapproximate the bulbospongiosus muscle and dartos fascia to prevent herniation.

Commentary by David L. McCullough

I generally prefer to perform the urethrectomy at a separate procedure 4 to 6 weeks after the cystectomy. This is better tolerated in older patients and gives one the luxury of studying the cystectomy specimen in minute pathologic detail to determine whether urethrectomy is really required. The fossa navicularis incision should be closed with a deep figure-eight absorbable suture because of its tendency to bleed. Patients should be warned that they will have ecchymosis of the penis and perineum. Two 0.25-inch Penrose drains can be brought out through separate stab wounds in the perineum and left for 24 hours, or one Jackson-Pratt drain can be placed in the wound for drainage as long as is necessary. As described before, a bulky cotton-fluff perineal dressing left in place for 24 hours is invaluable in preventing oozing. We begin sitz baths as soon as the drains are pulled; they afford great comfort to the patient.

If one has begun the procedure with a linear incision over the urethra and exposure is not optimal, it can be enhanced by converting it to a Mercedes-Benz incision by adding two incisions at 120 degrees to the original one. One of the most difficult aspects of the procedure is getting purchase on the most proximal urethra near the urogenital diaphragm. Several Babcock clamps placed around the catheter-containing urethra at that level are often helpful in obtaining additional traction, which enhances the proximal dissection. Plastic or metal self-retaining ring retractors are invaluable in exposing the entire field.

Pelvic Lymphadenectomy

OPEN TECHNIQUE

The limits for node dissection are: laterally, the genitofemoral nerve; medially, the bladder; cephalad, the bifurcation of the common iliac artery; and caudad, the endopelvic fascia. If a radiation dose of 5000 rads has been given, omit dissection in the area around the external iliac vessels.

Lymphadenectomy in the Male

1 **A,** *Position:* Lithotomy position with legs in gynecologic leg holders. Alternatively, use a hyperextended supine position. Insert a 22 F, 5-ml silicone balloon catheter. Drape sterilely with a barrier sheet, towels, and a half sheet under the buttocks. Place perileggings or Mayo stand covers over the legs. Apply a laparotomy sheet.

Incision: Make a midline incision from the symphysis to 5 inches above the umbilicus (see page 867), deviating it away from the stoma site. Enter the peritoneum near the umbilicus, insert two fingers, and complete the peritoneal opening cephalad. If the patient has had a previous partial cystectomy or cystostomy, excise that tract en bloc with the bladder.

Explore the abdominal contents systematically. This includes the liver, the undersurfaces of both diaphragms, the spleen and other viscera, the omentum, the paracolic gutters, and the peritoneal surfaces. Free adhesions. Take needle biopsy specimens of suspicious hepatic lesions. Palpate the para-aortic nodes with the hand medial to the descending colon. Inspect the pelvic viscera for metastatic spread.

Free the lower margin of the peritoneum from the posterior rectus sheath on each side; avoid tearing the inferior epigastric veins.

B, Develop a V-flap of peritoneum with its apex at the umbilicus to include the urachus and its arms at the external rings bilaterally, just medial to the cord structures.

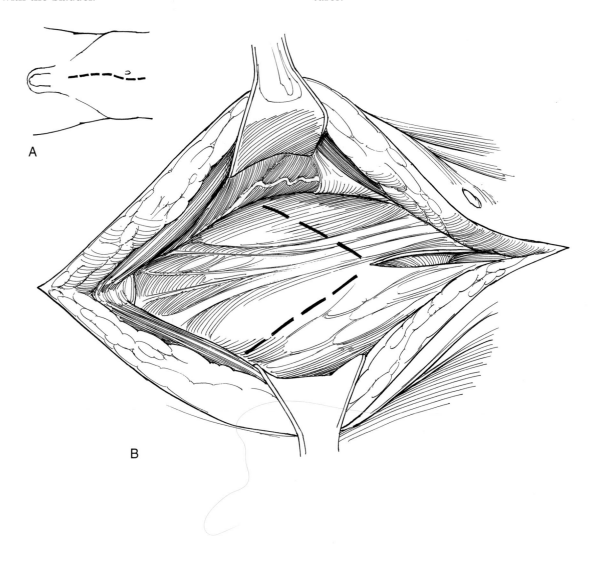

A

B

2 Preserve the inferior epigastric vessels. Grasp the apex of the peritoneum in a clamp for exposure.

3 Pass the index finger under the curving edge of peritoneum from the direction of the external iliac vessels, as shown. Alternatively, it may be easier to introduce the finger from above, beginning at the level of the common iliac artery. Sharply divide the elevated portion of peritoneum and adventitia anterior to the external iliac vessels, extending from above the bifurcation of the common iliac artery. Clip or fulgurate the tissue. Divide the vas deferens in the course of this incision. Ligate or clip the proximal end, and place a long silk suture on the distal end for later identification. This exposes the femoral canal and the external iliac vein. Locate the ureters bilaterally as they pass in front of the common iliac artery, and isolate them with small Penrose drains. They may be divided distally if one is certain of proceeding with cystectomy.

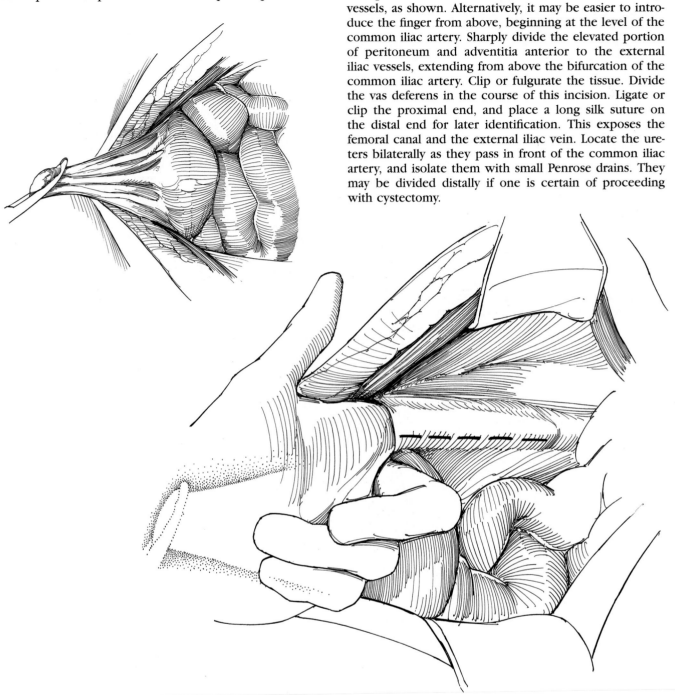

4 Place an opened gauze pad over the left hand and retract the iliac vessels medially and inferiorly. First, bluntly using closed scissors, clear the tissue from the psoas and iliopsoas muscles, then from the exposed posterolateral aspect of the common and external iliac veins. Watch for branches to the psoas muscle from these vessels.

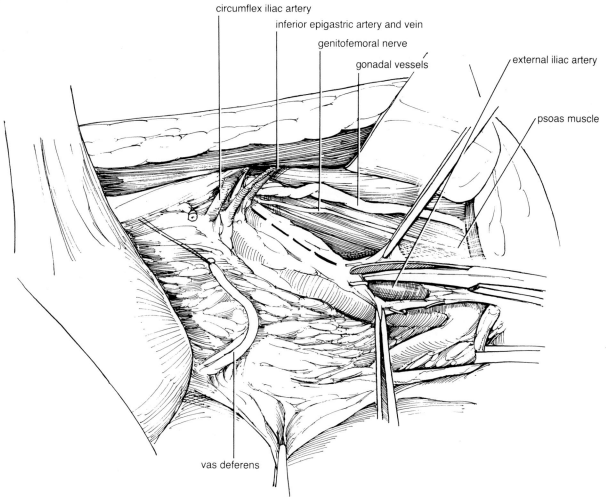

circumflex iliac artery

inferior epigastric artery and vein

genitofemoral nerve

gonadal vessels

external iliac artery

psoas muscle

vas deferens

5 On the right side, incise and reflect the adventitia along the lateral aspect of the external iliac artery from 2 cm above the bifurcation of the common iliac artery to the level of the inguinal ligament. Enter the subadventitial planes around the iliac artery and vein in order to strip the perivascular tissues cleanly from the vessels.

Expose and preserve the circumflex iliac and inferior epigastric vessels. Also preserve the genitofemoral nerve. Dissect the contents of the femoral canal immediately medial to the external iliac vein, and carefully clip or divide it between ligatures, to secure not only anomalous obturator vessels but also the major lymphatics from the leg.

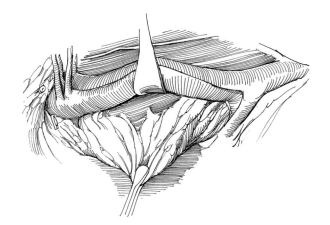

6 Continue dissection along the inferomedial aspect of the retracted external iliac vein to the level of origin of the internal iliac artery, exposing the underlying iliopsoas muscle. Watch for an obturator tributary to the external iliac vein, which is present in one quarter of cases. If one is found, ligate or clip it and divide it.

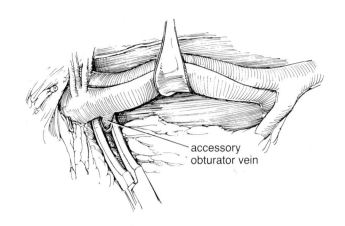

accessory obturator vein

7 Bluntly dissect the fat and areolar tissue from the fascia covering the muscles of the inferolateral pelvic wall around the obturator foramen to define the obturator nerve and vascular bundle. Retract the bladder medially to dissect in the obturator fossa, and gently pull out the important nodal tissue and fat, clearly exposing the obturator vessels and nerve. Tie the vessels near the pelvic wall, and divide them while protecting the nerve. If the obturator vessels escape clamping and ligation, pack absorbable hemostatic gauze into the obturator foramen to control bleeding. Bluntly mobilize the nodal tissue medially from the nerve as you retract it laterally. Do not bother to clamp and ligate the multiple small venous tributaries running from the pelvic wall; just divide them "long" near the nodal tissue.

Proceed medially to the termination of the obturator vein in the internal iliac (hypogastric) venous plexus, at which point ligate and divide it. Treat the obturator artery similarly. This cleans the posterior pelvic wall of nodal tissue and fat and exposes the internal iliac artery. Note a 2- to 3-cm fat pad loosely attached lateral to the rectum; bluntly pluck it out to expose an anatomic defect in the endopelvic fascia at the posteromedial border of the levator ani muscle and lateral to the rectum. If an exenteration is planned (see page 525), develop an avascular areolar plane bluntly posterior to the rectum and in front of the sacrum through this fascial defect. Remove the specimen, and orient it for the pathologist. Send suspicious nodes for frozen-section examination. Proceed with a similar procedure on the left side. Place Jackson-Pratt suction drains and close the wound.

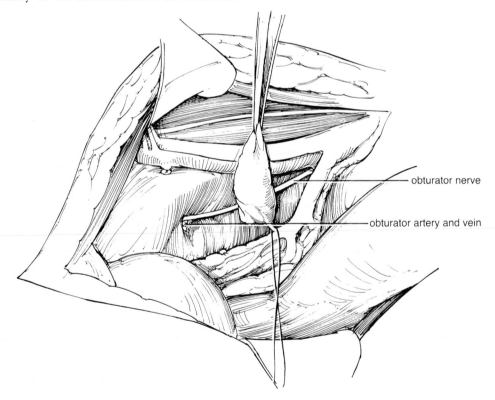

obturator nerve

obturator artery and vein

POSTOPERATIVE PROBLEMS

A *lymphocele* may form as the bowel falls down and seals off a portion of the peritoneal cavity. It is not common and is usually small but may become symptomatic. Locate it ultrasonically; then aspirate it and inject tetracycline. Laparoscopic drainage with formation of a window is an option for a large lymphocele, especially if it is infected or obstructs venous return from the legs. Open drainage is seldom needed. *Lymphedema* of the legs is not common if extensive dissection lateral to the iliac vessels is avoided in patients subjected to previous pelvic radiation therapy.

Thrombus formation may be reduced by early ambulation, made possible if ketorolac tromethamine (Toradol) analgesia is given instead of narcotics. Ambulation plus the use of pulsatile stockings is currently the most effective method of avoiding deep vein thrombosis (DVT). Although minidose heparin (5000 units subcutaneously every 12 hours) is safe, it is not necessary if the other measures are instituted, unless the patient is obese or has other risk factors. *Postoperative bleeding* is usually the result of failure to dissect and visualize the pelvic vasculature.

Obturator nerve injury occurs as a large fixed tumor is resected, rarely during a routine node dissection. Prescribe physical therapy; usually other muscle groups take over. It is possible for branches of the lateral femoral cutaneous and genitofemoral nerves to be injured, resulting in paresthesias in the upper thigh or in the groin and scrotum. Finally, *pelvic abscess* may result from a rectal injury.

Commentary by Jean B. deKernion

Pelvic lymphadenectomy is an integral part of radical cystectomy or partial cystectomy for bladder cancer. In these cases, the operation should indeed begin in the common iliac vessels and extend to the inguinal canal and the inguinal ligaments. However, when performed in conjunction with a radical prostatectomy, the operation should be more confined, excluding the tissue around the external iliac artery, and should extend only to the bifurcation. It should also be performed extraperitoneally.

Dissection of the tissue from the iliac artery is often facilitated by first entering the plane of dissection at the common iliac artery and sharply dividing the adventitia as well as the peritoneum and the fatty tissue for a distance on to the external iliac artery. A finger can then be insinuated in that plane and worked distally all the way to the area of the inguinal ligament. That tissue can then be fulgurated or clipped and divided, along with the vas deferens. This defines the lateral extent of the dissection on the pelvic floor, and all the tissue medial to that point is reflected from behind the pubic bone medially. This exposes the femoral canal and the external iliac vein.

The bundle of tissue emerging from the femoral canal must be carefully secured because all lymphatics from the lower extremity and the groin drain through this route. Similarly, at the superior extent of the dissection near the bifurcation of the iliac vessels, the tissue should be carefully clipped or fulgurated.

Dissection in the obturator fossa is greatly facilitated by retracting the bladder medially. Unless a pelvic exenteration is planned, it is not necessary to dissect much more posterior than the obturator nerve. If one is excising extensive lymphadenopathy (which is rarely indicated), the tissue in the fossa should be dissected down to the deep branches of the internal iliac vein.

At the bifurcation of the iliac vessels, the lymph node dissection should include skeletonization of the upper portion of the internal iliac artery. This provides a convenient point to end that part of the dissection and also allows proper identification and dissection of the superior vesical artery. The superior vesical artery helps guide the subsequent blunt dissection to identify all of the vessels emerging from the internal iliac, usually called the "lateral vascular pedicle." The artery is most easily identified by completing most or all of the lymph node dissection. The medial traction on the bladder is removed, and the bladder is grasped and lifted upward.

During dissection of the external iliac vein or the branches of the internal iliac, it is important to minimize retraction or compression of the vein, which may promote thrombus development. Occasionally, a branch into the vein is torn or a deep branch of the internal iliac vein is opened. This is best managed by grasping the opening with a small Allis clamp and suturing the defect with 5-0 vascular silk, causing as little narrowing of the lumen of the external iliac vein as possible. The obturator nerve should never be completely divided but is sometimes traumatized during the dissection. If the nerve is inadvertently divided, it should be approximated with several very fine wire sutures to promote at least some return of function (see page 63). Patients whose obturator nerves are damaged must be cautioned about the risks of driving, especially if the injury involves the right obturator nerve. Usually, with the aid of physical therapy, other muscle groups assume the role of the obturator and the injury becomes inconsequential except in the very athletic.

The use of postoperative drainage is imperative in a patient who has had a pelvic lymphadenectomy. We currently prefer Jackson-Pratt suction drains, but any drain is suitable.

DVT and pulmonary embolism are the most feared complications of major pelvic surgery. The use of pulsatile stockings, intraoperatively and postoperatively, has markedly reduced the incidence of thrombosis. In addition, most of our patients are now managed with ketorolac analgesic, with little or no narcotic analgesic. This enables them to ambulate and move actively immediately after surgery. DVT has now become an extremely rare complication of pelvic surgery at our institution. The use of minidose heparin (5000 units subcutaneously every 12 hours) is quite safe. We used this regimen in almost 300 patients undergoing lymphadenectomy as part of a radical retropubic prostatectomy, with no incidence of pulmonary embolism and only two cases of manifest clinical DVT. However, we have abandoned routine anticoagulation in favor of pulsatile stockings and ambulation. Patients who have several risk factors, such as a history of DVT and severe obesity, may still be candidates for the minidose heparin regimen.

Similarly, wound and pelvic infections occur rarely in the era of perioperative prophylactic antibiotics. Clinically detectable and significant lymphoceles are likewise extremely rare, occurring in less than 1 percent of patients. Lymphedema should also be a rare complication as long as the procedure is modified in patients with prior radiation therapy or other risk factors.

In summary, pelvic lymph node dissection remains an integral part of radical pelvic surgery for bladder and prostate cancer. Careful and thorough dissection, as defined in this chapter, is especially important in bladder cancer patients because prevailing evidence suggests that some patients with microscopic nodal metastases limited to the pelvis can be cured by the procedure. Extensive nodal metastases beyond the pelvis invariably indicate distant metastases with little hope for cure by any surgical technique. In addition to a curative potential in patients with minimal metastatic adenopathy, the procedure provides valuable staging information as a guide to subsequent systemic treatment in patients with extensive nodal metastases.

Lymphadenectomy in the Female

For cervical cancer, the limits of the dissection are the psoas muscle and pelvic wall veins laterally, the internal iliac artery and its continuation, the superior vesical artery medially, the obturator nerve posteriorly, the bifurcation of the aorta cephalad, and the femoral canal beneath the inguinal ligament caudad.

8 *Incision:* Work from the side of the table opposite the involved lymph nodes. Make a midline transperitoneal incision (see page 867) from well above the umbilicus, and carry it down over the symphysis pubis. Alternatively, stay extraperitoneally. The round ligament must usually be divided and care exercised to avoid the inferior epigastric vessels. Incise the parietal peritoneum lateral to the external iliac artery below the infundibulopelvic ligament; expose the ureter and keep it under direct vision at all times. Clamp, transect, and ligate the ligament with 2-0 SAS. Extend the peritoneal incision with the scissors down to the round ligament along the line of the external iliac artery. Clamp, clip, and divide the round ligament.

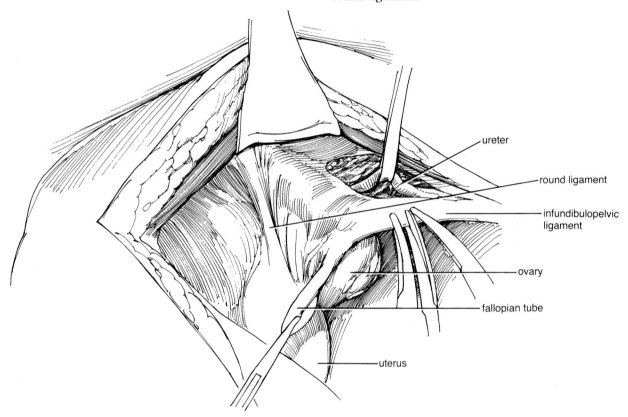

ureter

round ligament

infundibulopelvic ligament

ovary

fallopian tube

uterus

9 Start the node dissection at the junction of the internal iliac artery, clearing the tissue lateral to the external iliac artery first. Exercise care to avoid the genitofemoral nerve, which courses on the surface of the psoas muscle. Clamp this lateral tissue bundle, divide it, and ligate it proximally to close the lymphatic channels. Use the clamp on the distal end of the tissue for traction to allow dissection down the lateral border of the external iliac artery. Once the space is developed lateral to the artery, the index finger may be inserted behind the external iliac artery and vein and the nodal tissue gently dissected free of the side wall to the level of the obturator nerve. Include the nodal tissue medial to the artery as the dissection progresses down to the entrance of the femoral canal, where several nodes are found. Send the specimen from this area, properly oriented, for examination by frozen section.

10 Dissect the tissue from the medial surface of the iliac vein, and approach the obturator fossa. Locate the obturator nerve, uncover the obturator fossa lying inferiorly and medially, and dissect the tissue between the nerve and the superior vesical artery. Clamp, cut, and ligate this bundle close to the femoral canal. The veins there only loosely correspond to the arteries and are more numerous. Because they are easily injured behind and lateral to the obturator nerve, avoid dissecting into this area. Injury of the veins in the pelvic wall plexus can result in massive hemorrhage that can be very difficult to control. Apply pressure with your finger or a stick sponge; get some help to expose and control the vessel. Do not clamp blindly.

11 It may be desirable also to divide the superior vesical pedicle.

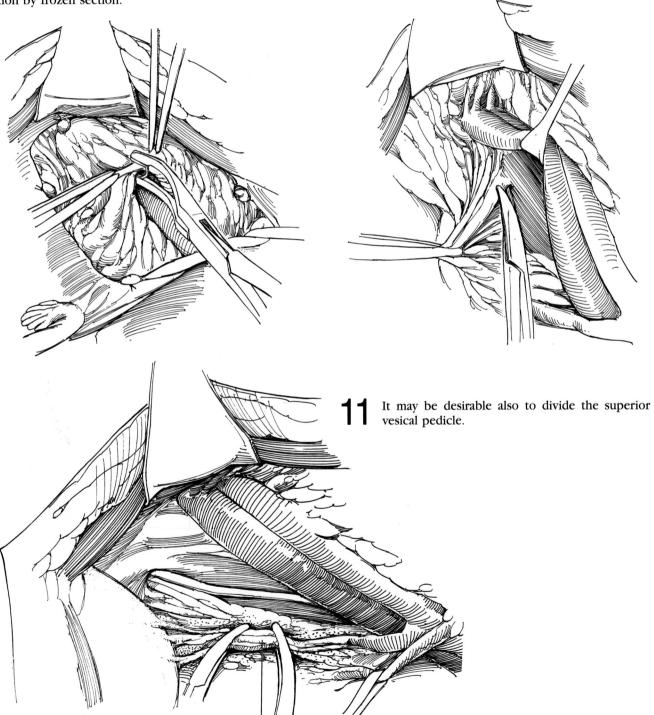

Superior vesical pedicle

12 Clamp, divide, and ligate the uterine artery. Clear the internal iliac nodes from the internal iliac artery and vein by successively dividing the medial branches. Repeat the procedure on the opposite side. Submit the specimens for frozen-section examination. If they are negative for malignancy, proceed with cystectomy (see page 505) or anterior exenteration (see page 525).

uterine artery

POSTOPERATIVE PROBLEMS

Wound infection is not common. If *lymphatic drainage* is found issuing from the wound, instill tetracycline into the tract. A *lymphocele* may form as the bowel falls down and seals off a portion of the peritoneal cavity. It is usually small but may become symptomatic. Locate it ultrasonically; then aspirate it and inject tetracycline. Laparoscopic drainage with formation of a window is an option for a large lymphocele, especially if it is infected or obstructs venous return from the legs. Open drainage is seldom needed. The incidence of lymphoceles has been greatly reduced in recent years by use of suction drains.

Edema of the legs is an uncommon problem but is more likely to occur if the patient has had pelvic irradiation. Sparing the lymphatic trunks by not dissecting lateral to the iliac vessels has reduced the incidence of this complication, but in the female with cervical carcinoma it is advisable to take all the lymphatic trunks because of the significant incidence of external iliac node metastases. Massive *venous bleeding* can occur if the important vessels are not visualized by an adequate dissection. *Major vein thrombosis* is reduced by early ambulation and sequential compression stockings.

Obturator nerve injury occurs when a large fixed tumor is being resected; rarely does it occur during a routine node dissection. If this prominent nerve is not identified and separated from the nodal tissue, injury is possible. Division of the obturator nerve is usually innocuous but may result in significant adductor weakness. *Paresthesias* in the groin, labia, and anterior thigh may appear if the lateral femoral cutaneous or genitofemoral nerves are injured. *Pelvic abscess* may result from a rectal injury. *Other complications* include prolonged ileus, urinary tract infection, and atelectasis.

LAPAROSCOPIC PELVIC LYMPHADENECTOMY

Section 11 contains a description of pelvic node dissection by the laparoscopic technique for carcinoma of the prostate. For carcinoma of the bladder, the limits of dissection are extended.

Mobilize both the sigmoid colon and cecum medially by dissection along the white lines. Dissect to the genitofemoral nerve laterally, and clear the tissue at the bifurcation of the external and internal iliac arteries and over the common iliac artery proximally. It is necessary to take precautions to protect the ureter.

LAPAROSCOPIC DRAINAGE OF PELVIC LYMPHOCELE

Induce pneumoperitoneum, and introduce an 11-mm trocar subumbilically, a second 11-mm trocar in the upper quadrant of the affected side, and a 5-mm trocar in the midline 6 cm below the umbilicus. Free any adhesions with the suction-irrigator (see page 525), and tilt the table to expose the lymphocele. Identify the ureter and other retroperitoneal structures.

Pick up the wall of the lymphocele in atraumatic forceps, and open it with either electrocautery or scissors. Aspirate and irrigate the interior of the lymphocele with antibiotic solution. Cut a very generous window in the wall with scissors. Inspect the interior, looking for septa that need to be penetrated. Carefully release the omentum and hold it in the cavity with clips. Inspect the abdomen, and leave the abdomen systematically.

Pelvic Exenteration

ANTERIOR EXENTERATION IN THE FEMALE

Instruments: Instruments are the same as those for radical cystectomy (see page 505). An Omni retractor (Minnesota Scientific) can provide both superficial and deep exposure.

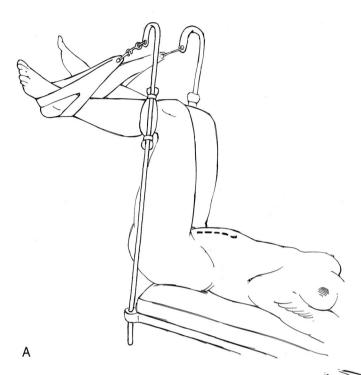

A

1 A, *Position:* If the urethra is involved, use St. Mark's position, a not-quite-full lithotomy position that is less taxing on the lower extremities during a prolonged procedure. Place the thighs abducted at 45 degrees to the body with the legs parallel to the floor, supported in cradles. If the urethra is not involved, the supine position is acceptable, with the legs placed in the frog-leg position so that the urethra and vagina may be approached at the level of the perineum during the procedure. If the entire rectum is to be taken, have the buttocks overhang the end of the table so that it may be excised perineally. Take great precautions against injuring the peroneal nerve or instigating the anterior compartment syndrome. After preparing and draping that includes the vagina, insert a balloon catheter into the bladder and drain it.

B, Complete the pelvic lymphadenectomy (see page 517). If no malignancy is found in the specimens, divide the ureters at their exit from the paracervical tunnel. (If the patient has had pelvic radiation, transect the ureters above the pelvic brim.) Send a portion for frozen-section examination; if findings are positive, resect more of the ureter and repeat the examination until the findings are negative. Ligate the distal ureteral stumps. Spatulate the ureters, insert an 8 F infant feeding tube proximally in each, and suture them in place. Open the space of Retzius by incising the peritoneal reflection over the bladder *(dashed line)*. Place a large hysterectomy forceps on each uterine cornu to include the round ligaments, fallopian tubes, and utero-ovarian ligaments to reduce back-bleeding and facilitate dissection.

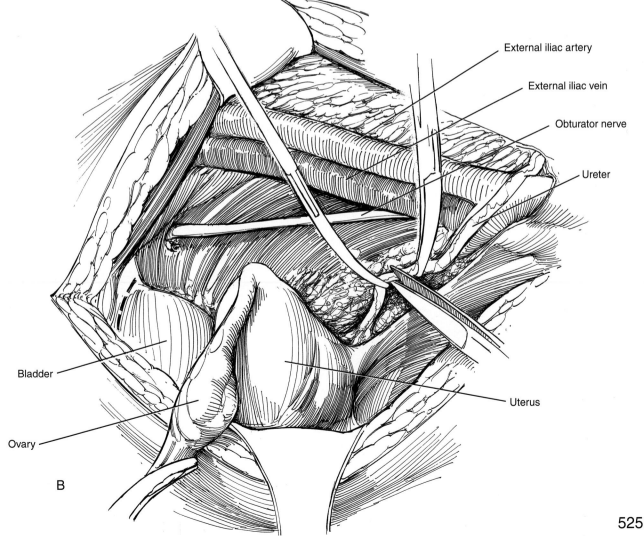

External iliac artery

External iliac vein

Obturator nerve

Ureter

Uterus

Bladder

Ovary

B

525

2 Dissect the anterior bladder wall to the level of the endopelvic fascia, exposing the entire urethra. Clear the fascia bilaterally, and incise it on each side to allow for better exposure of the urethra all the way to the perineum.

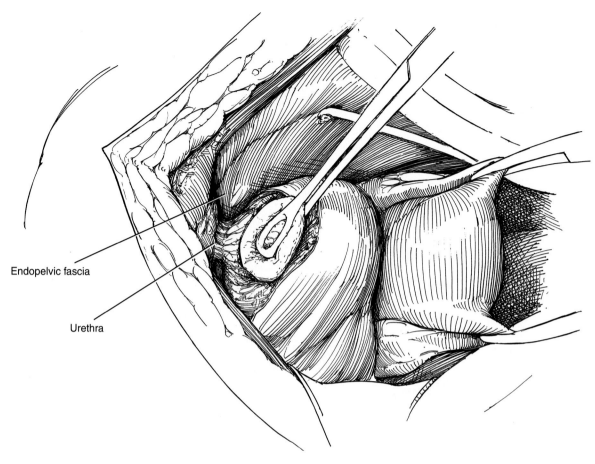

Endopelvic fascia

Urethra

3 Clamp, divide, and ligate the round ligament at the pelvic sidewall. Do the same for the broad ligament, including the ovarian vessels, to free the lateral and posterior attachments of the uterus, tubes, and ovaries. Incise the peritoneum in the cul-de-sac, and dissect the rectum from the posterior wall of the vagina for several centimeters. Place a stick sponge into the posterior fornix of the vagina, and apply pressure cephalad to define the extent of the vagina and aid in the dissection posterior to the vagina. Clamp, divide, and suture-ligate the uterosacral ligament on both sides.

4 Doubly clamp the right cardinal ligament with curved Kocher clamps; divide and ligate it. Keep well anterior to avoid the pelvic plexus. Do the same for the left cardinal ligament.

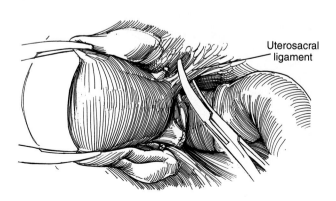

Uterosacral ligament

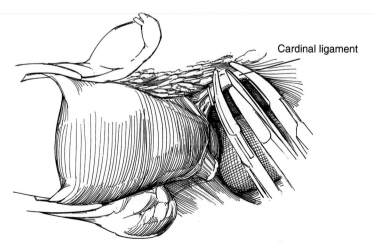

Cardinal ligament

5 Clamp, divide, and ligate the lateral vesical pedicles at the level of the incised endopelvic fascia with 2-0 nonabsorbable suture to expose the sidewall of the vagina. Place a stick sponge in the posterior fornix of the vagina, open the vagina over it with the cutting current, and incise the lateral wall for a short distance. Suture the cuff with a hemostatic running locking 1-0 CCG suture. Continue to cut and suture until the lateral vaginal wall is divided to within several centimeters of the endopelvic fascia. Identify and suture-ligate the dorsal vein of the clitoris. Dissect the urethra to the perineum and excise it. Divide the anterior vaginal wall several centimeters

above the perineum, and remove the entire specimen, including the urethra, bladder, and anterior vaginal wall with the uterus, tubes, and ovaries, en bloc. Close the posterior wall of the vagina by bringing it to the short anterior leaf. Place a warm pack in the area, and proceed with a urinary diversion procedure. Defer vaginal reconstruction until after recovery and healing.

Irrigate the pelvic basin. Insert a suction drain through a stab wound in the lower quadrant. Reperitonealize the floor of the pelvis. Use the omentum or sigmoid colon to fill the space, especially if total exenteration has been done.

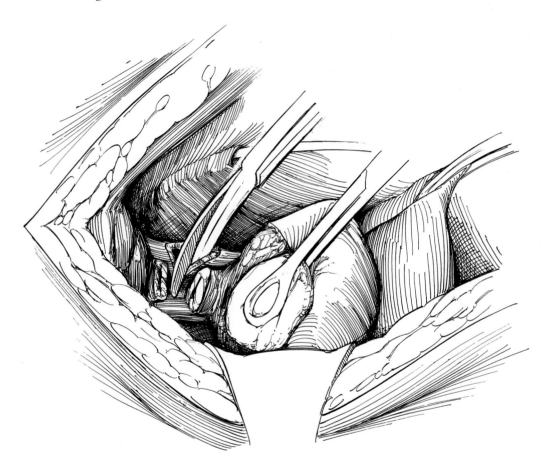

TOTAL PELVIC EXENTERATION IN THE FEMALE

6 Proceed as described through Step 4. Incise the sigmoid mesentery perpendicular to the bowel at a level that provides adequate circulation to the proximal segment. Divide the superior hemorrhoidal artery where it crosses the left common iliac artery. Transect the sigmoid colon between Kocher clamps placed below the superior hemorrhoidal artery, between it and the middle hemorrhoidal vessels. This prevents fecal spill. Oversew the end of the distal segment with a 1-0 SAS, removing the clamp. Alternatively, transect the colon with the gastrointestinal anastomosis (GIA) stapler.

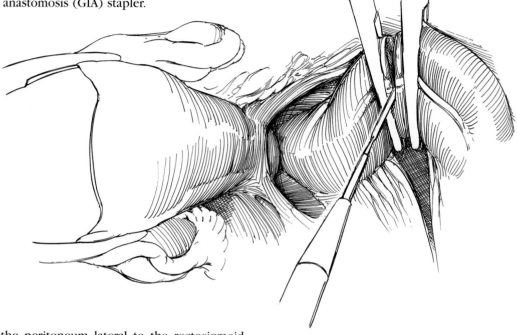

7 Incise the peritoneum lateral to the rectosigmoid, and slide a hand into the hollow of the sacrum behind the sigmoid to the level of the levators. Sharply incise any fibrous attachments. Elevate the segment, and clamp, divide, and ligate the lateral rectal stalks. Dissect distally to expose the endopelvic fascia and distal end of the coccyx. This frees the rectum posteriorly and laterally.

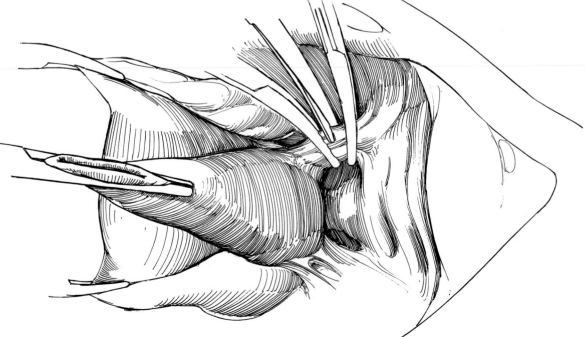

8 Progressively divide the urethra, vagina, and rectum, and remove the specimen. (If the operation is for vesical carcinoma, remove the urethra to the level of the perineum.) Oversew the ends of these three structures to provide hemostasis. Cover as much of the raw surface as possible with peritoneum, or bring an omental pedicle into the area and tack it to the pelvic sidewalls.

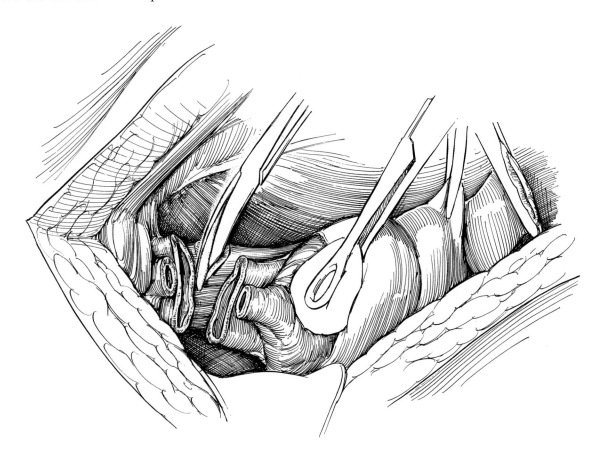

Rectal Resection

For removal of the entire rectum, approach the area perineally (not shown). Close the anus with a running silk suture. Make a circumferential incision, and incise the subcutaneous tissue. Divide the central tendon. Expose and incise the pubococcygeal muscle, and expose Waldeyer's fascia, the stout avascular structure running from the anterior sacrum to the anorectal junction. Incise this fascia sharply to allow placement of the hand in the sacral hollow.

Excise a circle of skin and subcutaneous tissue in the left lower abdominal quadrant, and incise the fascia, muscle, and peritoneum. Bring the distal end of the remainder of the sigmoid colon through the defect, and fashion an everting stoma (see pages 654 to 655). If ureteroileostomy is the method of urinary diversion with a stoma in the right lower quadrant, place the colonic stoma higher on the abdomen by the width of the stoma. Proceed with urinary diversion. Irrigate the pelvic cavity. Insert suction tubes through lower quadrant stab wounds. Reperitonealize the floor of the pelvis. Use the omentum or sigmoid colon to fill the space. An organic iodine pack may be left in the vagina. Close the abdominal wound in layers without Penrose drains, irrigating the subcutaneous layer before closing the skin.

Remove the pack in 2 days and the suction drains after urograms show no leakage.

TOTAL PELVIC EXENTERATION IN THE MALE

The indications for total pelvic exenteration in the male are few. It is seldom of value when vesical carcinoma is too advanced for removal by radical cystectomy. However, it may provide palliation or prolong life in patients with prostatic sarcoma, squamous carcinoma of the urethra, or seminal vesicular involvement from rectal carcinoma.

Prepare the patient as for radical cystectomy. Consider hypotensive anesthesia with continuous epidural block. Begin intravenous hydration with lactated Ringer's solution or 5 percent dextrose in 0.5 percent normal saline the afternoon before surgery. Shave the patient from the nipples to upper thighs. Apply elastic stockings. Use polyethylene glycol electrolyte solution (GoLYTELY) as a mechanical bowel preparation. Give oral neomycin sulfate and erythromycin base in three doses of 1 g the day before surgery and a parenteral antibiotic the morning of surgery.

Position (Step 1A): Place the buttocks on a sandbag overhanging the end of the table so that the rectum may be excised perineally. Place the patient in a 20-degree Trendelenburg position.

Preparation: Prepare the abdomen and perineum. Seal the anus with a purse-string suture. Apply drapes. Insert a 24 F urethral balloon catheter. Clip the catheter to the drapes under the leg so that it is accessible. Drape the perineum separately with a folded towel. Stand on the left side of the table.

Incision: Make a midline (see page 867) or left paramedian incision (see page 869), extending to the left of the umbilicus from above the umbilicus to the symphysis.

9 *Blood supply to the pelvis:* The inferior mesenteric artery supplies the lower portion of the left colon through the left colic artery and the sigmoid colon through the sigmoid artery. The sigmoid artery gives off the inferior left colic arteries and the superior rectal artery. It is divided beyond the take-off of the left colic artery. Note the relationship with the vascular supply to the pelvic organs, where the internal iliac can be temporarily clamped and the superior vesical artery ligated.

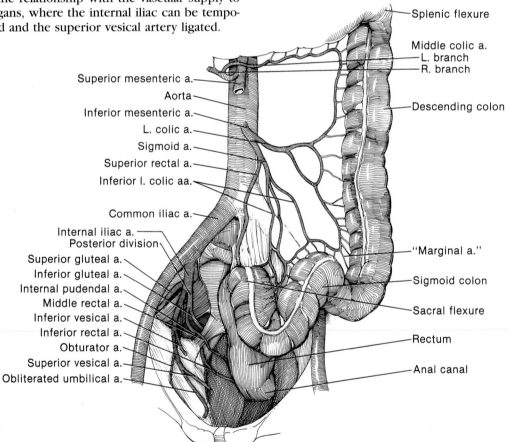

10 Make an incision in the posterior peritoneum over the external iliac artery that extends from the bifurcation, then runs beside the bladder, and ends near the sacrum. Divide and ligate each vas deferens. Proceed with bilateral pelvic lymphadenectomy (see page 517).

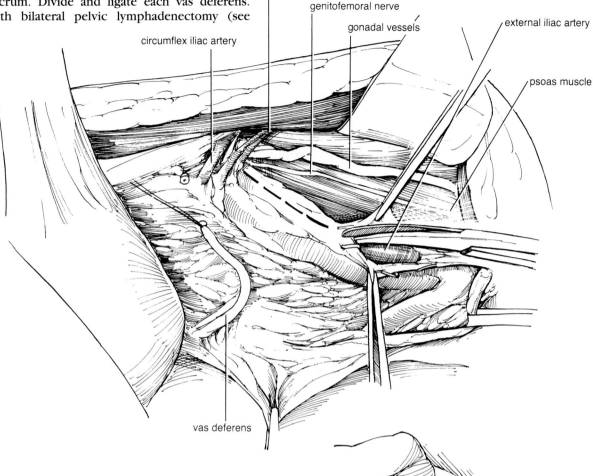

circumflex iliac artery

inferior epigastric artery and vein

genitofemoral nerve

gonadal vessels

external iliac artery

psoas muscle

vas deferens

11 **A,** Put a bulldog clamp on the internal iliac artery. Ligate and sever the superior vesical artery, its first anterior branch. Incise the peritoneum on either side of the sigmoid colon. Insert the index finger of the left hand behind the internal iliac artery; with the remainder of the fingers, retract the bladder. Run the index finger down to the endopelvic fascia between the vesical and rectal pedicles. Watch for veins extending from the bladder to the iliac vein; clip and divide them as they are exposed.

B, Pass a clamp behind the internal iliac artery distal to the take-off of the gluteal branch, draw a heavy suture through, and ligate the artery. Successively apply large clips to the superior vesical pedicle as you move the finger down between pedicle and rectum, and divide the pedicle. Mobilize the ureters laterally.

Free the sigmoid colon on the left side, starting in the iliac fossa, by incising the peritoneal folds and dividing its mesocolon. Continue the division of the peritoneum to reach that made for the node dissection. Ligate and divide the sigmoid mesentery over the sacrum. On the right side, divide the right leaf of the sigmoid mesocolon. Extend the peritoneal incision distally to the opening made for node dissection and proximally to the site chosen for division of the sigmoid colon, near its junction with the descending colon. Clamp, cut, and ligate the inferior colic arteries and the superior rectal artery and their veins. Place a hernia tape around the proximal sigmoid colon, and divide it proximal to the tie with the GIA stapler.

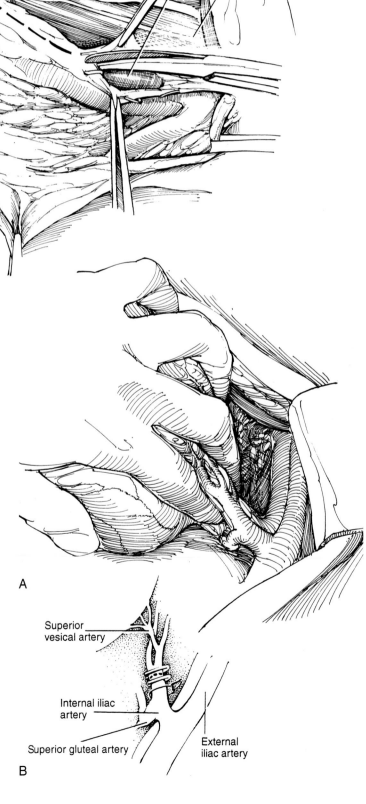

A

Superior vesical artery

Internal iliac artery

Superior gluteal artery

External iliac artery

B

12 With a hand in the sacral hollow, free the rectum posteriorly by sharp and blunt dissection.

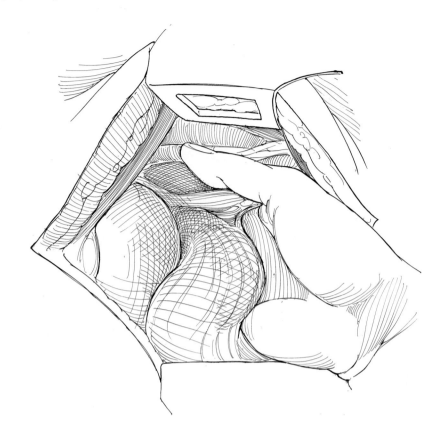

13 Draw the sigmoid anteriorly, and enter the plane behind the mesorectum. Develop it anterior to the hypogastric plexus, and dissect laterally to join the areas of previous node dissection. Continue the dissection lateral to the rectum, and divide the middle rectal arteries and veins. Dissect the rectum from the sacrum *(dashed line)*.

Dissect the ureters distally, divide them, and send specimens for frozen-section examination.

As done for radical cystectomy, divide the puboprostatic ligaments, divide the dorsal vein of the penis, and incise the endopelvic fascia. Divide the urethra (see page 509).

Mobilize, divide, and suture-ligate the lateral rectal pedicles if they were not divided earlier.

Move to the perineum. Suture the anus closed.

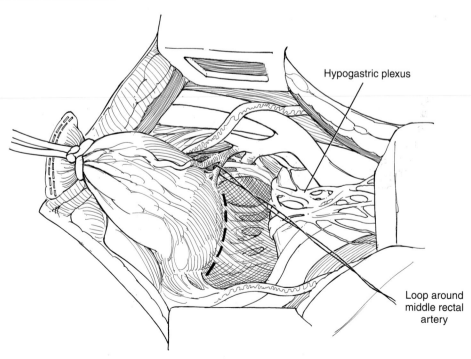

Hypogastric plexus

Loop around middle rectal artery

14 *Perineal structures:* The perineal body occupies the center of the perineum; it is the site of insertion of the anterior central tendon that joins the rectum. When this tendon is divided, the rectum can fall back and expose the pubococcygeal portions of the levator ani muscles that lie on either side of the rectum.

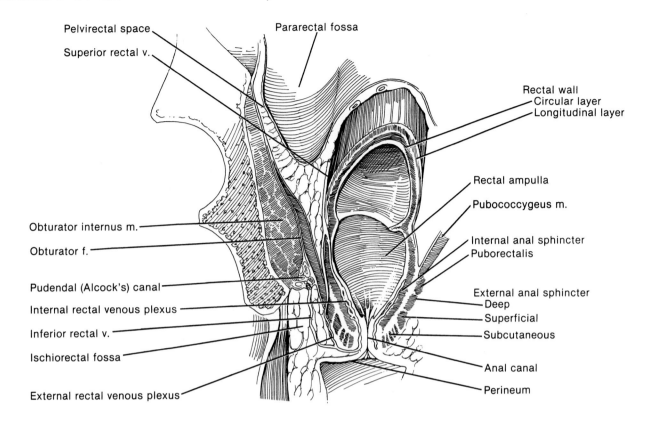

15 Make an elliptical incision around the anus. Incise the ischiorectal fat laterally, and divide the posterior central tendon. Expose the pubococcygeal portion of the levator ani. Open the pubococcygeus and iliococcygeus muscles adjacent to the coccyx, thus making a connection with the distal portion of the abdominal dissection, identified by a hand from above. Continue incising anteriorly, dividing the levator muscles lateral to the prostate until the symphysis pubis is reached, from which the insertion of the muscle is divided. Ligate and divide the posterior lateral rectal pedicles. Remove the specimen. Suture-ligate the prostatic veins and other vessels. Mobilize the omentum (see page 71), and place it in the pelvic defect to promote healing and to keep the small bowel from entering. Insert a flap of rectus muscle in the pelvic defect. Polyglycolic acid mesh may be substituted (Clarke-Pearson et al, 1988), formed into a sling from the sacral promontory to the pubis, but it is a less permanent solution.

Proceed with some form of urinary diversion. (Use of the left colon as a conduit saves one bowel anastomosis.) Form an end colostomy. Place a drain in the pelvis to exit through an abdominal stab wound or the perineal incision.

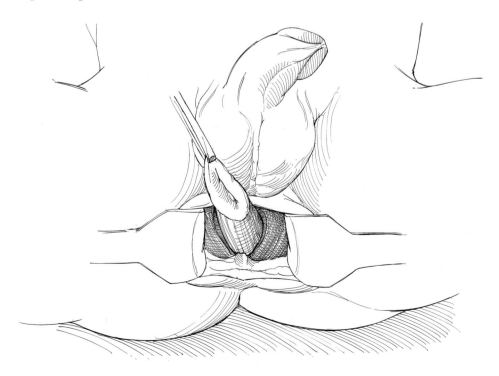

Alternative Exenteration in the Male

Proceed as for radical retropubic prostatectomy. Expose the urethra by dividing the endopelvic fascia, puboprostatic ligaments, and dorsal vein complex. Divide the urethra to expose the anterior surface of the distal rectum. If the colonic or bladder lesion is above the rectum, divide the rectum high enough to preserve the terminal segment and anastomose the colon end to end.

POSTOPERATIVE CARE

Withhold oral intake in anticipation of ileus; begin feeding when bowel sounds are of good quality and flatus has been passed. Consider parenteral nutrition. Remove the drain when drainage becomes minimal. Continue antibiotic coverage well into the period of recovery.

POSTOPERATIVE PROBLEMS

Bleeding from the large pelvic defect and from the retropubic area may be so severe that a pelvic pack is required for 2 days. Remove it under anesthesia, and insert a suction drain. *Thrombosis and emboli* arise from the manipulated pelvic veins, but prophylactic anticoagulation may lead to excessive blood loss. *Serous drainage* from the pelvic defect may become infected. This complication is minimized by adequate coverage of the pelvic floor, by prolonged suction drainage, and by adequate antibiotic coverage. *Delayed wound healing* may be expected if the pelvis was radiated. Problems from the urinary diversion may arise. A *fistula* may form with the small bowel, requiring parenteral nutrition. *Abscess formation* is more common in women, associated with vaginal dissection.

Commentary by W. Scott McDougal

Anterior exenteration, when performed for bladder malignancy in the female, should include the anterior vagina and the entire urethra. The posterior portion of the vagina may be preserved. However, when only the remnant vagina is used for reconstruction, a functional vagina cannot be constructed. If one is desired, a myocutaneous flap or muscle pedicle flap with a split-thickness graft applied is required for the anterior vaginal wall. An innovative technique involves the use of polyglycolic acid mesh for the anterior vagina. When omentum is placed over the mesh, the undersurface of the mesh re-epithelializes, resulting in a satisfactory anterior surface and a vagina of sufficient size. If an orthotopic bladder is contemplated in the female, the reconstructed remnant vagina provides needed support for the bowel segment. In that case, the urethra must be left in situ. It is transected at the bladder neck.

Total exenteration should be approached from the abdomen first. With large pelvic malignancies, the surgeon should begin the dissection in the hollow of the sacrum. The dissection should extend laterally, as these two areas, when free of tumor, allow for clean margins. On occasion the tumor grows posteriorly into the coccyx, which may be separated from the sacrum and taken with the specimen. If the tumor grows directly into the sacrum, its complete removal with attendant nerves creates considerable disability. For palliation, partial removal of these tumors followed by intraoperative radiation therapy has been employed. Dissection then proceeds from above and below, often simultaneously by two operating teams, thereby reducing operative time.

Excision of Vesical Diverticulum

Distinguish congenital diverticula, which occur in children in the absence of vesical trabeculation, from the acquired forms produced by obstruction. Treat the obstructive cause of the diverticulum first, usually by transurethral resection of the prostate in an adult male, a procedure that may be done at the same time as the diverticulectomy.

Intravenous urography may detect ipsilateral ureteral obstruction or bilateral hydronephrosis. Voiding cystourethrograms with oblique views and a postvoid film help define the extent of the diverticulum. A video urodynamic study may help define the voiding dysfunction, especially in patients with significant urinary retention. Cystourethrography can rule out strictures and bladder neck contracture, and cystoscopic examination within the diverticulum is necessary to rule out tumor because total diverticulectomy may be warranted if the entire wall cannot be visualized. Give specific antibiotics to clear the urine.

Consider simple endoscopic incision of the neck of the diverticulum with thorough fulguration of the mucosa. Vesical diverticula usually occur on the posterior wall of the bladder, overlying one or the other ureter. Thus, excising the entire diverticulum, including the desmoplastic wall that has formed as a reaction, is not a practical solution even if ureteral stents are in place. The most universally practical technique is removal of the lining extravesically. Another alternative is to invert the diverticulum into the bladder and excise it. The most hazardous method, because of the possibility of ureteral injury, is dissecting the entire diverticulum out and excising it extravesically. A combined intravesical-extravesical technique is possible. Closing the bladder opening and applying phenol to the diverticular mucosa in situ, then inserting a Penrose drain, are not recommended.

Instruments: Provide a Basic set, six to eight long fine Allis clamps, long Babcock clamps, peanut dissectors, long Metzenbaum and Lahey scissors, iris scissors, Potts and DeBakey forceps, Major retractors, an infant feeding tube, and a Malecot catheter.

EXTRAVESICAL EXCISION OF THE DIVERTICULAR LINING

This method is ideal for diverticula with wide openings.

1 **A,** *Position:* Place the patient supine with the pelvis slightly elevated by extending the table. Stand to the left. Insert a balloon catheter, and fill the bladder by gravity with sterile water.

Incision: Make a midline extraperitoneal incision from the umbilicus to well over the symphysis (see page 487) or a lower abdominal transverse incision (see page 490).

B, Bluntly dissect the peritoneum upward and the prevesical tissue laterally. Insert a self-retaining retractor.

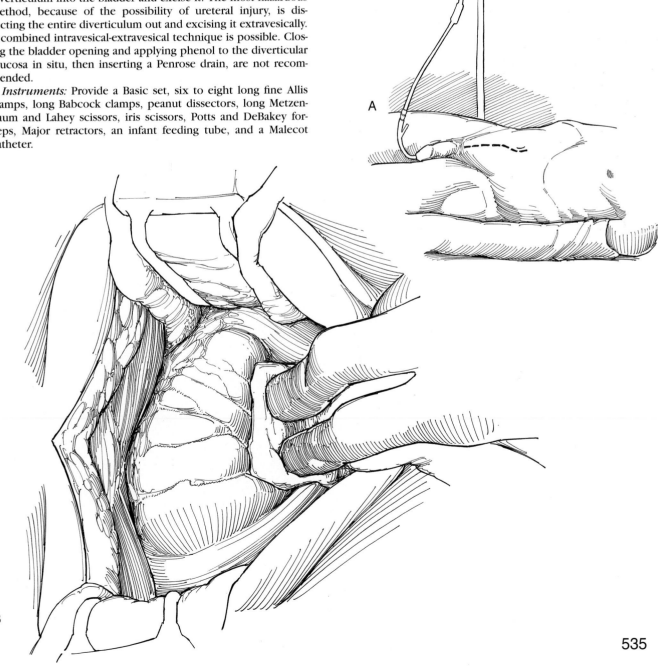

535

2 **A** and **B,** Open the bladder between stay sutures just wide enough to insert the index finger. Insinuate the left index finger into the diverticulum, forcefully if necessary. Flex the finger so that its tip can be palpated anteriorly in the incision; then dissect the peritoneum and perivesical tissue away from the bladder wall down to the palpable fingertip.

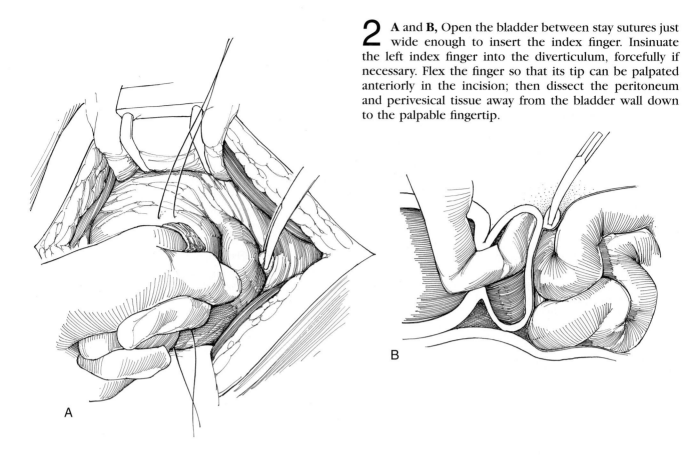

A

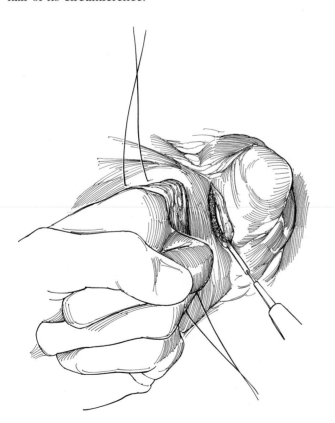

B

3 Divide the neck of the diverticulum against the finger with the cutting current sufficient to open half of its circumference.

4 Through this incision, divide the remainder of the mucosa connecting the diverticulum to the bladder. *Alternative approach* (Barnes): Instead of limiting the incision to the neck of the diverticulum, divide the bladder wall from the initial opening down to and into the mouth of the diverticulum. This gives a larger opening through which the lining can be manipulated and excised. Proceed with removal of the lining, as described in Step 6.

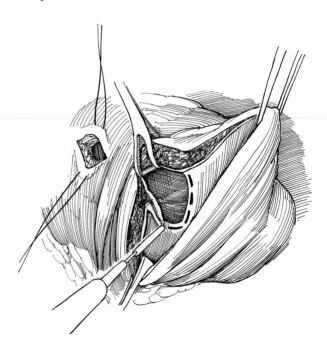

5 Grasp the uroepithelial edges of the diverticulum with fine Allis clamps. Start the dissection progressively and carefully around the circumference of the mouth with Lahey scissors. Traction on the clamps by the assistant must be controlled. Even though the uroepithelium is relatively thick and appears to have a good plane for dissection under it, it is easy to tear.

6 As the dissection continues with the scissors and peanut dissector, the floor of the diverticulum is gradually drawn up, allowing it to be separated visually from the lining. The ureter lies outside the sac, out of harm's way.

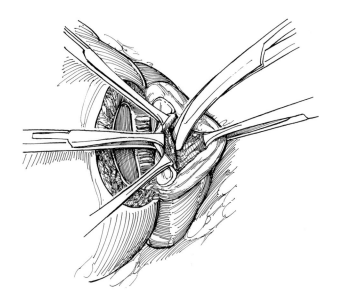

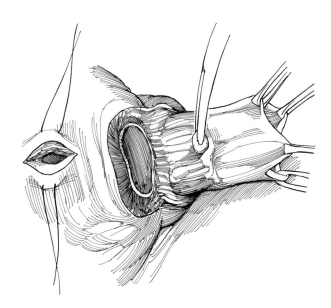

7 Place a running 3-0 plain catgut suture subepithelially around the bladder defect to invert the edge into the bladder. Cover this with a layer of interrupted 2-0 SAS to include the muscularis and adventitia.

8 Insert a 24 F Malecot catheter through a stab wound in the bladder and body wall, and suture it to the bladder and to the skin. For females, a balloon catheter through the urethra is adequate. Close the initial suprapubic vesical opening in two layers. Insert a Penrose drain into the remains of the diverticular sac. Close the wound in layers around the Penrose drain, placing a safety pin through it.

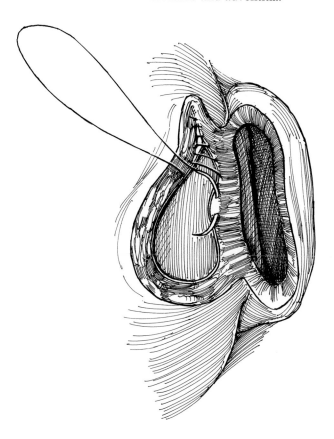

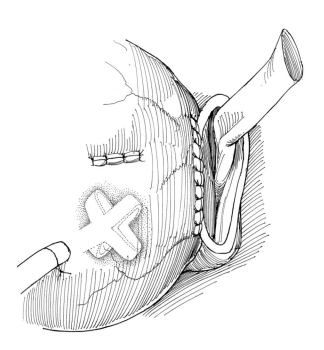

INTRAVESICAL INVERSION TECHNIQUE

The diverticulum must have an open mouth for this technique to be applied.

9 Open the bladder between stay sutures. Grasp the mucosa of the distal wall of the diverticulum through its neck with a curved clamp, and draw it into the bladder.

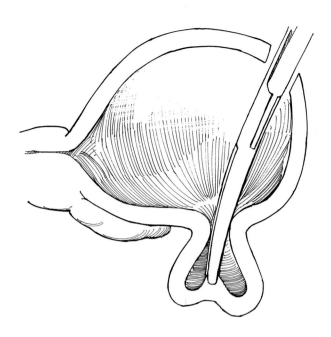

10 Insert ureteral catheters to be sure the ureter is not drawn up with the diverticulum. Place stay sutures on either side of the neck of the diverticulum and sharply divide it.

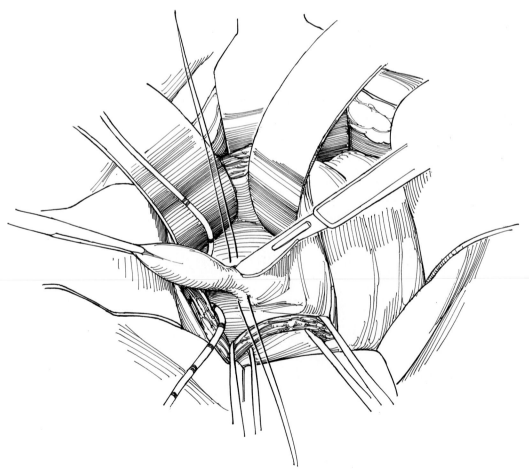

11 Close the muscularis with 2-0 CCG sutures while the stay sutures hold the defect in view. Close the mucosa with a 3-0 plain catgut inverting running submucosal suture.

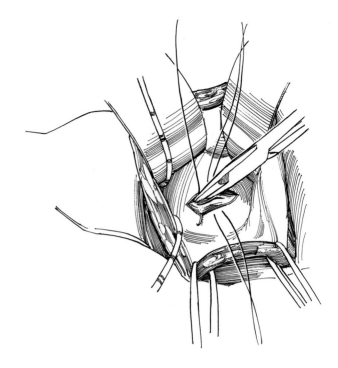

EXTRAVESICAL EXCISION TECHNIQUE

This technique carries a risk of injuring adjacent organs, especially the ureter.

12 Open the bladder and bisect it to the neck of the diverticulum. Insert a catheter in at least the ipsilateral ureter.

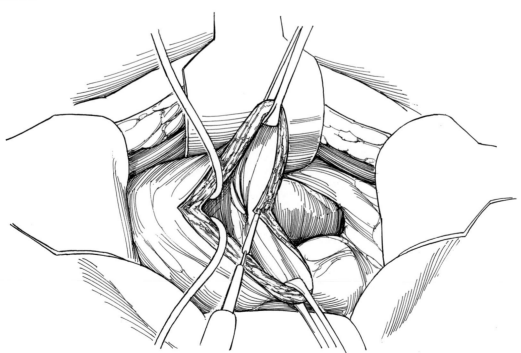

13 A and B, Pack the diverticulum with gauze. Free the entire diverticulum, beginning by dissecting and dividing the neck. Take great care not to injure the ureters. If the ureter is involved in the wall of the diverticulum, leave part of the wall in place or transect the ureter and reimplant it in the bladder.

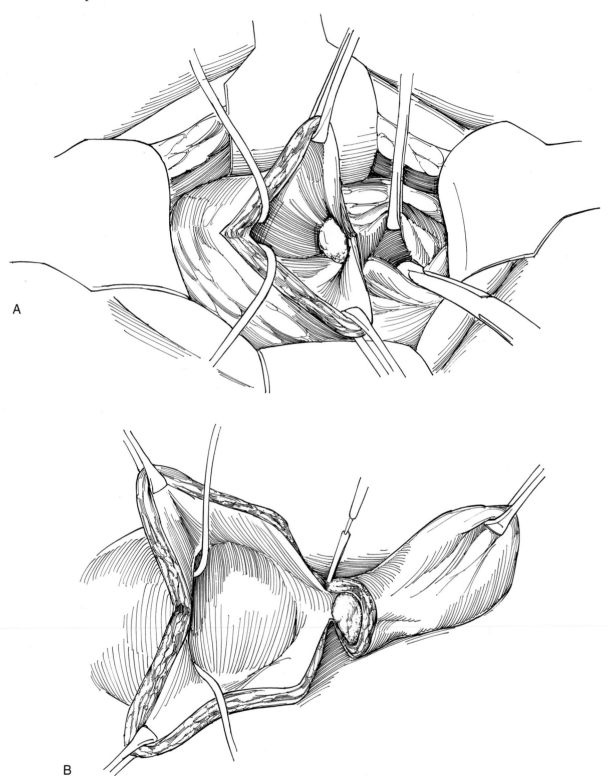

A

B

14 Insert a 24 F Malecot catheter through a stab wound. Close the bladder defect in layers. Drain the extravesical space.

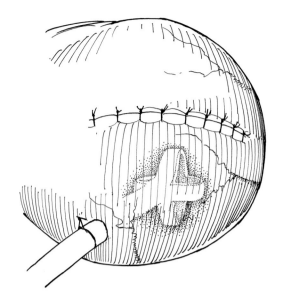

LAPAROSCOPIC DIVERTICULECTOMY (Parra-Jones)

This procedure is used for a diverticulum with a narrow neck. Induce pneumoperitoneum and insert four ports: a subumbilical 10-mm port, right and left paramedian 12-mm ports, and a 5-mm port above the symphysis. Insert a cystoscope, and use the light to identify the diverticulum. Dissect the peritoneum from the bladder and identify the ureter. After dissecting the diverticulum to its base, successively divide the neck with an endostapler. Check the closure cystoscopically. Grasp the specimen with gall bladder grasping forceps, and remove it through the 12-mm port. Fill the bladder to check for leaks.

POSTOPERATIVE PROBLEMS

Persistent leakage suggests vesical outlet obstruction and may be relieved by a longer period of catheter drainage. An *abscess* may form either within the remaining wall if only the lining is removed or in the potential space left after total excision. Adequate drainage and specific antibiotic therapy are important.

Ureteral involvement in the excision or closure may lead to hydronephrosis or a ureteral fistula. If flank pain or continuous drainage occurs, obtain an intravenous urogram and a cystogram. If ureteral catheters were placed intraoperatively, leave them as stents for at least 5 days; then watch the patient for signs of ureterovesical obstruction after removal. A follow-up intravenous urogram after 3 months is advisable in any case if the diverticulum lay near the orifice. If reimplantation is ultimately required, discard the terminal ureter and use a vesical hitch. *Rectal injury* rarely occurs.

Commentary by Gary D. Steinberg

The indications for vesical diverticulectomy include persistent infection, stone formation, ureteral obstruction, malignant transformation, and urinary retention. Before the diverticulum is treated, bladder outlet obstruction should be looked for and treated if present.

The majority of vesical diverticula that I have treated have been greater than 3 cm in size and located posteriorly. These are best managed with the combined intravesical-extravesical approach. The surgeon may be able to remove the entire diverticulum, but usually it is safer and easier to remove the mucosa of the diverticulum. With this approach, the risk of an inadvertent or unrecognized ureteral injury is greatly reduced. The important aspects of this approach are placing a temporary 5 F catheter in the ureteral orifice and packing the diverticulum with gauze or a radiopaque sponge. For removal of a tumor in

a diverticulum, it is important to obtain an adequate margin around the diverticular orifice. However, some believe that tumors in diverticula are best treated by cystectomy. After the diverticular orifice is circumscribed, the proper plane is developed by sharp and blunt dissection using the gauze-filled diverticulum as a landmark. Once the diverticulum has been completely excised, I close the bladder defect in two layers. If the ureter is involved in the wall of the diverticulum or has been skeletonized as a result of the dissection, it should be transected and reimplanted. Rectal injuries occur rarely during vesical diverticulectomy.

Vesical diverticula may be treated endoscopically, but one must be extremely careful not to perforate the bladder or diverticulum.

Cystolithotomy

Cystolithotomy is intended for patients with stones greater than 6 cm in diameter and for those with urethral disease. Remove the obstruction to outflow either before removing the stone by transurethral resection if prostatic enlargement is moderate or concomitantly by supra-retropubic prostatectomy (see pages 426 to 429).

Position: Place the patient supine with the penis draped in the field and covered with a towel. Insert a 22 F balloon catheter, and partially fill the bladder.

Incision: Make a transverse lower abdominal incision (see page 490) or a lower midline extraperitoneal incision (see page 487).

Follow the steps for suprapubic cystostomy on pages 625 to 628. Fill the bladder to capacity at the time of cystoscopy. After making the lower abdominal incision, grasp the transversalis fascia overlying the bladder in forceps, divide it with scissors, and sweep it laterally. Incise the detrusor muscle vertically with the electrocau-tery. Place two full-thickness stay sutures, and incise the detrusor between them. Insert a clamp into the bladder lumen, open it, and quickly replace it with the tip of the suction. Enlarge the opening with the index fingers. Grasp the stone with ring forceps and remove it. Inspect the base of the bladder for other stones.

Close the bladder with a running 4-0 plain catgut suture applied to the subepithelium (as for a subcuticular skin closure). Reinforce it with interrupted sutures of 3-0 CCG placed through the muscularis. Bring the transversalis fascia back over the bladder, and tack it in place to prevent adherence to the anterior body wall with resulting inhibition of contraction. Place a small suction drain or Penrose drain (avoid latex in patients with spina bifida because of the risk of an allergic reaction) to exit through the wound for a few days. Leave the catheter in place, and remove it in 8 to 10 days. Close the fascia with 3-0 CCG.

Bladder: Reconstruction

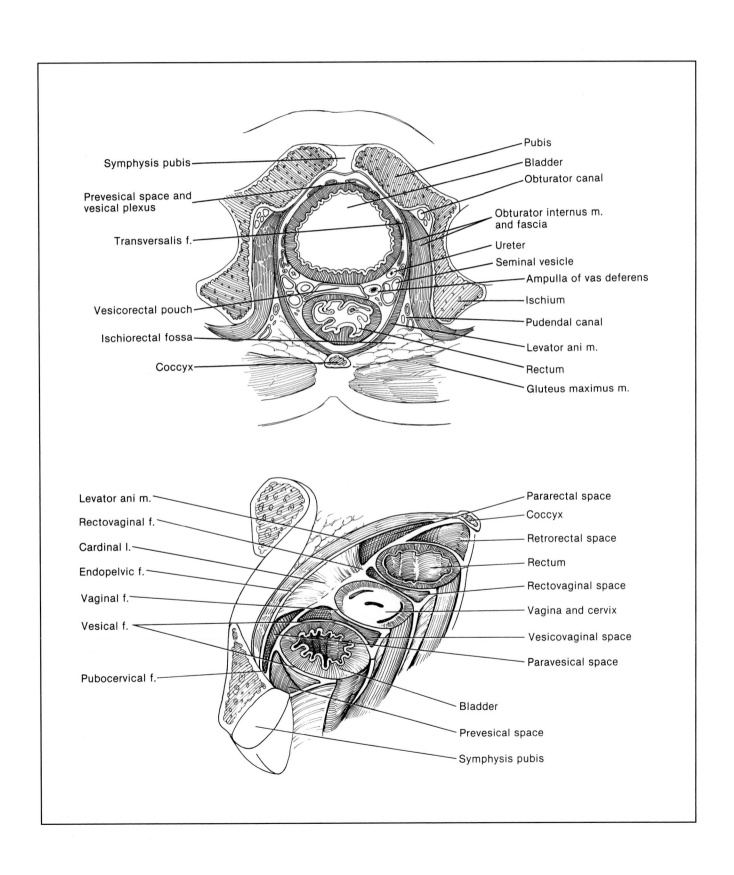

Symphysis pubis

Prevesical space and vesical plexus

Transversalis f.

Vesicorectal pouch

Ischiorectal fossa

Coccyx

Pubis

Bladder

Obturator canal

Obturator internus m. and fascia

Ureter

Seminal vesicle

Ampulla of vas deferens

Ischium

Pudendal canal

Levator ani m.

Rectum

Gluteus maximus m.

Levator ani m.

Rectovaginal f.

Cardinal l.

Endopelvic f.

Vaginal f.

Vesical f.

Pubocervical f.

Pararectal space

Coccyx

Retrorectal space

Rectum

Rectovaginal space

Vagina and cervix

Vesicovaginal space

Paravesical space

Bladder

Prevesical space

Symphysis pubis

Principles of Bladder Reconstruction

Reconstruction of the bladder centers on treatment of urinary incontinence: by elevating the bladder neck, by constricting the urethra, or by forming a new outlet. Success depends on proper evaluation of the cause; one type of operation is not universally applicable. Whether the approach should be retropubic or transvaginal or both depends in part on the type of defect and in part on the preference of the surgeon. The bladder, bladder neck, and urethra are suspended by the pelvic floor and by the several pelvic fascias. These fascial layers enclose compartments that contain the female structures. Reconstructive surgery is directed at manipulation of these elements. If that is not possible, the vesical neck itself can be reconstituted or an artificial sphincter may be placed. An approach to incontinence due to neurologic abnormality is nerve stimulation through dorsal rhizotomy.

In contrast to suspension procedures, repair of a fistula, whether to the vagina or bowel, requires meticulous technique if it is to succeed. The same advice applies to closure of the vesical neck.

REPAIR OF BLADDER RUPTURE

Make a lower abdominal midline incision (see page 487). Make a small peritoneotomy. If blood is found, search intraperitoneally for associated injuries. Do not enter an adjacent hematoma. Open the bladder vertically well above the bladder neck. For an *extraperitoneal* defect, close it with a single layer of 3-0 chromic catgut (CCG) sutures. Consider managing it with a urethral catheter, to remain for 14 days.

For an *intraperitoneal* rupture, close the defect in three layers with a running subepithelial stitch, interrupted muscular stitches, and interrupted peritoneal sutures. Insert a 28 F Malecot cystostomy tube to exit through a stab wound. Close the cystotomy incision in two layers. Insert drains, but remove them within 3 days for fear of infecting an adjacent hematoma. Close the fascia and skin. Remove the tube in 10 days.

Cystourethropexy

(Marshall-Marchetti-Krantz)

Urinary continence can be achieved by urethrovesical reconstruction in several ways: bladder neck suspension (Marshall, Pereyra), pubovaginal sling (McGuire), posterior urethral tube (Young-Dees, Leadbetter), detrusor tube with tunnel (Kropp), anterior tube (Tanagho), and artificial sphincter (Scott).

Demonstrate leakage on stress, and arrest it by elevation of the vaginal vault (the Marshall-Marchetti-Krantz [MMK] test). Be alert for detrusor instability as a principal cause of incontinence. Rule out residual urine and areflexic vesical dysfunction unless life-long intermittent catheterization would be tolerated. Apply pharmacologic and hormonal agents, in addition to exercises. For the mobile vagina with a cystocele, consider colposuspension (see page 549). If minimal cystocele exists, do a cystourethropexy by an open or a vaginal needle technique. For a fixed vagina or urethra (usually from failure of previous procedures), use a pubovaginal sling (see page 565). As a last resort,

insert an artificial sphincter (see page 580). Vaginal repair can be combined with a retropubic operation.

The object of cystourethropexy is to bring the bladder and urethra back into the pelvis by suturing the paraurethral vaginal tissue to the back of the symphysis pubis. Take care after irradiation or previous operations; the dissection may be difficult.

Instruments: Provide a Basic set, a GU long set, a Major retractor set, DeBakey forceps, vascular forceps, 10 Allis clamps, fiberoptic suction, long smooth forceps, stick and cherry sponges, six rubber-shod spring clamps, a 22 F 5-ml balloon catheter, 2-0 synthetic absorbable sutures (SAS) on round needles, a Jackson-Pratt drain with a large needle, and large and medium clip appliers. Preoperatively, have the patient douche with povidone-iodine solution and start antibiotics.

1 *Position:* Place the patient in a low lithotomy position with the pelvis elevated and the legs suspended by the feet. Prepare the perineum and vagina. Insert an 18 F 5-ml balloon catheter filled to 10 ml, with the end of the catheter in the operative field connected to a filling bag of water. Drape the perineum to allow vaginal access,

and station the second assistant there. Stand to the left of the patient.

Incision: Use a Pfannenstiel incision (see page 490) or a lower midline extraperitoneal incision carried well down over the pubis (see page 487).

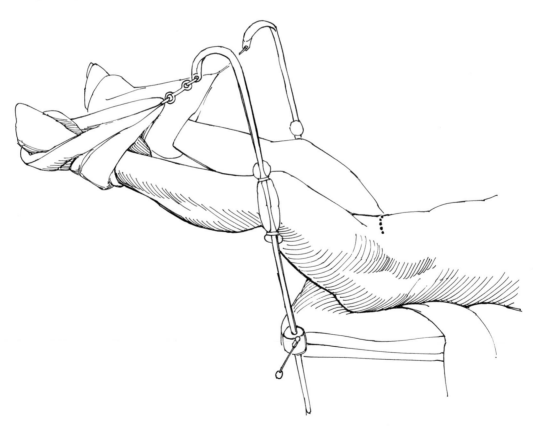

2 Incise the fascias transversely, and separate the rectus abdominis and pyramidalis muscles in the midline. Expose the retropubic space, and place a self-retaining retractor.

3 Fill the bladder with 200 ml of sterile water. Dissect the peritoneal reflection from the bladder. This also prevents the intestines from subsequently wedging between the bladder and body wall. Empty the bladder and push it posteriorly with a stick sponge; be very gentle. With a cherry sponge and long smooth forceps, pick the fat from among the veins in the space of Retzius. Displace the fat and contained small vessels laterally and cephalad from the surface of the vagina on either side of the urethra. Carefully grasp the friable veins with smooth forceps, cauterize them, and divide them with scissors. The bladder may be entered to aid the dissection; close it later in two layers.

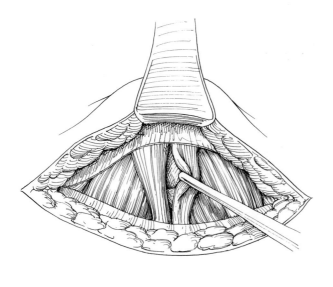

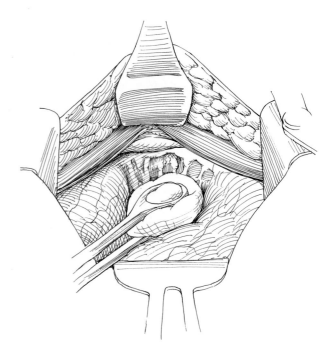

4 Continue careful blunt dissection first on either side of the bladder neck and then around the urethra, identified by the catheter and balloon, until the distal tissue starts to curve anterolaterally as it joins the endopelvic fascia. The assistant's two fingers in the vagina may help identify and visualize the white vaginal fascia, exposed by sweeping aside the overlying fat.

5 For the classic three-suture procedure, place a figure-eight 2-0 SAS or CCG mattress suture firmly into the paraurethral tissue and deep into the vaginal wall adjacent to the urethra on the right and left as low in the pelvis as the curve of the needle allows, but do not insert it close to the urethra itself. When the sutures are subsequently tied, they should elevate the vagina, not constrict the urethra. Catch the ends in rubber-shod clamps, and drape them caudally outside the wound to avoid later confusion when tying them.

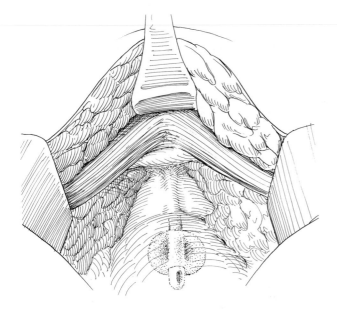

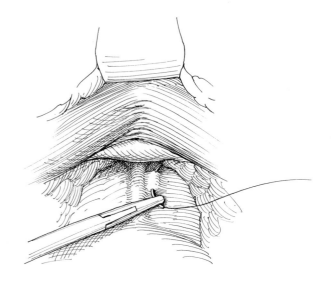

6 Place the second pair of sutures about 1 cm proximal to the first. Insert a third pair of sutures at the urethrovesical junction, as determined by palpation of the balloon. These last are the most important sutures; some surgeons place only this pair of sutures. Hold each with rubber-shod clamps. If the insertion of a suture provokes bleeding, pass it through again in the same place.

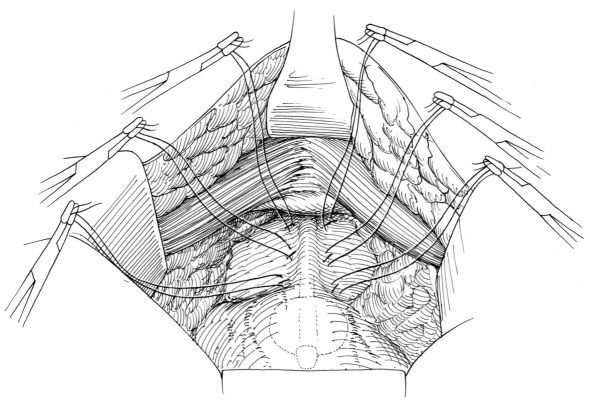

7 **A,** Grasp the needle of one of the pair of most distal sutures. Using a smooth rotation of the needle holder, insinuate the needle beneath the pubic periosteum (easily torn) and the extension of Gimbernat's ligament just a little more proximal than the site of origin of the suture on the vagina. Reclamp the suture. *Caution:* If the periosteum is flimsy, consider doing a colpourethropexy by placing the sutures in Cooper's ligament (see pages 551 to 554). Continue these maneuvers with each

successive suture. Open the bladder, if desired, and visualize the vesicourethral junction to be sure that the sutures do not obstruct or compress the urethra.

B, Tie the sutures, beginning distally. Avoid pulling them away from the periosteum. The assistant can help by elevating the vagina. Alternatively, perform cystoscopy on the patient and tie the sutures just tight enough to close the bladder neck.

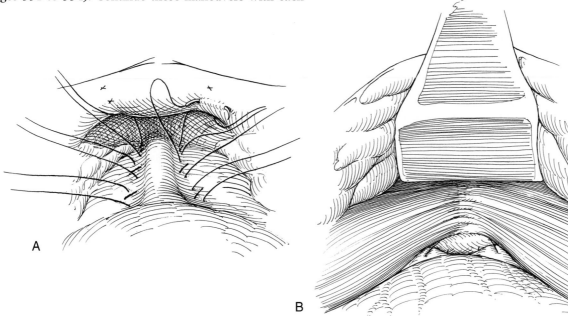

8 Place another pair of sutures more laterally above the bladder neck, and fasten these to the upper portion of the symphysis or to the insertion of the rectus muscle. Place a Penrose drain in the retropubic space, bringing it through the wound. Alternatively, a suction drain may be used, especially in secondary operations, although a small collection of blood is said to make the tissues in the repair more permanently adherent. If the bladder has been opened, place a cystostomy tube, to exit through a stab wound. Close the abdominal wound. Tape the catheter to the leg using tincture of benzoin and waterproof tape; inadvertent traction could destroy the repair. Allow the patient out of bed. Remove the drain in 2 or 3 days, but leave the catheter in place 3 to 5 days; remove it for a trial of voiding. If more than 100 ml of urine remains after voiding, replace the catheter overnight and then start the patient performing intermittent catheterization if appreciable residual urine persists. Continue antibiotic suppression. Tell the patient to avoid heavy lifting.

POSTOPERATIVE PROBLEMS

Inability to void is the most frequent complication, arising from sutures placed too close to the urethra or, if inserted too distally, causing a kink in the urethra. Previous scarring may be an important factor, as can overcorrection by excessive elevation and constriction. Resort to temporary intermittent catheterization. A punch cystostomy is rarely needed. Add bethanechol chloride, 25 mg orally four times a day. Adequate voiding usually returns within 2 weeks. If the inability to void persists for weeks or months, try dilating the urethra with a Kollmann dilator to 30 or 36 F, at the same time levering the dilator down to loosen the urethral fixation.

Surgical revision is occasionally necessary for persistent retention. It may be done by *transvaginal urethrolysis* (Foster and McGuire, 1993). Use a midline incision or, better, a vaginal incision, forming a U-shaped flap with the base oriented dorsally. Dissect the vaginal epithelium from the urethra and periurethral fascia, and separate the urethra from the surrounding tissue until the endopelvic fascia is reached and entered. Assess urethral mobility by traction on a balloon catheter. Insert adjacent fibrofatty tissue between the urethra and pubis, or mobilize a labial fat pad flap (Martius) (see page 590) and interpose it. Another approach (Webster and Kreder, 1990) is to divide the retropubic adhesions, aided by two fingers in the vagina. Completely free the urethra anteriorly, but leave the vaginal attachments. Place three interrupted 1-0 SAS at 1-cm intervals through the paravaginal fascia and vagina. These should be placed from the urethrovesical junction to 3 cm above it. Pass the sutures through the obturator fascia and muscle before tying them as an obturator shelf repair.

Dysfunctional voiding with detrusor instability may persist after operation. Try anticholinergic medication and retraining. The dysfunction may be due to overcorrection. *Enteroceles* occasionally appear after suspension because the vagina has been repositioned anteriorly.

Urinary infection is treated if it persists. *Wound infection* is not uncommon, although osteitis pubis is rare. Treat osteitis pubis with corticosteriods, analgesics, and bed rest. *Stone formation* can occur on nonabsorbable sutures (NAS). *Bleeding* arises from injury to the prevesical venous plexus or from the endopelvic fascia if the sutures are not tied before bringing them to the symphysis. Because drains are customarily placed, hematomas are not common, but the blood loss from the retropubic veins may be excessive and require replacement. *Urinary drainage* from an inadvertent opening in the bladder should respond to catheter drainage. *Ureteral obstruction* should be rare even in complicated cases (for which ureteral catheters would have been inserted). A tear into the vagina can be repaired intraoperatively.

Commentary by Victor F. Marshall

The old vaginal repairs were based on the idea that a vaginal hernia needed repair and the bladder neck needed to be plicated. We showed that fixation inside the pelvis would give the same or better results. Our whole idea was that the various plications did fix the bladder, for an improved mechanical advantage. This could be done from above or below, provided that enough muscle remained.

We found that gingerly picking the fat away from the friable veins during exposure of the urethra and vagina allowed them to be skeletonized and moved aside; rarely did they require fulguration or division. It took a few minutes longer but it saved blood, and I think it looked better.

We routinely went down to within 1 cm of the external urethral meatus, not hesitating to sharply incise the endopelvic fascia if necessary. We could insert three fingertips under the lower surface of symphysis. Despite traditional cautions not to get close to the urethra itself, we originally sutured into the top of the urethra! We moved laterally to provide wider support more than to prevent leakage. We never had a fistula that did not close spontaneously within 3 weeks, even in previously operated cases.

We used two ordinary clamps at each echelon: two straight, two Kelly, two Kocher, and two small Kelly clamps. We used rubber-shod clamps because we always took double bites with the needle on the vaginal side to get more tissue against the symphysis for eventual fibrous adherence. The double bite is shown in the original 1949 article. Place the suspending sutures as much as possible into the cartilage of the symphysis.

Colposuspension

(Burch)

Suspension of the urethra by the vagina (colposuspension) is more frequently performed than cystourethropexy for several reasons: It is not followed by osteitis pubis, Cooper's ligament offers better tissue than periosteum for suture placement, and denervation of the urethra is avoided. Although the initial success rate of needle suspension is similar (±85 percent versus ±92 percent), later follow-up shows colposuspension to give better results (±72 percent versus ±91 percent).

Demonstrate descent of the base of the bladder by lateral cystography with the patient both relaxed and straining. Observe leakage on straining (in the upright position) and its suppression by elevation of the vagina on both sides of the vesical neck (MMK test). Ascertain that the vagina has adequate mobility in the lateral fornices. Provide suppressive antibiotics.

1 *Instruments:* Instruments are the same as for cystourethropexy.

Position: Place the patient in the low lithotomy position with legs abducted. Prepare the perineum and vagina, and insert a 22 or 24 F 5-ml balloon catheter, keeping the end in the sterile field.

Incision: Make a transverse lower abdominal incision (see page 490) or midline lower abdominal incision (see page 487). Enter the retropubic space close to the pubic bone. Gently push the fat and veins up and laterally (this is a very vascular area). Expose the vaginal wall lying on either side of the urethra. *Caution:* Avoid dissection over the urethra itself (it is easily palpated because of the catheter).

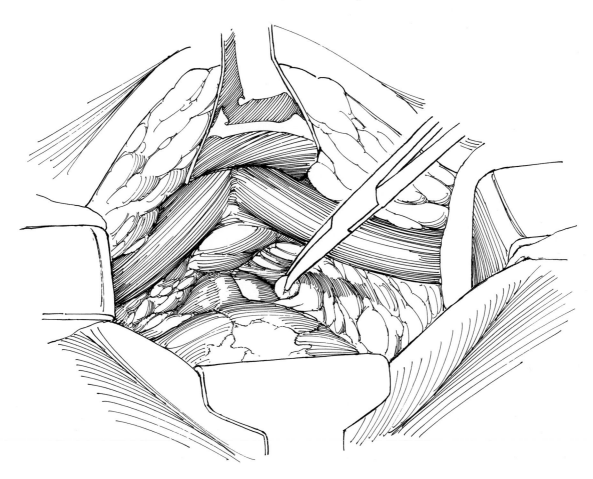

2 Identify the vesicourethral junction by palpating the balloon as it is gently pulled down. If in doubt, partially fill the bladder to define the rounded lower vesical margin. Do not dissect there; protect the detrusor fibers as they join the urethra.

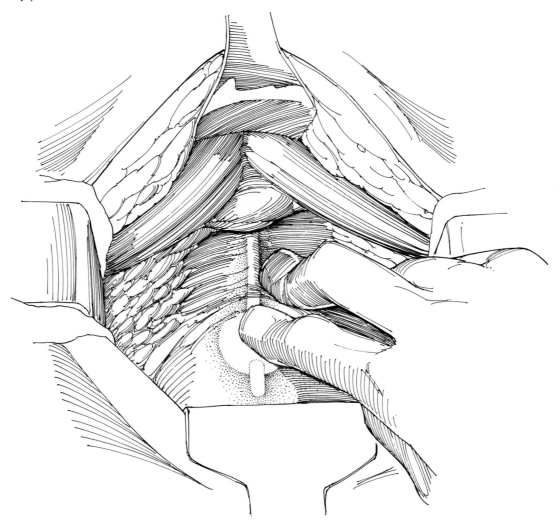

3 **A,** Start dissecting lateral to the lower margin of the sagging bladder and mobilize it upward, off the anterior vaginal wall. Two fingers in the vagina can help in determining how much mobilization is needed to return the bladder to its normal height. Be sure the bladder and its neck are free. In secondary operations, the dense adhesions that fix the low-lying bladder to the back of the pubis are divided sharply with great care, but enough to allow the bladder and vesicourethral junction to slide upward freely. *Caution:* Do not lacerate the vesical or (especially) the urethral muscle. If the lower margin of the bladder is still not clearly defined, open the bladder at the dome; a finger inside then defines its limits for easier dissection and mobilization.

B, Clear the fatty tissue from the lateral pelvic walls to expose each pectineal ligament (Cooper), consisting of a white band involving the periosteum of the superior ramus of the pubis along the pectineal line.

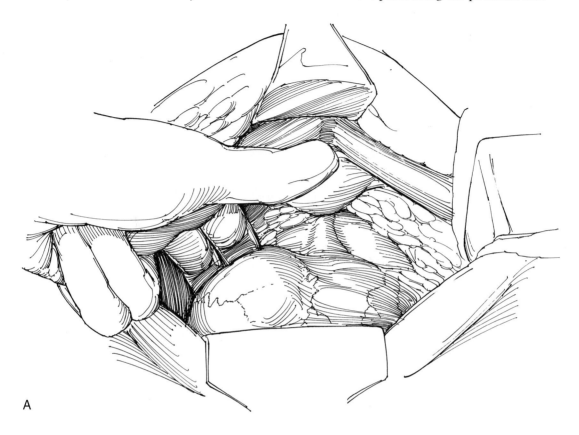

A

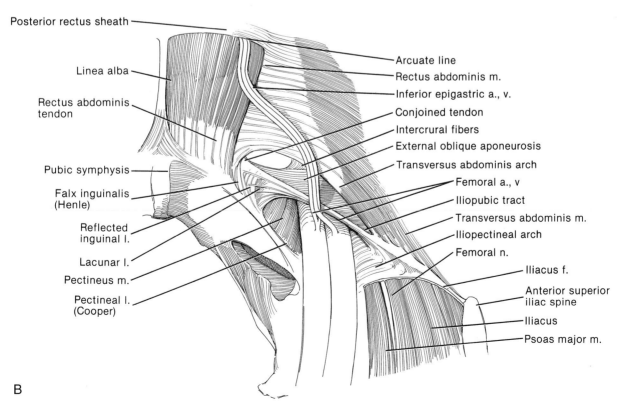

Posterior rectus sheath
Linea alba
Rectus abdominis tendon
Pubic symphysis
Falx inguinalis (Henle)
Reflected inguinal l.
Lacunar l.
Pectineus m.
Pectineal l. (Cooper)

Arcuate line
Rectus abdominis m.
Inferior epigastric a., v.
Conjoined tendon
Intercrural fibers
External oblique aponeurosis
Transversus abdominis arch
Femoral a., v
Iliopubic tract
Transversus abdominis m.
Iliopectineal arch
Femoral n.
Iliacus f.
Anterior superior iliac spine
Iliacus
Psoas major m.

B

4 Use 1-0 SAS on tapered needles. Place the first, more distal suture in the least vascular area of the vagina. Insert it on one side of the urethra as deeply as possible but, guided by the vaginal finger, not passing through the mucosa. It should be as far laterally in the anterior vaginal wall as possible and lie opposite the midurethra. Hold the ends of the suture in a rubber-shod bulldog clamp. Place a second suture similarly on the other side. *Caution:* This area is very vascular, and vigorous bleeding may require reinserting the needle to form a figure-eight tie or placing fine hemostatic mattress sutures; lesser bleeding stops when the fixation is complete.

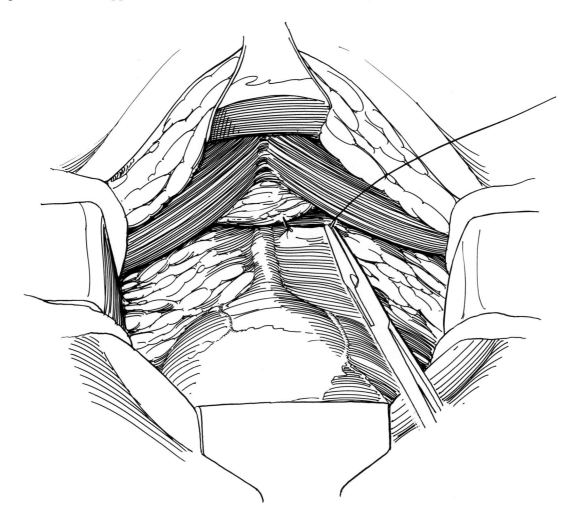

5 Place the third and fourth sutures (the key sutures) just below the reflection of the anterior bladder wall on the vagina at the level of the vesicourethral junction but well lateral to it.

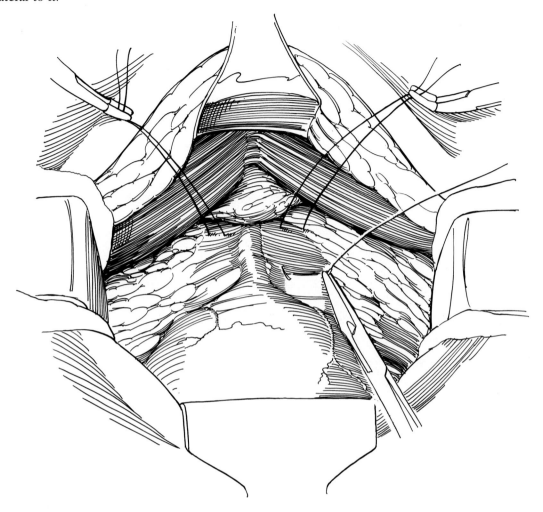

6 Expose Cooper's (pectineal) ligament on the pubic bone (see Step 3B). Because the sutures are not double armed, a curved needle must be mounted on the free end of the suture to insert that end. Place the first two sutures successively in the more medial portion of the ligament, such that when tied they lift the vagina directly upward and do not compress the urethra medially. Place a second set slightly more laterally.

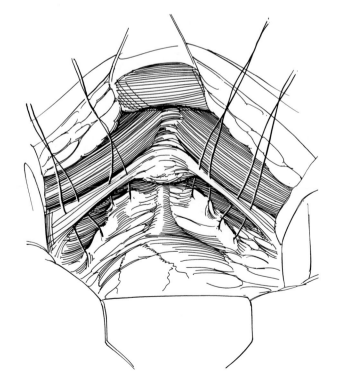

7 **A,** Have the assistant tie the sutures in succession from below upward, aided by vaginal elevation by your fingers.

B, Avoid tension. A space can properly remain between vagina and ligaments, a space that intra-abdominal pressure closes and allows adherence to the pubic bone, with subsequent fibrosis. Do not encroach on the anterior vesical wall. Place one or two Penrose drains. Replace the balloon catheter with a 16 F silicone one, to remain 5 days, during which time the patient stays in bed. The catheter is replaced temporarily, or intermittent catheterization is begun in the infrequent event that voiding is delayed.

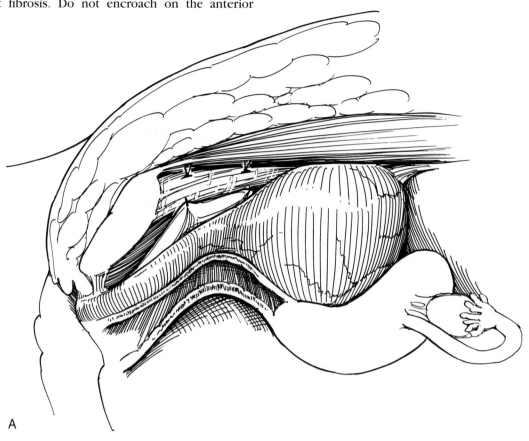

A

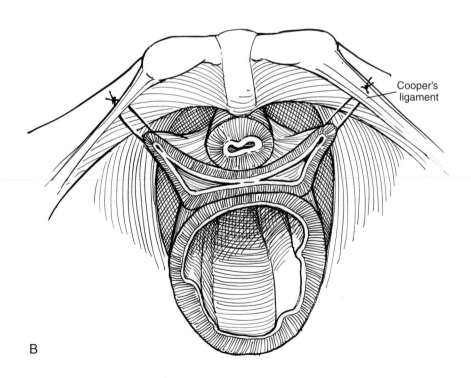

Cooper's ligament

B

ENTEROCELE REPAIR

8 **A,** An enterocele descends between the vagina and the rectum.

B and **C,** Open the peritoneum and elevate the anterior wall of the rectum. Place a purse-string stitch of 1-0 NAS around the pouch of Douglas that includes the uterosacral ligaments and the anterior wall of the rectum. Stay well medial to the course of the ureters.

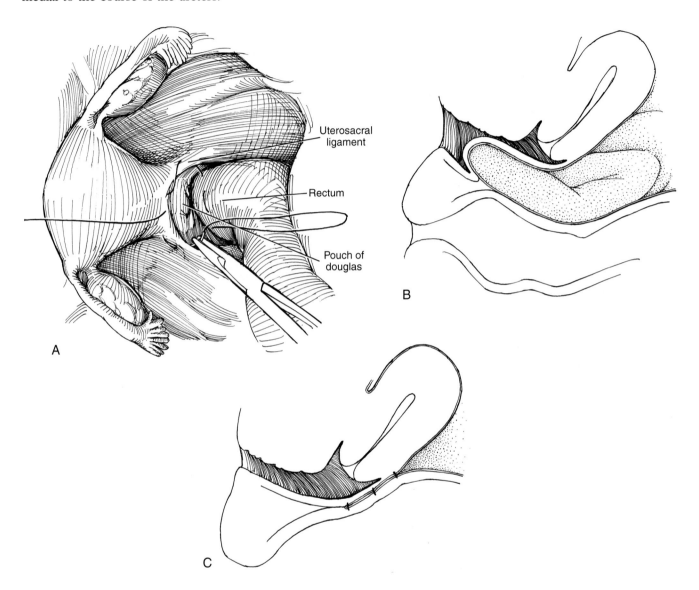

Uterosacral ligament

Rectum

Pouch of douglas

A

B

C

POSTOPERATIVE PROBLEMS

Delayed voiding is less of a problem with this technique than with needle and sling suspensions. However, urinary *obstruction* may be a problem with any anti-incontinence procedure. Treat retention by inserting a Kohlman dilator, expanding the urethra, and tilting the instrument posteriorly to loosen the sutures. This can be done progressively over a period of days, depending on the result, with the dilation going as high as 36 F. If that fails, perform transvaginal urethrolysis by dissecting the urethra from the pubic bone and resuspend the bladder neck from below (Raz). A *vesicovaginal fistula* may occur after injudicious placement of sutures, as well as *ureteral obstruction.* An *enterocele* may result from elevation of the bladder and consequent weakening of the posterior vaginal wall. However, if this appears likely during surgery, the pouch of Douglas can be closed with purse-string sutures placed in the pelvic peritoneum as described.

Commentary by Paul Abrams

My philosophy on colposuspension differs from the description in the text. I confirm genuine stress incontinence by urodynamics, allowing visualization of the bladder base on videocystometry and assessment of urethral function by a urethral pressure profile. At that investigation I assess vaginal mobility, making sure that there is some degree of anterior wall descent and sufficient mobility to allow a proper colposuspension.

Having cleared the fat, as described, I use a vaginal finger to identify the endopelvic fascia and to break through the fascia, mobilizing the periurethral veins with the fingertip, which, when clear of all other tissue, appears uniformly white. Using this technique, one can be sure of being clear of the bladder. In difficult cases, the bladder can be filled with dilute methylene blue, which helps with identification and certainly demonstrates any holes! Having mobilized the vagina, I place 3-0 NAS into the vaginal wall in the axis of the urethra, as opposed to the right-angle approach shown in Step 5. I try to ignore the bleeding, packing the first side while I dissect the second side with the identical technique. The bleeding almost always stops when the sutures are tied.

The next stage involves judgment as to the level at which the vagina comfortably meets the back of the pubis. I believe that colposuspension is the best operation when it offers tissue apposition between the vagina and the back of the pubis. I do not believe that bow-stringing is acceptable, tethering the vagina at "whatever level it wants to go." Most middle-aged women have good tissue at the back of the pubis between 1.5 and 3 cm from the midline. If the quality of the tissue appears doubtful, I would run the suture from the vaginal attachment at the back of the pubis up to the iliopectineal ligament for further security.

Once the sutures have been placed through the vagina and into the back of the pubis on both sides and I am satisfied that tissue apposition can be achieved, I tie the sutures one by one. Either a peanut dissector mounted on Nelson-Roberts forceps or a narrow Deaver retractor can be used to elevate the vagina at the point of suture insertion so that the sutures can be tied without tension. At the end of the procedure, it should be possible to get one fingertip between the newly created vaginal hammock and the underside of the pubic arch.

Using this technique, voiding dysfunction postoperatively is kept to a minimum. If one makes extreme attempts to mobilize the vagina and secure it to the iliopectineal ligament, marked distortion can be produced at the bladder neck. Some believe that this is instrumental in inducing postoperative detrusor instability by trigonal stretching.

My maxim in stress incontinence surgery is to prevent descent rather than to achieve elevation.

I use a 16 F suprapubic Foley catheter and a 20 F Silastic drain to the retropubic space.

Postoperatively, the suprapubic catheter is clamped as soon as the patient is comfortable to walk to the toilet. Once the residual urine is consistently less than 100 ml or less than 30 percent of the bladder capacity, the suprapubic catheter can be removed. Delayed voiding can be managed by sending the patient home with instructions to report when voiding is effective, as described above. Alternatively, the catheter can be removed after the patient has been taught intermittent self-catheterization, which should be continued until efficient voiding is established.

Complications include delayed voiding. This is less of a problem than with sling suspensions but more of a problem than with a needle suspension of the Stamey type.

Laparoscopic Colposuspension

(Vancaille-Schuessler)

TRANSPERITONEAL LAPAROSCOPIC SUSPENSION

Prepare the bowel and provide broad-spectrum antibiotics before the operation. *Anesthesia:* General. Insert bladder and nasogastric catheters. *Position:* Place the patient in a dorsal lithotomy position. Prepare the abdomen and vagina.

Insufflate the abdomen and insert a 10- or 11-mm trocar under the umbilicus, an 11-mm trocar midway between pubis and umbilicus, and two 5-mm trocars lateral to the rectus muscle half way between the umbilicus and the anterior superior iliac spine. Lyse pelvic adhesions.

Incise the retroperitoneum over the pubic bone medial to the left medial umbilical ligament. Expose the posterior surface of the pubic bone. Have the assistant hold the bladder aside. Enter the space of Retzius, and expose the pubic arch anteriorly and the urethra and vagina posteriorly. Use fulguration generously to prevent pooling of blood.

With two fingers in the vagina to elevate it, insert a 2-0 SAS via the suprapubic port into the fascia overlying the vaginal wall immediately lateral to the urethra, and then pass it through Cooper's ligament. Pull up on the suture to check the position of the vesical neck. Place a second suture on the other side of the urethra.

Form extracorporeal knots to tie the sutures, and tighten them to elevate the vesical neck with assistance from the vaginal finger. Alternatively, apply absorbable clips (LapraTy, Ethicon) as the vagina is held in position. Insert a second pair of sutures near the bladder neck. Close the peritoneum with the hernia stapler. Drains are not needed.

EXTRAPERITONEAL LAPAROSCOPIC SUSPENSION

An extraperitoneal approach is not suitable for patients with previous transverse lower abdominal incisions or extensive pelvic surgery.

Position: Place the patient supine after inserting a 24 F balloon catheter transurethrally, inflated to 5 ml. Prepare the lower abdomen and perineum. Provide a dissecting balloon, made from either the finger of a glove or an O'Conor drape (see page 994) or obtained commercially (Preperitoneal Distention Balloon System, Origin Inc., Menlo Park, CA).

Incision and exposure: Make a horizontal skin incision immediately below the umbilicus, and expose the anterior rectus sheath. Place two 1-0 SAS in the sheath at either end of the incision, and open it at the linea alba. Separate the bellies of the muscle with a clamp, insert the index finger between the muscle and the posterior sheath, and bluntly dissect a space for the balloon. Insert the balloon, positioning it at the arcuate line.

Inflation: Inflate the balloon with a sphygmomanometer pump with 800 or 1000 ml of saline or air. Deflate and remove the balloon. Insert a Hasson cannula and tie it in place. Inflate with CO_2 at high flow and 15 mm Hg pressure until the space can be seen to be adequately dissected for the operation (less for retropubic work and more for node dissection).

Trocar insertion: Insert a 30-degree 10-mm laparoscope. Add two additional trocars with the usual precautions, one 10- or 12-mm port midway between umbilicus and symphysis and a 5-mm port just above the symphysis, taking care not to enter the peritoneum. Alternatively, place these last two ports on either side of the lower abdomen.

Identify and expose the pubic bone by clearing the tissue across it from left to right (much of the dissection will have been done by the balloon). Dissect the fibrofatty tissue from the urethra and a portion of the anterior vaginal wall, palpating the intravesical balloon for orientation. Clip large veins as they are encountered.

Insert the index finger of the left hand (or sponge forceps) into the vagina. Place one or two 2-0 synthetic NAS in the vaginal wall just lateral to the urethra (see page 546) and bring them through the symphysis as a modification of the MMK operation (see page 547).

For a more effective suspension, expose Cooper's ligaments bilaterally and place a long suture through them on each side, to produce a modification of the culposuspension procedure of Burch (see page 549). While the vagina is elevated, tie the knots extracorporeally, using a "pusher" to place them, or clip them with synthetic absorbable clips (LapraTy). Check the suspension cystopanendoscopically.

Remove the trocar sheaths under direct vision. Close the fascial defects with 1-0 SAS. Allow the gas to escape before removing the Hasson catheter. Seal the umbilical defect by tying the stay sutures, and close the skin with a subcuticular suture. Leave the catheter in place overnight.

Postoperative problems include *retropubic bleeding* and *bladder perforation.*

Commentary by William W. Schuessler

Laparoscopic surgeons should be familiar with the basic principles of the open procedure. The intraperitoneal approach requires slightly more time but is more versatile. Very careful identification of the anatomy—the bladder neck, the vagina freed of fatty tissue, and Cooper's ligament on each side—is most important prior to positioning sutures on each side.

A curved ring forceps is used to elevate the vagina to the level of Cooper's ligament laterally, allowing the bladder neck elevation to be seen prior to positioning the first suture in the vagina on each side. A short 20-mm half-circle atraumatic needle with a 2-0 NAS at least 36 inches long should be used for the sutures. A curved-tip needle holder is a distinct advantage. Once the first suture is placed on the right side and tied, the second suture is placed distal to the first, again using the ring forceps to elevate the vagina. The second right-hand suture is not tied prior to repeating the procedure on the left. All the knots are first tied extracorporeally with a knot pusher and then reinforced with three throws of intracorporeal knots. After completion of the sutures, the vagina should be in contact with Cooper's ligament on each side, with the bladder neck just behind but not touching the pubic symphysis. The peritoneum should be closed with a hernia stapler when using the intraperitoneal approach.

Precise attention to detail allows duplication of the surgical principles of the open procedure in a reasonable amount of time. Laparoscopy allows postoperative morbidity to compare favorably with that for vaginal procedures. Long-term results should duplicate those of open colposuspension.

Vaginal Needle Suspension

BLADDER NECK SUSPENSION
(Pereyra-Raz)

The initial success rate of needle suspension is similar to that of colposuspension, although colposuspension probably holds better over time.

Start parenteral antibiotics and provide an organic iodide douche.

Position: Place the patient in the dorsal lithotomy position, with feet suspended in padded boots. Prepare the abdomen, perineum, and vagina. Place a balloon cystostomy tube using a curved Lowsley retractor (see page 628) and drain the bladder. Insert a weighted posterior vaginal speculum. Tack the labia back with silk sutures. Insert a balloon catheter through the urethra.

Dissection

1 Grasp the vaginal wall with an Allis clamp half way from meatus to bladder neck, and hold it up to stretch the wall. Inject 5 to 10 ml of saline solution under the anterior vaginal wall beneath the proposed inverted U-incision. Make an incision over the injected tissue so that the arms extend to the urethrovesical junction. Place tension on the balloon to help identify this level. Cut down to the shiny white paraurethral fascia.

2 Dissect laterally under the anterior vaginal wall at the level of the bladder neck (direct the scissors toward the shoulder of the patient) along the pubic bone and sliding over the surface of the paraurethral fascia. Cut against the pubic bone to begin freeing the attachment of the endopelvic fascia. This cut must be at the level of the urethra, not at that of the bladder neck, to avoid vesical perforation. Enter the retropubic space at this level, again pointing the scissors toward the shoulder of the patient.

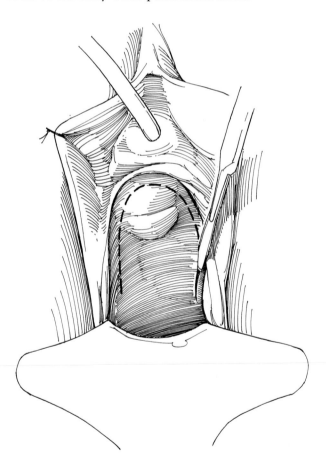

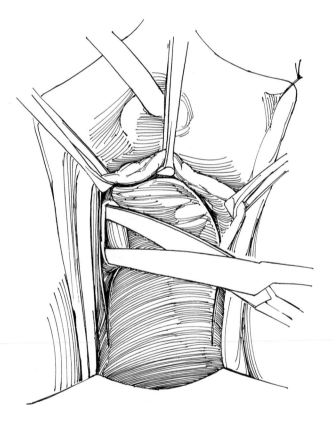

3 Use the index finger to free the adhesions in the retropubic space, separating the bladder from the pubic bone as far posteriorly as the ischial tuberosity.

Vaginal Suturing

4 *Bladder neck suspension:* Insert long forceps into the retropubic space to displace the urethra medially. Place a 1-0 Prolene suture on a heavy noncutting needle into the retropubic space to catch the urethropelvic ligament. Make two passes with the needle to secure it firmly to the ligament. Then pass the needle through the pubocervical fascia and the anterior vaginal wall, but do not include the vaginal epithelium. Make two passes with the needle to grasp the vaginal wall firmly, forming a helical suture line. Be sure to take adequate bites of tissue. Repeat the stitch on the other side.

Minimal cystocele: Extend the ends of the U-incision deeper into the vagina. Pass the helical suture once or twice again at the cephalic end near the cardinal ligament to elevate the cystocele along with the bladder neck.

Grade II and III cystoceles: Use two sets of helical sutures, one set at the bladder neck and the other at the base of the U-incision. Both sutures include the vaginal wall, the pubocervical fascia, and the medial portion of the endopelvic fascia (four-corner suspension, Raz).

Anterior vaginal wall sling: Insert long forceps into the retropubic space and expose the levator muscle. Pass a 1-0 Prolene suture on a heavy noncutting needle through the levator muscle with two passes to include the edge of the urethropelvic ligament, and then insert it through the anterior vaginal wall, excepting the epithelium.

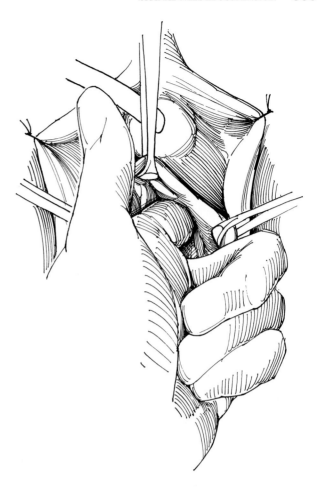

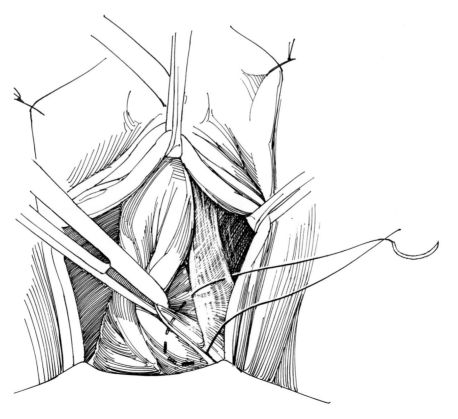

Needle Suspension

5 Make a puncture incision in the abdomen just above the symphysis pubis, and expose the rectus fascia. Insert the double-pronged suspension needle from above. With an index finger inserted from below through the retropubic space, guide the needle out the introitus. It is important to pass the needle under constant fingertip control to avoid injury to adjacent structures. Have the anesthetist inject indigo carmine intravenously, preparatory to the next step.

6 Thread both ends of the suture onto the needle, draw them out suprapubically, and place them in a clamp. Pass the needle again down the other side, draw out the sutures, and clamp them. Remove the urethral catheter. Insert a cystoscope to check for vesical penetration of the sutures and position of the suprapubic catheter. Make certain that elevation of the bladder neck is easy with traction on the sutures and that coaptation of urethra and bladder neck occurs. If elevation requires effort, return below and free the vagina more completely laterally. Be sure indigo carmine issues from the ureteral orifices.

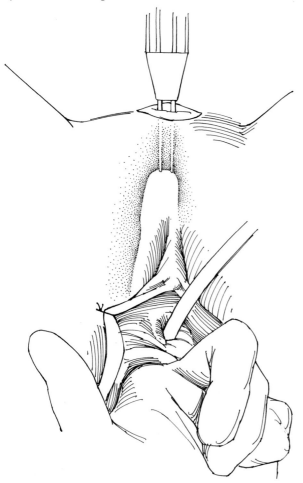

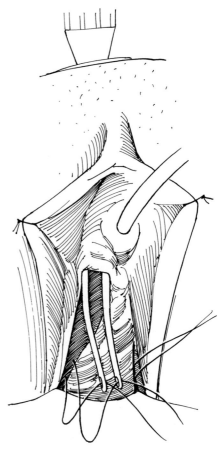

7 Close the vaginal incision with running 2-0 SAS. Always place a vaginal pack saturated with sulfonamide cream *prior* to tying the suspension sutures. Tie these sutures in pairs on each side, and, in addition, tie them to each other across the midline. If in doubt about the required degree of elevation, reinsert the cystoscope and observe the approximation at the bladder neck before tying the sutures. Reinsert the balloon catheter. Remove both pack and catheter the next day. Plug the suprapubic catheter, and have the patient check her own postvoid residual urine. Remove the suprapubic catheter when the volume is 60 ml or less.

MINIMAL CYSTOCELE REPAIR

8 If a minimal cystocele is present, make a vertical midline rather than a U-incision. Proceed with suspension as described. Trim the excess vaginal wall, and approximate the pubocervical fascia with multiple mattress sutures.

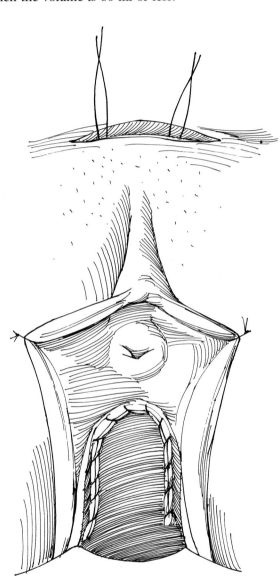

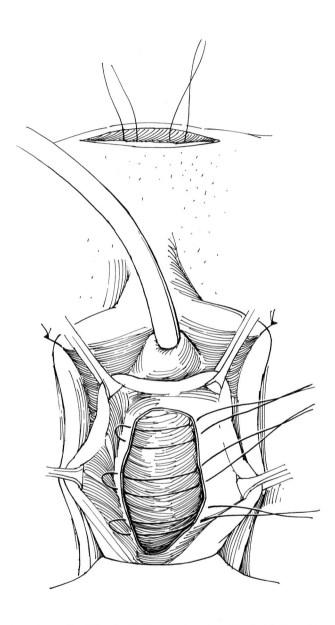

MAJOR VAGINAL REPAIR
(GRADE IV CYSTOCELE)

Repair may be necessary for a cystocele associated with genuine stress incontinence to avoid bladder neck obstruction after bladder suspension. Minimal or moderate cystoceles can be repaired at the same time as a needle bladder neck suspension is carried out.

Insert suprapubic and urethral catheters and empty the bladder.

9 Suture the labia back for exposure. Grasp the vagina with Allis clamps. Make a goal-post incision as shown. The crossbar should be at the level of the midurethra.

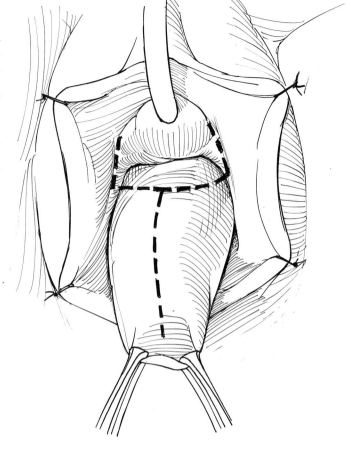

10 Insert a Scott ring retractor, and use the hooks for retraction. By sharp but superficial dissection, free the vaginal wall from the perivesical fascia as far as the pubocervical fascia laterally, the periurethral fascia anteriorly, and the cardinal ligaments posteriorly. Open the retropubic space with curved Mayo scissors. Place a layer of absorbable mesh on the exposed bladder base, and retract it upward to reduce the cystocele.

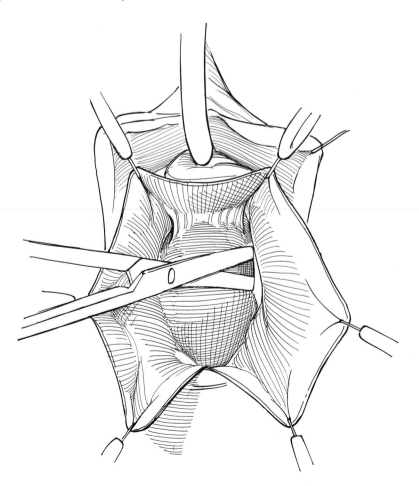

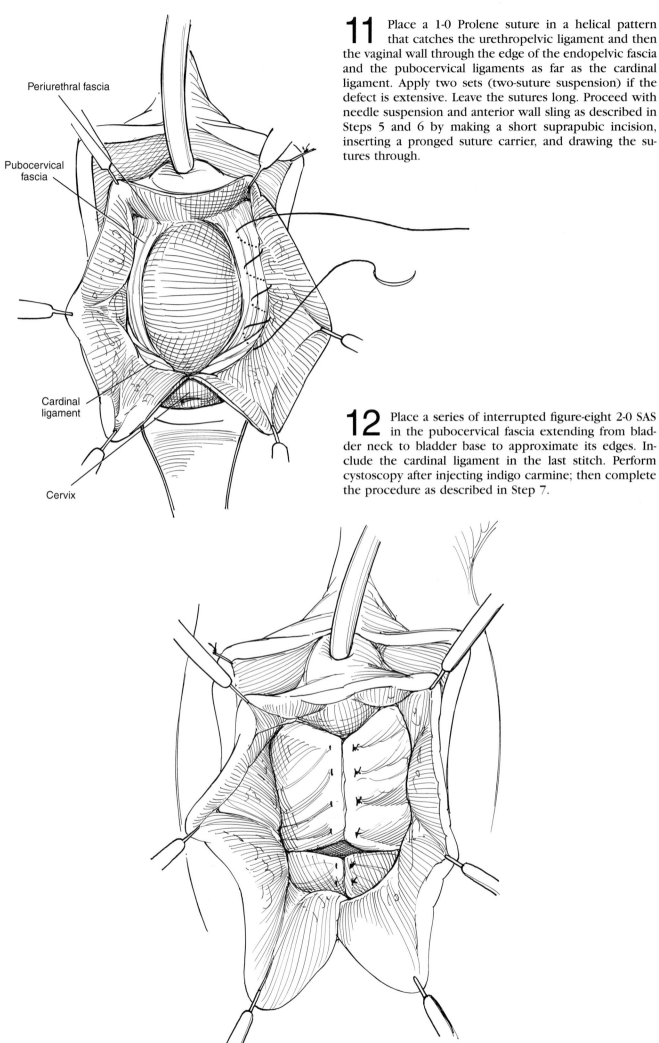

11 Place a 1-0 Prolene suture in a helical pattern that catches the urethropelvic ligament and then the vaginal wall through the edge of the endopelvic fascia and the pubocervical ligaments as far as the cardinal ligament. Apply two sets (two-suture suspension) if the defect is extensive. Leave the sutures long. Proceed with needle suspension and anterior wall sling as described in Steps 5 and 6 by making a short suprapubic incision, inserting a pronged suture carrier, and drawing the sutures through.

Periurethral fascia

Pubocervical fascia

Cardinal ligament

Cervix

12 Place a series of interrupted figure-eight 2-0 SAS in the pubocervical fascia extending from bladder neck to bladder base to approximate its edges. Include the cardinal ligament in the last stitch. Perform cystoscopy after injecting indigo carmine; then complete the procedure as described in Step 7.

563

POSTOPERATIVE PROBLEMS

Inability to void after prolonged suprapubic drainage may require a period of intermittent catheterization. Placing sutures too close to the urethra may be one factor. *Actual urinary retention* is rare and is managed by taking down one or both of the sets of sutures suprapubically. If this fails, the repair must be taken down entirely and repeated.

Detrusor instability is treated with anticholinergic medication, anticipating subsidence of the symptoms. *Persistent incontinence* occurs in less than 10 percent of cases. It is usually due to inadequate suspension secondary to insufficient mobilization of the urethra, vagina, and bladder neck, to placing sutures too high proximally or too far distally, or to poor quality of local tissue. If the intrinsic urethral mechanism is defective, elevation alone is insufficient and a pubovaginal or anterior vaginal wall sling procedure is required (see page 565).

Ilioinguinal nerve entrapment causes pain in the ilioinguinal dermatome, at first sharp and later dull, lessened by flexion of the hip. Block the ilioinguinal nerve (see page 76) with 0.5 percent bupivacaine for diagnosis and temporary relief. Successive blocks may eradicate the pain, or surgery may be required to release the trapped nerve (Monga and Ghoneim, 1994). *Protracted suprapubic pain* may be helped by infiltration of the area with a local anesthetic agent. *Dyspareunia* may occur, as can clitoral anesthesia.

Commentary by Schlomo Raz and Lynn Stothers

Patient selection for the various operations to correct stress urinary incontinence with or without anterior vaginal wall prolapse is critical in achieving a long-lasting result. As a general principle, we perform the anterior vaginal wall sling procedure for patients with anatomic incontinence and intrinsic sphincter dysfunction and do not perform the bladder neck suspension with only two sutures. The four-corner suspension for moderate cystocele should be performed in a highly selected group of patients with a lateral defect of support only. Performing this procedure in patients with a significant central defect in the pubocervical fascia or in patients with Grade IV cystocele results in a poor outcome. These cases require surgical correction of a central defect, a lateral defect, and support of the bladder neck and midurethra. Correcting the cystocele in this case without attention to the bladder neck and midurethra may result in postoperative stress incontinence in patients without clinical stress incontinence preoperatively.

Currently at the University of California, Los Angeles, we do not do bladder neck suspensions. We use the anterior vaginal wall sling for patients with hypermobility with or without minimal cystocele and intrinsic sphincter dysfunction. The procedure begins as the Pereyra-Raz bladder neck suspension but adds two more Prolene sutures. These sutures include three structures: the levator musculature, the edge of the urethropelvic ligament, and the anterior vaginal wall without epithelium. The vaginal wall sling created by burying the anterior vaginal wall is no longer done and has been replaced by the anterior vaginal wall sling. For severe (Grade IV) cystocele, we use a goal-post–shaped incision. This allows for four Prolene sutures to be placed. The more distal pair is placed exactly like the sling and includes the levator musculature. The second pair of sutures is as described and illustrated in the text. We use a Dexon mesh to help reduce the cystocele and better expose the edges of the pubocervical fascia, as shown in Step 12.

Technical considerations are important in these reconstructive procedures. We believe that an extensive urethrolysis in patients with prior surgery is important prior to placement of the permanent sutures. After the incisions in the anterior vaginal wall, dissection over the periurethral fascia reveals a shiny surface. If dissection is carried out too deeply and the urethropelvic ligament is entered, increased bleeding can occur. The vaginal incisions should be closed with care so that the Prolene suture is buried well below the absorbable sutures to prevent later exposure of the nonabsorbable sutures through the vaginal wall. The sutures should be tied down after a vaginal pack is placed, which helps to support the anterior vaginal wall while you tighten the sutures in the lower abdominal stab incision. After the permanent sutures are tied, it is important to free the edges of the subcutaneous fat before closing the abdominal wound. Failure to do so results in a dimpling of the skin over the permanent sutures, and the patient is able to feel the knots of the sutures under the skin, which can cause discomfort.

We have not had a single case out of more than 800 operations in which the patient was unable to void. It has not been necessary to reopen the abdominal wound and cut one of the sutures. Unless intrinsic sphincter damage pre-exists, persistent incontinence is rare. In 94 percent of cases, continence is achieved with the first operation.

Pubovaginal Sling

Test the patient urodynamically to be certain that the principal cause of incontinence is an incompetent urethral sphincter mechanism (Type III incontinence). This usually follows multiple surgical attempts but may also occur after pelvic trauma or radiation or accompanying some neurologic defects. Be certain that it is not the consequence of detrusor hyperactivity or vesicourethral malposition. Determine detrusor contractility because its absence means that the patient indeed requires perpetual intermittent catheterization. For girls with meningomyelocele and poor compliance or intractable uninhibited contractions and incontinence, perform augmentation cystoplasty in addition to the sling procedure.

Exhaust medical approaches using alpha-adrenergic and anticholinergic medications. Caution the patient or family about complications such as the possible need for intermittent catheterization, persistent untreatable detrusor instability, upper urinary tract damage, and urinary tract infection.

Arrange for a second surgeon to stand between the patient's legs. *Position*: Place the patient in the low lithotomy position. Use Allen stirrups with the legs suspended by the feet, which are firmly planted in the stirrups so that no pressure is placed on the calf. Prepare the lower abdomen, perineum, and vagina. Drape to provide access to the vagina. Place a balloon catheter in the bladder. A catheter may be placed suprapubically with a Lowsley retractor (see page 628) that can be left indwelling to allow the patient to check for residual urine during convalescence. Drain the bladder. Fill the balloon enough to allow palpation of the vesical neck.

1 *Retropubic operator:* Make a transverse lower abdominal skin incision (see page 490) 4 cm above the symphysis and 8 cm long. Expose and clear the areolar tissue from the rectus sheath. Incise the sheath transversely above the symphysis for a distance of 8 cm (the distance may be 5 to 15 cm, depending on the size of the patient). Lift up both edges and separate them from the rectus muscles superiorly and inferiorly, as is usually done for the transverse incision. Place stay sutures at each end of the lower flap, and cut a fusiform strip of fascia between them, the length determined by estimating the distance around the urethra and through and over the rectus muscle and fascia. The center of the strip should be at least 2 cm wide to provide broad urethral support. At each end, place a 2-0 nonabsorbable running horizontal mattress suture at right angles to the direction of its fibers. Cover the strip with moist gauze and put it aside. Alternatively, the strip may be harvested after the retropubic dissection.

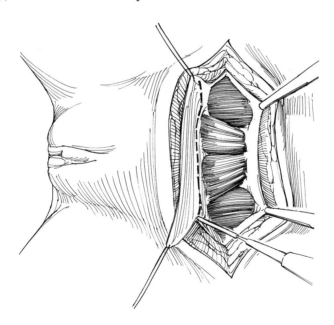

2 Form a tunnel starting digitally in the triangular space just lateral to the recti. With alternate blunt and sharp dissection, pass lateral to the anterior bladder wall and urethra. Continue the dissection until the endopelvic fascia of the pelvic floor is reached. In difficult cases, such as after multiple procedures, detach the rectus muscles from the symphysis for a short distance on either side of the midline and dissect with the point of the scissors directly on the periosteum of the symphysis pubis to its lower margin, while depressing the bladder. Opening the bladder at this point can facilitate the dissection but usually is not necessary.

3 *Perineal operator:* Insert a weighted vaginal retractor. Infiltrate the vagina with normal saline. Make a 2-cm vertical incision in the vaginal wall. (Alternatively, make a small inverted U-incision and reflect it posteriorly.) Dissect just beneath the vaginal epithelium using Metzenbaum scissors. It is important to enter the proper plane. Leave the white paraurethral fascia in place to keep away from the urethra and bladder, with the risk of subsequent erosion of the sling. Keep the scissors parallel to the perineum in order to enter the retropubic space in a safe and bloodless plane. Take a course lateral to the urethra in the direction of the patient's ipsilateral shoulder to reach the surface of the ischium. Using the fingernail to push the tissue from the periosteum, continue with digital dissection through the endopelvic fascia until you reach the retropubic space at the inferior margin of the pubic symphysis (see page 558). As an alternative, incise the pelvic floor and dissect with the fingers superiorly and laterally to develop the retropubic space. If help is needed with orientation to create the tunnels for the sling and to allow detection of vesical injury, open the bladder if that was not done.

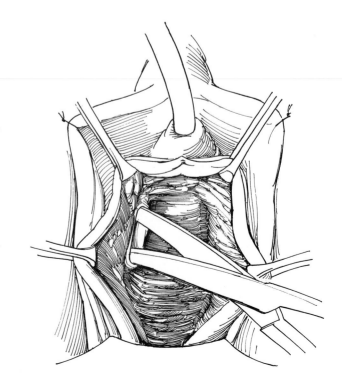

4 **A,** *Retropubic operator:* Free the urethra and, with guidance from a finger in the vagina, insert the scissors lateral to it on both sides to make an opening in the pelvic floor where it attaches to the symphysis. Be sure that the points of the scissors lead laterally and superiorly toward the anterior superior iliac crest. Enlarge the opening with a finger in this same direction.

Alternative (not shown): To avoid having to dissect the bladder neck retropubically from above (Step 2), free the bladder neck from below, insert a finger, and push the bladder neck medially to palpate the fingertip behind the rectus muscle. Make an incision in the rectus fascia slightly off the midline, keeping close to the pubis to avoid postoperative pain from motion of the abdominal wall. Insert a long clamp through the incision, and use the index finger to guide it into the perineal wound.

B, Insert the index finger of the left hand in the vagina. Grasp a curved clamp in the right hand with the concave side up, and advance it from above down the right side with the finger as a guide, keeping the curved side against the symphysis to avoid entering the bladder. The guiding finger in the vagina keeps the tip of the clamp from entering the vagina.

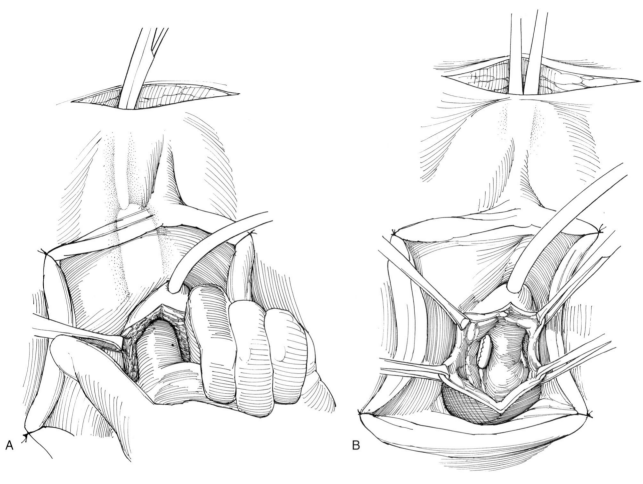

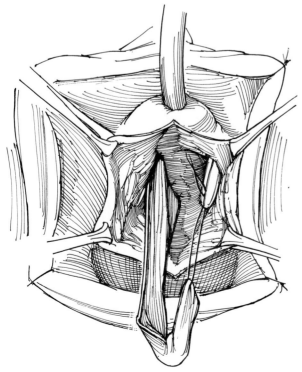

5 Grasp one end of the sling (or its stay suture) presented by the perineal operator, and draw it retropubically into the upper wound. Spread the middle of the sling, and tack it to the paraurethral tissues and perineal fascia, smooth surface down, with an absorbable suture to obtain as broad a bearing as possible. Repeat the procedure on the left side, passing the clamp down that side and drawing up the other end of the sling. Check for vesical injury by irrigating the catheter and draining the bladder completely. If blood is seen in the urine, perform cystoscopy of the bladder. If perforation has occurred, remove and replace the suture.

567

6 A, Suture one end to the rectus fascia, making a three-bite helix in the fascial strip with the 2-0 or 3-0 NAS. (Alternatively, pass a tonsil clamp through the belly of the rectus muscle on the right, and draw the end of the strip through it and the corresponding rectus fascia.) Draw the other end of the strip through muscle and fascia similarly on the left side. Have the perineal operator close the incision in the vaginal mucosa before the retropubic operator tightens the sling. Suture the end in place with 2-0 or 3-0 SAS placed as a three-bite helix. In addition, suture the strip to the fascia at the site of exit. This allows the strip to have an ovoid shape that keeps better tension on the urethra.

B, Trim any excess length from the strip. Tighten the sling until about 6 to 7 cm H_2O pressure is exerted on the urethra. This can be checked by endoscopic inspection or by profilometry. Another way is to insert the endoscope and increase sling tension until the proximal urethra is slightly compressed under the sling. Yet another method is to tighten the sling until no leakage occurs with gentle compression over the filled bladder. Obtaining correct tension requires considerable judgment because no exact criteria can be used, but endoscopic observation helps. "The appropriate tension is the minimum required to stop urethral motion" (McGuire). Suture the free end to the fascia with 2-0 or 3-0 NAS, again with a three-bite helix in the fascial strip. Another way to fix the sling is to place the sutures in each end using multiple stitches, then tie them together over Teflon bolsters. From below, tack the sling to the periurethral fascia with a fine absorbable suture and close the vaginal opening. Place a balloon catheter through the bladder wall if it was not placed initially. Close the bladder if it was opened, and close the suprapubic wound. Insert a Penrose drain. Place a vaginal pack, and remove it the next day. Remove the drain and the catheter after 2 days. Teach the patient intermittent catheterization.

Alternative technique 1 (Blaivas): After harvesting the strip, close the rectus fascia. Proceed to a vaginal approach. Make a short curved incision in the anterior vaginal wall that extends only through the vaginal epithelium, with its apex at the bladder neck as determined by palpation of the balloon. Dissect laterally to reach the periosteum of pubis or ischium and, using the fingertip, go through the endopelvic fascia into the retropubic space. This releases the vesical neck and posterior urethra. Palpate the tip of the index finger in the retropubic wound, and make a 2-cm incision in the rectus fascia. Insert a long curved clamp retropubically onto the index finger, and draw the tip out the introitus. Do the same on the other side. With traction on the stay sutures, guide the fascial strip up either side. Check the bladder neck cystoscopically. Insert a 12 F punch cystostomy under vision. Close the vaginal incision with interrupted 2-0 chromic figure-eight sutures. Tie the long sutures together in the midline so that little or no tension is placed on the sling. It is not necessary that the ends of the fascial strip extend through the fascia. Place a vaginal pack, to be removed the next day. The suprapubic tube allows for trials of voiding.

Alternative technique 2 (Ghoneim): Proceed as described in Steps 1 to 4. Before drawing the fascial strip sutures retropubically, cross them so that the sling almost completely encircles the urethra.

Alternative technique 3: The strip may be left attached to the symphysis (Millin technique) and passed entirely around the bladder neck ("cinch," Hanna, 1995); a 12-cm strip is required. In girls, a simple sling is adequate.

Alternative technique 4: For neurogenic incontinence in children, take a pedicle strip of anterior bladder wall based at the bladder neck, pass it to encircle the neck as for the cinch, and attach the end to the symphysis (Kurzrock et al, 1995).

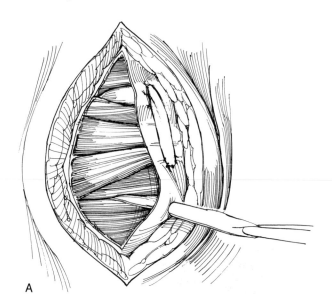

A

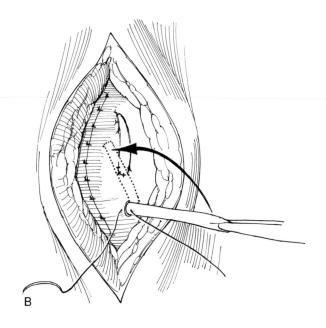

B

RECURRENT INCONTINENCE

For Type III stress urinary incontinence recurring after previous repairs, release the bladder from its bed through a suprapubic approach. Proceed with a fascial sling as described. Alternatively, set a 1.5-cm polypropylene strip in place perineally, and secure it with little tension to Cooper's ligament from above (Morgan et al, 1995). With mesh, watch out for urethral erosion, formation of a granuloma, and vesicovaginal or urethrovaginal fistulas. Provide temporary suprapubic drainage.

POSTOPERATIVE PROBLEMS

Urinary retention may be the greatest concern. It is usually the result of too much tension at the urethrovesical junction. Straining to void only pushes the bladder neck down, tightening the sling. The patient must learn to void by perineal relaxation with its accompanying reflex detrusor contraction. The options are intermittent catheterization, removal of the fascial sutures (as an outpatient procedure), or division of the sling vaginally to place dependence on the fibrosis that has developed. Another option is to turn down a vaginal flap, expose and divide the sling in the midline, and interpose a graft from the vaginal flap (Ghoniem and Elgamasy, 1995). Expect one third of patients to void at least by 7 days and one third within 3 months; the remainder require a longer term of intermittent catheterization. In one quarter of the patients, uninhibited detrusor contractions may persist postoperatively, but these usually respond to anticholinergic medication.

The sling may *erode* into the urethra or bladder, obliterating the lumen or producing a urethrovaginal fistula, or it may leave *incontinence* by not sufficiently compressing the urethra because of excessive scarring from previous procedures. Decline in bladder *compliance* may follow a sling operation. Patients with borderline compliance may benefit from concomitant augmentation.

OBSTRUCTIVE FASCIAL SLING NEEDLE SUSPENSION (McGuire)

This operation is designed for girls with myelodysplasia.

Through a midline vaginal incision, free the urethra and urethrovesical junction from the vaginal mucosa. Pass scissors through the pelvic floor on either side of the urethra.

Obtain a strip of rectus fascia through a suprapubic incision (Step 1). Fasten 2-0 polypropylene sutures to the ends of the strip with Teflon bolsters, and pass them on Stamey needles into the retropubic space. Check the path of the sutures endoscopically. Pull the sling into place, and draw the sutures up until the vesical neck is seen to be closed endoscopically. Tie them over pledgets. Remove the catheter and institute intermittent catheterization after 24 hours.

Commentary by Edward J. McGuire and Helen E. O'Connell

A pubovaginal sling may be used as a stand-alone procedure or in association with a variety of procedures such as augmentation cystoplasty, cystocele repair, or other repair of genital prolapse. The conditions that may be treated with a pubovaginal sling include Type III stress incontinence due to any cause, combined intrinsic sphincter deficiency and urethral hypermobility, urethral wall deficiency such as after urethral diverticulectomy surgery, pelvic trauma, and Foley catheter trauma. Because of the long-term success and robustness of a sling in relation to other treatments for stress incontinence, a sling may be the procedure of choice in certain patients with Type II incontinence. These include obese patients, those with chronic obstructive pulmonary disease, and athletes. No other suitable option is available for the combination of Type II hypermobility plus intrinsic sphincter deficiency, for Type III stress incontinence and a cystocele, for neurogenic Type III stress incontinence, or for a previous failed sling.

The most important issues to discuss in obtaining informed consent are the probability of short-term voiding dysfunction and the possibility of de novo urge incontinence postoperatively. In the early postoperative period, the incidence of voiding dysfunction is high even if voiding was normal preoperatively. In patients who were voiding normally preoperatively, a return to complete bladder emptying without intermittent catheterization is expected in virtually all cases. Detrusor instability may co-exist and require concomitant treatment. Approximately 60 percent of detrusor instability present prior to the sling procedure resolves. In a small proportion (less than 10 percent), detrusor instability occurs de novo postoperatively. Other potential complications are postoperative pain, urinary infection, wound hematoma, and, rarely, incomplete cure of stress incontinence and sling breakage.

Intravenous antibiotics are given prior to surgery. General or regional anesthesia may be used. Epidural anesthesia offers no particular advantage in sling patients.

Postoperative problems: Because of the high incidence of voiding dysfunction at least temporarily, intermittent catheterization is taught to all on a 4-hour and as required basis. Once the residual volumes are consistently less than 60 ml, the patient stops catheterization. Usually a few doses of parenteral analgesia are required. The sling sutures often cause asymmetric pain, which may take weeks to settle. It is important that exercise of the abdominal wall be avoided for the first 3 to 4 weeks so as not to break the sling. After that, the patient is free to do any exercise. Vaginal spotting is very common and relates only to the healing vaginal suture line. Wound problems other than pain are uncommon. Although incomplete cure of stress incontinence is rare, it may be the result. This type of incontinence responds very well to transurethral collagen injection therapy.

Trigonal Tubularization

(Guy Leadbetter)

Perform urodynamic studies to determine that the incontinence is due to low urethral closure pressure, usually with scarring and fixation of the urethra from previous operations, and that the detrusor is compliant.

Clear (or suppress) bacteriuria. Panendoscopy may show a treatable bladder neck stricture or residual obstruction, and cystometrography may show treatable detrusor hyperreflexia. Women with hyperactive neurogenic dysfunction are not candidates for this operation, but those with compliant bladders do well if intermittently catheterized postoperatively.

This operation and the Mitchell modification have an advantage over the intravesical lengthening technique (Kropp, see page 576) in that they allow spontaneous voiding.

Position: Place male patients supine with the pelvis slightly elevated over a rolled towel; for women, use a modified lithotomy position; and for infants, a frog-legged position is best.

After preparing and draping, insert a 16 F 5-ml balloon catheter and instill sterile water into the bladder to partially fill it.

Incision: Make a lower midline extraperitoneal incision (see page 487) or, preferably, a lower transverse incision (see page 490).

Reflect a limited area of the peritoneum from the anterior bladder surface, and dissect carefully in the space of Retzius to expose the proximal two thirds of the prostate. In females, expose the urethra to the level of the endopelvic fascia. In a patient who has had previous procedures, take care not to disturb the vessels on the anterior bladder wall. Dissect laterally around the vesicourethral junction, identified by the balloon on the catheter, avoiding the rectum or vagina and neurovascular bundle. Avoid mobilizing the more posterior aspects of the bladder and urethra, risking disturbance of the neurovascular connections.

1 Open the bladder in the midline all the way into the deep urethra. Insert 5 F silicone catheters into the ureters. Mobilize the ureters extravesically, taking care to bring them under the vas or uterine vessels so that they have a straight course after reimplantation higher in the bladder. Implant each ureter 3 to 4 cm more cephalad than the normal position, using a tunnel technique. A transtrigonal implantation (see page 793), as shown, may be a good choice.

2 Place a stay suture in the anterior urethral wall at the apex of the initial cystotomy. With curved scissors, cut through the entire thickness of the urethra and bladder wall, beginning just lateral to the stay suture and continuing through the site of the previous orifice and 1 to 2 cm beyond *(dashed lines in Step 1).* Alternatively, it may be easier to start the incision at the trigone and cut distally. The entire trigone must be tubularized because it will form the new sphincter. This incision leaves a posterior segment 1.5 to 2 cm wide and 4 to 5 cm long.

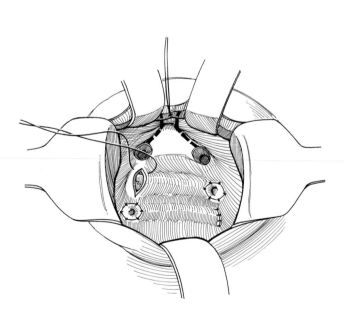

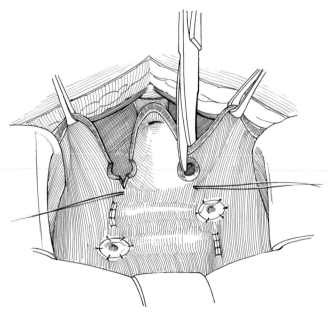

3 **A,** Place a 12 F or 14 F silicone catheter up through the urethra. The smaller size may preclude spontaneous voiding but ensures continence. Approximate the uroepithelium of the edges of the neourethra with interrupted sutures of 5-0 CCG, making the strip snug around the catheter. In fact, it is difficult to make it too tight. It may be easier to start by placing the most proximal suture and progress distally. If inserting the distal sutures in children is difficult, divide the symphysis and spread it with a pediatric rib spreader.

B and **C,** Imbricate the detrusor muscle in the neourethra by suturing one edge firmly to the undersurface of the opposite edge, then lapping that edge back to the first side (vest-over-pants technique). If the resulting bladder capacity is small, consider augmentation with subsequent intermittent catheterization.

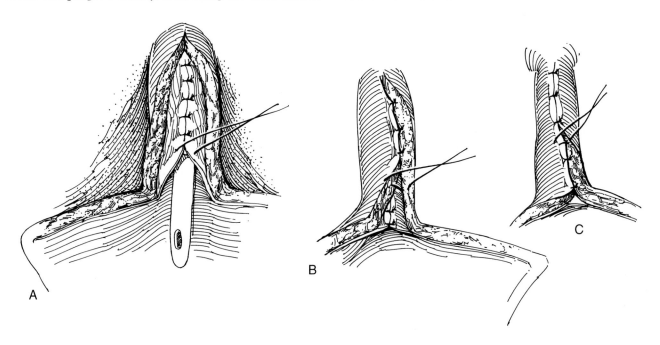

4 Insert ureteral stents bilaterally, and have them exit through stab wounds. Draw a 14 F or 16 F Malecot or balloon catheter out through the bladder and body walls, and fasten it to the skin with an NAS. An 8 F or 10 F balloon catheter may be left as a urethral stent if desired. Close the bladder defect with a running 4-0 or 5-0 CCG subepithelial suture, and with interrupted 3-0 or 4-0 CCG sutures to the muscle and adventitia. Close the wound around a Penrose drain. Remove the stents in 1 to 2 weeks and the suprapubic tube in 2 weeks.

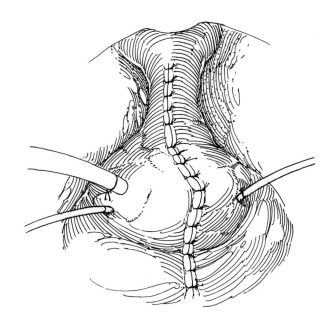

POSTOPERATIVE PROBLEMS

Urinary retention is rare; these patients always seem able to void unless the bladder has been augmented. In that case, intermittent catheterization may be needed. *Incontinence* may persist; if it is from poor vesical compliance, it requires bladder augmentation. For *low outlet resistance*, apply a sling procedure (see page 565) or implant an artificial sphincter (see page 580). *Ureteral obstruction* can occur as with any ureteroneocystostomy. Failure of the cystostomy site to close indicates *stenosis* in the new urethra.

Commentary by Guy W. Leadbetter, Jr.

Comments and tips gained from 30 years of experience with this operation: First, the procedure is often long and arduous and tests one's equanimity.

In a child, splitting the symphyseal cartilage and spreading the symphysis with a pediatric rib spreader may give better exposure and room for suturing, but never spread an adult symphysis, as this causes severe pain in the sacroiliac area postoperatively. In the adult it is better to remove a portion of symphysis if necessary. This trigonal flap method is contraindicated in adult males unless total prostatectomy has been done.

It is important to place sutures at the sites of the ureteral orifices to mark where the trigone is to be tubularized. It is all important for continence that the trigone be tubularized to make the new bladder neck.

Do not remove dog-ear flaps from the bladder after the urethral bladder incision has been made because this causes a decrease in bladder capacity and results in a noncompliant bladder. When reimplanting the ureters, it is important to be certain that they are brought out from under the vas or uterine vessels in order to allow a straight entrance into the bladder. If this is not done, the ureters are obstructed by the vas or vessels as the bladder fills.

Ureteral and suprapubic catheters are left in place for 7 to 14 days. This allows healing to occur in a urine-free field. I believe this prevents possible fibrosis or fistula formation, which may occur if urine leaks into the reconstructed bladder neck area.

MITCHELL DISASSOCIATION TECHNIQUE

This modification of the Young-Dees-Leadbetter procedure provides greater assurance of continence (Jones et al, 1993).

Make a full-thickness transverse incision in the anterior aspect of the urethra as far distally as possible. Extend this incision laterally on each side for three quarters of the urethral circumference. At that posterolateral point on each side, incise proximally as far as the ureteral orifice.

Progressively retract the bladder as the upper end of the incision is completed. This leaves a strip of urethra 1.5 cm wide. Detach the ureters.

Reimplant the ureters by the Politano-Leadbetter technique (see page 789). A Cohen implant may leave a ridge that can interfere with urethral catheterization and prevent later ureteral catheterization.

Tubularize the urethral strip in two layers over a feeding tube of appropriate size (5, 8, or 10 F), first with a running 6-0 SAS to the uroepithelium, followed by an interrupted 4-0 SAS. Add an occasional suture to support the muscularis.

Place a Malecot suprapubic tube, and fix a 5 F feeding tube by bringing a suture through the bladder and body walls. The procedure may be supplemented by a sling or suspension procedure. Close the bladder in two layers in the midline.

Vesical Neck Tubularization

(Tanagho-Flocks)

Clear, or at least suppress, bacteriuria. Panendoscopy may show a treatable bladder neck stricture or residual obstruction, and cystometrography may show treatable detrusor hyperreflexia. Patients with hyperactive neurogenic dysfunction are not candidates for this operation, but those with compliant bladders do well if they are intermittently catheterized. The wall of an atonic bladder is not suitable material for a tube, nor is that of a bladder subjected to previous cystostomies and anterior incisions.

Position: Place males supine with the pelvis slightly elevated; for females, use a modified lithotomy position; and place infants in a frog-leg position. After preparing and draping, insert a 16 F 5-ml balloon catheter and partially fill the bladder with sterile water.

Incision: Use a lower midline extraperitoneal (see page 487) or lower transverse (see page 490) incision.

1 Reflect a limited area of the peritoneum from the anterior bladder surface, and dissect in the space of Retzius carefully to expose the proximal two thirds of the prostate. In females, expose the urethra to the level of the endopelvic fascia. In a patient who has had previous procedures, take care not to disturb the vessels on the anterior bladder wall. Dissect laterally around the vesi-courethral junction, identified by the balloon on the catheter, avoiding the rectum or vagina and neurovascular bundle. Place four stay sutures to outline a flap on the anterior surface of the half-filled bladder, marking a 1-inch square beginning exactly at the internal meatus. The two distal sutures are in the prostate in males and in the urethra in females.

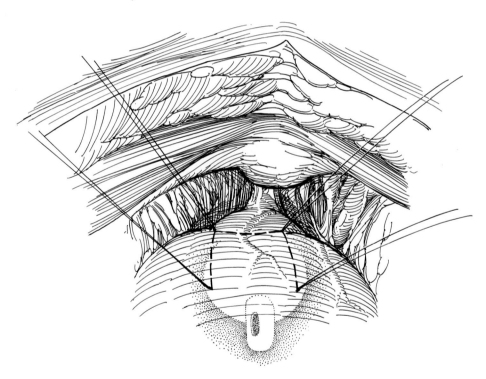

573

2 Make a full-thickness transverse incision across the bladder neck with the cutting current just below the distal sutures of the flap. Once the bladder is entered, extend the initial transverse incision at the vesical neck, cutting laterally inside the bladder. Identify the trigone and ureteral orifices. Cut deeply through the full thickness of the bladder at the apex of the trigone to expose the seminal vesicles and ampullae. Make the cut sufficient to allow the base of the bladder to slide upward for 1 or 2 cm.

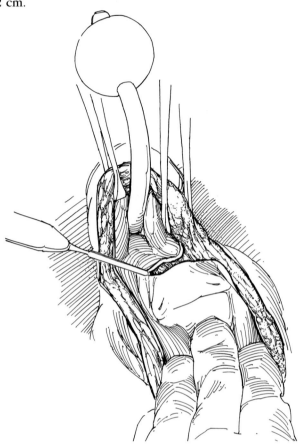

3 Make two parallel cuts running from the lower to the upper stay sutures. Reflect the flap upward. Insert a Malecot catheter as high as possible and to one side through the dome of the bladder, and lead it out through one lower abdominal quadrant (not shown). Anchor it to the skin with an NAS. Roll the bladder flap into a tube around the balloon catheter, and suture the sides together with full-thickness stitches of 3-0 or 4-0 SAS. Be sure to catch the retracted middle layer of the detrusor in each stitch. It may help to put one suture at the base of the flap and one at the apex and then fill in between.

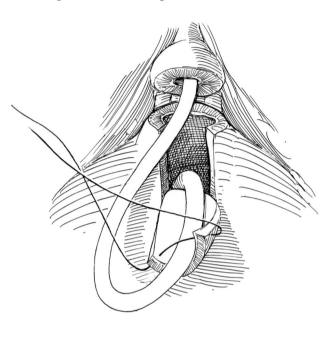

4 Attach the apex of the trigone to the base of the tube with a mattress stitch, and close the remainder of the defect in the bladder transversely.

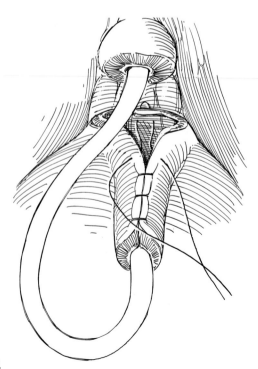

5 Anastomose the tube to the cut end of the urethra with five or six 3-0 or 4-0 SAS. Place all the sutures first, then pull them down and tie them successively. In males, insert two 3-0 or 4-0 CCG sutures into the anterior bladder wall close to the base of the tube and bring them through the lower rectus fascia. In females, use sutures in the vaginal wall as in a suprapubic vesical suspension (see pages 546 to 547).

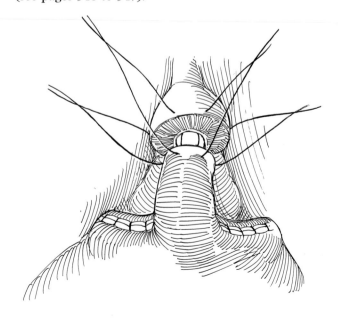

6 **A** and **B,** Alternatively, raise a transverse flap and suture it to the urethra in a corkscrew fashion (Flocks and Boldus, 1973). Or the bladder can be transected and a tube formed from the distal portion, which is then tunneled under the trigone to move the vesical neck into the bas-fond (Kropp; see page 576). Insert Penrose drains to the posterior suture line. Close the wound. Maintain cystostomy drainage for 3 to 4 weeks; then test for residual urine before removing the tube.

POSTOPERATIVE PROBLEMS

Persistent incontinence can occur in patients with noncompliant bladders or in those with tubes constructed from bladder wall of poor quality. *Strictures* can develop between the tube and the prostatic fossa, requiring internal urethrotomy. Postoperative instrumentation and catheterization can be difficult and must be done under direct vision.

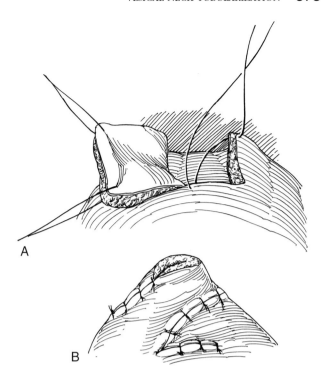

A

B

Commentary by Emil A. Tanagho

An anterior bladder tube can foster continence in boys and girls born with epispadias and also in girls with a short urethra (significant hypospadias) or a high urogenital sinus with a short urethral segment, which might have to be mobilized independently from the urogenital sinus and brought down to the vaginal vestibule. It can also be used in cases of trauma in which the urethrovesical segment is disrupted, especially in girls, and in selected cases of flaccid neurogenic bladder.

The rationale of the procedure is to incorporate in a bladder flap the ventral condensation of circular fibers that extend above the internal meatus for about 1 inch on the anterior bladder wall. Normally, if this area has not been violated before by surgery or trauma, the condensation of circular fibers raised in a flap and turned around into a tube has enough tonus to provide an occlusive effect and sphincteric function that can replace a nonexistent or traumatized normal sphincteric segment. Do not try to make the tube too long; it should be confined to the condensation of circular fibers in the anterior bladder wall. If it is less than 1 inch in length, the tube should be made shorter. The quality of the muscles in the tube rather than the length is what is important. The tube should not be occlusive but should be of adequate diameter to wrap easily around a 16 F catheter (in pediatric cases we usually fit it to a 10 F catheter). Bring the apex of the trigone to the base of the tube and re-create the bladder neck configuration, providing for a sharp transition from the large cavity of the bladder to the adequate lumen of the reconstructed tube. Extreme care should be taken in mobilizing the anterior bladder surface, keeping all the adventitial layers and blood vessels on it. During exposure, aim at the urethrovesical junction. Do not try to free too much of the anterior bladder wall because this might interfere with the blood supply to the flap. Mark the flap with the bladder half distended before starting the incision in order not to lose your orientation. The flap consistently looks narrower after it has been delineated and cut because of the contraction of the circular fibers in it; this is a good sign.

It is essential to handle the tissue with the utmost care in order not to devitalize any of the critical delicate muscle tissue. Accurate coaptation of uroepithelium to uroepithelium with full-thickness muscle-wall sutures is essential in both constructing the tube and establishing the anastomosis between the tube and the urethra. The procedure is suitable for both female and male patients. In cutting the bladder neck completely from the urethra, extreme care should be taken posteriorly not to enter the vaginal wall in girls and not to injure the seminal vesicle and vas in boys. However, a full-thickness cut into the bladder muscle wall is essential to permit the bladder to slide upward.

Closure of the rest of the bladder leaves two small dog ears. Do not attempt to smooth these because they round themselves and become absorbed into the bladder cavity with time to provide additional capacity. If there is a midline incision in the bladder from a previous cystostomy and if conditions are favorable, a one-sided tube can be used: The site of the previous midline incision can form one lateral margin, and the flap can be taken off center. Extensive previous surgery on the anterior bladder wall dooms the operation to failure. Proper suspension and support should be provided without putting tension on the tube and on the suture line between it and the urethra. Mobilize the bladder base and trigone upward to prevent formation of a sharp posterior angle, which can be obstructive. Suprapubic drainage should be adequate for at least 3 weeks, and the patient should be tested for adequate voiding with minimal residual urine before the suprapubic tube is removed. Temporary stenting of the reconstructed tube and site of anastomosis by urethral catheter is desirable for 10 days.

In selected patients with a flaccid neurogenic bladder, a tube can also be most effective. Its purpose is not to act as a sphincter but to provide resistance to permit continence between intermittent catheterization. Emphasis is on supporting the tube after its reconstruction to prevent it from being telescoped or crushed by the weight of the bladder above it. Thus, some kind of suspension is created using either the vaginal wall in girls or the anterior bladder wall in boys and small girls if the vaginal wall is not appropriate for suspension.

The surgeon has to be extremely aware of the major potential causes of failure of this technique: a devascularized flap leading either to contracture or sloughing and fistulization, too wide a flap becoming funneled and absorbed into the bladder cavity, too narrow a flap becoming a precursor for ischemia once it is wrapped into a tube around the catheter, inaccurate opposition of uroepithelium-to-uroepithelium sutures at the site of an anastomosis, and lack of proper suspension of the bladder after tube reconstruction.

Intravesical Urethral Lengthening

(Kropp-Angewafo)

An artificial sphincter or continent diversion should be considered as an alternative, especially because catheterization through the male urethra is generally not well accepted. The procedure is most often done for patients with meningomyelocele, who have poorly compliant bladders. For these patients, perform simultaneous bladder augmentation because a large-capacity, low-pressure reservoir is essential.

Insert a balloon catheter transurethrally, of a size that can eventually be used for intermittent catheterization.

Incision: Make a lower midline incision from umbilicus to symphysis (see page 487), but do not enter the peritoneal cavity. Expose the bladder neck and proximal urethra, identifying the neck by the catheter balloon.

1 **A,** Mark a rectangular bladder flap with stay sutures, with the base at the bladder neck. The length should be about 6 cm and the width 2 to 2.5 cm.

B, Incise the flap with the needle-tip cutting current. Draw the catheter into the bladder, and fold it back over the symphysis. Place an infant feeding tube in each ureteral orifice, and suture them in place with 5-0 SAS. Continue the incision posteriorly around the bladder neck. Incise the midline posterior bladder muscle completely so that the bladder neck–anterior bladder flaps can be converted into a tube, but preserve the outer posterolateral musculoadventitial fibers shown in Step 3 so that the bladder is not completely separated from the bladder neck. Dissect further beneath the bladder neck posteriorly to leave a smooth transition from the proximal urethra to the detrusor tube. If the track is angulated, take a wedge out of the posterior bladder neck to effect a smooth transition.

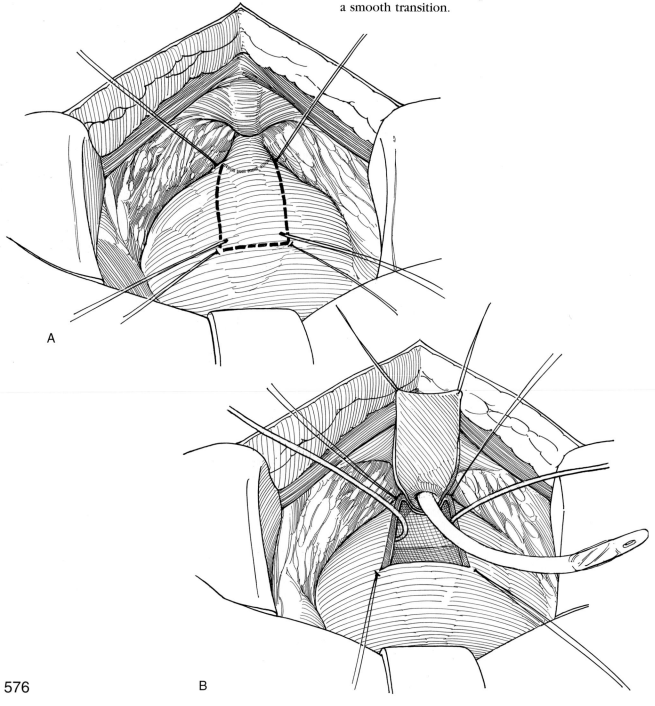

A

B

2 Roll the flap into a tube over the 20 F balloon catheter, and close it with a continuous subepithelial plain catgut (PCG) suture. Place interrupted sutures of 4-0 CCG in the muscularis, starting at the distal end. If the wall of the flap is too thick for tubularization, resect half of its thickness (Mollard et al, 1990).

3 With curved scissors, make two parallel tunnels, each running just medial to the respective ureteral orifices. Use both blunt and sharp dissection. Join the two tunnels by placing a blade of the scissors in each tunnel and cutting the remaining septum. It is easier to divide the bladder in the midline to a point 3 to 4 cm from the interureteric ridge; then begin subepithelial tunnels with sharp dissection from the new edge of the bladder opening. Continue the tunnel down to the interureteric ridge. Develop the distal portion under the ridge by working from the bladder neck up to the interureteric ridge. Form this part of the tunnel between the superficial and deep trigonal musculature. Re-enter the tunnel from above, and make it wide enough to easily accommodate the tubularized bladder strip. If it is not possible to fit the tunnel between the ureters, place it to one side and reimplant that ureter. (Reimplantation is also necessary for ureters showing reflux preoperatively.)

Insert the end of the new urethra into the flange of a Robinson catheter. Thread the previously placed stay sutures onto Keith needles, and pass them through the flanged end of the catheter from inside to outside. This draws the bladder tube into the flange, which acts as a guide to bring the tubularized bladder strip up through the subepithelial tunnel. Place sutures through the bladder musculature on either side of the tunnel at the bladder neck area and then through the bladder neck–proximal urethra and tie them. This effectively brings the bladder back down to the bladder neck. At the same time, pull the bladder down over the new tube to reach the former bladder neck. Amputate any excess tubing.

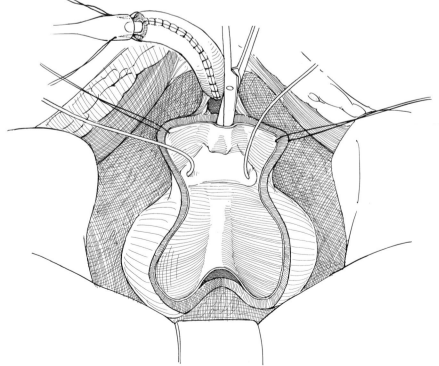

4 Bring the ureteral catheters out through stab wounds in the bladder (not shown). Secure the end of the urethral catheter (not shown) to the bladder wall in the fundus with interrupted 4-0 CCG sutures and to the former bladder neck with similar sutures. Open the peritoneum and proceed with vesical augmentation, or close the anterior bladder wall starting distally around the urethra with a running PCG subepithelial suture, reinforced with interrupted 4-0 CCG sutures. Alternatively, start the closure proximally.

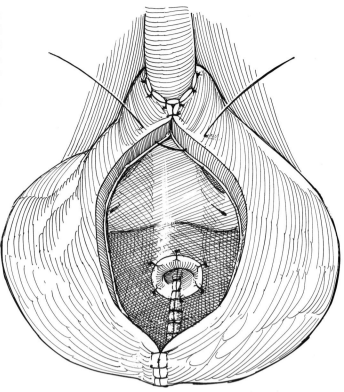

Postoperatively, most urine drains through the ureteral catheters. Remove the ureteral catheters on the fourth postoperative day. If augmentation has been accomplished, irrigate the suprapubic and balloon catheters alternately every 4 hours with 30 to 60 ml sterile water, and make sure that the family knows how to irrigate so that no mucus build-up can occur and cause plugging of the Foley and suprapubic catheters. In addition, instill 10 ml of Mucomyst twice a day, and clamp both catheters for 15 minutes to keep the mucus in a more liquid state. Discharge the child on the sixth or seventh postoperative day, to be seen weekly as an outpatient.

Readmit the patient for a short stay between 4 and 6 weeks postoperatively. Remove the balloon catheter and clamp the suprapubic tube. If the patient is performing catheterization easily, remove the suprapubic tube and discharge the patient.

Advise catheterization every 1 to 1.5 hours for the first several days, working down over the next 3 to 4 weeks to four to six times per day.

POSTOPERATIVE PROBLEMS

The arrangement does not have a safety valve, so *obstruction to catheterization* can be a serious problem. It may require cystoscopic manipulation, and, in boys, a perineal urethrostomy may be necessary. Leaving the urethral stent in place for 5 to 6 weeks reduces the problem. *Reflux* may develop postoperatively but may not require correction if catheterization is done frequently.

Commentary by Kenneth A. Kropp

We have recently reviewed our first 39 children with urethral lengthening followed from 42 to 163 months (median is 102.6 months). All but one were children with meningomyelocele who had failed to attain dryness on intermittent self-catheterization. All but 6 had a simultaneous bladder augmentation, and 5 of these 6 subsequently required augmentation. Nineteen of the 39 have not experienced any complications. Mucus has not been a problem for any after the early postoperative period. Thirty-three children (84 percent) have never had any difficulty with catheterization. Six children (16 percent) have experienced two or more episodes of difficulty, usually in the first few months. Placing a Foley catheter for 3 to 7 days solved most of these problems. With more than 50 children living in our area with urethral lengthening who catheterize themselves four to six times per day, we have not seen a single child present to our emergency room or office in the past 2 years who has had difficulty catheterizing. Thirty-one (80 percent) are completely dry day and night; 3 have rare leakage but require no pads; 3 leak rarely but wear a pad for security. Only 2 are back in diapers because of leakage.

INTRAVESICAL URETHRAL LENGTHENING
(Pippi Salle)

This technique is a modification of the Kropp procedure.

5 A, Insert a balloon catheter and partially fill the bladder. Make a midline lower abdominal incision (see page 487) or transverse incision (see page 490). Mark a 1-cm by 4- to 5-cm full-thickness flap on the anterior bladder wall with the base at the outlet. Mark the distal end with stay sutures. Incise the flap with the needle electrode. On the posterior wall of the bladder, mark two lines 1 cm apart and 4 to 5 cm long between the ureteral orifices to match the anterior flap. If necessary, reimplant the ureters by the transtrigonal technique (see page 793). Incise the uroepithelium and subepithe-lium of the posterior wall along the lines, and separate them laterally from the muscularis. Trim a strip of uroepi-thelium 1 to 2 mm wide from both sides of the anterior flap.

B, Insert an 8 F catheter, place the flap against the posterior bladder wall between the incisions, and run a suture on each side to approximate uroepithelium to uroepithelium. Attach the muscularis of the flap to the exposed muscle of the bladder wall with continuous sutures. Elevate the lateral epithelial edges, and bring them together over the new urethra with a continuous CCG suture. Insert a Malecot catheter. Augment the blad-der if necessary. Stent the ureters as needed. Close the bladder by starting with a short transverse suture line at the origin of the flap and continuing with a continuous suture. Insert a 5 F infant feeding tube, to remain 3 weeks before beginning intermittent catheterization. If a leak does occur, it will be where the bladder neck is closed over the tube.

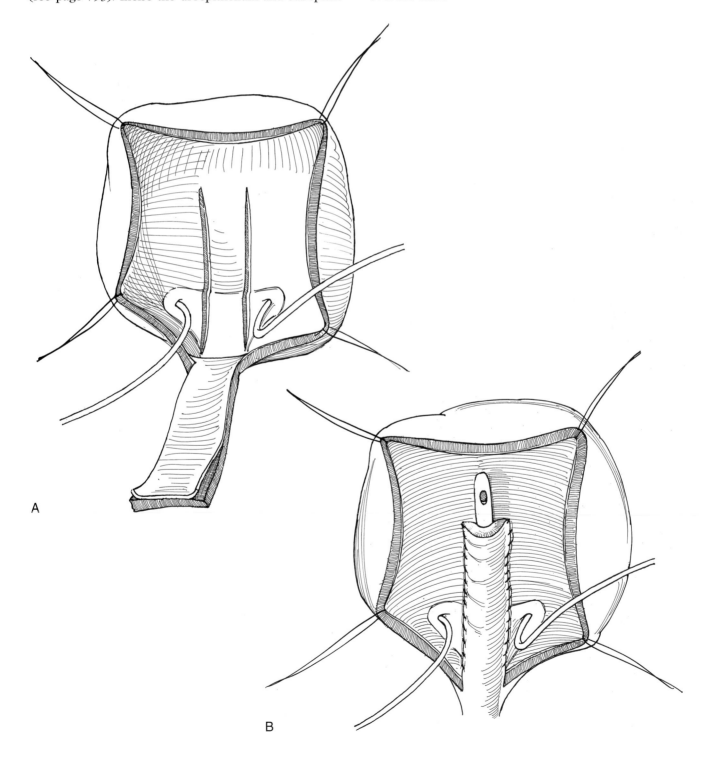

A

B

Insertion of Artificial Sphincter

TECHNIQUE FOR AS 800 ARTIFICIAL SPHINCTER

Perform uroflometry to detect outlet obstruction, and check residual urine. Do cystometrography to rule out uninhibited contractions. In some cases, urethral pressure profilometry is indicated. Perform cystography or cystoscopy to look for structural vesical abnormalities and to help select the best site for cuff placement. A video urodynamic evaluation gives the most information.

Have the patient shower preoperatively with organic iodine soap solution. Treat urinary tract infection, and give perioperative cephalosporin. Shave the patient in the operating room. Prepare for 10 minutes with iodophor solution, including the perineum and external genitalia (and vagina in women). Restrict traffic and reduce room contamination to a minimum because most prosthetic infections are caused by airborne *Staphylococcus epidermidis*. Spray the wound throughout the operation with a dilute antibiotic solution.

Instruments: Provide a Basic set, a GU fine set, a Scott retractor with small and large stays, a baby Deaver retractor, skin hooks, Babcock clamps, Lahey clamps, large right-angle dissecting scissors, four curved and four straight mosquito clamps shod with silicone tubing, DeBakey forceps, two pairs of Cushing forceps (smooth and toothed), Hegar dilators, a headlight, a soft adjustable stool, an artificial sphincter (AS 800) in three sterile packages (pump, preparation package with sizer and blunt needles, and connectors), one bowl for 11.5 percent Cysto-Conray II, one bowl for dilute antibiotic solution (50,000 units bacitracin, 1 g neomycin, and 300 ml saline), dilute methylene blue solution, two basins with 1500 ml of water to wash gloves, nonpenetrating towel clips, a silicone sheet to block the

anus, a 14 F 5-ml silicone balloon catheter with syringe, lubricant and plug, a scrotal supporter, 2-0 Prolene sutures for connectors, 4-0 CCG sutures with an RB-1 needle, two 0.5-inch Penrose drains, and vacuum suction and tubing.

Be sure to flush all air from the components of the system, and be careful not to let any blood enter the system. Handle the components carefully with vascular forceps to avoid damaging the silicone, and discard any component that becomes scratched.

Bladder Neck Placement of Cuff

Place the device at the bladder neck in women and children and in men who wish to maintain fertility by preserving antegrade ejaculation. This route has the advantages of being more physiologic, less prone to erosion, suitable for patients with small bulbar urethras, and less irritating with intermittent catheterization. Avoid placing a cuff around a reoperated bladder neck. If it is used around bowel, add extra fluid to the reservoir because the wall shrinks. The abdominal approach is not recommended after previous retropubic operations or trauma; if it is used, however, do not hesitate to open the bladder for dissection.

Position: For men, use a low lithotomy position. For women, keep the thighs parallel to the floor to permit vaginal access. Insert a 24 F 5-ml balloon catheter to allow better assessment of the urethrovesical junction. A firm vaginal pack may help to avoid entering the vagina; alternatively, access to the vagina for digital examination during the dissection can also be protective.

Incision and approach: Stand on the left of the patient. Make a low midline (see page 487) or a low transverse (see page 490) incision. Transect the insertion of the rectus muscles if necessary for exposure (see page 493).

1 Palpate the balloon of the catheter through the vesical wall. Incise the visceral extension of the endopelvic fascia on either side, taking care not to injure the underlying veins. Grasp the tissue posterior to the catheter between the thumb and index finger of the left hand. Establish a plane between the bladder neck and the underlying rectum (or vagina). Push the neurovascular bundle laterally. It may be helpful to open the parietal extension of the endopelvic fascia to allow lower placement of the cuff.

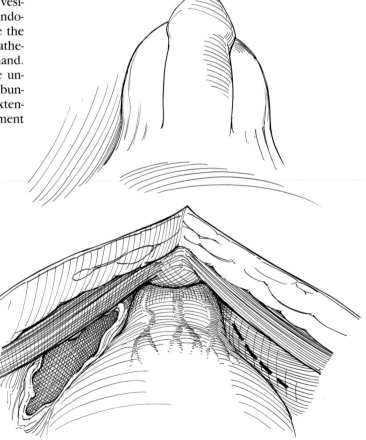

2 In the male, palpate the vas deferens posteriorly and pinch the trigone anteriorly to separate it from the vasa. (In the female, insert the thumb and index finger of the left hand and palpate the trigone and catheter balloon anteriorly.) With right-angle scissors held against the finger, alternating with a right-angle clamp, dissect between the bladder neck and the ejaculatory mechanism. Work from one side, then the other. If difficulty with the dissection is encountered, open the bladder through an incision well above the bladder neck. Secure venous hemostasis. (In the female, dissect through the urethrovaginal septum with the right-angle clamp and expand the opening to 2 cm.) Pass an umbilical tape through the tunnel to improve exposure for the control of venous bleeders. Fulgurate or place interrupted catgut sutures; clips are inadvisable at a site where metal could erode into silicone rubber.

Check for trigonal leaks by filling the wound with water and instilling air into the bladder through the catheter. Repair defects with a two-layer closure, and check again for leaks. Remove the balloon catheter. (In the female, inspect the vagina and repair any injury with a horizontal mattress running suture.) If the rectum has been entered, close the opening in two layers, place a drain, and abandon the operation.

With a large right-angle clamp beneath the bladder neck, draw the cuff sizer through the tunnel.

3 Measure the circumference with the markers on the tape while drawing it relatively snugly against the bladder neck. An alternative method of measurement is to pass a hernia tape accompanied by a length of heavy suture through the tunnel, clamp only the tape when it is snug, cut it distal to the clamp, and use the segment for measurement, leaving the suture in place for passage of the clamp and sizer. Add 0.5 to 1 cm to the measured length to allow for postoperative edema. While measuring with the sizer in males, one should keep the caudal edge at the top of the prostate. Measurements greater than 10 cm suggest that too much areolar tissue remains. In females, the cephalad edge should lie just above the bladder neck as previously determined by palpation of the catheter balloon. Do not make the cuff too tight; that would cause difficulty in voiding. If the bladder is open, insert the fifth finger into the bladder neck and tighten the cuff sizer so that the fingertip can just pass through.

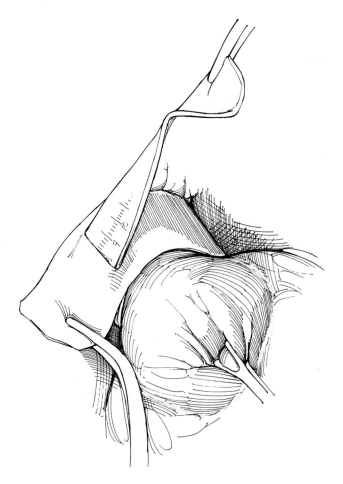

4 Select a narrow-back, surface-treated inflatable cuff 4.5 cm wide. Clear the cuff of air by replacing it with isosmotic contrast solution. Replace the sizer tape with the cuff by tying it to the heavy suture placed previously and drawing it through the tunnel. Pass the tubing through the opening in the cuff, and snap the end of the cuff in place.

Irrigate the wound vigorously when making connections. Be very careful that blood or serum does not enter the tubing where it can block the one-way valves.

Pass a large clamp from the subcutaneous tissue through the (usually right) rectus abdominis muscle and anterior sheath above the inguinal canal, and draw the tubing from the cuff through the muscle. Alternatively, use the supplied blunt tubing needle and work from inside out. Bluntly dissect a place for the reservoir in the prevesical space beneath the muscle and anterior to the peritoneum, and draw the tubing through the rectus as done for the cuff tubing. Fill the balloon with 20 to 22 ml of isotonic contrast medium (11.7 percent Cysto-Conray II) or physiologic saline. Make temporary connection between balloon and cuff to "charge" the cuff; then refill the balloon. Be certain that the balloon does not make contact with the cuff, where the silicone could become eroded.

5 Run a Hegar dilator, a large curved clamp, or long scissors down into the (usually left) scrotum or labium, and create a space under the dartos. Insert the pump with the aid of a nasal speculum, and milk it into a position accessible to the patient. Insertion in the labium should be in a low and not too superficial position. Trim the tubing to the proper length, fill the cuff and balloon to the recommended volume of 20 ml, and connect it with stainless steel quick connectors, the black tubing connecting tubing to pump and the clear tubing connecting the cuff to the pump. (For revisions, do not use quick connectors on used tubing; use plastic connectors and tie them in place with two 3-0 NAS at each end.) Place the connections subcutaneously to make them accessible in case revision is required.

Obtain complete hemostasis (no drains will be placed). Close the rectus fascia with a running horizontal mattress monofilament suture that is kept away from the prosthesis. Activate the device, and allow the cuff to fill while closing the subcutaneous tissue. Test the device by counting the number of pumps needed to empty the cuff. The cuff should not contain more that 1.5 ml (one or two pumps); if it does, do not hesitate to open the wound and replace it with a smaller cuff. Wait 10 minutes and recheck cuff filling. Fill the bladder, remove the catheter, and gently press suprapubically to be sure that continence has been achieved. Deactivate the cuff by pressure on the poppet valve. Close the wound in layers, providing two layers for the subcutaneous tissue without drainage. Replace the catheter and leave it in place for a day; after that, use intermittent catheterization if necessary.

Caution the patient about sitting (perineal compression). Continue parenteral antibiotics for 4 days and oral antibiotics for 2 weeks. Six to 12 weeks postoperatively, check for urinary infection, and make a radiograph of the cuff full and empty. Activate the cuff by firm pump pressure to displace the poppet valve, and allow the fluid to flow through the pump to fill it. Teach the patient how to manage the device, and encourage him to deactivate it at night if he is continent in bed.

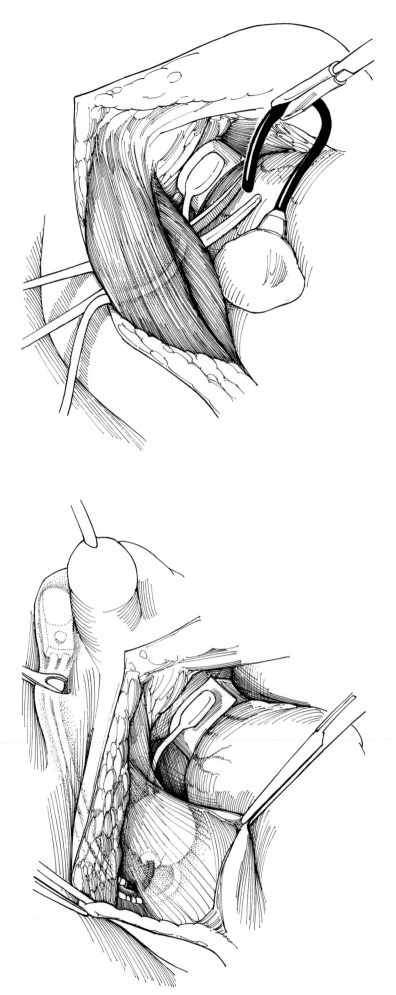

Bulbar Urethral Placement of Cuff

For males, especially after prostatectomy, pelvic operations, or trauma, this is an easier operation than vesical neck placement. For persistent severe incontinence, two cuffs may be placed around the bulbar urethra.

Instruments: Use the same instruments listed for bladder neck placement. Provide a model AS 800 urinary sphincter; make a urethral balloon catheter from an 18 F Robinson catheter with a finger cut from a rubber glove and attached by a silk tie.

6 *Position:* Use the extreme lithotomy position with the thighs parallel to the ceiling. Insert the prepared balloon catheter into the bulbar urethra and inflate it with air.

Incision: Use a midline perineal incision, incising vertically onto the bulbospongiosus muscle.

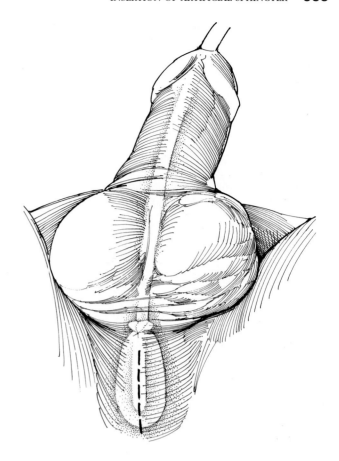

7 Dissect laterally under the bulbocavernosus muscle to make a passage 2 cm wide. Stay close to the tunica albuginea of the cavernous bodies to avoid exposing the contained urethra and to keep the muscle intact to protect the urethra from the cuff. Take special care at the 12-o'clock position, where the tissue is thin and friable. Removing the balloon helps with exposure there. Test the urethra for leaks by urethral instillation of saline mixed with a few drops of methylene blue. If the urethra has been entered, repair the injury with 5-0 SAS, move the proposed cuff site, and delay activation.

8 Enlarge the space around the urethra bluntly, working proximally to enable the cuff to be placed as high and as near to the crura as possible. Measure the circumference by passing the cuff sizer; alternatively, pass a Robinson catheter (as shown) or hernia tape around it, clamp it at the intersection, and trim the ends to determine the length of cuff needed. A 4.0- to 4.5-cm cuff is standard.

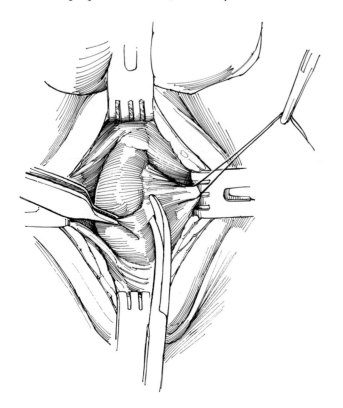

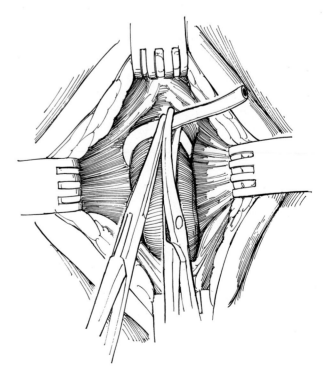

9 Select the appropriate cuff and draw it under the urethra, tab end first. Pass the tubing through the opening in the tab and snap it in place.

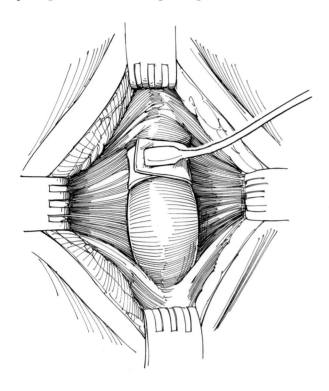

10 For *wheelchair-bound patients*, place a silicone-covered malleable stainless steel metal strip over the cuff and tie the sutures lying within its back. The strip prevents compression of the cuff when the patient is sitting. An alternative is to free more of the bulb by dividing the central tendon and placing the cuff in a higher position.

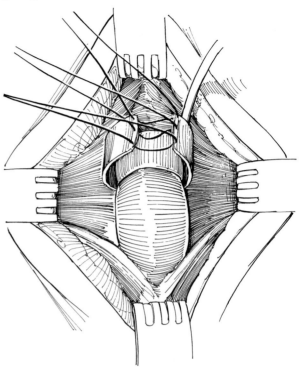

11 Make a short incision over the left external inguinal ring, and enlarge it toward the perineum with a finger. Place the cuff tubing on a tubing needle, and pass it subcutaneously out the inguinal incision.

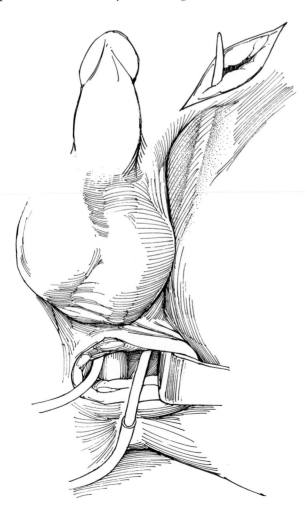

12 Bluntly dissect a pocket in the left scrotum and place the pump in it.

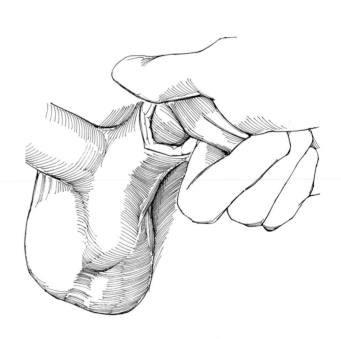

13 With the index finger through the external inguinal ring, break through the floor of the inguinal canal. It may be necessary to use Metzenbaum scissors there. Digitally create a space between the bladder and the pubic ramus.

Select a reservoir with an appropriate pressure range (61 to 70 cm for most patients, although the 51- to 60-cm reservoir is safer for high-risk patients). In any case, the pressure should be lower than the patient's diastolic blood pressure. Insert a tubing passer through the inguinal ring, and have it exit through the external oblique muscle 1 inch above the ring. Pull the balloon into place. Fill it with 20 ml of solution, and make temporary connection with the cuff to "charge" it; then refill the balloon.

Close the external oblique layer around the external ring.

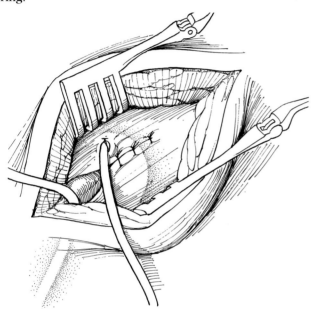

14 Connect the cuff to the control assembly tubing with a right-angle connector to reduce the chance of kinking. Connect the control and reservoir tubing with quick connectors (or with plastic connectors tied in place with 3-0 Prolene sutures). Set the pump in the "off" position. Fill and empty the cuff.

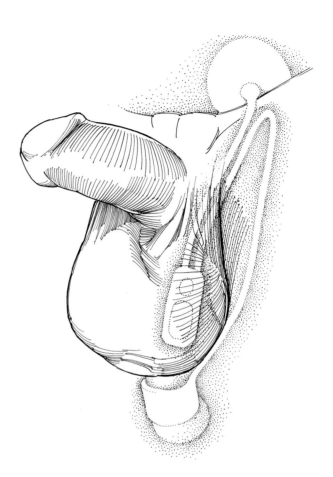

To test for continence, fill the bladder and remove the catheter. Inflate the cuff. Place a stack of towels on the abdomen and press down as hard as possible. There should be no leakage. Open the pump and check for good flow. Alternatively, inflate the distal urethra using cystometrographic equipment, and observe the pressure at which fluid or CO_2 flows retrogradely (direct sphincterometry). Do urethral pressure profilometry if available; it should show an occlusion pressure between 60 and 90 cm H_2O. Pump the cuff empty and deactivate the system. Spray the wound with antibiotic solution again, and close it in layers, using 4-0 running subcuticular SAS for the skin. Do not place drains. Insert a balloon catheter.

Continue parenteral antibiotics for 48 hours; then substitute oral broad-spectrum antibiotics for the next week. Maintain deactivation at least until the patient can comfortably manipulate the device. However, if revascularization of the cuff site is required, wait for 8 to 10 weeks. If the tissues are atrophic or affected by radiation, prolong the period of deactivation. Remove the catheter after 1 or 2 days; leave it longer if the cuff site required repair. Cycle the apparatus every 2 hours for the first 3 or 4 weeks to avoid formation of a sheath around the balloon. Have the patient avoid tight-fitting clothes that could displace the pump.

POSTOPERATIVE PROBLEMS

Infection is the greatest hazard. For this reason, maintain strict asepsis perioperatively and postoperatively. Most prosthetic infections are caused by *Staphylococcus epidermidis*, probably from airborne contamination. Culture the urine if there is doubt about infection or if catheterization becomes necessary for any reason. Myelomeningocele patients have a high rate of infection of the prosthesis with both gram-positive and gram-negative bacteria; they require assiduous attention to clear bacteriuria. If a dental procedure is required in any patient, prophylactic coverage is essential. When the devices become infected by bacteria carried by the bloodstream, it is usually at the area of least vascularity, which is the cuff. If incorporation of bowel is needed for bladder augmentation, enlarge the bladder at a first stage and place the device at a second stage to reduce the chance for contamination.

Watch for fever, swelling, or drainage from the incision or cuff site and erosion of the pump or cuff, indications that the device must be removed. In an occasional case, prompt evacuation and irrigation of the infected area with antibiotic solutions can save the device.

Cuff erosion into the urethra is heralded by burning perineal pain and also by swelling in the scrotum or labium at the site of the pump. Check by cystoscopy, and, if erosion is present, proceed with removal. If the infection is purulent, the rest of the device must also be removed. Place a catheter for 2 weeks to permit healing, and return in 6 months to replace the cuff. For bulbar replacement, move the cuff away from the previous site. To facilitate cuff replacement at the bladder neck, if the area is not infected, close the opening in the bladder neck primarily, irrigate the wound, and loosely place a silicone strip 2 cm wide in the bed of the cuff. Alternatively, approach the bladder neck transperitoneally and bring omentum into the former site of the cuff. In an occasional case, evacuation of the collection in the periurethral area, diversion of urine, and irrigation with antibiotic solutions can save the device.

For *persistent incontinence,* check for *leakage* of the inflating fluid during inflation and deflation, detecting its absence by radiography. Leakage is most likely to arise from the lower surface of the cuff, but because the cuff is so difficult to replace, be sure to exclude leaks from connectors and from the stem of the reservoir. *Recurrent incontinence* may be the result of an alteration in detrusor function or an inefficient cuff. Cuff erosion may be a cause for the return of incontinence. Perform urethroscopy to detect it.

Pressure atrophy under the cuff, allowing incontinence, may be expected in only a few patients now that the cuff has been redesigned, and care is taken to place the cuff around the thickest portion of the bulb. Filling the reservoir to 22 ml instead of 18, pressurizing the cuff, and then removing and replacing the remaining fluid with 20 ml of solution may compensate for atrophy initially. If atrophy is suspected as the cause, try raising the pressure in the reservoir, although this results in little increase in cuff pressure and may lead to cuff erosion.

Proximal cuff replacement: To determine that atrophy under the cuff is responsible for the incontinence, rule out all other causes. Perform panendoscopy and retrograde urethrography to identify failure of urethral coaptation; urodynamic studies may be helpful to rule out detrusor-related causes. Check for normal pumping action, and rule out malfunction or leakage in the device. If atrophy has occurred, move the cuff proximally (Couillard et al, 1995). Excise the right-angle connector to the cuff, open the pseudocapsule, and remove the cuff. Place a new one proximally on the bulbar urethra. Retain the proximal rim of the capsule to support it. Slit the bulbocavernosus muscle surrounding the proximal bulb, expose the urethra, and place a new 4.5-cm cuff. Close the bulbocavernosus muscle over the cuff, incorporating the proximal lip of the pseudocapsule in the distal suture. Pass the tubing from the cuff over the symphysis with the tubing passer, and make connections in the suprapubic area. Irrigate thoroughly with bacitracin/kanamycin solution. Deactivate the sphincter, and drain the bladder with a 16 F balloon catheter for 24 hours. Maintain antibiotic coverage for 7 to 10 days. Reactivate the sphincter in 6 weeks.

Mechanical problems, such as leaks, kinks in the tubing, and malfunction of the pump, are uncommon with the newest devices. *Intermittent action* on inflation or deflation may be caused by particulate matter that remained in the system. Kinks in the tubing may produce the same result.

Upper tract damage may be a problem in children. Check for *reflex bladder activity* or reduced detrusor *compliance* as a cause by performing cystometrography and cystography. Children with meningomyelocele must be followed carefully; they usually require vesical augmentation after 4 or more years. *Minor complications* are few. For *urinary retention,* be sure that the cuff has been deactivated. Intermittent catheterization may be required at first. Have the patient with a bulbar cuff do it gently with a small catheter after deactivation (the bladder neck is resistant to the catheter). If retention is to be prolonged, place a suprapubic tube. *Hematomas* may form in the scrotum or labia, displacing the pump. Occasionally a very large hematoma requires drainage. *Constriction* of the urethra with difficulty emptying, difficulty catheterizing, or upper tract deterioration may occur as the child reaches puberty, but increasing the size of the cuff is not beneficial.

Commentary by Rodney A. Appell

In the treatment of urinary incontinence due to intrinsic sphincteric deficiency (ISD), one of the goals is to establish a normal voiding pattern while allowing the patient to become dry between voidings. Treatment is designed to close the outflow channel. However, this may result in inability of the patient to empty the bladder completely or at all. Of the treatments designed for ISD, only implantation of the artificial urinary sphincter (AUS) allows the obstruction to be relieved at the time of voiding so that the actual voiding pattern is normalized and the desired state of dryness is achieved. It is not sufficient to state that patients with ISD are natural candidates for the AUS; they must also have adequate manual dexterity, mental capacity, and motivation to manipulate the pump mechanism each time they need to urinate.

Mechanical reliability of the device has improved significantly following various manufacturing changes, including nonkinkable tubing, surface treatment of the narrow-back cuff, and the ability to deactivate the device using the poppet valve located in the pump itself.

Bulbar urethral placement in the male has revolutionized the ability to help men with postprostatectomy incontinence, with an overall continence rate greater than 90 percent achieved by implantation. In most men following radical prostatectomy, there is atrophy of the bulbospongiosus muscle, allowing the cuff to be placed around it as it "contains" the urethra, giving another source of "padding" to help prevent erosion of the urethra while not affecting continence results. However, in neurogenic cases such as myelodysplasia, where the bulbospongiosus is still significant, it should be incised so that the cuff can be placed directly around the urethra and the bulbospongiosus muscle can then be closed over the cuff as "padding" to prevent cuff compression when the patient is sitting rather than the malleable strip described in Step 10.

In females the most difficult part of the surgery is negotiating around the bladder neck/posterior urethra because the urethrovaginal septum is not a true surgical plane. Proper positioning of the cuff is the most important aspect of the surgery and can be the most challenging. The procedure described in the text and figures is the original retropubic approach described by F. Brantley Scott; I believe it can be improved by using a device he invented called a cutter clamp. This device is positioned in the area of the proposed cuff site and allows the passage of a cutting blade from one arm of the clamp to the other through the urethrovaginal septum, after which the right-angle clamp, used to stretch the tissue to accommodate cuff placement, can be appropriately guided without trauma to the urethra, bladder neck, or vagina.

I facilitate placement of the cuff by a transvaginal approach that is similar to placement of a suburethral sling. An inverted U-incision is made in the anterior vaginal wall to expose the bladder neck and posterior urethra. The endopelvic fascia is taken down from its insertion on the underside of the pubic bone to allow entrance of the surgeon's finger into the extravesical space on either side of the bladder neck. This is followed down laterally to the ischial spine on both sides, leaving only a small, weak attachment anteriorly of the bladder neck and posterior urethra, which is easily taken down by spreading either Metzenbaum scissors or a right-angle clamp on the underside of the symphysis pubis. A Satinsky clamp or renal pedicle clamp can then be passed completely over the top of the bladder neck and the sizer tape grasped and placed in position to make the measurement for cuff size. After placement of the cuff in this manner, a small inguinal incision (the same one described for placement of the balloon and pump in the male undergoing bulbar cuff AUS placement) can be used to place the other components. The advantage of this approach is simplified positioning of the cuff around the bladder neck under direct vision. The main concern has been increased risk of infection by a transvaginal approach, but this has not been a problem; fear can be allayed by knowledge that synthetic slings have been placed per vagina for years without undue risk of infection. Decreased tissue trauma and the judicious use of antibiotics, including coverage for anaerobes, have made this approach successful. Of the alternative treatments available for females with ISD, all appear to be successful in approximately 90 percent of cases. Because the primary goal in treatment of females with ISD is to allow coaptation of the mucosa of the proximal urethra and bladder neck without obstruction, this goal is best attained by using the AUS because it alone can permit intermittent urethral compression, allowing the patient to reduce urethral resistance voluntarily during voiding.

Vesicovaginal Fistula Repair

Timing of Repair

Proceed as soon as the patient has recovered enough to physically allow reoperation, usually within 2 or 3 weeks. Otherwise wait a minimum of 3 months to allow the inflammation to subside. For small fistulas less than 2 to 3 mm in diameter, try fulgurating the lining by inserting a Bugbee electrode into the tract vaginally or cystoscopically and applying minimal current; then leave a catheter in place for 2 to 3 weeks.

Preliminaries

Perform intravenous urography to be sure that the upper tract is normal. A displaced or partially obstructed ureter suggests a ureterovaginal fistula, in which case retrograde ureterography is needed to be certain such a fistula is not missed. Perform cystoscopy on the patient (a finger in the vagina can be visualized cystoscopically through large defects), and ascertain the relation of the fistula to the ureteral orifices. Examination of the vagina with the cystoscope may also be useful. For detection of small fistulas, pack the vagina and instill dilute methylene blue intravesically. Blue stain on the pack proves the presence of a vesicovaginal fistula. If the pack is not stained, the diagnosis is ureterovaginal fistula unless reflux is present. If all else fails because the fistula is so minute, place the patient in the knee-chest position, fill the bladder with air, and perform cystoscopy of the vagina looking for air bubbles. Alternatively, perform vaginography with the introitus occluded by a balloon, or instill air in the vagina and look for bubbles cystoscopically. If, on intravenous urography, the ureter appears involved and preliminary tests for vesicovaginal fistula are negative, suspect a ureterovaginal source for the leakage.

Caution the patient about the chance for successful closure (90 percent for an initial repair), the possibility of ureteral injury, the possibility of change in vaginal caliber, and the chance for changed voiding habits in the postoperative period.

Approaches

Remember that the first operation is the one most likely to succeed. Select an approach with which you feel comfortable. The *vaginal approach*, with the patient in the lithotomy position, is easiest on the patient. Increased visualization and easier access are found with the jack-knife (Kraske) position (Step 17), although administration of anesthesia is more difficult. Previous attempts at closure or prior radiation may preclude a vaginal approach.

An *abdominal approach* is better for fistulas at the apex of the vaginal vault; for those larger than 1 cm, especially with indurated margins; for multiple fistulas, unless adequate exposure can be obtained by a Schuchardt incision (Steps 18 to 20); and for patients with intra-abdominal conditions that require procedures such as cystoplasty.

Have the patient douche with povidone-iodine solution the night before surgery. Give gentamicin and ampicillin intravenously 1 hour before the operation. Apply intermittent compression stockings.

TRANSVAGINAL REPAIR

Instruments: Provide a Basic pack, a GU fine set, a cystoscopy set, a weighted posterior vaginal retractor, a Lowsley prostatic tractor, a 4 F tapered ureteral catheter, an 8 F 3-ml balloon catheter, and a 24 F 5-ml silicone balloon catheter. Have a tray attached to the foot of the table for easy access to instruments, and provide a stool for the surgeon.

If the fistula is close to the orifices, place ureteral catheters cystoscopically.

1 *Position*: Use the overflexed lithotomy position. Prepare and drape the patient. Place a suprapubic catheter by the Lowsley tractor technique (see page 628). Consider inserting ureteral catheters if the defect is near the trigone. Suture the labia to the inner thighs, or retract them with the hooks of a Scott ring retractor. Place a weighted posterior vaginal retractor. If more exposure is needed, make a Schuchardt relaxing incision (Steps 18 to 20) at the 5- or 7-o'clock position. Place a tenaculum or two heavy sutures in the cervix for traction. Insert a 4 F tapered ureteral catheter directly through the fistula from below or, if that is not possible, cystoscopically from above. Or try traversing it with a lacrimal probe. Dilate the tract with straight sounds until it is large enough to accommodate an 8 F balloon catheter inserted from below, to be used for traction. Infiltrate the area with 1:200,000 epinephrine solution. Incise the vaginal mucosa and perivesical fascia around the fistula well outside the scarred tissue. Using a delicate technique to avoid further tissue damage, develop a plane between the mucosa and fascia and another between the fascia and the bladder wall.

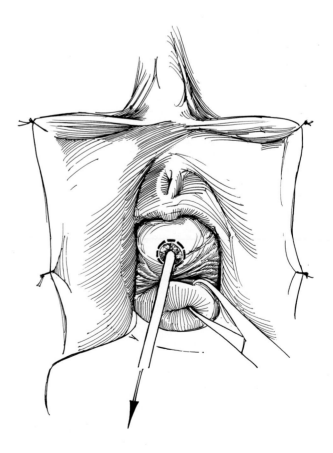

2 Thoroughly mobilize the bladder wall, but do not excise the fistula. Rather, trim its edges and use the scarred margins for placement of sutures.

Alternative: Develop a peritoneal flap (Raz) by dissecting along the anterior vaginal wall until the anterior cul-de-sac is reached and mobilizing the peritoneal edge from the back wall of the bladder without opening into the peritoneum. After closing the vesical opening (Step 10), tack the double flap over the repair with interrupted 2-0 SAS.

3 Close the vesical defect vertically with one layer of carefully placed interrupted 3-0 CCG sutures, inverting the scarred edges. *Alternatively,* close the defect transversely with a running locking 3-0 SAS that includes the full thickness of the vaginal wall and some of the bladder wall. Add a vertical row of Lembert sutures (see page 38), folding the surface upon itself.

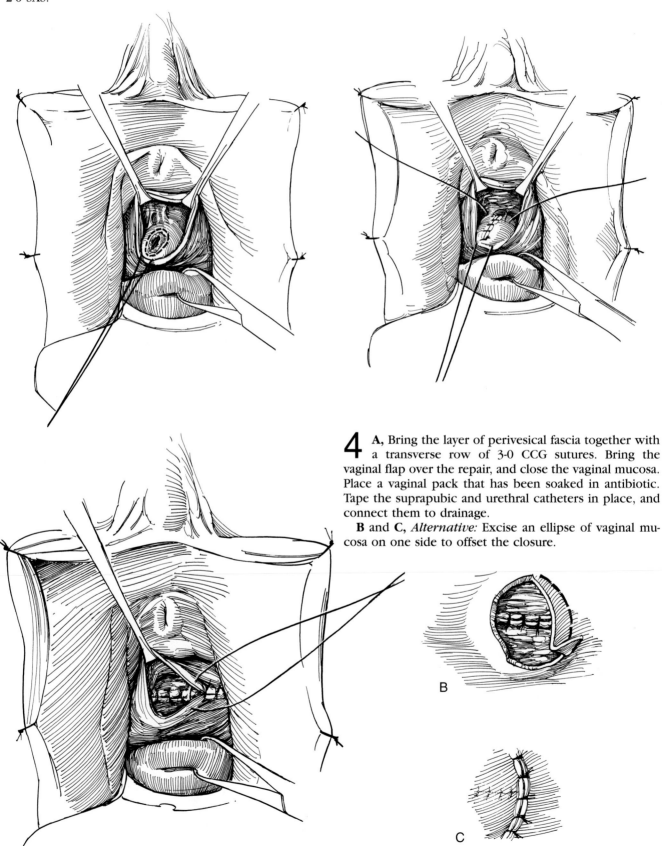

4 **A,** Bring the layer of perivesical fascia together with a transverse row of 3-0 CCG sutures. Bring the vaginal flap over the repair, and close the vaginal mucosa. Place a vaginal pack that has been soaked in antibiotic. Tape the suprapubic and urethral catheters in place, and connect them to drainage.

B and **C,** *Alternative:* Excise an ellipse of vaginal mucosa on one side to offset the closure.

INVERTED U-INCISION FLAP REPAIR

5 An inverted flap not only gives more exposure for the repair but also completely covers the area of the defect, especially if a portion of the vaginal mucosa is excised proximally. Place a suprapubic tube with the Lowsley tractor technique (see page 628) and a urethral balloon catheter. Infiltrate the anterior vaginal wall with saline, and raise a U-shaped flap with the apex adjacent to the fistula. Insert a balloon catheter through the fistula. Dissect the vaginal wall around the fistula, and trim it in the area superior to the fistula so that with closure the suture lines do not overlap. Trim the edges of the fistula

(Step 9). Put traction on the catheter to allow closure of the fistula transversely with a running locking 3-0 SAS through the full thickness of the vaginal wall and including part of the bladder wall. Withdraw the catheter as the last stitches are placed. Reinforce the closure with interrupted inverting 3-0 Lembert sutures (see page 38) placed vertically in the prevesical fascia (not shown). Test the closure by instilling dilute methylene blue through the cystostomy tube. If the closure looks tenuous or is a repeat procedure, insert a Martius labial flap (Steps 13 and 14). Bring the vaginal flap over the suture line and approximate it with interrupted 3-0 SAS. Pack the vagina with povidone-iodine gauze.

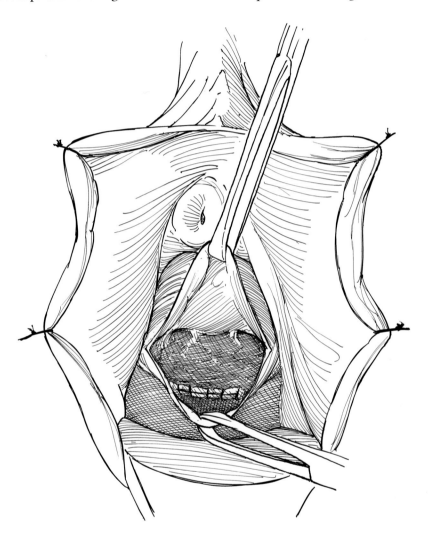

Care after Vaginal Repair

Suture the suprapubic catheter to the skin and tape it to the abdomen. Firmly tape the urethral catheter to the leg if it is to remain. Connect both catheters to bag drainage by sterile technique. Continue antibiotic coverage. Discharge the patient in 3 to 4 days, after giving instruction on the care of the catheter and the risks of vesical overfilling. Provide anticholinergic medication. Stop the medication after 10 to 14 days, wait a day, remove the urethral catheter, and perform voiding cystourethrography through the suprapubic tube. If healing is satisfactory, clamp the catheter for a trial of voiding. (Expect frequent voiding because the bladder has contracted after long disuse.) When urinary control is regained and residual urine is less than 100 ml, remove the suprapubic tube. Provide local or parenteral estrogens. Instruct the patient to abstain from

intercourse for 6 weeks. For bleeding, pack the vagina and place the patient at bed rest.

COLPOCLEISIS
(Latzko)

Consider partial colpocleisis if the fistula lies in the vault of a deep vagina. Perform a Schuchardt incision for access (Steps 18 to 20). Extensively excise the scar tissue of the vaginal wall around the fistula both proximally and distally. Invert the vesical opening into the bladder lumen in two layers. Obliterate the vaginal vault by approximating the edges of the denuded area of the vaginal wall with two transverse rows of interrupted sutures.

INSERTION OF FLAPS

Closure with Bulbospongiosus Muscle Flap (Martius)

6 Close the bladder defect, leaving the vagina open to receive the flap. Mark a vertical incision in the labium minus.

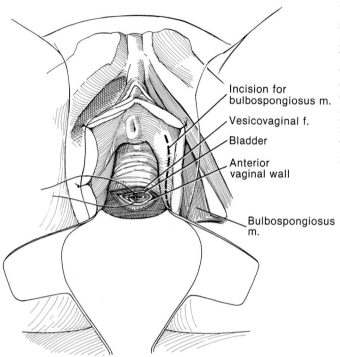

Incision for bulbospongiosus m.

Vesicovaginal f.

Bladder

Anterior vaginal wall

Bulbospongiosus m.

7 Incise the labium minus vertically, and expose the bulbospongiosus muscle with its covering of fat. Mobilize both muscle and fat with part of the vestibular bulb on its posterior pedicle. The complex is supplied by the deep perineal branch of the external pudendal artery that enters the muscle near its point of origin (see page 244). Divide the muscle anteriorly and check its viability. Bluntly tunnel along the upper portion of the descending pubic ramus beneath the vaginal vault, and draw the muscle flap to the site. Suture it over the repair with 3-0 SAS. For additional security, fasten it to the periosteum of the opposite pubic ramus. Close the labial incision over a small Penrose drain, and close the vaginal wound by approximating the full thickness of the vaginal wall.

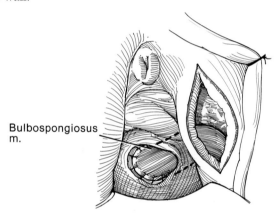

Bulbospongiosus m.

Closure with Labial Fat Pad Flap

Instead of mobilizing the bulbospongiosus muscle itself, dissect through the subcutaneous fat to reach the labial fat pad overlying the muscle. Preserve the blood supply from the pudendal vessels that enters posteriorly, and proceed as in Step 7.

If the fistula is associated with Type II urinary incontinence, place *suspension sutures* and insert a Martius graft beneath them. If a defect is present in the vaginal surface, leave a patch of labial skin attached to the Martius graft, and use it to fill the defect.

Closure with Island Flap (Lehoczky)

Make a Schuchardt episiotomy incision (Steps 11 to 13). Proceed to close the fistula as described in Steps 1 to 4. Raise a 3- to 4-cm skin island from the labium majus on the side opposite the episiotomy, to include the underlying adipose tissue and the internal pudendal artery and pudendal nerve (Lehoczky island flap). Make a tunnel under the bulbocavernosus muscle, and suture the island in the defect. Close the episiotomy and the donor site. Leave a catheter in place for 2 to 3 weeks.

Closure with Gracilis Myocutaneous Flap

Prepare the left (or right) leg from the lower abdomen to below the knee. Also prepare the vulva and vagina. Drape the area appropriately. A cystostomy tube may be placed. Insert a 22 F 5-ml balloon catheter urethrally. Place a weighted retractor.

8 **A,** First trim the rim of the fistula. Enter the plane of cleavage between the bladder and the anterior vaginal wall, and continue dissecting until the bladder is freely mobilized so that the edges of the fistula can be brought together without tension. Dissect especially deeply on the left side where the new muscle will enter. With large fistulas, this much mobilization may not be possible and dependence must be placed on the transplanted muscle. Place a vaginal cystostomy (see pages 628 to 629) unless the fistula is near the bladder neck, in which case insert a 24 F 5-ml balloon catheter through the urethra, or, preferably, place a suprapubic cystostomy (see page 625).

B, Close the fistula in one layer with interrupted 4-0 SAS (extra layers merely add extra suture material without adding strength).

Raise a gracilis myocutaneous flap (see page 50).

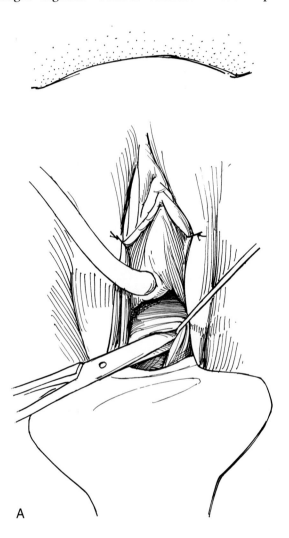

A

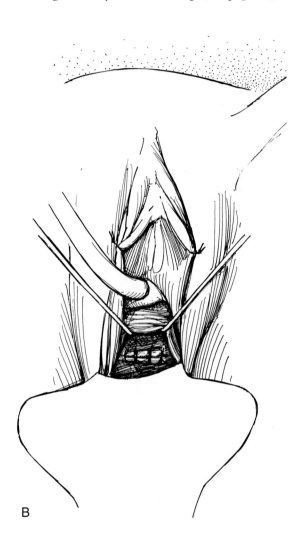

B

9 Bluntly make a subcutaneous tunnel from the incision on the leg to that in the vagina. Pass a long curved clamp to retrieve a silk suture presented at the vaginal edge. Thread it on a large Mayo needle, and stitch the traction suture to the distal end of the gracilis. Draw the muscle through the tunnel. Adduct the leg so that the muscle reaches the vaginal area. Trim the tendon and excess muscle from it. Suture the muscle to the bladder edge over the defect with interrupted 3-0 SAS. Place further sutures to attach it to the opposite pubic ramus and thus stabilize it. Return to the incision in the leg, and tack the posterior surface of its proximal end to the adductor magnus and the lateral edge to the adductor longus to support the blood supply. Close the vaginal wound and the incision in the leg. Apply a light pressure dressing; avoid a vaginal pack. A gracilis flap may also be placed over the repair from an abdominal approach (Fleischman and Picha, 1987) by bringing the flap through the urogenital diaphragm and endopelvic fascia.

CLOSURE WITH SEROMUSCULAR FLAP (Mráz and Sutorý)

After dissecting the bladder from the vagina, obtain an 8-cm segment of ileum with a long mesentery. Open the bowel and scrape the mucosa from it. Coagulate the larger bleeders; place the bowel in a warm towel for a few minutes to control the ooze. Bring the patch between the bladder and vagina with the denuded side against the bladder, and secure it to the margins of the defect with 3-0 SAS. Spread the patch out and tack it to the bladder with a widely spaced continuous suture. Close the vaginal defect in layers if possible. Place suction drains to remain 4 to 5 days and a balloon catheter to be removed in 6 weeks.

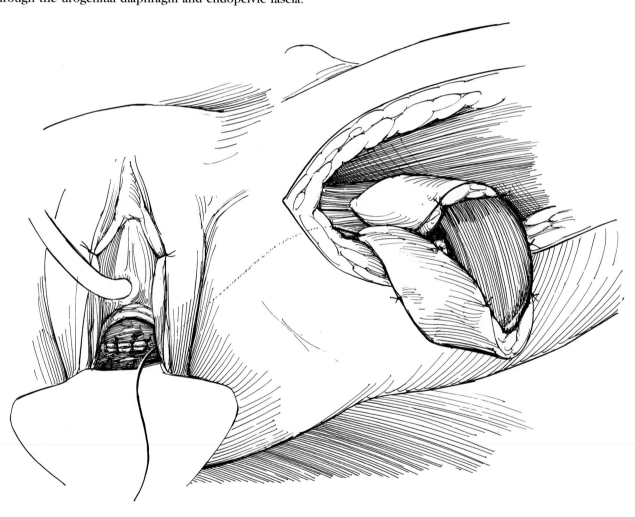

PRONE (JACK-KNIFE) POSITION
(Kraske)

This position provides excellent visualization of the operative field, although it does make anesthesia more hazardous.

10 **A,** Place the patient prone with the hips elevated on pillows, the thighs flexed and padded, and the knees supported.

B, Hold the fatty upper thighs apart with 3-inch adhesive strips, raise the posterior vaginal wall with a Sims speculum, and suture redundant labial tissue laterally.

Follow the illustrations shown in Steps 8 to 12 *inverted,* and proceed with repair.

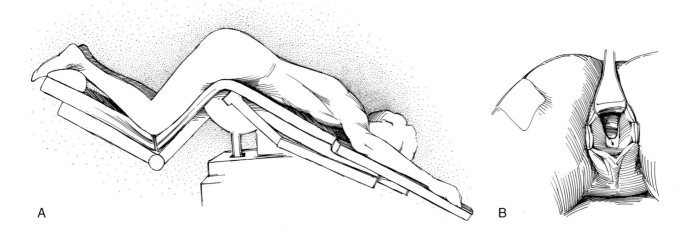

A   B

SCHUCHARDT PERINEAL INCISION

This paravaginorectal displacement incision can provide wider exposure for vaginal and uterine surgery.

11 Infiltrate broadly along the route of the incision *(dashed line)* with 0.5 percent xylocaine and 1:200,000 epinephrine, inserting the 22-gauge spinal needle half way between the anus and the left (for right-handed surgeons) ischial tuberosity. Make a curved incision through the skin starting at the 4-o'clock position on the margin of the hymen and ending at the site of the needle entry half way between the anus and the ischial tuberosity. For wider exposure, the incision can be extended to the midline posterior to the anus, taking care not to disturb the anal sphincters. Insert the index finger of the left hand deeply into the vagina posteriorly to protect the rectum. Have the assistant insert a finger of the left hand laterally to place tension on the posterolateral vaginal wall. Place a retractor on the right side (not shown). Extend the incision up the vaginal wall by having the assistant apply firm digital tension on the left lateral wall while you pull the posterior vaginal wall downward.

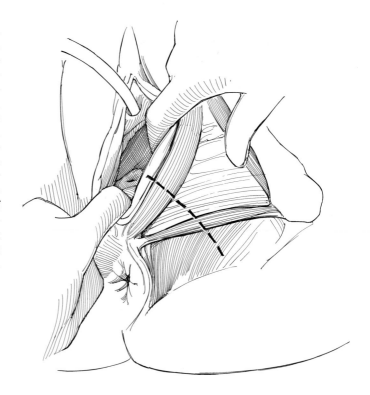

12 Deepen the incision, extending it into the vagina with an electrosurgical knife by dividing the tissues in a posterolateral direction. Fulgurate vessels as the incision proceeds across the bulbocavernosus muscle and the urogenital diaphragm. Spread the tissues bluntly to expose fibers of the pubococcygeal portion of the levator ani muscle. Enter the pararectal space above the levator ani with the blunt end of the knife. For greater exposure, identify the pubococcygeus muscle and divide it *(dashed line)*; then enter the ischiorectal fossa.

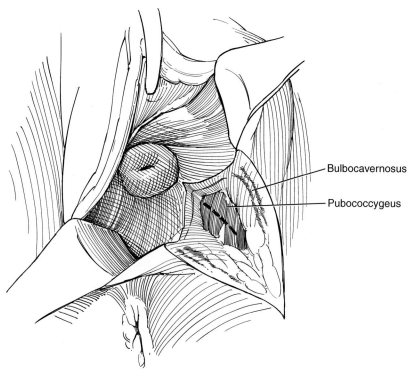

Bulbocavernosus

Pubococcygeus

13 After the fistula has been repaired, approximate the pubococcygeus muscle with a few 2-0 SAS. Close the vaginal portion by placing deep sutures in the vaginal wall. Bring the bulbocavernosus muscle together with sutures that also include the levator muscle and fibers of the urogenital diaphragm to obliterate the dead space. Close the perineal incision in layers, and approximate the perineal skin with interrupted NAS.

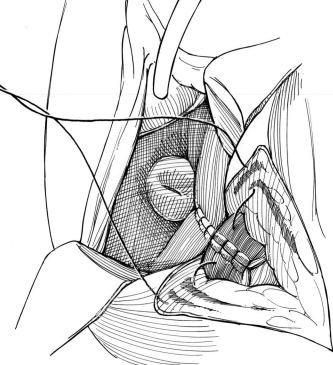

TRANSVESICAL REPAIR
(Mundy)

Instruments: Provide a Basic set, a GU plastic set, angled needle holder, vascular forceps, a weighted speculum, lateral retractors, Heany retractors, baby Deaver retractors, a Balfour or Turner-Warwick ring retractor, a fiberoptic suction tip, nonperforating towel clips, a table extension, gynecologic leg holders, a padded stool, a 2-inch hard rubber ball, an Ingram catheter, a 12-gauge butterfly needle and vacuum tube, whistle-tip ureteral catheters, an 18 F 5-ml silicone balloon catheter and bag, and 3-0 synthetic absorbable, T-16, and 2-0 silk CE-6 sutures.

Position: Place the patient in the low lithotomy position with legs spread and supported and the table tilted into moderate Trendelenburg position. Prepare and drape the perineum and vagina, in addition to the abdomen. If the defect is near the ureteral orifices, place ureteral catheters endoscopically or intraoperatively. Insert an 18 F 5-ml silicone balloon catheter to fill the bladder if that is possible. Insert a rubber ball in the vagina, or pack the vagina tightly with gauze.

14 **A,** *Incision:* Make a vertical midline incision (see page 487) in case omentum will be needed for large defects, or use a transverse lower abdominal incision (see page 490). Insert a Balfour or ring retractor.

B, Open the bladder. Place a stay suture above and below the fistula. Incise the full thickness of the bladder wall above and below the fistula with a #10 knife blade to the depth of the vaginal wall. Join the ends of the incisions *(dashed lines)* to circumscribe and excise the bladder wall portion of the fistula.

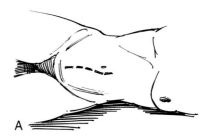

A

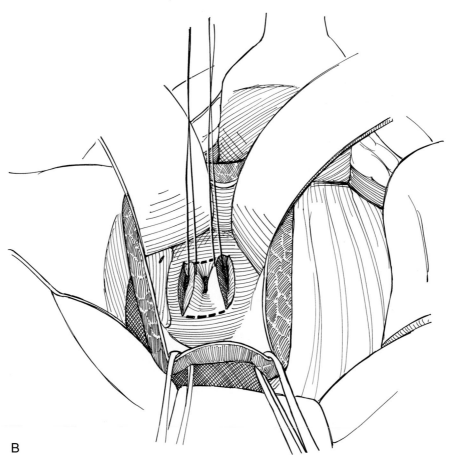

B

15

A, Free the bladder from the vaginal wall for a distance of 1 to 2 cm with Lahey scissors. Lift up on the tract, and excise the diseased vaginal wall circumferentially *(dashed line)* against the pack or ball being held up in the vagina by an assistant.

B, Invert the vaginal mucosal layer with interrupted 3-0 SAS. Free a middle layer of combined perivaginal and perivesical tissue with the scissors. It must be dissected far enough that no tension is present on closure. *Note:* In a radiated bladder, if the ureteral orifice lies near the defect, do not hesitate to reimplant the ureter.

Intermediate and detrusor layers: Close this intermediate layer with interrupted 3-0 SAS in a line perpendicular to the first closure. Alternatively, tack the omentum over the vaginal suture line. The omentum may be found adherent to the vaginal vault or may require mobilization (see page 71). Approximate the detrusor with interrupted 3-0 SAS, and close the vesical urothelium with a running subepithelial 4-0 PCG suture. Place a 22 F Malecot catheter through a stab wound in the bladder and body wall, and insert a Penrose (or vacuum) drain. Close the bladder with a running subepithelial 4-0 PCG suture, with interrupted sutures to the muscle. Close the abdominal wound. Fasten the suprapubic tube to the skin and attach it to drainage, which must be meticulously maintained free of obstruction. Provide broad-spectrum antibiotics, and give anticholinergics for bladder spasm. At 10 days, perform voiding cystography, after discontinuing anticholinergic medication the previous day. If the closure is seen to be intact and, after a period of voiding with the tube clamped, residual urine is determined to be less than 100 ml, remove the suprapubic tube. In postmenopausal women, provide estrogen cream for vaginal application.

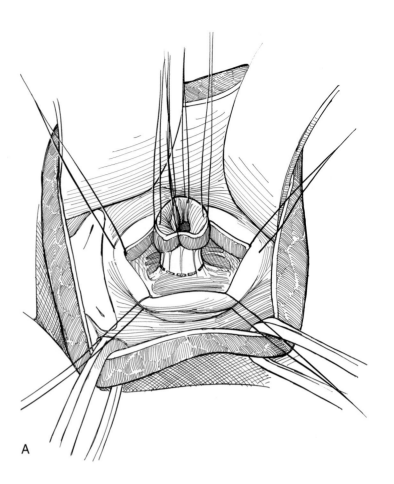

A

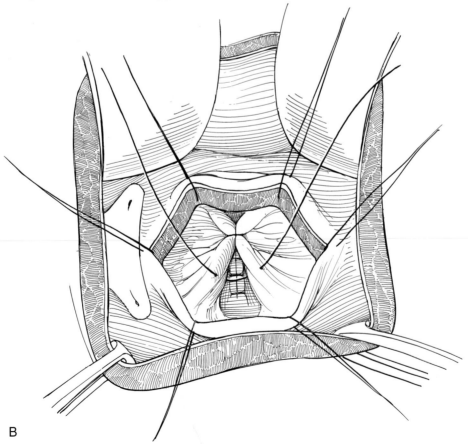

B

TRANSPERITONEAL TRANSVESICAL OPERATION
(O'Conor)

Position: Place the patient as in Step 1A.
  Incision: Make a vertical incision, one that allows access to the omentum if it is needed.

16 Open the peritoneum and bluntly push it from the dome of the bladder. Pack the small bowel out of the way. Open the bladder over the dome between stay sutures. Bisect the bladder wall and overlying peritoneum down to the edge of the fistula, placing stay sutures to elevate the bladder as the division progresses.

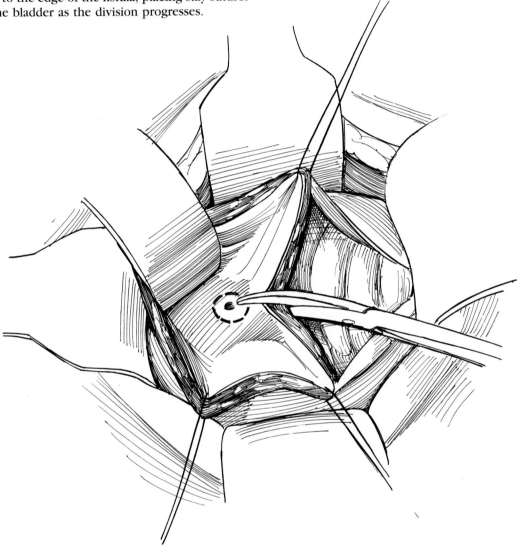

17 Cut the peritoneum transversely at the level of the fistula to form a pedicled flap for use in closure. Use a probe to localize the fistula if it is small. Separate the bladder from the vagina widely on either side of the fistula. Place the nondominant index and middle fingers in the vagina to help define the proper plane. Alternatively, have the assistant exert upward pressure on a rubber ball or pack in the vagina to facilitate this dissection. Or, if it is possible to put a balloon catheter through the fistula into the vagina, inflate it for traction during the dissection. Excise the fistula completely as it becomes exposed.

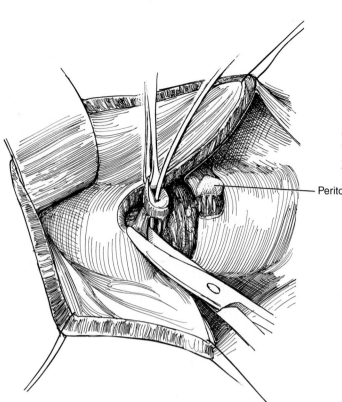

Peritoneal flap

18 Continue freeing the bladder from the vagina widely to allow mobility for separate closure. Close the vagina in two layers vertically or transversely with inverting interrupted 3-0 SAS. Avoid tension.

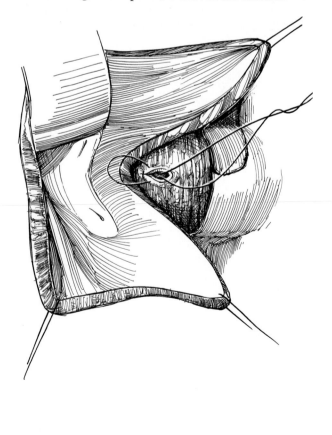

19 Swing the peritoneal flap into the defect, and suture it in place to retroperitonealize the repair. If it is inadequate, elevate a long peritoneal flap or use a free peritoneal graft.

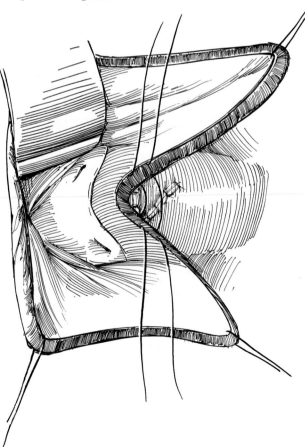

20 Close the bladder uroepithelium-subepithelium with a running 3-0 PCG suture, and approximate the muscularis and adventitia from the outside with interrupted 3-0 SAS. Be sure that there is no tension because success depends on the effectiveness of the bladder approximation, not on the vaginal closure. If the repair is tenuous or if the area has been radiated, bring the omentum behind the right colon for an omental graft, and tack it between the bladder and vagina in the area of the defect. A fistula from radiation necrosis, however, is best managed with a musculocutaneous graft (Steps 15 and 16). Remove the ureteral catheters. If they were not placed, ask the anesthetist to inject indigo carmine intravenously to check ureteral patency. Although a balloon catheter may suffice, a suprapubic tube is safer and is less likely to press on the suture line. Insert a 22 F Malecot catheter through a stab wound in the bladder wall, and place a Penrose (or vacuum) drain, both to exit through stab wounds in the body wall and be sutured to the skin. Close the bladder in two layers with a continuous subepithelial suture and interrupted sutures to the muscularis placed from the outside. Close the wound in layers. Remove the urethral catheter in 5 days, if one was placed, and take the suprapubic tube out in 2 weeks. Advise the patient against sexual intercourse for 6 weeks.

Alternative: To avoid closing a long posterior vesical incision that could compromise vesical function and capacity, do not bisect the bladder. Instead, incise the peritoneum in the vesicouterine pouch, and establish a plane between bladder and vagina by sharp dissection. Do this before or after opening the bladder. Insert catheters into the ureters and a small Foley or Fogerty catheter through the fistula into the vagina. Continue the retrovesical dissection for at least 1 or 2 cm beyond the fistula. Trim the edges of the fistula just enough to remove inflammatory tissue, but not to try to débride it of all scar tissue. Complete the operation as described in Step 7.

ABDOMINAL PLACEMENT OF A GRACILIS FLAP
(Fleischmann and Picha)

With the patient in the lithotomy position, expose and close the vaginal and vesical defects from above (Steps 3 to 6), with or without splitting the bladder. Continue dissecting behind the bladder and ureter. Incise the endopelvic fascia for 3 cm on one side. Working from above and below, create a tunnel that traverses the urogenital diaphragm and joins the retropubic space with the incision in the upper thigh. With the tendon still attached for traction, bring the gracilis muscle through the tunnel so created. Close the bladder in two layers. Trim the muscle, fold it anteriorly, and fix it in place against the bladder, between it and the vagina. Suture its fascial sheath with 4-0 SAS to a site above the bladder closure.

Insert suction drainage. Postoperatively, keep the leg adducted. Allow the patient out of bed with assistance after 3 days. Remove the stents after 7 days and the suprapubic catheter after 8 days. Finally, remove the urethral catheter when drainage has ceased.

CLOSURE WITH RECTUS ABDOMINIS MUSCLE FLAP

Make a midline incision and raise an inferior rectus abdominis flap (see pages 54 to 57), leaving it attached to the inferior epigastric artery and vein. Make a vertical 5- to 6-cm incision in the most lateral aspect of the posterior rectus sheath around the site of take-off of the inferior epigastric artery. Extend the incision through the peritoneum so that the flap can be passed into the abdominal cavity. Close the posterior rectus sheath loosely around the pedicle.

Feed the flap between the bladder and vagina, and tack it in place with 2-0 SAS. Close the defect in the anterior rectus sheath, and close the wound.

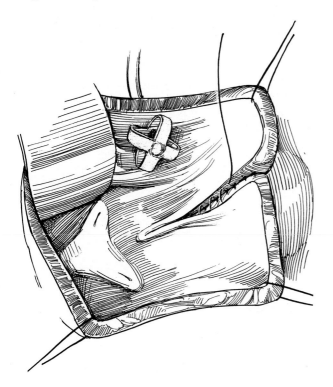

REPAIR OF COMPLEX FISTULAS

Approach the fistula abdominally and transvaginally. Excise all abnormal (postradiation) tissue. Close the defect by a rotational bladder flap, if feasible, and seal the area with omentum. If it is impossible to restore the integrity of the bladder, cover the defect with omentum and allow spontaneous re-epithelialization. Alternatively, perform augmentation cystoplasty.

REPAIR DURING VAGINAL HYSTERECTOMY
(Hernandez)

This approach is used for repair of laceration of the bladder occurring during vaginal hysterectomy.

Give indigo carmine and observe ureteral efflux. Insert ureteral catheters, and place a suprapubic balloon catheter retrogradely (see page 628). Use an extreme Trendelenburg position, and place a weighted speculum and a Scott retractor. Pass a balloon catheter through the defect, and make traction on it. Insert two stay sutures in the corners of the defect, and remove the catheter. Mobilize the bladder from the vagina with the aid of saline infiltration. Invert the bladder epithelium with absorbable running sutures placed from each end. Approximate the perivesical fascia with running sutures at right angles to the first row. Check watertightness by filling the bladder with dilute methylene blue. Abdominally, mobilize a peritoneal flap and cover the repair. (Alternatively, perineally mobilize a Martius flap, Steps 6 and 7.) Trim the anterior edge of the vaginal incision, and advance the posterior edge over the repair. Place a pack for 48 hours. Perform cystography on the 12th day to check the repair, and remove the catheters sequentially.

POSTOPERATIVE PROBLEMS

Vaginal bleeding responds to vaginal packing and bed rest. *Bladder spasms* should be treated vigorously with anticholinergic medication to avoid stress on the suture line. *Infection* is avoided by administration of antibiotics. *Urinary frequency* usually subsides spontaneously, aided by anticholinergic medication. *Incontinence* may appear after repair; it must be evaluated to be sure it is not due to recurrence of the fistula. *Obstruction* at the ureteral orifice can occur, especially after repair of large fistulas, and requires percutaneous nephrostomy; do not attempt to intubate it from below. Reimplantation of the ureter may be required. *Reflux* may be produced by the repair. It usually stops spontaneously but in any case is rarely harmful to the upper tract. *Leakage* should be detected before the catheter is removed by performing voiding cystourethrography. If it appears later, it requires replacement of a catheter for 2 or 3 weeks, with the hope of spontaneous closure. Other, uncommon complications include dyspareunia, vaginal narrowing, and difficulties at labor. *Recurrence of the fistula* requires waiting for complete healing and a secondary repair that brings in a flap of healthy tissue.

Commentary by Gary E. Leach

I prefer the vaginal approach to vesicovaginal fistula repair in almost all situations without an enforced waiting period prior to repair. An abdominal approach to repair is considered when another simultaneous abdominal procedure is required (such as augmentation cystoplasty), when adequate vaginal exposure cannot be obtained (which is rare), or when the fistula is so small that its exact location cannot be confirmed with certainty. Also, because approximately 10 percent of vesicovaginal fistulas are associated with a ureterovaginal fistula, I routinely perform bilateral retrograde ureterography perioperatively because a ureterovaginal fistula may exist even in the presence of a relatively normal intravenous pyelogram.

Because most vesicovaginal fistulas occur after hysterectomy, they are usually located at the vaginal cuff. Exposure of the fistula tract is greatly enhanced by catheterizing the fistula from the vaginal side with either a small Foley catheter or a Fogarty catheter, then utilizing the catheter to place traction on the fistula site. Exposure is also enhanced with use of the Scott ring retractor with its elastic hook stays as well as use of a vaginal relaxing incision when required. A 24 F suprapubic Foley catheter is initially placed, utilizing the Lowsley tractor as well as inserting an 18 F urethral Foley catheter. If there is any concern regarding the proximity of the fistula to the ureters, ureteral catheters are inserted prior to fistula closure.

When the fistula is at the vaginal apex, the vaginal flaps used for the closure are oriented with the base of the flap at the bladder neck and the apex of the flap adjacent to the fistula at the vaginal cuff. None of the fistula tract is excised, but, rather, the margins of the fistula are incorporated into the first layer of tension-free closure with a running absorbable suture after adequate mobilization between the bladder and vaginal wall. The second layer of reconstruction is the prevesical fascia, which is approximated over the fistula site with 3-0 absorbable interrupted sutures. At this point, if any question remains regarding the integrity of the closure, the bladder is filled with methylene blue–stained fluid and the closure site is carefully observed. When there is any concern about the strength of the closure, a Martius labial fat pad graft is mobilized (without the underlying muscle), tunneled into the vagina, and fixed between the prevesical fascia and the vaginal wall flap. This final vaginal wall flap is advanced over the closure without tension to avoid any overlapping suture lines.

Both the suprapubic and urethral catheters are placed to gravity drainage. Oral anticholinergics are given to paralyze the bladder for 7 to 10 days, at which time cystography is performed to confirm closure of the fistula before the catheters are removed.

Closure of Vesicosigmoid Fistula

Gas in the bladder on computed tomographic (CT) scan is strongly suggestive of a communication with the bowel. Culture the urine (usually a mixed flora with microaerophilic bacteria). Cystoscopy detects the fistula in two thirds of cases as an edematous, erythematous area, usually posteriorly high on the left side of the bladder or occasionally at the dome. Attempt to pass a spiral-tipped ureteral catheter into it; if successful, inject contrast. Cystography shows the fistula in one third of cases.

Oral charcoal is sometimes useful, as is the detection of vegetable fibers in the urine, but instilling methylene blue in the bladder and looking for it in the feces is more often effective. A Hypaque enema may be helpful to detect diverticular bowel disease and may demonstrate the communication. In the absence of diverticula, suspect malignancy and obtain a CT scan.

Prepare the bowel. Give urinary antibiotics. Correct malnutrition.

1 **A,** *Position:* Place the patient supine, in the Trendelenburg position. Insert a 22 F 5-ml balloon catheter, and fill the bladder with 100 ml of sterile water. Clamp the catheter.

Incision: Make a midline or paramedian transperitoneal incision (see pages 867 and 869). Examine the abdominal contents: If you find a large walled-off inflammatory mass, do not enter it but perform a transverse colostomy, converting to a two-stage operation.

B, Mobilize the descending and sigmoid colon by incising the fascial fusion layer along the white line of Toldt. Identify the loop of sigmoid colon involved.

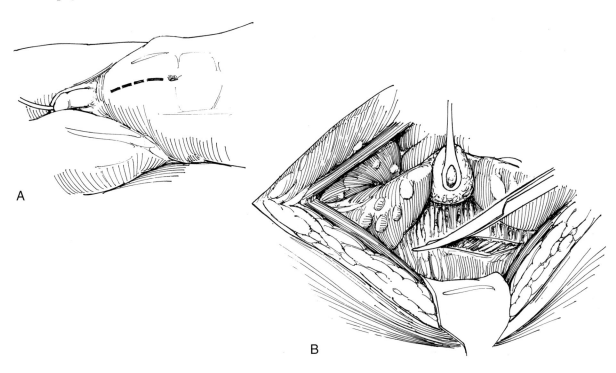

A

B

LESIONS WITH MINIMAL INFLAMMATORY REACTION

2 Pinch off the fistulous tract with thumb and forefinger.

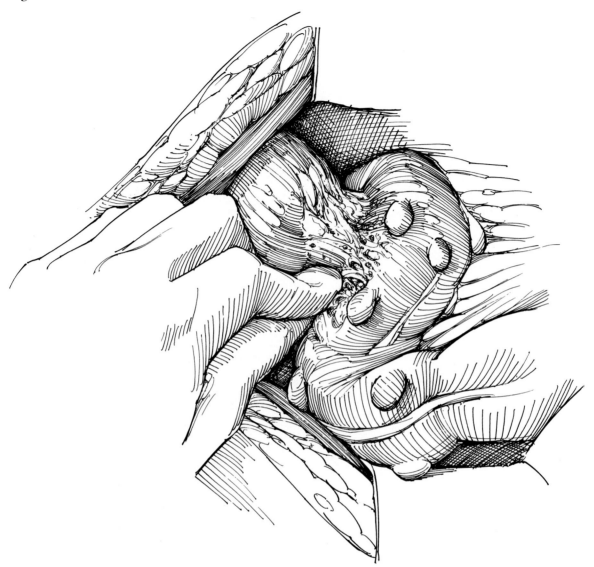

3 Débride the defects in bladder and bowel back to healthy tissue. Close the bladder in two layers by placing a submucosal continuous 3-0 PCG suture and an interrupted 2-0 CCG suture in the muscle and adventitia.

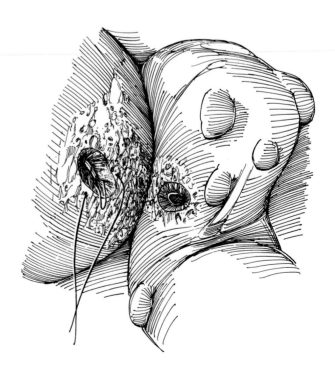

4 A, Trim the edges of the bowel defect well back into normal tissue. Place a stay suture at each side of it.

B, Pull the defect transversely.

C, Close the mucosa and submucosa with a Connell suture (see page 37).

D, Approximate the muscularis and serosa with inter-rupted Lembert sutures (see page 38). Consider placing omentum between the repair sites (see page 71). Close the peritoneum. Drain the wound with a large Penrose or suction drain. Place a balloon catheter in the bladder. In 10 days perform cystography; if it is negative for extravasation, remove the catheter.

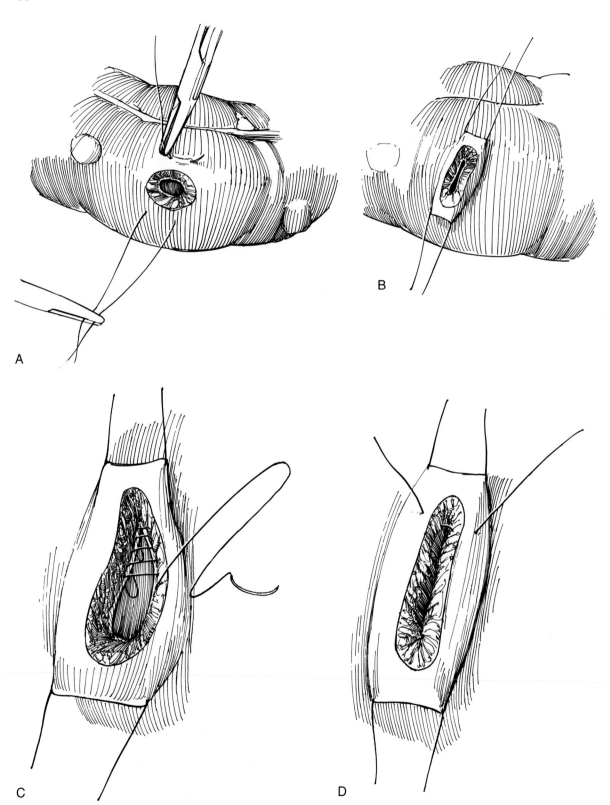

LARGE INFLAMMATORY MASSES

Resection of the involved colon is required for large inflammatory masses.

5 Separate the colon from the bladder either bluntly or by resection of an adequate portion of the bladder wall with the cutting current. Débride the edges and close the vesical defect in two layers, as described in Step 3. A suprapubic tube may be inserted, but at least provide balloon catheter drainage for 5 to 7 days postoperatively.

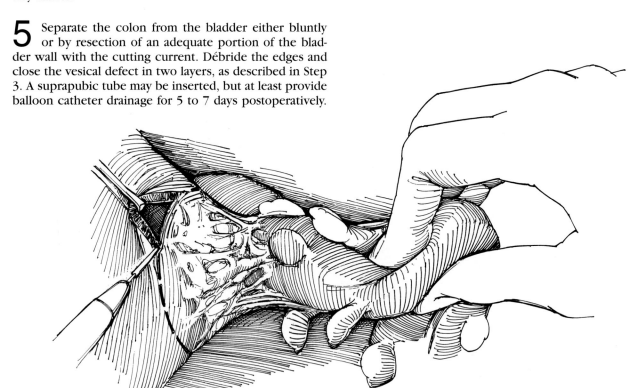

6 Divide the retroperitoneum on the white line.

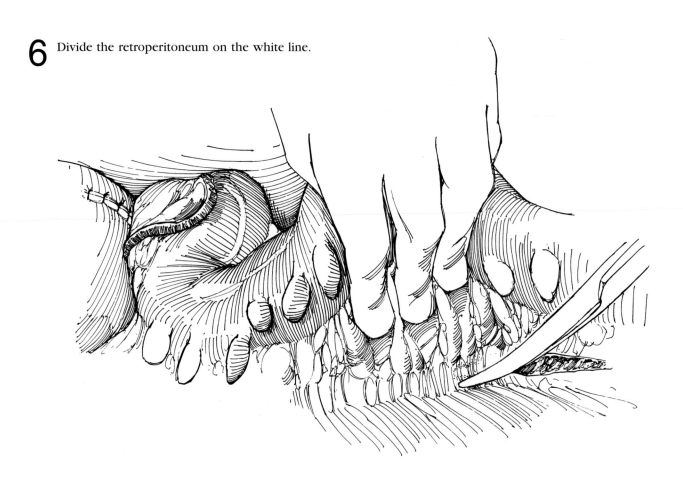

7 Select the sites for bowel transection. The segment should include all of the sigmoid colon to the rectosigmoid junction, lying approximately at the sacral promontory. Encircle the sites with 14 F Robinson catheters held on clamps.

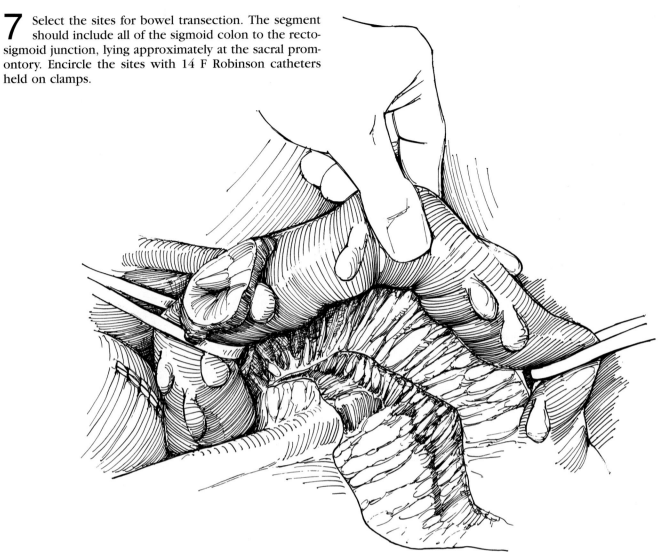

8 Make a curvilinear incision on the medial surface of the sigmoid mesentery. Clamp the exposed vessels as the mesentery is divided. These vessels are more delicate than those on the small intestine; use greater care when handling them.

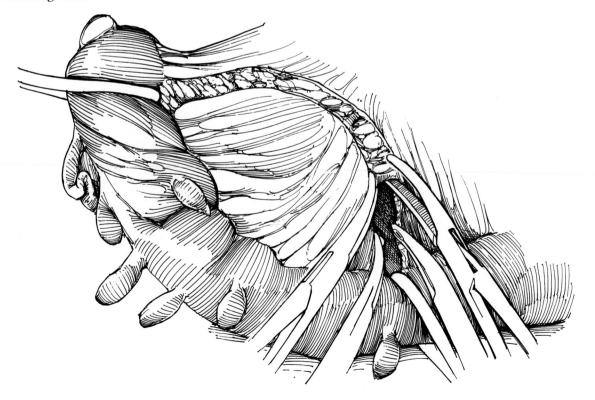

9 Place a Kocher clamp across the bowel just above the lower line of excision and a noncrushing intestinal clamp below on the bowel that is to remain. Divide the bowel with the cutting current. Similarly clamp and cut the proximal end of the segment, and remove the resected bowel.

COLORECTAL ANASTOMOSIS, OPEN TECHNIQUE

For another suture technique, see pages 736 to 737.

10 Note that the colon is constructed as a tube within a tube, defining the two layers for closure. Place a series of interrupted 4-0 silk sutures posteriorly to approximate the seromuscular layers constituting the outer tube. Tie them after all are in place. Hold one of them at either end in a clamp to stabilize the bowel. (For anastomosis by stapling technique, see page 66.)

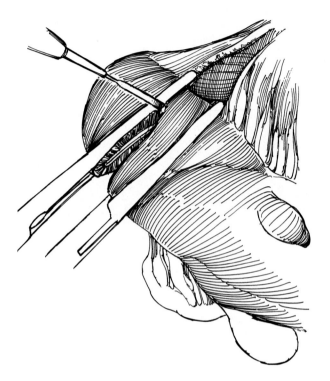

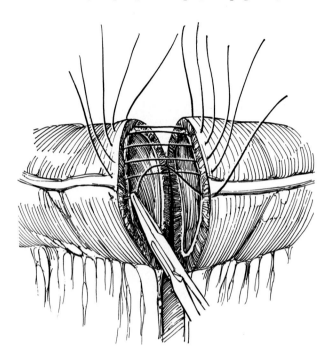

11 From inside the bowel, run a continuous 3-0 PCG suture down the mucosa and submucosa, locking every third or fourth stitch.

12 Turn the angle by placing the suture from the inside on the same side.

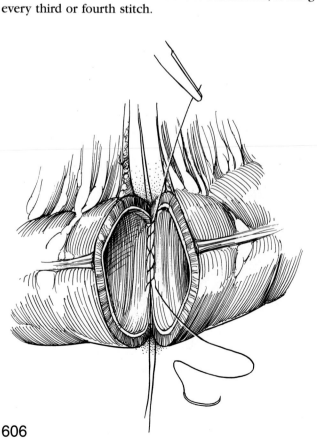

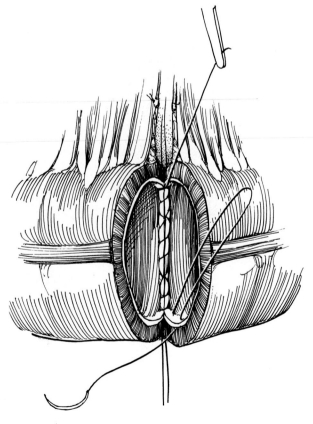

13 Insert the suture in the opposite mucosal angle from the outside, and have it exit from the inside (Connell technique, see page 37).

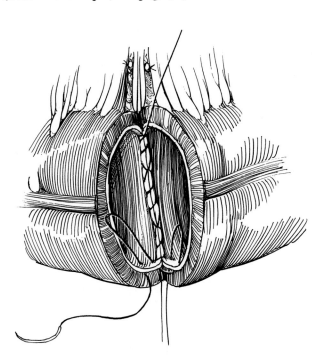

14 Place another Connell stitch on the original side. Draw the suture taut and invert the mucosal angle.

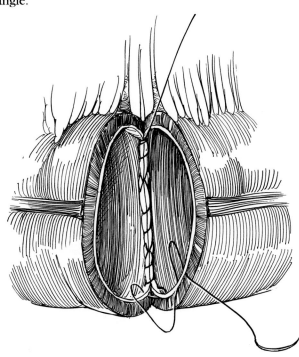

15 Continue the mucosal suture up the anterior surface as a simple through-and-through stitch to meet and tie to the other end of the suture.

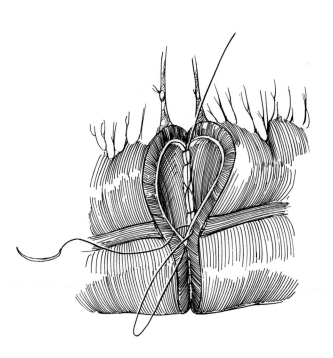

16 Place interrupted 4-0 silk sutures to approximate the seromuscular layer anteriorly. These stitches should also catch some of the submucosa.

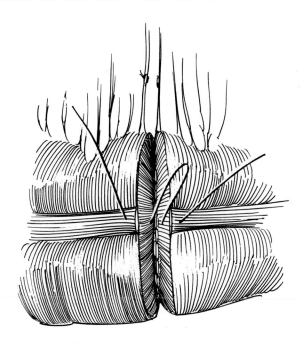

17 Close the mesentery with 4-0 silk sutures. Invaginate the bowel at the anastomosis with thumb and forefinger to check for patency. If possible, bring the peritoneum over the vesical defect. Use an omental sleeve (see page 71) if the inflammatory reaction was gross and the repair difficult. In such a case in a male, place a cystostomy. Drain the suprapubic area with a Penrose drain through the wound. Place a sump drain to the bowel anastomosis, and bring it out a stab wound. Tack the colon laterally along the white line with 4-0 silk sutures. Irrigate the wound thoroughly. Close the peritoneum and the wound. Insert a 22 F 5-ml silicone balloon catheter into the bladder, to remain 5 to 7 days.

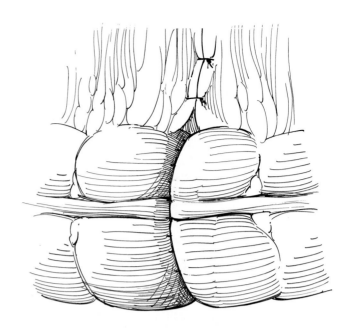

POSTOPERATIVE PROBLEMS

Wound infection and its persistence as an *abscess* are the most common postoperative problems. Their incidence is reduced by copious wound irrigation, prolonged adequate drainage, and liberal antibiotic coverage, including agents against microaerophilic organisms. *Anastomotic leaks* are infrequent, usually related to large pelvic abscesses.

Commentary by James F. Glenn

Vesicosigmoid fistula is the most common of the enteric fistulas of the urinary tract. However, it must be remembered that fistulas of the renal pelvis and ureter also occur, although rarely, and occasionally a vesicovaginoenteric fistula.

The causes of vesicosigmoid fistula include diverticulitis with an inflammatory mass, malignancies of either bowel or bladder, radiation necrosis, previous surgery, and traumatic injury. Precise definition of the cause of the fistula is necessary in planning the appropriate course of management.

Characteristic presentation of vesicosigmoid fistula includes symptoms of pneumaturia, fecaluria, and chronic or recurring urinary tract infection, frequently with multiple organisms. The most common physical findings of abdominal tenderness and mass are not always manifest.

Diagnostic maneuvers include cystoscopy and cystography, as noted above, as well as the use of oral charcoal or methylene blue instillation in the bladder. An additional maneuver requires thorough cleansing enemas, followed by instillation of methylene blue into the rectum with concomitant cystoscopy.

Almost invariably, the fistula is visualized within the area of intense inflammatory reaction on the dome or posterolateral surfaces of the bladder. The techniques of repair as described and illustrated previously are appropriate in the varying circumstances of the particular fistula. In the presence of an inflammatory process, I undertake prolonged antibacterial treatment and extensive bowel preparation; reduction of the inflammatory mass facilitates surgery. Even with the smallest of fistulas and minimal inflammatory reaction, my preference is for primary resection of the involved area of the bladder, as well as resection of the involved segment of the sigmoid. Simple closure of the bladder and the colon carries a definite risk of recurrence of fistula. Because most vesicosigmoid fistulas are of inflammatory origin, interposition of omentum between bladder and bowel is highly desirable, and mobilization of the omentum may require superior extension of the abdominal incision.

As final words of caution, it should be acknowledged that fistulas secondary to radiation injury may involve a great deal more tissue than is visually apparent, and the repair of fistulas secondary to malignancy may require massive extirpation and, on occasion, both fecal and urinary diversion.

Closure of Female Vesical Neck

Provide continent diversion or place a suprapubic cystostomy. Clear the urine of infection if possible, and provide antibiotic coverage.

The simplest method (and an effective one, if well executed) is to open the bladder, make a circumferential incision around the bladder neck to remove a divot of uroepithelium, and then close the muscularis and subepithelium with two layers of purse-string absorbable suture. However, adequate removal of

the uroepithelium may be quite difficult. More security may be obtained by inverting the urethra, as is done with the combined approach. The key to success is to be sure that all of the uroepithelium has been removed so that both the urethral and vesical surfaces are in contact and are able to fuse. Omental interposition gives added security.

Perform a continent diversion procedure or install a suprapubic cystostomy.

VESICAL APPROACH WITH URETHRAL INVERSION

1 Through a lower transverse abdominal (see page 490) or lower midline incision (see page 487), enter the retropubic space and free the urethra by dividing the pubourethral ligament and dissecting it distally from the vagina with the aid of a finger in the vagina. Elevate the urethra from the vagina by sharp dissection with a knife to include the urethral adventitia. The longer the segment freed by sharp dissection, the easier the closure. Divide the urethra, and ligate the distal end with a 3-0 SAS. Ligate the proximal end loosely and leave the proximal suture long.

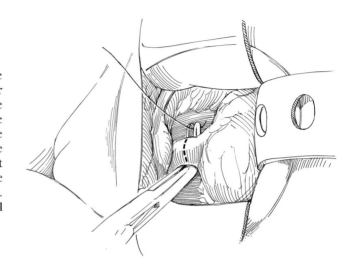

2 Open the bladder and visualize the outlet. Insert ureteral catheters for safety. Place four 3-0 traction SAS through the uroepithelium, closely surrounding the vesical neck. With a hooked knife, cut through the uroepithelium circumferentially 1 to 2 cm away from the outlet, and free up the epithelial margins with scissors.

3 Trim the freed uroepithelium flush with the outlet, being certain that all of the lining at the outlet is removed. Insert a curved clamp into the transected urethra, insinuate it through the previously loosely tied end, and grasp the suture that was left long. Pull on it to invert the urethra into the bladder. Trim excess urethra.

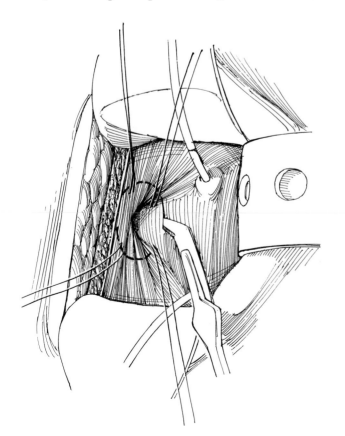

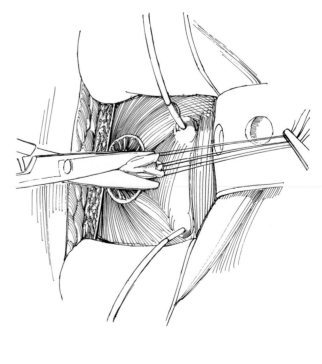

4 **A,** Close the end of the trimmed urethra with inverting 4-0 SAS, and tack it to the surrounding detrusor.

B, Place a 4-0 purse-string SAS 1 cm from the urethra to invert the urethral uroepithelium as the suture is tied. Place a second circumferential suture 1 cm outside the first and tie it. Close the uroepithelium of the bladder over the repair with interrupted 4-0 PCG sutures. Insert a Malecot catheter to exit through a stab wound. Close the bladder and the wound. Further security may be had by excising the urethral uroepithelium perineally and obliterating that space (Steps 5 to 7).

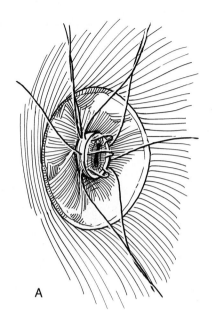

A

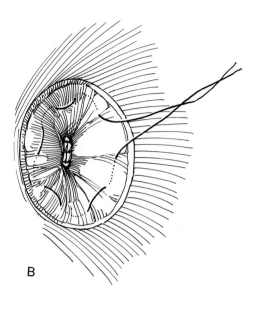

B

URETHRAL APPROACH

This approach avoids a formal abdominal incision, yet inverts the urethra into the bladder. Provide a cystostomy (see page 625).

5 With the patient in the dorsal lithotomy position, fix the labia laterally with stay sutures, and place a small posterior retractor in the vagina. Place four traction sutures around the meatus that extend through the urethral subepithelium. Alternatively, run a purse-string suture around the meatus. Incise the meatus circumferentially. With sharp dissection, enter the plane between the urethra and the vagina. Free the urethra from the vagina to the level of the bladder neck. Dissect it from the retropubic tissue also to the level of the bladder neck by dividing the endopelvic fascia laterally and entering the retropubic space. It is essential to divide the pubourethral ligament anteriorly to mobilize the urethra fully up to the vesical neck and to expose the base of the bladder.

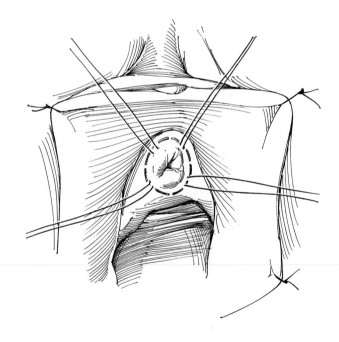

6 Invert the urethral meatus into the urethra by placing three end-on 2-0 mattress SAS in the urethral wall to hold it inverted. Then insert a 2-0 purse-string SAS around the vesical neck, and invert the urethra into the bladder. *Alternatively,* trim the urethra and close it with an inverting purse-string suture. A second purse-string suture may be inserted.

7 Approximate the periurethral fascia with several 4-0 SAS, and close the uroepithelium vertically with interrupted 4-0 CCG sutures. Pack the vagina to reduce the chance for formation of a hematoma.

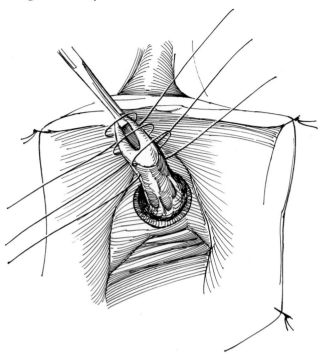

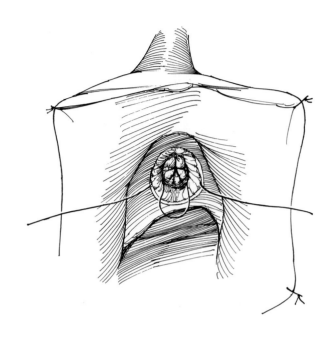

TRANSVAGINAL APPROACH
(Zinman)

This method provides greater exposure for excision.

8 With the patient in the dorsal lithotomy position, fix the labia laterally with stay sutures, and place a small posterior retractor in the vagina. Incise the vaginal epithelium widely around the urethra, extending the incision as far posteriorly as the introitus, and continue as an inverted U by forming wings into the vagina beyond the bladder neck.

9 Free the vaginal flap from the urethra and posterior bladder neck after injecting normal saline beneath the anterior vaginal wall to help delineate the plane.

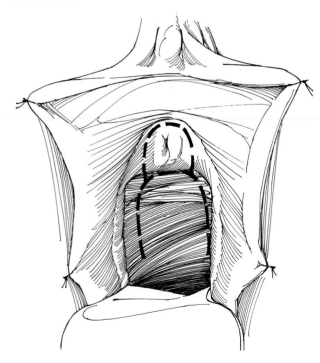

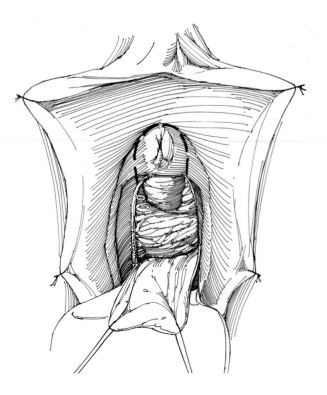

10 Continue the dissection around the urethra and bladder neck. Separate the bladder neck from the endopelvic fascia and from its retropubic attachments, including the pubourethral ligaments, staying close to the vesical wall. Trim the urethra flush with the vesical neck.

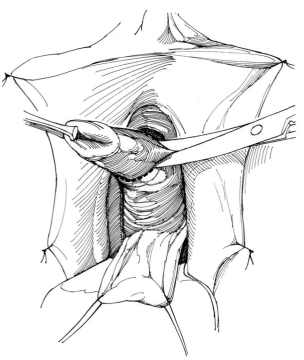

11 Close the vesical neck with a running 3-0 PCG suture placed subepithelially in a vertical direction. Over this, place a running 3-0 SAS.

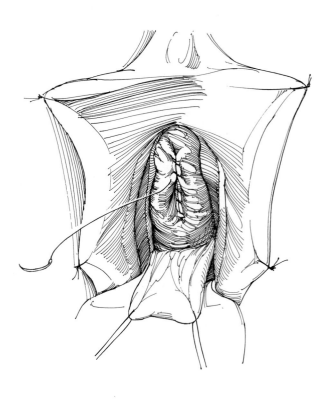

12 Reinforce this suture line with a transversely placed running 3-0 SAS to the perivesical fascia and superficial layer of the bladder wall, to move the repair behind the symphysis.

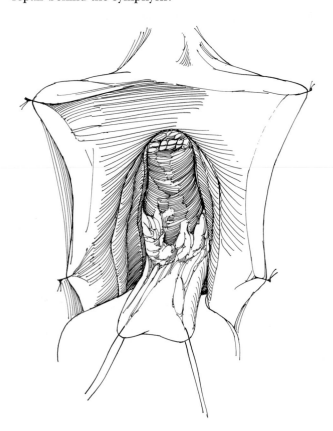

13 Bring the vaginal flap forward to cover the urethral defect, and tack it in place with four or five 3-0 subcutaneous SAS. Run a 3-0 SAS with an occasional lock stitch to fasten the flap to the defect. *Alternatively,* bring a vascularized labial fat pad into the defect before suturing the flap (see page 590). Test for watertightness. Pack the vagina over strips of petroleum jelly gauze.

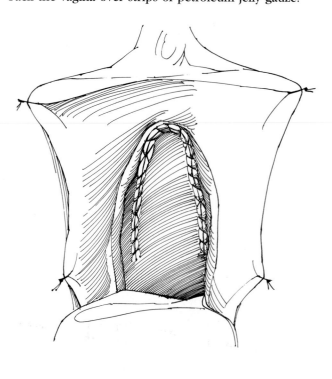

FUNCTIONAL CLOSURE WITH PUBOVAGINAL SLING

Secure and place a pubovaginal sling as described on page 565. Suture one end of the fascial sling to the rectus fascia with multiple interrupted 2-0 or 3-0 NAS. Bring the other end of the strip through muscle and fascia similarly on the left side. Draw up firmly on the suture, and fasten the end to the fascia with 2-0 or 3-0 NAS, making a three-bite helix in the fascial strip with the suture.

POSTOPERATIVE PROBLEMS

Leakage may appear immediately if the bladder has not been continuously decompressed. It may occur later as the sutures are resorbed and areas of injured tissue break down. Prolonged suprapubic drainage sometimes allows the fistula to close.

Commentary by Roger C. L. Feneley

Closure of the vesical neck is not the simple operation that it may appear because it can be followed by persistent urinary leakage from a vesicovaginal fistula. The first attempt to close the vesical neck provides the optimal opportunity to achieve a successful outcome. In a personal series of these patients, the majority have been severely disabled and confined to bed or a wheelchair; their urinary incontinence has usually been related to a neuropathic bladder disorder that was managed initially by long-term urethral catheterization. Complications of this include a chronic urinary tract infection, persistent leakage or bypassing of urine around the catheter, and spontaneous extrusion of the balloon catheter, which can dilate, damage, and eventually destroy the urethra.

Vesical neck closure is performed to resolve the incontinence problem. In the presence of a chronic urinary infection, invagination of the urethra into the bladder without opening the bladder is the preferred option. The essential step involves division of the pubourethral ligament by sharp dissection so that the urethra is fully mobilized up to the vesical neck. The urethra cannot be invaginated into the bladder if it is tethered to the ligament, and failure to free the urethra carries a high risk of subsequent urinary leakage through a vesicovaginal fistula. Before proceeding with the closure, it is prudent first to establish a suprapubic cystostomy by a percutaneous method to ensure patient acceptance of the re-sited catheter.

BLADDER NECK CLOSURE IN MALES (Rentzepis and Stone)

Through a lower midline incision, expose the bladder neck and incise it longitudinally. Insert infant feeding tubes into the ureteral orifices. Divide the posterior bladder neck transversely, draw it forward, and dissect it free from the prostate to a point well behind the bladder. Place a suprapubic catheter (or construct a catheterizable stoma). Close the distal end of the prostatic urethra with 2-0 SAS. Close the bladder neck with two layers of the same suture. Insert a pedicle of omentum (see page 71) or a rectus abdominis flap (see pages 54 to 57) between the prostate and the bladder neck. Provide a suction drain.

Excision of Urachus

PATENT URACHUS

Perform excretory urography or voiding cystography. Ultrasonography is not helpful. Before proceeding with repair, test for outlet obstruction.

1 *Position:* Have the patient lying supine. Insert a balloon catheter, and fill the bladder to carry the anterior bladder wall up to the abdominal wall and move the peritoneum cephalad. If possible, place a fine tube into the bladder through the urachus. Try a stiff 3.5 F polyethylene pediatric feeding tube, a pigtail ureteral catheter, or even a lacrimal duct probe. If nothing passes, stain the tract by instilling methylene blue for subsequent identification of the lumen.

Incision: Place a lower transverse incision in a skin fold well above the symphysis *(dashed line)*. In infants, because of the high position of the bladder, the incision can be placed nearer the umbilicus. A midline incision is an alternative *(dotted line)*.

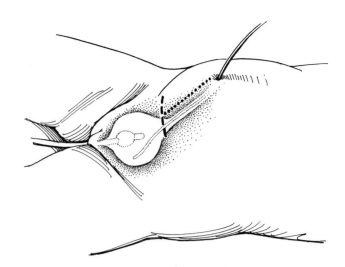

2 Divide the fascial junction between the rectus abdominis muscles vertically, and enter the preperitoneal space. Identify the high-lying dome of the bladder in this space, but do not enter the peritoneum.

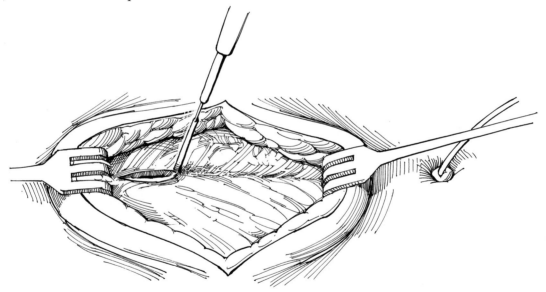

3 Expose the dome of the bladder, and carefully free the connective tissue between the vesical adventitia and the peritoneum to expose the two obliterated umbilical arteries with the urachus lying between them. Bluntly dissect the urachus free at a convenient level, and encir- cle it with a vascular tape or Penrose drain. Continue to sharply dissect the urachus down to the bladder. Place two stay sutures in the bladder wall adjacent to its termination.

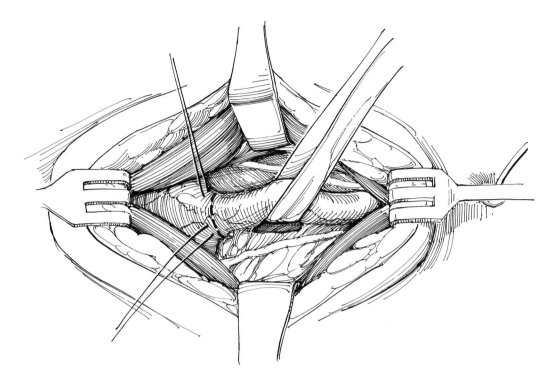

4 Divide the urachus within the bladder wall in order to remove a small cuff. This is to avoid the (remote) possibility of the development of adenocarcinoma. Use progressive cuts so that, while the area is suspended by the urachus, a 4-0 PCG continuous suture can be inserted to invert the vesical uroepithelium. Add interrupted 3- or 4-0 SAS to approximate the muscle. Elevate the upper end of the wound with retractors, and dissect the urachus from the closely adherent peritoneum as far as the umbilicus. Excise the urachus along with the ends of the umbilical arteries and remove the specimen. It is not necessary to remove the last bit of the urachal stoma. Close the umbilical defect in two layers from inside, preserving as much as possible of the umbilicus for cosmetic reasons.

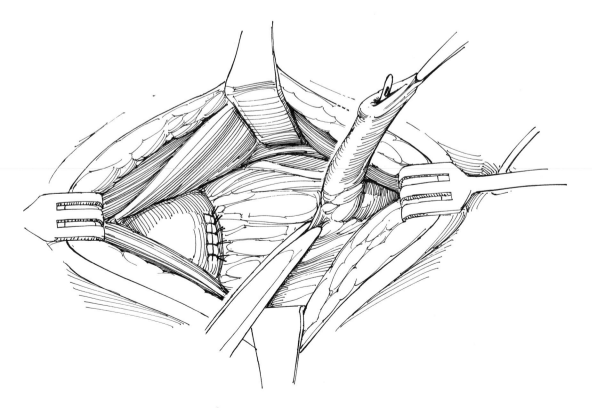

5 Place a drain through a stab wound to the bladder region. Approximate the rectus muscles loosely, and close the incision in layers. Remove the drain in 3 days if the wound is dry. Leave the catheter indwelling for 7 days.

A large acontractile *urachal diverticulum* at the apex of the bladder is resected in the same way as is done for the caudal end of a patent urachus.

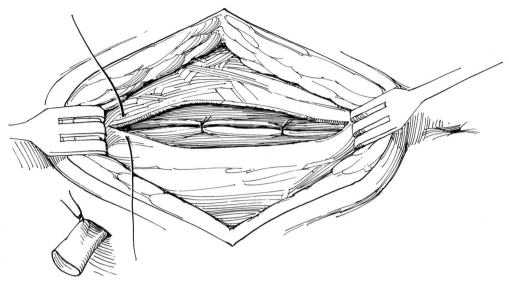

URACHAL CYST

Perform an ultrasound study; if it is not diagnostic, perform a CT scan.

For a urachal cyst, use the same technique as for the patent urachus. The exception is the large infected urachal cyst, which should be initially drained percutaneously and excision delayed until antibiotic therapy reduces the inflammation. Carefully dissect the bulging cyst from the surrounding tissues and from the peritoneum behind it. Bowel may be adherent. Divide its attenuated attachment to the bladder and ligate it. Dissect the narrow upper end from the umbilicus. Drain the area with a Penrose drain.

URACHAL SINUS

Perform a sinogram. Ultrasonography may be helpful.

6 *Incision:* Make a circumferential cut around the stoma of the sinus to preserve as much of the umbilicus as possible. It may be necessary to remove the entire umbilicus as shown. Place Allis clamps on the stoma, and sharply dissect the tract to its termination. Ligate the obliterated hypogastric arteries as they are encountered. If the sinus ends within the bladder wall, resect a cuff. Drain the area because a sinus tract is usually infected.

URACHAL CARCINOMA

Excise the umbilicus with the underlying peritoneum and the posterior rectus fascia as far as the medial umbilical ligaments. Include the dome of the bladder with the specimen to obtain a margin of 2 cm from the tumor. Check the cut margin of the bladder wall by frozen section. Proceed with bilateral pelvic lymphadenectomy.

Follow the patient with regular cystoscopic examinations and cytology, as well as with CT scanning.

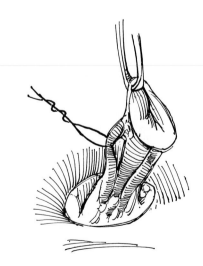

POSTOPERATIVE PROBLEMS

Persistent *urinary drainage* may require replacement of a catheter to drain the bladder. *Wound infection* around the umbilicus is usually superficial.

Sacral Laminectomy and Dorsal Rhizotomy for Placement of Pacemaker

Perform a complete urodynamic work-up, including a trial of percutaneous sacral root stimulation. Have the patient prepared with antibacterial showers, perioperative antibiotics, and proper skin preparation.

Instruments: Provide a Basic set, a laminectomy pan, a dural pan, Rhoton neurosurgical instruments, vasovasostomy instruments, a surgical or a binocular loupe microscope, a round periosteal elevator, large square-edged rongeurs, ball and perforating drills, a Cloward punch rongeur, dull nerve hooks, a nerve stimulator, bipolar electrocoagulator, rake retractors (sharp, small), calipers, neuropaddies and thrombin, absorbable sponge, bone wax, a bulb syringe, a urethral catheter, a tuberculin syringe with 27-gauge needle, and a 0.5-inch Penrose drain.

Have the patient bathe with antibiotic soap for 3 days preoperatively.

1 *Position:* Place the patient prone with the abdomen on a pillow and the table flexed 45 to 90 degrees. To straighten the lumbodorsal curve, use an orthopedic table (Chick or Wilson-Krane). Insert laminectomy rolls at all pressure points; wrap the legs and pad the knees. Be prepared to level the table for insertion of the neurotransmitter. Place urodynamic catheters intraurethrally to record bladder and mid and proximal urethral pressures to monitor striated and smooth sphincteric mechanisms. Connect the catheters, test by recording, and fix them firmly in place. Prepare the lower back, upper thigh, and perineum with povidone-iodine scrub and coating. Cover the area with a transparent adhesive drape so that the region of the external sphincter remains visible. Avoid administration of atropine or neuromuscular blockade.

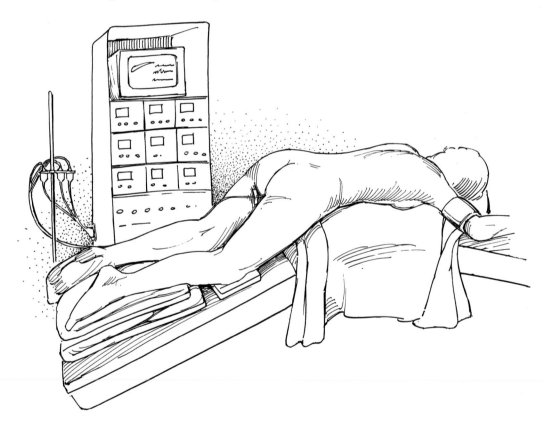

SACRAL LAMINECTOMY

2 **A,** Palpate the spinous process and the posterior superior iliac spine. The foramen of S2 lies 1 cm medially and 1 cm caudally from this prominence. The S3 foramen lies 1 to 1.5 cm lateral to the midline of the sciatic notch.

B, The roots lie directly beneath the area of sacrum to be resected.

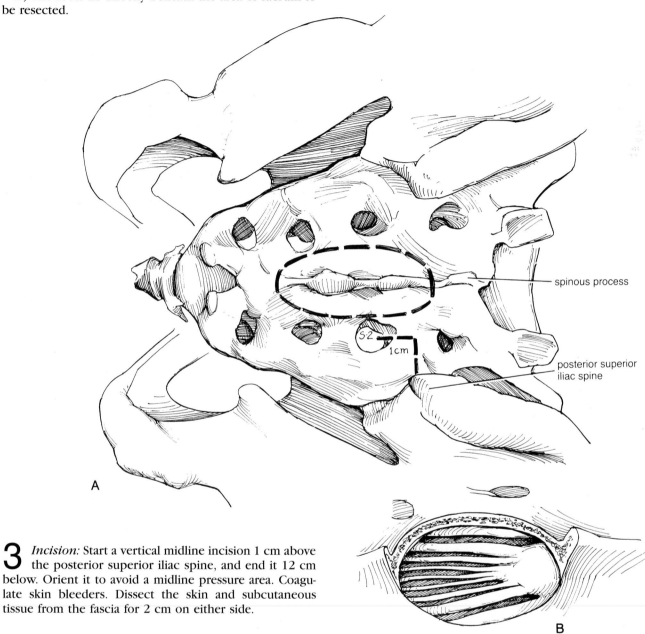

spinous process

posterior superior iliac spine

A

B

3 *Incision:* Start a vertical midline incision 1 cm above the posterior superior iliac spine, and end it 12 cm below. Orient it to avoid a midline pressure area. Coagulate skin bleeders. Dissect the skin and subcutaneous tissue from the fascia for 2 cm on either side.

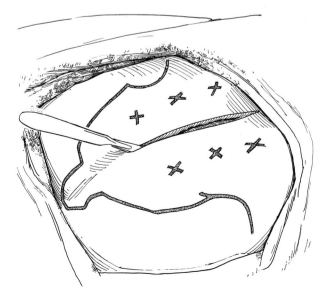

4 Use the cutting current (or a Shaw knife with a heated blade to reduce bleeding) to cut directly over the palpable spinous processes through the fascia and gluteal tendon. Continue down each side of the processes, staying very close to the bone. Push the muscle and periosteum from the surface of the sacrum, using a gauze dissector to minimize bleeding.

5 With the help of a round periosteal elevator, try to remove the periosteum along with the muscle. When one side is done, pack the space with a moist gauze pack. Divide the interspinous ligaments at either end of the section to be resected.

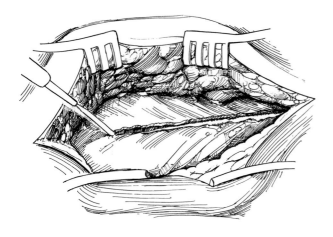

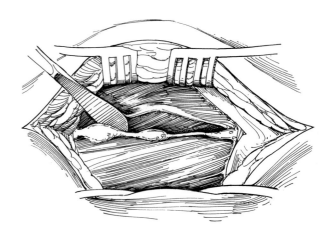

6 Remove the exposed spinous process with heavy rongeurs.

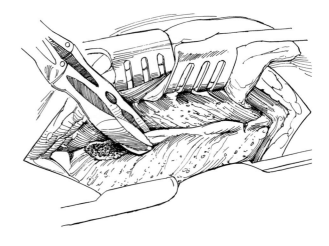

7 **A** and **B,** Open the lamina in the midline or in the angle between the stump of the resected spinous process and the adjacent vertebral arch with a perforating drill to barely expose the yellow ligamentum flavum. Control the drill very deliberately. As the deep bone table is reached, the drill catches on the edges and becomes harder to rotate. Stop at this point.

C, With a ball drill, enlarge this opening enough to admit the punch rongeur. As drilling proceeds, inspect the bone periodically to determine when the full thickness of bone has been penetrated. Seeing and palpating intraspinal fat helps.

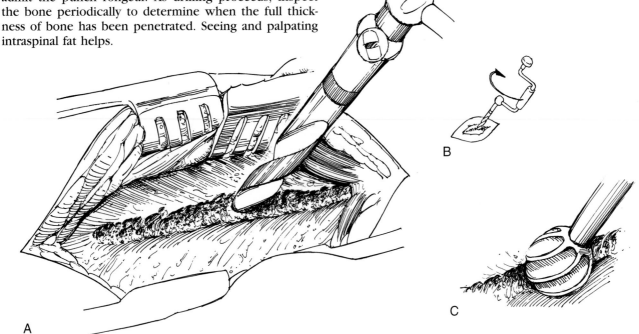

A

B

C

8 Remove a rectangle of the vertebral arches by taking small bites with the punch rongeur after depressing the tissue overlying the nerves with a nerve dissector. Be sure to hold the tip of the rongeur up against the inner table. Continue to the distal end of the dura (usually at the level of the S1 vertebral body), the level of the filum terminale. Remove this dorsal table all the way to the lateral margins of the canal. Rub bone wax into the cut lamina to control bleeding, and lay down neuropaddies soaked in bovine thrombin or 4 × 4-inch gauze squares along the soft-tissue edges of the wound. Take care not to injure the delicate veins among the fatty tissue that fills the spinal canal. Bleeding, especially during exposure of the roots, can be profuse and should be controlled using bipolar coagulating forceps on identifiable bleeders in addition to compression from neuropaddies soaked in epinephrine.

Identification of the Sacral Roots

9 Remove fat very carefully from around the nerves with suction and forceps. If one area starts to bleed, place neuropaddies and work elsewhere. Identify the S2 and S3 roots on both sides with the nerve stimulator. S2 is usually at the upper limits of the laminectomy and is usually larger. On stimulation, S2 causes inward rotation of the leg with little perineal activity but strong urethral sphincteric response. S3 produces both detrusor and sphincter contraction, as well as plantar flexion of the great toe or entire foot and contraction of the anal sphincter. S4 contracts the levator ani. Establish which gives the best detrusor and sphincteric responses. Place colored rubber barriers to identify and shield each nerve.

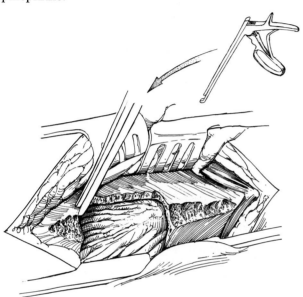
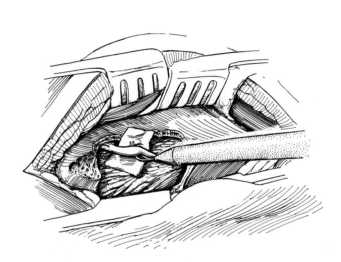

10 **A** and **B,** Optional: Inject saline through a 27-gauge needle into the epineural space, keeping the needle parallel to the nerves.

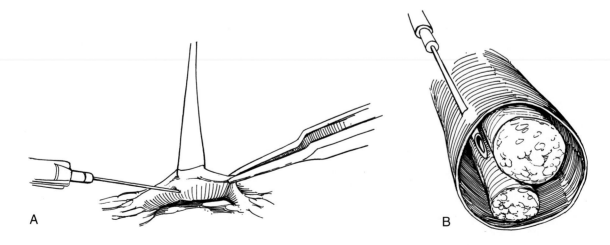

A

B

11 **A,** Open the epineural space with microscissors, and identify the plane between the dorsal and ventral roots. Bleeding can be profuse from the small veins accompanying the nerves. Control it with bipolar coagulating forceps for identifiable bleeders and neuropaddies to compress the others.

B, Place the stimulator on the dorsal and the ventral root under vision to identify each. Observe the simultaneous recordings of detrusor and sphincter activity as well as the reaction of the anal sphincter. Start stimulating S2 on one side and then the other. Do the same for S3. If S4 has shown significant response, test it also. If one particular root responds poorly, it need not be considered further. Compare these results with the preoperative ones; they are usually quite similar.

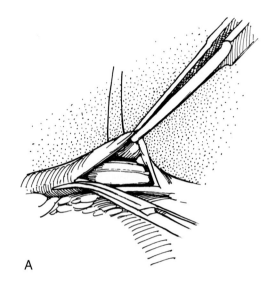

A

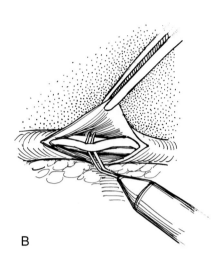

B

DORSAL RHIZOTOMY

12 **A,** Separate the dorsal from the ventral components of the S2 and S3 nerves under magnification. Rotate the selected sacral root using traction with forceps on the epineurium over the ganglion, and place the epineurium under tension to visualize the plane of separation between the ventral root and the ganglion. Incise the perineurium, and develop a plane between the ventral root and at least the proximal half of the ganglion using microscissors. This separation is easy if the right plane is entered.

B, Divide the dorsal root, and lift up the ends to aid completion of the separation. Clip both ends. Remove a segment to expose the ventral root for application of the electrode. Both dorsal roots of S2 and S3 may be divided, or one of each may be left intact to preserve potency. Leave the electrode terminals there for later connection. Alternatively, proceed with placement of the wires. Protect the back wound, rotate the patient onto the side opposite that of the leads, prepare the abdomen, make an extension of the subcutaneous tunnel to McBurney's point, and pull the wires through. Develop a pocket for the receiver, connect it to the wires, seal the joints with silicone glue, and close the skin over it.

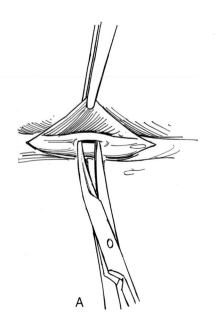

A

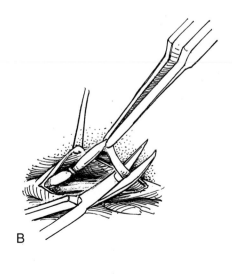

B

Wound Closure

Approximate the muscles and fascia over the defect with 2-0 interrupted SAS in two layers. Bring the subcutaneous tissue together, and close the skin with interrupted sutures.

For *sphincteric stimulation*, the pudendal nerve may be divided unilaterally, its urethral or pudendal branches selectively divided, and an electrode placed in the wide end of the chest tube and drawn through the tunnel. Retest each electrode.

If the receiver was not placed at the time of laminectomy, wait 5 days to insert it and to activate the electrodes.

POSTOPERATIVE PROBLEMS

Hematoma and *wound infection* can occur. If a cerebrospinal fluid leak is present, *meningitis* may result. The ventral root may be inadvertently damaged. Twisting of the electrode from scarring or tension on the cable may cause traction on the nerve.

Commentary by Richard A. Schmidt

The neurologic approach to treatment of voiding dysfunction remains very much an unexplored frontier, especially for urologists. However, new advances in its treatment will most certainly evolve from the rapidly expanding research into function of the nervous system. Urologists need to be prepared to apply these principles that new research will provide, to assess the integrity of the innervation to the bladder and sphincter, and to become trained in surgical access to the sacral nerve roots. As a beginning, a variety of techniques used in previous decades need re-evaluation in this era of urodynamic monitoring—percutaneous blocks; chemical, heat, and high-frequency lesions of peripheral nerves; selective surgical rhizotomy for spasticity and pain; and neurostimulation for bladder evacuation and continence. Of all these approaches, the last continues to offer the greatest promise.

There are two basic types of stimulation units. The Brindley device is self contained for activating multiple lead contact sites. It is passive and requires that a coil be placed over the stimulation unit. The Itrel Two design (Medtronic) allows activation of only one electrode at a time. It is self powered and can be activated with a magnet. The Brindley unit has more power and programming flexibility but requires much more sophistication in hand manipulation. Both devices produce electromicturition in suitably screened patients.

SECTION
15
Noncontinent Urinary Diversion

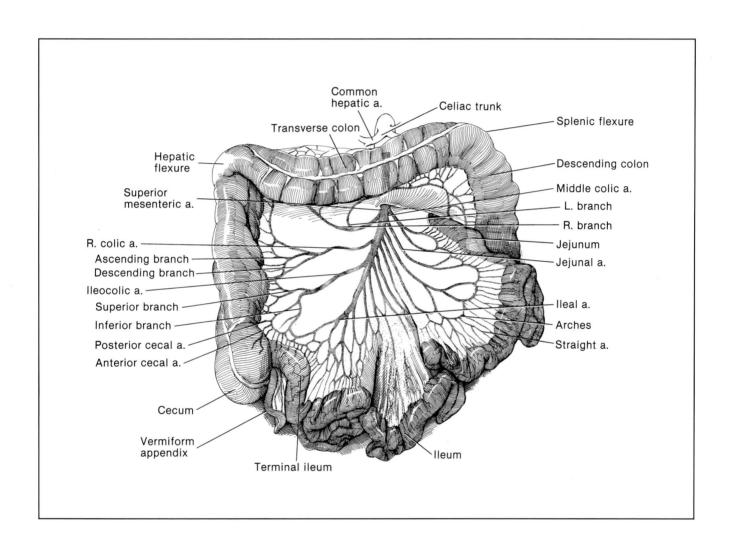

Principles of Noncontinent Diversion

Because most diversions are potentially reversible, it is no longer necessary to distinguish between temporary and permanent diversion.

Diversion from the Bladder

A *cystostomy* provides direct drainage for the bladder, especially after open operations on the bladder, but for the long term the catheter may be irritating, and continuous drainage and infection may result in a small bladder. For temporary drainage in the male, a *perineal urethrostomy* diverts the urine effectively from the urethra, but usually, if a urethral catheter is inadvisable, a cystostomy is preferable in children. For more permanent diversion, a *vesicostomy* provides effective drainage at the price of poor stomal position, a tendency for stomal stenosis, and infection and stone formation.

Diversion for the Upper Tract

Percutaneous nephrostomy drainage and *indwelling ureteral stents* can allow relief of obstruction without formal surgical intervention, but in infants and children the need for good drainage is imperative and the quality of the endodrainage is often inadequate. A *nephrostomy* gives the most direct drainage but is associated with so much infection and concomitant renal damage that it is reserved for more extreme circumstances and is seldom considered, even for short-term diversion. A percutaneous nephrostomy is usually better. Because the ureter and pelvis are dilated, a cutaneous ureterostomy or cutaneous pyelostomy is feasible. *Cutaneous (end) ureterostomy* is a simple form of urinary diversion but is more often permanent unless done in the distal ureter. A prerequisite is a ureter dilated to at least 1 cm in diameter, thick walled and well vascularized. Be certain that a cutaneous ureterostomy is made low enough in the ureter that it does not interfere with later reconstruction. This procedure can be appropriate for temporary diversion in infants but is seldom applicable in adolescents with normal ureters because of the high incidence of stricture from ischemia of the cutaneous portion of the nondilated ureter.

Pediatric loop nephrostomy has the advantages of good drainage and ease of closure when no longer needed. If it is sited high in the flank, drainage is optimal but appliances are difficult to maintain. If lower, drainage may be satisfactory for less compromised renal units and maintenance of appliances is simplified, but later reconstitution may be more difficult. An end cutaneous ureterostomy may be preferable.

During a difficult operation on the lower ureter, a *ureterostomy in situ* may be used as a last resort. Intubate the ureter, and bring the tube retroperitoneally to the skin. After a tract has formed, the tube may be changed, but it must be done quickly to prevent loss of the tract.

Urinary conduits formed from intestine have the advantage of relative freedom from stenosis, but late complications, especially stricture at the site of ureteral anastomosis, as well as stomal problems, have reduced their use. They have largely been replaced by forms of continent diversion, avoiding the need to wear an appliance. Whether the ileum makes a better conduit than the sigmoid or the transverse colon has not been determined. Colon conduits do have the advantage of allowing formation of a nonrefluxing ureteral anastomosis.

Ureteroileostomy is a standard procedure with good short-term results, although reflux can occur with stasis. The stoma may be a problem, and a device must be worn. A *high ileal conduit* may be useful in children. The *colon conduit,* whether the usual sigmoid conduit or the transverse colon conduit, is associated with few stomal problems, and the ureteral anastomosis can be made antirefluxive. It may serve well for the long run. The *sigmoid conduit* has certain advantages: It provides a greater length for high positioning of the stoma; it need not be isoperistaltic; it allows formation of a nonrefluxing ureteral anastomosis; and it results less frequently in stomal stenoses.

Although a sigmoid or transverse colon conduit can be constructed so that reflux with renal deterioration is less than with other systems, it is less acceptable for social rather than medical reasons than those procedures that produce continence. For temporary diversion before major vesical augmentation, the sigmoid conduit is useful. Only after extensive pelvic irradiation, rarely seen in children, is the transverse colon conduit preferred. It does have the additional advantage of requiring shorter lengths of ureter obtained away from the radiated field.

Follow-up

No matter what form diversion takes, long-term surveillance is essential to identify dysfunction before the kidneys are irreversibly damaged. Intravenous urograms and sonograms, urine cultures, retrograde loopograms, and repeated determinations of serum electrolytes are indicated at regular intervals.

COMPLICATIONS OF NONCONTINENT DIVERSION

Bacteriuria is common, but *symptomatic infection* requiring treatment is less frequent. A normally functioning system keeps itself free of infection. The corollary is that recurrent symptomatic infection suggests malfunction of the conducting structures. *Pyocystis* is an extreme form of infection, restricted to the totally diverted bladder and occurring most commonly in girls. Antibiotics and lavage of the bladder with saline solution with or without an antiseptic usually suffices, especially because the condition is usually self limiting. Overdilation of the urethra with a Kollmann dilator can be effective, but opening the bladder into the vagina may be necessary in a few stubborn cases. *Stomal problems* begin with improperly fitting appliances. This is often associated with encrustation and stomal stenosis, the latter less often seen if a tongue of skin is incorporated in the stoma. *Parastomal hernia* from too large a fascial defect usually requires taking the stoma down, repairing the defect, and bringing the bowel out at a new site, preferably on the opposite side. *Residual urine* in the conduit may be secondary to a narrow stoma, but usually it appears later as a result of reduced peristaltic activity in the loop. Replacement of the segment may be required.

For further discussion, see pages 661 to 662.

Cystostomy

Direct drainage of the bladder may be accomplished suprapubically by an open procedure, by an instrumental technique using a Lowsley tractor placed transvesically, or by a punch technique with a trocar. An alternative in women is a vaginal approach. A perineal urethrostomy may be selected occasionally (see pages 630 to 631).

SUPRAPUBIC CYSTOSTOMY

Antegrade Approach

1 *Position*: Supine. Fill the bladder with sterile water until it is just visible or palpable suprapubically.

Incision: Depending on the site of previous suprapubic incisions, make a short vertical or a more concealable transverse incision through the skin and subcutaneous layers well above the symphysis pubis so that the tube is accessible to the patient. Provide a larger incision if the area has been approached previously because exposure of the bladder wall is more difficult.

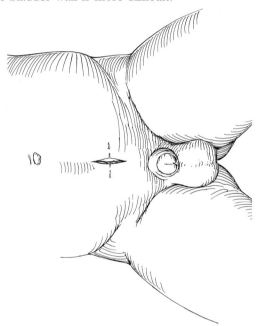

2 Expose the rectus fascia in the midline by pushing back the covering subcutaneous tissue. Incise the fascia transversely.

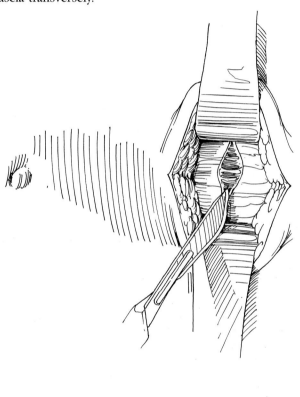

3 **A,** Enter between the recti and separate them bluntly. Hold the muscles back with two U.S. Army retractors to expose the prevesical fat.

B, Starting directly behind the symphysis, bluntly push the peritoneal fold upward. This may not be easy if the area has been approached before. Expose minimal bladder surface. The vascular pattern and tissue characteristics of the bladder are usually unmistakable. If in doubt, insert a fine needle and aspirate, or pass a curved sound through the urethra and palpate the tip.

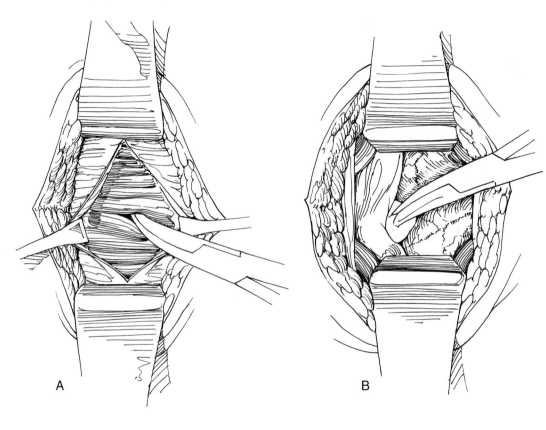

A

B

4 Place two 3-0 chromic catgut (CCG) stay sutures into the bladder wall well above the symphysis. Alternatively, grasp the wall with two Allis clamps. Fulgurate obvious crossing vessels. With suction at hand, incise the bladder vertically between the sutures with the cutting current, and enter the bladder.

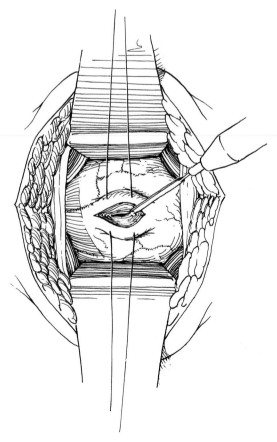

5 Position two Allis clamps to grasp the full thickness of the wall. While the urine is still running out, insert a silicone Malecot catheter, stretched on a Mayo clamp to reduce the diameter of the wings. Alternatively, insert a balloon catheter and inflate it. Withdraw the catheter slightly to be sure the catheter tip does not touch the trigone.

6 Close the bladder tightly around the catheter with full-thickness 3-0 CCG sutures. If the bladder wall is thin, use mattress sutures. Fasten the catheter to the bladder wall by looping and tying the ends of one of the sutures around it. For permanency, place a purse-string suture around the exit site of the catheter from the bladder. Use this suture to anchor the site to the posterior surface of the rectus fascia and thus stabilize the exit route.

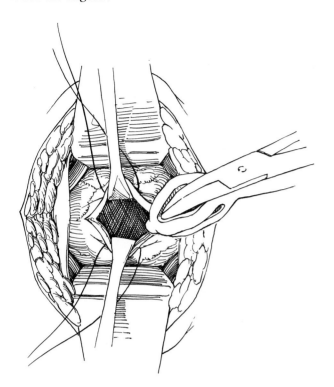

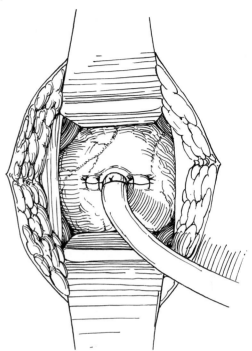

7 Make a stab wound in the skin near the incision well above the symphysis, and force a curved clamp through it to emerge beneath the rectus muscle. Trim the end of the tube obliquely to form a point. Grasp the pointed end, and pull the catheter out through the body wall.

8 Close the fascia around a Penrose drain with 3-0 CCG sutures. Close the skin. Fasten the catheter to the skin with a heavy silk suture, and tape it to the abdomen with waterproof tape over tincture of benzoin. Connect the catheter to sterile drainage at the table. For a more permanent cystostomy, having anchored the bladder to the rectus fascia with the long ends of a purse-string suture (described in Step 6), lead the catheter directly through the wound.

Alternative method to insert a cystostomy tube into an empty exposed bladder without formally opening it: Pick up the double thickness of the bladder between thumb and forefinger and stretch the wall. Insert a curved clamp through both layers. Grasp the tip of a balloon catheter, draw it through the first layer of the wall, and inflate the balloon inside the bladder. Suture both sites (Shaw, 1993).

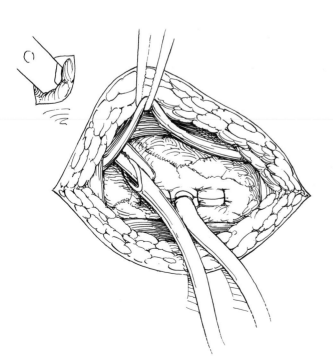

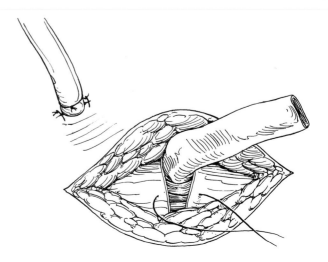

Vesical Lithotomy

Stones that cannot be removed by shock wave or with instruments are best removed by an open operation. This is especially true for stones in a male patient with a neurogenic bladder, for whom urethral instrumentation is not advisable.

Proceed as for suprapubic cystostomy, but insert a Mayo clamp into the opening, aspirate the contents, and insert two fingers to make the opening somewhat larger. Remove the stones under vision. Irrigate the bladder to remove stone fragments that could occlude the suprapubic catheter. Insert a Malecot catheter that exits through a stab wound. Because infection may cause problems, drain the prevesical space with a Penrose drain that exits from a separate stab wound.

Retrograde Approach

This is a rapid method of placing a balloon catheter in females before a gynecourologic procedure.

9 Insert a curved Lowsley prostatic tractor (or curved sound with a hole near the tip) through the urethra until it can be palpated directly over the symphysis. Keep the retractor against the anterior wall of the urethra and as close to the symphysis as possible; avoid leverage against the urethra. Cut down on the tip of the tractor to let it emerge suprapubically. Grasp the tip of a Malecot or balloon catheter in the blades of the tractor, or suture the tip to the blades. Draw the tractor and catheter out of the urethra, and regrasp the catheter tip with a Mayo clamp. Position the catheter in the bladder by countertraction on the clamp on the tip. Test the position by irrigation, and inflate the balloon. Draw the catheter to bring the balloon against the abdominal wall for tamponade, and tie a wet 4 × 4-inch gauze pad around it to hold it in position until the end of the operation. After completing the operation, suture the catheter to the skin with heavy silk and tape it to the body wall.

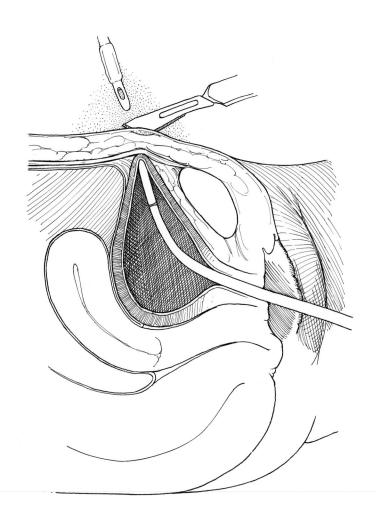

TROCAR CYSTOSTOMY

This procedure is not advisable in patients with previous suprapubic surgery because of the risk of injury to the bowel.

Instrument: A disposable trocar-cystostomy kit (Cystocath or Malecot kit). Partially fill the bladder through a urethral catheter. At a site 1 to 2 cm above the upper border of the symphysis, inject 1 percent lidocaine into the skin through a 24-gauge needle, followed by infiltration of the subcutaneous tissue and rectus sheath with a larger and longer needle, such as an 18- or 20-gauge spinal needle, directed at an angle caudally. Aspirate as the needle is advanced. When urine is obtained, cross-clamp the needle at the surface, withdraw it, and use the distance from clamp to tip to determine the depth needed for penetration of the trocar.

Make a stab incision in the skin, angling the trocar caudally. Insert it into the bladder a few centimeters beyond the measured length. Withdraw the trocar, leaving the catheter in place. If the catheter has a balloon, inflate it and draw it against the anterior bladder wall. In any case, suture the catheter to the skin with a heavy nonabsorbable suture (NAS).

VAGINAL CYSTOSTOMY

A vaginal approach may occasionally be better than a suprapubic one after repair of urethrovaginal and retrotrigonal fistulas because contact of the catheter with the urethra and bladder neck is avoided. Do not leave the catheter in for more than 1 week because epithelialization of the tract can occur, leading to a permanent fistula.

10 **A,** Place the patient in the lithotomy position and prepare the perineum. Insert a weighted speculum in the vagina.

B, Draw the cervix down with tenaculum forceps. Insert a long curved Kelly or Mixter clamp through the urethra to the base of the bladder, concave side down. Open the clamp slightly in the midline, and press it posteriorly against the anterior fornix close to the cervix until it can be felt in the vaginal vault. Make an incision in the midline between the blades through vaginal and bladder walls to allow the tip of the clamp to emerge into the vagina.

11 Grasp the tip of a 24 F 5-ml silicone balloon catheter with the clamp, draw it into the bladder, and release it. Close the vaginal incision with one or two 3-0 CCG sutures that pass through the full thickness of vaginal wall above and below the catheter. Inflate the balloon.

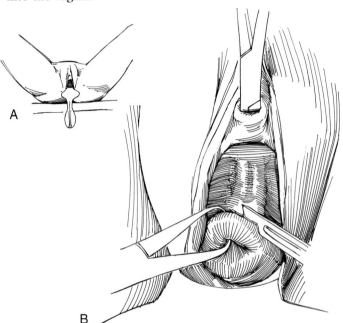

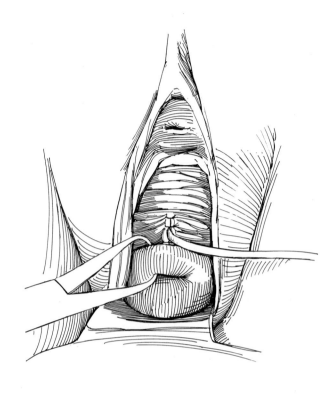

POSTOPERATIVE PROBLEMS

Obstruction requires irrigation. If that fails, obtain a cystogram to see if the end of the catheter is displaced. *Urgency* and pain can be distressing, caused by contact of the catheter on the trigone. Retract the tube and refasten it to the skin. *Inadvertent removal* of the tube can occur if it is not sutured to the skin and retaped regularly with fresh tape over tincture of benzoin. *Urinary infection* is delayed but not necessarily prevented by maintaining closed drainage and giving suppressive antibiotics. *Calculi* may form from the scaly phosphates released upon deflation of a balloon catheter after it has been in place too long. Avoid this by changing the catheter at intervals determined by the degree of encrustation found on the old catheter. *Peritonitis* is a rare complication, secondary to puncture of the bowel during introduction of the tube.

Persistent drainage after removal of the tube usually responds to urethral catheter drainage. If the tract has epithelialized, it does not close until the surface has been denuded by applying a silver nitrate stick, by curetting, or by screwing a new wood screw through the opening and forcibly withdrawing it.

Commentary by Roger R. Dmochowski

Suprapubic cystostomy is useful in a variety of urologic procedures. Open cystostomy, as described in this chapter, is very useful in patients with prior abdominal surgery with the potential of bowel adhering to pelvic structures and the potential entry into bowel from attempted percutaneous techniques.

In patients who have not undergone prior procedures, the prepubic space is often very easily developed bluntly to expose the anterior surface of the bladder. In patients who have undergone prior procedures, it is often helpful to keep the bladder distended to facilitate dissection in the correct plane and avoid entry into either the superficial dorsal vein complex or the peritoneum. Apical sutures at either end of the suprapubic cystostomy itself are useful to prevent further tearing of the bladder wall during manipulation such as with vesicolithotomy. If the incision is made in the anterior wall of the bladder in the sagittal plane, it is very important to have an apical suture present at the distal end of the incision to prevent laceration into the bladder neck and sphincteric mechanism. It is most useful to bring the tube itself out through a separate stab incision and to provide drainage with a Penrose drain, also through a separate stab incision, especially in the presence of infection.

Percutaneous placement of a suprapubic tube has been greatly improved by the special equipment developed for this purpose. Larger trocar catheters are now available for direct percutaneous installation. Utilizing equipment developed for fascial dilation in percutaneous renal procedures, it is now possible not only to establish bladder access but also to dilate the tract with fascial dilators to a large enough size to accommodate larger Foley catheters for longer-term drainage. These fascial dilators may be used either with or without fluoroscopy; however, again great care must be taken in patients who have had prior pelvic surgery and therefore are at greater risk of bowel adherence to pelvic structures.

It is often helpful to use cystoscopic visualization of catheter placement to ensure placement of the catheter in the appropriate area of the high anterior bladder wall or dome for adequate drainage purposes. This also helps reduce morbidity due to trigonal irritation from the catheter when it is not placed in a snug position against the anterior bladder wall.

Perineal Urethrostomy

GROOVED SOUND TECHNIQUE

Provide a biopsy set; curved grooved (Gouley) sounds, sizes 12 to 14 F for boys and 18 to 24 F for adults; three small Allis clamps; 3-0 plain catgut (PCG) sutures; and a balloon catheter already mounted on a lubricated stilet.

1 Insert a grooved sound of suitable size until its tip rests in the prostatic urethra. Have your assistant lever *(upper arrows)* the curved portion caudad toward the perineum *(lower arrow)*.

2 Grasp the sound and urethra through the perineum with the left thumb and index finger. Do not let go!

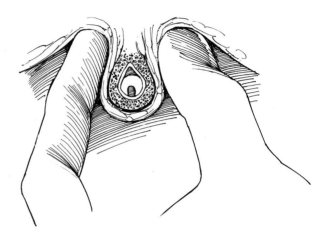

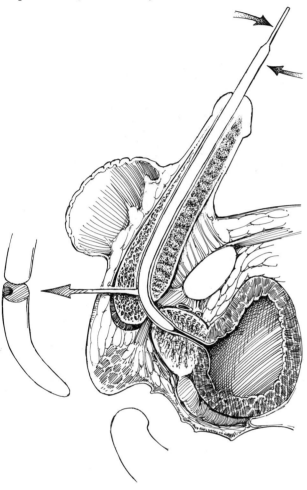

3 Incise the perineum, inserting the point of a #15 blade knife into the groove over the curve of the sound. Lengthen the stab wound anteriorly; then invert the knife and extend it posteriorly. Compress the urethra between the thumb and index finger to evert the urethra.

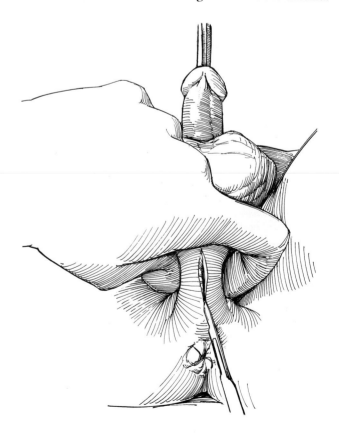

4 **A,** Insert one blade of an Allis clamp into the groove of the sound to catch the uroepithelial edge. With the other blade catch the spongy tissue as you close the clamp.

B, Secure the opposite edge in the same way with a second clamp. Substitute a third clamp if the epithelial edge is not caught cleanly by the clamp the first time on either side.

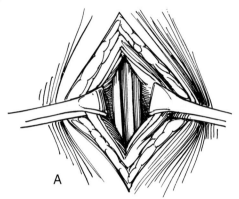

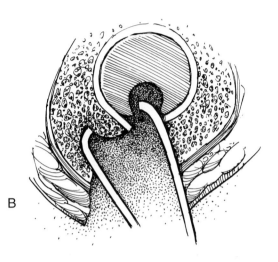

5 Release the grip on the sound and urethra. Have your assistant slowly withdraw the sound. As its tip clears the incision, insert the tip of the catheter inverted on its stilet into the urethra. Once it has entered the urethra, rotate it 180 degrees and pass it into the bladder. Replace the Allis clamps with 3-0 CCG traction sutures.

6 If the urethrostomy is to be *permanent* as shown, place one or two PCG sutures to close the urethral wall and corpus spongiosum. Insert these *proximal* to the exit site of the catheter so that the urethral lumen cannot be compromised. Close the skin similarly. If the urethrostomy was *temporary*, tie the 3-0 CCG traction sutures together. In adults, be sure to place a small rubber drain (a piece of rubber glove is suitable) into the area of the urethra. Close the skin around it with 3-0 PCG sutures. Remove the drain in 24 hours.

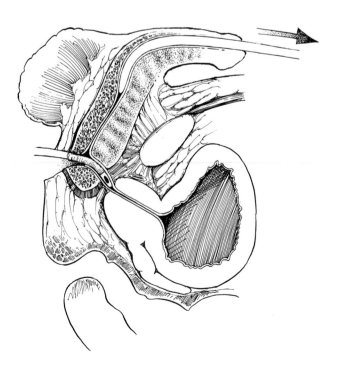

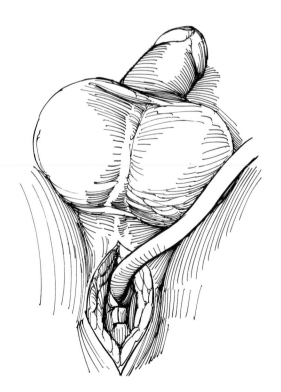

Commentary by Philip B. Clark

Perineal urethrostomy is a useful procedure to have up one's sleeve, and every urologist should know how to perform it. I have used it in preference to Otis urethrotomy whenever the anterior urethra looked narrower than normal to avoid producing that urologic humiliation, a postoperative stricture, with my resectoscope. Almost invariably, therefore, I would use it to insert a resectoscope, and I would insert a catheter only after the resection of prostate or bladder tumor is complete. An added bonus of perineal urethrostomy is the wonderful mobility of any instrument introduced via this route; it becomes as mobile as it would be in a woman. Perineal urethrostomy, therefore, is preferable to Otis urethrotomy for patients with tight suspensory ligaments, penile prostheses, or anterior bladder tumors that are difficult to reach. It is a simple and useful temporary procedure and remarkably free from complications.

For permanent urethrostomy, I prefer to mobilize the bulbar urethra and divide it sufficiently far forward to be able to bring out a stump that projects 2 cm from the skin surface; this is the only foolproof method I know of avoiding a stricture after this operation.

Differences in technique: I use an ordinary metal sound. Although Ambroise Paré used grooved sounds for perineal lithotomy in 1585, we do not seem to have them in England yet! I grasp the sound through the perineum with my fingers, and then encircle it and the urethra with a pair of Littlewood forceps (these resemble towel clips). This frees my left hand to allow me to continue operating normally. I use monofilament stay sutures to pick up the urethra and skin, instead of small Allis clamps, because these are at less risk of becoming dislodged during any subsequent transurethral resection and they are needed to hold the edges of the urethra apart while the catheter is inserted. Do not remove the Littlewood forceps until the stay sutures have been inserted. These stay sutures are taken out at the end of the procedure; I do not insert any other sutures or any drain; the wound is left entirely open.

Postoperatively, remove the catheter at the normal time. The patient at first passes urine through both the urethrostomy and the urethra, but the urethrostomy closes spontaneously within a few days. A dressing should be kept on the perineum and the patient should have a bath twice a day, but this is the only special treatment needed.

Difficulties: In an obese person you may not be able to find the cut edges of the urethra immediately and may need to insert stay stitches on each side to hold the tissues apart until the urethral mucosa itself can be identified.

Complications: Postoperative bleeding: This is very rare; the bleeding point may need to be oversewn. *Infection:* This too is very rare provided that no attempt is made to close the wound. *Urinary leakage:* Because no attempt is made to close the wound, all these incisions leak. The narrower the anterior urethra, the longer they leak. Yet they all heal eventually. Most patients are dry within 3 or 4 days. The longest any patient has leaked is about 10 days. *Urethral stricture:* Perineal urethrostomy prevents strictures; it does not cause them! *Wound implant:* The only serious complication during 25 years' experience with this procedure has been a wound implant in a patient in whom I used this route to reach an anterior bladder tumor. He was treated by local excision of the implant followed by radiation therapy; he died later of unrelated causes.

Vesicostomy

ADULT VESICOSTOMY
(Lapides)

Vesicostomy may be suitable for semipermanent urinary diversion in an adult with a spastic neurogenic bladder who, even with vesical augmentation, cannot be catheterized urethrally either by themselves or by an attendant.

Insert a 22 F 5-ml silicone balloon catheter and fill the bladder with 300 ml of water.

1 *Position:* Supine.
First incision: Make a typical transverse lower abdominal incision (see page 490), exposing the anterior surface of the bladder. Mobilize the peritoneum well upward.

Second incision: Select a site high enough on the abdomen and away from scars or depression that would interfere with adherence of a collecting device. Grasp the edge of the rectus fascia, and pull it down level with the skin. Make an inverted U incision through the skin measuring 3.25 cm in width and length, with its apex 1 inch below the umbilicus.

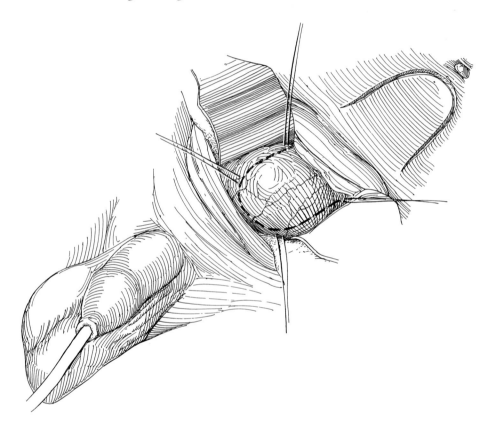

2 Cut out an adequate circle of rectus fascia behind the skin bridge. Avoid making it so large as to allow herniation. Raise a bladder flap of similar size from the anterior bladder wall, with the base upward, after marking the flap with stay sutures when the bladder contains 300 ml. Make the base wider than the apex, and preserve the blood supply.

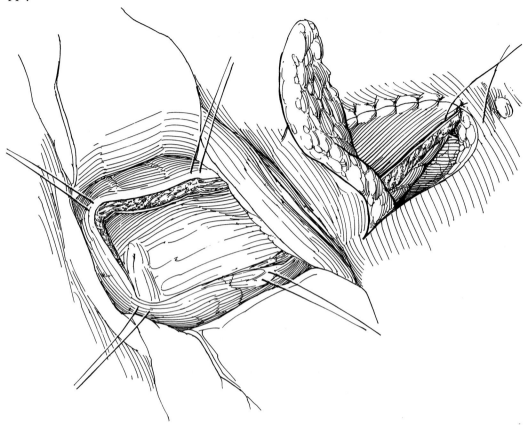

3 Pass the bladder flap beneath the skin bridge, and suture it to the upper skin edge with 2-0 NAS. Pass the skin flap down behind the bridge, and suture it to the upper edge of the bladder incision. Suture the lateral edges of the skin flap to the lateral edges of the bladder flap. Provide adequate Penrose drainage in the perivesical space. Close the abdominal incision with interrupted CCG sutures or synthetic absorbable sutures (SAS). Attach the catheter to sterile gravity drainage.

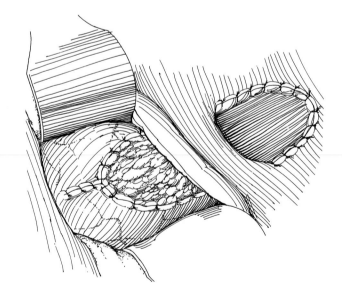

Closure of Vesicostomy

4 Insert a 5-ml balloon catheter into the stoma for traction. Mark an ellipse on the skin. Incise the skin, and divide the subcutaneous tissue with the cutting current down to the adventitia of the bladder caudad and to the dermis cephalad.

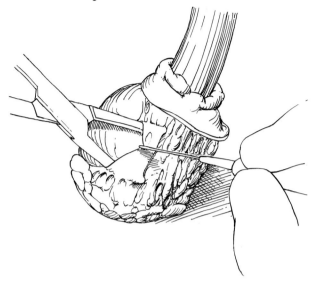

5 Insert an 18 F Malecot catheter into the bladder. Divide the protruding portion of the stoma, including the previously inverted skin flap.

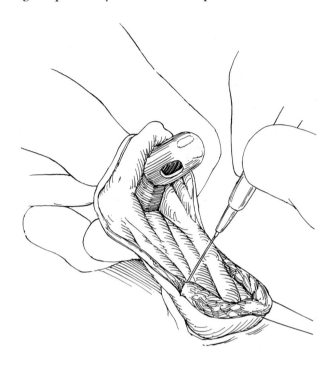

6 Close the vesical defect with an inner layer of a running 3-0 PCG subepithelial suture, reinforced with interrupted 2-0 CCG sutures to the bladder wall. Replace the bladder beneath the fascia.

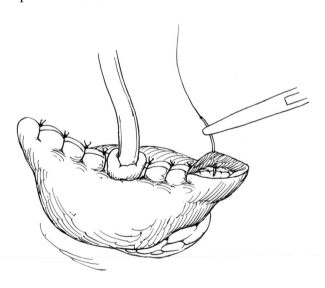

7 Bring the catheter to the surface through a stab wound and close the wound in layers, without drainage.

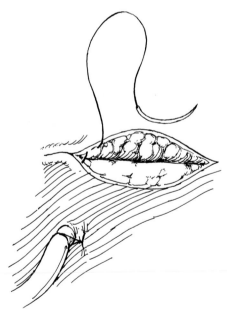

Check renal function and visualize the bladder cystoscopically at yearly intervals.

PEDIATRIC VESICOSTOMY
(Blocksom)

Vesicostomy is a useful form of temporary urinary diversion in infants who are in need of urinary tract rehabilitation and delayed reconstruction. Consider vesicostomy in ill infants and in neonates with posterior urethral valves or severe reflux and in children with a neurogenic bladder associated with meningomyelocele, who require particular attention to avoid pressure sores.

Insert a small catheter, and fill the bladder until it is quite full and palpable.

8 *Position:* Supine.
Incision: Make a very short (2-cm) transverse incision midway between the symphysis and umbilicus, over the dome of the bladder (stay at least 2 cm above the symphysis). The incision should be just large enough to admit the little finger; too large or too low an incision encourages vesical prolapse. Incise the rectus fascia transversely, and separate the muscles bluntly.

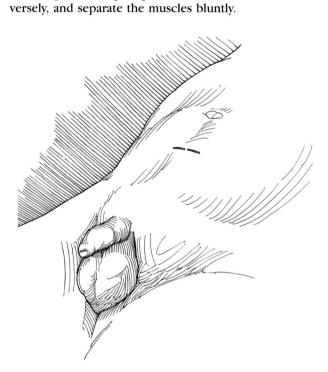

9 Remove small triangles from the fascia, and trim some of the muscle to make an opening for the stoma.

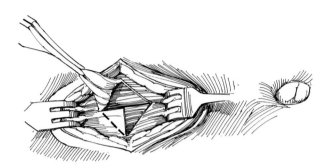

10 Expose the bladder and place several traction sutures in the anterior wall to draw it inferiorly. Peel the peritoneum from the dome, mobilizing it until the obliterated umbilical arteries and urachus are identified, marking the end of the dissection.

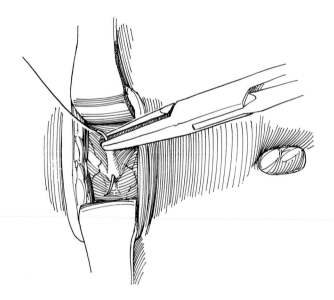

11 **A,** Pull the bladder into the wound so that the posterior wall is at skin level and the urachus is exposed.

B, Divide the urachus. Open the bladder by circumscribing the urachus.

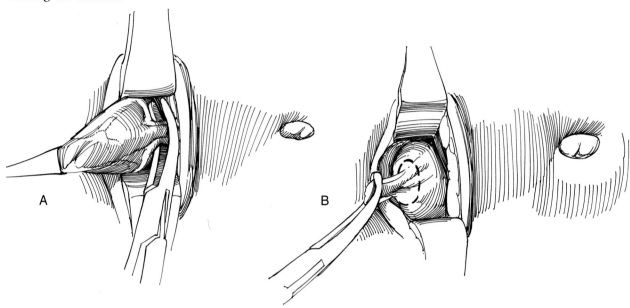

12 Suture the anterior and posterior walls of the bladder to the rectus fascia with at least six 3-0 SAS to tubularize the stoma. Close the lateral fascial defects around the outside of the bladder to achieve a 24 F lumen at the internal stoma. Too wide a stoma in a child with a bladder wall of normal thickness allows prolapse. The thick bladders associated with meningomyelocele do not tend to prolapse. Approximate the subcutaneous tissues.

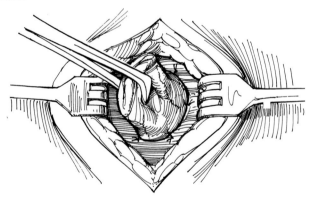

Postoperative Problems

For *stenosis of the stoma*, try regular dilation. If that program fails, incise the fibrous band on the inferior edge of the stoma and move a triangle of skin from the abdomen into the edge. *Prolapse of the bladder* occurs when the stoma originates too low on the bladder so that the upper portion, which is covered with peritoneum, is forced against the site of the stoma. Close the bladder at the original site, and make a new vesicostomy at a higher level.

13 Suture the full thickness of the bladder to the subcuticular layer with 5-0 SAS. The stoma should not admit the fingertip but should calibrate to 24 F. This ensures that the fascial defect is narrow enough to avoid prolapse of the posterior wall of the bladder through the stoma. Close the remainder of the incision. Apply petroleum jelly gauze and diapers.

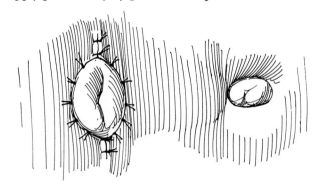

Closure of the vesicostomy: To evaluate how the bladder will function after closure for compliance, emptying, and continence, insert a Bard gastrostomy button to occlude the tract and allow a trial of intermittent catheterization. Excise the vesical epithelial tract. Place a cystostomy tube to exit through a stab wound. Close the bladder in two layers (5-0 PCG subepithelially, 4-0 SAS to the wall). Approximate the fascia and the skin around a Penrose drain. In infants with valves, it may be expedient to fulgurate the valves through the vesicostomy stoma prior to its closure, thus using the same anesthetic. In these cases, place a urethral catheter for a few days to avoid stricture of the urethra from the absence of urine flow.

BLADDER TUBULARIZATION

A large bladder, even with a previous open vesicostomy, may be converted into a continent reservoir with a catheterizable stoma. The tube, constructed from bladder wall, may be developed posteriorly beginning at the trigone (posterior flap tube) for attachment at the umbilicus or formed from the anterior wall (anterior flap continent vesicostomy) for exit in a labium. Tube length and coaptation of the tube within the bladder (flap-valve) are responsible for continence.

Posterior Flap Tube (Klauber)

14 **A,** Outline a flap on the anterior wall of the bladder 9 cm long and tapering from 3 cm at the tip to 5 cm at the base near the dome. Divide the vesical urothelium on either side down the posterior wall.

B, Construct a tube around a 16 F catheter with a continuous 4-0 SAS, leaving the last 1 cm open.

C, Suture the medial urothelial edges on the posterior wall to form a tube (flap-valve), and close the lateral edges to cover.

D, Close the anterior bladder wall, and connect the tube to the skin at the umbilicus.

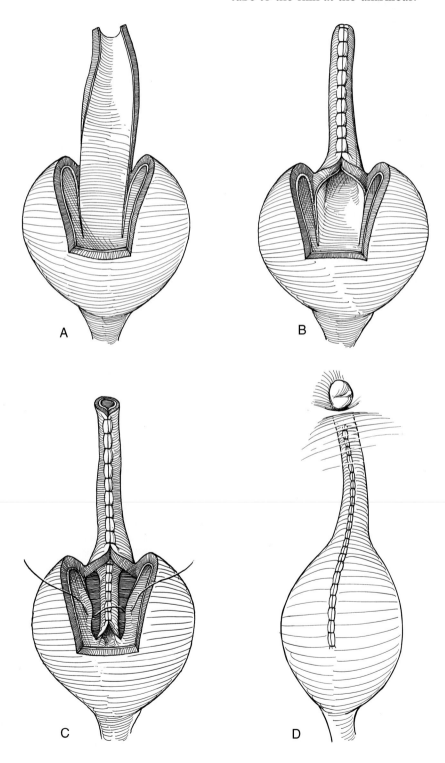

Posterior Flap Tube for Revision (Klauber)

This procedure is used for continent revision of adult (Steps 1 to 3) or pediatric (Steps 8 to 13) vesicostomies.

15 **A,** Expose and mobilize the bladder and vesicostomy tract through a subumbilical incision, and open its anterior wall. Make two parallel incisions 2.4 cm apart and 13 cm long through the exposed posterior wall from the stoma to a point above the trigone, and free the strip.

B, Insert a 24 F silicone balloon catheter, and form a tube from the strip of bladder with a continuous 3-0 CCG suture. Close the defect remaining in the posterior wall of the bladder with a similar suture.

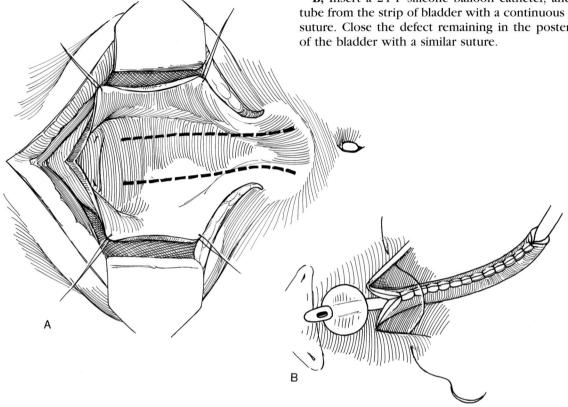

16 **A,** Approximate the anterior bladder wall. Tack the new tube to the fascia during wound closure so that it will neither prolapse nor recede, and suture the new stoma to the skin.

B, Complete the closure of the abdominal wall. Remove the catheter and start clean intermittent catheterization in 12 days.

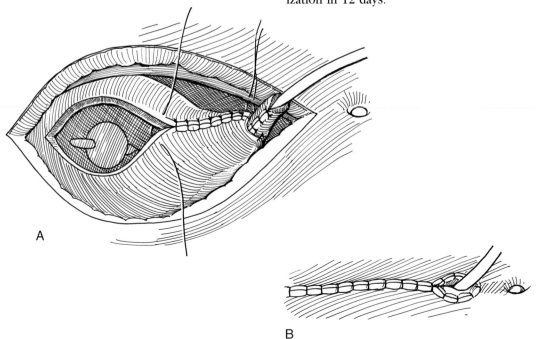

Anterior Flap Continent Vesicostomy (Naudé)

This operation is especially applicable to patients with uncorrectable vesicovaginal fistulas. Close the bladder neck (see pages 609 to 613) and also the vesicovaginal fistula, if present (see page 587), resecting the pubis if necessary to achieve closure. Interpose the omentum (see page 71).

17 **A,** Outline a flap on the anterior wall of the bladder 9 cm long and tapering from 3 cm at the tip to 5 cm at the base to one side of the bladder neck. Construct a tube around a 16 F catheter with a continuous 4-0 SAS. Leave the last 1 cm open. Bluntly fashion a tunnel subcutaneously to exit in the right labioclitoral fold. Cut a 1.5 × 1.5-cm U-shaped skin flap in the fold. Pull the tube through the tunnel.

B, The tube should lie behind the symphysis, with a narrow angle between tube and bladder. Anastomose the tubularized bladder flap to the labial skin edges, and insert the U-shaped skin flap in the ventral portion that was not closed. Insert a tube in the bladder through the new vesicostomy. Augment the bladder if small. Close the bladder in layers with perivesical drainage. Remove the drains on the 5th day, the suprapubic tube on the 7th day, and the catheter from the new tube on the 10th day after proving the suture line intact by cystography. Start intermittent catheterization with a soft coudé or silicone catheter.

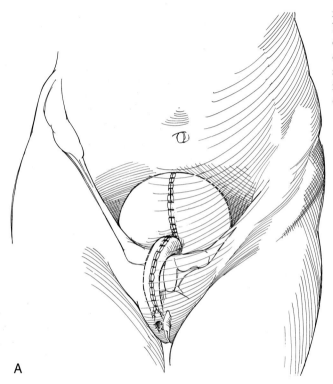

A

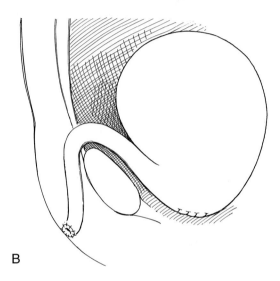

B

ILEOVESICOSTOMY
(Schwartz and McGuire)

This procedure is for patients with high spinal lesions who cannot perform intermittent catheterization.

18 Mark the stoma site. Make a midline or Gibson incision. Expose the posterior surface of the bladder, and make an inverted U-shaped incision to form a wide-based bladder flap. Isolate 10 to 15 cm of ileum (see pages 651 to 654), and spatulate the antimesenteric border of the proximal end for a distance of 4 to 6 cm. Create a nipple on the skin with the distal end (see pages 654 to 657). Insert a 22 F catheter with extra holes. Anastomose the proximal end of the loop to the bladder, starting posteriorly with a running 4-0 SAS. Close the urethra if required (see page 609). Close the incision without drainage. Check for watertightness at 2 to 3 weeks by cystography, and ascertain that the leakpoint pressure is less than 30 cm H_2O.

POSTOPERATIVE PROBLEMS

Watch for *inadequate decompression* of the upper tracts. The trial of catheter drainage preoperatively shows what to expect immediately after operation, but the ureteral orifices may become obstructed from edema, inflammation, or spasm of the detrusor, requiring percutaneous nephrostomy. If that fails, consider loop ureterostomy.

Dermatitis, when it occurs, is treated with antifungal and antibacterial agents, urinary acidification, and protective skin coatings. *Prolapse* of the posterior wall of the bladder is caused by placing the bladder incision too low and not fixing the dome. Revision is necessary to make a new opening in the most cephalad part of the dome and to narrow the fascial defect. *Vesical epithelial eversion* and *squamous metaplasia* are managed at the time that the vesicostomy is closed.

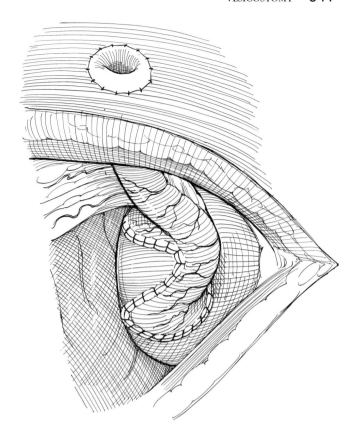

Stomal stenosis seldom is a problem because an opening of 8 F is not obstructive, but obstruction may occur in some thickened bladders, evidenced by residual urine, infection, and signs of backpressure on the upper tracts. Dermatitis also may narrow the lumen. Sometimes the stoma can be kept open by dilatation with an eyedropper, but revision may be necessary. *Bladder capacity* usually increases after vesicostomy. Finally, advise the patient to stay thin.

Commentary by Johannes H. Naudé

The incontinent vesicostomies are designed to provide low-pressure, free drainage of the bladder while avoiding prolapse of the bladder through the vesicocutaneous fistula. The principles for achieving this are fully described in the accompanying text. In infants with posterior urethral valves and a vesicostomy, the valves can easily be ablated with the use of a flexible cystoscope passed through the vesicostomy. In this manner, the incidence of urethral stricture, a most unfortunate complication, can be eliminated. Mothers of infants with vesicostomies need much support and reassurance regarding the unsightly and distressing dermatitis so often associated with this procedure.

The continent, hidden vesicostomy (Naudé) provides a catheterizable, not readily visible stoma and a more normal body image. The procedure was developed for the management of vesicovaginal fistulas with destruction of old continence mechanisms. It has also found application in pediatric neurogenic bladder (in lieu of an artificial sphincter) and in carcinoma of the urethra. Continence is maintained by compression of the neourethra against the pubis by the transmission of abdominal pressure through the bladder to the neourethra. To ensure a good blood supply, the neourethral flap is not based centrally, but to one side of the bladder neck.

Exact dimensions of the flap vary with patient size and anatomy, but one does well to make it longer than anticipated and then trim it to size during final placement. Redundant mucosa (more than that required to encircle a 16 F catheter) is trimmed away, preserving the underlying muscle and blood vessels. The flap is tubularized with a running mucosa-to-mucosa suture of 4-0 SAS material. Denuded muscle is folded over this suture line and sutured in waistcoat manner with interrupted sutures. To prevent fistula formation, opposing neourethral and bladder suture lines are avoided by the interposition of other tissue, usually omentum.

Continence has been incomplete in 20 percent of cases and has been corrected by perineourethral injection of Teflon. Complete failure can be salvaged by the continent, catheterizable stomata associated with the Mitrofanoff, Indiana, and Benchekroun procedures.

Complications have included stomal stenosis, managed by intermittent self-dilation, stone formation (endoscopically treated), and spontaneous rupture of the bladder in poorly compliant patients who have had augmentation cystoplasty. Advantages of the procedure include device-free continence and a good body image, the preservation of the normal ureterovesical junction, and avoidance of the complications of bowel in the urinary tract. These advantages are shared with the Klauber procedure. It can, however, be performed in bladders of small capacity, with additional augmentation cystoplasty.

Cutaneous Ureterostomy and Pyelostomy

Cutaneous ureterostomy is the least desirable form of permanent diversion but may be the only solution in special cases.

URETEROSTOMY IN SITU

This may be a simple way to provide temporary upper tract diversion from a dilated ureter until a more definitive procedure can be completed. More often, it is resorted to when the ureter is damaged during operations associated with poorly controlled bleeding when immediate repair is not practical.

Make a short incision above the anterior superior iliac spine, and identify the dilated ureter through the retroperitoneum. Make a small puncture wound in the ureter; immediately insert a 6 F infant feeding tube or a single pigtail catheter before the ureter collapses, and pass the catheter to the renal pelvis. Tack the catheter to the ureteral wall. Make a stab wound in the flank below the incision and draw the catheter through it. Fasten it securely to the skin with a silk suture. After 2 or 3 weeks, the stent can be replaced, but this must be done quickly after removing the initial catheter to avoid losing the tract.

A similar technique may be used if a ureter is injured during an operation and cannot be repaired at once.

END CUTANEOUS URETEROSTOMY

End cutaneous ureterostomy may be done in patients with poor bladder function who are not candidates for augmentation or substitution. Interposition of a short ileal segment may be a better solution, especially when the ureter is not dilated. In addition, some patients with intractable bladder symptoms from malignancy may be candidates for this operation.

For a ureter to be brought to the skin and remain free of stenosis, it should have become dilated with resultant increase in vasculature. The blood supply to the free end of a normal-caliber ureter is so tenuous after passage through the abdominal wall that it necroses and stenoses. The ureter in obese patients sometimes does not reach the skin surface, and even if it does, it exits so far posteriorly under the rib cage that a collecting device does not adhere. Because cutaneous ureterostomy can often complicate subsequent surgical procedures, it should seldom be considered as a first choice. In any case, the midportion of the ureter should not be disturbed.

Before operation, select one or two sites on the lower abdomen suitable for retaining a collecting device, avoiding the area near the ribs.

Incision: A transverse lower abdominal (see page 490) or Gibson incision (see page 495) is suitable. Approach the ureter extraperitoneally, but in adults it may be necessary to have the ureter traverse the abdominal cavity, even though intraperitoneal disease may make an intra-abdominal approach more difficult. Dissect extraperitoneally to reach the ureter over the sacral promontory. Place a Penrose drain around it, and free it all the way to the bladder to enable the end to reach the anterior abdominal wall, but do not attempt to straighten it by adventitial dissection. Dissect the ureter very carefully, keeping well outside the adventitia to preserve as much as possible of the blood supply coming from the upper end. Clamp and divide it. Ligate the stump, and insert a stay suture in the free end.

1 **A,** The site for the stoma may have to be reconsidered if the ureter is short.

B, If both ureters are involved, consider a double stoma (Step 3A to E).

C, Alternatively, make a ureteroureterostomy with a single cutaneous opening (Steps 4 and 5). A cutaneous pyelostomy (see page 646) is available for temporary diversion with a dilated pelvis.

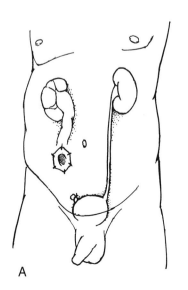

A

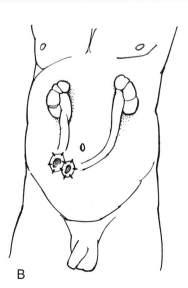

B

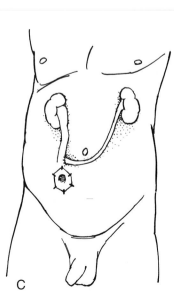

C

Formation of Cutaneous Stoma

V-Flap Technique

2 **A,** For connection of the ureter to the surface of the abdomen, incise the skin in the shape of a U or V. Make a direct tract through subcutaneous tissue, rectus sheath, and peritoneum, as for an ileal conduit (see pages 654 to 655), taking care to keep the body layers lined up. Draw the ureter through the opening without tension for at least 3 cm. Incise the lateral, less vascular side to spatulate it.

B, Insert a 4-0 SAS through the apex of the skin flap into the apex of the ureteral slit and tie it. Pass a similar suture through each angle of the skin incision, then through the free corners of the ureter, and tie them.

C, Place five or six everting sutures around the circumference, tie the sutures; then complete the attachment to have the end of the ureter at the level of the skin, or better, to form a little nipple so that appliances stay on better. Stenting is not necessary when the ureter is dilated.

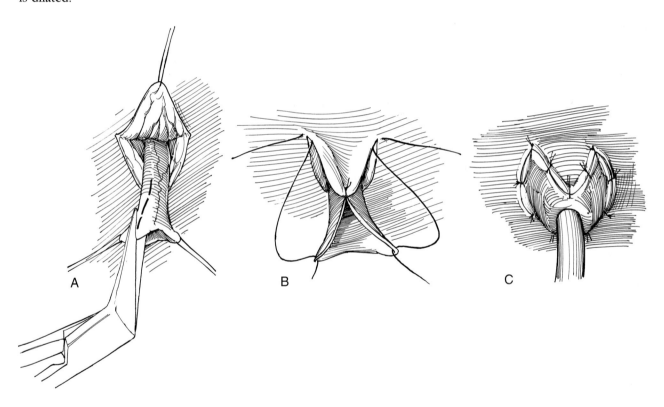

A   B   C

Square Flap Technique
(J. Smith)

First make an incision over the site equal to twice the length of the proposed nipple. Extend it at each end at right angles for a distance equal to slightly more than half the circumference of the ureter. Continue it, again at right angles, back to the midpoint. Raise the two flaps. Move the base of the flaps toward each other to place one flap on each side of the extruded ureter. Incise the skin at the end of the defects, and form rotational flaps to cover the raw surface. Suture the flaps to the ureter and to each other with interrupted 4-0 SAS.

TRANSURETEROURETEROSTOMY WITH CUTANEOUS STOMA

If two ureters are involved, rather than forming a double stoma, bring the more dilated one to the skin and perform transureteroureterostomy (see pages 838 to 839) on the other, transabdominally or extraperitoneally, as shown in Figure 1C.

3 *Incision:* Make a midline transabdominal incision (see page 867). Pack the intestine into the upper abdomen. Lift up the parietal peritoneum over the more normal ureter near its crossing of the iliac vessels, and open it with Lahey scissors as far caudally as possible. Encircle the ureter with a small Penrose drain well outside the adventitia, free it distally, and clamp it. Place a traction suture through the proximal end before cutting and ligating the distal stump with an absorbable suture.

Open the parietal peritoneum over the more dilated ureter, and expose a section of it. Under vision, digitally dissect a channel from one retroperitoneal incision to the other, and draw the smaller ureter through it with a curved clamp.

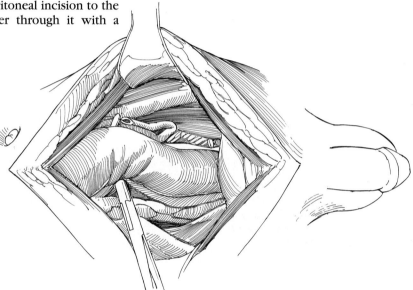

4 Dissect the larger ureter to the bladder; cut it, place a stay suture, and ligate the stump. Continue the retroperitoneal dissection that was begun over the larger ureter around the lateral and anterior body wall to the site selected for the stoma.

Form an opening for the stoma, but make it only through the subcutaneous tissue and muscles and not into the peritoneum. Connect the dissection through the body wall with the previous retroperitoneal dissection. Through the opening, insert a large clamp that passes beneath the peritoneum to grasp the stay suture on the larger ureter, and bring it out through the skin. Be sure the ureter is not angulated.

Trim the smaller ureter to the proper length to meet the more dilated one, cutting it obliquely. Make a 2-cm longitudinal incision in the dilated ureter, and proceed with transureteroureterostomy (see pages 838 to 839).

Bring a Penrose drain extraperitoneally through a stab wound in the skin below the stoma. Close the parietal peritoneal incisions, and close the abdomen. If necessary, spatulate the protruding ureter, and then suture it to the skin as described on page 643. Stents are not necessary.

A bilateral single stoma loop cutaneous ureterostomy that avoids having the end of the ureter as a stoma (Namiki and Yanagi, 1995) can be constructed by looping one ureter to a cutaneous position to make a stoma on the skin, and anastomosing the opposite ureter to the end of the first, end to end.

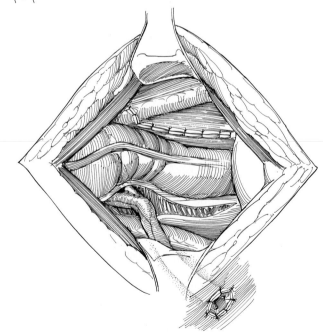

DOUBLE-BARRELED CUTANEOUS URETEROSTOMY

If both ureters are dilated, they may be combined into a single stoma with a Z-plasty.

5 Approach the ureters extraperitoneally.
A, Make a Z-shaped incision in the skin in a previously selected site.

B, Trim the subcutaneous fat from the flaps.

C, Remove a minimum amount of deep fat to avoid inversion of the skin at the site of the stoma. Excise a button of anterior rectus sheath. Make an X-shaped incision in the transversalis fascia and peritoneum.

D, Draw the ureters through the opening and trim them to length. Spatulate each ureter by incising its lateral border.

E, Suture the flaps into the V's with 3-0 SAS.

Alternatively, make a simple stoma by suturing the incised ureters together, slightly everting them, and suturing them to the skin as shown in Step 1B.

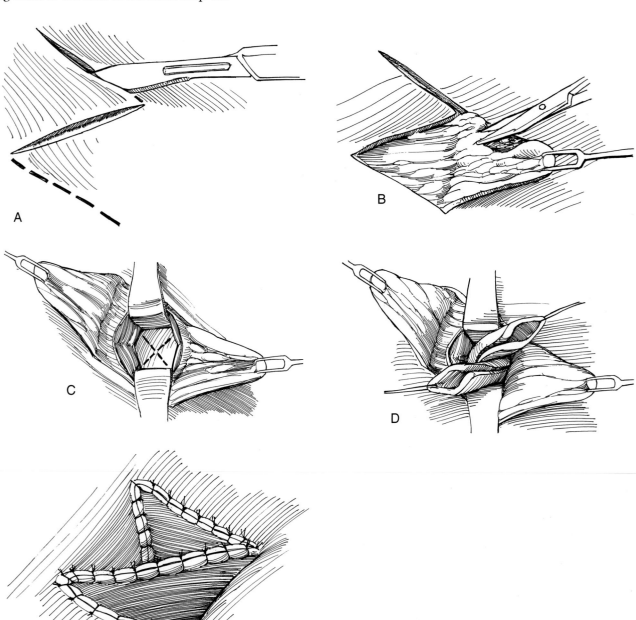

CUTANEOUS PYELOSTOMY

Cutaneous pyelostomy may be a useful procedure in the presence of obstruction and severe infection. A large extrarenal pelvis is required.

Incision and dissection are done as described for cutaneous loop ureterostomy, except that instead of actually mobilizing the proximal ureter, merely trace it to the renal pelvis. Rotate the kidney anteromedially.

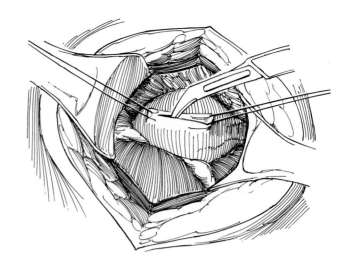

6 Place two traction sutures in the posterior surface of the dilated pelvis, well above the ureteropelvic junction. Incise the pelvis with a hooked blade for 3 cm.

7 Place several 3-0 or 4-0 SAS between the pelvis and body wall to relieve tension. Suture the full thickness of the pelvis to the skin with interrupted sutures. Do not leave the opening too large or the pelvis may prolapse.

For closure, encircle the connection to the skin and dissect the redundant pelvis, staying clear of the ureteropelvic junction. Trim the edges and close the defect with a running 4-0 SAS, with occasional locked stitches.

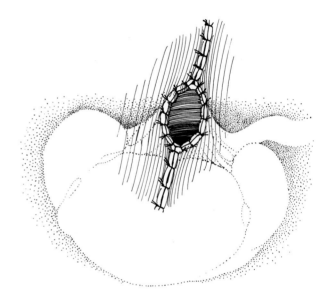

POSTOPERATIVE PROBLEMS

Stenosis at the skin level is almost the rule when a nondilated ureter is brought out because of relative ischemia of the ureteral tip or tension. Try dilation, and then treat it with intubation with a round-tipped silicone tube. A meatotomy can be done by bringing a flap of skin into a notch in the ureter. Surgical revision seldom helps because the 3 cm of extra ureteral length necessary to construct a new stoma is seldom available. Instead, an alternate form of supravesical diversion must be applied. Other causes of obstruction of the ureter are angulation and narrowing as it passes through the peritoneum or fascia, corrected by freeing the ureter and placing it in a wider bed. *Pyocystis* or empyema of the bladder not infrequently can occur after total proximal diversion, especially if the bladder is denervated. Overdilatation of the urethra followed by regular catheterization and irrigation often provide long-term relief. In females, the urethra may be split. If these measures are not successful, cystectomy may be advisable unless reconstruction is planned.

Commentary by Hrair-George J. Mesrobian

Although the indications for end cutaneous ureterostomy and pyelostomy have dwindled over the past decade, they still do have a place in the urologic armamentarium. The main indications for end cutaneous ureterostomy in children are poor bladder function due to a variety of congenital anomalies such as posterior urethral valves and bladder exstrophy and the emergence of increasing hydronephrosis. In adults, the main indications for end cutaneous ureterostomy occur in conjunction with advanced pelvic malignancies and kidney transplantation.

The ability to perform a transureteroureterostomy (TUU) with one cutaneous stoma is quite attractive to the patient and the urologic surgeon alike. In children and thin adults, the procedure can be performed entirely retroperitoneally through a Pfannenstiel incision. The donor ureter is dissected extraperitoneally near the hiatus and mobilized proximally. The recipient ureter is dissected in a similar fashion. It is possible to create a retroperitoneal tunnel in front of the vessels using gentle blunt and sharp dissection. With the help of a Satinsky clamp, the donor ureter can then be transposed to the opposite side. This obviates opening of the peritoneum. In our experience, it is also essential to construct the ureteral stoma first, prior to performing the TUU. By doing so, one can place the anastomosis at a predictable location and not risk distortion during the construction of the TUU. When the ureter is not dilated, one should not hesitate to maintain intubation of the cutaneous ureterostomy all the way up to the renal pelvis with a double-J stent. This stent can be changed periodically.

When a cutaneous pyelostomy becomes the procedure of choice, it is important to remember that during the incision of the pelvis, one should stay as far away from the ureteropelvic junction as possible. This procedure provides the urologic surgeon an opportunity to take biopsy samples of the kidney, which can have prognostic significance. Finally, if a future reconstructive procedure is contemplated, it is worthwhile to preserve enough length of the distal ureter on one side to allow its use as a Mitrofanoff stoma for intermittent catheterization.

Ileal Conduit

(Bricker)

Because of a high incidence of stomal problems, an ileal conduit is seldom the first choice for urinary diversion. Select other forms of cutaneous urinary diversion. First, the ileal stoma usually becomes inflamed and scarred and does not enlarge as the child grows, thus requiring frequent revisions. Second, because of reflux of mucus, kidney stones appear during adolescence. An alternative is a cutaneous ureterostomy with transureteroureterostomy if the ureter measures at least 1 cm in diameter (see pages 838 to 839). A stoma formed from large bowel, such as with a sigmoid conduit (see page 664) or even a transverse colon conduit (see page 667), may be more stable, and the ureters can be inserted with an antireflux technique. Consider an ileocecal conduit that allows end-to-side ureteral anastomosis and maintains the antireflux protection of the ileocecal valve (Zinman).

An ileal conduit does have the advantage that the proximal end may be attached at any site along the upper urinary tract and the distal end may surface anywhere on the abdomen. Later, undiversion can be readily accomplished by attaching the conduit to an augmented bladder or continent reservoir (see pages 733 to 734).

1 Select a site on the surface of the abdomen for the stoma where the skin is not rolled into folds while the patient is either sitting or standing. The stoma should not be near the umbilicus (unless it is through it), the edge of the rectus muscle, a bony prominence, or an abdominal scar. Mark the site with a ballpoint pen or scratch it with a needle. An even better plan is to have the patient wear the partially filled appliance for a day or two before operation to be sure that the placement is optimal and to start to become accustomed to it. Although the standard location for a stoma is just below the center of a line between the umbilicus and the anterior superior iliac spine, this is often too low, especially in children with myelodysplasia, in whom an umbilical stoma or even an epigastric one is easier to manage. An enterostomal therapist can be helpful not only in positioning the appliance but also in counseling the patient and allaying concerns. Obtain an intravenous urogram and blood chemistry studies. Prepare the bowel (see page 6).

Instruments: Provide four Kocher clamps, curved mosquito (Providence) clamps, a Kelly clamp, Adson forceps, tenotomy scissors, a Balfour retractor, 5 F and 8 F infant feeding tubes, a plastic rod, 4-0 silk sutures with detachable needles, 4-0 and 5-0 CCG ureteral sutures, 2-0 and 3-0 SAS, and a Penrose drain.

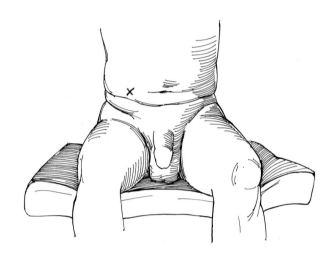

URETERAL MOBILIZATION

Position: Place the patient supine. After the operation is underway, have the anesthesiologist place a nasogastric tube.

Incision: Make a midline transperitoneal incision (see page 867). Free adhesions and explore the abdomen.

2 Unless the retroperitoneal area has already been exposed during cystectomy, make a vertical incision lateral to the sigmoid mesocolon where it joins the parietal peritoneum to expose the left ureter. Dissect medially over the left iliac vessels to locate the ureter. It is found lifted up with the peritoneum. Free the left ureter with a right-angle clamp, and encircle it with a Penrose drain for traction. Dissect it well down into the pelvis without disturbing its adventitial circulation.

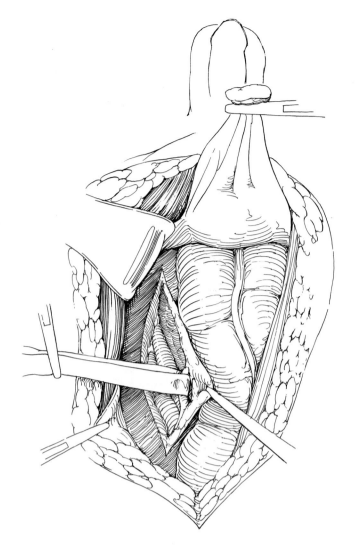

3 Clamp the ureter distally, insert a fine traction suture in its anterior proximal surface, and divide it against the clamp with a knife. Ligate the distal stump with a 3-0 CCG suture, cut long so it may be identified later. Then dissect the ureter proximally so that about 8 cm is free. Repeat the procedure on the right side. There the ureter lies retroperitoneally just over the iliac vessels and so not only is easier to find but also requires less mobilization.

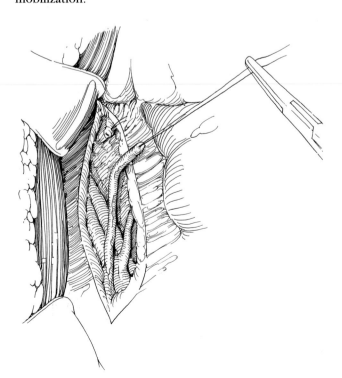

4 Tunnel gently between the two peritoneal openings with the index and middle fingers of each hand, staying beneath the superior hemorrhoidal vessels, to create a channel for the left ureter to allow it to sweep over in a smooth arc from the left to the right side. Draw it through by its stay suture with Péan forceps. Take great care that the ureter is not angulated or twisted.

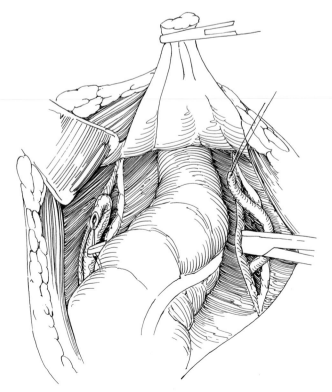

PREPARING THE LOOP

5 Adjust the light behind the mesentery, and select a suitable segment of ileum near the ileocecal junction by visualizing the mesenteric vessels. An avascular area is usually found slightly more proximal than shown. If a suitable segment is not found, use a more proximal segment of ileum or consider a transverse colon conduit (see page 667). Place a temporary stay suture of 4-0 silk on a detachable needle in the bowel 10 to 15 cm from the ileocecal valve and beyond the ileocecal arcade, the distance depending on the size of the patient. Select a loop of ileum that contains one or two distinct vascular arcades, as shown. Move the stay suture several times if necessary. Because it marks the distal end of the segment, tie a knot in the end for identification and thus prevent inadvertent reversal of the loop.

Measure the segment. It should be long enough to reach the skin level plus another 2 cm. In adults, the length of a Kocher clamp is usually about right. If a Turnbull loop stoma is to be formed, add 8 to 10 cm more. Place a second stay suture to mark the proximal end. Re-examine the loop and its arcades, moving the stay sutures as necessary to provide an adequate segment containing one or preferably two major vascular arcades. Hold both stay sutures in clamps. (The *technique for clearance of mesentery from bowel* is described on page 683 under the heading "Technique.")

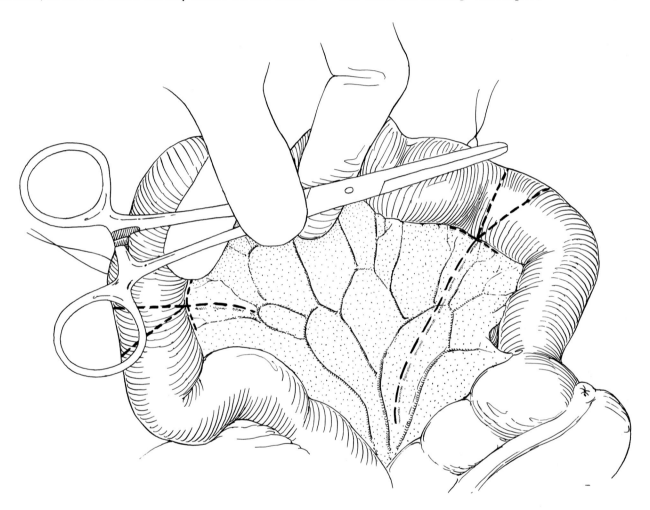

6 For a *sutured anastomosis,* place Kocher clamps at 45-degree angles on the ends of the bowel that will be anastomosed in continuity, and place them at right angles on the ends of the proposed loop. Divide the bowel with the cutting current, leaving a protruding 2-mm edge, which is then fulgurated. (Be sure to keep the adjacent bowel against the wound to ground it during fulguration.) Discard the excised wedges; a sterile pan technique is not necessary because the ileal contents are essentially sterile. For a *stapled anastomosis,* apply the GIA stapler as described in Step 14. Drop the isolated segment into the pelvis, and cover it with a moist laparotomy pad.

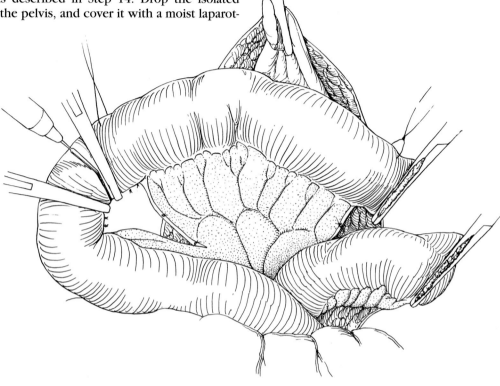

ILEOILEAL ANASTOMOSIS

Single-Layer Closed Technique

7 Hold the clamps so that the cut ends are apposed. Place 4-0 silk detachable sutures into but not through the submucosa about 3 mm apart. The wall should be seen to blanch when the tougher submucosa is partially penetrated. If they are placed too deeply, they catch the sutures on the opposite side and occlude the lumen, but they do not hold if placed too superficially. When one side is completed, bundle the sutures into a clamp, turn the bowel over, and place the sutures in the opposite side. Be certain that the sutures at the mesenteric angles are well placed; this is where leakage is most likely to occur. Again bundle the sutures in a second clamp. Slowly manipulate and withdraw the clamps as your assistant gently supports the ends of the sutures.

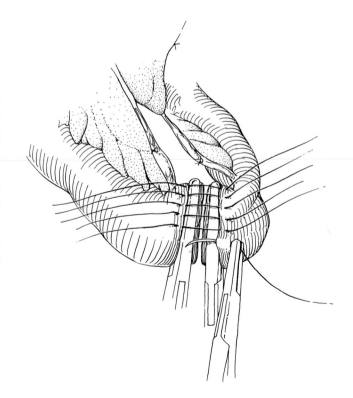

8 Tie the sutures in pairs as they are lifted on a clamp by the assistant. Do not cinch them too tight. If the edges do not automatically invert, have the assistant hold a slightly open clamp under the suture loop and press a blade against each bowel edge as the knot is tied. Do not hesitate to put in extra sutures.

9 Check the patency of the anastomosis first by inspection as the two bundles of uncut sutures are drawn apart, and then by palpation of the lumen with the thumb and forefinger. If you are concerned about cross-suturing, remove a few sutures and look inside, cut the offending sutures, and replace them. Cut the ends of the remaining sutures.

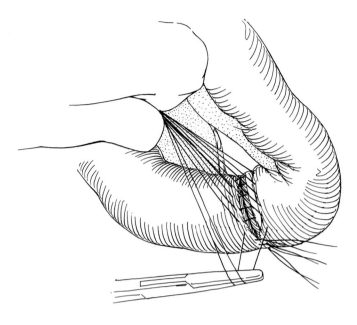

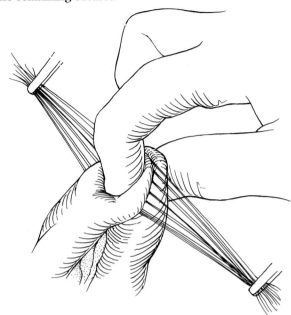

Single-Layer Open Technique

10 A and B, Appose the ends of the ileum with vertical mattress sutures of 3-0 silk placed in four quadrants to catch 3 mm of serosa and submucosa and a little mucosa. Tie these sutures, and add interrupted sutures that catch the submucosa between.

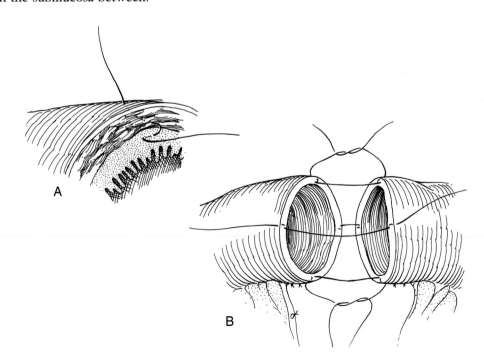

Two-Layer Closure

Approximate the posterior bowel wall from the outside with interrupted seromuscular sutures of 3-0 silk. Turn the bowel over.

11 Place full-thickness continuous sutures of 3-0 or 4-0 CCG to invert the mucosa of the posterior wall.

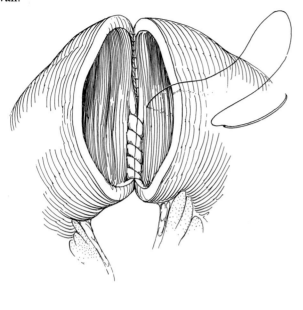

12 Continue this suture on the anterior wall and corners with a Connell stitch (see page 37).

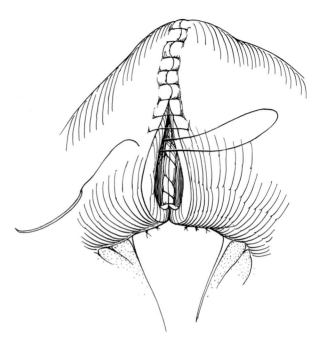

13 Complete the anastomosis with interrupted 3-0 silk sutures on the anterior seromuscular surface.

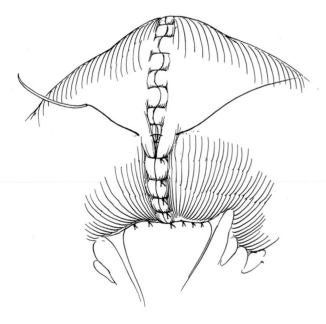

14 Close the mesentery on both sides with fine silk, taking care to incorporate only the delicate peritoneal surface. Annoying hematomas occur if a vessel is caught and breached. Test the anastomosis for patency (Step 8).

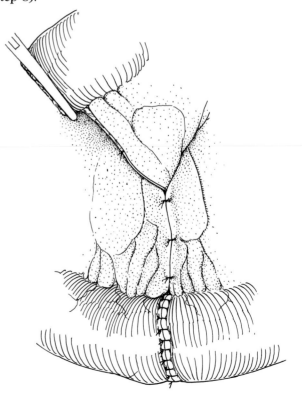

Stapled Technique

15 Select a segment of ileum and divide the mesentery (Step 5). Place a GIA stapler at the distal site and push the lever home, thus placing two rows of staples and dividing the bowel between. Repeat the procedure at the proximal site.

16 Trim the antimesenteric corner from both staple lines. Rotate one loop of bowel 180 degrees, and insert a blade of the GIA stapler all the way into each lumen. Connect the handles of the blades, and close the lever to make two rows of sutures with an opening between. Check the serosal side of the staple lines for hemostasis, and reinforce it as needed with horizontal, inverting mattress sutures of 4-0 silk.

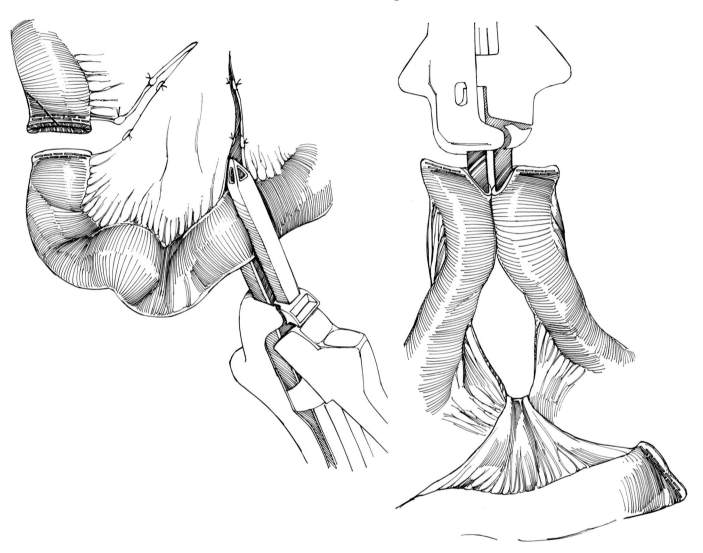

17 Place a stay suture at the end of each row of staples. Then apply the TA 30 stapler over the remaining opening to overlap the original rows of staples; drive in the staples.

18 Close the mesentery. Check for hemostasis on the serosal surface, and reinforce it with horizontal, inverting mattress sutures of 4-0 silk.

The completed procedure is shown. It is performed in a sequence: (1) formation of the stoma; (2) implantation of the right ureter; (3) implantation of the left ureter; (4) resection of excess length from the proximal end of the loop; and (5) closure of the proximal end of the loop. The stoma is formed first before anastomosing the ureters to allow them to be inserted in an optimal position.

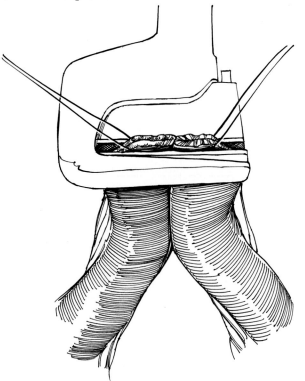

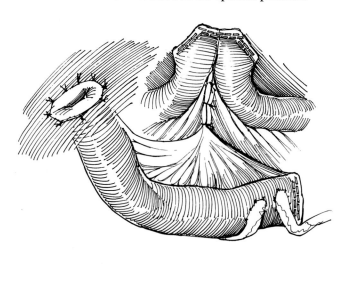

FORMATION OF A STOMA

19 **A,** On the right side of the incision, draw the fascia and peritoneum in line with the skin using Kocher clamps. Alternatively, place heavy sutures through all layers of the abdominal incision. At the site that was marked previously, grasp the skin with a Kocher clamp, lift it, and sharply cut off the elevated mound with a

knife, removing a circular piece slightly smaller than the diameter of the ileum.

B, Grasp the subcutaneous fat with a Kocher clamp, and circumscribe it with the electrosurgical blade, taking care to angle the cut inward to remove a narrow core. Avoid undermining by taking too much fat because the subcutaneous tissue stretches as it is elevated; removing too much subcutaneous tissue encourages inversion of the stoma.

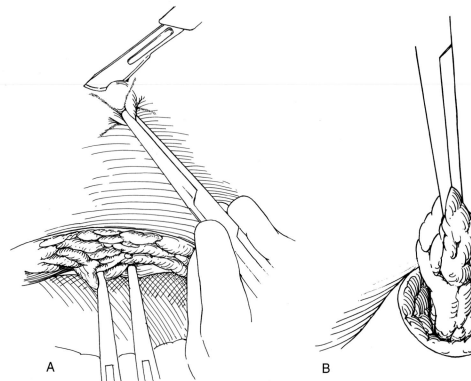

A

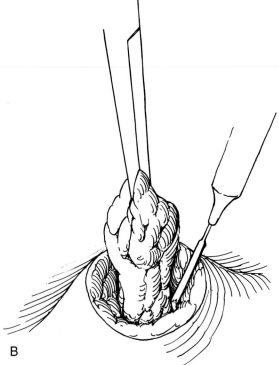

B

20 **A,** Incise the anterior rectus fascia with a cruciate cut with the cutting current.

B, Alternately, remove a disc of fascia.

Separate the rectus muscle bluntly, and divide as little of the muscle as possible to help avoid a parastomal hernia. Hold the muscle apart with U.S. Army retractors. Hold the left hand inside the abdomen to prevent injury to the bowel, and remove a disc of the posterior fascial layer and the peritoneum, or merely incise it in a cruciate fashion. One or two fingers should readily pass through all layers. Insert a Kocher clamp into the stoma, and grasp and clamp the end of the loop as the assistant simultaneously releases the original clamp. Draw it out to the surface, but be sure it lies without tension 2 to 3 cm above the skin surface.

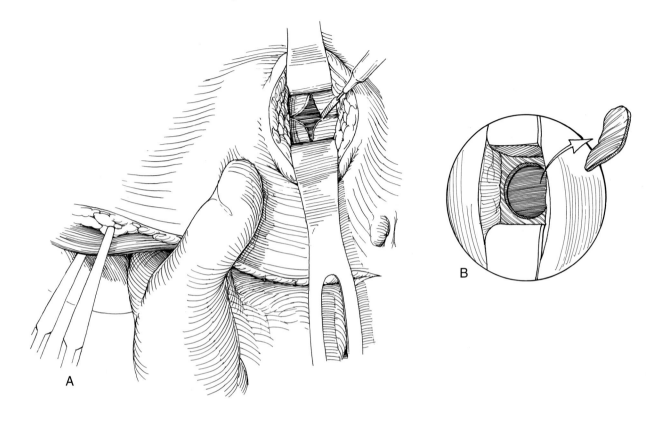

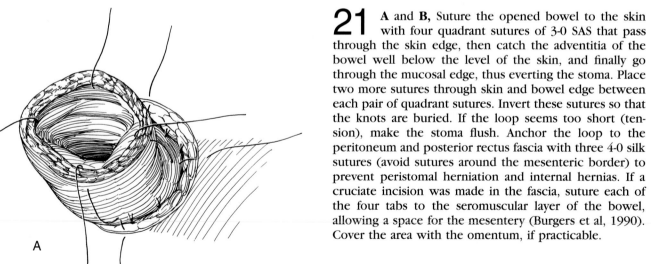

21 **A and B,** Suture the opened bowel to the skin with four quadrant sutures of 3-0 SAS that pass through the skin edge, then catch the adventitia of the bowel well below the level of the skin, and finally go through the mucosal edge, thus everting the stoma. Place two more sutures through skin and bowel edge between each pair of quadrant sutures. Invert these sutures so that the knots are buried. If the loop seems too short (tension), make the stoma flush. Anchor the loop to the peritoneum and posterior rectus fascia with three 4-0 silk sutures (avoid sutures around the mesenteric border) to prevent peristomal herniation and internal hernias. If a cruciate incision was made in the fascia, suture each of the four tabs to the seromuscular layer of the bowel, allowing a space for the mesentery (Burgers et al, 1990). Cover the area with the omentum, if practicable.

Umbilical Stoma

Preserve the cup of the umbilicus, and anastomose the bowel to the juncture of the umbilicus with the fascia.

NIPPLE VARIATIONS

It is advisable to avoid a circular anastomosis of bowel to skin. Simply interposing skin as an inverted V at the 6-o'clock position reduces the possibility of stricture. Certain plastic techniques can reduce the incidence of stomal stenosis. These techniques are even more useful when redoing the stoma.

Z-Incision Stoma

22 **A,** Make a Z-incision in the skin at the stomal site.

B, Raise two flaps.

C, Incise the mucosa and submucosa of the bowel, or the entire thickness of the bowel, on either side.

D, Insert the flaps in the defects and suture them in place with 3-0 SAS.

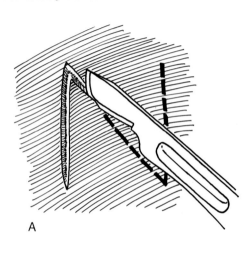

A

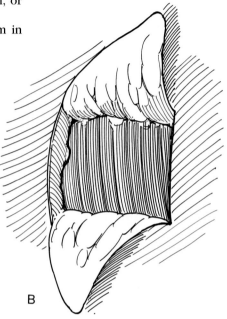

B

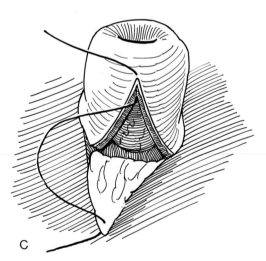

C

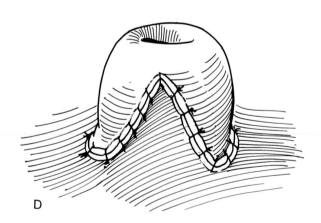

D

Loop Stoma
(Turnbull)

This procedure is useful for obese patients with a short mesentery. Initially provide a longer (8 to 10 cm) ileal segment.

23 **A,** Close the distal end of the conduit as described for the proximal end in Steps 31 and 32. In obese patients, carefully undercut the mesentery of the distal end to obtain adequate mobility. Pass a clamp bluntly through the most mobile and well-vascularized part of the mesentery in order to loop it with a Penrose drain.

B, Draw the bowel loop through the body wall for at least several centimeters without tension or twisting.

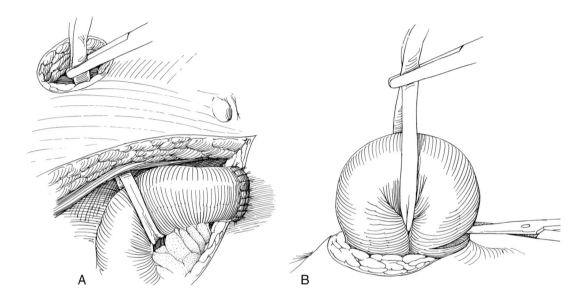

A   B

24 **A,** Replace the Penrose drain with a plastic rod. Open the loop transversely four fifths of the distance along the exposed bowel, nearest the defunctionalized (distal) limb. Reach inside the opening with an Allis clamp and pull out the mucosa.

B, Suture the mucosa to the subcuticular layer of skin with interrupted 4-0 SAS, catching the seromuscular layer of the bowel to evert the stoma. The defunctionalized portion requires only superficial sutures. Fasten the rod in place with two silk sutures; withdraw it 1 to 2 weeks postoperatively.

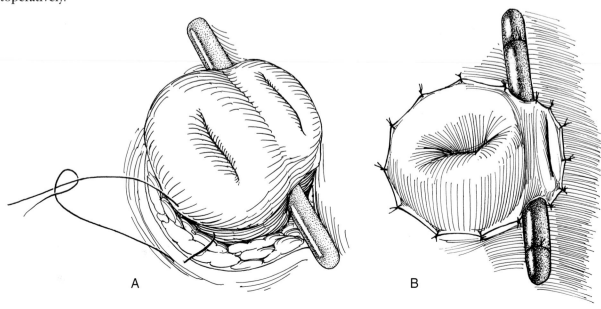

A   B

URETERAL ANASTOMOSIS

Ureteral implantation is best performed after the loop is in place so that kinking can be avoided.

Direct Anastomosis, Right
(Cordonnier)

Close the left parietal peritoneal opening with 4-0 silk sutures.

25 Cut the right ureter obliquely to freshen the end, and spatulate it (*dashed line*) to provide a larger lumen for anastomosis.

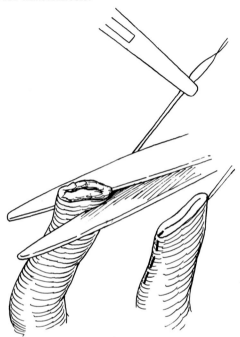

26 Place a 4-0 SAS through the adventitia and muscularis of the ureter 2 cm from the end, and stitch it on the antimesenteric border of the ileum.

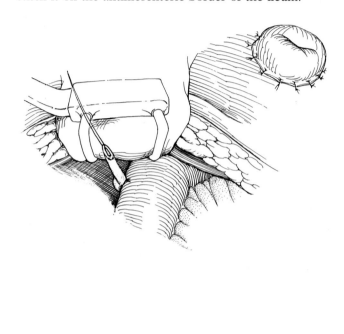

27 Pinch the bowel between the thumb and forefinger of the left hand, and incise through the muscularis with a #15 blade, exposing the submucosa with its fine vessels.

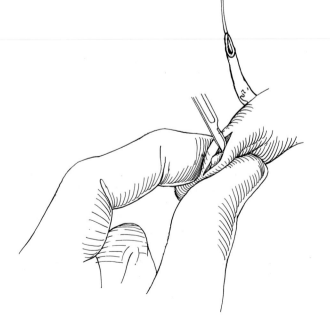

28 Grasp a bit of the extruded submucosa with smooth Adson forceps, and trim it, along with the underlying mucosa, with tenotomy scissors. Remove as little as possible; the opening always enlarges. Insert a mosquito clamp into the bowel lumen to check that an opening has been made into the lumen.

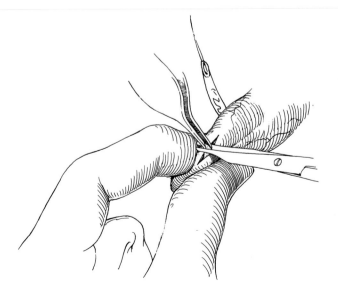

29   **A,** Place a 4-0 or 5-0 SAS or catgut suture through the apex of the bowel opening (from outside in), then through the apex of the ureteral spatulation (from inside out). Use the stay suture for manipulation; do not grasp the tissue with forceps. Incorporate a little mucosa, more muscularis, and adequate serosa in the stitch. Tie the suture.

B, Place sutures similarly half way along each side and tie them.

A stent may be inserted if you have concern over the quality of the tissues. However, stents can be obstructive, they take time to insert, and they may come out too soon. Without them, leaks are uncommon. If a stent is to be used, mount a 5 F or 8 F infant feeding tube on a Péan clamp and pass it through the ileal stoma and out through the opening in the bowel. Irrigate it clear of mucus. Take it up in a Kelly clamp, and introduce it into the ureter until resistance is felt as it reaches the kidney. Irrigate again to test the position of the tip. Immediately fasten the tube to the skin with a silk suture; it is later cut short to fit within the collecting bag. Alternatively, a double-J stent may be inserted.

C, Place a fourth suture through the bowel and the tip of the ureter as it is manipulated on the stay suture. Cut the stay suture. Place three more sutures from the muscularis of the ureter to the serosa of the bowel.

D, These sutures invert the anastomosis slightly into the bowel and provide a double layer for watertightness.

Perform the same maneuvers with the left ureter. Make certain that it passes beneath the colon in a smooth curve. Insert it 1 to 2 cm more proximally on the loop than the right, at a site where it is easily accommodated and not angulated.

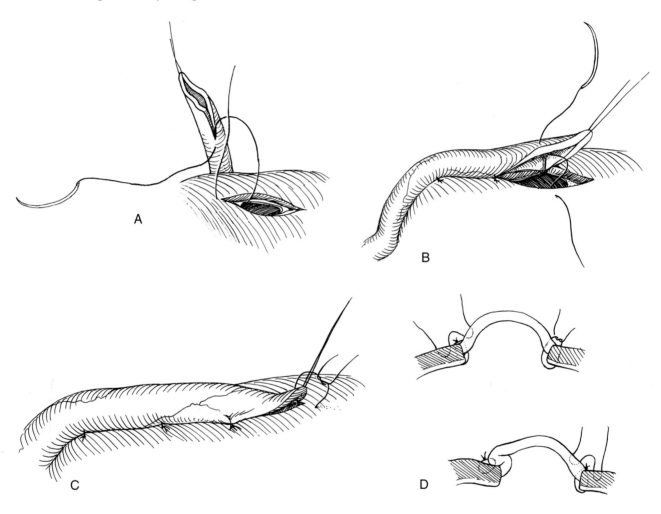

Split-Cuff Nipple Ureteral Anastomosis (Sagalowsky)

This alternative technique is simple and prevents reflux.

Spatulate the ureter for a distance of 1 cm. Place a 4-0 CCG stitch at the apex of the spatulation, leaving it long to aid in manipulation. Place a stitch through a corner of the spatulation and then through the adventitia of the ureter 1 cm proximally. Turn the corner back as you tie the suture. Repeat the procedure on the other corner to form a nipple, but place the suture in the adventitia a few millimeters away from the first to prevent constriction of the ureter at the base of the nipple. Add two or three additional sutures to close the side of the nipple. Insert the nippled ureter into the bowel segment through a stab wound, and fasten it by a series of interrupted sutures from the edge of the nipple to the bowel mucosa and submucosa. Reinforce the connection outside the segment with a few sutures from ureteral adventitia to bowel serosa.

TRIMMING AND CLOSURE OF THE PROXIMAL END OF THE LOOP

Spread the loop so that it makes an easy curve from the stoma to the area from which the ureters emerge. If there is excess bowel, apply a second Kocher clamp distal to the one placed initially and trim the excess.

30 Insert stay sutures in the mesenteric and antimesenteric margins. Place a row of detachable 4-0 silk sutures over the Kocher clamp. Pass these through the serosa and muscularis, and incorporate the firm submucosa. Slightly open and then manipulate the clamp to free it while keeping traction on the stay sutures.

31 Tie the end sutures first to invert each end. Have the assistant lift the crossing suture with a mosquito clamp, at the same time depressing the two edges of the bowel, while you tie the suture.

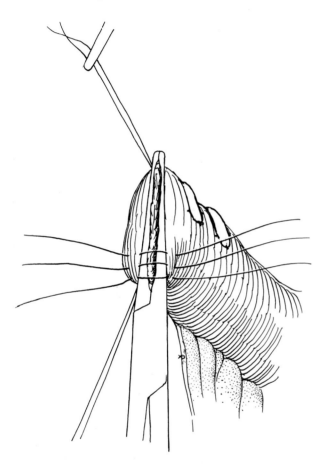

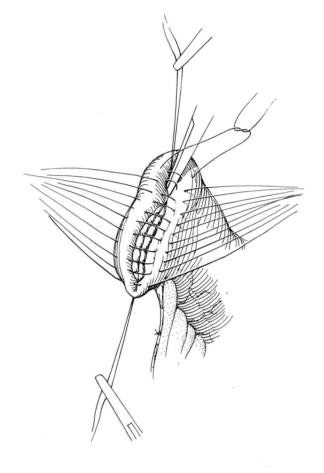

32 The loop is shown of the proper length, with the two ureters emerging from beneath it from the defect in the parietal peritoneum.

33 Pull the medial peritoneal flap over the ileal stump and ureters, and fix it with interrupted 4-0 silk sutures. Continue these sutures up along the edge of the mesentery to prevent an internal hernia. Survey the conduit. If it is dusky, apply warm packs. If in doubt about its circulation, excise it and start over.

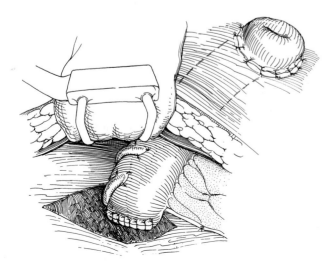

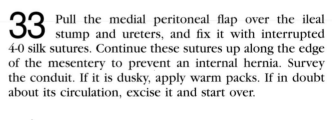

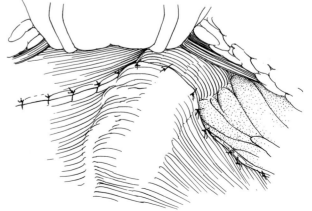

CONJOINED URETER TECHNIQUES

Side-by-Side

34 **A,** Do not close the proximal end of the loop. Spatulate each ureter for a distance equal to the diameter of the ileum. Join their posterior edges side by side with a fine running absorbable suture.

B, Anastomose the joined ureters to the open bowel with two running 4-0 SAS, placing an occasional lock stitch.

C, Reinforce the anastomosis with a second layer of five or six interrupted sutures.

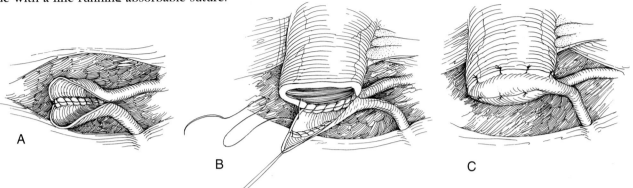

End-to-End
(Wallace)

35 **A,** Spatulate each ureter for a distance slightly more than the diameter of the ileum.

B, Join their posterior edges with two running 4-0 CCG sutures, starting in the middle and continuing around each end (only one suture is shown).

C, Continue the sutures to join the back walls of the bowel and ureter, taking care to invert the angles. Then complete the closure anteriorly. Reinforcing sutures may be added.

An alternative technique can provide a nonrefluxing ileal conduit (Grossfield). After isolating the ileal segment, make a 5-cm enterotomy just distal to the afferent limb and intussuscept the ileum through it. Fix the intussusception to itself with two rows of staples from the GIA stapler, and fix it to the back wall with a third set. Place a polyglycolic acid collar at the base of the nipple valve, and close the enterotomy in two layers.

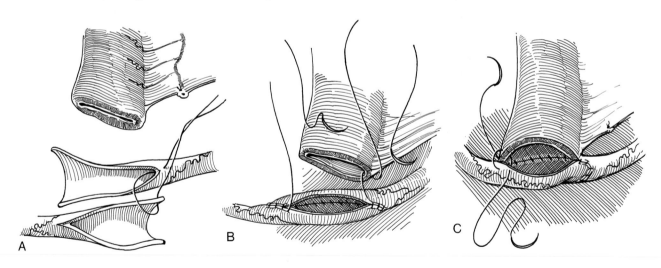

Closure

Proceed with closure. Trim the stents and apply a collection appliance in the operating room. Drain the wound with suction drainage, and remove the drains as soon as it is dry.

POSTOPERATIVE PROBLEMS

Anuria after surgery is usually secondary to operative fluid shifts, so a challenge with mannitol is the first step.

Wound infection or dehiscence may occur, although neither is common. Malnutrition, which should have been corrected preoperatively, can be an important factor. Running monofilament sutures with adequate bites of rectus fascia can prevent disruption. *Paralytic ileus* is usual and resolves quickly if gastric decompression is maintained, but intestinal obstruction may occur from herniation of the bowel into the mesenteric "trap." Continuation of decompression with a long (Baker) tube usually permits resolution, but reoperation is occasionally necessary.

Intestinal fistulas can occur from the site of the ileoileal anastomosis as a result of local ischemia from interference with the mesenteric arcades, and the whole segment can become necrotic if the mesentery is carelessly tacked to retroperitoneum or if it is subjected to too much tension. The vascular supply can be judged by the color of the stomal mucosa. *Leakage* at the ileoileal anastomosis is usually due to tension and to rough handling of the tissue. Leakage can also occur at the suture line that closes the proximal end of the loop. Leakage from the ureteroileal anastomosis is uncommon. The source can be determined by testing the fluid from the drains because urine has a higher urea content than blood. Intraperitoneal absorption causes the blood urea nitrogen level to rise relative to the creatinine. Do a loopogram. If the leakage is minimal, place a double-lumen suction tube (a Malecot catheter containing an infant feeding tube connected to low suction) to allow healing. Alternatively, insert a tube into the kidney percutaneously or place stents antegradely. If an appreciable urinoma has formed and the patient is ill, reoperation with resection of the anastomosis and reimplantation at a new site is required. This is not an easy procedure, but attempts at resuturing seldom succeed. Prompt reoperation with insertion of a gastrostomy and replacement of the loop is usually required.

Redundancy of the segment is usually secondary to obstruction at the stoma or at the body wall. For correction, not only should the loop be shortened but the cause of the obstruction must be corrected.

Obstruction at the sites of ureteral anastomosis is rare; it need not be considered if stents are in place and can be irrigated. Ureteral dilatation may result from *ureteral stenosis* from technical error or may appear late, cause unknown. Revision is necessary unless the ureter is atonic, in which case a new anastomosis does not help.

Place a catheter in the stoma to check for obstruction at the level of the body wall. If all attempts fail and no urine is recovered, place percutaneous nephrostomies. Obstruction usually develops within the first 2 years, but it may occur much later. It is due to devascularization of the terminal ureter and is usually unsuspected. Regular follow-up is necessary to avoid this complication, with sonograms, scans or intravenous pyelograms, and loopograms at regular intervals.

Before reoperation, an attempt may be made at balloon dilatation of the anastomosis through a percutaneous nephrostomy tract, but this is seldom successful because of the fibrous cause of the stricture. Repair entails an approach extraperitoneally through a modified Gibson incision or transperitoneally. Dissect retroperitoneally, but stay away from the stoma. Incise the ureter and bowel at the site of the anastomosis, and perform a Heineke-Mikulicz transverse closure. Alternatively, take an ellipse from the ureter, incise the ileum above the stricture, and suture the defects side to side. It is also possible to detach the ureter and either reanastomose it or do a ureteroureterostomy.

Hyperchloremic acidosis, similar to that with ureterosigmoidostomy, may infrequently occur. It is usually associated with obstruction at the stoma, either from stenosis or from infrequent emptying of the drainage bag with the associated back pressure. Catheterization of the conduit is immediately corrective; revision of the stoma or shortening of the loop may be needed for the long term. It should be noted that jejunal conduits have greater problems with electrolyte imbalance, characterized by azotemia and hyponatremic hypochloremic acidosis, and should be used only if no other bowel is available.

Renal calculi appear later, usually in alkaline urine harboring urea-splitting bacteria. Shorten the loop, increase water intake, give thiazides, add bicarbonate, and inhibit the infection with antibiotics. Removal is usually reserved for stones that are obstructive. *Pyelonephritis* occurs with increasing frequency the longer diversion is present, as a result of a combination of back flow and bacteriuria. Antibacterial therapy for symptomatic attacks and attention to better drainage will help.

Stomal Problems

Disturbances around the stoma are very common and are often directly related to the quality of stomal care. *Peristomal dermatitis* occurs frequently and may lead to stomal stenosis. The cause may be an improperly located or constructed stoma, an appliance that does not fit, poorly tolerated adhesive, alkaline urine, or inadequate stomal care. It starts with skin inflammation and progresses to ulceration and encrustation. Hyperkeratosis, scarring, and stenosis are the final result. *Stomal ischemia* is usually temporary, but if it persists it requires stomal revision with resection of a short segment. If the whole loop is ischemic, remove it, ligate the ureters, and place percutaneous nephrostomies. Wait 3 months and repeat the whole operation.

Stomal stenosis occurs at the circular mucocutaneous junction. The Z-flap technique or an end-loop stoma lessens the chance of stenosis. Everted (nipple) stomas have a lower incidence of stenosis. It usually occurs at the skin level, secondary to the effects of dermatitis, but can result from fascial angulation or ischemia of the terminal portion of the bowel. Alignment at the time of formation and prevention or correction of peristomal dermatitis are the remedies. Correction is needed if the stoma does not admit a 30 F catheter, if the residual urine is more than 10 ml, or if luminal pressure is greater than 20 cm H_2O.

Revision of the stoma: Circumscribe the stoma close to the mucosa, and excise it because the redundant bowel can be readily mobilized through the defect. Free the bowel for 10 to 12 cm through the body wall by dissecting intraperitoneally and dividing adhesions, resect the terminal portion with its mesentery, and tack the bowel to the fascia. Form a new nipple stoma by interposing a V-flap of skin to prevent further circular contraction. If the adjacent skin is badly scarred, form several Z-plasties or insert a spiral flap (David). Most important is to follow with improved care with the help of an enterostomal therapist.

Stomal prolapse results from inadequate fixation of the loop to the peritoneal-fascial layers, and the treatment is similar to that for stenosis. *Parastomal hernias* usually occur on the mesenteric side secondary to inadequate fixation of the conduit at the peritoneal opening. They can make fitting the appliance difficult and may lead to incarceration of the bowel. Free the stoma and distal loop as done for stomal stenosis. Excise the peritoneal sac, fix the loop internally, and close the defect in the fascia. If this is not feasible, relocate the stoma to the opposite side. This can be done without opening the abdomen: Pass the end of the loop from the old stoma to the new one on ring forceps. Resect *excessive length* of the loop through the stomal site by progressively dividing the mesenteric arcades as they join the bowel.

Appliances: If it becomes impossible to keep an appliance attached because of body configuration, move the stoma up or down on the same side, place it at the umbilicus, or move it across the abdomen. Sometimes the entire loop must be mobilized or a new conduit constructed to reach the new site.

Commentary by Panayotis P. Kelalis

At least as far as pediatric urologists are concerned, the ileal conduit (Bricker operation) is an operation for the history books. Only with exceptional problems when the surgeon is challenged with shortness of bowel should the use of ileum be considered for urinary diversion. In cases in which the ileal conduit is still employed, presumably in older patients in association with removal of the bladder, it is, I believe, preferable that the ileal conduit be brought to the left ureter rather than

the ureter to the conduit. In these situations, especially if associated with postoperative radiation therapy, the incidence of stricture can be reduced. Unfortunately, in my experience, problems with the stoma when the large bowel is used are also present. I believe that a skin interposition with an inverted V at the 6-o'clock position after spatulating the bowel segment in this area does much to prevent stricture and stenosis in the future. I have employed this routinely with good success.

Laparoscopic Ileal Conduit

Prepare the bowel, and insert bladder and nasogastric tubes. Mark the site of the stoma. Cystoscopically insert ureteral stents.

Induce pneumoperitoneum. Place the umbilical port. Insert four 10-mm ports, plus one 12-mm port for the stapler, spaced to allow access to both sides of the cavity.

Place long sutures, differently colored for identification, to tag the limits of the ileal resection; bring the ends through two right-sided ports.

Free the colon on both sides by incising the white line of Toldt. Manipulate the stent to identify one ureter. Encircle it with a vessel loop, and bring the loop to the surface. Elevate the ureter, and dissect it bluntly and sharply into the deep pelvis. Doubly clip the ureter, and divide it between clips. Repeat the procedure on the opposite side. Determine the length of bowel required by holding one end against the anterior abdominal wall and the other against the sacral promontory.

Place an ENDO GIA-30 or 60 stapling device across the bowel from the antimesenteric border. (Refer to pages 64 and 653 to 654 for stapling details.) Staple-transect it. With the same stapler, transect 1 to 2 cm of the mesentery. Make this a limited cut to minimize injury to a major vessel in the mesentery. Repeat the procedure at the other end of the segment. Deposit the loop caudally into the pelvis, avoiding rotation.

Trim the antimesenteric corner of each suture line with endoscopic scissors. Hold both ends, and pass the jaws of the ENDO GIA stapler into each limb of bowel. Be sure nothing is caught between the limbs before firing the stapler. Fire two loads for the ENDO GIA-30 or one for the ENDO GIA-60.

Close the end of the anastomosis with an ENDO GIA. Clip the mesenteric defect closed.

Bluntly (and gently) tunnel the left ureter under the sigmoid colon, being certain that it does not become twisted. Spatulate each ureter with the endoscopic shears. Elevate the bowel wall at the site of anastomosis, and cut a small opening. Fasten the ureter to the bowel with a 4-0 SAS, and run a separate suture to approximate the back side. Bring the distal end of the loop and the trocar out through the port in the right lower quadrant, and pass a guide wire and then a stent up each ureter through a cystoscope. Suture the front wall of the ureters with a 4-0 running absorbable suture.

Secure the stoma to the fascia and skin. Place a straight catheter with multiple holes in the loop. Place two suction drains through the lower quadrant ports under vision. Cover the anastomosis with the omentum. Terminate the procedure sequentially.

Commentary by Louis R. Kavoussi

To date, only a limited number of cases of laparoscopic ureter-oileostomy have been reported owing to the technical challenge of intracorporal reconstruction. As has been demonstrated in the text, a bowel anastomosis can be safely performed with the endoscopic stapling devices. The first aspect of this procedure is isolating the segment of bowel. A cloth or metal ruler can be placed in the abdomen to measure the correct length of bowel to be excised. Paper rulers tend to disintegrate in the moist environment of the peritoneal cavity. It is likewise crucial to try to demonstrate that a vascular arcade is present. This may be accomplished by disconnecting the laparoscope light and placing it behind the suspended segment of bowel. Unfortunately, in patients with a fatty mesentery, the brightness of this light may not be sufficient to demonstrate an arcade adequately.

The technique described is applicable primarily in very thin patients in whom the ureters can be pulled through the stoma site. With the availability of automated suturing devices, such as the Endostitch (U.S. Surgical, Norwalk, CT), intracorporal reconstruction is now possible.

Once the bowel is isolated, the distal end can be brought up through the stoma site. A right-angle clamp can then be passed through the stoma, and the site of the ureteroileal anastomosis can be selected under direct laparoscopic control. A feeding tube can be passed via the right angle and threaded up each ureter. The ureter can then be spatulated, intussuscepted into the loop, and fixed to the serosal surface. Longer follow-up and a larger series utilizing laparoscopic techniques to create urinary diversions are required to assess the ultimate benefit to the patient.

Sigmoid Conduit

BLOOD SUPPLY TO THE COLON

Conduits may be formed from one of the several divisions of the colon, each with a distinct source of blood, as illustrated on pages 680 to 681.

The ascending and most of the transverse portions of the colon are supplied by the ileocolic, right, and middle colic arteries (see page 680). The descending and sigmoid portions of the colon are supplied by the left colic, sigmoid, and superior rectal arteries (see page 681). Because the rectum after cystectomy receives its blood supply principally from the superior rectal artery, this vessel must be preserved when forming a sigmoid conduit.

For obese patients, a transverse colon conduit (see page 667), created by a similar technique, may be preferred, especially if the ureters have been shortened.

SIGMOID CONDUIT

1 **A,** *Incision:* Make a midline transperitoneal incision (see page 867). Usually place the stoma on the left, except when replacing an ileal conduit, in which case the previous stomal site can be used. Unless already divided as part of the cystectomy, isolate and divide the ureters below the pelvic brim. Incise the lateral attachment of the sigmoid colon along the white line.

B, Choose a segment of sigmoid colon longer than needed, as it shortens after division (6 to 8 inches is usually enough). Be sure it has a broad-based blood supply, but avoid interference with the superior rectal artery if a cystectomy has been done. Place a double set of stay sutures in the bowel at each end, one pair above and the other below the sites of division. Mark the distal end of the segment with a knot in its stay suture. Incise the peritoneum on the anterior surface, and divide and individually ligate the crossing mesenteric vessels. Mobilize the sigmoid colon from its lateral and posterior attachments as far as the sacral promontory medially and the inferior mesenteric artery superiorly. Release the splenic flexure if greater length is required because the loop must be rotated 180 degrees after it is created. Also, sufficient length is needed for reanastomosis. Unless a cystectomy has preceded the diversion, divide the superior rectal branch of the inferior mesenteric artery to give increased mobility to the distal end of the loop. Make the cut in the proximal mesentery very short.

Clear the ends of the bowel of appendices epiploicae and mesenteric fat. Divide the bowel with a knife; clamps are not needed. Wash out the lumen.

Open the parietal peritoneum over each ureter, and divide it low in the pelvis between a clamp and a stay suture. Make a tunnel bluntly under the sigmoid mesentery, and bring the right ureter to the left side.

2 Place the bowel segment to the left of the sigmoid colon. (If the stoma is to be on the right, leave the segment on that side.) Rotate the segment 180 degrees clockwise so that the proximal end is near the exit site of the ureters.

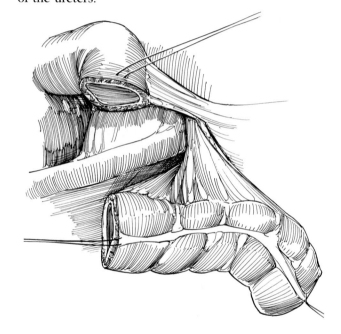

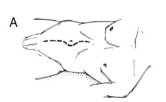

A

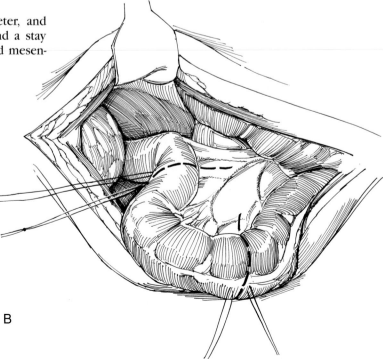

B

3 Close the proximal end with a Parker-Kerr stitch (see page 39) of 3-0 CCG plus a layer of 4-0 silk Lembert sutures (see page 38). Alternatively, use staples.

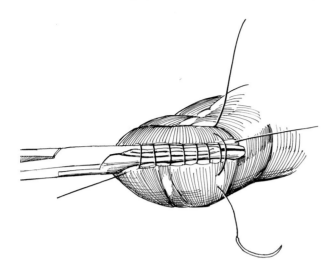

4 Restore continuity to the sigmoid colon with a running Parker-Kerr stitch of 3-0 CCG and interrupted Lembert sutures (see page 38). Alternatively, use staples (see page 64).

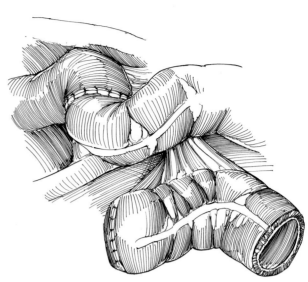

5 Bring the right ureter under the sigmoid colon through a retroperitoneal tunnel. Anastomose the ureters to the colon by one of the methods described for ureterosigmoidostomy (see page 717), making long (6 to 8 cm) tunnels and undermining the muscularis well laterally for each. Place 5 F infant feeding tubes as stents. Take care not to constrict the ureter when closing the tunnel; be able to insert a right-angle clamp alongside it. If insertion is restricted, incise the serosa and muscularis laterally as a T. Taper large ureters (see page 804). If one or both are very dilated, consider ureteroureterostomy (see page 804) with implantation of the single normal or tapered ureter into the bowel.

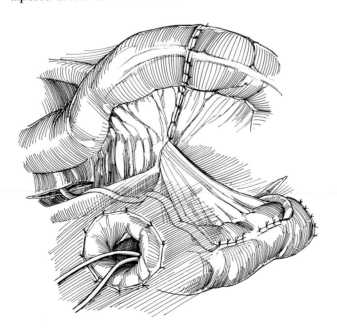

6 Construct a stoma by everting the end of the colon as a short nipple (see page 655). Fix the colon to the psoas muscle. Suture the distal end of the segment firmly to the anterior peritoneum at the site of exit (not shown) to prevent prolapse. Extraperitonealize the conduit with the lateral peritoneal flap. Close the wound with or without drainage.

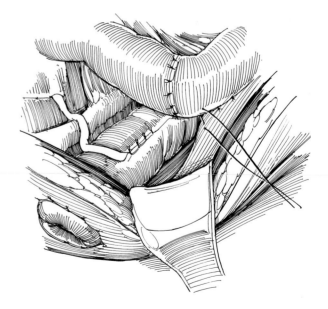

POSTOPERATIVE PROBLEMS

Compared with the ileal conduit, one formed from the sigmoid colon has fewer complications. Although *early leakage* is less common, *ureteral stenosis* is more likely to occur, making stenting advisable. Compared with ureteroileal strictures, those at the ureterocolic anastomosis are more easily dilated endoscopically. *Stomal problems* are seen less often, but the *antireflux mechanism* of the ureteroileal anastomosis may fail, accelerating renal deterioration.

Commentary by Klaus-Peter Jünemann

The development of large bowel conduit diversion was based on long-term experience with Bricker's ureteroileocutaneous diversion. Owing to the open refluxing system and stomal stenosis (up to 42 percent) with subsequent pressure increase and reflux, the long-term follow-up of patients subjected to ileal conduit diversion reveals chronic pyelonephritis and renal deterioration in up to 20 percent. In contrast, the ureterocolonic implantation in colon conduit diversion provides an antireflux effect, and the incidence of stomal stenosis is markedly reduced. This results in a lower complication rate on long-term follow-up, particularly in the upper urinary tract.

For these reasons, sigmoid conduit diversion is always indicated in children or young patients who require low-pressure urinary diversion, that is, children with meningomyelocele and a dilated upper system that demands a surgical procedure comprising antireflux implantation of both ureters. The sigmoid conduit has become an excellent alternative to the ileal conduit in cases in which future urinary conversion is already planned at the time of the initial surgical intervention, that is, bladder augmentation at an adolescent age, and in patients with Crohn's disease who are candidates for or wish to be fitted with a "wet stoma" urinary diversion.

Surgical procedure: Our experience has shown that a lower midline paraumbilical incision generally suffices to expose the sigmoid colon. If a greater length is required, the incision can always be extended to achieve release of the descending colon from the splenic flexure. It is important to choose a segment approximately 15 cm long because it subsequently shrinks. In cystectomy patients, great attention must be paid to careful and filigreed isolation of the sigmoid segment so that the remaining blood supply to the rectum—the superior rectal artery—suffers no adverse effect. During mobilization of both ureters, the blood supply must be considered in order to avoid or at least lower the risk of ureteral stenosis at the implantation site. Bipolar coagulation could prove helpful in this respect. At our institute, the ureters are always dissected down to the entrance into the bladder before division. This always ensures adequate ureteral length for ureteroileal anastomosis.

As in the ileal conduit procedure, mobilization of the ureters and isolation of the colon are easily performed, whereas achievement of an antireflux effect by implantation of the ureters can be a tricky procedure. We prefer the "open end" technique. Close to the proximal end, the conduit is opened within the tenia libera at the antimesenteric side at a length of about 4 cm. I have found the placement of four stay sutures, two opposite one another at a distance of 1 cm, and the other two in a longitudinal direction approximately 2.5 to 3 cm distally, advantageous for the formation of the submucosal tunnel. The dorsal wall of the conduit is perforated and a short length excised between the proximal stay sutures for insertion of one ureter. In order to construct the submucosal tunnel, the intraluminal site of the sigmoid conduit can be stretched by carefully pulling the proximal and distal stay sutures, thus allowing excellent preparation of the submucosal tunnel with small scissors without perforating the mucosa. At the end of the tunnel, the colonic mucosa is incised and the ureter is pulled through the submucosal tunnel and anchored with 4-0 Maxon in the 6-o'clock position with inclusion of the seromuscularis of the colon in this fixating stitch. Completion of the open-end ureteral anastomosis and closure of the mucosa above the ureteral entrance should be made with 5-0 Maxon absorbable suture material. Intraluminal fixation of the ureteral stent should be performed with 4-0 PCG suture because our experience has shown that, occasionally, stronger or other suture material does not dissolve on the 10th and 11th days when the feeding tubes should be removed. The implantation site of the second ureter should be positioned 2.5 to 3 cm laterally and slightly proximal to the former implantation site.

Tips, shortcuts, and cautionary measures: It is sometimes difficult to detect the blood supply of the sigmoid, making correct location and incision of the mesentery and ligation of the crossing mesentery vessels problematic. Should this be the case, a cold light source can be positioned behind the mobilized and raised colon, thus enabling identification of the sigmoid arteries emerging from the inferior mesentery artery.

Delicate preparation of the mesentery window is mandatory because severe complications can arise from hematomas within the mesentery. Staples can be used for reanastomosis of the colon and for closure of the proximal end of the sigmoid colon without increasing the risk of anastomotic leakage.

Commentary by Paul C. Peters

Richard Mogg of Cardiff popularized the use of the sigmoid conduit in modern times. He had noted the presence of a redundant sigmoid colon when performing urinary diversions on the sons of Welsh coal miners suffering from spina bifida. These children had large redundant sigmoid colons. It occurred to Mogg that he could use these colons to substitute for the conventional ileal conduit. Mogg and others thought that a better ureteral reimplant could be done into the colon (suburothelial tunnel) and that the incidence of renal reflux and scarring might be less than in the conventional ileal loop diversion. Also, a stoma made from the colon was larger and tended less to become stenotic than did the ileal stoma. With the passage of time, renal scarring has been shown to occur in conduits with or without demonstrable reflux and in colonic or ileal conduits (Kristjansson et al, 1995). Stomal problems do occur, although less frequently than with the ileal stoma.

Currently, we reserve the use of the colon conduit as an alternative to the ileal conduit. We use it preferentially for disease of the small bowel, such as regional enteritis (Crohn's disease), short small bowel for any reason, and bowel disease in patients who already have sigmoid colostomy and need a urinary diversion. We do not currently do a "wet" colostomy and only occasionally perform ureterosigmoidostomy in some exstrophy patients with insufficient bladders and some patients undergoing pelvic exenteration. Continent diversions have further decreased the need for colon conduits.

Transverse Colon Conduit

Creation of a transverse colon conduit, performed by a technique similar to that for a sigmoid conduit, may be preferred for obese patients, especially if the ureters have previously been shortened. It is especially applicable after pelvic irradiation.

Prepare the bowel and sterilize the urine if possible. Provide high-calorie and high-protein supplements. Mark the preferred stomal site(s) with the patient in a sitting position. It may be well to mark four possible sites, two in the lower quadrants and two in the upper, so that the stoma may be placed through whichever provides the easiest egress for the segment. Instruments and postoperative problems are similar to those for ileal conduit (see page 647) and sigmoid conduit (see page 664).

1 **A,** *Incision:* Make a midline incision (see page 867).
B, Transilluminate the transverse mesocolon in order to choose a suitable 10- to 15-cm segment, and place stay sutures to mark it. Dissect the greater omentum from the superior surface of the transverse colon. Incise the mesocolon, making the cut longer on one side (left side shown) for increased mobility.

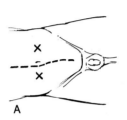

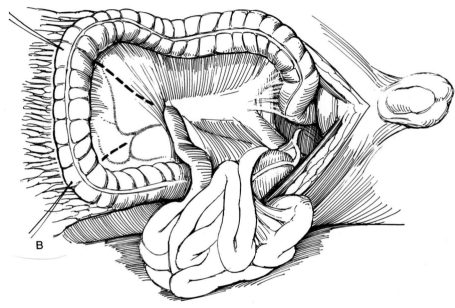

2 Divide the colon and reanastomose it superior (or inferior) to the segment by a suture technique (see pages 736 to 737) or with staples (see page 66). Approximate the mesentery with a few 3-0 silk sutures. Choose the portion of the conduit that appears better suited as the stomal end, and close the opposite end (see page 665). Fix the closed end securely to the adjacent parietal peritoneum near the midline. Incise the parietal peritoneum over the ureters. Mobilize the ureters, and lead them into the peritoneal cavity side by side through a suitably sited peritoneal incision. (If a ureter is too short, consider anastomosing the pelvis directly to the colon.) Trim the ureters obliquely to the proper length and spatulate them.

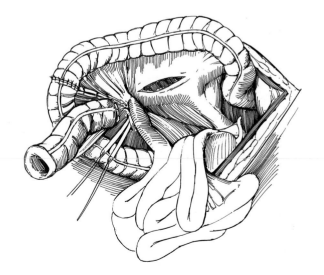

3 Incise the conduit along a tenia and anastomose the ureters with 4-0 CCG sutures, using a submucosal tunnel technique (see pages 718 to 719). Place stents if the ureters are small, if they are large and aperistaltic, or if the quality of the tissue is in doubt. Bring the inferior peritoneal flap up to cover the anastomoses.

4 Choose the site for the stoma among those marked that provides the easiest egress for the segment. Fashion a stoma (see page 655). Close the wound and place a temporary appliance.

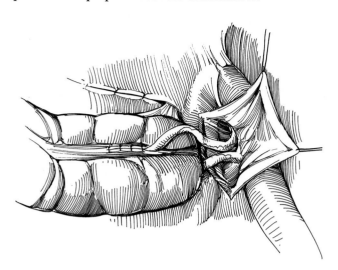

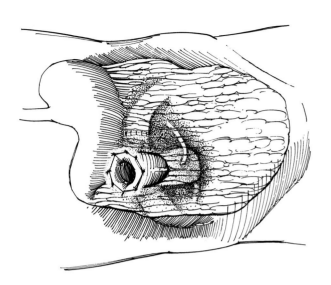

ASCENDING COLON CONDUIT

Divide the ascending colon beyond the cecum and again 20 cm distally. Restore colonic continuity. Bring the ureters out from the retroperitoneum in the right lower portion of the pelvis. Close the proximal end of the colon, and fix it to the retroperitoneum. Anastomose the ureters by a nonrefluxing technique (see pages 718 to 719). Bring the other end of the colon to the skin as a stoma in the right lower abdominal quadrant.

ILEOCECAL ANTIREFLUXING CONDUIT (Libertino and Zinman)

Isolate the cecal segment of the right colon with the ileocecal junction attached. Wrap the cecum around the terminal ileum to form a valve, and place the spatulated ureters side to side in the proximal end (Wallace technique, see page 661).

Loop Ileostomy and Colostomy

A colostomy constructed from transverse or descending colon has been the standard form of fecal diversion in the past, but a loop ileostomy has now taken its place because it is easier to do and provides better diversion, at the cost of the need to manage liquid fecal material.

LOOP ILEOSTOMY

For temporary fecal diversion because of problems in the distal colon or rectum, create a loop ileostomy as an effective substi-tute for a colostomy. (A sigmoid colostomy is an alternative.) The ileum is smaller than the colon, the procedure is simpler to perform and take down, and the stoma is easier to cover with a bag.

With the patient sitting, mark a stoma site at the summit of the infraumbilical fat mound, overlying the middle of the rectus muscle.

1 **A,** Approach the ileum through a midline incision, usually already created. Make an opening for the stoma as described on pages 654 to 655. Pass a small Penrose drain through the mesentery of the ileum about 15 cm from the ileocecal junction, and draw the loop through the opening. A plastic rod may be substituted for the Penrose drain but is not essential.

B, Incise the ileum for four fifths of its circumference on the distal end, 1 cm above the skin. Place 4-0 CCG sutures through the full thickness of the ileum and then through the subcutaneous tissue and tie them. Remove the Penrose drain or rod in 5 days.

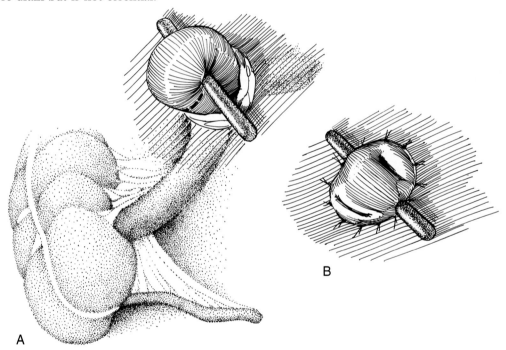

COLOSTOMY

A colostomy may be considered if the lower bowel is inadvertently entered during pelvic surgery.

2 **A,** Make a short transverse incision in the left lower quadrant through all layers of the body wall.
B, Expose enough of the descending colon to be able to select a mobile portion. Pass a fine clamp through the mesentery close to the colon in the center of the selected portion, and draw a narrow Penrose drain through to loop the colon as a sling.

3 Pass a clamp through the abdominal incision, grasp the ends of the drain, and gently pull on them while coaxing the colonic loop through the opening. Grasp the protruding colon with a moist sponge, and pull it out until the mesenteric slit is seen.

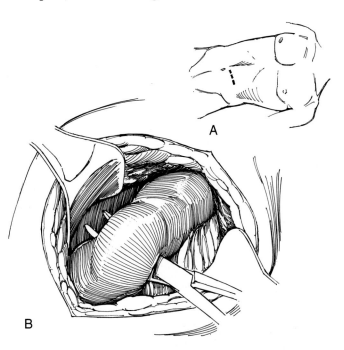

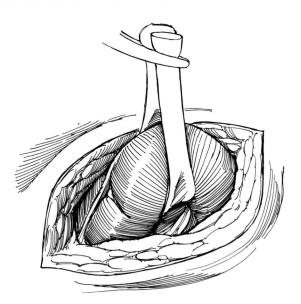

4 Run a plastic rod through the mesenteric defect. Fix the colon to the parietal peritoneum with two silk sutures that pass successively through the colonic serosa, the parietal peritoneum, and the posterior fascia. Suture the bowel at either end through the tenia to the skin edges with silk sutures. Tack the rod to the skin with braided silk sutures.

5 Two or 3 days later, open the bowel longitudinally, first with a knife and then with electrocautery, because entering intact bowel with a cautery may spark an explosion of colonic gas. No further sutures are needed; the bowel is now adherent. As an alternative, especially in the presence of distention, open the colon longitudinally and immediately after wound closure at the end of the first stage of the operation, and fasten the mucosal edges to the skin with interrupted sutures of 3-0 CCG. The distal end of the loop may be occluded by a row of staples. In either case, leave the bridge in place for 5 to 6 days.

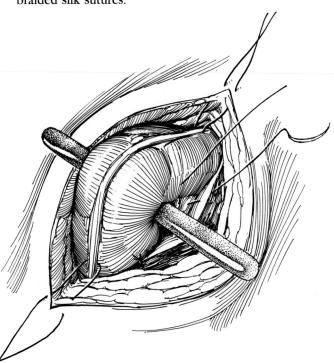

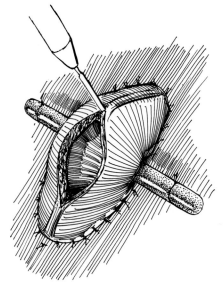

CLOSURE OF COLOSTOMY

If it has not been occluded with staples, cleanse the defunctionalized distal portion by copious lavage, using saline and then antibiotic solution.

6 Place a running suture to close the lumen of the colon. Incise the junction of the skin and the bowel, and free the colostomy edge. Enlarge the skin opening at either end for 1 or 2 cm. Separate the two limbs of the colostomy from the layers of the body wall by sharp dissection while maintaining traction on the loop with a Penrose drain through the mesentery. Locate the fascia, and free the colon from it by a spreading motion with the scissors; incision of the fascia is seldom necessary. Identify the mesocolon, and lyse its adhesions to the parietal peritoneum. Apply a noncrushing intestinal clamp and a Kocher clamp to each limb. Divide the colon below each Kocher clamp. Proceed with end-to-end anastomosis with sutures (see pages 736 to 737) or with staples (see pages 65 to 66). As an alternative, merely freshen the edges of the colostomy opening, and close it with a two-layer technique without excising a segment. Remove the Doyen clamps. Close the mesocolonic defect, and drop the colon into the abdomen.

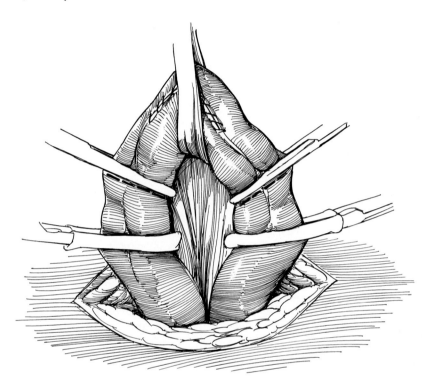

7 Start closure of the abdominal wound by placing a 1-0 polypropylene suture at each end of the wound to include the peritoneum and deep fascia and tying them. Run each suture to the center and tie them; make the knot with seven square throws.

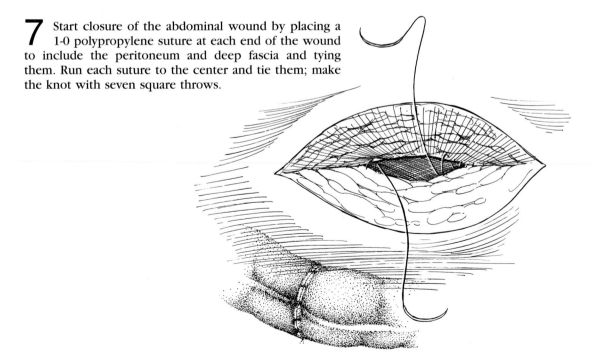

8 Place interrupted 1-0 SAS to close the anterior fascial layer. Insert three or four vertical mattress sutures of 3-0 polypropylene through the skin and subcutaneous tissue; cut them 15 cm long and tie the ends together, leaving them loose. Dress with petroleum jelly (Vaseline) gauze and a dry dressing. Alternatively, omit the skin sutures, and use only sterile skin strips.

On the fifth postoperative day, cut the knots from the ends of the skin sutures and tie them. The delayed closure reduces the chance of a wound infection. If there is any inflammation, do not close the wound but allow it to heal by second intention.

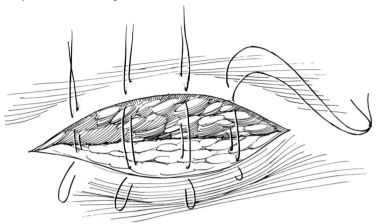

Commentary by Theodore R. Schrock

A loop ileostomy provides effective fecal diversion if constructed as described. The incision in the intestine must be on the mucous fistula side nearly at the skin level, and about 75 to 80 percent of the circumference should be incised. These details allow the functioning side of the stoma to be everted, so the ileostomy looks like an end stoma rather than a loop. If the intestinal incision is too far proximally, the stoma is flat, the appliance fits poorly, and the ileal contents tend to leak beneath the seal. I prefer to place a plastic ileostomy rod through the mesentery after the loop has been exteriorized. Rods made for this purpose have a T-bar across both ends. One of the bars straightens for insertion through the mesentery and then can be returned to the T configuration to hold it in place without sutures. I agree that the rod can be removed in 5 days in most instances. I like to wait 2 months before taking down a loop ileostomy; before that interval, the bowel is soft and the serosa is easy to injure as it is detached from the abdominal wall. Take-down of a loop ileostomy usually does not require reopening of the main abdominal incision. If the edges of the loop are trimmed, the defect is closed transversely rather than by resecting the segment.

A loop transverse colostomy, in fact a transverse colostomy of any kind—loop or divided—is an operation mainly of historic interest. Transverse colostomies are bulky and odorous, the output is liquid, and they tend to develop prolapse and parastomal hernias. If the entire descending colon and rectum must be resected to treat the condition, it is best to complete the total colectomy and construct an end ileostomy rather than an end transverse colostomy. If temporary fecal diversion is required for some problem involving the distal colon or rectum and the sigmoid colon is unsuitable for the purpose, it is nearly always preferable to create a loop ileostomy rather than a loop transverse colostomy.

Gastrostomy

Gastrostomy avoids the disadvantages of nasogastric suction because it is more comfortable for the patient and does not interfere with respiration or respiratory secretions. However, it does not necessarily prevent aspiration. The disadvantages are that it takes more operating time and it can allow intraperitoneal or cutaneous leakage of gastrointestinal contents.

Incision: Make a vertical upper abdominal incision to the right of the midline.

1 Select a dependent area of the stomach that is nearly free of vessels, as high on the anterior wall as is convenient. *Alternatively*, choose a site in the dependent portion of the greater curvature, approximately 5 to 6 cm away from the pylorus (marked X). Place one purse-string suture of 2-0 silk 1 cm distant from the proposed site and a second purse-string suture 2 cm from the site. Make a stab wound incision with a #15 blade. A short incision with a small opening is best because the opening in the mucosa always enlarges to admit the catheter. Aspirate the stomach contents.

2 Insert a suitable size (20 F to 26 F) Malecot catheter (will drain better) or a de Pezzer catheter (less readily displaced) stretched on a curved clamp, or place a balloon catheter, to a depth of 1 or 2 inches. Tie the inner suture while pulling the wings of the catheter up against the stomach wall. Have your assistant gently press the catheter in to invert the gastric wall, but not so much that the catheter slides deeper. Tie the outer suture.

Alternative: Elevate the stomach wall with a Babcock clamp, and make the stab wound and insert the catheter before placing the two purse-string sutures.

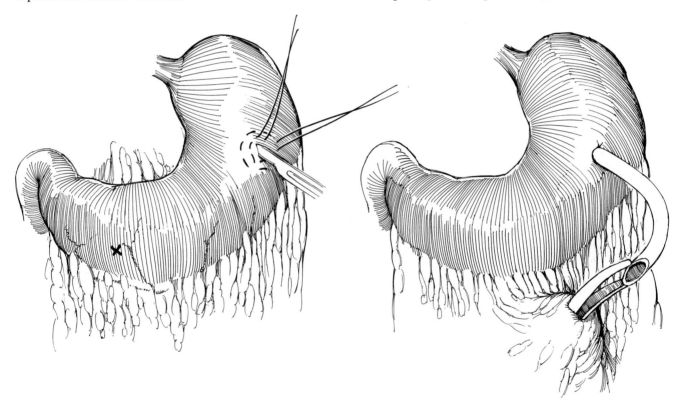

3 Lift the omentum up and fold it back to cover. Pass a clamp through it to grasp the tube and bring it through the omental opening. Let the stomach fall back to its normal position. It is not necessary to bury the catheter in the wall of the stomach beyond the purse-string, but it may be worthwhile to try to anchor the site of the purse-string to the undersurface of the abdominal wall, although the path of the tube intra-abdominally is sealed off quickly by adjacent tissues. Cut the end of the catheter obliquely. Grasp the end in a clamp, and pull it through a short stab wound in the left upper quadrant. Suture it in place with a 2-0 braided silk suture so no tension occurs between stomach and abdominal wall. Close the abdominal wound.

Start feeding immediately.

Postoperative Problems

Stoppage of drainage, usually associated with nausea, may be the consequence of a balloon catheter, if placed, falling into the duodenum. Deflate and reinflate the balloon.

Commentary by Donald D. Trunkey

Nasogastric suction is used less frequently than it was 30 years ago. Multiple studies show a high complication rate, and only a small percentage of patients require gastric drainage in the postoperative period. However, gastrostomy continues to be used primarily in patients with head injuries and neurologic disease states. It must be emphasized that gastrostomy may not decompress the patient's stomach adequately, and aspiration can still take place. This is particularly true in the neurologically impaired patient. In contrast to the technique described, I prefer to put the gastrostomy in the dependent portion of the greater curvature, approximately 5 to 6 cm away from the pylorus. I do not use an omental wrap and prefer to tack the serosa of the stomach to the peritoneal surface beneath the left rectus where the tube exits the abdominal cavity. This dependent drainage and anterior gastropexy may reduce the incidence of reflux and aspiration.

Appendectomy

In the past, routine removal of the appendix at the time of urinary diversion was advocated to prevent diagnostic confusion between appendicitis and a urologic disorder related to the operation. It was found that appendectomy did not add morbidity in these cases, but routine appendectomy can no longer be justified because the appendix may be needed for urinary tract reconstruction. Appendectomy is contraindicated during retroperitoneal lymphadenectomy because it increases the incidence of infection (Leibovitch et al, 1995). Appendectomy for acute appendicitis may be done laparoscopically.

Concurrent Appendectomy

1 Look for the ileocecal fold, the bloodless fold of Treves, on the antimesenteric border of the terminal ileum; it is an excellent landmark to allow easy and accurate identification of the base of the appendix.

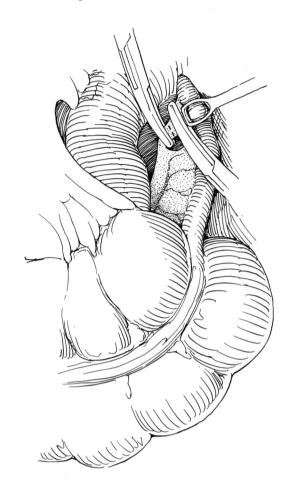

2 Divide the mesoappendix and tie both sides. Grasp the end of appendix with a Babcock clamp to assist in the dissection. Free adhesions. Pass a fine curved clamp through the mesoappendix below the most distal vessels; then doubly clamp the vessels in the mesentery and divide them to the base of the appendix. Tie the vessels on the mesenteric side with 3-0 SAS or silk. It is not necessary to tie those on the side of the appendix.

Place a 3-0 silk purse-string suture that enters into the submucosa of the cecum around the base of the appendix.

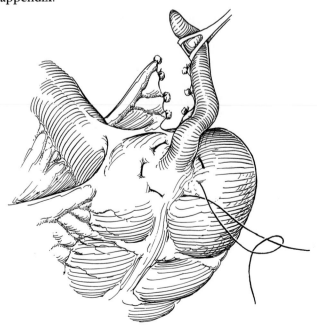

3 Crush the appendix at the base with a Kocher clamp; then milk the contents distally with the aid of the clamp, and reclamp adjacent to the base. Place a 2- or 3-0 CCG suture around the site of the crush, tie it, and cut it, leaving 0.5-cm ends. (Alternately, staple the base with the TA-30 4.8-mm stapler if the instrument is already on the table.)

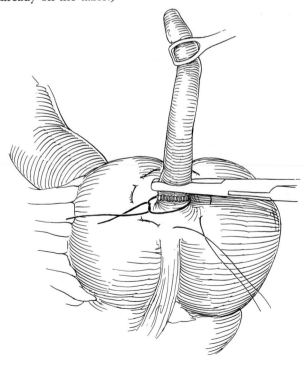

675

4 Divide the appendix proximal to the clamp. If the bowel has been prepared, it is not necessary to treat the stump further. Otherwise, coat the cut end with alcohol or organic iodide solution. Place the appendix and attached clamps in a basin to be taken off the table.

Put a clamp on the tie, and tuck the appendiceal stump into the cecum. Tie the purse-string suture.

5 Place a figure-eight 4-0 silk suture to invert the stump.

Inversion technique (Lilly-Randolph; Arango): With a normal appendix, inversion avoids possible contamination of the wound. Divide the vessels of the mesoappendix, clearing them down onto the serosa. Pinch the end of the appendix to soften it. Press a metal probe against the tip, and gently intussuscept the appendix. Withdraw the probe, and place an absorbable suture around the appendix near the base to ensure that it subsequently sloughs intraluminally. Place a silk Z or purse-string suture to invert the base. Reinforce this suture with several interrupted sutures.

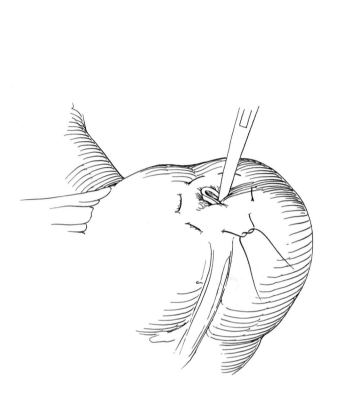

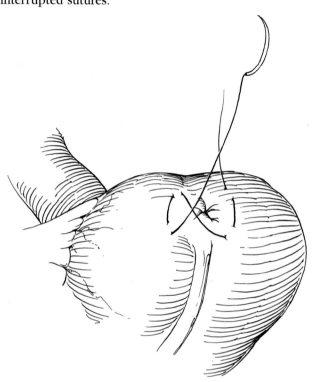

Commentary by Carlos A. Pellegrini

Laparoscopic appendectomy: The main modification that the technique of appendectomy has undergone over the last 5 years has been that caused by the introduction of videoendoscopic techniques. It is possible today to remove the appendix through the laparoscopic approach. I have used this method extensively and believe that evidence from other groups is increasing that laparoscopy is useful in patients who present with acute appendicitis because it allows a very thorough diagnostic approach to the acute abdomen and provides for a means of treating the disease with a minimally invasive technique. As for the diagnostic aspects, laparoscopy offers a unique way to examine the entire abdomen, particularly in patients who have not had previous operations. In women in whom the differential diagnosis with pelvic inflammatory disease is important, laparoscopy also offers diagnostic advantages. Therapeutically, laparoscopy offers the possibility of removing any diseased organ such as

the gallbladder, treating a perforated ulcer, performing closure of a perforation of the bowel, or removing the appendix.

From a technical standpoint, the laparoscopic technique can be performed using three entry sites: one for the telescope and two for the left and right hands of the surgeon. With these, most appendices can be easily removed. Of particular interest is that when the appendix is in a retrocecal position, the laparoscopic technique allows the surgeon to reach the appendix relatively easily by mobilizing the entire cecum and the ascending colon. The postoperative course of patients who have undergone laparoscopic appendectomy compares favorably with that of those who have had the open technique, although the differences are not as remarkable as with, for example, cholecystectomy. It is, however, probably the procedure of choice in most instances today.

SECTION

16

Continent Diversion

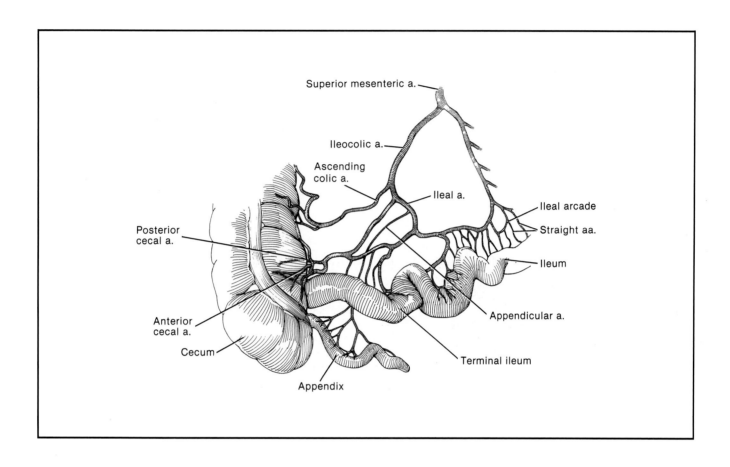

Superior mesenteric a.

Ileocolic a.

Ascending
colic a.

Ileal a.

Ileal arcade

Straight aa.

Posterior
cecal a.

Ileum

Appendicular a.

Anterior
cecal a.

Cecum

Terminal ileum

Appendix

Principles of Continent Diversion

Incorporation of intestine into the urinary tract can provide a urinary conduit if both urethra and ureterovesical junctions are gone (noncontinent diversion), it can provide a continent reservoir (continent diversion), it can enlarge the bladder if both the urethra and the ureterovesical junctions are present (augmentation), or it can replace the entire bladder down to the urethra (substitution) (Table 1). All require a bowel supplement of adequate capacity at physiologic pressure.

Because of the risk of overfilling and rupture, the ideal system for continent diversion would have a pop-off mechanism that prevents filling beyond 600 ml or 60 cm H_2O of pressure. The conduit should be easy to catheterize, and the stoma should be relatively inapparent. If feasible, the urethra would be kept as the safety valve.

BLOOD SUPPLY TO THE BOWEL

To use bowel in reconstructive urologic procedures, its blood supply must be kept clearly in mind. Two major blood vessels supply the large and small bowel. The *superior mesenteric artery* gives off in succession, working clockwise, the jejunal and ileal arteries to those structures; the ileocolic artery to the cecum, first part of the ascending colon, and the terminal ileum; the right colic artery to the main portion of the ascending colon; and the middle colic artery to the right part of the transverse colon. The *inferior mesenteric artery* provides the left colic artery to a limited part of the transverse colon and the descending colon, the sigmoid artery to that organ via inferior colic arteries, and the superior rectal artery to the rectum.

The circulation of the large bowel differs from that of the small bowel. The small bowel has a microcirculation that supports it after its straight arteries have been resected. In the large bowel, the straight arteries do not give off collateral vessels that spread longitudinally along the bowel wall so that more of the vascular supply must be preserved.

Table 1. Procedures for Bladder Diversion, Augmentation, and Substitution

Noncontinent diversion: neither urethra nor ureterovesical junctions present (Section 15)
Ureterostomy (cutaneous, loop); pyelostomy
Pediatric loop ureterostomy
Ileal conduit
Pediatric high ileal conduit
Sigmoid conduit
Transverse colon conduit

Continent diversion: neither urethra nor ureterovesical junctions present (Section 16)
Ileal reservoir—open: Kock pouch
Cecoileal reservoir
   Intact: Gilchrist, Mansson, Stevens
   Open: Mainz, Penn pouch, LeBag, Indiana pouch
Appendiceal urethra
Ureterosigmoidostomy, intact

Augmentation: urethra and ureterovesical junctions present (Section 17)
Ileocystoplasty—open: Tasker patch, Goodwin cup, hemi-Kock
Colocystoplasty—intact or open
Cecocystoplasty—intact or open
Ileocecocystoplasty—open: Mainz pouch, LeBag, Indiana pouch

Substitution: urethra present (Section 18)
Ileal bladder substitution
   Intact: Camey
   Open: Camey, Ghoneim-Kock
Ileocecal bladder substitution
   Intact: Mansson, Stevens
   Open: Mainz pouch, LeBag, Indiana pouch

Blood Supply to the Ileocecal Region and Appendix

1 The more proximal part of the ileum is supplied by a system of ileal arcades terminating in long straight arteries that supply the entire circumference. In contrast, the terminal ileum has a distinct and highly variable blood supply. It lies at the center of the loop formed between terminal branches from the superior mesenteric artery to the ileum and the ileocolic artery, a major branch of that artery. The network that branches from this loop provides the opportunity for several forms of distribution. The trunk of the ileocolic artery as it terminates gives off branches in several sequences, one being ascending colic artery, ileal artery, appendicular artery, and anterior and posterior cecal arteries. Alternatively, the ileal artery may be given off prior to the ascending artery, or the ileocolic artery may bifurcate into trunks to terminate as the anterior and posterior cecal arteries after releasing branches to the other structures.

Recurrent arteries may originate near the ileocecal junction from one of the cecal arteries or from the ileocolic arcade. These arteries that run along the antimesenteric border of the ileum can be important for the vascularity of the last 3 to 5 cm of ileum, where the straight vessels from the ileal arcades not only may be scanty but may be short and can supply only the superior half of the

ileal circumference. Contrary to previously held opinion regarding the risk of devascularization of the last few centimeters of ileum during bowel resection, a terminal type of vascularization that could leave the distal segment devascularized is not found. Sufficient straight vessels are present, and these are supplemented by recurrent arteries from the cecal circulation. Only a short segment that lies 1 or 2 cm from the valve is at risk.

The *surgical significance* of these details of arterial supply is that the mesentery must first be examined to see the orientation of the branches of the loop. For ileocecocystoplasty, it is especially important to look for a high bifurcation of the ileocolic artery so that the artery itself is ligated, not its branches; this leaves intact the arcades of the ileal artery and the ascending colic artery. Finally, the mesentery must be detached by dividing the terminal arterial branches very close to the ileum to preserve the smaller arcades.

The appendicular artery originates directly from the ileocolic artery (or its ileal branch) or from the cecal artery. Usually only one artery is present, but there may be two. The base of the appendix may be supplied by the anterior or posterior cecal arteries. The appendicular vein accompanies the artery to the cecal vein, which drains into the ileocolic vein. Chains of lymph channels and nodes along the arteries drain the lymph to the celiac nodes.

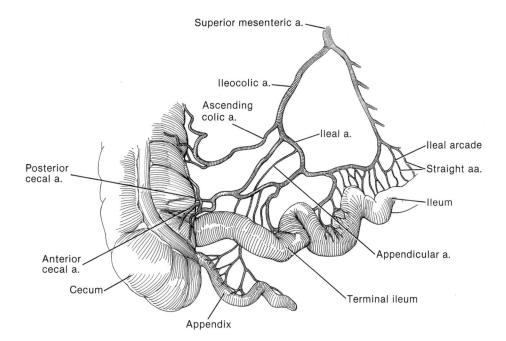

Blood Supply to the Ascending and Transverse Colon

2 Arterial blood to this part of the colon, a derivative of the midgut, is delivered by the superior mesenteric artery. Three branches are involved: the ileocolic artery, as the lowest branch of the right-side system; the right colic artery; and the middle colic artery as far as the hepatic flexure.

The *ileocolic artery* divides into a superior and an inferior branch. The superior branch joins the descending branch of the right colic artery. The inferior branch divides into the ascending colic artery that supplies the lower part of the ascending colon, the anterior and posterior cecal arteries that supply the cecum, the artery to the appendix, and an ileal artery that supplies the terminal ileum.

The *right colic artery*, which originates from the superior mesenteric artery cephalad to the ileocolic artery, divides into a descending branch that joins the ileocolic artery and an ascending branch that joins the middle colic artery. They supply the hepatic flexure as well as that part of the ascending colon not supplied by the ileocolic artery.

The *middle colic artery*, after leaving the superior mesenteric artery below the pancreas, divides into right and left branches. The right branch supplies the right half of the transverse colon and joins the right colic artery. The left branch supplies the left half of the transverse colon and joins the inferior mesenteric system through the left colic artery. Venous drainage is through the superior mesenteric vein.

Peripheral mobilization of the portion of bowel to be used allows the arteries to be identified so that they may remain intact and be encased in an adequate mesenteric fold.

The blood supply to the large bowel is more tenuous than that to the ileum and jejunum. Few anastomoses exist between the small terminal arteries, and the supply to the mesenteric side is greater than that to the antimesenteric border, especially because the long arteries become appreciably reduced in caliber as they pass under the antimesenteric taeniae.

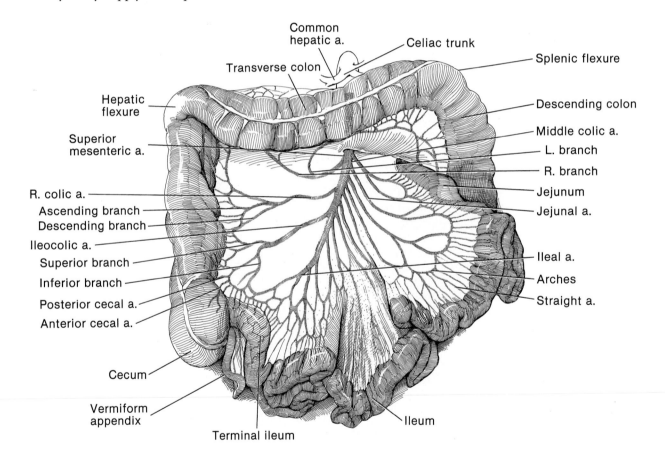

Blood Supply to the Jejunum and Ileum

As derivatives of the midgut, the jejunum and ileum are supplied from the superior mesenteric artery. This artery emerges from the aorta 1 cm below the celiac trunk and passes ventral to the left renal vein to give off 12 to 15 jejunal and ileal arteries. As these arteries divide and each member of the pair joins an adjacent branch, they form arches. The divisions continue until, especially in the more distal ileum, as many as 5 arches are developed to form an arcade. From the arches, short terminal arteries called *straight arteries* join the bowel, distributed more or less equally to each side. There they spread between the serous and muscular coats and give off multiple branches to the muscle. Successive vessels usually supply opposite sides of the bowel. After passage through the muscle layer, they join a plexus in the submucosa which supplies the glands and villi of the mucosa. The veins follow a similar course to the arteries and drain into the superior mesenteric vein. The mucosal lymphatics form a plexus in the mucosa and submucosa which drains the villi and the solitary lymph follicles in the wall. Lymph vessels (lacteals) drain either the muscle or the mucosa.

Blood Supply to the Descending and Sigmoid Colon

3 The inferior mesenteric artery supplies the remainder of the large bowel, the part that is not supplied by the superior mesenteric artery. Its first branch, the left colic artery, supplies a limited part of the transverse colon near the splenic flexure and the first part of the descending colon. The next branch, the sigmoid artery, after giving off the superior rectal artery, splits into two or three inferior left colic arteries that supply the sigmoid colon. The anastomoses between these arteries appear to form a "marginal artery" near the mesenteric margin of the colon. During resection of the right colon, because the anastomosis between the left colic artery and the left branch of the middle colic artery may be highly variable, the main trunk of the middle colic artery should be left to supply the transverse colon up to the left colic flexure. By dividing a major vessel close to its origin, circulation through the arcades formed by the marginal artery can be exploited. Venous drainage follows the arteries to the inferior mesenteric vein.

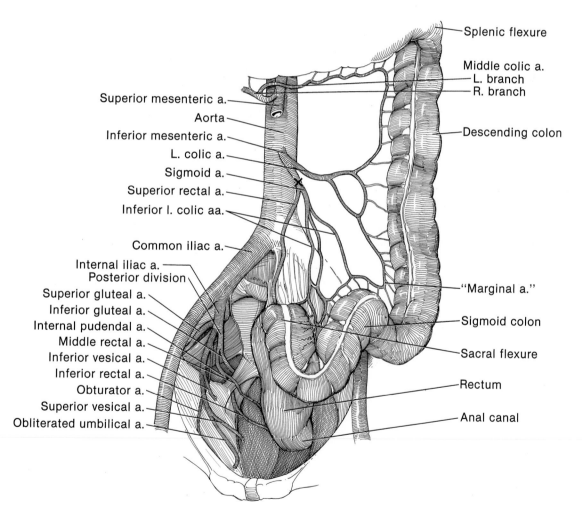

Blood Supply to the Rectum

The rectum and upper half of the anal canal receive blood from the most distal branch of the inferior mesenteric artery, the superior rectal (hemorrhoidal) artery. These structures are also supplied by the middle rectal (hemorrhoidal) artery, a branch of the posterior division of the internal iliac artery, and the inferior rectal artery, a branch of the internal pudendal artery. Venous drainage accompanies the arteries; that going with the superior rectal artery drains into the portal system. The lymphatics from the rectum accompany the superior rectal and inferior mesenteric arteries to the aortic nodes, whereas those from the anus drain to the superficial inguinal nodes.

INDICATIONS AND CONTRAINDICATIONS TO CONTINENT DIVERSION

The purpose of continent diversion is to improve the quality of life of patients who have lost a usable bladder. It may well not improve renal function or prolong survival. Ultimately, the patient must make the choice between simple conduit diversion and more complicated continent procedures, with older patients favoring the former and younger ones the latter, an overall ratio of 50:50.

Continent urinary diversion is contraindicated in some patients: those who have insufficient bowel secondary to intestinal or mesenteric adhesions, previous resection, or disease of bowel; those who would suffer adverse effects of loss of bowel length, especially children with neurogenic bladders, in whom resection of the ileocecal region can result in loose stools with fecal incontinence; those who have had prior radiation to the intestines; and those who are inadequately motivated and/or skilled to take care of the new system, which may require intermittent self-catheterization.

ELEMENTS OF CONTINENT DIVERSION

Continent diversion requires a reservoir, a stoma that does not leak yet can be catheterized, and usually an antireflux mechanism. Different parts of the bowel, including the stomach, can be used as the reservoir. Continence can be achieved by forming a one-way conduit by ileal intussusception, plicated terminal ileum, or tunneled ureter or appendix. The antireflux mechanism depends on the type of ureteral implantation.

Detubularization. Detubularized bowel segments provide a greater capacity at lower pressure and require a shorter length of intestine than do intact segments. The function of bowel as a reservoir is determined by its geometric configuration, accommodation, compliance, and contractility (Hinman, 1988). Geometric capacity depends on the fact that the volume of a reservoir rises with the square of the radius. Thus, folding the bowel once doubles its capacity, and folding it twice increases it four times. Accommodation follows the La Place relation: As the viscus fills, the stress on the wall increases, which permits the pressure to remain constant. Because the bowel is viscoelastic, it demonstrates compliance as it fills. Contractility is reduced by folding because the several components no longer contract synchronously.

SELECTION OF A BOWEL SEGMENT

Urinary reservoirs for vesical augmentation and substitution, as well as for continent urinary diversion, require adequate capacity at physiologic pressure.

The upper urinary tract must be protected by antireflux mechanisms constructed from intussuscepted bowel segments made by forming a flap-valve in the intestinal wall, by tunnel implantation of the ureters, or by providing a long proximal loop.

In selection of a segment, other factors than capacity and pressure need to be considered: tolerable electrolyte reabsorption and loss, accessibility of the segment, simplicity of the procedure, need for an antireflux mechanism, carcinogenic risk, and special requirements and age of the patient.

The preference of the surgeon is important in the selection because no objective data indicate that one region is better than another. The colon allows implantation of a normal ureter using an antireflux technique. Combining ileum with cecum based on the ileocecal artery allows formation of a mobilizable reservoir of good capacity free from mass contraction and an ileal arm to substitute for any loss of ureteral length. However, exclusion of the ileocecal segment from the intestinal tract in patients with neurogenic bladders who rely on constipation for rectal continence may result in loose stools and fecal incontinence, as well as later vitamin deficiency. After extensive pelvic radiation, a transverse colon conduit may be required. A segment from the stomach can be useful, especially in a patient with compromised renal function in whom electrolyte reabsorption would exacerbate the problem. The stomach is elastic; half of it can provide a reservoir with a 300- to 500-ml capacity.

SELECTION OF PROCEDURE

Several choices are now available for continent reservoirs (see Table 1), and more are being devised almost yearly. The list of eponyms provided in Table 2 may be helpful.

A continent reservoir constructed entirely of ileum, such as the Kock pouch, has the advantage of avoiding use of the ileocecal region but may be technically more difficult. Some form of cecoileal reservoir, despite its functional disadvantages, is the technique most often selected, especially after cystectomy, whether for malignancy or congenital vesical abnormality. The Mainz pouch uses ileum to gain capacity at low pressure, whereas the more easily constructed Indiana pouch must incorporate most of the ascending colon, although an ileal patch can reduce the amount of colon needed. The appendix interposed for a catheterizable stoma, as is done in the Penn pouch, is an alternative to using intussuscepted or plicated ileum. Ureterosigmoidostomy may be an alternative in adults without long life expectancies.

UNDIVERSION

Transforming an ileal conduit to a continent reservoir is often desirable, but it is not suitable for very young children (even though their parents may desire it) and for those without adequate motivation. Poor renal function is not an absolute contraindication, because undiversion may not only provide a better

Table 2. Eponyms for Reservoirs, Augmentations, and Substitutions

Camey	Detubularized U-shaped ileal bladder	769
Florida	Ileocecal pouch	700
Ghoneim	Modified rectal bladder	725
Goodwin	Ureterosigmoidostomy, transcolonic	720
Hautmann	W-shaped neobladder, sutured	772
Indiana	Ileocecal pouch	698
Kelalis	Ureterosigmoidostomy, spatulated	720
Kock	Hemi-Kock pouch	773
Kock	Ileal reservoir	686
Leadbetter	Ureterosigmoidostomy, closed	717
Mainz	Ileocecal pouch	693
Mainz II	Sigma rectum pouch	724
Mitchell	Gastric reservoir	705
Montie	W-shaped neobladder, stapled	773
Penn	Ileocecal pouch	699
Studer	Cross-folded pouch	774
Zingg	S-pouch	774

life but delay the time of renal transplantation. Several techniques similar to those used for initial construction of a continent reservoir are available that open the ileal loop and add it to the opened cecum.

PREOPERATIVE ASSESSMENT

The function of the bladder must be assessed with voiding cystourethrography and then cystoscopy under anesthesia. A small catheter can be placed percutaneously so that the patient can fill his bladder and report on volume, sensation, and continence.

POSITIONING OF STOMA

The stoma of a continent pouch, because it does not require coverage with an appliance, may be placed in a lower position, below the belt (bikini) line but not so low that it cannot be easily catheterized by the patient while sitting. Do not be concerned about skin folds. The umbilicus may be preferable because that area of the abdomen is thinner, it has less chance for parastomal hernia because of the backing by the rectus sheath, and the stoma is easier to catheterize, especially for the patient in a wheelchair. Preoperatively, mark the standard site and warn the patient that a ureteroileostomy may be all that can be done.

TECHNIQUE

Anastomosis of the bowel can be accomplished by one of several techniques listed in Table 3. Stapling has the advantage of being faster and provides safe closure and anastomoses. To avoid stone formation in the butt ends of conduits, either use suture closure or place a second row of absorbable staples distal to the metal staple line. The ureters may be anastomosed to the bowel by the several techniques listed in Table 4. Stent either with infant feeding tubes or, for interchangeability, with a 90-cm end-hole single-J stent. Insert soft silicone suction drains because leaks may occur at the anastomosis. Consider heavy stay sutures in obese patients and those with poor nutritional status.

Prevention of reflux from the reservoir may not be important if the chamber is large and maintains a low pressure. Although all of the antireflux techniques are successful, the tunnel techniques probably have a higher incidence of late stenosis than do the direct techniques.

Table 3. Bowel Anastomoses

Ileoileal	
Dividing ileal arcades	683
Sutured	
Single-layer closed technique	650–651
Single-layer open technique	651
Two-layer closure	652
Stapled	
End-to-end	64–65, 653–654
End-to-end, triangulated	64–65
Side-to-side	67
Ileocolic	
Sutured	
End-to-end	744
End-to-side	66
Colocolonic	
Sutured	
End-to-end	606–608, 736–738
End closure	738
Stapled	
End-to-side	66
Colorectal	
Sutured	
End-to-end	606–608

Table 4. Ureterointestinal Anastomoses

Ureteroileal	
Direct	658–659
Conjoined ureter	661
End-to-end	661
Camey	770–771
Ureterogastric	705
Ureterocolonic	
From margin	694
Closed technique	718–720
Closed technique with ureteral spatulation	720
Transcolonic technique	720–723
Serosa-lined extramural tunnel	775

Pointers in Technique

Division of Mesenteric Vessels. Preparing the bowel for anastomosis requires clearing the terminal portion of its mesentery.

With a fresh #15 blade, delicately divide the thin peritoneal layer of the mesentery on each side parallel to the bowel for a distance of 1 to 3 cm. Take care not to divide crossing vessels of the arcades as the bowel is approached. Keep the incision about 2 mm away from the bowel, and expose the straight vessels running from the arcades to the bowel. Insinuate a small curved clamp under the first straight artery that is encountered, and lift it from the mesenteric fat. Open the clamp with the curved side against the bowel, and clamp the vessel in its tip. Have your assistant place a clamp similarly on the mesenteric side. Cut between with the knife. Pass a 4-0 silk suture in a clamp around the vessel on the bowel side, and tie it with a square knot; do the same for the other end of the vessel. Continue these maneuvers until sufficient bowel is cleared to allow anastomosis. Be careful not to tear the vessels because a hematoma from subadventitial bleeding is very difficult to control. If a clamp slips and a hematoma starts to develop, compress the site for 5 minutes between finger and thumb, and then secure it with a fine stick tie.

Bowel Relaxation. Spasticity of the bowel or a thick short mesentery may lead to incorporation of more bowel than necessary when suturing the segment, thus reducing the reservoir capacity. Administering papaverine relaxes the bowel (Malkowicz et al, 1989). For normotensive patients, mix 300 mg of papaverine in 500 ml of saline and give an initial dose of 20 to 50 mg by slow infusion until a fall of 10 to 15 mm Hg occurs; then provide a maintenance dose of 1 to 5 mg/min up to the total of 300 mg. Calcium chloride reverses the effect.

Ureteral Implantation. Anastomose the ureters to the reservoir in as low a position as possible so that they do not kink as it is distended. Be certain that the left ureter takes a smooth curve. With large reservoirs, direct anastomosis without tunneling or other antireflux mechanism may be satisfactory and less likely to stenose.

Appendectomy has been done routinely in the past with diversion or supplementation because of the risk that appendicitis would affect the new system or would confuse the differential diagnosis of an intra-abdominal complication. Now that the appendix is appreciated as a continent stoma, it is no longer regularly removed, at least in children who might be expected to require further reconstruction, even though it is not associated with an increased risk of wound infection.

COMPLETING THE PROCEDURE

Do a definitive procedure at the first attempt, preferably through a very long midline incision, including transureterostomy with stenting if necessary. To use an omental wrap in preventing adhesions, place a cuff if an incontinence device is going to be needed later, and remove all abnormal tissue except the bladder, which may later be used for constructing a bladder neck, for the formation of a new urethra, or for future mucosal grafts. Good advice for re-do cases is to take the original diversion completely apart, then put it together using all your talents. The greatest error is not doing enough. For conversion from an existing conduit, take down the peritoneal adhesions and dissect the conduit from the abdominal wall. Excise the previous small bowel anastomosis, including the site of the mesenteric division. Be familiar with more than one technique so that you can adapt to the circumstances found at surgery. As it becomes more obvious that obstruction after an antireflux procedure is a more serious complication of ureteral anastomosis (8 percent) than reflux from a large, low-pressure reservoir, the tendency is to make shorter tunnels for ureteral implantation.

POSTOPERATIVE PROBLEMS

Postoperative leakage can be reduced if the bladder is filled to capacity before closure and the leaks are sutured. Leaks may be managed conservatively if the area is drained adequately. A percutaneous nephrostomy may be enough to divert the urine and allow healing of the defect. Decompress the conduit or reservoir even if stents are in place because they do not divert all the urine. Be certain that mucus is not blocking the outlet. Suction drainage (Jackson-Pratt) is better than Penrose drainage because it allows measurement of output, is associated with less contamination, and keeps the patient dry. However, suction drainage itself may prolong leakage because it diverts the urine from its intended course or, by contact of the tip of the drain with the anastomotic site, it prevents closure of the leak. Silastic single-J stents placed intraoperatively reduce the incidence of leakage.

Should *dehiscence of the ureteral anastomosis* occur, caused by inadequate mobilization of the ureter (tension), too much mobilization (ischemia and kinking), or failure to construct a watertight uroepithelium-to-uroepithelium anastomosis, conservative management usually fails and reoperation is needed.

Urinary retention from inability to insert the catheter (it becomes caught in folds in the conduit) is an emergency. Pass a coudé catheter or insert a flexible cystoscope and a wire over which a catheter can be passed.

Mucus collection requires vigorous irrigation in the immediate postoperative period but becomes less of a problem with time. Daily irrigation is then usually sufficient.

Bacteriuria is almost the rule after pouch diversion involving intermittent catheterization, but clinically important infections are the result of increase in the bacterial population from infrequent or incomplete emptying or from refilling from reflux. Training is necessary to teach the patient how to empty to the last drop, by aspiration if necessary. Urease produced by several types of bacteria, particularly *Proteus mirabilis*, fosters stone formation. Give antibiotics if pain is experienced in the region of the pouch associated with increase in contractions and incontinence. *Pyelonephritis* suggests upper tract obstruction and requires immediate sonography or intravenous urography. Giving antibiotics at the time of stent removal is good practice.

Early ureteral strictures at the site of anastomosis that are detected soon after operation in the absence of a stent may be due to edema or possibly to angulation at the site; a hematoma may compress the ureter. Percutaneous nephrostomy is necessary. *Ureteral obstruction* occurs later from local fibrosis after an early leak, although it may be caused by persistent cancer within or outside the ureter at the anastomotic site or by a stone. It may appear in the first 3 to 6 months, and the incidence increases with time. Obstruction is evidenced by pain, septicemia, upper tract dilation on radiographic studies, and an abnormal furosemide renogram. Try dilating the stricture endoscopically with a balloon, or incise and stent it. These procedures may also be done antegradely but fail in half the cases. Open repair with excision of the stricture and reanastomosis of the ureter is then necessary: Expose the ureter transabdominally where it joins the reservoir, resect the intramural portion which could become malignant, and reimplant the ureter by a tunnel technique (see pages 717 to 719). Alterna-

tively, approach the obstruction through the reservoir (Helal et al, 1995): Insert a ureteral stent antegradely, and fill the reservoir through a balloon catheter. Make a midline incision, and open the reservoir to expose the stented ureteral meatus. Place a traction suture and circumscribe the orifice. Bring 4 to 5 cm of ureter into the pouch, and excise the distal segment. Spatulate the end, turn it back on itself, and suture it with multiple fine sutures to the vesical epithelium. Leave a single-J stent in the ureter that exits from the reservoir with a balloon catheter, and place a suction drain adjacent to the repair. Because strictures may occur late, long-term follow-up is mandatory.

Spontaneous intraperitoneal rupture of a reservoir is a serious problem, especially as conduits are being made more leakproof. It is unfortunately not rare, and also, unfortunately, it is often overlooked until the patient, usually a child, is gravely ill. Voluntarily allowing the reservoir to overfill may lead to repeated ischemia at a weak point in the bladder, perhaps in the presence of peritoneal adhesions that induce a seromuscular tear. The patient must be warned of the virtue of frequent emptying and the dangers of overfilling. It is advisable that the patient not only wear a medical alert bracelet that states the situation but also has access to an 18-gauge needle to allow direct puncture of the reservoir in an emergency. By selecting patients who are willing and able to assume responsibility for care of the diversion, complications are fewer. For treatment, immediately decompress the pouch and, in most cases, explore the abdomen to drain the infected urine and repair the defect.

Deterioration of the upper urinary tracts occurs in as many as one fifth of patients if they are followed long enough. It is due to pyelonephritis, stenosis at the ureteral anastomosis, electrolyte imbalance, reflux, and calculi. *Renal calculi* are associated with chronic upper tract infection, and calculi in the reservoir or conduit accompany foreign bodies, usually metal staples, in the presence of stasis. Hypocitraturia, common in these patients, may be an important factor. Administer potassium citrate on a regular basis to reduce the incidence. It is possible to manipulate or fragment the stones through the stoma, albeit with some risk to the continence mechanism; direct puncture into the reservoir is an alternative. Finally, *carcinoma* may develop, although less frequently than after ureterosigmoidostomy.

Electrolyte imbalance with hyperchloremic acidosis and metabolic acidosis is especially prevalent in patients with initially poor renal function and requires oral bicarbonate supplements, at least for the first 6 months to 1 year. For patients unable to tolerate the sodium load, give nicotinic acid or chlorpromazine to inhibit chloride resorption from the intestine. Alternatively, substitute stomach for the bowel segment. *Osteomalacia* or renal rickets occurs from the chronic acidosis, more often in female patients, with the onset of joint pain and myopathy in addition to lethargy. Correct the acidosis and provide calcium supplements. Be especially alert for this complication in children.

Stone formation in the reservoir may eventually occur in as many as one fifth of patients. Some are related to foreign bodies (sutures and staples), some are metabolic (calcium oxalate), and many are related to bacteriuria. Regular irrigation of the pouch and increased intake of fluids can reduce the incidence. Other measures include prophylactic antibiotic therapy and acetohydroxamic acid therapy. Check for hypocitraturia in acidotic patients with struvite stones, and replace the citrate if indicated.

Stone removal: Remove the stones *transstomally* by endoscopic techniques aided by a guide wire; do the extraction carefully to avoid injury to the stomal continence mechanism. Use an electrohydraulic lithotriptor if necessary. A transstomal technique is not proper for the delicate narrow lumen of a Mitrofanoff stoma. Rather, approach those stones *percutaneously*, a technique also useful for large stones. Distend the pouch with saline, and insert the instrument where the pouch is closest to the anterior abdominal wall and away from the mesentery (the site determined by computed tomography if necessary). Leave a balloon catheter through the puncture site for a week, and insert a catheter through the stoma when the balloon catheter is removed to allow the hole to close. An open technique is seldom necessary.

Short bowel syndrome appears as diarrhea, malabsorption of bile salts, and vitamin B_{12} deficiency. *Vitamin B_{12} deficiency* may also appear after the terminal ileum is harvested. The deficiency needs to be detected by obtaining vitamin B_{12} or methylmalonic acid levels at regular intervals so that life-long parenteral supplementation may be given if needed. Carotene and folate levels also may be reduced and require supplementation. *Magnesium deficiency* may become evident with the onset of neuromuscular dysfunction and personality disorders.

Clostridium difficile infection is secondary to antibacterial suppression of normal flora, fostered by bowel stasis, and transmitted through spores from colonized patients or the hands of attending personnel. It is heralded by fever and diarrhea postoperatively, and overgrowth can result in pseudomembranous colitis. Diagnose it by finding polymorphonuclear leukocytes in the stool, detecting the cytopathic toxin in the stool by latex agglutination immunoassay, and obtaining a *C. difficile* blood titer. For treatment, stop the offending antibiotic and give oral metronidazole (Flagyl) first; if needed, give oral vancomycin.

For *stomal problems*, revision may be necessary. A good enterotherapist and a supportive ileostomy association are invaluable to prevent their development.

REOPERATION

Difficulty with catheterization requires reoperation with revision of the efferent conduit. *Incontinence* is due to failure of the nipple valve. If the leak is from a pinhole fistula secondary to failure to close the site of the aligning pin, close the defect at reoperation with a suture. For prolapse of the valve, repeat the intussusception with staples, and fix it to the wall of the reservoir with staples or sutures. Shortening of the nipple secondary to ischemia or effacement from overfilling requires reforming the intussusception. In some cases, a new segment must be used. After repair, fill the reservoir to check for leaks and to test the effectiveness of the continence mechanism. Also be sure that the conduit can be easily catheterized.

Intussusception following abdominal or retroperitoneal surgery on the intestinal tract is a rare complication and presents as prolonged ileus followed by symptoms of small bowel obstruction. The pain is not colicky and a mass is not felt, perhaps because the site of intussusception postoperatively is high (ileoileal or jejunojejunal). Immediate reoperation is required.

Ileal Reservoir

(Kock Pouch)

Evaluate the upper urinary tract by ultrasonography and intravenous urography. Determine renal function. Patients with deteriorated upper tracts are not candidates for diversion into continent reservoirs because of excessive reabsorption (serum creatinine should be no greater than 3 mg/100 ml). An ileal reservoir does adapt by decreasing the absorption of chloride and potassium, a fact not true of colonic reservoirs. Be certain that the patient is able to perform intermittent catheterization. Treat existing urinary tract infection, and start prophylactic antibiotics. Mark the stoma site with the patient sitting (see page 647). Prepare the bowel carefully. For bladder cancer, proceed with cystectomy, during which the ureters can be mobilized.

Instruments: Provide a PI 55 stapler with 4.8-mm staples, removing the six staples nearest the straight arm beforehand; a 30 F Medina tube; Prolene mesh; polyglycolic acid (PGA) mesh cut in 2-cm strips; two 8 F infant feeding tubes; 3-0 synthetic absorbable sutures (SAS); 1-0 nylon, 1-0 PGA, and 2-0 chromic catgut (CCG) sutures.

1 **A,** *Position:* Supine, slightly hyperextended.
Incision: Make a midline incision. Mobilize the ureters early, and ligate them so that they are dilated by the time the anastomosis is done.

B, Divide the mesentery between the terminal branch of the superior mesenteric artery and the ileocolic artery in the avascular plane of Treves. It is not necessary to carry the division to the base of the mesentery to provide adequate mobility for the efferent limb of the reservoir. Divide the bowel, leaving the terminal part of the ileum to provide for vitamin B_{12} absorption. With a sterile flexible centimeter tape, measure four segments along the bowel and mark each with a silk suture: 17 cm for the efferent conduit, two 22-cm segments for construction of the pouch, and a 17-cm segment for the afferent limb (13 cm for patients with existing ileal conduits and up to 25 cm for those with short ureters). In an obese patient, make the efferent segment longer than 17 cm.

Alternative (Kock): Use 15 cm for the efferent conduit (somewhat more in the obese patient), 2 15-cm segments for the pouch, and 15 cm for the afferent limb, for a total of 60 cm instead of 78 cm, because the reservoir enlarges during maturation. In patients with an existing ileal conduit, it may be possible to construct an intussusception valve in the conduit and insert the loop into the reservoir, for a saving of 15 cm of ileum. Tie these stay sutures loosely and trim the ends.

Incise the mesentery at the distal end to a depth of 8 cm and at the proximal end for a few centimeters. Divide the bowel between clamps 5 cm apart. Resect and discard the 5 cm of ileum proximal to the segment, along with a wedge of mesentery, to allow for mobility to be able to separate the pouch from the small bowel anastomosis. Close the proximal end of the segment (see page 38). Anastomose the ileum to restore continuity (see pages 650 to 652). Close the defect in the mesentery with a fine running catgut suture. If there is an existing ileal conduit, leave the end of the ileum open for anastomosis to the proximal end of the conduit.

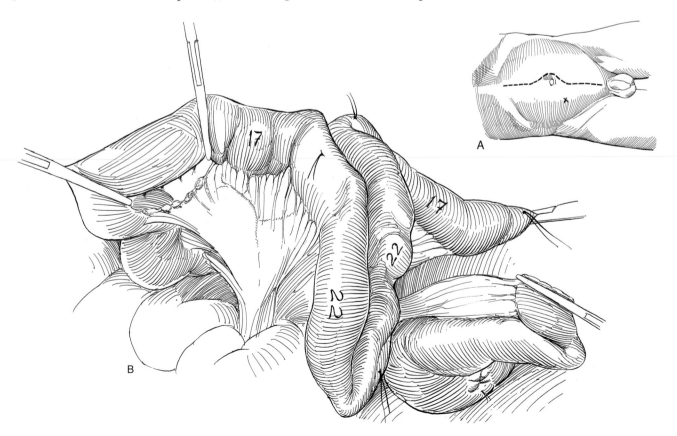

2 Lay the isolated segment on a moist laparotomy tape in the shape of an inverted U. The bend of the U should coincide with the marking suture that was placed between the two 22-cm segments. Sew the two sides together with a running locking 3-0 SAS such that the serosa 2 to 3 cm lateral to the mesentery is apposed. Insert a large plastic tube. With the electrocautery, incise the bowel onto the tube in a line 1 cm lateral to the serosal suture, first on one side and then on the other.

Alternative (Kock): To use less bowel in the suture line, omit the serosal layer, open the bowel, and place a single running suture as shown in Step 3. Extend the incision into the efferent loop for 3 cm and into the afferent loop in a curve for approximately 2 cm to allow the nipples to be staggered and to prevent the staples from involving the posterior suture line.

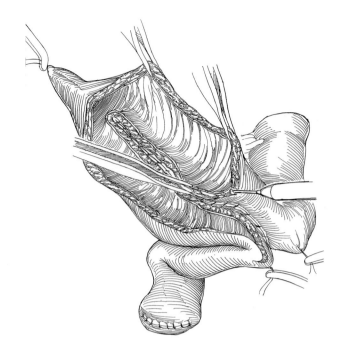

3 Oversew the edges of the back wall of the incised bowel with two layers of a running 3-0 SAS. The suture line must be watertight. (A second surgical team may then enter the field so that another surgeon, sewing one of the layers in the opposite direction, can speed this part of the procedure.)

Clear the mesentery cleanly from the proximal end of both limbs, the portions that will be intussuscepted, for a distance of 6 cm using Adson forceps and the electrocautery. Leave a little fat on the mesentery.

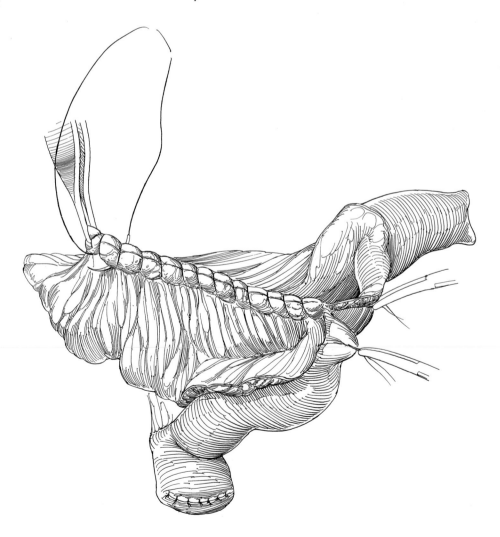

4   Pass a Mayo clamp through the mesentery of the
    efferent limb at a point one arcade beyond this
opening (about 8 cm), and draw a 2-cm strip of PGA
mesh through it. It is customary to do the same on
the afferent limb, although it may not be necessary (Mc-
Loughlin, 1991).

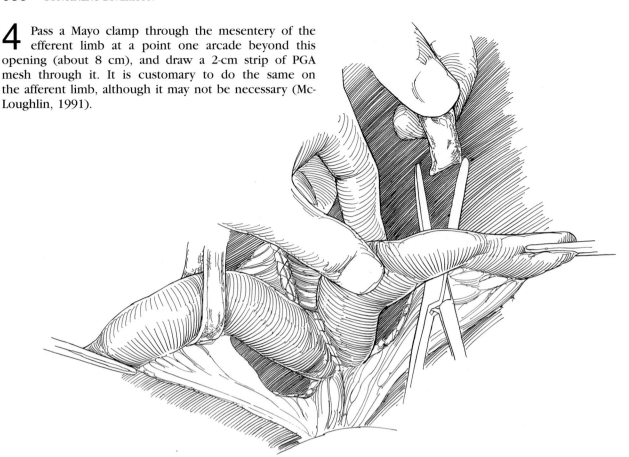

5   Create a nipple in both the afferent and efferent
    limbs. **A** and **B**, Insert two Allis clamps up the lumen
for two thirds of the way to the mesh, and grasp the
mucosa to intussuscept the ileum into the open pouch
to form a nipple.

6   Use a TA 55 stapler with 4.8-mm staples. Have the
    scrub nurse remove the six staples lying adjacent to
the straight arm before the operation, or choose a custom
staple cartridge from V. Mueller in which the six staples
have been removed at the factory. Use the pin in the
stapler to provide alignment. After stapling, be sure to
close the pinhole with 3-0 SAS. While suspending the
nipple with an Allis clamp, place three parallel rows of
staples within the anterior 270 degrees. Insert the stapler
to its full 5.5-cm length, thus ensuring a nipple at least 5
cm long. At the same time, be sure that the last staple is
at least 1 cm away from the mucosal edge so that the
pouch can subsequently be closed.

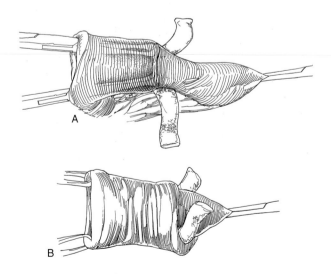

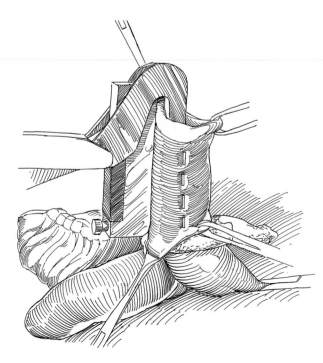

7 Place a fourth row of staples posteriorly to fix the nipple to the back wall of the pouch. Use the full row of staples. Insert the anvil up the inside of the nipple near the mesentery from outside the pouch; this fixes one wall of the nipple to the back wall of the pouch. Place a figure-eight nonabsorbable suture (NAS) at the tip of each nipple to further fix it to the back wall. Fibrin glue insinuated between the two layers of the nipple may be an effective substitute for some of the staples (Henriet et al, 1991).

8 *Alternate method:* Make an opening in the back wall at the site to which the nipple should extend, insert the anvil from outside the bowel, extend it up the nipple, and then staple it full thickness to the back wall of the pouch. Close the entry hole. Add a fixation suture.

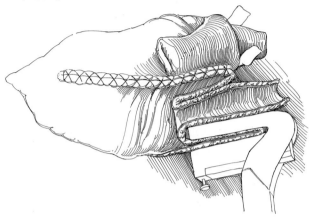

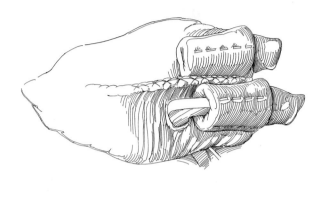

9 Insert a 30 F Medina tube through the efferent nipple. Soak the PGA mesh strip in tetracycline solution (250 mg in 10 ml normal saline), which will stimulate reaction around it. Sew it circumferentially to the serosa of the pouch and the respective limb of ileum with interrupted figure-eight 2-0 CCG sutures. The tube prevents the collar from being too tight. Trim the redundant mesh.

10 Complete the fixation with a distal row of similar sutures. Usually do the same for the afferent limb.

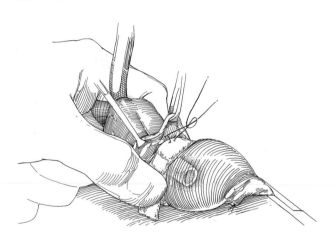

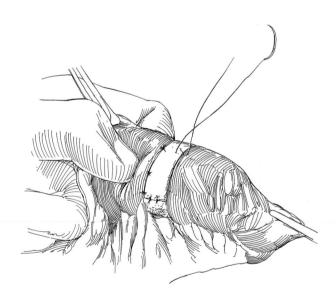

11 **A,** Close the pouch by folding it in the opposite direction from which it was opened. First pass a 3-0 SAS through the apex of the flap, then through the notch between the limbs, and tie it. Run this suture half way to the base, then across the base.

B, Finally, run it back again and tie it. Do the same for the three other quadrant sutures so that each one closes a quarter of the defect in two layers.

Alternative (Kock): First appose the apex of the plate to the notch between the limbs with a 3-0 SAS. Use this suture to connect the intestinal walls from the notch to one corner and a second suture running from the notch to the other corner.

Prepare the ureters, and anastomose them as described for the ileal conduit (see pages 658 to 659 and 661). Before the final sutures are placed, pass 8 F infant feeding tubes, with many extra holes cut along their length, to the renal pelves, and place the other ends in the pouch. Close the trap at the base of the mesentery with 4-0 silk sutures.

12 Adjust the site of the stoma in the lower quadrant or the umbilicus so that the efferent limb has a straight course to the surface. **A and B,** Remove a plug of skin smaller than for ureteroileostomy at the stoma site. Make a vertical incision in the fat and anterior rectus fascia, split the muscle, and incise the peritoneum sufficiently to admit two fingers.

Alternative: For an umbilical stoma, preserve the cup of the umbilicus, and anastomose the bowel to the juncture of the umbilicus with the fascia.

Pass a 1-0 SAS through the rectus fascia medial to the pouch, then through the width of the PGA mesh strip, then back through the strip at a distance of one quarter of the circumference, and finally through the rectus fascia of the corresponding quadrant. Repeat the procedure on the lateral side of the stoma.

Secure a strip of Prolene mesh 1 cm wide to the posterior abdominal fascia, lateral and slightly cephalad to the opening in the fascia. Bring this strip through the window of Deaver in the pouch mesentery adjacent to the PGA mesh. Pull up on the two sets of 1-0 SAS to embed the PGA mesh in the rectus muscle. Test for a straight run into the pouch with the index finger and

with the Medina tube (if there is any difficulty, redo the fixation). Fix the PGA mesh strip to the abdominal wall medial to the pouch with a 1-0 nylon suture. This permanent mesh acts as a strut to prevent a parastomal hernia and to fix the base of the efferent nipple to the abdominal wall, which also greatly facilitates catheterization.

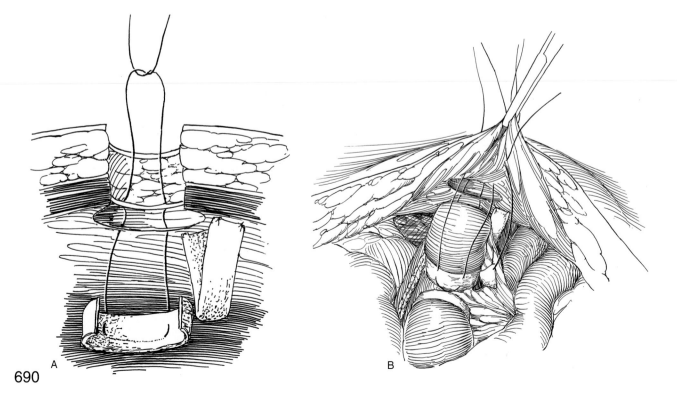

13 Trim any redundant ileum, and make a flush stoma by suturing the mucosa to the subcuticular layer with interrupted 3-0 SAS.

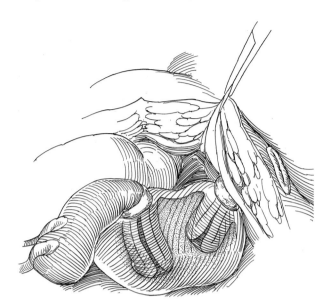

14 Insert a 30 F Medina tube into the stoma, keeping the drainage holes away from the efferent nipple and the end of the tube away from the suture line. Test it by irrigation and by observing free exchange of irrigant during respiration. Suture it to the skin with two 1-0 nylon sutures.

Mobilize the omentum on the left gastroepiploic artery (see page 71), and place it around the pouch. Draw two 2-inch Penrose drains through separate stab wounds. Fasten them to the psoas muscle a few centimeters from the pouch with 3-0 CCG sutures. Insert a Hemovac drain and a Jackson-Pratt drain. Flush the wound with water, and close it in layers.

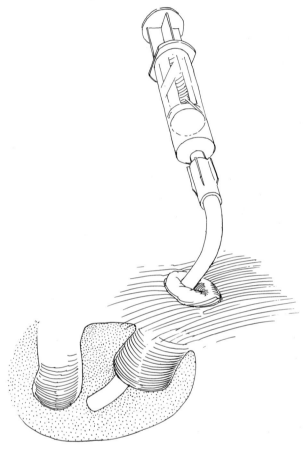

For *bladder substitution,* the Kock pouch may be anastomosed to the urethra after rotating it 90 degrees so that it reaches the urethra at the end of the suture line. In this situation, a continence valve is not needed.

POSTOPERATIVE CARE

Have an experienced nurse irrigate the Medina tube every 4 hours with 60 ml of normal saline to prevent obstruction from mucus. The patient should soon learn self-irrigation. After 2 days, remove the sutures holding the Medina tube, and place an ileostomy flange to hold the tube in place so that it can be rotated by the nurses to prevent it from pressing against any one portion of the reservoir wall, thereby producing ischemia and necrosis. At that time, remove the Hemovac and Jackson-Pratt drains.

Have the patient readmitted to the hospital at 3 weeks, and administer aminoglycosides parenterally. Inspect the pouch with a cystoscope, and remove the stents. Fill the pouch with contrast medium for cystography. Perform intravenous urography. Do not replace the Medina tube if the pouch is intact. At this time, remove the Penrose drains. Teach the patient self-catheterization beginning at 2- to 3-hour intervals, and instruct him or her to keep the catheter always at hand. Continue oral antibiotics for another month or two, and consider suppressive medication thereafter. Treat urea-splitting colonization aggressively. The catheterization interval can be extended 1 hour per week until intervals of 6 hours during the day and 8 hours at night are reached.

POSTOPERATIVE PROBLEMS

Leakage of urine from the Penrose drain for a period of time after operation is not uncommon. Check the placement of the Medina tube by irrigation or radiography. The drainage usually ceases in time. Drain a *urinoma* percutaneously, and consider insertion of percutaneous nephrostomy tubes if it persists.

Efferent valve malfunction causes the most trouble from this operation, occurring in 10 percent of cases. It results in incontinence and difficulty with catheterization. The incontinence is the result of a fistula secondary to ischemic erosion between the valve and the pouch. Treat it by creating a new efferent limb and valve after rotating the pouch because direct closure of the fistula usually is not possible. More commonly, incontinence arises because the intussusception fails to hold. Correction involves intussuscepting the nipple again and repairing it with more rows of staples, a new sling, and refixation to the abdominal wall. The valve may also prolapse, but this may be corrected through the stoma.

Difficulty with catheterization occurs when the pouch comes loose from the abdominal wall and migrates to one side. The entering tip of the catheter impinges on the fascial edge and cannot be advanced. In an emergency, if a soft coudé catheter cannot be manipulated through the angulation, aspirate the pouch with a needle. Occasionally, a catheter can be passed after the body wall has been relaxed by general anesthesia. After recovery from the acute episode, the pouch must be reattached to the abdominal wall.

Afferent valve malfunction is less frequent than that of the efferent valve, so reflux into the upper tracts is not a common complication. *Stenosis of the afferent valve* where it opens into the pouch may rarely occur. Try endoscopic balloon dilation. If that fails, treat it like a meatal stricture (see page 114): Open the pouch, engage the stenotic opening in a clamp, and sharply divide it. Suture the inner and outer edges of the mucosal lining together. *Ureteroileal stenosis* can occur, producing upper tract obstruction.

Urinary tract infection is not common, although bacteriuria is the rule. *Calculi* were a problem on exposed staples, but the incidence has been greatly reduced by omitting Marlex collars and using shorter staples. *Hyperchloremic acidosis* is rare but can occur, especially in patients with impaired renal function. Loose bowel movements are uncommon; if present, they clear after a while. *Vitamin B_{12} deficiency* occurs in about 30 percent of patients if they are observed long enough. Supplements should be provided at 5-year intervals.

Commentary by Nils G. Kock

The dynamic revolution of urinary diversion and orthotopic bladder reconstruction during the past three decades has greatly changed the life situation of patients needing cystectomy and those with severe malfunction of the lower urinary tract.

Currently cystectomy is not necessarily followed by uncontrolled urinary outflow—that is, incontinence—for the lifetime of the patient. When the urethra can be used for orthotopic bladder reconstruction, this should be the first option, but where this is not possible, continence still can be achieved by diversion of the urine either to the augmented and valved rectum or to the skin surface via a continent intestinal reservoir.

Various types of intestinal reservoirs have been advocated and different parts of the gastrointestinal tract used for construction of the pouch, and it is therefore difficult for the surgeon to decide which method is preferable.

The optimal intestinal reservoir for urinary storage should fulfill the following requirements:
1. Low pressure even at large volumes
2. Minimum reabsorption of urinary constituents
3. Minor sequelae from harvesting the intestinal segment

The ileal reservoir seems to have the lowest pressure at the largest volume. Owing to the remarkable morphologic changes of the ileal mucosa after exposure to urine, the reabsorption decreases with time. Hyperchloremic acidosis is uncommon, and bicarbonates are generally not needed. The ileal reservoir expands to the needed volume, meaning that only the amount of intestine necessary for the surgical construction must be harvested.

These characteristics of the ileal reservoir are not only a prerequisite for achieving continence and convenient emptying intervals but also a qualification for preservation of the upper urinary tract.

To date it is not possible to categorically recommend one type of bladder substitute over another, although I believe that data in favor of the ileal spheric reservoir are slowly accumulating.

Ileocecal Reservoir

MAINZ POUCH

Urologists who know more than one technique are equipped to adapt to unanticipated findings.

Locate the stomal site before operation. Patients may prefer to catheterize the penis, perineum, or umbilicus, the last being especially suitable for the obese or wheelchair-bound patient.

1 **A,** *Incision:* Stand on the right side of the table. Make a long midline incision (see page 867). Mobilize the cecum and ascending colon all the way beyond the hepatic flexure.

B, Starting from the cecum, measure 10 to 15 cm on the ascending colon and mark that point with a stay suture. Measure and mark three segments on the ileum starting at the ileocecal valve: 10 to 15 cm, 10 to 15 cm, and 20 to 25 cm. Divide the mesentery of the ascending colon above the ileocolic artery and the mesentery of the ileum at the most proximal stay suture; then divide the bowel at each end.

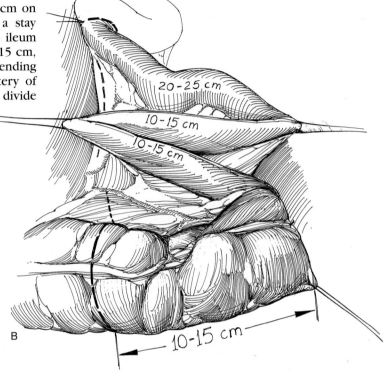

2 Spatulate the antimesenteric border of the ileum, and anastomose it to the cecum with staples using the EEA and TA 55 staplers as described on page 66. Let the loop drop behind the anastomosis; do not leave it anterior to the anastomosis as is done with ureteroileostomy.

3 Irrigate the bowel segment and open the cecum and ileum on the antimesenteric border with scissors, but leave the proximal 20 to 25 cm of ileum intact to provide for the construction of nipple and stoma.

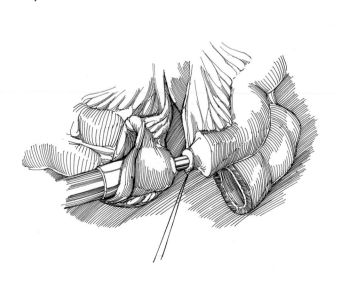

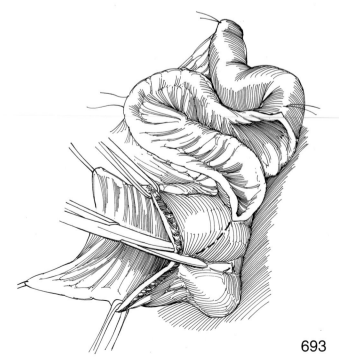

4 **A,** Suture the medial edge of the ascending colon to the first part of the ileum; then suture that first ileal segment to the second, as identified by the marking stay sutures. Use a single row of through-and-through running 4-0 SAS swaged on a straight needle. Mobilize the left ureter to the level of the lower pole of the kidney, insert a stay suture, and pull it through retroperitoneally below the duodenum. The right ureter needs less dissection and remains retroperitoneally.

B, Mark the site of *ureteral implantation* with four stay sutures through the mucosa and submucosa placed at the margin of the opened segment to tent the edges.

Enter the free edge between submucosa and mucosa with blunt-tipped scissors, and form a 4- to 5-cm pocket. Invert the scissors, and cut down on the tip with a knife.

C, Insert a clamp through this opening, and direct it back to the free edge. Grasp the ureteral stay suture, and draw the ureter into the tunnel. Spatulate it, fasten the tip to the submucosa and muscularis with a deep stitch, and approximate the edges epithelium to mucosa. Tack the ureter at its site of entry into the tunnel. Repeat the procedure for the second ureter. Place a 6 F or 8 F infant feeding tube in each, and bring the ends of the tubes out through the intact portion of bowel.

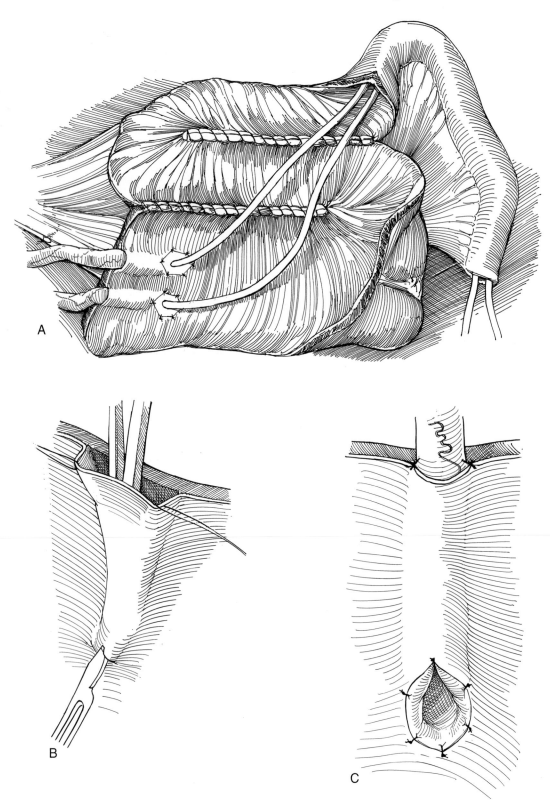

Intussuscepted Ileal Valve

5 Make a 6-cm window in the mesentery midway in the unopened segment, and make a smaller window half way out from the midpoint.

6 Invaginate the bowel with two Allis clamps, and place three or four rows of 4.8-mm metal staples by inserting the TA 55 stapler from outside the pouch at the base of the intussusception into the space between the inner and outer walls.

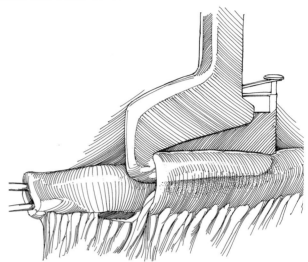

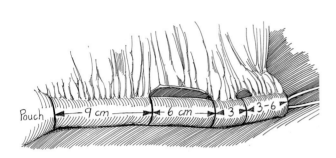

7 Close the anterior wall of the pouch in a single layer with a running stitch of 3-0 SAS. At the sites of ureteral exit, take care to close only the mucosa and to use interrupted sutures in that area.

8 Stretch the ileal spout lengthwise because it will have contracted during the operation. Run a 2-cm strip of PGA mesh through the second mesenteric window and around the ileum. Fix it in place with multiple interrupted 3-0 SAS on both sides. Make an opening in the body wall (see pages 708 to 709), the umbilicus, or the right lower quadrant within the future hair line. Place three mattress sutures in the mesh, and fasten them to the external oblique or rectus fascia.

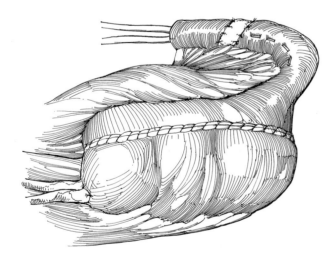

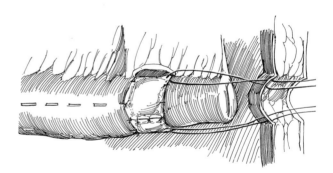

9 Trim excess ileum and suture the ileum flush with the skin with sutures that include mucosa and submucosa, then some muscularis proximal to the edge, and finally the skin edge. Remove the retractor after the intussusception has been sutured in place, to allow the abdominal wound to assume its normal alignment for a trial of catheterization of the new stoma.

Irrigate and test for leaks. Drain the pouch with a 26 F 5-ml balloon catheter, and drain the site of ureteral anastomosis with a Jackson-Pratt drain on gravity drainage. Cycle the reservoir with 20 to 30 ml of saline three times a day while the patient is in the hospital. Remove the stents one at a time in 10 days and the catheter in 2 to 3 weeks. If a suprapubic tube is used, be sure to keep it clamped when the urethral catheter is removed so that urination prevents the anastomosis from sealing.

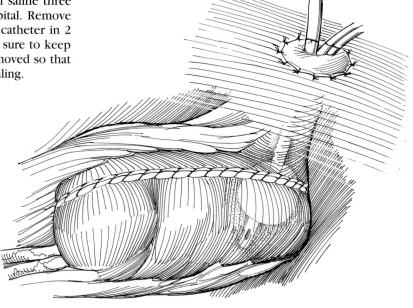

Intussusception Through the Ileocecal Valve

10 Open the loop of ileum and the cecum as shown in Step 3, but preserve the portion of cecum containing the ileocecal valve.

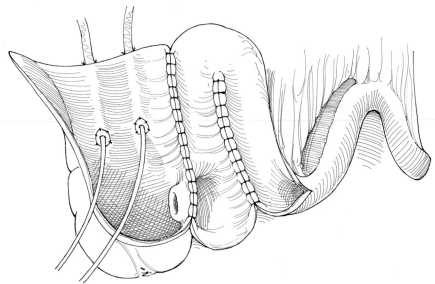

11 Intussuscept the ileum, and fix it with two rows of staples. Denude a portion of mucosa over the intussuscepted segment.

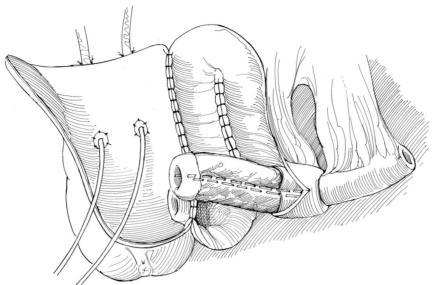

12 Draw the intussuscepted ileum through the ileocecal valve, and fix it with a third row of staples. Proceed as in Steps 7, 8, and 9.

Alternative (Mraz et al, 1994): Construct a flap-valve from an 18-cm segment of ileum by bringing 4 cm of the end that has been cut diagonally through an opening in the cecal wall. Anchor it circumferentially to the wall intraluminally at the site of entrance. Make two parallel mucosal incisions in the wall of the cecum, each beginning beside the site of ileal entrance. Suture the edges of the diagonal cut to the mucosal edges, making a flap-valve.

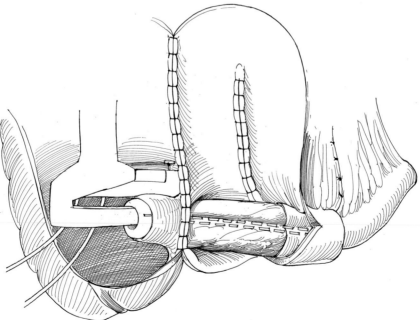

MAINZ POUCH WITH APPENDICEAL STOMA

Check the appendix to be sure that it has not been inflamed and is of adequate length and caliber.

Proceed through Steps 1 to 4, but do not open the last 4 cm of the cecum. Close the pouch (Step 7). Clean the mesentery of the appendix to skeletonize the vessels while preserving the appendicular artery on a branch of the anterior or posterior cecal artery. As shown on page 711, form a trough in the cecum that ends at the base of the appendix by incising the seromuscular layer of the taenia libera to the depth of the mucosa. Turn the appendix up, and embed it in the trough. Close the seromuscular layer over it with 2-0 SAS.

Make a V-plasty in the umbilicus to form a funnel for connection of the skin to the appendix. Attach the pouch to the anterior abdominal wall to keep the course of the appendix straight.

IN SITU TUNNELED BOWEL FLAP TUBES

Techniques other than intussusception are available to achieve continence (Lampel et al, 1995). *Seromuscular bowel flap tube:* Make a tube from a seromuscular bowel flap in the lower pole of the cecum, anastomose one end to an opening in the cecum, bury it in the cecal wall, and bring the other end to the skin as a stoma. *Full-thickness bowel flap tube:* Raise a full-thickness flap from the wall of the cecum, and form it into a tube. Close the resulting defect in the cecum, and place the tube in a submucosal tunnel extending laterally on the cecum.

INDIANA POUCH

Mobilize the left ureter adequately, preserving the adventitia, and pass it cephalad without twisting to the level of the inferior mesenteric artery and through the mesentery of the reservoir. The right ureter can be freed less extensively.

13 **A,** Isolate a 25- to 30-cm segment of cecum and ascending colon plus the entire hepatic flexure in addition to 8 to 10 cm of terminal ileum. Be sure not to make the reservoir too small. Split the ascending colon and cecum down its antimesenteric border to within 2 cm of the caudal tip. For more complete *detubularization,* open the bowel the full length of the taenia libera, and encircle the appendiceal base as an appendectomy (Ahlering et al, 1991).

B, Perform ileocolostomy by a suture technique (see page 744) or by a staple method (see page 66). Insert the ureters by a submucosal technique.

C, Place a Malecot catheter through the wall of the lowest part of the complex in a position to allow direct exit through the abdominal wall. Close the U-shaped defect by folding the distal portion of the colon into the proximal end and suturing it in place with a running 3-0 SAS to the mucosa and some of the muscularis. Add a serosal Lembert stitch (see page 38) with occasional lock stitches. Leave the ileum to form the cutaneous conduit with tapering, as shown in Step 18 or 19.

Alternatively, if the cecum and ascending colon prove to be too short or especially narrow in diameter, take an additional 15- to 20-cm segment of ileum, open it, and place it as a patch over the open cecum to augment the reservoir. Or take a longer segment of ileum and use the proximal part for an intussuscepted conduit (Bellevue pouch). Alternatively, tunnel the appendix into a taenia to serve as the conduit (see page 711) and so release the terminal ileum for use as a patch.

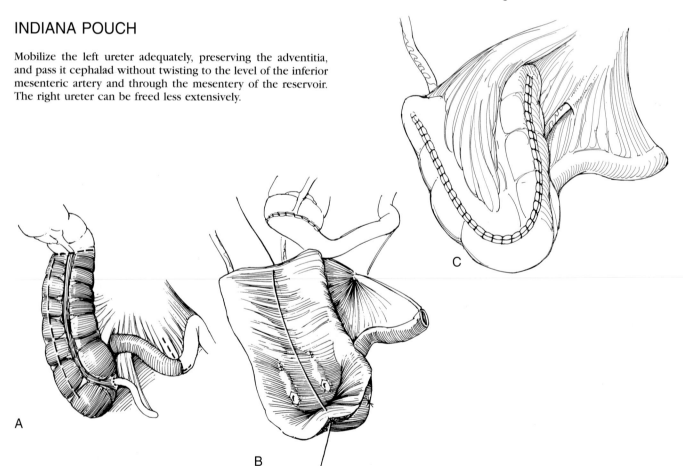

PENN POUCH WITH APPENDICEAL STOMA
(Duckett)

14 Open 30 cm of colon on the mesocolic tenia and 20 cm of ileum on its antimesenteric border to prepare a cecal pouch. Fold the ileum into a U, and suture the edges with 3-0 running SAS. Insert the ileal patch into the cecal defect. Fold the distal end of the cecum to complete the pouch. If the mesoappendix is mobile and vascularized, excise the base of the appendix, taking a generous disk of cecum while preserving the mesentery of the appendix. Close the cecal defect in two layers. Implant the ureters into the cecum by an antireflux method (see pages 718 to 720).

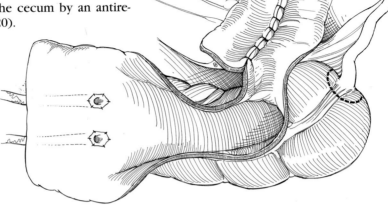

15 Rotate the appendix on its mesentery, and trim its tip. Calibrate it with a bougie à boule, continuing to trim the end until an adequate lumen is reached. Create an 8-cm trough in the most accessible taenia of the seromuscular wall of the ascending colon, laying back flaps and exposing submucosa for a width of 2 or 3 cm. The trough can be widened by grasping the bowel wall on either side and gently pulling it open. Open the mucosa at the distal end of the groove, and anastomose the opened tip of the appendix with interrupted 4-0 SAS. Close the lateral seromuscular flaps over the appendix with 3-0 SAS, taking care not to constrict its mesentery in the tunnel. Three to 4 cm within the tunnel is sufficient to produce continence.

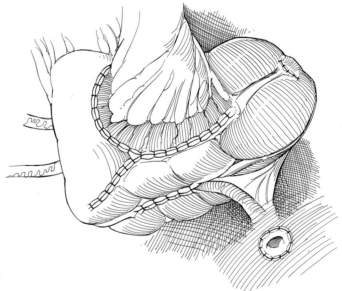

Lead the base of the appendix through the body wall in an appropriate site in the left lower quadrant, and suture it to the skin. Alternately, shorten the appendix and place it with a V flap in the umbilicus to hide it. Hitch the cecum and ascending colon to the retroperitoneum so that the appendix and its mesentery are not kinked. If this procedure is used for bladder augmentation, fix the bladder to the psoas muscle so that the appendiceal mesentery does not move during bladder filling. Place a Moreno tube to drain mucus from the pouch, of a size not so large that it stretches the appendix. Close the wound appropriately.

The appendix may be buried without detachment from the cecum, as described above under "Mainz Pouch with Appendiceal Stoma," or reinforced at its junction with the cecum (Bissada, 1993), although it may then be more difficult to catheterize.

FLORIDA POUCH
(Lockhart)

16 This pouch has a configuration similar to that of the Indiana pouch but has a greater capacity because it includes more colon and becomes more spherical. Incise the parietal peritoneum and gastrocolic ligament to mobilize the right colon, the hepatic flexure, and the right half of the transverse colon. Leave the middle colic artery within the left portion of the transverse mesocolon. Reconstitute the colon by a lateral anastomosis between ileum and transverse colon, end to end (see page 744) or end to side (see page 66).

A, Open the colonic segment on the antimesenteric border. Fold it into a U shape, and suture the inner edges with a running locking 3-0 SAS.

B, Anastomose the ureters to the colon by a standard technique (see pages 718 to 720). Suture the lateral edges of the colonic U to form a large-bore tube, and then close the end of the tube with sutures. Reduce the diameter of the ileum (Step 18 or 19), and bring it through the abdominal wall.

Alternatively, before opening the colonic segment, fold it double and attach the adjacent walls with interrupted sutures. Insert the GIA stapler into the double-barrelled end, and fire the staples for a side-to-side anastomosis (see page 67). Place a suture on either side at the apex of the staple line to hold the mucosa, reinsert the stapler, and divide a second portion of the septum as in the Olsson technique (Step 17). Repeat the stapling to the end of the U. Proceed with closure of the loop.

Conversion from a ureteroileostomy (Florida pouch II, Pow-Sang): Partially open the end of an ileal conduit on the antimesenteric border, and apply it as a patch to the open lower end of a Florida pouch. Taper the unopened portion to achieve continence, and bring the end to the skin.

For a variation of the Florida pouch (Marshall, 1988), use a longer segment of ileum that is folded on itself, opened, and attached to the opened cecum to form an S shape before closure.

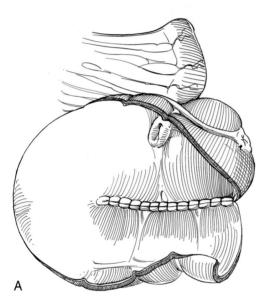

A

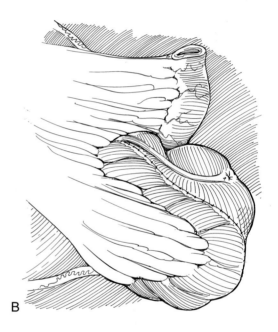

B

STAPLED CONTINENT RESERVOIR
(Olsson)

This is a prototypical stapling technique for reservoir formation. It is made possible by development of absorbable staples for a 75-mm GIA stapler that delivers two sets of staggered polyglactic and polyglycolic blend copolymer staples and cuts between the pairs.

17 **A**, Secure an appropriate length of ascending colon, ending at the junction of the right and middle colic blood supply, along with 10 cm of attached ileum as described in Step 10*A*. Perform a lateral anastomosis of the ileum to the colon with GA and TA staplers (see page 66). Make a small opening in the dome of the cecum.

B, Resect the distal staple line in the colon, and fold the segment of large bowel on itself, keeping the antimesenteric border in contact. Load the GIA stapler with absorbable sutures, and introduce one limb through the cecal port and the other into the open end of the colon. Fire the stapler.

C, Before releasing the stapler lock, put traction on the stapler to withdraw the lining and evert it. Place Babcock clamps on the distal ends of the staple lines to hold the unstapled end of the septum in view while reapplying the stapler. To prevent overlap of staple lines, make a short cut with scissors in the uncut septum just beyond the last staple, and then reapply the stapler. Insert sutures to close the defects on either side caused by the cuts. A third application of the stapler is usually needed to cross the apex of the folded bowel.

D, The folded ascending colon is now continuous with the cecum. Proceed with ureteral anastomosis, placement of stents, and formation of an ileal stoma with formation of a buttressed ileocecal valve or construction of an appendiceal stoma. Close the residual opening at the base of the pouch with an absorbable TA staple or with a running absorbable suture.

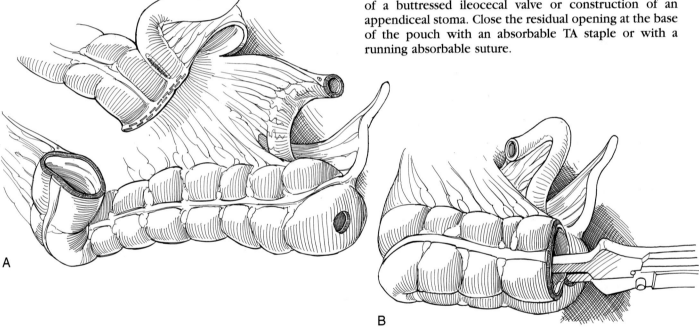

A

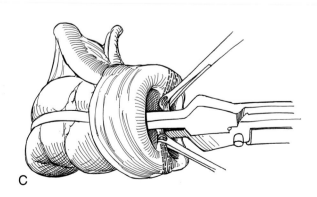

C

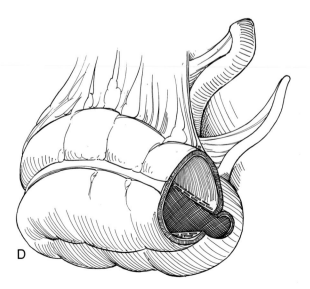

B

D

Commentary by Carl A. Olsson

The use of absorbable staples in the construction of colon conduits facilitates the procedure and substantially shortens operative time. Ordinarily, after resecting the bowel segment, Heineke-Mikulicz reconfiguration requires spatulation along the antimesenteric border and the application of multiple runs of absorbable sutures to create the pouch. This process usually consumes the better part of an hour. In contrast, the staple technique allows the surgeon to complete the entire pouch construction within 10 minutes. Furthermore, because no spatulation is required, bothersome blood loss at the bowel edges is not experienced.

All of the salient features of the technique are well described. Remarkably little in the way of a learning curve is associated with absorbable staple pouch construction. The only feature I would emphasize is to try not to stretch the bowel along the arms of the stapler before activating the unit. The frugal surgeon should keep in mind that each stapling device costs $350.

Stretching the bowel along the stapler lens leads to the need for more applications than the three described.

We recently reported on similar technology being utilized in the construction of orthotopic sigmoid neobladders. The procedure is carried out in precisely the same fashion, except that the two stapled ends of resected sigmoid are brought together, their stapled butts excised, and neobladder formed by serial applications of absorbable staples along the antimesenteric borders. A buttonhole is cut in the dome of the sigmoid pouch for urethral anastomosis. The resultant open superior end may be closed after ureterointestinal anastomosis, using a running absorbable suture or an absorbable TA stapling device.

Thus far, we have been fortunate in experiencing no complications as a consequence of stapled reservoir construction. There have been no urinary leaks or calculus formation. The patient should be warned that particulate remnant staples are often passed in the urine from 2 to 6 weeks postoperatively.

GASTROILEOILEAL POUCH
(Lockhart)

This pouch is best for patients with short bowel syndrome, acidosis, and an ileocecal segment made unusable by radiation damage.

Obtain a segment of stomach (see pages 758 to 760) and a 32-cm length of ileum (see pages 649 to 650). Divide the ileum into two segments, 20 to 22 cm and 12 to 14 cm. Open the long segment on its antimesenteric border. Fold it into a U shape, and anastomose it to the gastric segment with a running 3-0 SAS. Taper the short segment around a 14 F red rubber catheter with nonabsorbable staples (see Step 19) for 9 to 10 cm and absorbable sutures (see Step 18) for the remainder. Implant the short tapered segment into the gastric wall in a 3- to 4-cm submucosal tunnel. Reimplant the ureters into the gastric segment submucosally from inside (see page 720). Stent with a single-J stent; place a Malecot catheter in the reservoir and a 12 F straight catheter in the conduit.

CONDUITS FOR CONTINENT RESERVOIRS

Sutured Continent Conduit

18 A and B, Insert a 12 F Robinson catheter in the terminal ileum and ileocecal valve, and place Lembert sutures of 3-0 silk 0.5 cm apart for the entire length. Place a second layer, a running 3-0 silk suture. Fill the pouch to a volume of 300 to 400 cm. Remove the catheter, and press firmly on the reservoir to test for continence.

If there is leakage, reinforce the suture line with interrupted 3-0 silk sutures at the ileocecal valve area. Insert a 12 F and a 14 F catheter to test for ease of catheterization.

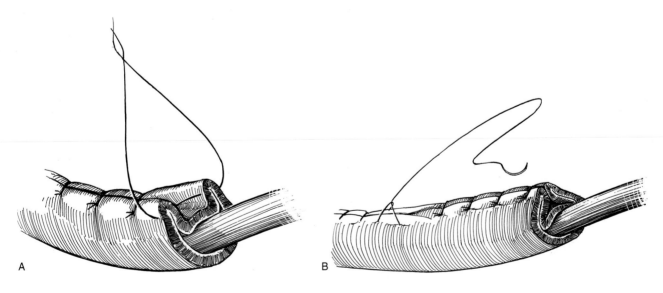

A   B

Stapled Continent Conduit
(Bejany and Politano)

19 To form a narrow conduit from the terminal ileum, place the GFIA 90-mm stapler on the antimesenteric border firmly against a 14 F Robinson catheter. It is usually necessary to apply the stapler more than once because the staple line should extend right down to the ileocecal valve. At the ileocecal valve, angle the stapler to cut off that portion. During the stapling process, make traction along the long axis of the terminal ileum to make sure that the catheterizing channel is straight and without folds. With the catheter in place, several interrupted sutures may be inserted in the angled cut at the ileocecal junction to maintain the continence mechanism of the ileocecal valve, not necessarily to "nipple" the terminal ileum into the cecum. Remove the catheter after filling the reservoir. There should be no leakage into the terminal ileum.

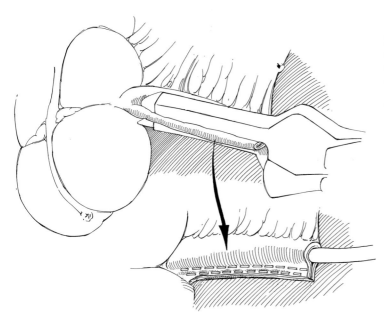

ILEOCECAL VALVE RECONSTRUCTION
(Fisch)

This procedure is for patients who have had extensive resection of the bowel. The technique reduces short bowel syndrome by increasing transit time and preventing cecoileal reflux.

After closing the ascending colon, incise the tenia libera longitudinally for 6 to 7 cm beginning 1 cm from the end. Bluntly dissect the muscularis from the mucosa. Make a 2-cm incision in the exposed mucosa distally. Prepare the terminal portion of the ileum by spatulating it and removing the serosa and fat from the terminal 4 or 5 cm. Anastomose the full thickness of the ileum to the colonic mucosa, and cover it with the seromuscular layer of the colon to force the end of the ileum into the colonic lumen and create a submucosal tunnel 4 cm long.

POSTOPERATIVE PROBLEMS FROM URINARY RESERVOIRS

Immediate Problems. Whichever form of continent diversion is used, it is extremely important before the patient leaves the operating table to prove that the continence mechanism is effective and that the conduit can easily be catheterized with suitable catheters of various types at various degrees of reservoir filling. If there is any difficulty catheterizing a conduit in the operating room, it will be that much harder later. Leaving a silicone catheter indwelling, sutured to the skin, is good insurance for the first week.

Late Problems. Bacteriuria is inevitable in systems requiring self-catheterization, but pyelonephritis is rare. *Reflux* is present in a small number. *Ureteral obstruction* is more common and may require balloon dilation or revision. *Mucus secretion* is greater in reservoirs of cecum than of ileum, requiring more frequent and vigorous irrigation over a more prolonged time. In contrast, the ileal mucosa tends to atrophy. Mucus is often obstructive and requires weekly irrigations with sterile water or bicarbonate solution. Occasional obstruction during catheter drainage may be overcome if the patient coughs. *Stomal stenosis or eversion* may require revision of the stoma. *Stone formation* is secondary to residual urine and may be managed by direct-vision lithotripsy or percutaneous techniques. The *metabolic changes* of increased serum chloride and decreased bicarbonate occur frequently. An occasional patient must be managed by ingestion of bicarbonate, more frequent emptying of the reservoir, and continuous drainage at night. Loss of potassium is not a problem. Renal function must be monitored. These metabolic problems improve after 6 months.

Commentary by Randall G. Rowland

In my experience, several factors are needed for success with an Indiana pouch. In addition to judicious patient selection, several technical points are important. In order to make a functional, low-pressure reservoir that allows the patient to stay dry for 4 or more hours, at least 25 to 30 cm of cecum and ascending colon must be used and complete detubularization must be accomplished by incising the cecum to approximately 2 cm from its most dependent portion. The preparation of the efferent limb and continence mechanism (ileocecal valve) is done with the reservoir opened. After plication of the ileocecal valve area over a 12 F catheter, resistance should be felt as one passes an 18 F catheter through this area. If there is difficulty passing the catheter beyond mild resistance, one or more of the plication sutures should be removed from the end of the suture row closest to the stoma site. If no resistance is felt with catheter passage, additional sutures are needed. They should extend in the direction of the stoma and be made wider in the areas where sutures have already been placed. These maneuvers should create resistance as the 18 F catheter is passed.

Usually the ureters are implanted after the reservoir has been closed. This approach allows the surgeon to lead the ureters to the pouch in a manner that allows smooth alignment with the taenia. The left ureter must be mobilized to the level of the lower pole of the kidney or renal pelvis to provide adequate length, taking care to avoid devascularization. The ureter is passed through the retroperitoneum cephalad to the origin of the inferior mesenteric artery and then through the mesentery to the reservoir. The reservoir can be detubularized and closed in two manners. A traditional technique is that described in the text. I personally close the pouch with a single layer of absorbable 3-0 synthetic braided suture. Every third suture is locked to prevent shortening of the suture lines.

A new method of detubularization and closure uses GIA and TA absorbable staples. This technique rapidly accomplishes detubularization of the segment. With the use of absorbable staples, stones have not been a problem.

Meticulous long-term follow-up must be performed to detect silent complications that could cause deterioration of renal function or metabolic abnormalities. Intravenous pyelography and/or ultrasound studies are needed to watch for upper tract obstruction. Electrolytes, blood urea nitrogen, creatinine, and hemoglobin should be followed. Patients should be urged to perform at least daily irrigation of their reservoir to help avoid stone formation on inspissated mucus. In a patient who has had good function of the pouch and suddenly develops incontinence, a pouch infection should be suspected. Sterile catheterization for a culture should be performed. Usually treating "pouchitis" promptly resolves the alteration in function and continence of the pouch.

Commentary by Jorge L. Lockhart

Difficulty in creating a right colonic reservoir often stems from the extent of adhesions present around the hepatic flexure and ileocecal areas. When the outer surface of the colon adheres to the liver, it is better mobilized by first dividing the gastrocolic ligament and dissecting the transverse colon. The right colon can then be dissected in a retrograde fashion. Preservation of the ileocecal segment is essential for creating a functional anti-incontinence segment and a satisfactory ileotransversostomy. Dissection of these segments may be especially difficult in re-operations and on heavily radiated patients.

Creation of these reservoirs can be greatly facilitated by using absorbable staples as described in Step 17. Ureteral reimplantation has been performed utilizing direct or tunnelled techniques, depending on the surgeon's preference. At present, we favor the direct reimplantation, while trying to avoid tension and to create a long ureteral spatulation. It is advisable to mobilize the left ureter up to the lower pole of the kidney and then bring it to the right hemiabdomen above the inferior mesenteric artery. Such a maneuver prevents angulation and minimizes the likelihood of obstruction. The anti-incontinence mechanism is developed utilizing plicating or stapling techniques previously described. When we find a patent appendix of adequate length, we use it as a catheterizable segment. The surgeon should be familiar with all the previously described alternatives for the creation of an anti-incontinence system.

Patients are discharged as soon as they resume bowel function. We prefer to bring the ureteral stents through the stoma to drain into a collecting bag. Home care manages only the cecostomy tube and urostomy bag until readmission for pouch activation. The gastroileal pouch is an alternative in selected patients. Because patients undergoing this procedure have a tendency to electrolytic neutrality (opposite to hyperchloremic metabolic acidosis observed with ileal and colonic reservoirs), we prefer this technique for children and young adults.

Gastric Reservoir
(Mitchell)

1 Harvest a wedge from the stomach (see page 757). If staples were placed to obtain the gastric wedge, remove them. Rotate the wedge 180 degrees so that the anterior surface of the stomach becomes the posterior surface of the reservoir when moved to the pelvis. Fold the wedge to delineate the posterior surface for ureteral implantation.

2 With curved tenotomy scissors, form two oblique tunnels 2 to 3 cm long on the posterior wall in the layer beneath the gastric mucosa, and draw the ureters through them (see pages 720 to 723). Place a deep 3-0 SAS into the gastric muscularis and through the tip of the spatulated ureter for fixation. Suture the epithelial edges of the ureter to the gastric mucosa with fine interrupted sutures. If the reservoir is to be placed to the native urethra, continue the closure of the edges of the flap after insertion of a Malecot catheter into the reservoir. If a gastric urethra or Mitrofanoff procedure is to be done, leave the reservoir open for ease of implantation.

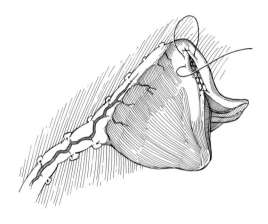

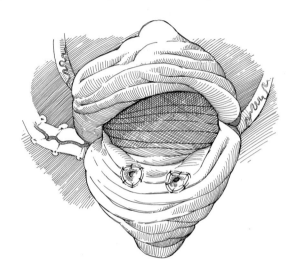

Stomach Tube Conduit

3 Mark and cut a strip 2 cm wide from the anterior arm of the flap that is long enough to reach the abdominal wall or perineum easily. Form it into a tube over a 14 F catheter.

4 Intussuscept the base of the tube for a short distance into the reservoir to increase resistance. Fix the tube in place with several NAS. Close the reservoir. Bring the open end of the tube to the skin of the anterior abdominal wall, and fix it in place. Insert a Malecot catheter. Fill the reservoir, and test with catheters to make absolutely certain that the conduit is both catheterizable and continent.

An *artificial sphincter* could be inserted around a gastric nipple, although there has been little experience with this arrangement. After formation of the nipple (Steps 3, 4, and 5), make a window in the gastroepiploic mesentery, and place the cuff on the nipple far enough from the end to allow it to traverse the abdominal wall. Suture the stoma to the skin. Arrange the reservoir and pump.

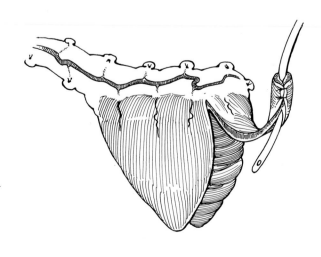

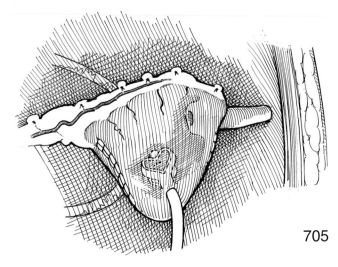

5 *Alternative technique* (Gosalbez et al, 1993). **A,** Resect a rectangle of stomach from the greater curvature, keeping its attachment to the distal end of the vascular pedicle. Form it into a tube.

B, Insert the distal end of the tube submucosally into the stomach portion of the reservoir or augmentation, or insert it into the wall of the residual bladder.

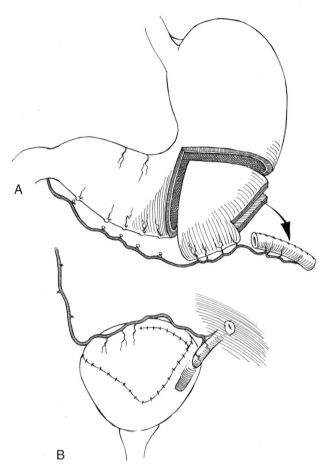

Mitrofanoff Adaptation

6 To form a Mitrofanoff valve, tunnel the appendix (or the residual ureter) through the wall obliquely into a 2- or 3-cm gastric submucosal tunnel. Fix it in place as for ureteral implantation. Bring the end of the appendix through the body wall, and fix it to the skin. Suture the wall of the stomach to the abdominal wall around the appendix and the cystostomy tube as for a gastrostomy to avoid leakage when the cystostomy tube is removed and to provide ease of catheterization. Complete the closure.

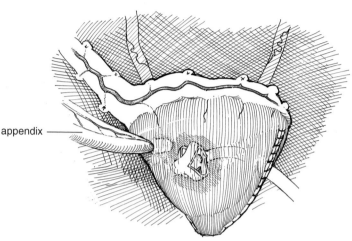

appendix

POSTOPERATIVE PROBLEMS

Metabolic acidosis, manifest as hypochloremic hypokalemic acidosis, may occur in patients with diminished renal function, especially if they are volume depleted. Administration of histamine blockers and, if necessary, omeprazole, a drug that blocks the hydrogen-potassium-adenosine triphosphatase pump, is usually effective.

Commentary by Richard C. Rink

One of the most important aspects in the use of gastric segments in lower urinary tract reconstruction is patient selection. Our initial indications for the use of stomach were significant compromise in the renal function of patients in whom it was not feasible to use intestinal segments, such as children with short gut syndrome and a history of significant radiation to the bowel. As with many surgical procedures, over time the indications have expanded. However, some significant disadvantages have been noted that are unique to the stomach. Our current recommendations are to return to the above-noted original indications. It is now well documented that the hematuria/dysuria syndrome occurs in at least one third of patients after gastrocystoplasty, and this can be particularly troubling to the patient with normal sensation. Severe hypochloremic alkalosis has also been noted in a small group of patients. In our experience this has occurred primarily following a viral illness with associated chloride loss from vomiting. The patient and family must be aware of these potential problems. The use of stomach is contraindicated in patients with significant salt-wasting nephropathy, delayed gastric emptying, or prior history of ulcers.

Several technical points for gastrocystoplasty or creation of a gastric reservoir should be stressed. The gastric segment chosen for the reservoir must be distal enough on the gastroepiploic artery to reach the pelvis easily. Tension or angulation of this vessel may result in compromise of the vasculature. If the segment requires greater length to reach the pelvis, further mobilization of the right gastroepiploic artery to its origin may be necessary. Length may also be gained by dividing some of the proximal branches off the gastroepiploic artery where they enter the isolated gastric segment. Initially we used a small triangular wedge of stomach but have recognized the need to take a larger gastric segment, particularly for creation of a complete reservoir. This is now done in a more rhomboid shape with the base along the greater curvature being at least 10 to 12 cm in children and longer in adults. The segment should not extend all the way through the lesser curvature, as this may injure branches of the vagus nerve to the remainder of the stomach. Significant bleeding from the stomach can be prevented by prospectively ligating the small branches from the left gastric artery where they enter the stomach near the proposed isolated segment just off the lesser curvature.

Stapling techniques have been popularized for excising the gastric segment to prevent bleeding and spillage of gastric contents. However, this requires excision of the staple lines later and may waste gastric tissue. We continue to excise the segment between bowel clamps, particularly when requiring a larger segment, as in those needing a complete gastric reservoir. To create a gastric reservoir, ureteral reimplantation as well as some form of implantation for a continence mechanism, such as a Mitrofanoff procedure, is necessary. We have found submucosal tunnels to be most easily created from inside while the gastric segment is open. Occasional stay sutures may help identify that portion of the gastric segment appropriate for the site of implantation. The ureters and the Mitrofanoff tube must be

secured where they enter the stomach. Implantation of the ureters into stomach is easily performed in a manner similar to reimplantation into the native bladder.

The vascular pedicle must be secured rather than left free-floating in the abdomen. We have had at least one patient develop a volvulus around the pedicle. Either this pedicle can be fixed to the posterior peritoneum near the root of the small intestine after first bringing it through windows in the transverse mesocolon and terminal ileum, or the right colon can be completely mobilized and the entire pedicle placed within the retroperitoneum.

It is important to secure the gastric reservoir in place. If the continence mechanism of the reservoir is not in the patient's native urethra so that catheterization can occur through a continent abdominal wall stoma, the reservoir should be secured to the abdominal wall at both the catheterizable stoma and cystostomy tube. This immobilizes the reservoir and thus prevents difficulties with catheterization.

The management of these patients in the postoperative period is not significantly different from that of those with any other continent urinary reservoir. The native stomach can be drained by nasogastric suction. We use an H_2 antagonist in the immediate postoperative period and continue this for the first 3 to 4 months. Although mucus production with stomach segments is less significant than with intestinal segments, we still encourage the patient or parents to irrigate the reservoir two to three times a day in the early postoperative period and then once daily forever. The cystostomy tube is left in place for 3 weeks before beginning intermittent clean catheterization. The tube is then clamped and intermittent clean catheterization started at 2-hour intervals during the next few days, increasing to every 4 hours during waking hours and 8 hours at night. As the drawings indicate, gastric tubes can be used as a nipple valve or as a Mitrofanoff tube to create the continence mechanism. It should be noted that our group and others have noted skin irritation or excoriation when stomach segments have been brought to the skin. A similar problem can occur following gastrocystoplasty if the patient is incontinent. It is imperative for continence to be achieved in any patient in whom stomach has been used. We would not choose a catheterizable gastric tube to bring to the abdominal wall if other tubular structures, such as ileum or appendix, were available. We have not had problems combining gastric and intestinal segments in this manner.

Rhythmic uninhibited contractions of the gastric segment during filling have been noted in a high percentage of patients by our group and others. We see less problem with these now than early in our experience because a larger segment of stomach is used.

The use of stomach has allowed lower urinary reconstruction in patients who were not previously candidates for such surgery using intestine. However, the surgeon and patient must understand the operative and postoperative risks involved with these procedures.

Appendicovesicostomy

(Mitrofanoff)

Access to a continent reservoir for intermittent catheterization can be obtained by submucosally implanting the appendix, thus providing both a flap-valve for continence and a catheterizable stoma. The same principle can be applied for the use of a segment of tapered ileum, ureteral remnants, or uterine tube. If a ureteral remnant is available, the technique for its use is simpler and the complications fewer, making that tissue preferable to appendix. Because these stomas do not leak even with high intravesical pressure, the risk of spontaneous perforation is high unless another route is present that responds to a lower leak pressure. For that reason, closure of the vesical neck may not be advisable unless the patient actually has stress incontinence.

Prepare the bowel. Insert a balloon catheter into the bladder transurethrally.

1 **A,** *Incision:* Make a midline lower abdominal incision (see page 487).

B, Before opening the peritoneum, prepare the lateral vesical space generously on the right. Divide the spermatic cord, vas, and obliterated hypogastric artery to gain adequate exposure. Mobilize the cecum and the terminal ileum on their mesentery to allow placement of the end of the appendix at the desired site, such as at the umbilicus.

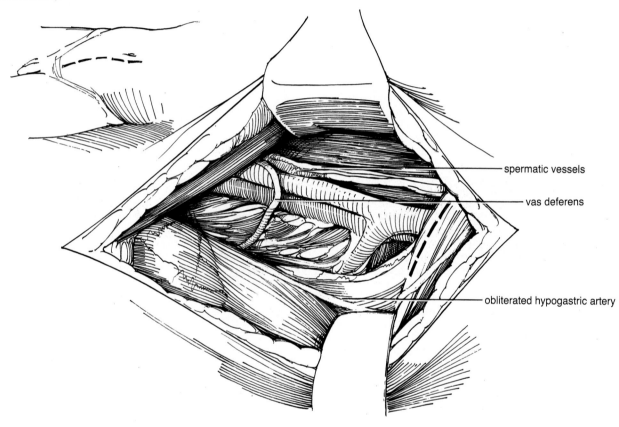

spermatic vessels

vas deferens

obliterated hypogastric artery

2 **A,** Insert stay sutures at the base of the appendix, and incise the wall circumferentially to take a cuff of cecum with the appendix. Separate the appendiceal mesentery for a short distance from that of the cecum, preserving all of the appendiceal blood supply. Because of the mobility of the cecum, it is not necessary to move the appendix away from it. Close the cecal defect left by the appendix with an inner running 3-0 SAS and an outer layer of interrupted Lembert 3-0 SAS (see page 38).

B, For a short appendix or an obese patient, make the appendix longer by incorporating some of the cecal wall. Apply the stapler across the cecum a short distance from the base, taking care to preserve the vascular pedicle to the appendix. Fashion this cecal portion into a tube to allow the appendix to reach the abdominal wall.

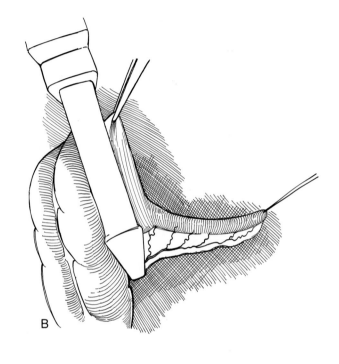

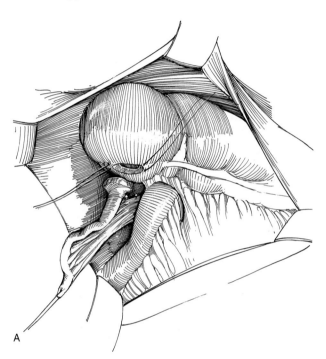

3 Extraperitonealize the appendix through a small opening in the peritoneum behind the ileocecal junction. Close the peritoneum with a running suture. For umbilical placement it is not necessary to extraperitonealize the appendix; fix it and the cecum intraperitoneally.

Trim back the appendiceal tip successively with Mayo scissors until an adequate lumen is exposed as checked with a catheter of the appropriate size. Irrigate the lumen with antibiotic solution to clear it of fecoliths.

If the decision has been made to close the bladder neck, open the bladder in the midline down to the vesical neck and extend the incision transversely so as to transect the neck completely. Close it solidly (see page 609). Because a pop-off valve is very desirable, a better alternative may be to achieve continence by sling or tubularization.

Drain the bladder with a suprapubic Malecot catheter. Leave an infant feeding tube through the appendix for 2 or 3 weeks, at which time the patient is taught intermittent catheterization. Do a cystogram at 4 weeks, and at that time remove the cystostomy tube.

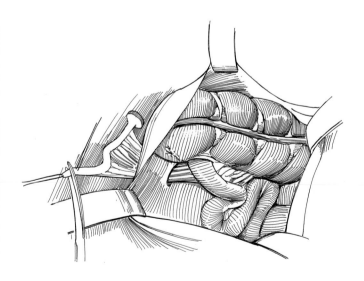

Implantation into the Bladder

4   **A** and **B**, In the posterolateral wall of the bladder, develop a wide submucosal tunnel beginning well above the right ureteral orifice, as in the Cohen procedure (see page 793). Implant the appendix and its mesentery in the tunnel, being certain that the blood supply is not constricted. Proceed with bladder augmentation.

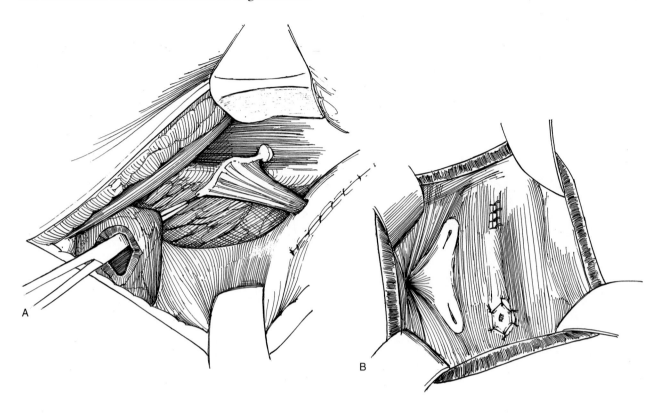

A

B

5   Pass the appendiceal base through an opening in the abdominal muscles large enough to accommodate a finger. Make a small opening the diameter of the cecal cuff in the skin in the edge of the future hairline in the right lower quadrant. Alternatively, make a circumferential incision around the umbilicus, leaving a short flap of skin on one side that fits into a notch in the end of the appendix to prevent stenosis. Suture the appendiceal base to the skin with 3-0 CCG sutures. Hitch the bladder to the anterior abdominal wall around the site of exit, and fix it in four places with sutures to prevent kinking of the appendix and to compensate for its limited length. At the same time, protect the appendiceal mesentery. Insert a catheter through the appendix before closing to be sure that it passes easily and leave it in place.

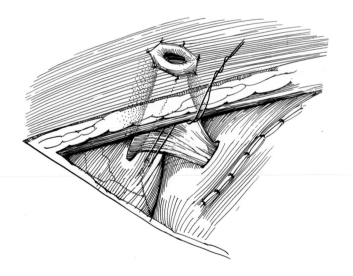

Implantation into Bowel Segment

This procedure is used, for example, in forming a Mainz pouch with appendiceal stoma (see page 698).

6 Clean the mesentery of the appendix to skeletonize the vessels while preserving the appendicular artery on a branch of the anterior or posterior cecal artery.

Make a T incision in the cecum, and create a trough by incising the seromuscular layer of the tenia libera to the depth of the mucosa. Place stay sutures, and free the flaps on either side. Make a vertical incision in the submucosa and mucosa at the distal extremity of the trough, and anastomose the tip of the appendix (or ureteral remnant) to the mucosa with 4-0 interrupted SAS. Suture the seromuscular flaps with similar sutures to cover the appendix. Bring the proximal end of the appendix through the abdominal wall as a stoma.

Implantation into Bowel Segment, Alternative Technique (Keating)

7 **A**, In the absence of adequate tenia in which to insert an appendiceal valve, form a submucosal trough in the bowel or in the bladder.

First, pass the appendix (or ureteral remnant) through the body wall and fix it to the skin, utilizing a V-shaped, laterally based skin flap. Place a finger into the augmentation, reservoir, or bladder to elevate it against the abdominal wall. Tack it in place with NAS.

Place four stay sutures such that a 5 × 5-cm area of bowel or bladder can be stretched flat (not shown). Make an incision through the mucosa, and open it to form a trough. Lay the appendix or ureter in the trough, and anastomose the tip mucosa to mucosa. Approximate the lateral edges of the incision with interrupted 4-0 SAS to bury the appendix.

B, *Alternative:* Make two parallel incisions through serosa and muscularis 2 to 3 cm apart. Place the appendix between them, and bury it in a tunnel by approximating the lateral margins of each incision with interrupted 3-0 SAS.

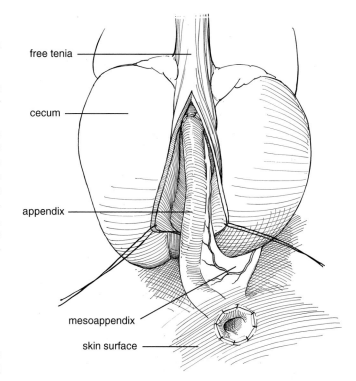

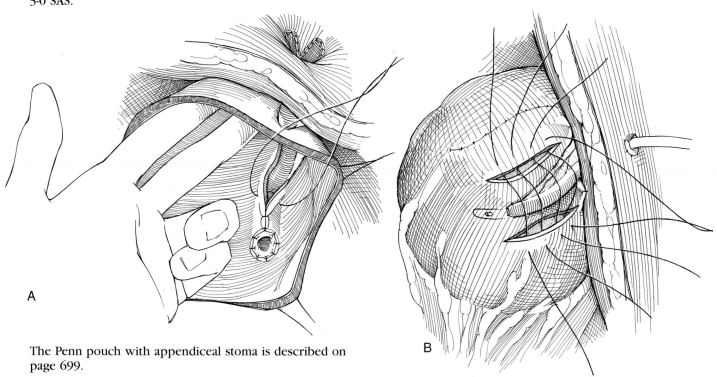

A

B

The Penn pouch with appendiceal stoma is described on page 699.

OTHER APPLICATIONS OF THE MITROFANOFF PRINCIPLE

The Mitrofanoff principle can be applied using other structures besides the appendix and ureteral remnant. Uterine tube, and even small bowel that has been tailored, may be implanted in a subepithelial tunnel into the bladder or an intestinal reservoir.

Ureteral Remnant for Implantation

The ureter is a good substitute for the appendix. The lower end of the ureter may remain after a transureteroureterostomy and an antireflux procedure that was performed in two stages.

A ureteral conduit is especially suitable when one end of the ureter is well vascularized, as after cutaneous ureterostomy or previous ureterointestinal anastomosis.

8 **A,** Select the ureter that was implanted in the skin and has had time to gain a blood supply from the distal end. Divide it in its midportion. Insert the proximal end of its distal segment in the bladder or pouch, and anastomose the distal end of its proximal segment to the contralateral ureter, which in turn is reimplanted in the bladder (or into an augmentation) with an antireflux technique.

If the ureter was previously implanted in a bowel conduit and is to be used as a catheterizable stoma after the segment has been converted into a reservoir, test its vascularization by placing a bulldog clamp across it and observing the color of the distal portion. Then form a tunnel for it and bring it to the skin. Perform ureteroureterostomy on the other end.

B, *Alternative without ureteroureterostomy:* From a cutaneous ureterostomy that has been in place long enough for the distal end to become vascularized, divide the ureter. Leave one end attached to the skin to provide an entrance for intermittent catheterization, and insert the other end of the distal segment into the reservoir or bladder with a tunnel of the same proportions as for ureteroneocystostomy to provide a nonrefluxing (leak-proof) valve. Insert the proximal end into the reservoir or bladder by a nonrefluxing technique.

It is also possible to form a pedicled graft of ureter by preserving the ureteral branch from the internal iliac artery. Divide the distal end, place a rubber-shod clamp on the proximal end, and check for viability (a Doppler stethoscope helps).

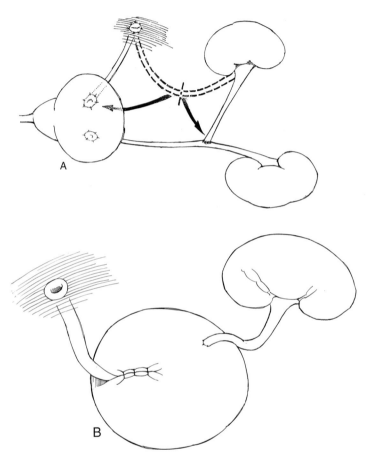

Implanted Tapered Small Bowel (Adams-Bihrle; Figueroa)

This alternative is used in the absence of the appendix or ureter.

Isolate a 10-cm segment of ileum (see pages 649 to 650), and taper it over a 12 F catheter. Use the stapler combined with trimming the redundant margin for the distal four fifths (see page 703) and a suture technique for the proximal fifth (see page 702) to avoid staples in the pouch. Remove the fat and serosa from this portion, and place it through a generous hiatus in the pouch. Raise the mucosa and submucosa either extraluminally or transluminally to form a tunnel. Pass the end of the tapered ileum through, and suture it in place. Form an abdominal stoma (see pages 654 to 657, Steps 19 to 24). Stent the conduit with a 12 F red rubber catheter, and drain the pouch with a Malecot catheter.

The fallopian tube, if long enough, may be mobilized on an ovarian pedicle and placed like an appendix.

APPENDICOCECOSTOMY FOR ANTEGRADE COLONIC ENEMA (ACE PROCEDURE)
(Malone)

Deliver the cecum and appendix through a right McBurney incision.

9 Turn the appendix with its vessels onto the cecum, and imbricate the cecal wall over it. A better technique (not shown) is to form a series of windows in the mesentery between the terminal branches of the appendiceal artery. Pass the imbricating sutures through them successively, thereby leaving the artery itself outside the tunnel.

Deliver the appendiceal stump onto the skin through the previously selected site. Fix the cecum to the anterior abdominal wall. Connect the trimmed end of the appendix to a broad-based lateral skin flap to allow recession of the anastomosis. Start daily colonic washout in 10 days, and remove the catheter in 2 to 3 weeks.

Alternative (original) technique: Resect the appendix as for the Mitrofanoff procedure, and reverse it before placing it submucosally in a tenia. Anastomose one end to the cecum and the other to the skin.

Leave a 12 F catheter in the stoma, and start tap water instillations after the patient has had a bowel movement. Have the patient gradually increase the volume until the flush is successful in preventing fecal incontinence. Complications include stomal stenosis, especially if the appendix is brought to the umbilicus, and difficulty with catheterization, the latter partially resolved by using flexible endoscopy to replace the catheter.

POSTOPERATIVE PROBLEMS

Necrosis of the base of the appendix requires revision but is usually limited to the cecal cuff. *Urinary fistulas* pose a larger problem, either from leakage into the urethra at the site of vesical neck closure or at the vesical suture line anteriorly. *Reflux* can also be a problem and should be corrected at an earlier stage. If it begins after operation, the incidence of upper tract dilation can be reduced by vesical augmentation. *Mucus* is a problem even if the bladder has been augmented with stomach. Mucus from the appendix falls into the base of the bladder, where it is not completely evacuated by intermittent catheterization; it fosters infection and obstructs the catheter. *Bladder calculi* are common, perhaps secondary to mucus that passes down into the pouch from the appendix, and are not reached by the catheter. Regular thorough irrigation is required.

Stenosis at skin level is the most common problem, occurring in one third of the patients. Try dilation with Teflon dilators or with balloon dilators under radiologic control, but formal revision is usually required. Some Mitrofanoff arrangements need to be converted to another form of urinary diversion. *Rupture* may result from traumatic catheterization or acute or chronic overfilling in the absence of a safety valve.

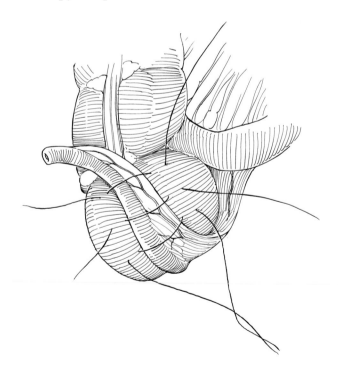

Commentary by Paul Mitrofanoff

If reflux is present, it requires correction in a preliminary stage, but it is usually a symptom of bladder hypertonicity that requires bladder augmentation. The decision to perform an enterocystoplasty to enlarge the bladder has to be made at the first stage if the bladder is too small and hypertonic or later if reflux or upper tract dilatation appears. This enterocystoplasty seems to be necessary in about one half the cases of neurogenic bladders that are retained for urinary storage.

Specific technical points: A large peritoneal dissection of the right lower quadrant is necessary to place the appendix and its mesentery under the peritoneum in the best way. This dissection is easier to perform before opening the peritoneum.

Good vascularization of the appendix is, of course, essential. If it appears jeopardized during the operation, another solution must be used: ureterovesicostomy or intestinal stoma associated with an enterocystoplasty.

I believe that the bladder should be opened for three reasons: (1) to close the bladder neck, (2) to select the best place to implant the appendix, and (3) to help accomplish the bladder hitch to the anterior abdominal wall. This hitch is useful to avoid kinking of the appendix between the abdominal muscles and bladder and also if the appendix is short.

The closure of the bladder neck is necessary in almost all the cases, the neck being left open only if it appears to be totally continent but self-catheterization is impossible owing to an orthopedic situation. In girls, this closure could be easily carried out in a later stage using a perineal approach.

It is better to carry out the enterocystoplasty in the same stage as the vesicostomy. Sometimes, however, the symptoms of the bladder hypertonicity develop with the passing years after closure of the bladder neck. The bladder must then be enlarged without delay.

Complications: Different types of complications can occur, complications with the appendix such as stenosis of the cutaneous stoma or appendicular kink blocking the catheterizations. A limited reoperation is sufficient to resolve these problems. Urinary leakage from the cutaneous stoma requires a more difficult reoperation to lengthen the submucosal tunnel of the appendix and to restore continence. However, it is essential to check if this leakage is not due to a high bladder pressure requiring an augmentation.

Vesicourethral fistula, urinary infections, dilation of the upper tract, and reflux are possible. They are almost always symptoms of too small a bladder with too high a pressure. Anticholinergic drugs are usually insufficient, and enterocystoplasty is necessary.

Bladder lithiasis is favored by the presence of the intestinal mucus. Such stones are often well tolerated, and their removal is usually easy to perform. Prevention should associate an increased diuresis and catheterizations with a large catheter, 14 F when possible, trying to have the child perform complete emptying each time by siphoning. A weekly bladder wash can be useful. More severe is a spontaneous rupture of an enteroplasty. It is probably due to catheterizations being done too infrequently, leading to an overdistended bladder. It is essential to teach patients to respect a timetable, with at least four catheterizations a day.

Ileal Hydraulic Valve Conduit

(Benchekroun)

After formation of an ileocecal reservoir (see page 693), secure a separate 14-cm segment of ileum proximal to the 8-cm terminal portion that was left attached to the cecum during the formation of the pouch.

1 Insert two Allis clamps into the lumen, and grasp the rim of bowel at the proximal end. Pull this end into the lumen to invaginate it completely, forming a double-walled tube (like an inkwell). The serosa, rather than the mucosa, now lines the conduit.

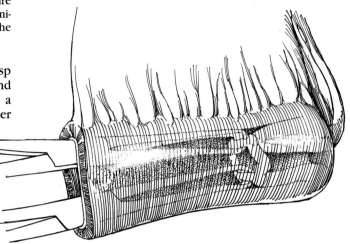

2 Suture the mucosa of the inner and outer bowel edges together in a watertight fashion on the *ventral* side half way around the circumference with a running 3-0 SAS. Reinforce this with a serosa-muscularis suture. Place a single full-thickness mattress suture on the *dorsal* side half way between the terminations of the running suture, thus leaving two distinct openings between the layers of the inverted ileum. This opening on either side of the suture allows the space between the two layers of ileum to fill with urine from the reservoir to compress the lumen throughout the entire length of the central portion of the ileum to shut it like a valve. Also, any mucous secretions from the ileum can return through it to the reservoir.

Suture the double end to the opening in the bladder or bladder augmentation in two layers with 3-0 SAS.

3 Make an opening through the body wall somewhat larger than for an ileal conduit (see pages 654 to 657) and form a stoma, suturing the adventitia of the bowel to the skin. A peristomal skin flap (see page 656) may be inserted to reduce the opportunity for stomal stenosis. Place a Levine tube through the stoma, to remain for up to 3 weeks.

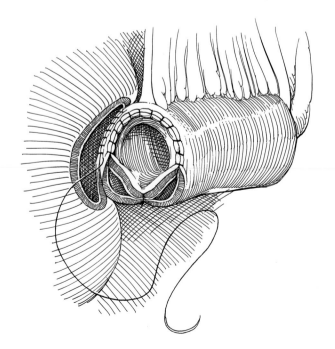

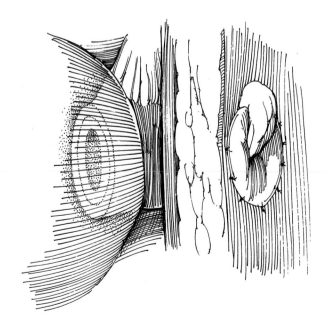

POSTOPERATIVE PROBLEMS

Fistulas between the conduit and the skin may occur if more than the serosa is sutured to the fascia and skin. An indwelling catheter may allow healing, but the valve usually must be replaced. *Stomal stenosis* results from poor stomal care and infrequent catheterization. It may be relieved by dilation and prolonged catheterization; it can be mitigated by inserting a V of skin at the time of construction but may require refashioning of the stoma. *Pouch overdistention* causes the Benchekroun valve to overfill and distort the mechanism, resulting in inability to catheterize the stoma. It can be relieved by needle aspiration of the pouch and a period of catheterization to restore the valve to normal.

Deintussusception, resulting in difficulty with catheterization or incontinence, is secondary to poor fixation of the invaginated ileum.

Commentary by Abdelatif Benchekroun

The ileal valve can be adapted to all types of reservoirs, according to the indications in the patients involved. *Ileocecal reservoir:* The "hydraulic valve" can be inserted in an ileocecal reservoir by placing it over the distal end of the cecum (ascending colon) and using the terminal ileum for ureteral implantation. *Detubularized ileocecal reservoir:* Since 1991 we have systematically detubularized the cecoileal segment and inserted the hydraulic valve at the cecal part of the reservoir. The afferent ileal loop can be used to construct an antireflux hydraulic valve if the ureters are dilated. A valve-in-continuity can be formed in a Hautmann or Kock pouch by inverting the 14-cm efferent loop and converting it into a hydraulic valve. This is done through a transverse ileotomy made 12 cm from the end and folding the loop upon itself within the bowel lumen. The usual half-circle anastomosis is performed through the transverse ileotomy, which is then closed. The valve is exteriorized in the right iliac fossa and the stoma formed by suturing the adventitia of the bowel to the skin. The ureters are implanted into the reservoir by the LeDuc-Camey method.

Sigmoid bladder: The loop is isolated and closed distally. The ureters are implanted by the Leadbetter antireflux technique. The ileal valve is placed on the proximal end of the segment and exteriorized. This procedure has few indications, but in two cases we did it to transform a wet colostomy into a continent sigmoidostomy and colostomy and in one case for a man with right colonic agenesis. *Rectal bladder bypass:* The valve can also be used for bypassing the rectal bladder. After the rectum is sectioned, the valve is attached to the margins of the proximal rectotomy and the stoma placed in the left iliac fossa.

Transverse colonic reservoir: In one case with a short cecum, we used the transverse colon as the reservoir after closing one end and putting the valve on the other. *Continent cystostomy:* This technique consists of preserving the vesical reservoir, excluding the bladder neck, and apposing the ileal valve on the bladder dome. The cutaneous stoma can be either median or pararectal.

Ureteral implantation may be done to incorporate the principle of the hydraulic valve to prevent reflux. The distal ends of the two ureters are spatulated for 2 to 3 cm and anastomosed side to side to create a wide common opening. Through a transverse ileotomy made 8 cm from the ureteroileal anastomosis, a 4-cm long invagination is created by pulling the ureteroileal anastomosis intraluminally. The invagination is maintained by attaching the ureteroileal anastomosis to the proximal lip of the transverse ileotomy by a three-quarter circumferential continuous suture. The ileotomy is closed with a continuous suture.

During the past 20 years we have successfully performed continent urinary diversion in 260 cases, 30 of which were children younger than 15 years of age.

Cautions and pitfalls: Concerning the abdominal fixation of the valve, your needle must take only the serosa. Ureteral stents must be exteriorized through the reservoir and not through the stoma. When the hydraulic valve is made, the two posterior openings must be loose to allow free passage of urine between the reservoir and the valve. Sometimes you need to excise a cuneiform part of the inner layer to enhance the passage of urine outside this layer.

Postoperative problems: The incidence of most complications has decreased. A *valve fistula* may be avoided by not transfixing the walls of the hydraulic valve during fixation to the skin. An indwelling catheter may allow the fistula to heal. This complication is rare in our recent series for two reasons: We no longer exteriorize the ureteral stents through the hydraulic valve, and we monitor the stoma to avoid its distention by mucosal secretions and its erosion by the catheter.

The valve may *evaginate*, as shown by ileal mucosa extruding from the stoma if the evagination is exterior or by leakage with a normal-appearing stoma if the evagination is interior. Continence may be restored in two ways: by repeating the invagination, using the same steps described under the heading "Detubularized Ileocecal Reservoir," or, if that is not possible, by constructing a new valve from a 12-cm length of ileum. We think low pressure in the reservoir reduces the frequency of spontaneous evagination. Stomal stenosis seldom occurs and is treated by dilation and prolonged catheterization.

Ureterosigmoidostomy

Ureterosigmoidostomy is probably the oldest and technically easiest means of continent diversion. It diverts the urine without the need for external appliances. Despite its limitations of electrolyte imbalance, potential for upper tract damage, and association with later development of adenocarcinoma near the ureteral anastomosis, the procedure still has a place in certain cases. It is not suitable for a patient with neurogenic bladder dysfunction because of the associated anal malfunction, but it may be used for children with vesical exstrophy.

Whether the ureters should be implanted in the sigmoid as distally as possible to reduce resorption or higher to allow later conversion to a sigmoid conduit without redoing the ureterocolonic anastomoses, should the ureterosigmoidostomy fail, has not been decided.

In children, this procedure is most successful in achieving postoperative urinary continence when performed on those who are already continent of feces, but these patients, being young, have more time to develop neoplasms in the colon.

Determine if the anal sphincteric mechanism is intact by digital palpation, by anal stimulation, and by having the patient hold warm watery mush for a couple of hours. If there is doubt, perform the ureterosigmoidostomy in two stages, first making a nonrefluxing sigmoid conduit. When the child is older and assessment is more accurate, evaluate the function of the conduit and anal sphincter tone. With anal continence, anastomose the conduit to the intact sigmoid colon, establishing a continent internal urinary diversion (Kroovand). Perform an intravenous urogram to be sure that absolutely no ureteral dilation is present, which is a contraindication to this operation.

Place the patient on a liquid diet for 24 hours, and prepare the bowel with balanced saline solution (GoLYTELY). Provide two cleansing enemas with neomycin solution the day before operation. Give intravenous cephalosporin 6 hours preoperatively, and continue for 72 hours. It may be advisable to install a central venous line.

CLOSED TECHNIQUE OF URETEROCOLONIC ANASTOMOSIS (Leadbetter)

1 *Position:* Supine, in slight Trendelenburg position. Insert a large rectal tube with extra holes as high as possible, and tape it near the anus with waterproof tape placed over tincture of benzoin or suture it para-anally. The right-handed surgeon stands on the right side of the patient.

A, *Incision:* Make a midline transabdominal incision. With exstrophy, the incision must be well off the midline over one belly of the rectus muscle. If the bladder is to be removed, do it first, leaving the transected ureters to drain freely. Have a nasogastric tube inserted, and palpate it in the stomach. Free any adhesions. Pack the small bowel in the upper end of the abdominal cavity. Move the rectosigmoid junction to the right, and incise the parietal peritoneum where it touches the taenia to be sure that the anastomosis can be reperitonealized.

B, Elevate the left peritoneal flap and expose the left ureter. Carefully mobilize it sharply and bluntly from its bed, preserving the adventitial vessels. Watch for vessels entering laterally below the pelvic brim and medially above it; clamp, cut, and ligate them or control them with bipolar coagulation. Continue releasing the ureter to as close to the bladder as possible to provide a long ureter for a low anastomosis. Place a 4-0 silk stay suture in the ureter; then clamp it distal to the suture with a right-angle clamp, and divide and ligate it. If the ureter is small, it may be ligated just proximal to the site of division to allow it to dilate before anastomosis. Repeat the procedure on the right side by moving the sigmoid colon to the left. Incise the adjacent peritoneum at the site of contact with the colon; on this side the retroperitoneal incision can be made somewhat more medially. Expose and free the right ureter as was done on the left.

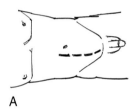

A

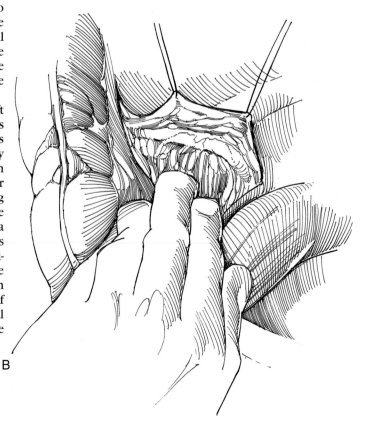

B

2 With the left thumb and forefinger, grasp the sigmoid colon at its junction with the rectum to elevate the tenia libera. Incise the peritoneal coat and muscularis for 5 to 6 cm with a #15 blade until the white submucosa is expressed.

3 Separate the muscle from the submucosa with a curved mosquito clamp for at least 1 cm on either side of the incision to provide seromuscular flaps to cover the anastomosis.

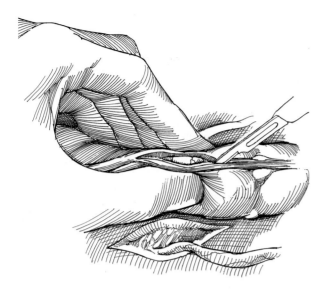

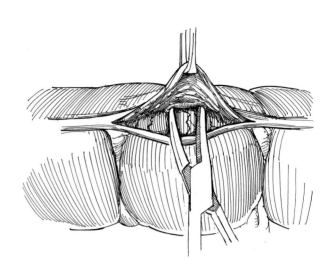

4 Tack the medial flap of the posterior peritoneum adjacent to the bowel incision on the right to the serosa with 4-0 or 5-0 SAS.

5 Hold up a bit of the submucosa in fine forceps, and excise the elevated tip to leave a 3-mm opening into the bowel. Mucus exudes; if not, insert the tip of a small curved clamp to be sure the bowel has been entered. The opening enlarges surprisingly during the anastomotic procedure.

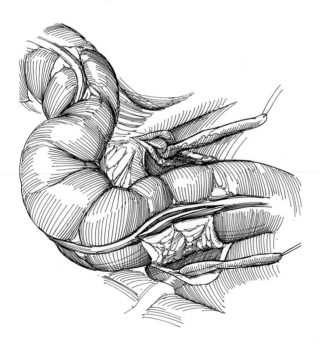

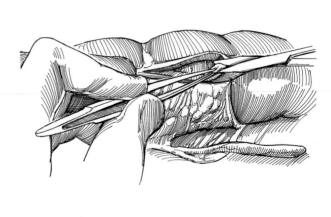

6 Trim the ureter to the proper length to avoid kinking (in the figure it is too long). Spatulate it and replace the stay suture. Place a 4-0 or 5-0 SAS through the mucosa and submucosa of the bowel from outside in, then through the apex of the ureteral cut from the inside out. Place a second suture next to the first, and tie both of them.

7 Run each suture down each side, locking a stitch occasionally, and tie them together at the tip.

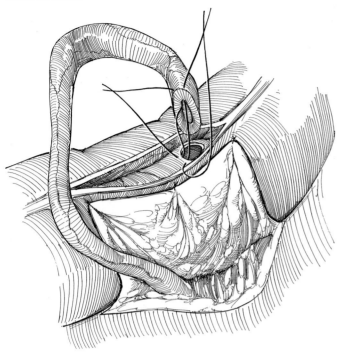

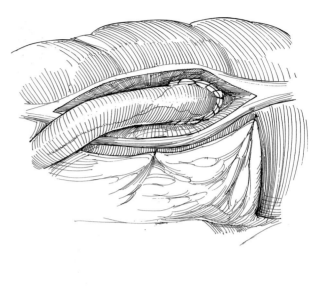

8 Approximate the seromuscular layer over the anastomosis with interrupted 4-0 or 5-0 SAS, taking care not to constrict the site of ureteral exit (leave the hiatus twice the diameter of the ureter). Bring the area of closure to the lateral flap of peritoneum, and suture it in place with 4-0 or 5-0 SAS.

9 Repeat the procedure on the left side. Stents are usually not necessary. Close without drainage.

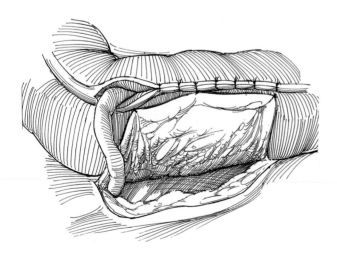

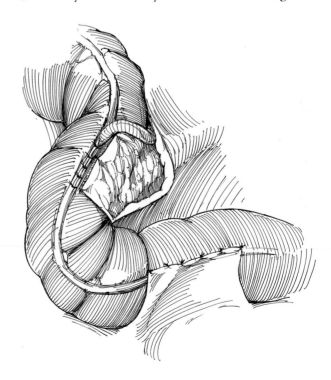

CLOSED TECHNIQUE WITH URETERAL SPATULATION
(Kelalis Modification)

At Step 5 of the closed (Leadbetter) technique, spatulate the ureter.

10 **A,** Incise through the muscular coat of the colon for 1 or 2 cm, just enough to expose the submucosa. Pick it up in Adson forceps, and trim a very small button of mucosa and submucosa with fine scissors.

B, Anastomose the mucosa of the ureter to the mucosa at the opening in the bowel using interrupted 4-0 or 5-0 SAS in a watertight fashion. Incorporate the anastomosis into the bowel by placing a series of sutures over the ureter, starting the stitch laterally and exiting from the bowel wall about 1 cm from the taenia, then entering on the other side 1 cm from the tenia and exiting laterally. Tie the sutures successively from the distal end, making sure that the ureter is not constricted at the hiatus.

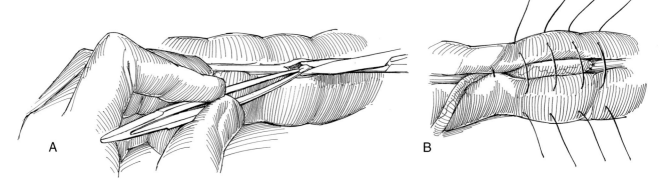

TRANSCOLONIC TECHNIQUE
(Goodwin)

11 **A,** *Incision:* Lower midline (see page 867).
B, Retract the sigmoid colon to the left, and incise the peritoneum over the right ureter just below the crossing of the iliac vessels, where it is most easily identified; continue the incision to as low a point as possible.

MODIFIED RECTAL BLADDER
(Kock-Ghoneim)

22 **A,** Make a 15-cm longitudinal incision in the taenia libera on the anterior wall of the rectum, extending from the rectosigmoid junction to a point 3 to 5 cm distal to the peritoneal reflection. Clear the mesentery from the distal 10 cm of sigmoid. Grasp the wall of the sigmoid with Babcock clamps introduced through the rectal opening, and intussuscept it into the rectum for a distance of 5 cm. Fasten it with a row of staples on either side of the mesentery and in the opposite quadrants. Apply an additional row to fix the nipple to the rectal wall. Anastomose the ureters by the transcolonic technique with stents (Steps 11 to 17).

B, Isolate a 20-cm segment of ileum, open it, fold it into a U shape, and suture the medial borders. Apply the flap to the rectal defect. Form a transverse colostomy, to be maintained for 6 to 8 weeks. Insert a rectal tube. Remove the stents in 10 days, but leave a rectal tube in place for 3 weeks.

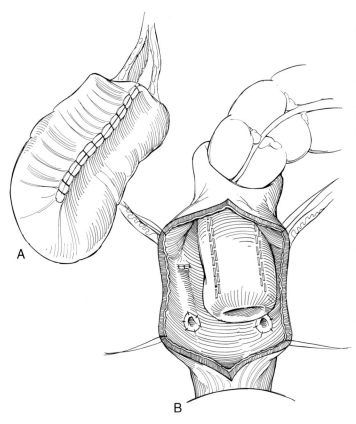

A

B

OTHER ALTERNATIVES TO URETEROSIGMOIDOSTOMY

One alternative to simple ureterosigmoidostomy for vesical exstrophy is the Boyce-Vest operation, in which the base of the closed bladder is anastomosed to the adjacent bowel wall below a colostomy. This variation may produce better long-term results at the cost of a permanent colostomy.

Another alternative to standard ureterosigmoidostomy to prevent reflux is the valved S-shaped rectosigmoid pouch (Sundin and Mansi, 1993): Detubularize the intact rectum and sigmoid colon and form an S-shaped pouch, into which intussuscept 10 cm of the colon proximal to the pouch.

POSTOPERATIVE PROBLEMS
Immediate Problems

Oliguria and anuria are most often the result of inadequate intraoperative fluid replacement and hypotension. Try challenging with furosemide. Perform ultrasonography to detect hydronephrosis; if it is present, place percutaneous nephrostomies at once before anastomotic leakage can occur.

Leakage at the anastomosis is signaled by fever and signs of peritonitis. Immediate reoperation is mandatory, although small leaks have been known to close spontaneously if the rectum is well drained. A *pelvic abscess* may develop after the first 5 or 10 days and requires drainage. Do an ultrasound study (or a computed tomographic scan) to detect it.

Peritonitis, formerly a frequent complication and cause of death, now seldom occurs if the bowel is well prepared, suitable broad-spectrum antibiotics are given, and the anastomoses are extraperitonealized. *Incontinence,* especially at night, is common, even though many of the children had anal continence before diversion.

Later Problems

When chronic urinary tract infections with *pyelonephritis occur,* the cause is often ureteral obstruction or reflux. Perform an enema with water-soluble contrast medium. Deterioration of the upper tracts is the result of infection in a high proportion of patients. Early *obstruction at the ureteral anastomotic site* can be avoided by using a meticulous epithelium-to-epithelium technique, but late stenosis is frequent enough to require at least yearly intravenous urography at first so that reoperation can be done at the first evidence of upper tract obstruction or deterioration. *Pyohydronephrosis* is not a rare sequela to ureterosigmoidostomy, often requiring nephrectomy after a mean interval of 16 years in one large series (Kälbe et al, 1990).

Significant *hyperchloremic acidosis* is usually seen only in patients with existent or developing renal impairment. It may be prevented by a low-chloride diet with added sodium and potassium as bicarbonate or citrate. In fact, regular ingestion of an elixir of potassium citrate is advisable. Titrate the dose to keep the serum bicarbonate level nearly normal. Treat the decompensated patient with a rectal tube, fluids, and additional sodium and potassium bicarbonate. Frequent evacuation of urine and retention of a rectal tube at night may reduce reabsorption and also avoid the not-unusual nocturnal incontinence. Rectal irritation (proctitis) and perianal excoriation are common. Some cases are converted to another form of diversion.

Adenocarcinoma may occur at the site of anastomosis after an average interval of 25 years, with an incidence of 5 percent. The stools should be screened for blood every 3 months and colonoscopy done yearly starting on the fifth anniversary. If the ureterosigmoidostomy is converted to a ureteroileostomy or to cutaneous diversion, be sure to excise the terminal ureter and an adjacent cuff of colon in an effort to avoid later development of adenocarcinoma at the initial anastomotic site.

REVISION OF URETEROCOLIC ANASTOMOSIS

Perform colonoscopy on the patient to determine if the obstruction has a malignant cause. Provide a mechanical bowel preparation, and give perioperative intravenous antibiotics. Insert a large rectal tube, and fix it pararectally. Expose the ureter transperitoneally, and mobilize it to its junction with the taenia. Incise the taenia longitudinally, and dissect the ureter with a button of colonic mucosa. Trim the ureter, and send the end for pathologic examination. Select a new site, and implant the ureter by the Leadbetter technique (Steps 1 to 9). Alternatively, if one implant is functioning well, insert the obstructed ureter into it (transureteroureterostomy, see pages 838 to 839). If operation is for ureteral reflux, incise the taenia proximal to the anastomosis to the depth of the mucosa, and lay the ureter in the longer tunnel that is formed. Consider ureteroureterostomy for bilateral cases, implanting the better ureter into the bowel.

Alternatively, consider reconstructing the lower urinary tract (undiversion) or converting the ureterosigmoidostomy to another form of continent diversion. If renal function has deteriorated, provide free drainage with a conduit such as an ileal conduit (see page 647) or a nonrefluxing sigmoid conduit (see page 664). In either case, resect a 10-cm segment of the colon, including the ureterocolonic anastomosis, to reduce the risk of malignancy.

Commentary by Mohamed A. Ghoneim

Several of the technical modifications that are described reflect a need to circumvent the disadvantages of the conventional ureterosigmoidectomy.

The incidence of ureteric obstructions following a submucosal tunnel reimplantation ranges between 10 and 15 percent, whether a closed or open technique was used. Attention to technical detail may reduce this incidence. However, the best technique for ureterointestinal anastomosis is a wide spatulated mucosa-to-mucosa anastomosis. This can be achieved if the ureters are implanted in an independent ileal nipple valve (hemi-Kock) pouch.

The urodynamic properties of the rectal reservoir can be improved in terms of volume/capacity by patching with ileum (Kock-Ghoneim) or folding the sigmoid (Hohenfellner). These techniques should reduce the incidence of nocturnal incontinence.

The extent of electrolyte imbalance and the resulting metabolic acidosis are proportional to the surface area of bowel exposed for reabsorption of urine. Evidence has been provided that limitation of this area can be achieved by creating a colorectal intussusception valve (Kock-Ghoneim). However, this procedure requires a temporary colostomy. If this option is not desired, prophylactic alkali therapy is required. The potential danger of carcinogenesis must be considered if the patient's expected span of life is long, such as in cases of ectopia vesicae. The use of an ileal intussusception valve for reflux prevention removes the ureter from colonic mucosa. It is theoretically possible that this reduces the incidence of development of an adenocarcinoma at the anastomotic site.

Two developments may reduce the need of diversion into the large gut. Arap's procedure for reconstruction of ectopia vesicae is one. In addition, several published reports indicate that orthotopic bladder substitution in women following cystectomy is feasible and has good functional results.

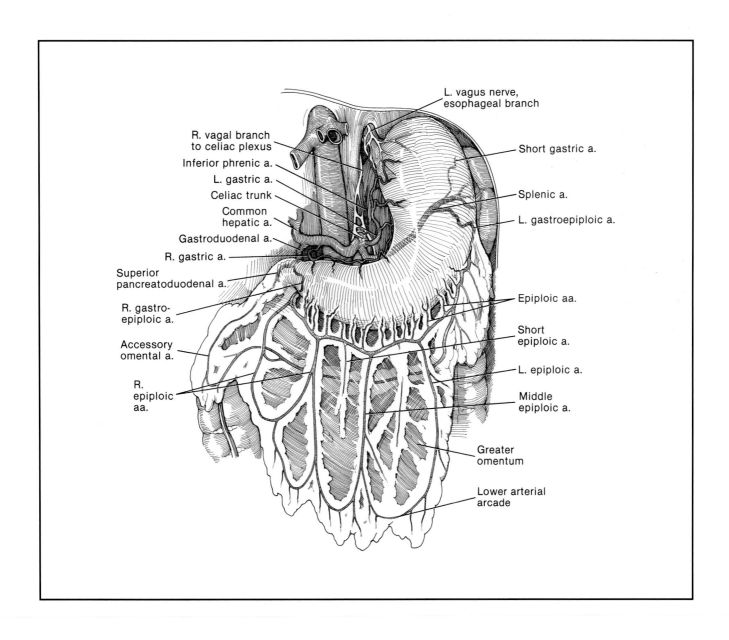

Principles of Bladder Augmentation

Augmentation cystoplasty is usually done for reduced bladder compliance or for detrusor hyperreflexia-instability in patients with spinal cord disease, myelodysplasia, interstitial cystitis, idiopathic detrusor instability, radiation cystitis, neurogenic bladder, and a few other states. The ileum, parts of the colon, the stomach, and the dilated ureter are sources for tissue (Table 1). A fascial sling may be added to improve continence. An increase in bladder capacity of 400 percent can be expected. In patients with a dysfunctional vesical neck, place an encircling rectus fascial wrap with or without narrowing to tighten the vesical neck (Walker et al, 1995); then establish intermittent catheterization.

Augmentation is preferable to substitution. It results in less disturbance of metabolism because it requires resection of a smaller amount of bowel, especially if the terminal ileum and cecum are used for substitution. Preservation of the trigone obviates problems with ureterointestinal anastomosis. Augmentation also has a lower rate of complications.

Complications include the development of stones and incontinence. Revision of the augmentation is seldom necessary. Pyelonephritis is not uncommon, small bowel obstruction occurs less frequently, and rupture of the reservoir occurs even less often.

Enuresis is a common and very distressing complication, probably resulting from an obtunded sensation of fullness of the bladder combined with perineal relaxation during sleep.

Table 1. Bladder Augmentation

	Page
Ileocystoplasty	
Ileocystoplasty	729–731, Steps 1–5
Hemi-Kock procedure	732, Steps 6 and 7
Conversion of ileal conduit for augmentation	733–734, Steps 8–10
Sigmoidocystoplasty	
Sigmoidocystoplasty	735–740, Steps 1–13
Cecocystoplasty and Antireflux Cecocystoplasty	
Cecocystoplasty	742–748, Steps 1–13
Antireflux cecocystoplasty	749–752, Steps 14–19
Ileocecocystoplasty	
Ileocecocystoplasty	753–756, Steps 1–9
Gastrocystoplasty	
Gastrocystoplasty	757–762, Steps 1–8
Appendicovesicostomy with gastric augmentation	762
Ureterocystoplasty	
Ureterocystoplasty	763, Steps 1 and 2
Autoaugmentation	
Autoaugmentation by seromyotomy	765, Steps 1 to 3
Laparoscopic autoaugmentation	766

Ileocystoplasty

Determine the patient's renal function; it must be adequate to cope with urine absorption from the bowel. Evaluate vesical residual urine and capacity, detrusor contractility and compliance, and urethral function to select the appropriate augmentation procedure and to decide whether an increase in outlet resistance by bladder neck reconstruction or artificial sphincter placement or a reduction in resistance is needed. Obtain an intravenous urogram and a voiding cystourethrogram to assess bladder size and configuration. Serum creatinine helps define upper tract function. Cycling the bladder may be useful to increase its capacity and make the attachment of bowel easier.

Preoperatively, consider the need for and feasibility of intermittent catheterization after augmentation, making sure that the urethra is continent, patent, and accessible. Teach the patient how to perform self-catheterization. Especially consider the motivation of the patient for reconstruction, which must be strong to warrant operation. If capacity is limited or the outlet relaxed, warn the patient of the possibility of incontinence.

The ureters may be left in the bladder or may be reimplanted into the bowel via tunnels, with or without transureteroureterostomy. Implantation of the dilated ureter into the intussuscepted ileum is least desirable. In general, tunnels are preferable to nipples. Reimplant the ureter into the bladder whenever possible, although not at the cost of using ischemic ureter or reimplanting under tension.

ILEOCYSTOPLASTY, CUP PATCH (Goodwin)

Instruments: For stapled anastomoses, provide an autosuture set with TA 55 4.8-mm and 3.5-mm and EE-A staplers.

1 **A,** *Position:* Supine.
Incision: Standing on the left side of the patient, make a lower midline transperitoneal incision (see page 867). Tilt the head of the table down, and pack the intestines. Insert a ring retractor. Check the mobility and mesenteric length of the terminal ileum. The bladder may be opened at this time (proceed to Step 4), or the bowel segment may be prepared first.

B, Choose a 20- to 25-cm loop of ileum; leave the terminal 15 to 20 cm of ileum in place. Mark the ends and the center with stay sutures as for ileal conduit (see page 649). Draw the center of the loop over the dome of the bladder to be sure it reaches the anterior part of the proposed vesicoileal anastomotic line. Divide the ileum between Kocher clamps. The mesentery, which should be well vascularized, needs to be divided for a shorter distance than for ureteroileostomy. Reapproximate the ileum in front of the loop (sutured: see page 652; stapled: see pages 653 to 654), and close the mesentery. Irrigate the loop with saline solution until clear, then with 1 percent neomycin solution (keep the solution away from the peritoneum), and finally with air. Divide the ileal segment along its antimesenteric border with straight Mayo scissors, or with the cutting current if the loop is kept broadly in contact with the body to avoid thermal damage to the mesentery. Trim the corners.

Alternatively, before opening the bowel, shape it into a loop and suture the adjacent serosal surfaces together with a running 4-0 chromic catgut (CCG) suture.

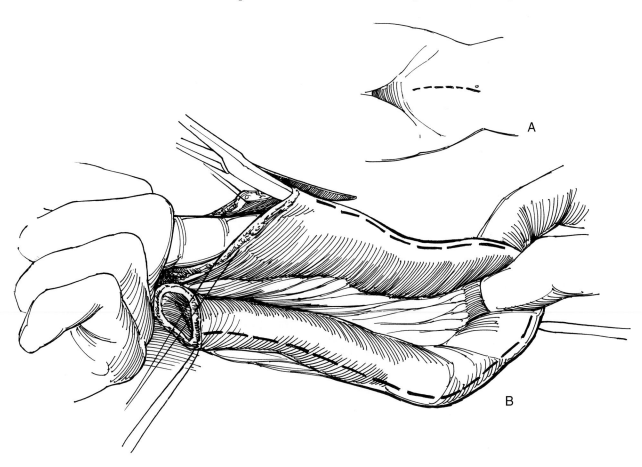

2 Suture the adjacent mucosal edges with a continuous 3-0 CCG or synthetic absorbable suture (SAS). Use an atraumatic tapered needle through all layers of the bowel. Because the bladder contracts, place stay sutures to allow the bowel to be bunched. Also, tie the running suture at least once on the outside to control gathering of the suture line. Fold the open end of the segment over itself.

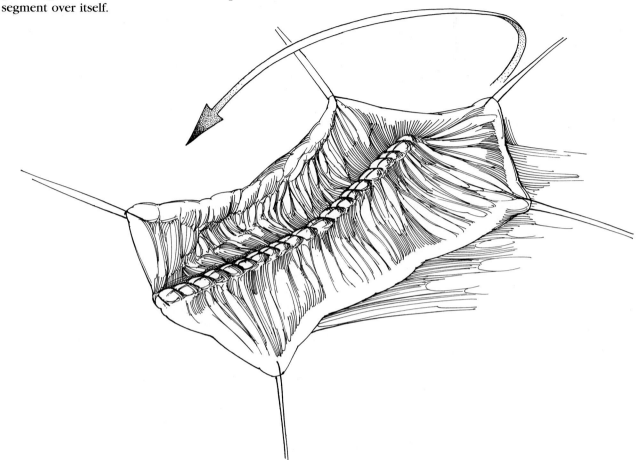

3 Suture the segment along each margin to form a cup. If a larger opening is desired for anastomosis to the bladder, do not suture the edges together for their entire length. Watch for interference with the blood supply.

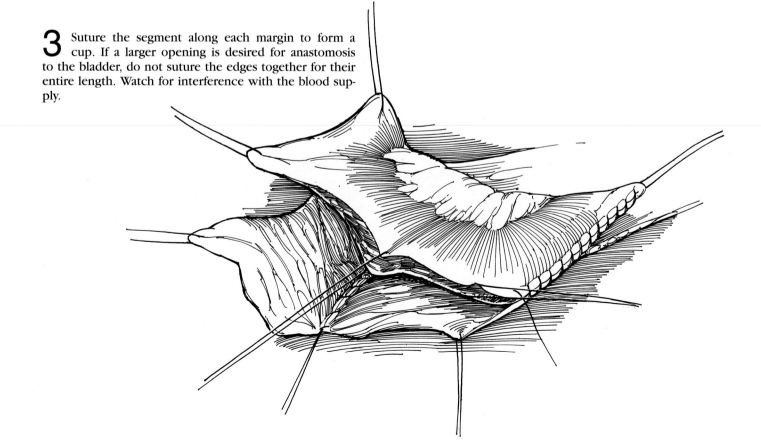

4 Grasp the bladder at the apex adjacent to the peritoneal reflection. Sharply divide the peritoneum and transversalis fascia laterally on both sides, and open the cleavage plane as far as the ureters and superior vesical pedicles. Open the bladder sagittally as far posteriorly as possible, using the cutting current. Fulgurate the smaller vessels, and ligate the large vessels with 4-0 CCG. Make generous lateral cuts to lay the bladder flat, thus maximizing defunctionalization by eliminating noncompliant or hypercontractile elements. These cuts also increase the template for anastomosis of the bowel to the bladder.

Alternative: Use a coronal incision carried within 1.5 cm of the bladder neck. In this case, insert ureteral catheters early to avoid injury to the ureters, and use Lahey scissors to complete the incision anterior to the ureteral orifices to leave an adequate margin for the bowel anastomosis.

Insert infant feeding tube catheters to identify the ureters, and place a Malecot cystostomy tube through the bladder wall away from the future suture line. If the bladder is very small, the tube may be placed through the new augmentation, as shown, although this solution is less satisfactory.

Place the posterior rim of the ileal cup adjacent to the posterior apex of the bladder incision. It helps to place stay sutures in the edge of the bladder to divide it into quarters. Starting posteriorly, run a 3-0 CCG suture through all layers up each side to form a watertight closure. Tie the sutures several times during insertion to prevent gathering, and take extra care where the suture lines meet. Reinforcement with 2-0 CCG sutures may be helpful, especially posteriorly where tension can exist.

A YV-plasty at the vesical neck should be considered only when intermittent catheterization is not planned. An artificial sphincter may then be applied; the chance of contamination is minimal because ileal contents are sterile.

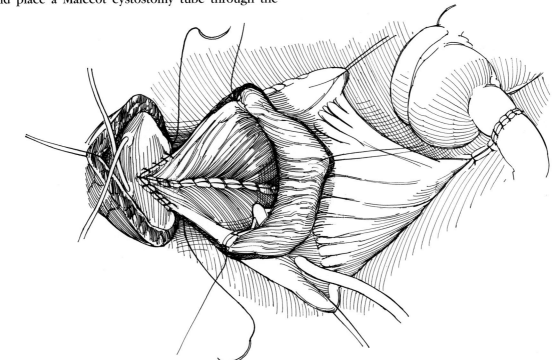

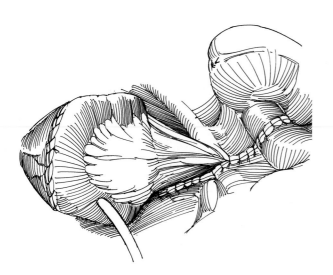

5 Remove the ureteral catheters, and close the mesentery. Fix the mesentery of the segment to the posterior peritoneum to prevent an internal hernia.

Free the omentum from the transverse colon; first tack it posteriorly and then wrap it around the repair to cover the suture lines. Insert a straight 22 F silicone urethral catheter, fill the bladder with saline, and test the watertightness. Reinforce the suture line at the site of leaks. Place one (or two, if the anastomosis is tenuous) Jackson-Pratt drain(s) for suction drainage. Take cultures from the peritoneal cavity and wound. The catheter may remain in the bladder for extra security during the immediate postoperative period. Close the wound in layers around the drain(s).

Postoperative Care

Provide antibiotic coverage for 10 days. Watch for mucous obstruction of the catheter by hourly checks of output and careful irrigation. Remove the Jackson-Pratt drains on the 5th day and the suprapubic tube on the 14th. It is good practice to check the area by sonography the following day. Intermittent catheterization may be necessary for a period of time.

HEMI-KOCK PROCEDURE

6 Follow Steps 1 to 5 of ileocystoplasty, resecting a loop of ileum 40 to 45 cm long. (For an orthotopic bladder replacement, use a 55- to 60-cm segment.) Open the distal 30 cm of ileum on the antimesenteric border.

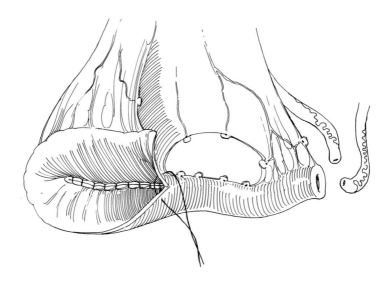

7 Fold the opened flap upon itself, and close it with a running 3-0 SAS to form a pouch. Clear the mesentery from half of the more proximal segment (8 cm), and intussuscept the ileum to form a nipple (see page 688). Incise the full thickness of the outer wall of the nipple, denude the adjacent muscle in the pouch, and suture the two surfaces together with 3-0 SAS. A collar made of a 1-cm strip of polyglycolic acid mesh soaked in tetracycline may be placed where the ileum enters the intussusception for further stabilization. Anastomose the pouch to the remainder of the bladder. Conjoin the ureters, and implant them in the proximal end of the ileum (see page 661), inserting stents. Suture the pouch to the levator ani muscles on both sides. Insert a balloon catheter through the conduit, and secure it and the stents to the skin.

Postoperatively, monitor drainage from the ureteral catheter every 6 hours. If it declines, irrigate the catheters. After 2 weeks, perform cystography at minimal pressure (15 to 20 cm H_2O). If leakage is seen, leave both catheters in place another week, and repeat the study.

The hemi-Kock pouch may be applied to the rectum below a rectal intussusception to create a *valved augmented rectum.*

The technique used for constructing the W-shaped neobladder (see pages 772 to 773) can be applied to augmentation by anastomosing the neobladder to the opened bladder instead of closing the caudal end of the W complex.

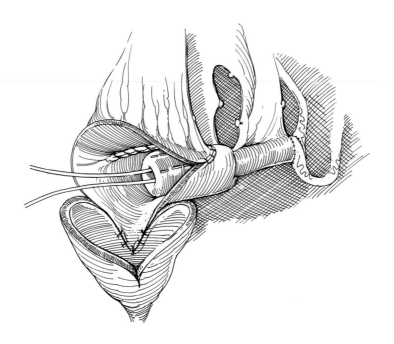

CONVERSION OF ILEAL CONDUIT FOR AUGMENTATION
(Hanna)

8 **A,** Dissect the ileal conduit from its bed. Circumcise the stoma *(dotted line)*, and discard the distal end of the ileum. Open the loop on the antimesenteric border.

B, Trim the ileum obliquely *(dashed lines)*. Free the ureters, and close the defects in the ileum in two layers. Reanastomose the ureters by the Camey technique (see page 770), and stent them with 5 F infant feeding tubes.

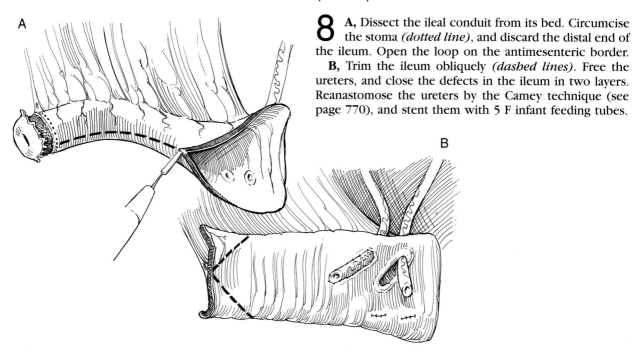

9 Isolate a new segment of ileum 30 to 33 cm long, and open the proximal two thirds along the antimesenteric border. Free the mesentery from the terminal 8 cm, and create a 5-cm intussusception. Externally, fix the exiting bowel with 3-0 silk sutures. Internally, make three seromuscular incisions in the posterior wall of the nipple, in the opposite side and near the tip of the nipple, and make corresponding incisions in the bowel wall. Approximate the incisions of the nipple and the bowel wall with 3-0 CCG sutures, with a technique similar to fixation of the intussuscepted ileocecal valve (see page 749).

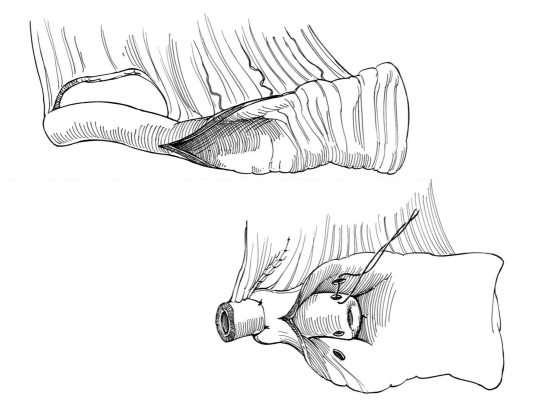

10 Suture the patch from the previous conduit to the new pouch with a continuous suture of 3-0 CCG. For extra capacity, fold the new, opened loop back upon itself, suture the edges, and then fold the patch into a cup (see Step 1). Fix the pouch to the abdominal wall near the stomal site with catgut sutures. Excise the umbilicus, and form a flush stoma. Arrange for the stents to exit from the stoma to divert the urine. Insert a perforated catheter, and irrigate it regularly to prevent accumulation of mucus. Remove the ureteral stents at 2 weeks. Before discharge, teach the patient how to irrigate the bladder daily. Perform cystography through the cystostomy tube at 2 weeks to ascertain the integrity of the anastomoses. Clamp the tube; if the patient can either void or perform intermittent catheterization, remove it. Even if the patient is able to void, it is advisable to check the bladder by catheter once a day for a couple of weeks to detect accumulation of residual urine. Query the patient about the frequency of bowel movements.

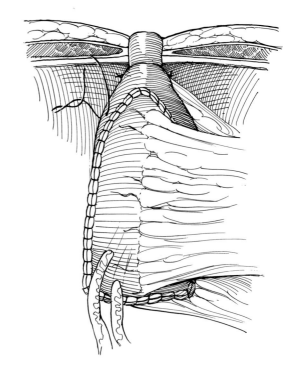

POSTOPERATIVE CARE AFTER AUGMENTATION

Maintain nasogastric suction until good-quality bowel sounds are heard. Watch for jejunal paralysis with fluid levels in the left upper quadrant on radiography; if paralysis is present, delay feeding. Have the system irrigated with normal saline three times a day to clear the mucus. The broad-spectrum antibiotics may be stopped after 5 days and the drains removed when drainage ceases. If infection appears, treat it according to the operative cultures. Be cautious with nephrotoxic drugs because of the resorptive characteristic of the ileum in the presence of residual urine. If diarrhea occurs that is twice as frequent as preoperatively, check for bile acid dysfunction with ^{75}Se-labeled homocholic acid–taurine (SeHCAT). If it is poorly retained, provide anion-exchange resins (Barrington et al, 1995). If reoperation is necessary, the new bladder can be easily identified if filled with dilute methylene blue.

Commentary by Anthony Richard Mundy

There are two types of cystoplasty: (1) augmentation cystoplasty, in which the aim is to turn an overactive hypercontractile or poorly compliant bladder into a substantial docile reservoir, usually in patients with detrusor hyperreflexia due to spina bifida, spinal cord injury, or detrusor instability; and (2) substitution cystoplasty, in which a much larger segment of bowel is used to replace the entire bladder with much the same aims, usually in patients having a cystectomy for transitional cell carcinoma of the bladder. In both, the procedure is indicated after failed medical or other less radical treatment. The usual alternatives when surgery is contemplated are ileal conduit urinary diversion, particularly in patients with bladder cancer, and continent urinary diversion, in patients with either bladder cancer or neuropathic bladder dysfunction.

The most important factor in selection is the patient's motivation to use clean intermittent self-catheterization and otherwise cope with the requirements of long-term follow-up.

Although renal function should ideally be normal, in many instances abnormal renal function is due to abnormal bladder function, particularly when it is the consequence of outflow obstruction. In such circumstances cystoplasty may be corrective and therefore may lead to an improvement in renal function or, more commonly, to a delay before further decline into renal failure.

The key to a satisfactory result in any cystoplasty procedure is preparation of the bladder in augmentation cystoplasty and performance of the cystectomy in substitution cystoplasty. For augmentation cystoplasty, the natural bladder must be adequately bisected in whatever plane is chosen (it is irrelevant) so that the two halves of the bladder are separated and cannot function to produce a coordinated contraction. In the cystectomy prior to substitution cystoplasty, every care should be taken to preserve the neurovascular bundles innervating the corpora cavernosa and also to preserve as much as possible of the urethral sphincter mechanism to maintain continence and prevent stricture formation.

Having prepared the "recipient site" adequately, one must ensure that an adequate length is available of whatever piece of bowel is chosen. Again, it is probably irrelevant what segment of bowel is used or how it is reconfigured so long as it is sufficient to give an adequate capacity. Many surgeons prefer ileum because colonic anastomoses are more prone to problems, but the ileum does not always reach into the pelvis, particularly in patients with neuropathic bladder dysfunction. In children, colonic anastomoses are less prone to problems.

When opening the bowel prior to reconfiguration, I always pass a length of suction tubing down to stretch out the antimesenteric border and then cut down using coagulation diathermy. This opens the bowel with little or no bleeding.

When doing an augmentation cystoplasty, I usually use a straight "clam" ileocystoplasty, in which a simple patch of bowel rather than a cup is used to hold the bisected bladder halves apart. The hemi-Kock procedure, although commonly performed using a rather longer piece of ileum for substitution cystoplasty, is really only a means of incorporating an antireflux ureteric anastomosis into an enterocystoplasty. For a substitution cystoplasty, I prefer to use the right colon from the ileocaecal valve to the middle of the transverse colon; for an antireflux mechanism, I prefer a tunnel procedure and so have little use for the hemi-Kock procedure.

Most of these points are personal preferences, but careful patient selection based on the willingness and proven ability of the patient to use clean intermittent self-catheterization, adequate preparation of the bladder or bladder outflow prior to cystoplasty, and use of an adequate length of bowel of sufficient mobility are all of fundamental importance regardless of personal preferences in technique.

Sigmoidocystoplasty

1 *Position:* Place the patient supine. For female patients, prepare and drape the perineum so that a catheter can be inserted aseptically during the procedure. Instruments and preliminaries are the same as those for ileocystoplasty.

Incision: Stand on the patient's left side. Make a lower midline transperitoneal incision, from just above the umbilicus to the symphysis. Alternatively, if you are confident that an ileal or sigmoid patch can be used, make a transverse skin incision combined with a vertical midline incision in the fascia, a more cosmetic but more limiting approach. Pack the small intestine into the upper abdomen. Because the appendix may be needed as a cutaneous conduit, do not perform a preliminary appendectomy.

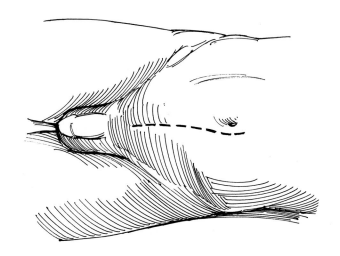

2 Backlight and study the *colonic vasculature* for the distribution of the sigmoid artery from the inferior mesenteric artery, and select a length of sigmoid colon at least 20 cm long, preferably 25 cm or more, that is mobile and has a very broad mesentery. Be sure to take enough bowel. It may be necessary to free the colon at the white line of Toldt for adequate visualization.

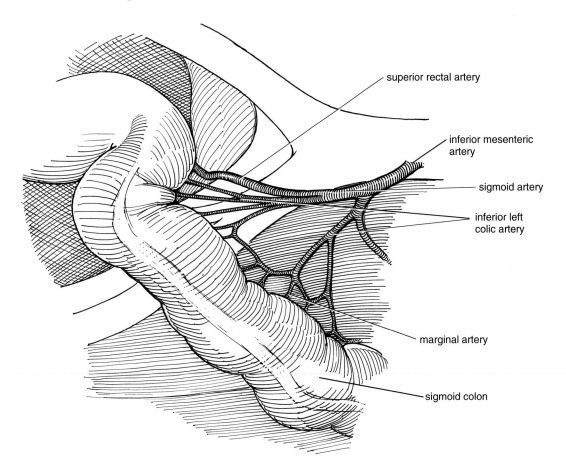

superior rectal artery

inferior mesenteric artery

sigmoid artery

inferior left colic artery

marginal artery

sigmoid colon

3 *Isolate the loop* of sigmoid colon from the retroperitoneum with scissors along the white line. Mark the selected length with silk stay sutures. Pull the proximal end down to be sure that the bowel can be reanastomosed without tension. Divide the mesentery, but not as deeply as for a sigmoid conduit (see page 664). Divide the bowel between two pairs of Kocher clamps. If the bowel has been properly prepared, it is not necessary to fulgurate the exposed mucosa.

4 *Colon-colon anastomosis, suture technique* (for alternative suture technique, see pages 606 to 608; for a stapling technique, see page 66): Make sure that the colon is anterior to the isolated segment. Place noncrushing intestinal clamps (Doyen) 2 cm proximal to each Kocher clamp, and remove the Kocher clamps. Insert a posterior row of six or eight interrupted inverting horizontal mattress sutures of 4-0 silk.

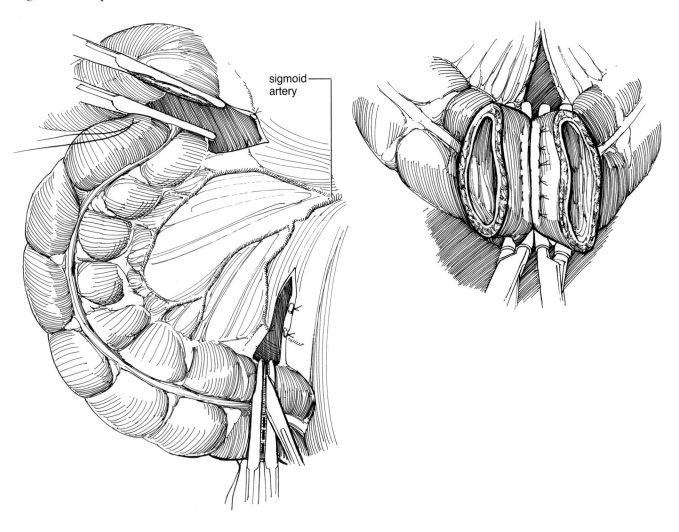

5 Start one double-armed or two single-armed 4-0 polypropylene sutures posteriorly in the center of the luminal side. Run the sutures in opposite directions. Take 3 mm of tissue in each bite, and keep the stitches close together.

6 Tie each suture in continuity near each corner to prevent purse-stringing. Construct the corners carefully, using one suture at a time, going from mucosa to serosa on one side and serosa to mucosa on the other (half-Connell suture, see page 37). Then tie another in-continuity knot at each corner anteriorly. Continue with an inverting suture from each end, going in and out on one side and in and out on the other (Connell suture, see page 37). Tie the sutures in the midline. Remove the Doyen clamps. As an alternative to the running 4-0 polypropylene sutures, place a layer of inverting interrupted 4-0 silk sutures. Use of interrupted sutures in the inner layer prevents possible purse-stringing, with resultant narrowing at the anastomosis.

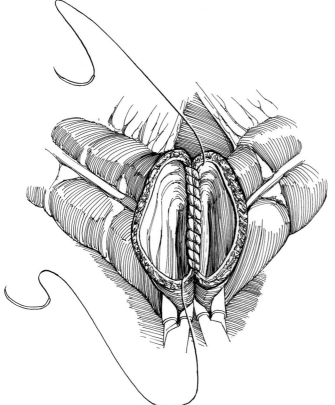

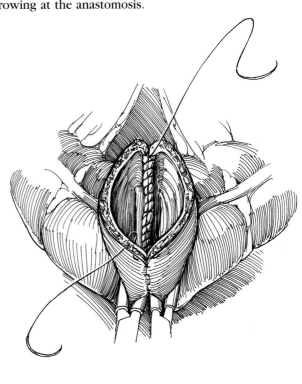

7 Place an anterior layer of interrupted inverting sutures of 3-0 or 4-0 silk through the serosa and superficial muscularis.

8 Close the mesocolon with interrupted 4-0 CCG sutures. The sigmoid loop lies lateral to the sigmoid colon.

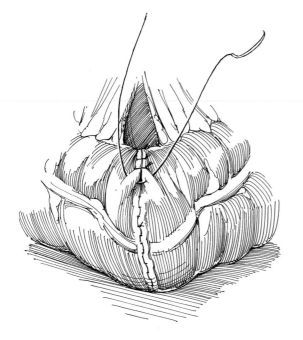

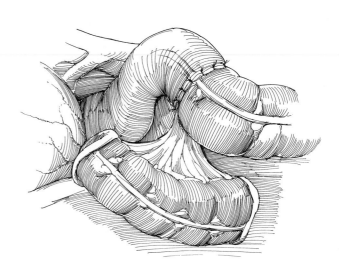

9 *Closure of proximal end.* **A,** Place stay sutures at the mesenteric and antimesenteric borders of the proximal end of the segment. With the Kocher clamp still on the end of the segment, place a running inverting 3-0 CCG suture to invert the mucosal edge (Parker-Kerr suture, see page 39).

B, Remove the bowel clamp, and pull the suture tight as the assistant helps invert the edge; then run the suture back to its origin and tie it. It may be well to place a second simple running 3-0 *non*absorbable suture (NAS) over this closure to ensure watertightness. Repeat the process at the distal end.

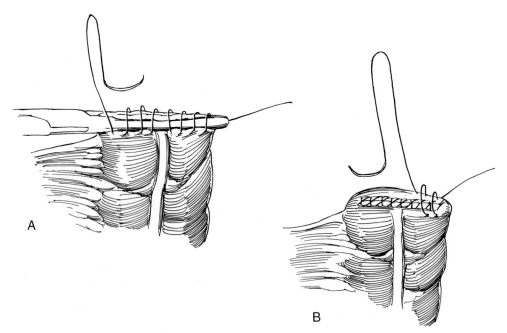

A

B

10 *Open the segment* along the antimesenteric border to within 1 cm of the suture line at each end. Isolate the segment with laparotomy pads, and carefully cleanse it with 0.25 percent neomycin-soaked sponges. Alternatively, irrigate it well over a basin. The sigmoid cap is then ready for placement on the bladder.

Dissect the peritoneum from the dome and posterior wall of the bladder. If this cannot be done, incise the peritoneum vertically over the fundus of the bladder to expose the anterior and posterior aspects. *Open the bladder* between stay sutures in a sagittal plane, approaching the trigone posteriorly and the bladder neck anteriorly. The bladder opening should equal the length of the opening in the segment when it is stretched out by its stay sutures. If the bladder wall is totally resected, as for interstitial cystitis, insert ureteral catheters for guidance. In other cases, such as with neurogenic bladder dysfunction, it is usually not necessary to resect bladder tissue. The bladder incision, however, must be extensive enough to prevent formation of a diverticulum or an hour-glass–type bladder. The ideal configuration after application of the cap is spherical. A transverse orientation of the segment, shown here, may fit better, but rotating the bowel into a sagittal orientation, as shown in Step 11, may be preferable because in this orientation tension does not develop on the mesentery with bladder filling. In fact, the mesentery may become more relaxed.

Begin the *anastomosis of bowel to bladder* in the midline posteriorly, running a 3-0 CCG locked suture posteriorly, including all layers of bladder and bowel.

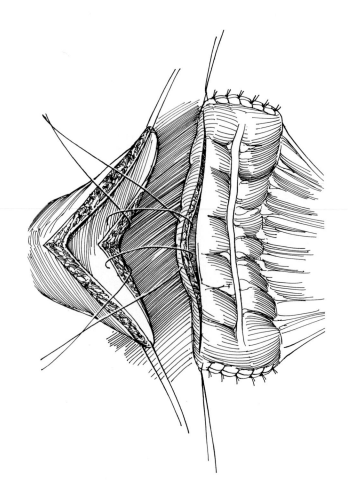

11 Run this suture to the apex of the lateral wall or what used to be the dome of the bladder on each side. Do the same for the contralateral side. Place a second running 3-0 SAS over this suture line to ensure a watertight inverted closure. If the bladder is very small, first suture the sigmoid cap to the bladder in the sagittal plane posteriorly and anteriorly; then close the bowel on each side as the lateral walls of the new bladder. The bladder may contract with time, leaving a rim at the bladder neck.

Place a 12 F or larger single-lumen plastic catheter in the urethra, and secure it by a 2-0 silk suture tied to its

tip and brought through the bladder wall. Alternately, use a balloon catheter. Place a Malecot catheter (except in children with possible latex allergy, for whom use a plastic catheter) in one quadrant of the bladder, to be brought through the body wall later; avoid bringing tubes through the wall of the bowel. The size of the Malecot catheter depends on the patient's size. For small children, size 18 F is the smallest that is acceptable; sizes 22 F to 24 F are ideal because the smaller sizes more easily become plugged with mucus in the postoperative period. Fasten the tube at the bladder wall with a 3-0 plain catgut suture.

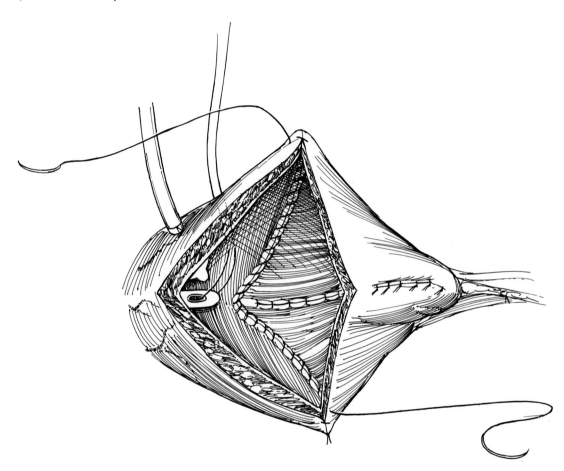

12 Close the anterior suture line in the same way as the posterior closure except in reverse order, beginning in front and proceeding around both sides. Bring the cystostomy catheter through a stab wound in the body wall, and suture it to the skin. Bring both ends of the silk suture in the urethral catheter through the abdominal wall with a straight needle, and tie them over a cotton pledget or a button. Place a 0.25-inch or 0.50-inch Penrose drain, the size depending on that of the patient, in the prevesical space, and bring it out through a separate stab wound. Do not drain patients with ventriculoperitoneal shunts. It may be wise to insert a silicone balloon catheter transurethrally to doubly protect from mucus accumulation. Close the wound in layers, and stitch the Penrose drain to the skin.

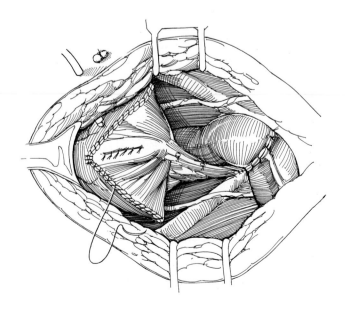

POSTOPERATIVE CARE

At first, irrigate the cystostomy at least three times a day with normal (or 3N) saline to prevent obstruction by mucus. Perform a cystogram in 1 week, and remove the urethral catheter if the anastomoses are intact. After another week or two, clamp the suprapubic tube and start the patient on self-catheterization. When you personally know that this program is being carried out in a satisfactory manner, remove the suprapubic tube after another 1 or 2 weeks, but have the patient continue irrigating at the time of catheterization to remove mucus. At first the bladder is small. Anticholinergic agents and frequent catheterization are required. For the long-term, have the patient use a catheter of generous size, because mucus plugs a smaller catheter and leads to subtle retention. Even if the patient voids, a check for residual urine is necessary at intervals.

S-SIGMOIDOCYSTOPLASTY
(R. Gonzales)

The open sigmoid may be folded into a cup (see pages 730 to 731), or, if the ureters are short and dilated to a degree that they require a long tunnel, it may be folded into an S shape, as described here.

13 **A,** Select a 25-cm segment from the lower portion of the sigmoid colon, and check it for mobility. Incise the mesosigmoid, and resect the segment. Reanastomose the colon, leaving the isolated segment medially. Irrigate the loop and open it on its antimesenteric border, leaving the proximal few centimeters intact to receive the ureters. Form the bowel into an S shape, and suture the two sets of adjacent edges with running polyglactin sutures. Anastomose the ureters to the straight segment by the closed technique. Anastomosing both ureters independently is usually preferable to performing ureteroureterostomy as illustrated. Open the bladder widely in the sagittal plane.

B, Suture the base of the S to the posterior end of the bladder incision. Place a Malecot catheter in the bladder (use a plastic catheter in children with myelomeningocele), and continue to suture colon to colon up the anterior wall. Close the mesocolon.

Cup-plasty: Open the sigmoid segment. Insert the ureters by the transcolonic technique (see pages 720 to 723). Fold the apex of the inverted U down, and suture it to the anterior corner of the bladder incision as a cup (see pages 730 to 731). Run these sutures laterally around the free edges.

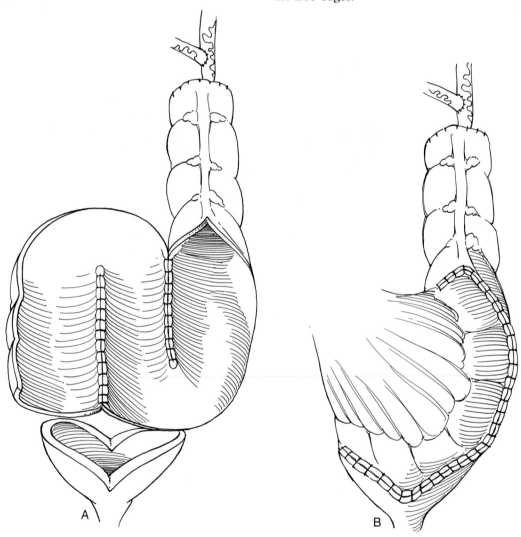

POSTOPERATIVE PROBLEMS

Mucus is formed profusely at first, but after 3 or 4 weeks the quantity subsides to manageable proportions.

Colicky pain suggests *intestinal obstruction*; a silent abdomen suggests *ileus*. *Adhesions* may cause intestinal obstruction soon after the operation; other causes may be an anastomotic stoma that is too narrow or a hernia through an unclosed defect in the mesentery. Take lateral or upright films of the abdomen, and look for gas-fluid levels proximally and for empty bowel distally.

Leakage from the bowel anastomosis can occasionally occur owing to ischemia from resection of too much mesentery. Place a long nasogastric tube, provide hyperalimentation, and continue suction drainage. If it persists for 10 to 14 days, reoperate. *Ischemia and necrosis* of the segment, seen as a dusky stoma during closing, come from tension on the mesentery, from hematoma, or from inadvertent ligation of a major vessel. The bowel remains intact for a week or two, but intervention is needed if the circulation has not recovered by that time. Perform endoscopy of the segment to see how much is involved; if it is only the terminal few centimeters, enough ileum may be pulled out to make a new stoma. Otherwise, another segment of ileum must be attached or a new loop must be created.

If the ileocecal region is used for augmentation, deficiency of vitamin B_{12} can be expected. A supplement must be given yearly. Bone demineralization from metabolic acidosis may result in osteoporosis. Follow the patient with serum electrolyte determinations. *Upper tract deterioration* is possible, especially in patients who are negligent in self-catheterization. *Rupture* of the augmented bladder occurs with overfilling. *Malignancy* must be watched for by yearly cystoscopy with biopsy of questionable areas; urinary cytology may help.

Commentary by Mitchell C. Benson

The patient, male or female, is placed with the break in the table approximately two fingerbreadths above the pubic symphysis. A three-way catheter is inserted after preparation and draping. In females the perineum is included, and in males the penis is included in the operative field. The three-way catheter allows the bladder to be sterilely inflated during the procedure without the inconvenience of repeatedly clamping the catheter and manually injecting irrigant. Despite preoperative intestinal assessment, I am never confident that any particular segment of bowel will be available; therefore, I always make a midline incision. One may encounter adhesions, a short mesentery, or unsuspected pathology. A transverse incision may limit exposure and make the procedure far more difficult. The sigmoid colon is my large bowel segment of choice because loss of a sigmoid segment has the least effect metabolically and functionally upon the patient. Cecal cystoplasty entails loss of the ileocecal valve and should be avoided whenever possible, especially in the younger individual. In my experience, backlighting the sigmoid segment prior to incision of the white line of Toldt may be very difficult. If the sigmoid appears and feels grossly normal, I recommend mobilization of the selected sigmoid loop by incision of the white line prior to illumination of the vascular pedicle.

Being sure to take enough bowel cannot be overemphasized. This applies to colonic mobilization (tension-free anastomosis to bladder and tension-free colonic anastomosis) and to the patch (sufficient size to result in adequate capacity and low pressures). I do not believe that fulguration of the exposed mucosa following bowel division is necessary, even if one still uses a hand-sutured anastomosis. This fulguration risks devitalizing the edges and in my opinion potentially increases the risk of leak. Anastomotic bowel suturing in elective large-intestinal reconstructive surgery is becoming an unnecessary art. The track record of stapled anastomoses is so good (fast and reliable) that hand sutures are being used less and less often.

Step 8 shows the isolated segment of sigmoid colon lateral to the anastomosed large bowel. In my experience (depending upon individual anatomic variation), the segment sometimes lies with less tension when brought medially. This should be determined prior to bowel-bowel anastomosis. Following isolation of the sigmoid segment, I irrigate the segment over a kidney basin lying on top of clean pads to eliminate any residual bowel contents. I do not irrigate with an antibiotic solution. Rather, I rely upon my preoperative mechanical and antibiotic bowel preparation.

I disagree with the technique used in this description for sigmoid cystoplasty. The author closes both ends of the sigmoid with running sutures and then opens the segment along its antimesenteric border. I favor using the entire segment as a patch with the ends left open. This has the advantage of increasing the volume of the augmented bladder and decreasing the risk of cul-de-sacs, which may not empty well. Furthermore, it may—at least in theory—reduce the risk of hour-glass anastomotic contraction because no portion of the patch is left intact.

The author recommends colon-to-bladder anastomosis with a running locked 3-0 CCG suture, followed by a second layer of 3-0 absorbable suture. I recommend a heavier suture and personally use a single-layer 2-0 polyglycolic acid suture as used in neobladder construction. This still results in a watertight anastomosis and saves considerable time.

The use of a small urethral catheter and a large Malecot catheter in Step 11 may not be necessary, depending upon the indication for bladder augmentation. For the adult patient with a high-pressure, contracted neurogenic bladder, I favor the use of a suprapubic tube and a urethral Foley catheter (18 F to 20 F). For the patient with a small normal-pressure bladder (posttraumatic, iatrogenic), a single 22 F to 24 F Foley catheter suffices. In young children, I use a single-lumen plastic urethral catheter secured with a suture.

When possible, I favor reinserting the urethral catheter for 24 hours at the time of suprapubic tube removal. This allows for a more rapid closure of the tract and reduces the risk of perivesical abscess formation.

Cecocystoplasty and Antireflux Ileocecocystoplasty

CECOCYSTOPLASTY

Study the patient urodynamically before planning the operation. This procedure is not suitable for a patient with a relaxed bladder neck because contractions of the bowel may open the neck and cause incontinence. Perform a meglumine diatrizoate (Gastrografin) enema to detect disease in the colon.

Prepare the bowel. If conversion is being made from ureterosigmoidostomy, place a rectal tube.

1 *Position*: Place the patient supine.
Instruments: Use the same instruments as for ileocystoplasty; add a TA-40 or TA-50 stapler.

Incision: Make a lower midline transperitoneal incision from epigastrium to pubis (see page 867). Stand on the left side of the table for most of the operation, although initial mobilization of the ascending colon may be more easily undertaken from the right. Examine the peritoneal contents, and pack the intestinal contents superiorly.

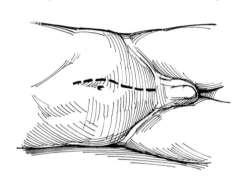

2 Mobilize the ascending colon from the right gutter with scissors along the white line of Toldt to the level of the hepatic flexure, and free the terminal ileum and cecum from their peritoneal attachments over the sacral promontory. Include the use of the hepatic flexure in the event of a substitution. Continue the peritoneal dissection medially to the ligament of Treitz, and separate the right colon and small bowel from the retroperitoneal surface.

Direct the operating light behind the bowel to study the ileocecal blood supply in order to select an appropriate vascular pedicle. Identify the ileocolic and right colic arteries coming from the superior mesenteric artery (see page 679), and divide the mesentery between them almost to the origin of the right colic artery. The stump of the ascending colon is dependent on the ileocolic artery. Be careful not to cut the marginal vessel to the distal colon when dividing the short proximal stem of the right colic artery. If the mesenteric pedicle is unusually short or if the pelvis is very deep, divide one or two additional perpendicular mesocolic vessels to obtain more freedom for the ascending colon. The segment depends on the ileocolic artery for its blood supply.

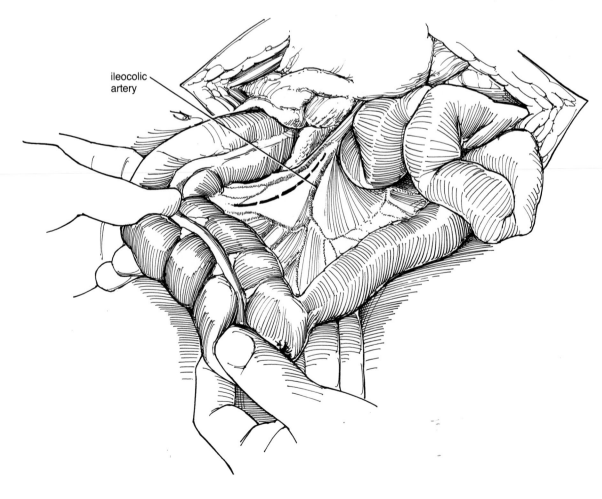

ileocolic artery

3 Divide the colon as close to the right colic artery as possible, either between Kocher clamps or with the GIA surgical stapler. Examine the mesentery to the cecum and terminal ileum to determine how much ileum must be taken to provide a very adequate pedicle for the cecum, usually 15 to 20 cm. Place a stay suture, and divide the mesentery on the other side of the ileocolic artery. Divide the ileum between Kocher clamps, or use the GIA stapler. Anastomose the ileum to the ascending colon using sutures (see page 744) or staples (see page 66).

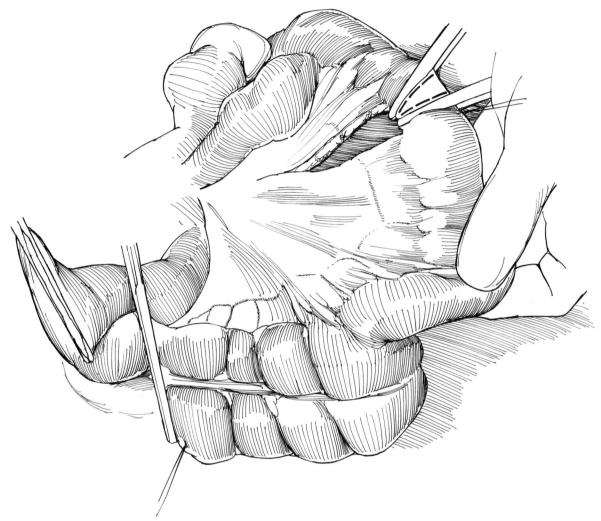

End-to-End Sutured Ileocolic Anastomosis

4 **A and B,** Place four stay sutures of fine CCG in the quadrants of the opening, two posterolaterally and two anterolaterally. Make a slit in the ileum on its antimesenteric border to equalize its diameter with that of the colon, or, if the difference is not too great, take larger bites of tissue on the colonic side during anastomosis. Leave the ears of extra bowel alone. Do not clear the

mesenteric fat from the bowel. Place a 4-0 NAS through the ileal and colonic mesentery 2 cm from the edge; leave it untied.

Start suturing at the mesenteric side. Place a vertical mattress suture of 4-0 CCG through all layers of the bowel, returning the needle only through the mucosa. Do not use forceps; depend on the stay sutures for manipulation. Continue closing the mesenteric half of the anastomosis.

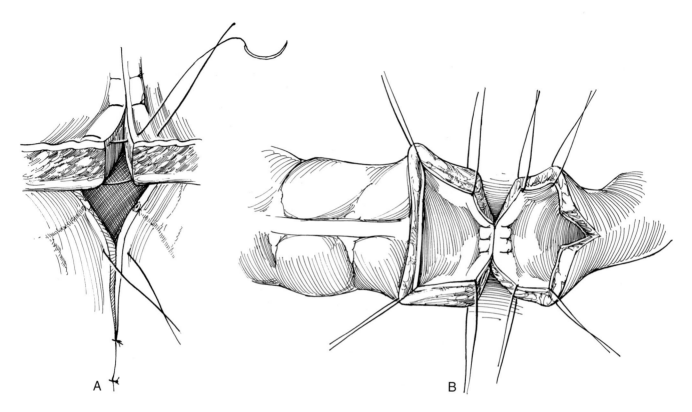

A   B

5 For the anterior half, place interrupted sutures of 4-0 CCG through all layers except the mucosa; this brings the mucosa in apposition inside the lumen. Cut each suture short.

6 Place a seromuscular layer of 4-0 NAS as a second layer anteriorly; it may be carried well laterally, using the original mesenteric suture to rotate the bowel. Complete closure of the mesenteric defect. Alternatively, do an end-to-side anastomosis using GIA and TA 40 or 50 staplers (see page 66). Drape the omentum over the anastomosis, and tuck it into the fornices of the pelvis to keep the bowel from touching the raw surfaces.

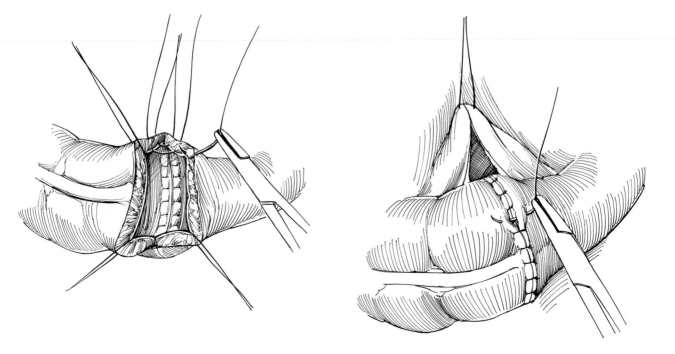

7 Make a small window in the posterior peritoneum, and pass the segment through it into the right gutter. Tack the mesentery that remains inside the peritoneal cavity to the posterior peritoneal surface to prevent an internal hernia. Close the margins of the window around the pedicle. Rotate the segment 180 degrees counterclockwise. Palpate for arterial pulsations in the mesentery to assess the viability of the intestinal segment.

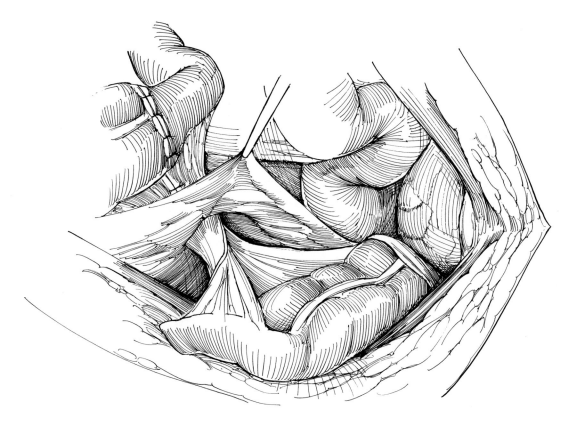

8 **A,** Discard the terminal ileum by dividing its blood supply close to the bowel wall and by dividing the ileum 2 cm from the cecum. Alternatively, keep the segment of terminal ileum attached in case you need to connect it to a continent pouch.

B, Close the stump with a full-thickness running suture of 2-0 CCG.

C, Invert the stump into the cecum with a layer of 3-0 SAS. Take care not to let the needle enter the cecum.

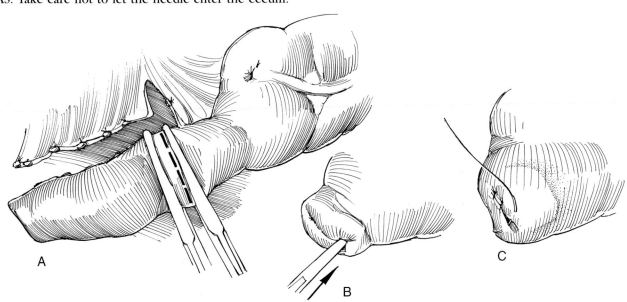

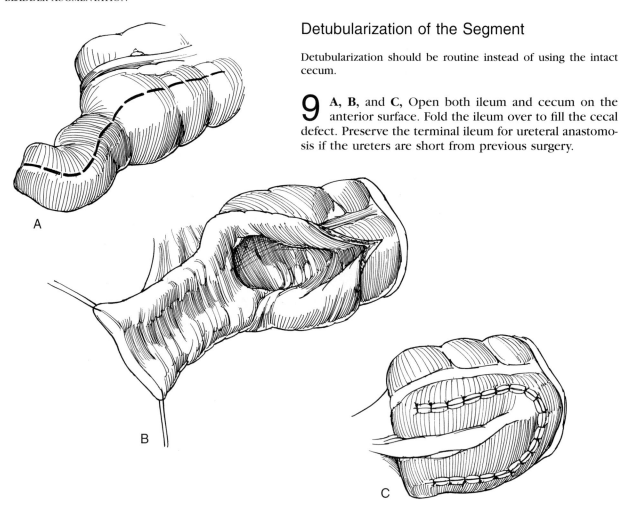

Detubularization of the Segment

Detubularization should be routine instead of using the intact cecum.

9 **A, B,** and **C,** Open both ileum and cecum on the anterior surface. Fold the ileum over to fill the cecal defect. Preserve the terminal ileum for ureteral anastomosis if the ureters are short from previous surgery.

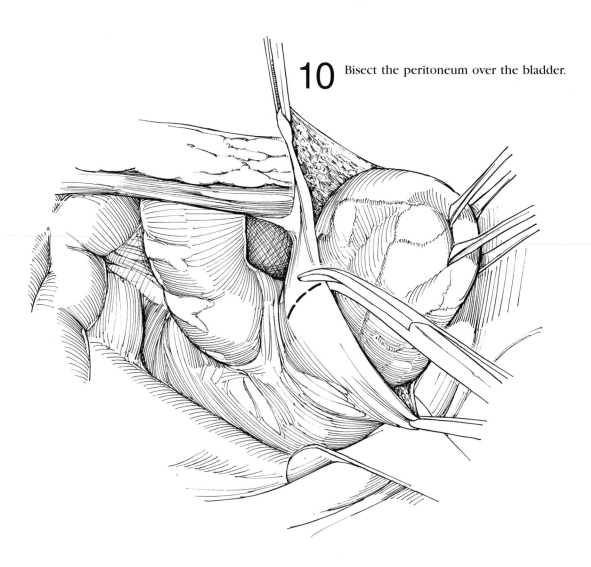

10 Bisect the peritoneum over the bladder.

11 Incise the bladder in a sagittal plane from the trigone to the deep anterior wall, a distance at least equal to the stretched diameter of the cecal lumen, and place four stay sutures. Be sure to place a catheter in each ureter for identification (not shown). Trim the crushed edges of the cecum caused by a Kocher clamp or stapler, and flush the bowel with 1 percent neomycin-bacitracin solution.

12 Stretch the opening to the cecal pouch to fit the bladder defect. If necessary, increase its circumference by making two short lateral incisions in it. Install a good-sized Malecot catheter through a stab wound in the anterolateral surface of the bladder because mucus is obstructive. If the remaining bladder is too small to accommodate the tube, bring the cystostomy tube out the dome of the reservoir. Start two sutures of 3-0 CCG posteriorly, including the mucosa and submucosa of the colon and the urothelium of the bladder.

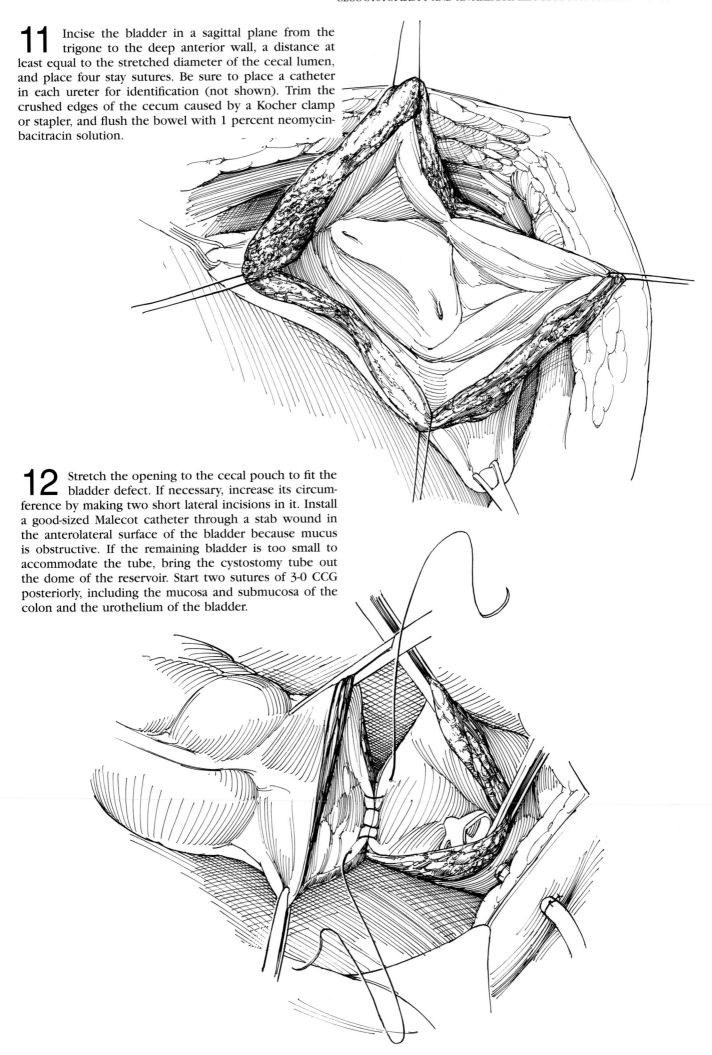

13 Run the sutures up each side, and tie them anteriorly. Place a second seromuscular layer of 2-0 CCG sutures. Alternatively, place four quadrant sutures and run a full-thickness suture from each quadrant, taking care to keep the knots outside and the mucosa inverted. Avoid purse-stringing. In a female, suspend the vagina on the round ligaments and tack it to the lateral pelvic wall to keep the bowel segment out of the cul-de-sac, where it could become obstructed. Suspend the new augmented bladder in either the right or left fossa or the midline, by suturing it to the posterior body wall.

Even though it is usually preferable to have the suprapubic tube exit through the bladder, having it exit through the dome of the bowel helps hold the pouch in place so that it does not fall into the cul-de-sac.

Consider inserting an artificial sphincter if the outlet is incontinent and the reservoir capacity and compliance are expected to be adequate with a pressure consistently below 35 cm H_2O, the ureteral pressure. This is not an option if the bladder neck has been subjected to a prior operation. In that event, perform a careful bladder neck closure (see page 609), and construct a continent self-catheterizing stoma.

Lavage the pelvis copiously with normal saline. Place a Penrose or Jackson-Pratt drain to the area. Close the peritoneum and body wall in layers, bringing the cystostomy tube through a stab wound and sewing it to the skin with braided silk. If the ureters have been anastomosed, bring the stents through stab wounds in the bladder and body wall. Because of the copious production of mucus, in addition to the cystostomy tube, insert an adequate silicone balloon catheter (or a straight catheter held by a suprapubic rein) transurethrally, and tape it to the leg.

Postoperative Care

Monitor the patient closely; considerable fluid loss occurs during the procedure and instability of fluid-electrolyte balance is to be expected. Wait 5 to 7 days before resuming oral feeding. Stop broad-spectrum antibiotics after 24 hours to reduce the chance of superinfection. Irrigate the cystostomy tube frequently to prevent plugging by mucus. Remove the drains 2 days after drainage stops, but continue irrigation three times a day. Remove the cystostomy tube on the 14th day, after performing cystourethrography to detect leakage and to ascertain that the patient can void. If the anastomosis is intact, remove the urethral catheter 2 days later. In 2 months, perform intravenous urography and cystography, and determine the serum creatinine level.

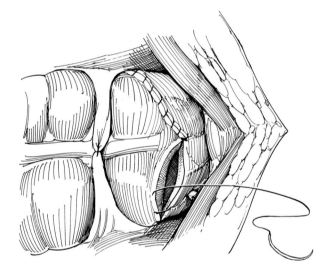

ANTIREFLUX ILEOCECOCYSTOPLASTY

Check for the presence of an adequate urethral continence mechanism. Serum creatinine level should not be higher than 2.2 mg/dl. Proceed as for cecocystoplasty through Step 8, thereby preserving 15 cm of the terminal ileal segment for use as an antireflux valve. Divide the ureters close to the bladder after inserting a stay suture in each. Ligate the ureteral stumps with 3-0 CCG sutures. Bluntly dissect a tunnel retroperitoneally, and bring the left ureter to the right side.

Ileocecal Valve Mechanism

14 **A, B,** and **C,** The ileocolic valve should have been evaluated by a preoperative barium enema to assess its competency. If reflux was noted at relatively low pressures, then a more secure nipple-type antireflux procedure should be planned (Step 15). If the ileocecal valve was found to be competent, insert three layers of interrupted seromuscular sutures of 4-0 silk to invert 3 to 4 cm of the terminal ileum into the cecum.

Test for obstruction from the supplemented valve by inserting an 18-gauge needle into the ileum and filling it with saline with a three-way stopcock and syringe, using a length of clear intravenous tubing on the stopcock for a manometer. The saline should flow through at very low pressure. Test the competence of the ileocecal valve by transcecal instillation of saline.

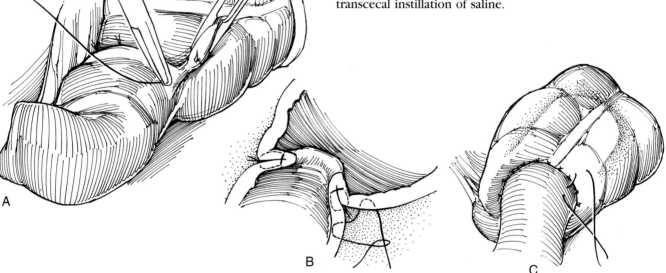

15 *Alternative 1*: Instead of supplementing the valve, prepare a 6- to 8-cm window in the ileal mesentery as for the intussusception described on page 688 for the Kock pouch. Draw the ileum through the ileocecal valve with Allis forceps.

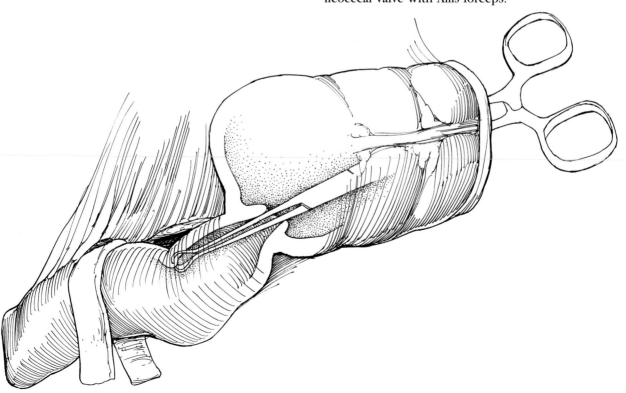

16 Fasten the ileum to the cecum with the aid of a strip of polyglycolic acid mesh and sutures.

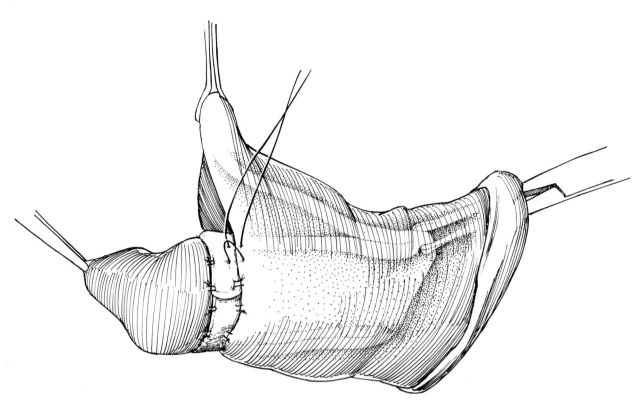

17 *Alternative 2*: A method that may be simpler and just as effective and that avoids devascularizing the bowel is to turn the cecum back to expose the nipple. Fix the nipple to the cecal wall by incising the wall of the nipple through the muscularis and the cecal wall into the muscularis for a distance of 4 cm. Approximate the two raw surfaces with a row of 3-0 polydioxanone sutures applied to the serosa and muscularis. Supplement this with some NAS around the site of entrance of the ileum.

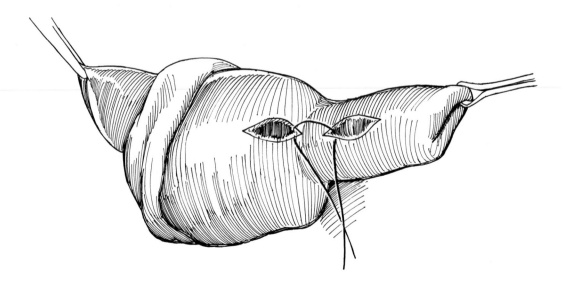

Preparation of Bladder

18 Bisect the peritoneum over the bladder, or leave it in place to help make the closure more secure. Halve the bladder from just proximal to the bladder neck anteriorly to the midtrigonal area posteriorly. If reflux or hydronephrosis is present, resect the trigone as well and reimplant the ureters.

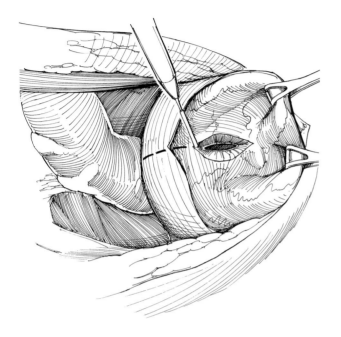

Ureteral Implantation

19 Place two silicone single-J tubes through the body wall and the anterior bladder wall preparatory to stenting the ureteroileal anastomoses. Insert a Malecot catheter through a stab wound in the anterolateral surface of the bladder to enable clearance of potentially obstructive mucus. Select a convenient site along the ileal segment for insertion of the ureters. Excess ileum is resected later.

Proceed with ureteral implantation, as described for the ileal conduit (see pages 658 to 659): Mobilize the ureters down to the trigone, and free the left one carefully as far as the kidney so that it may be pulled through retroperitoneally below the duodenum. Spatulate the right distal ureter, and anastomose to the right side of the ileum. Make a deeper spatulating incision in the left ureter, and use it to close the proximal end of ileum. During construction of each anastomosis, after the proximal suture is placed, hold a stent on a long clamp and insert it up the cecum and through the intussusception into the ileum. Or it may be easier to pass an extra feeding tube down through the intussusception and out the cecum and tie the stent to it to guide it through the ileocecal valve; then cut the tie, pull the stent back to the level of the anastomotic site, and advance it up the ureter. Pass the stents out through the bladder wall, or the colic taenia if the bladder has been subtotally resected, and fix them to the skin with silk sutures.

An alternative method is to resect the ileum and turn in the stump, as depicted in Step 8 and following. Then connect the ureters to the cecum with an antireflux technique (see pages 718 to 719 and 720 to 722).

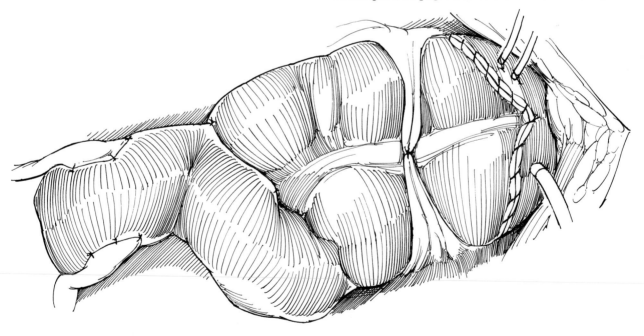

Closure of Ileum

Trim excess ileal length by dividing and ligating the vessels in the mesentery and by dividing the bowel beyond a Kocher clamp. Close the ileum in one layer with 4-0 silk pull-off sutures, as described on page 660. Tack it to the dome of the cecal segment unless it was already fixed, as previously described. When the ureters have been destroyed and ureteral substitution is required, start with a longer piece of terminal ileum so as to be able to anastomose the upper ureter or pelvis to it (see page 842).

Anastomosis to Bladder

Trim the crushed edges of the cecum caused by the Kocher clamp or stapler. Adjust the size of the cecal opening to fit that made in the bladder by slitting the antimesenteric border. Suture the cecum to the bladder opening after rotating it counterclockwise 180 degrees so that the mesenteric margin of the bowel fits into the interureteric ridge in the midline posteriorly. Start two sutures of 3-0 CCG posteriorly to include the mucosa and submucosa of the mesenteric edge of the colon and the urothelium of the bladder. Run them up each side, and tie them anteriorly. A second seromuscular layer of 2-0 CCG may be placed. Alternatively, use the anastomotic technique described for colocystoplasty (see pages 736 to 737).

Place Penrose drains to the area for adequate drainage. Close the peritoneum and body wall in layers. Bring the cystostomy tube and stents through stab wounds, and sew them to the skin with braided silk. Insert a 5-ml silicone balloon catheter of suitable size through the urethra. Attach the stents and catheters to drainage.

Postoperative Responsibilities

Adjust fluid and electrolyte levels assiduously. Irrigate the bladder through the cystostomy tube three times a day to evacuate mucus. Withdraw the drains after the drainage declines. Remove the ureteral catheters on the 10th postoperative day and the cystostomy tube on the 14th day after obtaining a gravity cystogram. Finally, take out the urethral catheter after testing for voiding.

Commentary by Leonard M. Zinman

The controversy over which intestinal segment is the ideal for augmentation or substitution cystoplasty continues. Ileum and right colon in the detubularized reconfigured form both achieve the goals of a low-pressure, large-volume receptacle, but the right colon possesses unique anatomic qualities that make it especially suitable for enterocystoplasty. It has a very mobile and dependable blood supply, a larger capacity, a low incidence of intrinsic pathology, an ileocecal valve that can be modified to serve as a reliable antireflux barrier, and a large amount of terminal ileum to accommodate short or absent ureters. There is general agreement that detubularized segments result in reservoirs with larger volumes and lower pressures, offering improved continence and upper tract preservation by virtue of longer intervals between emptying. The entire right colon, with an average bowel length of 25 to 30 cm, can be readily transferred to the base of the bladder or urethra without any restrictions when the right colic artery stem has been divided.

Patients undergoing this procedure should have a preoperative double-contrast barium enema or colonoscopy if they are over 50 years of age or have a history of some form of colonic disease. If stool guaiac measurements are abnormal, a colonoscopy is in order. Barium enema also identifies the relative competence of the ileocecal valve in the event that an antirefluxing ureteroenteric procedure is being considered. The concept of achieving an antirefluxing ureteral anastomosis in a low-pressure receptacle has been challenged in recent years, but a long-term study is needed before assuming a complacent view of free reflux in patients undergoing augmentation and spontaneous voiding. The patient with a normal ureterovesical junction may not require ureteral reimplantation if the trigone remains intact. A dilated freely refluxing or obstructed ureter, often noted in the hyperreflexic or unstable bladder, can be safely reimplanted using the technique of a modified ileocecal valve with its low resistance and low incidence of stenosis. This greatly simplifies ureterointestinal implantation and takes advantage of the nonobstructive sphincteric action of the ileocecal valve, which acts as an antirefluxing barrier in its unmodified form over 80 percent of the time. Direct tunnel-type reimplantation into the cecal wall introduces a higher incidence of anastomotic stricture than that seen with a direct ileal implantation. The short segment of ileum can also be used as a continent stoma in the event that augmentation is performed in conjunction with bladder neck closure, therefore using the intact trigone to avoid a ureteroenteric stricture. The optimal procedure for severe urinary incontinence from a neurologically impaired sphincter is the implantation of an artificial urinary sphincter in a male or a pubovaginal fascial sling that is designed to be obstructive, with the need for intermittent self-catheterization. All patients with noncompliant bladders or marginal bladder volumes who undergo these high resistance–producing procedures should routinely have augmentation cecocystoplasty to avoid the development of progressive detrusor instability with hyperreflexic activity which inevitably occurs.

The bladder preparation and pathology for which augmentation and substitution cystoplasty is performed have a signifi-

cant impact on the result of this type of reconstruction. It cannot be overemphasized that the results of enterocystoplasty, once a bowel segment of sufficient length has been properly isolated and reconfigured, depends to a great extent on the disease for which the procedure is being performed. The absence of a urethral stricture, the potential for a continence mechanism, and a creatinine clearance greater than 40 ml/min are essential requirements.

Bivalve clam cystoplasty in the sagittal plane from just proximal to the bladder neck to the interureteric ridge produces the optimal preparation for incorporation of an open bowel segment to achieve a large-volume, low-pressure urinary reservoir and prevent the diverticulum effect seen in the past with cylindrical segments. There is a chronic and unpredictable 20 to 30 percent risk of having to perform self-catheterization for effective emptying in the non-neurogenic bladder. This may very well be the result of an excessively capacious bladder or, more likely, intrinsic colonic wall dysfunction resulting in urinary retention. Only a small fraction of patients with interstitial cystitis are candidates for enterocystoplasty. These are patients with decreased bladder capacity, cystoscopic and histologic evidence of disease, and a clinical response, transitory though it may be, to bladder hydrodistension. These patients rarely respond to simple augmentation but require bladder substitution with an ileocecal neobladder and a direct anastomosis to the bladder neck or proximal urethra without any attempt to alter surgically the intrinsic sphincteric function.

The most immediate potential complication of cystoplasty with the use of the ileocecal bowel segment is inefficient voiding. Neuropathic bladders require evacuation by self-catheterization routinely, but for the non-neuropathic bladder patients, spontaneous voiding occurs, especially if the trigone is intact. Mucus collections persist chronically but eventually become finely dispersed and therefore clinically insignificant. The two serious metabolic consequences of using the segment of terminal ileum and excluding the ileocecal valve from the bowel are protracted diarrhea and vitamin B_{12} deficiency, which can result in an irreversible peripheral neuropathy without the classic preceding macrocytic anemia. The diarrhea is now known to be transitory in 15 percent of the patients with normal bowel function. The ability of the large colon capacity to adapt to loss of the entire ileocecal segment and the valve is now well established. Patients who have had extensive small bowel resection or prior abdominal radiation and those suffering from a neurologic disorder are at significant risk for developing persistent diarrhea, most of which can be readily managed by the use of cholestyramine. Vitamin B_{12} deficiency can be identified early enough if routine screening blood levels are obtained every 6 months, beginning 3 years after the terminal ileal resection, when liver stores for this vitamin begin to dwindle.

Enterocystoplasty has been used predominantly in a younger population of neurologically impaired patients, with dramatic short-term salvage. Life-long surveillance of these patients is required before complete understanding of the potential effects of the metabolic, infectious, and neoplastic complications can be achieved.

Ileocecocystoplasty

(Mainz)

Check on the competence of the ileocecal valve by instilling meglumine diatrizoate (Gastrografin) as an enema at relatively high pressure.

Bisect the bladder wall (see page 738). It is usually necessary to resect a portion of it to accommodate the bowel supplement.

Instruments and preliminaries are the same as those for ileocystoplasty.

1 **A,** *Incision:* Make a midline lower transperitoneal incision (see page 867). Mobilize the cecum and right colon. It usually is necessary to release the hepatic flexure to enable the cecum to reach the bladder. Follow the instructions for the ileocecal reservoir (Mainz) on page 693, but with different measurements for the ileum. Starting from the cecum, measure up to 15 cm on the ascending colon, and mark that point with a stay suture. Measure and mark two segments on the ileum starting at the ileocecal valve, each 10 to 15 cm in length. Divide the mesentery of the ascending colon above the ileocolic artery and the mesentery of the ileum at the most proximal stay suture; then divide the bowel at each end. Reanastomose the ileum to the large bowel with sutures (see pages 736 to 738) or with staples (see page 66). Irrigate the bowel segment. Open the colon along the taenia libera on the antimesenteric border and into the ileum through the ileocecal valve, using the electrocautery to reduce bleeding.

B, Place stay sutures on each of the three segments, and fold them into an S shape. Connect the two adjacent edges of the colon and ileum with running 3-0 SAS. Similarly suture the remaining ileal segment to its mate.

Alternative: For a smaller supplement using less bowel, take only one 10- or 15-cm length of small bowel and suture it to form a U.

C, Check again to be sure that the mesentery is long enough to allow the bowel plate to reach the resected edge of the bladder. If the mesentery is not long enough, rotate the bowel plate 180 degrees counterclockwise to be able to make an anastomosis to the posterior end of the bladder incision.

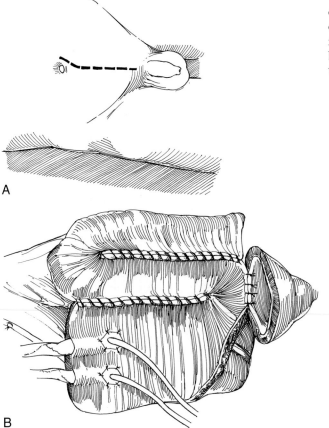

A

B

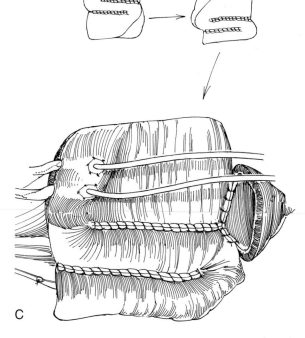

C

2 Place a single row of through-and-through interrupted 3-0 synthetic sutures to connect the lower edge of the bowel plate to the bladder posteriorly.

Anastomose the ureters either into the ascending colon or into the inverted cecum, depending on the rotation. Elevate the mucosa and submucosa at the upper margin of the pouch, and insinuate Lahey scissors between that layer and the muscularis (see page 694). Make a 4- or 5-cm tunnel, and cut down on the tip of the scissors. Pass a clamp retrogradely, and draw the stay suture on the ureter into the lumen. Place one deep 3-0 SAS at the apex of the spatulated ureter and finer sutures to attach uroepithelium to mucosa. Insert two 90-cm J stents or 5 F or 8 F infant feeding tubes into the ureters.

Place a 16 F Malecot catheter in the bladder through a stab wound, and bring the ureteral stents out through separate stab wounds. Complete the anastomosis of the bowel and bladder by a single row of through-and-

through interrupted 3-0 SAS that ends anteriorly. Close the anterior wall of the pouch with a through-and-through running 4-0 SAS. Take care to close only the mucosa at the site of ureteral entry to avoid constricting the ureter.

Insert a 22 F silicone balloon catheter transurethrally, and drain the area of bladder and ureteral anastomosis with two drains placed on gravity, not suction, drainage. Test the suture lines by filling the neobladder; even though watertight closure of the pouch is not essential, major leaks should be closed with additional sutures. Suture the cystostomy tube and stents to the skin.

Postoperatively, culture the ureteral urine repeatedly. Remove the stents one at a time in 10 days and the balloon catheter in 2 to 3 weeks. Remove the cystostomy catheter after cystography shows no extravasation and spontaneous voiding occurs with less than 50 ml of residual urine.

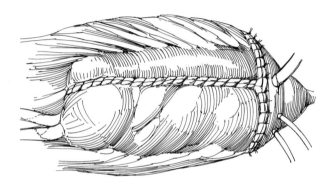

POSTOPERATIVE PROBLEMS

The problems are similar to those associated with other forms of bladder augmentation with bowel. Because the ileocecal region is used in this cystoplasty, deficiency of vitamin B_{12} can be expected. A yearly supplement must be given. Bowel control should not be affected, nor should malabsorption be a problem, especially if only one segment of ileum is used. *Metabolic acidosis* with resulting bone demineralization and osteoporosis is possible.

SPHINCTER PLICATION

Ileocecal Plication Technique (Nissan-Zinman)

3 Insert a 30 F catheter in the isolated ileocecal segment retrogradely through the ileocecal valve. Intussuscept the ileum into the cecum, and fix it with three or four 3-0 NAS.

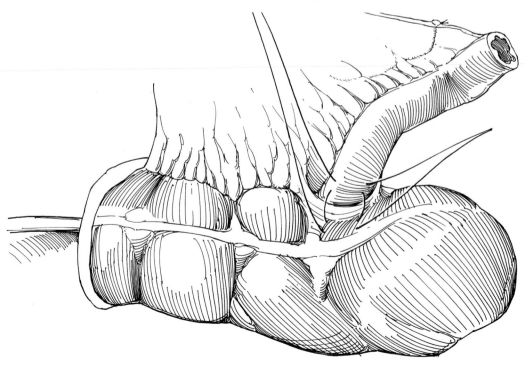

4 Wrap the redundant cecum around 6 to 8 cm of terminal ileum to enclose two thirds of ileal circumference. Fasten the ileum in place with a row of four or five 3-0 NAS. Test the effectiveness of the valve by gravity instillation of saline tinted with methylene blue. The valve can be reinforced with another row of sutures if it is shown to leak.

Internal Fixation Technique (Hendren-King)

5 Clear the mesentery from the terminal ileum for 8 cm. Open the cecum along the anterior taenia. Incise the serosa of the ileum on the antimesenteric border.

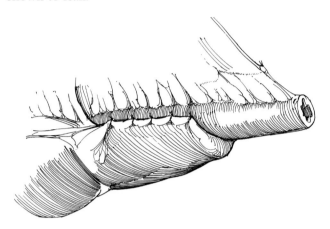

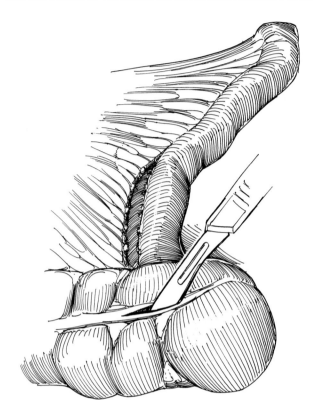

6 Draw 8 cm of the ileum into the cecum to make a 4-cm nipple. Incise the full thickness of the posterior wall of the ileal nipple with electrocautery for a distance of 3 cm. Similarly incise the facing cecal mucosa into the muscularis. Suture the apices of these incisions together with a 3-0 SAS.

7 Proceed down each side of the defects with interrupted sutures.

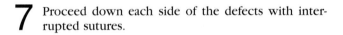

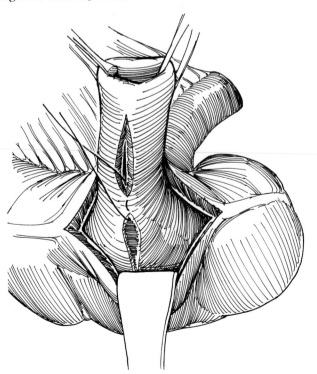

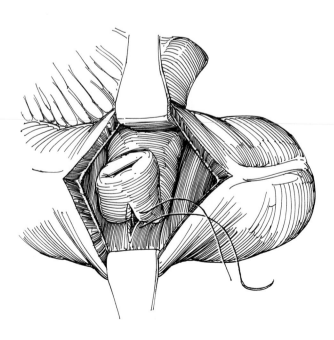

8 Close the cecotomy, and tack the ileum to the cecum with 3-0 adventitial NAS at the site of entry.

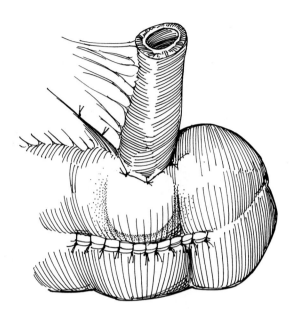

Ureteral Anastomosis

9 With any cecoileal antiregurgitation method, join the spatulated ureters and anastomose them to the ileum with interrupted fine absorbable sutures (see page 661). Alternatively, anastomose the right ureter to the side of the ileum (see pages 658 to 659), and, after widely spatulating the left ureter, anastomose it to the open end of the ileum. Stent the ureters with infant feeding tubes or single-J catheters led through the remains of the bladder wall or through the anterior taenia. Place a cystostomy tube in the bladder, to remain 3 weeks. Postoperatively, do not allow the bladder to overfill until the ileum bonds to the cecum.

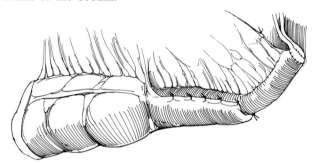

Commentary by Julio E. Pow-Sang

The surgical technique here described to obtain an orthotopic ileocecal-colonic bladder substitution meets all the requirements of a good-quality, anatomically and physiologically satisfactory voiding system. The detubularization and cross-folding spherical reservoir have several advantages: (a) a maximized volume–surface area ratio, producing less area with more volume capacity; (b) compliance with damping effect because of crossed antiperistaltic waves; (c) sensation of voiding at a determined volume-pressure filling point; and (d) a spherical reservoir that minimizes the amount of isolated intestinal segment as well as the area available so that metabolic advantages are obtained with less chance of malabsorption syndrome, fluid and electrolyte imbalance, or long-term metabolic complications.

Most of the reservoir techniques use 40- to 60-cm-long ileal segments. By either the M or W folding procedure here proposed, no more than a 30-cm ileal segment is required instead. It has been proven that a 30- to 40-cm-long ileal segment is enough for good volume and good compliance. Higher volumes by longer isolated ileal segments would go into a floppy bladder with significant residual urine. Low pressure (20 cm H_2O) in the reservoir versus high pressure in the outlet mechanism during filling is obtained in this procedure.

A gentle dissection of the membranous urethra and a nerve-sparing resection of the bladder-prostate complex are highly recommended, if possible. Postvoid dripping does not occur;

gentle pressing of the bulbar urethra after voiding aids in avoiding postvoid dripping.

Potassium and calcium metabolism impairment may occur with hyperkalemic-hyponatremic acidosis, and lately osteoporosis and/or osteomalacia has developed. Sodium bicarbonate prevents this situation. We must take into consideration that hypochloremic acidosis is present when ileal segments are used for diversion, whereas hyperchloremic acidosis occurs in colonic segments. Sodium reabsorption occurs more in colonic than in ileal diversions, and hyperchloremia may be present when cecal continent segments are used for diversion.

Reflux or obstruction of the ureteral-ileal anastomosis may produce infected urine, leading to renal insufficiency. Reflux is produced by overdistention when reservoir pressure is greater than ureteral pressure and when the antireflux system is not functioning.

Conclusions: All these techniques have been developed during the last 20 years; we expect to have, in the near future, a 10-year follow-up in order to know the real long-term range of morbidity of these procedures. Last but not least, the median 2 percent rate of operative mortality for these procedures and the 20 percent rate of mortality by progression of the disease in patients undergoing this type of surgery because of transitional cell carcinoma of the urinary bladder must be considered when making the decision to perform a urinary diversion.

Gastrocystoplasty

(Mitchell)

Using stomach for enlarging the bladder is especially suitable for patients with chronic renal insufficiency with acidosis in whom the gastric segment acts as a chloride pump with net chloride and hydrogen ion transport into the urine to prevent further acidosis. It is also useful in patients with a short bowel, such as cloacal exstrophy, and in those who have had pelvic irradiation that has compromised the bowel. Rule out patients with a history of stomach abnormalities such as ulcer disease and problems with gastric emptying.

Examine the urethra and bladder neck cystoscopically to be sure they can accommodate intermittent catheterization. If the patient has not been able to perform periurethral intermittent catheterization satisfactorily preoperatively, consider placing a Mitrofanoff conduit at the time of augmentation.

Place the patient on a liquid diet for 48 hours, and give magnesium citrate 24 hours before operation. A more complete bowel preparation allows for other options at surgery. The patient may be admitted the day of surgery, but make certain that the stomach is empty. Attempt to sterilize the urine. Cover with preventive antibiotics.

1 *Position:* Place the patient supine with the legs separated. Prepare the entire abdomen. Also prepare the perineum, and pack the rectum with sponges soaked in a non-iodine antibacterial solution.

Incision: Make a midline transperitoneal incision (see page 867) extending from xiphoid to pubis. Expose the bladder through the lower part of the incision, and open it sagittally in the midline ("bivalve"). The incision should extend from the bladder neck anteriorly to the trigone posteriorly. Control bleeding by electrocautery. Insert infant feeding tubes of suitable size into each ureter.

By preparing the bladder first, acid spillage from the stomach is reduced. In myelomeningocele patients with shunts, it may be better to open the bladder only after the gastric patch has been prepared to avoid prolonged drainage of urine into the abdominal cavity.

Extend the incision cephalad, and open the peritoneum. Reimplant the ureters and prepare the bladder neck area for sphincter or sling, if indicated.

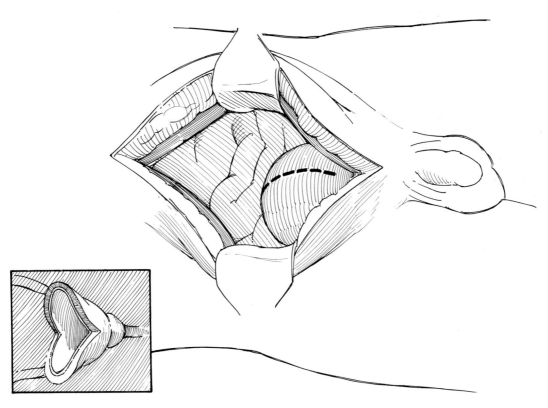

2 *Right-sided pedicle:* Draw the stomach into the wound with large Babcock clamps placed on the greater curvature. Examine the right and left gastro-epiploic arteries over the greater curvature of the stomach. The left gastroepiploic artery arises from terminal branching of the splenic artery. The right gastroepiploic artery is a branch of the gastroduodenal artery. Together they form the gastroepiploic arterial arch. The left gastroepiploic artery is not infrequently found to merge into the greater curvature or to taper to a small caliber, whereas the caliber of the right is more constant. For this reason, the right vessel is usually used to supply the flap.

Select as large a wedge as possible for the augmentation, one that encompasses at least one third, or even as much as one half, of the stomach. Because the right gastroepiploic artery is the base, place the wedge toward the left side of the stomach in order to have as long a pedicle as possible. While placing traction on the Babcock clamps, outline the proposed wedge with a marking pen. It should be about 14 cm wide along the greater curvature, with wings about 10 cm long, stopping short of the lesser curvature.

Incise the greater omentum 2 to 3 cm distal to the gastroepiploic artery on the right side with the electrocautery while clamping and tying the larger vessels to open the lesser sac. Divide the short arteries to the stomach, starting at the right side of the proposed wedge and working to the right (see page 71). Do this by passing a curved mosquito clamp through the omentum on each side of the first short artery to the right of the right arm of the wedge, elevating it, and drawing a 4-0 SAS under it. Tie the suture. Clamp and divide the artery close to the stomach; then ligate the end of the vessel in the clamp. Avoid traction on the gastroepiploic vessel to prevent arterial spasm (if it occurs, apply papaverine and warm saline). This technique also avoids retraction of the proximal (omental) end of the artery, which could quickly produce a potentially harmful interstitial hematoma.

Continue with the remaining branches, avoiding mass ligation and contact with the gastroepiploic arterial arch itself, to reach the gastroduodenal origin of the arch. Because an undivided branch can be easily torn when the flap is pulled into place, preserve a 5- to 7-cm band of omental vessels intact to protect the pedicle from avulsion. On the left side of the patch, leave the omentum attached to the pedicle so that it may descend with the patch; the omentum may subsequently be used to cover the repair.

Inspect the right gastroepiploic artery to be sure it has good pulsations before clamping and dividing the left gastroepiploic artery on the other side of the wedge.

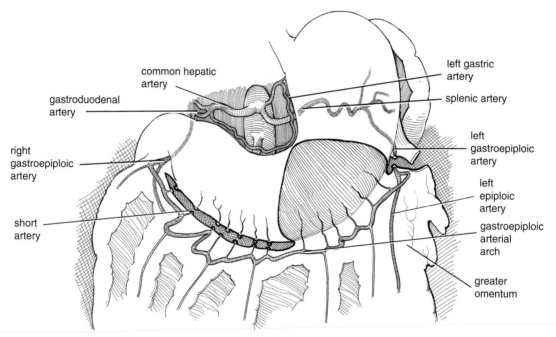

3 Incise the omentum on the left parallel to and 2 cm distal to the gastroepiploic artery, ligating the epiploic vessels as they are divided.

Closed technique: Insert the 70- or 90-mm gastrointestinal anastomosis stapler (GIA 70 or 90) in two places, and resect the wedge of stomach. Be careful not to damage the vascular pedicle when the instrument is placed at the right side of the wedge. If the stomach has a saccular shape, instead of taking a wedge, staple off the bottom by placing the GIA 90 stapler transversely along the greater curvature (Step 5). The stapler may prevent some gastric spillage and blood loss, but stomach tissue is lost during excision of the staple lines.

Open technique: Place a pair of bowel clamps on both sides of the gastric wedge. Ligate the branches of the gastric vessels of the lesser curvature near the apex of the wedge to prevent significant bleeding. Pack the area with laparotomy tapes to minimize spillage. Excise the wedge, taking care not to injure the vascular pedicle. Time may be saved by this open technique because it is not necessary to cut the staples out, but blood is lost during reconstitution of the stomach. First back the bowel clamp off the stomach wall, and run the inner layer on the back wall of the stomach closure to act as a hemostatic closure and to prevent inversion of a large portion of the stomach wall.

Place a moist laparotomy tape around the wedge before placing it in the pelvis; similarly protect the pedicle itself.

Make the pedicle as long as possible by dissecting near the gastroduodenal junction. If greater length is needed, divide a few more vessels distally on the patch

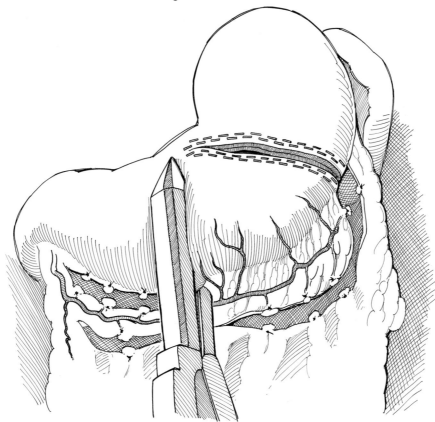

Left-Sided Pedicle

4 Divide the short arteries starting at the left side of the proposed wedge, and continue to just distal to the origin of the left gastroepiploic artery, near its origin from the splenic artery.

Crescent resection (Raz et al, 1993): To avoid opening the stomach, place the GIA stapler across the greater curvature, avoiding the antrum, and fire it. Reinforce the staple line on the stomach with 3-0 silk sutures. The patch is passed to the bladder and anastomosed in the same way as a wedge.

5 Pack the area to prevent contamination from oral pathogens. Open the stomach along the staple line with the cutting current. Close the stomach in two layers: Place a posterior seromuscular row of interrupted 3-0 silk sutures, tie them, and then remove the staples, at least those remaining on the anterior wall suture line.

Place a through-and-through layer of running locked stitches of 3-0 SAS to approximate the inner mucosal-submucosal layer. Insert a nasogastric tube, and position it in the antrum just proximal to the suture line.

Pass the flap on its pedicle under the transverse mesocolon along the root of the small intestine.

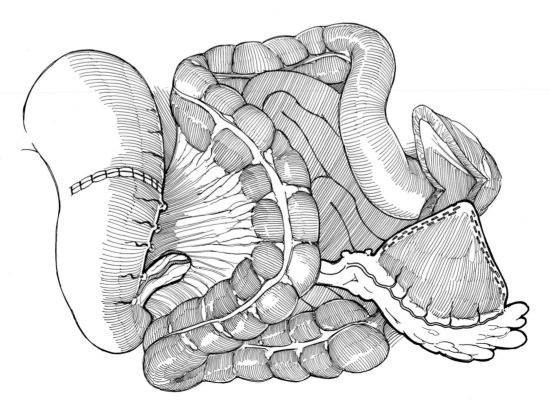

6 Pass the flap through an opening in the mesentery of the small intestine. (Alternatively, elevate the right colon and place the entire pedicle beneath its mesentery, thus placing it in the retroperitoneum.) Avoid rotating the flap on the mesentery. If the flap does not reach the bladder, free more of the vessels connecting the gastroepiploic artery to the duodenum. Recheck the pulsation in the artery in the pedicle.

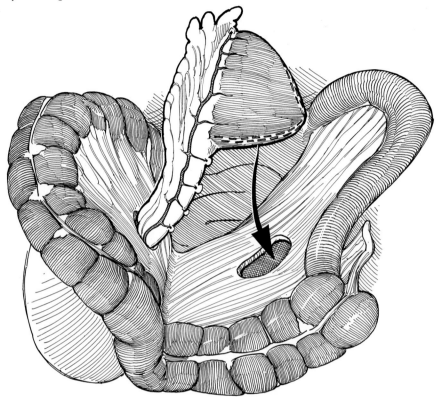

7 The ventral side of the stomach flap lies anteriorly. Rotate the flap 180 degrees in the coronal plane so that the apex of the former anterior surface can be fastened to the vesical neck while the apex that lay dorsally can extend to the trigone.

Remove the staples progressively to limit bleeding. Anastomose the posterior flap to the posterior wall of the bladder by running a full-thickness locked 3-0 CCG suture from the trigone up each arm to the dome from inside the bladder. Reinforce them with a second layer of seromuscular 3-0 SAS placed from the outside. If the ureters have been divided, anastomose them to the posterior flap by a tunnel technique (see pages 718 to 722). Make transverse incisions, which make tunneling with tenotomy scissors easier. Place ureteral stents.

Insert a Malecot catheter of a caliber adequate to handle mucus (at least 16 F) through the bladder wall (or through the patch, if necessary, although with that route more leakage can be expected when the catheter is removed). If the ureters have not been reimplanted, remove the feeding tubes from them.

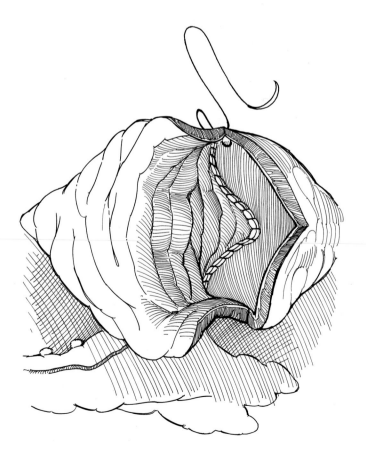

8 Insert a urethral catheter for added protection during the postoperative period, and fix it transvesically onto the anterior abdominal wall with a stitch through its tip, tied over a bolster.

Close the anterior portion with a running locked 3-0 CCG suture from the inside and a running 3-0 SAS from the outside. Test the suture line by filling the bladder, placing additional sutures if needed. Check to see if filling disturbs the blood supply to the pedicle, and inspect the gastroepiploic artery in the pedicle again. Look for angulation at the gastric antrum when the right gastroepiploic artery is used as the pedicle. It is better to free the gastroepiploic vessels so that tethering by short vessels to the gastric antrum is not possible. Also check the distal end of the gastroepiploic artery for angulation where it enters the flap. Divide one or two of the most proximal short vessels to the flap if necessary. This can be done without harm to the blood supply to this particular portion of the flap, and it protects the blood supply to the entire flap.

Fasten the pedicle to the posterior peritoneum to prevent injuring it and to avoid an area for bowel herniation. The omentum may be tacked to the posterior peritoneum alongside the pedicle as it runs along the root of the small bowel.

Fix the pedicle to the posterior peritoneum along the root of the small bowel, or close the opened peritoneum over it with a running 3-0 CCG suture. Alternatively, elevate the entire right colon, and place the pedicle in the retroperitoneum behind the bowel and its mesentery. Place the left side of the omentum over the small bowel (and, if long enough, over the anterior suture line), and use the portion from the left side that is attached to the patch to cover the posterior anastomosis. Drains are not necessary. Distend the bladder again for a final check.

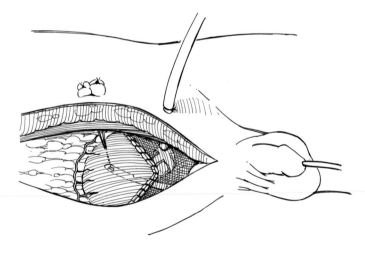

Maintain nasogastric suction until the patient passes gas; then start easily digestible liquid feedings. Give an H_2 blocker at the time of operation, and continue its administration for 2 months. Check the suture lines with a cystogram. Discharge the patient with the suprapubic catheter in place and on suppressive antibiotics. Have the patient return 1 or 2 weeks later to have the tube clamped so that either intermittent catheterization or voiding may begin. Open the tube at night because of the initial low bladder capacity. If intermittent catheterization goes well and nocturnal incontinence is not a problem, remove the tube 1 week later. Check the result in 2 or 3 months by ultrasonography and cystography. Be patient; gastric segments may take as long as 6 to 8 weeks to expand. Do not allow overdistention, which increases gastrin production.

APPENDICOVESICOSTOMY WITH GASTRIC AUGMENTATION (Burns-Mitchell)

If problems with urethral catheterization are anticipated, insert the appendix into the system to provide a catheterizable stoma. A portion of the cecum can be included with the appendix to give extra length for placement of the stoma in the umbilicus.

Dissect the appendiceal blood supply, and apply a GIA stapler across the terminal portion of the cecum. Trim the tip and irrigate the appendix. Implant the tip end into the anterior flap (or into the posterior portion if that gives a straighter channel) by the external tunnel technique (Barry; see pages 797 to 798). When forming the tunnel, fill the reservoir for better exposure of the mucosa.

POSTOPERATIVE PROBLEMS

The *hematuria-dysuria syndrome*, with penile burning from hyperacid urine, is treated with a histamine H_2 receptor antagonist such as ranitidine. Omeprazole can be given for the short term, but it can cause concern as maintenance medication. Giving the patient an antacid tablet after meals clears the penile burning quickly (Bogaert). Urinary pH should be checked regularly. Remember that overdistention increases gastrin secretion, especially if the antrum is included in the graft.

Asymptomatic infections do not need treatment. *Electrolyte imbalance* in the form of hypochloremic metabolic alkalosis can be detected by monthly determinations for the first 6 months. It may become serious if the child has an episode of vomiting or diarrhea with resultant salt loss; immediate replacement is mandatory. In any case, maintain the child on a normal intake of salt. If the antrum is included in the flap, it may respond to distention by increasing gastrin secretion, which in turn increases chloride and acid secretion from the stomach body, so that increased electrolyte loss from the gastric segment may be expected.

Postoperative *bowel obstruction* may come from adhesions secondary to spillage of gastric acid. Inadequate gastric *emptying* is treated with metoclopramide. *Excess mucus production* is a minor problem. *Perforation* can occur.

Commentary by Mark W. Burns, III

The evolving role of this operation is very important. From 1989 to 1992, we performed more than 50 gastrocystoplasties in Seattle. In the last 3 years we have done fewer than 6. I have gone back mostly to ileum, with the occasional autoaugmentation. Mike Mitchell has been using a demucosalized gastric flap versus peritoneum over an autoaugmentation. The reasons for our changes are interesting. We have not abandoned the gastrocystoplasty and, in fact, have had some of our best successes with it. The gastric segment, however, is not as docile as small bowel, and improvement in filling pressures (i.e., compliance) may take longer to come about. The problem of hematuria-

dysuria (in 36 percent of patients) is real, and it can be difficult to wean these children off ranitidine. The other potential problem, which is less often discussed, is the fact that stomachs develop cancer (and ileum seldom does). What effect will hydrochloric acid plus nitrogenous urinary waste have over 60 years in these children? The eventual incidence of cancer may be prohibitive—we just do not know. Our position has changed: We once said that stomach may be the tissue of choice for bladder augmentation in children. We now believe that it should be used only as a last resort when no other tissue is suitable.

Ureterocystoplasty

When the dilated tortuous megaureter is used to enlarge the bladder, it has an advantage over bowel of being free of mucus and the problems of electrolyte absorption. A ureter with ipsilateral nonfunction or a megaureter long enough to provide vesical augmentation and still allow reimplantation with tapering is expendable.

Prepare the bowel in case the ureter proves to be inadequate.

Incision: Make a single midline transperitoneal (see page 867) or a lower abdominal transverse (Pfannenstiel) (see page 490) incision. Alternatively, to stay out of the peritoneum, use two incisions, a dorsal lumbotomy (see page 896) and a transverse lower abdominal (see page 490) incision.

If the ipsilateral kidney is to be preserved as shown in Step 1, use only the lower portion of the ureter for augmentation, and perform a transureteroureterostomy on the proximal segment (see page 834). Alternatively, taper and reimplant the ureter (see page 803). If the ipsilateral kidney is functionless, remove it by dividing the renal vessels near the parenchyma and carefully dissecting the pelvis from it while preserving as much of the ureteropelvic blood supply as possible.

1 Dissect the ureter from the retroperitoneal tissues, keeping its segmental blood supply intact—that coming from the aorta, from the iliac and vesical vessels, and especially from the gonadal vessels. If previous surgery has been done on the distal ureter, preserving the proximal supply is all the more important. Use optical magnification. Do not disturb the connections between the ureter and the bladder at the ureterovesical junction. Divide the ureter at a site that leaves enough length for anastomosis to the contralateral ureter.

Open the ureteral segment on its anterolateral border, and extend the incision through the ureterovesical junction. Stay in the coronal plane to preserve all of the blood supply entering there, vessels upon which this section of the ureter depends. Continue the incision in the posterior wall of the bladder, then over the anterior wall (as for the clam augmentation; see page 731). With ureteral duplication, reimplant the ipsilateral ureter.

2 **A,** Double the ureter upon itself to form a U-shaped cup. Insert a suprapubic catheter in the bladder, not in the ureter (not shown).

B, Apply the cup-patch to the bivalved bladder with running locking 3-0 SAS (see page 731). Place a drain to the perivesical area. Connect the cystostomy tube to drainage; remove it in 10 to 14 days after cystography shows that the suture line is intact.

When the megaureter is not sufficiently dilated to provide adequate augmentation, perform a ureteroureterostomy. Ligate the lower end of the now-defunctionalized ureter, and bring the stump subcutaneously where it can be distended progressively with saline (Atala et al, 1996). At a second stage, open it and apply it as a patch. This preliminary dilation may not be necessary; the folded ureter, especially if it includes the renal pelvis, may dilate once it is in place (McKenna and Bauer, 1995).

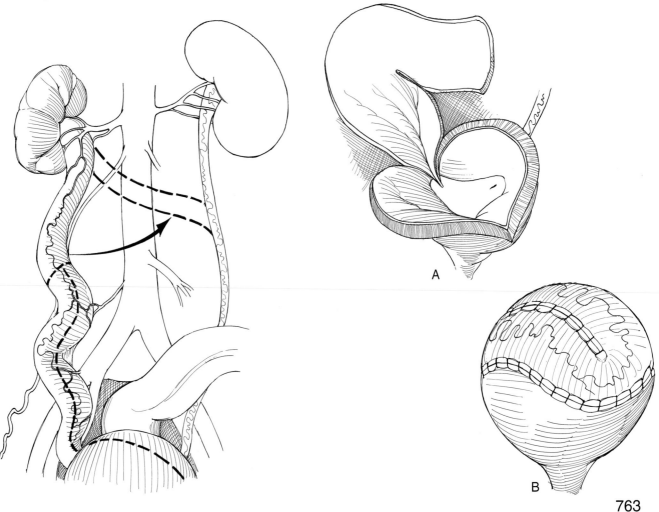

Commentary by Bernard Churchill

Preoperatively the surgeon should make sure that the patient has had a bowel preparation in case a stand-by enteric augmentation is necessary.

Avoid nitrous oxide anesthesia to minimize ileus and distention, which would place unnecessary pressure on the long delicate vascular pedicles in the postoperative period. This is an important adjunct.

The decision should be made as to whether the patients will at any time during their lifetimes require the peritoneum for peritoneal dialysis. If so, an extraperitoneal approach using a posterior lumbotomy incision for removing the kidney and a Pfannenstiel incision is desirable. If the patient is in no danger of renal failure, then a transperitoneal approach expedites the procedure.

Great care must be taken in mobilizing the bowel; the entire trick of the operation is to preserve the blood supply of the ureter. Although these megaureters have significantly increased blood supply because of their increased workload associated with inefficient ureteral transportation, it is imperative to preserve their integrity, starting with mobilization of the bowel.

The key vessel in each case is the gonadal vessel, which supplies the bulk of the ureter. It must be meticulously identified and preserved. Delicate dissection using magnification is indicated.

In doing the nephrectomy, it is important to stay as peripheral as possible so that the branches to the pelvis coming off the renal vessels can be preserved. Surprisingly, these usually go down to the bladder.

This technique differs significantly from that of a standard augmentation in that the intestinal tract is not used. Thus, bowel integrity is preserved, and well-described problems associated with enteric complications are avoided. Studies show that improvement in bladder storage using enteric augmentation is comparable to that for ileal augmentation.

Pitfalls: Almost all of the pitfalls are associated with ischemic injury of the ureter during mobilization. Preservation is the key technical step. Full understanding of the blood supply of the ureter and careful individualized strategy in mobilizing to maintain it result in a large segment of viable ureter, which provides the best biomaterial for augmenting the bladder.

Autoaugmentation

AUTOAUGMENTATION BY SEROMYOTOMY

Bladders with poor compliance and hyperreflexia but with only modestly reduced capacity are candidates for autoaugmentation.

Position: Supine. Insert a two-way urodynamics catheter connected to a Y-tube with a saline filling bag held at a height of 30 cm above the bladder.

Incision: Make a transverse lower abdominal incision (see page 490). Dissect the peritoneum from the dome of the bladder.

1 With the electrocautery set for coagulation, incise through three quarters of the thickness of the detrusor with a vertical midline incision over the entire dome. Separate the remaining detrusor fibers with a hemostat to expose the suburothelial layer. Release the clamp on the catheter, and allow the bladder to fill. Control any leaks with fine figure-eight sutures.

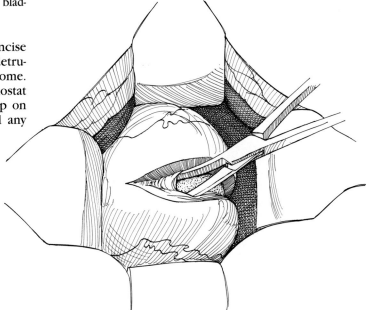

2 Grasp the edge of the detrusor with two Allis clamps on each side for countertraction during the submucosal dissection. Bluntly and sharply dissect laterally in the plane between muscle and urothelium until half of the wall is peeled back. Fill and drain the bladder intermittently to aid the dissection. Close any holes created by oversewing with 5-0 or 6-0 SAS. Excise the detrusor flaps.

3 Hitch each of the posterior edges of the bladder to the respective psoas muscles (see page 818) with 3-0 SAS. Drain the bladder with either a urethrally placed balloon catheter or a suprapubic tube emerging from an area of intact bladder wall. Place a Penrose drain paravesically.

Perform cystography in 1 week; if no extravasation is seen, remove the catheter and have the patient resume intermittent catheterization or voiding.

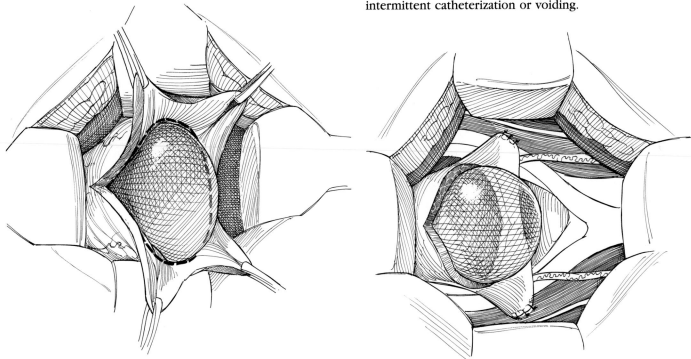

LAPAROSCOPIC AUTOAUGMENTATION

Create a pneumoperitoneum of 10 mm Hg. Insert one 10-mm trocar below the umbilicus, two in the right and left lower quadrants in the midaxillary line halfway between the umbilicus and the iliac crest, and a fourth in the right lower quadrant medial to the other trocar. Insert a balloon catheter, and fill the bladder with normal saline to which a vial of methylene blue has been added to help identify the mucosa. Alternatively, distend a balloon in the bladder to reduce the immediate consequences of puncture of the epithelium. Be sure to check for leaks by filling with saline after removing the balloon.

Incise the peritoneum over the dome of the bladder, and excise the perivesical fat. Clip the right and left medial umbilical ligaments to allow the bladder to fall posteriorly. Incise the serosa and muscularis with a harmonic scalpel in the sagittal plane to expose the mucosa. Dissect the muscularis from the mucosa with a ureteroscope using electrodissection and blunt dissection with the beak of the instrument. A few muscle strands may be left behind. Oversew any punctures; postoperative leakage produces harmful perivesical fibrosis. The fibrin glue Tisseal may be applied over the exposed epithelial layer to reduce leakage. Evacuate the bladder. Place a Penrose drain through one of the ports, and sew it in place. Close the portal sites with 2-0 SAS. Leave the urethral catheter in place for 1 week. Perform cystography to check for leaks, and remove the catheter if the repair is intact.

Commentary by Patrick C. Cartwright

The surgical concept of bladder autoaugmentation is simple—create a large augmenting bulge while preserving the urothelium. This avoids the problems associated with making bowel part of the urinary tract. Although this operation continues to be modified, I think that the idea of preserving urothelium will persist.

Some points on preparation and technique must be stressed. Prepare the patient as for an enterocystoplasty because this procedure may be required if the dissection proves technically inadequate and no bulging occurs. The patient (or parents) should be counseled as to this possibility.

We now use intraoperative cystometrics to evaluate the adequacy of the autoaugmentation. After the bladder is exposed, we insert a two-channel urodynamics catheter via the urethra and generate a pressure-volume curve before dissection. New curves can then be generated as the procedure progresses to assess changes. We expect at least a 30 to 50 percent increase in volume at 20, 30, and 40 cm H_2O during filling, with shifting of the filling curve to the right (better compliance). This catheter is left in to fill and empty as needed to aid the dissection.

The dissection should not be hurried; it can be tedious, especially if the bladder is deeply trabeculated. With a fine hemostat or tenotomy scissors, the plane between urothelium and muscle is defined. Do not overspread the blades, as this tears the underlying urothelium. If a perforation does occur at the edge of the dissection, a small amount of muscle is left at this site and the dissection is continued around it. This small amount of muscle is helpful to buttress closure of the perforation. When the procedure is nearly completed, the rim of detrusor may be split in several areas down toward the bladder neck, further releasing the epithelium to bulge. We now consider the psoas hitches optional. Finally, all bleeders should be carefully controlled because blood at the surgical site induces additional fibrosis.

During the recovery period, it is important periodically to distend the autoaugmentation to avoid contraction. This can be done by filling to a predetermined volume twice daily and clamping the catheter for 30 minutes. Constant pressure may be achieved by elevating the catheter drainage tubing to 30 to 40 cm above bladder level. At 7 days, if cystography shows no leakage, the catheter is removed and intermittent catheterization is begun.

Eventual fibrosis over the autoaugmented segment is the major concern in terms of limiting the augmenting effect over time. In 25 children (mostly myelodysplastic) in whom we have done long-term follow-up, we judge overall success as good in 50 percent, fair in 25 percent, and poor in 25 percent. In adults, Kennelly and his associates (1994) have reported uniformly good outcomes in patients with various diseases, and Stöhrer et al (1995) in Germany have demonstrated marked improvement in capacity and compliance in spinal injury patients.

Interesting variations are being investigated. Dewan and Stefanek (1994) have described covering the urothelium with a demucosalized pedicled gastric patch. In a similar mode, Gonzalez and co-workers (1995) and Lima and associates (1995) have demucosalized sigmoid and used it as backing to buttress the repair. They report little fibrosis, and early outcomes are encouraging.

Additional experience will provide clues as to which patients respond best and which techniques give the most reliable outcome. At present, we choose autoaugmentation for patients who have poor bladder compliance, but *not* a severe reduction in bladder capacity. If it does not provide adequate augmentation, enterocystoplasty can be pursued without difficulty.

SECTION

18

Bladder Substitution

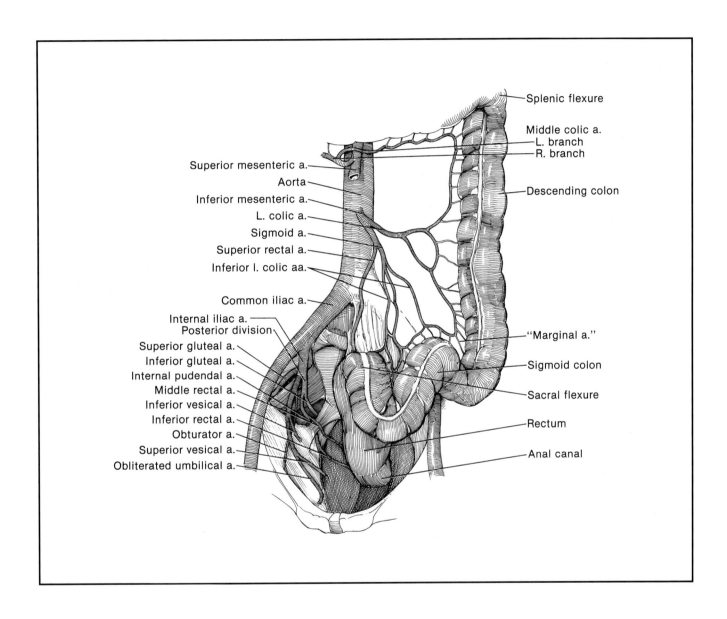

Principles of Bladder Substitution

Substitution is less desirable than augmentation because it results in more metabolic disturbance by requiring resection of more bowel, especially if the terminal ileum and cecum are used. Also, the trigone cannot be preserved, which results in problems with ureterointestinal anastomosis, and substitution is attended by more complications.

Enuresis is a common, very distressing complication, probably resulting from an obtunded sensation of fullness of the bladder combined with perineal relaxation.

Difficulty in voiding may result. Orthotopic bladder substitution requires that the patient strain to empty, and straining causes reflex contraction of the pelvic musculature and subsequent obstruction of the release of urine. Place patients initially on intermittent catheterization until they can demonstrate effective voiding. It may be useful to provide training in perineal control with biofeedback and allow only those patients who can relax the perineum during straining to stop intermittent catheterization (Kakizaki et al, 1995).

The several techniques available for bladder substitution are listed in Table 1.

Table 1. Techniques for Bladder Substitution

		Page
Ileal		
Camey	Detubularized U-shaped ileal bladder	769, Steps 1–4
Hautmann	W-shaped ileal neobladder	772, Step 5
Montie	Stapled technique	773, Step 6
Kock	Hemi-Kock pouch bladder	773, Step 7
Zingg	Ileal S-pouch bladder	774, Step 8
Studer	Cross-folded ileal bladder	774, Step 9
Ghoneim	W-shaped bladder	775, Step 10
Ileocecal		
Mainz	Ileocecal replacement, male	776, Steps 1–2
Light	Ileocecal replacement, female	777
Colonic		
Goldwasser	Right colon substitution	778, Steps 1–2
Reddy	Left colon substitution	779, Steps 3–4
Olsson	Stapled sigmoid neobladder	780
Gastric		
Mitchell	Gastric bladder replacement	781, Steps 1–3

Ileal Bladder Substitution

If the vesical tumor involves the urethra far beyond the bladder neck or if the urethra has been divided too far distally to allow continence, consider forms of diversion other than bladder substitution. Perform biopsy of the posterior urethra preoperatively to rule out carcinoma in situ in the periurethral glands. Be sure that the patient is otherwise in an optimal state of health, without serious adverse factors, and is psychologically attuned to his or her future situation.

Prepare the bowel. Give prophylactic antibiotics perioperatively.

Incision: Make a midline transperitoneal incision (see page 867). Expose the urethra.

DETUBULARIZED U-SHAPED ILEAL BLADDER (Camey)

Instruments are the same as those for radical cystectomy.

Incision: Make a midline incision and proceed with radical cystectomy (see page 505) in the male to the step of carefully cutting the dorsal vein of the penis between stitches at the prostatic apex and dividing the urethra. Dissect with preservation of the cavernous nerves in favorable cases, and obtain good hemostasis to prevent hematomas.

1 A, Partially transect the membranous urethra, and place eight sutures in it preparatory to ileal anastomosis. Do not compromise the cancer surgery just to avoid impotence in males.

B, Continue dividing the urethra just below the apex of the prostate in the male or at the vesicourethral junction in the female, while placing sutures in the posterior urethral wall. Take a biopsy specimen for frozen-section examination. Proceed with ileocystoplasty only if bleeding is controlled and the total length of membranous urethra remains intact. If a frozen-section examination shows positive margins, consider urethrectomy.

Select a 60- to 65-cm loop of terminal ileum, the midportion of which reaches the urethra without tension. If this is not possible, use another method of substitution. After being sure that the mesentery is long enough for the bowel to reach the urethra, divide the ileum at the ends of the segment and re-establish ileal continuity (see pages 649 to 654).

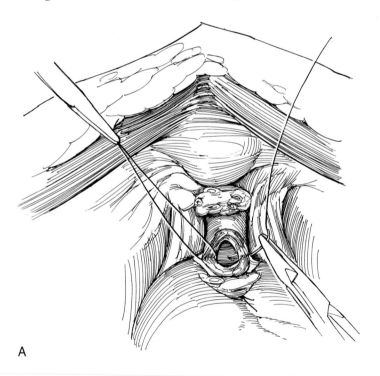

A

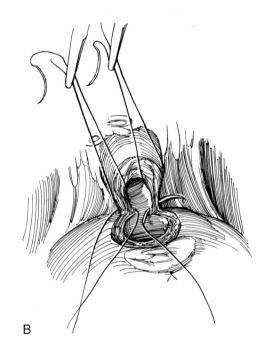

B

2 Completely open the ileum on the antimesenteric border, directing the line of the incision nearer the mesentery on the anterior wall around the site for the urethral anastomosis. Place marking sutures at the points selected for the ureteroileal implantations (marked **X**) and for the ileourethral anastomosis. Place one running layer of 2-0 synthetic absorbable suture (SAS) inside from right to left, creating a broad flat plate of ileum. Make a 1.5-cm incision in the antimesenteric border of the segment 10 cm to the right of center. Anastomose the ileum to the urethra using the eight prelaid sutures. Insert the posterior sutures first, and push the openings together while gradually tightening the sutures. Do not cut the sutures until they are all in place and tied. Hold the lateral sutures in clamps. Complete the ileourethral anastomosis with the remaining sutures.

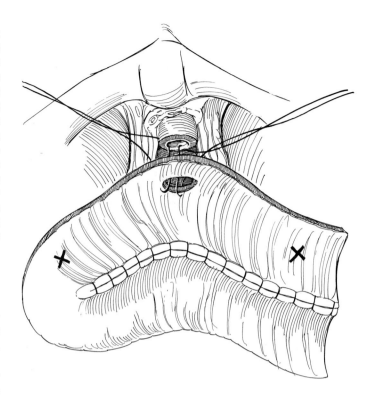

3 *Camey-LeDuc technique of ureterointestinal anastomosis:* **A,** Starting 1.5 cm from the end of the open bowel, divide the mucosa on the posterior wall longitudinally for 3 or 3.5 cm to expose the muscularis. Insinuate a curved clamp through the wall at the proximal end of the furrow from inside to outside to make a tunnel large enough for the ureter to pass through loosely.

B, Pull 3 cm of ureter into the lumen, and secure the adventitia of the ureter to the serosa outside with three 4-0 SAS.

C, Cut the ureter obliquely, and fix the tip to the mucosa and muscularis at the distal end of the furrow with three 3-0 SAS. Complete the anastomosis with lateral mucosa-to-adventitia sutures. Avoid angulating the ureter where it enters the ileum; that could lead to ureteral obstruction. Leave the ureter lying superficial to the ileum. Repeat the procedure with the other ureter at the other end of the loop.

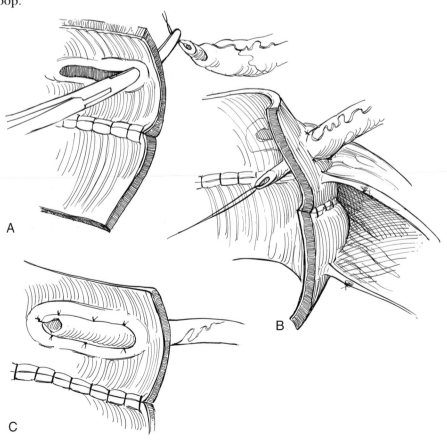

4 Cut extra holes in the ends of two lengths of 8 F silicone tubing, and insert each in the ureters as far as the renal pelves. With the help of a urethral catheter, pass the other end of each stenting tube through the ileourethral anastomosis and out the urethra. Leave a multifenestrated 20 F catheter through the urethra.

Fold over the upper edge of the ileal plate, and close the neobladder with a running 2-0 SAS. Fix the ends of the pouch to the pelvic wall. Close the wound, bringing drains through stab wounds. Tape and stitch the three catheters to the penis or vulva.

Alternative: Bring the ureteral catheters through the ileal wall distal to the ureteral implantation and then through the abdominal wall. Then fix the ileal wall to the retroperitoneum surrounding the exit site.

Postoperatively, provide for good diuresis to dilute the mucus and avoid occlusion of the ureteral stents. Irrigate the ileal bladder through the catheter four or five times every 3 hours with 30 ml of saline to evacuate the mucus. Maintain prolonged parenteral nutrition even after passage of gas. Remove the drainage tubes as soon as the volume drops, no later than the 12th day. At the same time, remove the ureteral catheters, but obtain a urine culture and perform cystography. If leakage occurs, let the ureteral stents remain for another week. Remove the urethral catheter 2 days later.

Conversion of Camey I ileal bladder: Because of the high incidence of incontinence in existing tubular bladder substitutes, convert them to low-pressure systems by detubularization (Carini et al, 1994). Incise the antimesenteric border of the loop for two thirds of its length, leaving the ends containing the ureteral anastomoses intact. Suture the medial margins together to form a posterior plate. Fold the plate over anteriorly like a cup, and suture it to the free anterior edges.

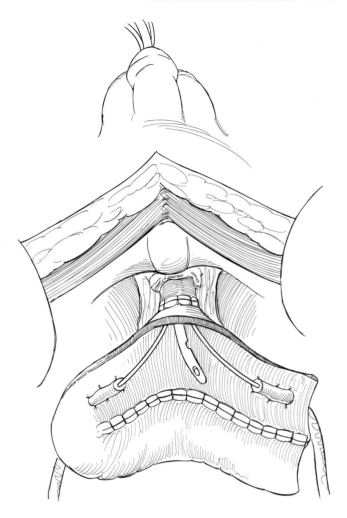

Commentary by Maurice Camey

Contrary to radical prostatectomy, continence following substitution ileocystoplasty cannot count on bladder neck reconstruction and bladder compliance. It needs the whole anatomic functional length of the membranous urethra and intact external sphincter. Therefore, we do not ligate the dorsal vein in front of the membranous urethra, as we do for radical prostatectomy. The right-angle clamp may take a part of the muscular structures and shorten the functional part of the membranous urethra, even though its transection has been done at the right place just below the prostate apex.

We emphasize perfect hemostasis of the pelvis following cystoprostatectomy before performing bladder substitution. Indeed, every pelvic collection (blood or lymph) tends to break out in the most dependent structure, the ileourethral anastomosis, and may thus create a fistula.

When performing the antireflux ureteroileal implantation and when fixing the extremities of the plasty, take care not to create a ureteroileal angle that can induce ureteral obstruction.

Irrigating every 4 hours (four or five times a day) with 30 ml of saline is necessary to evacuate mucus in order to avoid its accumulation, with resulting high pressure and leakage at the suture line.

The ureteral catheter can be pulled out through the ileal wall (7 to 8 cm below the ureteral implantation) and through the abdominal wall, if the catheter is not greater than 8 F. The ileal wall then must be fixed to the retroperitoneum with two sutures surrounding the exit of the stent.

Our experience of 30 years, starting in 1958, has demonstrated the effectiveness of this U-shaped tubular plasty applied on the pelvic wall (Camey I). Between 1987 and 1991, 110 detubularized U-shaped cystoplasties were carried out. Of 109 patients who survived the procedure, 101 (92.6 percent) recovered normal daytime continence without any leakage, and 81 patients (74.3 percent) achieved nocturnal continence. Nocturnal continence is achieved with only one or two awakenings. We advise these patients to void at least once a night to prevent bladder distention followed by retention.

W-SHAPED ILEAL NEOBLADDER

Sutured Technique
(Hautmann)

The larger number of folds (four) generated by this technique makes the bladder more spherical, resulting in increased capacity with less contractility.

Perform cystoprostatectomy and lymphadenectomy. Leave six double-armed 2-0 SAS on the urethral stump to prevent the urethra from retracting into the pelvic floor. To preserve continence in women, save the urethropelvic ligaments and the paraurethral vascular and nerve plexuses, and dissect the urethrovesical junction from the anterior vaginal wall.

5 Arrange four lengths of ileum marked with stay sutures in a total length of 60 to 80 cm in the shape of a W, and check that one of the loops can reach the urethra. Mark that point with a suture. If not, select another portion of ileum. Leave 20 to 30 cm attached to the cecum. An alternative is to select only three segments of ileum but also to open the cecum and part of the ascending colon to complete the complex. Resect the loop, and perform ileoileal anastomosis. With Babcock clamps, arrange the ileum in the shape of a W (or an M if one particular loop reaches the urethra more easily). Irrigate the loop to clear the mucus, and open it along the antimesenteric border. Suture the three adjoining edges together with running 3-0 absorbable sutures to form a flat plate that folds upon itself to form a large chamber.

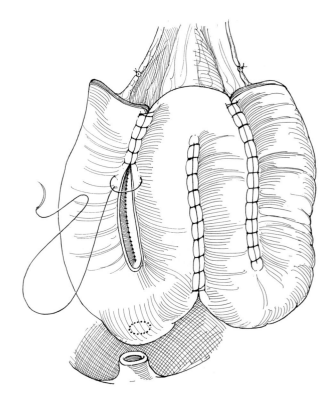

Make a small opening in the selected loop at the site of the marking suture. Insert a 22 F three-way catheter. Anastomose the bowel to the urethra by passing the inner end of the previously placed suture through the opening and inserting the outer suture 5 to 7 mm distal through the wall, tying the knots inside the bowel. If the bowel does not reach the urethra, try removing the retractors and straightening the table. If that fails, close the opening in the bowel and make a new one nearer the tip of the flap. Partially close the anterior wall of the new bladder with a running 3-0 SAS.

Implant the ureters into the ileal plate by pulling the right one through into the lumen of the lateral segment from the right and the left one through the left lateral segment after it has traversed the mesocolon. Implant them in a trough covered by mucosa (Camey), as shown in Step 3. Fix them to the adventitia outside where they enter the reservoir. Stent the ureters, and place a cystostomy tube. Fold the pouch, and close it with a running 3-0 SAS.

A similar technique may be used for bladder augmentation (see pages 729 to 731). Resect a portion of the bladder. Do not close the caudal end of the W complex, but anastomose it to the open bladder.

Stapled Technique (Montie)

6 Obtain a 50-cm ileal segment, and align it as a W. Via enterotomies, staple the limbs together with a PolyGIA device using absorbable staples. Close the enterotomy with a TA 55 instrument. Be careful not to overlap absorbable staples. Repeat the procedure for the middle and proximal segments. Make a short enterotomy at the bottom of the distal segment for anastomosis to the urethra. Insert the ureters into the afferent and efferent limbs by a direct end-to-side technique (see pages 658 to 659). Postoperative care and complications are similar to those with other neobladders.

HEMI-KOCK POUCH FOR BLADDER SUBSTITUTION

Follow the steps of ileocystoplasty (see page 729) by resecting a loop of ileum 55 to 60 cm long. Open the distal two thirds on the antimesenteric border (see page 730).

7 Fold the opened flap upon itself, and close it with a running 3-0 SAS to form a pouch (see page 730). Clear the mesentery from half of the more proximal segment (8 cm), and intussuscept the ileum to form a nipple. Incise the full thickness of the outer wall of the nipple, denude the adjacent muscle in the pouch, and suture the two surfaces together with 3-0 SAS. A polyglycolic acid mesh collar may be placed for further stabilization. Implant the ureters in the proximal end of the ileum (see pages 658 to 659), inserting stents.

Fold the free end upon itself to cover the ventral surface. Suture it closed semitransversely. Push the corners of the pouch downward between the leaves of the mesentery, bringing the posterior aspect of the reservoir anteriorly. Anastomose the base of the pouch to the urethra, and connect it as described on page 770. Fasten it to the levator ani muscles on both sides. Insert a balloon catheter, and secure it and the stents to the skin.

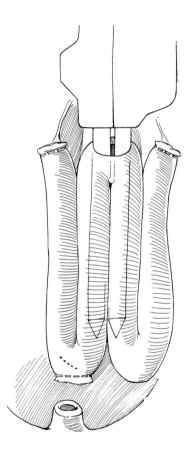

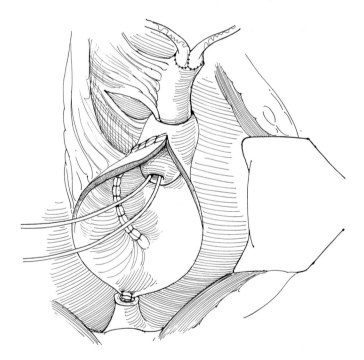

ILEAL S-POUCH BLADDER
(Zingg)

8 Take a 60-cm ileal segment, and open the distal 36 cm on the antimesenteric border. Fold the open ileum into three 12-cm segments in the form of an S and suture them together. Intussuscept the unopened ileum into the open pouch, and stabilize it with a nylon mesh band. Insert the ureters near the end (see pages 658 to 659). Suture the distal end of the pouch to the urethra, and close the remainder of the pouch wall.

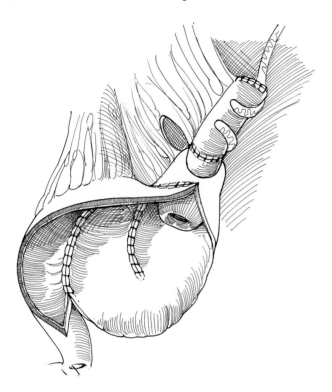

CROSS-FOLDED ILEAL BLADDER
WITH PROXIMAL ILEAL CONDUIT
(Studer)

9 Beginning 15 cm from the ileocecal valve, close the end of the isolated segment with seromuscular running 4-0 SAS. Open approximately 40 cm of the distal portion of the ileum on the antimesenteric border. Oversew the two medial borders of the open distal part of the ileal segment in a U shape with a single seromuscular layer of continuous 2-0 SAS. Fold the bottom of the U over between the two ends of the U. Before closing the pouch completely, insert ureteral catheters into the afferent limb of the ileum, and bring the ends through the side of the pouch. Digitally determine the most caudal portion of the reservoir, and make an opening. Anastomose the opening to the urethra with six 2-0 SAS, and tie the sutures after an 18 F catheter has been inserted. Insert a 12 F cystostomy tube, and bring it, with the stents, through the wall of the pouch.

After the reservoir is in place, form an isoperistaltic afferent tubular limb to prevent reflux. Divide the ileum 18 to 20 cm above the pouch at the level of the divided ureters. Spatulate the ureters, and anastomose them end to side (see pages 658 and 661) to the proximal end of this unopened segment. Introduce the inlying stents into the ureters. Restore bowel continuity. Bring the stents through the anterior abdominal wall, and place suction drains in the pelvis. Remove the stents in 7 to 10 days and the cystostomy tube in 10 to 12 days if no leakage is seen by pouchography. Remove the urethral catheter on the 14th day.

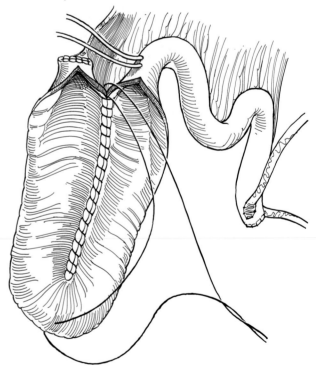

W-SHAPED BLADDER WITH SEROSA-LINED EXTRAMURAL TUNNEL IMPLANTATION
(Ghoneim)

10 Isolate a 40-cm length of ileum, open the antimesenteric border, and arrange it as a W. Join the serosa 2 cm from the medial edges of the flaps on each wing with running seromuscular 3-0 synthetic nonabsorbable sutures (NAS), thus forming two seromuscular-lined troughs. Place the spatulated ureters in the troughs, and anastomose them to the bowel mucosa at the end of the trough. Close the trough over the ureter with interrupted 4-0 SAS, thus forming an extramural serosa-lined tunnel. After closing the anterior wall of the pouch, anastomose the dependent portion to the urethra.

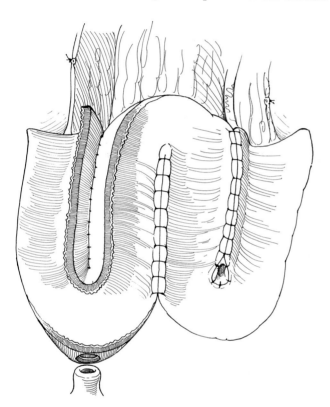

REANASTOMOSIS OF THE POUCH TO THE URETHRA FOR STRICTURE

For stenosis at the junction of the pouch with the urethra that does not respond to endoscopic treatment, approach the anastomosis retropubically. Pass a sound through the urethra from below, and dissect a stump 1 cm in length for the anastomosis.

If that is not possible, approach the area perineally (see page 451) to obtain a stump of adequate length. Because incontinence results, insert an artificial sphincter (see page 580).

POSTOPERATIVE PROBLEMS

Obstruction from edema at the ureteroileal junctions may cause flank pain, low-grade fever, and decreased renal function, which may be due in part to ileal stasis and resorption and drug toxicity. *Small* bowel obstruction is not common, but prolonged ileus can be a problem. *Lymphoceles* may form and require laparoscopic drainage because of pressure on the new bladder.

Ileourethral stenosis is usually treated with dilation. *Ileourethral fistulas* may respond to prolonged catheter drainage, but a few require surgical correction. *Wound infection* and pelvic abscesses may require surgical drainage. *Bacteremia, septicemia,* and *septic shock* are usually associated with displacement of catheters, for which percutaneous nephrostomy may be required. *Incontinence* is more likely if the neurovascular bundles are not preserved during cystectomy but is a special problem if the bowel is hyperactive. *Urinary retention* is more likely than incontinence (an incidence as high as 70 percent). It may be of late onset and require life-long self-catheterization.

Ileocecal Bladder Substitution

ILEOCECAL BLADDER SUBSTITUTION, MALE (Mainz)

The determination that the cecum can reach the urethral stump cannot be made until the cecum and ascending colon have been completely detached from the lateral pelvic wall, usually including release of the hepatic flexure. However, only very rarely are the ileocecal vessels not long enough. If the connection would be tenuous, consider a bladder composed entirely of small bowel (see page 769). This is a good time to send the ends of the ureters for frozen-section examination.

Proceed as described for the ileocecal reservoir (see page 693), but make the ileal segment 20 to 25 cm shorter and omit formation of the nipple (Steps 5 to 9).

1 Excise a buttonhole of serosa and muscularis in the lowest part of the cecum or ascending colon, depending on the position after the rotation, and open the mucosa. Place a few 4-0 interrupted SAS to evert the mucosa out to the serosa. This allows direct contact of mucosa with urethral epithelium and reduces the chance of stricture at the site of anastomosis. For the actual anastomosis, first place six or eight 4-0 SAS (only two are shown) in the end of the urethra (sutures were probably placed at the completion of the cystoprostatectomy). Pass the medial sutures successively through the opening in the bowel, and insert the corresponding outer sutures through the wall 5 to 7 mm proximally. Tie the knots outside the open neobladder.

2 Bring the left ureter under the mesocolon to the right side. Anastomose both ureters from inside the bowel by forming submucosal tunnels (see pages 770 to 771), with an additional tacking suture where the ureter enters the colon. Intubate them with J stents or infant feeding tubes that are brought out through the wall of the pouch and the skin, not through the urethra. Close the anterior wall with a full-thickness running 4-0 SAS. Perform a psoas hitch (see page 818). Place a 24 F Malecot cystostomy tube. Insert a 20 F silicone balloon catheter in the bladder through the urethra. Close the anterior wall of the pouch. Test for leaks. Fix the cecum behind the symphysis to approximate the site of exit of the cystostomy tube to the anterior abdominal wall. Place vacuum drains to the area.

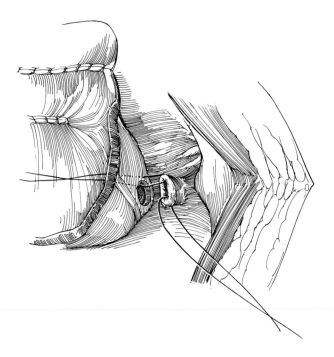

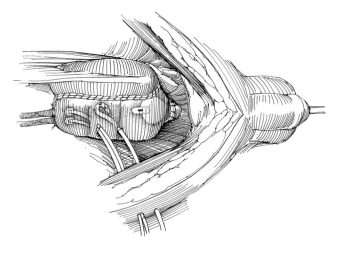

Have the reservoir irrigated with 50 to 100 ml of normal saline three times a day to clear the mucus. Remove the stents one at a time in 10 days, after culturing the urine from each kidney. At 3 weeks, perform cystography. Clamp the cystostomy tube at the time the urethral catheter is removed. Have the patient measure residual urine by self-catheterization. Check the serum electrolytes immediately before discharge, at 1 month, and then every 3 months. Determine vitamin B_{12}, folate, and magnesium levels yearly. Perform intravenous urography or ultrasonography at the same interval.

Other reservoirs such as the Indiana pouch (see page 698) can be similarly anastomosed to the urethra.

ILEOCECAL REPLACEMENT WITH ARTIFICIAL SPHINCTER, FEMALE
(Light)

Isolate 24 cm of cecum and ascending colon with 20 cm of attached ileum based on the ileocecal artery. Use the GIA stapler. Restore continuity with an end-to-side anastomosis (see page 66). Open the small bowel on the antimesenteric border and the colon along the taenia libera, leaving the terminal 4 cm intact. Staple the medial border of the colon to the cephalad margin of the ileum with absorbable staples.

Rotate the terminal end anteriorly, and staple the distal part of the free edge to the cecal end, leaving a large opening for later ureteral implantation. Make a short opening in the mesentery at the junction of the tubularized and detubularized portions, introduce the cuff sizer, and constrict the bowel so that the fifth finger inserted from above just passes through the lumen. Allow the tubing to pass anterior to the bowel reservoir. Remove some of the staples from the tubularized portion, and anastomose the opening to the stump of the urethra with full-thickness interrupted 3-0 chromic catgut (CCG) sutures.

Form a tunnel from the left through the base of the mesentery of the descending colon. Implant the ureters by the transcolonic technique (see pages 720 to 723). Insert a 24 F balloon catheter into the reservoir and test for leaks.

Form a space subcutaneously on one side of the abdominal incision for the connectors. Pass the cuff tubing into this space with the tubing passer. Fill a 61- to 70- or 51- to 60-cm H_2O balloon with 22 ml of Cysto-Conray II solution, and place it in the abdomen so that its tubing also exits to the subcutaneous space. With long scissors, create a subcutaneous space into the labium majorum on that side, and insinuate the pump. Connect the tubing with "quick connects," keeping them subcutaneously. Close the abdominal incision. Deactivate the device. If possible, avoid inserting abdominal drains.

Have the patient irrigate the catheter. Perform cystography at 3 weeks to check on healing; then remove the catheter, stop antibiotics, and activate the sphincter. Advise the patient on the need for abdominal straining to empty the colonic bladder.

POSTOPERATIVE PROBLEMS

Complications with bladder substitutions are similar to those with an ileocecal reservoir. *Deep pelvic thrombosis* and *lymphoceles* occur, as does *partial bowel obstruction. Leakage* from the urethral anastomosis subsides with more prolonged catheter drainage. In addition, *incontinence* may result from improper selection of a patient with sphincteric incompetence. *Ureteral strictures* at the anastomotic site can usually be managed by simple dilation. *Hyperchloremic metabolic acidosis* is common but usually improves with time.

Commentary by Joachim W. Thüroff

After the cecum and ascending colon have been detached from the abdominal wall up to right colonic flexure and the ascending colon has been divided between the middle and right colonic arteries, the cecum reaches the ureteral stump without problems. The anastomosis should be performed between the ureteral stump and the deepest point of the pouch, usually at the lateral aspect of the cecal pole. Attempts to anastomose an appendiceal stump to the urethra have led to voiding difficulties, mostly because of kinking of the appendiceal stump. Eversion of the intestinal mucosa at the buttonhole incision is essential to prevent anastomotic strictures. An increased incidence of anastomotic strictures has been seen with the use of polyglyconate sutures at this site, whereas strictures are not seen when 4-0 polyglycolic acid sutures or CCG sutures are used.

In bladder substitution, ureteral stents and the cystostomy catheter are brought out through the anterior wall of the pouch and the skin rather than through the urethra. A 10 F pigtail cystostomy catheter is sufficiently large for pouch irrigation and monitoring of residual urine after removal of the transurethral catheter. With this size of catheter, fistula formation after removal is of no concern. A transurethral 22 F silicone balloon catheter is left in place for at least 3 weeks. After removal of the transurethral catheter and initiation of spontaneous voiding, the cystostomy catheter is used for a few more days for monitoring residual urine. When residual urine is less than 50 ml, a transurethral catheter is inserted before the cystostomy tube is removed and left for another 24 hours to prevent fistula formation from the cystostomy tract.

Colonic Bladder Substitution

RIGHT COLON SUBSTITUTION
(Goldwasser)

Position: Supine. *Incision:* Make a midline incision and proceed with radical cystectomy (see page 505). Leave the ureters as long as possible, but check the ends for malignancy by frozen-section examination. Incise the peritoneum on the white line lateral to the ascending colon, and divide the hepatocolic ligament. Mobilize the entire right colon by carrying the incision around the cecum and continuing medial to the small bowel mesentery to reach the ligament of Treitz. Elevate the colon from the great vessels and the duodenum. Before proceeding further, determine if the lowest portion of the cecum can reach the pelvic floor; if not, consider an ileal substitute.

1 **A,** Isolate a segment of large bowel containing the cecum, the ascending colon, and the right side of the transverse colon to the level of the middle colic artery by incising the mesentery in the avascular plane between the right and middle colic arteries. Divide the small bowel mesentery near the cecum to include the ileocolic artery with the segment. Divide the colon. Divide the ileum, and perform an ileocolostomy (see page 744). Irrigate the segment.

Clear the mesentery from the stump of the ileum, and resect the stump. Close the ileocecal defect with two running layers of 3-0 SAS or with the TA 30 stapler. Also consider removing the appendix (see page 675). Bring the segment through the mesenteric opening so that it lies in the right gutter lateral to the site of anastomosis.

B, Open the colon on the antimesenteric side through the anterior (free) taenia, leaving the last 5 cm unopened. Pass the left ureter under the sigmoid mesentery. Implant the ureters in tunnels in the proximal half of the bowel segment and stent them (see pages 718 to 720, 720 to 723, and 775). Implant the right ureter longitudinally and the left ureter transversely to the long axis of the bowel (not shown). Insert infant feeding tubes in the ureters.

Urethral Anastomosis. Select a site on the cecum for the urethral anastomosis, depending on the position after the rotation. If it is difficult to bring the bowel down, sacrifice the right colic artery close to its origin. In the lowest and somewhat anterior part of the cecum or ascending colon, excise a buttonhole of serosa and muscularis, and make a small incision in the mucosa. Place several 4-0 interrupted SAS to bring the mucosa out to the serosa so that the mucosa is in direct contact with the urethral epithelium. This reduces the chance for stricture. For the actual anastomosis (see page 770), first place six or eight 4-0 SAS in the end of the urethra (sutures that usually are placed at the completion of the cystoprostatectomy). Pass the inner sutures successively through the opening in the bowel, and insert the corresponding outer sutures through the wall 5 to 7 mm proximally. Tie the knots inside the open neobladder. Insert a urethral balloon catheter and a Malecot cystostomy tube. Bring the stents and cystostomy tube through separate openings in the neobladder.

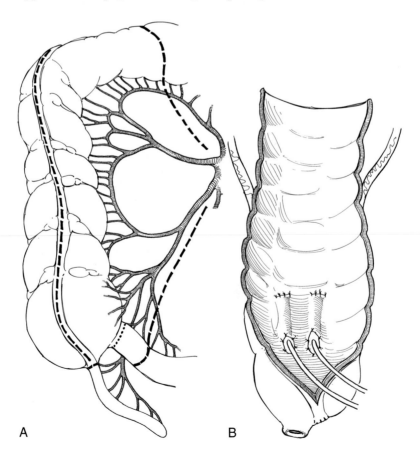

A   B

2 Fold the distal portion of the segment over, and place two layers of running 3-0 SAS to complete the closure. Alternatively, apply the TA 55 or TA 90 stapler.

Place two suction drains, and bring the stents and Malecot cystostomy tube through separate stab wounds in the right lower quadrant. Reperitonealize the bowel, and cover the area with the omentum before closing the abdominal incision.

The *Indiana pouch* for continent urinary diversion (see page 698) is formed in a similar way. For the *Florida pouch* (see page 700), the segment is opened fully before being folded back upon itself.

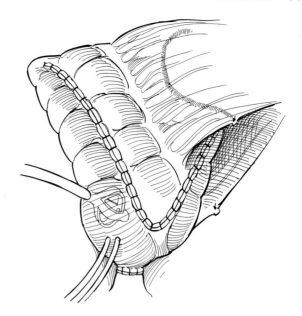

LEFT COLON SUBSTITUTION
(Reddy)

3 **A,** *Incision:* Midline. Explore the abdomen. During cystectomy, take care to preserve the left internal iliac artery, and avoid extensive dissection of the pelvic floor. Place traction on the sigmoid colon to be certain that it reaches the deep pelvis. Isolate a 30- to 35-cm length of sigmoid and descending colon supplied by the sigmoid branches of the inferior mesenteric artery (see page 735). Avoid cutting deeply into mesentery. Reapproximate the colon (see pages 736 to 738). Check again for mesenteric length; if it is not adequate, release the splenic flexure.

B, Form the bowel into a U, and tag the midpoint to mark the site for the urethral anastomosis. Flush the segment with antibiotic solution. Incise the bowel along the posteromedial (mesocolic) taenia, near the mesenteric border.

Implant the ureters through the posterolateral (omental) taeniae of each arm of the U by a transcolonic technique (see pages 720 to 723), and stent them with infant feeding tubes. Alternatively, implant the ureters by the closed technique before the bowel has been opened (see pages 718 to 720). Place a few interrupted aligning sutures to approximate the medial edges of the open U; then close the posterior wall with running 3-0 SAS.

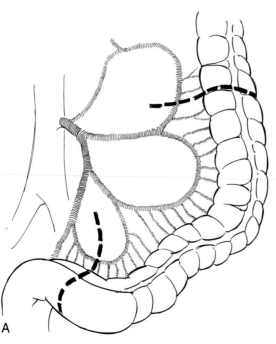

A

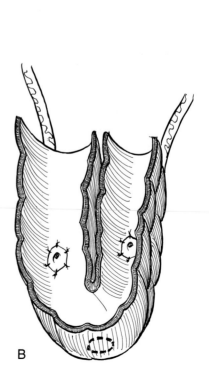

B

4 Place a similar running suture to close the anterior edges. Insert a 24 F Malecot catheter into the lumen. Bring the stents through the anterior wall, and close the cephalad end of the segment. Test for leakage.

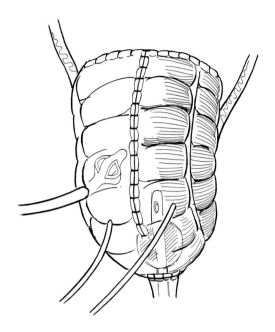

Urethral Anastomosis (see Step 1B): Make a 1-cm opening in the serosa-muscularis at the dependent site previously marked, and make a small opening in the mucosa. Tack the mucosa to the serosa to evert it. Insert a 24 F balloon catheter through the opening. Anastomose the reservoir to the urethra with six interrupted SAS. Place two Penrose or suction drains, one on either side; cover the site with omentum; and close the abdominal incision. Tack all tubes to the skin.

STAPLED SIGMOID NEOBLADDER (Olsson)

A technique similar to that used for ileocecal reservoirs can be used in the construction of a sigmoid neobladder. Proceed as described on page 693, except bring the two stapled ends of resected sigmoid together, excise their stapled butts, and form a neobladder by serial applications of absorbable staples along the apposed antimesenteric borders. Place Babcock clamps on each side of the distal staple line, and invert the bowel to allow continued application of staples. Make a small incision at the apex of each staple line to allow for subsequent application of staples. If a small portion remains open, close it with figure-eight SAS. Cut a buttonhole in the dome of the sigmoid pouch for urethral anastomosis. Close the resultant open superior end with a running absorbable suture or absorbable TA staples after making stented ureterointestinal anastomoses. Bring the stents and a suprapubic tube through the wall of the bowel and abdominal wall. Anastomose the urethra to the opening in the bowel with the aid of a balloon catheter inflated to 10 ml. Close the remaining opening in the colon with staples or a running suture. Insert a suction drain to the region of the anastomosis.

POSTOPERATIVE CARE

Irrigate the cystostomy at least three times a day at first with normal (or 3N) saline to prevent mucous obstruction. Remove the stents and drains in the first 10 days, and discharge the patient to return in 4 weeks. At that time, perform cystography and remove the urethral catheter if the anastomoses are intact. Clamp the suprapubic tube and have the patient void, an act that may require Valsalva assistance. If progress is made, remove the suprapubic tube. Instruct the patient to perform intermittent catheterization in case of obstruction by mucous plugs. At first the bladder is small. Check for residual urine as necessary at intervals, and monitor serum electrolytes and creatinine.

Commentary by Pretap K. Reddy

Left colon bladder substitution is technically simple. The intraoperative time can be further reduced by means of two techniques: For an end-to-end anastomosis I now use the Valtrac ring (Davis and Geck), a biodegradable anastomotic ring that is placed into each colonic end with a purse-string suture and the ends of the ring snapped on to complete the anastomosis. For constructing the bladder substitute, I hand sew the detubularized edges of the colon with a running stitch of 3-0 SAS on a 1.5-inch Keith needle.

Postoperatively, I remove the ureteral stents and the balloon catheter at 2 weeks and keep the bladder substitute drained through the suprapubic Malecot catheter for an additional week. After 3 weeks, the patient does a trial of voiding at home. If that is successful during the course of a week, the patient then returns on the fourth postoperative week for removal of the suprapubic tube.

Gastric Bladder Replacement

(Mitchell)

1 Obtain a stomach segment as described for gastro-cystoplasty (see page 757). Instead of forming an anastomosis of the segment to the bladder, remove the staples and suture the apex of the posterior wedge to the urethra with 4-0 SAS, molding it to form a tube. Partially tubularizing the flap before starting the anastomosis may be desirable to aid in anastomosis.

Ureteral Implantation (illustrated on page 705). Make a pair of 2-cm oblique tunnels in the plane under the gastric mucosa, and draw the ureters through them. For fixation, place a deep suture at the apex of each spatulated ureter that includes stomach muscularis, and then suture the edges of the ureter to the gastric mucosa.

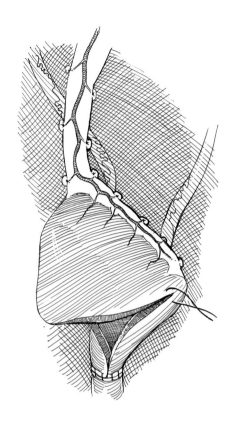

2 Insert a Malecot catheter into the reservoir. Close the edges of the flap, and complete the suturing of the apex of the pouch to the urethra with interrupted 3-0 CCG sutures. Suture the wall of the stomach pouch to the abdominal wall as for a gastrostomy (see pages 673 to 674) to protect the exit site of the catheter.

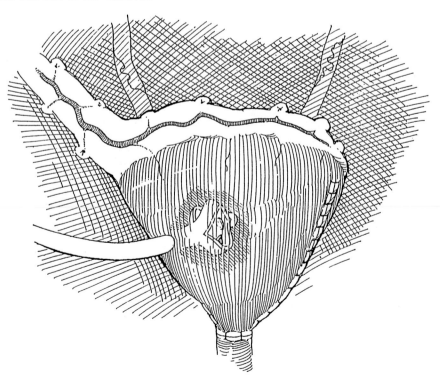

GASTRIC NEOURETHRA

If urethral supplementation or replacement is required because of loss of the native urethra, construct one from a portion of the stomach.

3 **A,** Mark and cut a strip 2 cm wide from one arm of the flap. Form it into a tube over a 10 F catheter.
  B, Slightly intussuscept the base of the tube into the reservoir to promote urethral resistance. Anastomose the distal end to the remains of the urethra.

POSTOPERATIVE PROBLEMS

Painful urination and *perineal pain* are treated with a histamine H_2-receptor antagonist. A postprandial antacid tablet reduces the stimulus for acid secretion (Bogaert, 1995). For low urinary pH and irritative symptoms, irrigate the bladder with phosphate buffer. In patients with renal failure, severe salt loss may occur during episodes of diarrhea and vomiting and require intravenous replacement.

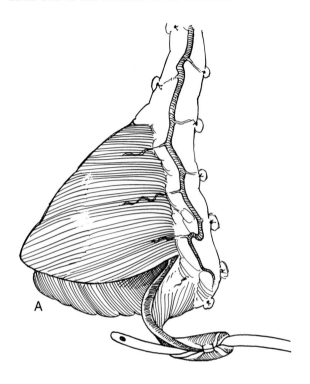
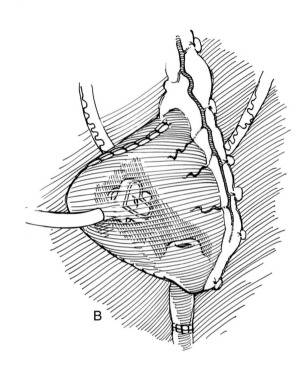

Commentary by Michael E. Mitchell

The gastric reservoir has proven to be a valuable addition to the surgical reconstruction in patients with complex problems, including those with classic exstrophy and cloacal exstrophy, some with severe cloacal malformations, and some who have had extensive radiation therapy for pelvic tumor. A short segment of small intestine may be added to the reservoir to balance salt loss by adding a resorptive surface and by increasing the volume of the reservoir without significantly reducing the length of the intestine.

Gastric tissue can facilitate reconstruction because the ureters are easily tunneled into the wall to prevent reflux. The nature of gastric tissue also provides several options for continence mechanisms. The appendix, ureter, or even tapered small bowel may be tunneled successfully into the gastric reservoir to construct a continent catheterizable channel. Furthermore, as illustrated in this chapter, it is possible to construct a tube from the gastric reservoir to form a catheterizable channel. A nipple is constructed in a manner similar to that of a Janeway continent gastrostomy. Hematuria-dysuria is not a problem in continent-reservoir patients; however, the possibility of salt loss

should be considered, particularly in the patient with short bowel syndrome.

Regarding technique, I find it easiest to position the new reservoir prior to reimplantation of the ureters. Therefore, it is usually best to anastomose the tip of the flap to the urethra before reimplanting the ureters. It is helpful to nipple the tip of the ureters to prevent stenosis. The suprapubic tube should be positioned such that the gastric bladder wall can be sutured to the abdominal wall, like a gastrostomy, to prevent leakage after removal of the tube. If it is necessary to create a catheterizable channel out of stomach, great care must be taken to make a nipple at the base to ensure continence and a straight channel to ensure ease of catheterization.

Mucus is usually not a problem after surgery, but initially the bladder should be irrigated at least daily. Because of acid production by the gastric mucosa, patients should be placed on H_2 blockers initially. Omeprazole is probably *contraindicated* in this group because it has greatest effect on stomach mucosa locally and therefore increases serum gastrin, which selectively increases acid production of the gastric bladder, resulting in dysuria and hematuria.

SECTION
19
Ureteral Reconstruction and Excision

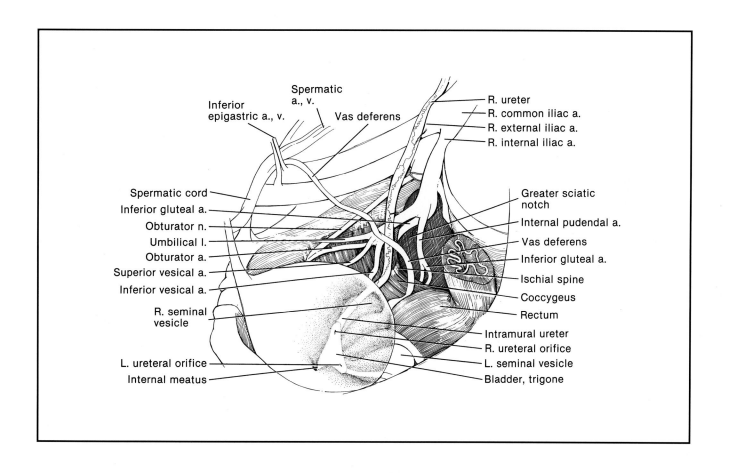

Inferior epigastric a., v.

Spermatic a., v.

Vas deferens

R. ureter
R. common iliac a.
R. external iliac a.
R. internal iliac a.

Spermatic cord
Inferior gluteal a.
Obturator n.
Umbilical l.
Obturator a.
Superior vesical a.
Inferior vesical a.
R. seminal vesicle

Greater sciatic notch
Internal pudendal a.
Vas deferens
Inferior gluteal a.
Ischial spine
Coccygeus
Rectum

L. ureteral orifice
Internal meatus

Intramural ureter
R. ureteral orifice
L. seminal vesicle
Bladder, trigone

Principles of Ureteral Reconstruction

A repertoire of procedures is needed when the ureter must be resected or reinserted. Reimplantation into the bladder is most direct but not always possible. Mobilization of a wing of the bladder and anastomosis to the other ureter are alternatives. If such procedures are not applicable, fall back on mobilization of the kidney, autotransplantation, or ureteral substitution with bowel.

The anatomic arrangement of the ureteral sheath, muscular coat, and blood vessels is important to surgical manipulation.

Ureteral Wall

1 The ureter is encased in a loose *ureteral sheath*, a layer of the intermediate stratum of the retroperitoneal connective tissue lying just under the peritoneum to which it is adherent.

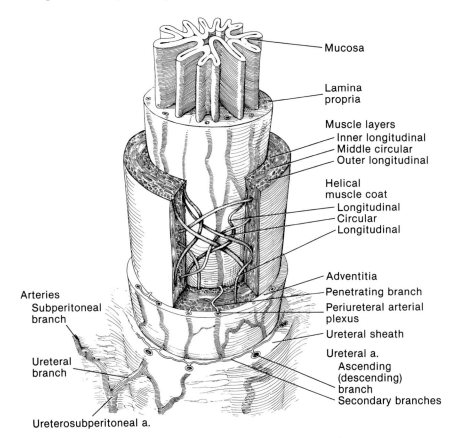

- Mucosa
- Lamina propria
- Muscle layers
  - Inner longitudinal
  - Middle circular
  - Outer longitudinal
- Helical muscle coat
  - Longitudinal
  - Circular
  - Longitudinal
- Adventitia
- Penetrating branch
- Periureteral arterial plexus
- Ureteral sheath
- Ureteral a.
  - Ascending (descending) branch
  - Secondary branches

Arteries
- Subperitoneal branch
- Ureteral branch

Ureterosubperitoneal a.

Proximally, both the ureteral sheath and the adventitia are continuous with the corresponding layers of the renal pelvis.

Distally, the sheath and adventitia are more prominent in the terminal portion of the ureter, where they join Waldeyer's sheath formed from the deep trigone as it extends from the bladder wall around the ureter. In the female, the sheath is closely associated with the uterovaginal and vesicovaginal plexuses of veins within the parametrium, making the ureter more difficult to free during operations on the uterus. There it is susceptible to injury and devitalization, as well as to subsequent fixation in fibrous tissue. After destruction of the ureteral sheath, adherence of the ureter to adjacent structures may result in functional obstruction. The sheath supplements the adventitia to act as a barrier to periurethral neoplastic and inflammatory processes. This is best appreciated after retroperitoneal inflammation, when the sheath is found to be composed of a series of onion-skin layers that allow some peristaltic movement of the ureteral wall to continue. The *adventitia* is loosely attached to the underlying muscularis, leaving it free to move.

The *muscular layers* are formed from smooth muscle cells arranged in bundles interspersed with collagen fibers. On cross-section, three layers are seen—inner, middle, and outer—but they actually are arranged in interlacing helices. Nexuses connect the individual smooth muscle cells that allow the spread of electrical excitation from one cell to the next. Nerves play only a modulating role in ureteral activity.

The transitional epithelium with multiple layers of cells lies directly on a relatively thick but loosely arranged fibroelastic layer, the lamina propria, there being no submucosa as such.

The *uretero-subperitoneal arteries* are supplied by several retroperitoneal vessels. Proximally the supply is from the renal artery, the aorta, and the gonadal arteries. Distally, the most frequent sources are the superior and inferior vesical arteries, but ureteral vessels also arise from internal iliac arteries, vessels that provide the richest supply to the lower portion of the ureter. The middle portion of the ureter between the lower pole of the kidney and the brim of the pelvis is the most poorly vascularized.

A uretero-subperitoneal artery divides into a subperitoneal and a ureteral branch. The ureteral branch has ascending and descending branches in the ureteral sheath that enter the adventitia through secondary branches. The secondary branches pass to a deeper layer to penetrate the adventitial coat of the ureter and there form a freely anastomotic periureteral arterial plexus that extends for the entire length of the ureter. The ureteral arteries branching from the uretero-subperitoneal vessels usually divide into long ascending and descending branches. These branches anastomose with descending branches from above and with the ascending branches from below.

This vascular arrangement does not limit the sites of division of the ureter because the anastomoses within a sectioned ureter prevent ischemia. On the other hand, interference with the arterial plexus jeopardizes the viability of the end of the ureter, whether the damage occurs directly during surgery or as the effect of electrocoagulation or infection. Viability of the distal ureter may be especially tenuous in secondary operations on the previously mobilized or resected ureter.

The preservation of the ureteral trunks in the ureteral sheath is essential when operating on long segments of the ureter, as when transplanting a kidney or tapering a megaureter. However, in about one quarter of the cases, the vessels do not have long branches but immediately form plexuses and therefore are more readily rendered avascular by division.

The subperitoneal arteries from the uretero-subperitoneal vessels supply the periureteral tissue and also provide some distribution to the peritoneum. They freely anastomose with neighboring vessels as they contribute blood to the ureter. Separation of the ureter from the peritoneum by division of the arterial twigs may compromise ureteral blood supply, especially in the lower ureter.

MANAGEMENT OF INTRAOPERATIVE INJURY TO THE URETER

Ureteral injury during a difficult abdominal operation may be less likely to occur if the ureters are stented at the beginning. If ureteral catheters are not placed, a plugged balloon catheter in the bladder allows detection of hematuria. The injury from cross-clamping the ureter in situ for an appreciable length of time should be treated with insertion of a double-J stent for at least 10 days, but if the ureter has already been isolated, resection and anastomosis are advisable, accompanied by insertion of a Penrose drain (see pages 835 to 836). Inadvertent ligation of a ureter, even if recognized immediately, usually warrants ureteral stenting. If the involved segment is obviously ischemic, it is better to excise and anastomose it. If the ureter is cauterized, inspect it for damage to the adventitial vessels. Such ischemic tissue must be excised.

A severed ureter requires spatulation and anastomosis over a stent, but avulsion or extensive damage makes the use of a psoas hitch (see page 818) or bladder flap (see page 822) necessary. Ureteral injury is suspected postoperatively from the presence of flank pain and tenderness in the costovertebral angle, low-grade fever, and ileus. Ultrasonography and urography may reveal the site and extent. Retrograde passage of a double-J stent should be tried first, with or without a guide wire. Percutaneous nephrostomy is an alternative, to await the dissolution of obstructing absorbable sutures. If the patient is in good condition, consider immediate surgical correction.

Ureteroneocystostomy

Perform antireflux surgery for demonstrated reflux after infection has broken through on suppressive antibiotics; for persistent, severe reflux with previous episodes of pyelonephritis; and for anatomic abnormality of the orifice. In adults requiring ureteral reimplantation for injury or tumor, the need for an antireflux procedure has not been demonstrated, and a simple direct anastomosis may have fewer problems.

Obtain a voiding cystourethrogram and a renal scan to assess for renal scarring. Ultrasonography can be useful as a screening procedure.

For *primary reflux* in a single system, grade the reflux. It may not be necessary to observe the orifice cystoscopically because its position correlates well with the grade of reflux. Treat Grades 1 through 4 conservatively unless infection persists or parenchymal loss or scarring supervenes. Consider endoscopic submucosal injection of polytetrafluoroethylene (Teflon) or gluteraldehyde cross-linked bovine collagen. For Grade 5, reimplant the ureter or, in duplex systems, perform pyelopyelostomy (see page 812) or transureteroureterostomy (see page 834).

For *secondary reflux,* assess vesical urodynamic status for evidence of neurogenic or non-neurogenic bladder dysfunction. Correct it by drugs and training or intermittent catheterization before considering surgical treatment of the reflux because implantation into such bladders is often unsuccessful. Every attempt should be made to obtain normal detrusor dynamics before operation.

Selection of Technique

A transvesical technique is used for small trigones or large ureters, especially in infants. The traditional intra-extravesical (Politano-Leadbetter), the distal tunnel advancement (Glenn-Anderson), and the cross-trigonal (Cohen) techniques are suitable for most cases because simple advancement may be done rapidly with minimal dissection. These techniques are preferred for bilateral cases because they do not interfere with perivesical nerves and thus reduce the risk of postoperative urinary retention. The extravesical (Lich-Gregoir-Hodgson) or external tunnel (Barry) technique can be used successfully not only for unilateral "virginal" cases but also for more complicated ones, including those with an extravesical diverticulum. It can be adapted as a laparoscopic technique (Steps 22 and 23). For megaureter, the techniques of ureteral tapering (Hendren) and folding are used. For thick-walled bladders, the ureter can be dissected extravesically, repaired, and pulled through the original hiatus, to be advanced subepithelially as in the Cohen technique.

Each technique has advantages and disadvantages: Blind extravesical passage of the ureter as in the Politano-Leadbetter technique carries the risk of obstructing the ureter by kinking. The Glenn-Anderson advancement technique avoids this problem and is a good choice for the laterally placed ectopic ureteral orifice even though the reflux may persist more often than after other techniques. The Cohen technique is easily performed and has a low rate of complications, but it does require a longer ureter and has the limitation of making future catheterization difficult, even with flexible cystoscopes. The extravesical techniques are useful, especially with large ureters.

For *ureteral injuries and stenosis,* performing ureteroureterostomy in the lower ureter is usually technically difficult and not infrequently fails. The following are suggested protocols: (1) If the obstruction is low, do a ureteroneocystostomy with or without a psoas hitch (see page 797). (2) If it is higher, make a bladder flap (see page 822). (3) If it is merely crushed, stent the ureter. Remember that a fibrotic or contracted bladder may be unsuitable for implantation or for flap procedures. Consider performing ureteroureterostomy (see page 834) or autotransplantation of the kidney (see page 830) to bridge the gap. As a last resort, a ureteroileostomy (see page 647) or even a cutaneous ureterostomy (see page 642) or nephrectomy may have to be done. In any case, avoid excessive ureteral mobilization and tension on the anastomosis. A nonrefluxing anastomosis may not be essential in an adult, thus making the anastomosis technically easier.

If the contralateral orifice is not entirely normal in appearance but does not reflux, simply advance that ureter intravesically. For bilateral megaureters, especially at reoperation, consider making a long reimplantation with a psoas hitch for one ureter and performing a transuretero-ureterostomy for the other.

Perform cystoscopy before open surgery to allow complete evaluation of the genitalia and urethra, the contralateral orifice, and missed duplication or ectopia.

TRANSVESICAL APPROACHES

Ureteral Mobilization

Insert a balloon catheter with a Y connector, clamp the outlet, and partially fill the bladder.

1 *Position:* Place the patient supine, and insert a silicone catheter into the bladder through the urethra. Partially fill the bladder with saline.

Incision: For primary operations, make a small transverse lower abdominal incision in a skin crease (see page 490); for secondary operations, a vertical abdominal incision may be required (see page 487), although in many cases the transverse incision may be quite adequate. Incise the bladder vertically; then enlarge the opening with two index fingers. A figure-eight suture may be placed where the incision in the bladder approaches the retropubic space to prevent tearing the vesical neck during the procedure.

Place four stay sutures around the margin of the cystostomy, and drape them over the retractor for exposure (not shown), or place lateral retractor blades inside the bladder. Insert a moist pack in the bladder dome to be held with a Deaver retractor or with the fourth blade of the retention retractor. Avoid rubbing the bladder wall, which causes edema.

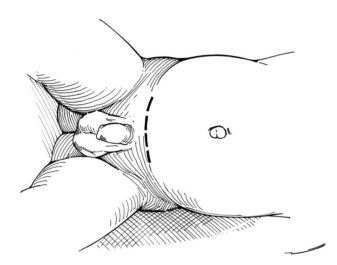

2 Insert a 3 F to 5 F infant feeding tube in the ureter, and suture it to the orifice with a purse-string 4-0 synthetic absorbable suture (SAS).

Alternative: Place a 3-0 plain catgut (PCG) suture deeply into the trigone at the orifice beneath the feeding tube and tie it over the tube, a technique that may be preferable if the distal ureter will not be resected later. To decrease bleeding and facilitate dissection, inject a solution of 1 percent lidocaine with 1:100,000 epinephrine through a 26-gauge needle around the ureter along the proposed subepithelial tunnel starting at the orifice.

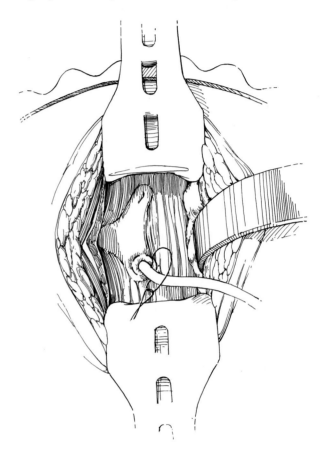

3 Gently lift the tube to draw the ureteral orifice into the bladder. Cut through the epithelium around the orifice with a hooked blade or sharp scissors, leaving a ring of bladder epithelium on the ureter.

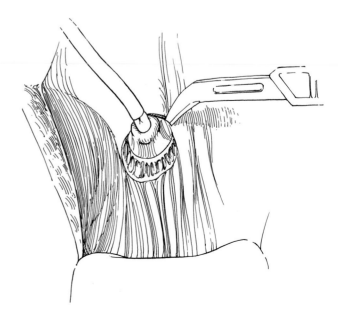

4 **A,** With tenotomy scissors held at right angles to the ureter against the ureteral wall, sharply divide the superficial trigonal muscles, which are clearly seen medially and inferiorly as the ureter is elevated.

B, Develop a plane inferiorly next to the ureteral adventitia, and bluntly and sharply free the ureter of all attachments to Waldeyer's sheath. Mobilize enough ureter by pushing the adherent peritoneum away with a peanut dissector to ensure tension-free repositioning. Preserve the ureteral adventitia because stripping it results in ureteral ischemia and necrosis. Watch for vessels tributary to the ureter. Avoid kinking, twisting, or J-hooking the ureter.

C, Insert traction sutures through the bladder wall medially and laterally to open the hiatus, and elevate the hiatus with a narrow Deaver retractor. Do not use forceps. Bluntly dissect between the ureter and bladder wall under vision with a large right-angle clamp or a Küttner dissector to free the peritoneal attachments. At least 4 cm of the ureter should be exposed. Avoid devascularization or perforation of the ureter. Be sure the clamp does not pass through peritoneum or bowel.

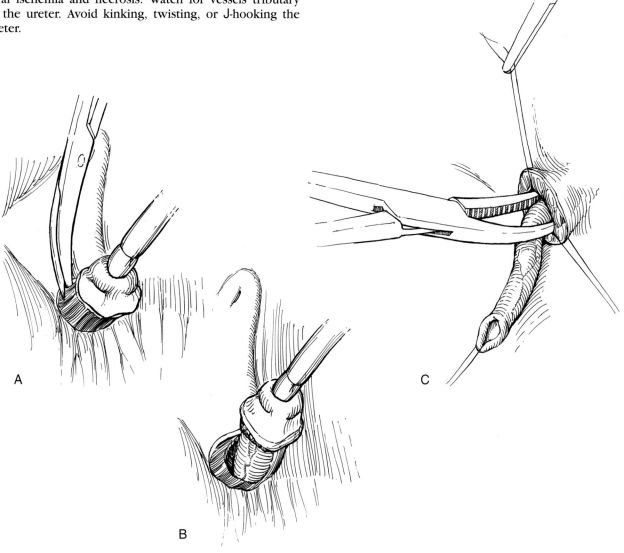

A

B

C

Intra-Extravesical Technique (Politano-Leadbetter)

5 **A** and **B,** Insert a long Mixter clamp into the hiatus, and dissect along the outer surface of the bladder wall. Elevate the tip against the wall at a point at least 2.5 cm cephalad and slightly *medial* to the hiatus, the distance dependent on the size of the ureter. A 3:1 or even 5:1 ratio of tunnel length to ureteral diameter is needed. Avoid placing the new hiatus any more lateral than the original. Incise onto the clamp, making sure that the opening is large enough to accommodate the ureter.

C, Catch the ureteral traction suture, and also the stent if it is still in place, in a right-angle clamp, and draw it up through the tunnel and out the new hiatus. Pull the ureter into the bladder through the retrovesical tunnel, checking to be certain it is not kinked or twisted. Close the bladder wall behind the original hiatus with interrupted 3-0 or 4-0 SAS. If a longer tunnel is needed, incise the hiatus cephalolaterally and close the bladder wall below the ureter.

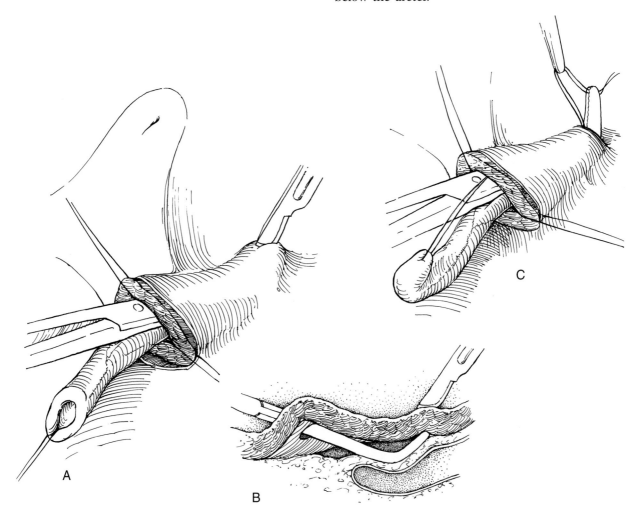

6 **A,** Dissect a subepithelial tunnel from the new to the old hiatus by cutting and spreading with small curved (tenotomy) scissors or scissors with a 135-degree angle. It may be easier in some cases to start dissection distally. If the roof is torn, merely tack it back after implanting the ureter. It is even possible to incise the intervening epithelium and dissect it back as two flaps to be approximated subsequently over the ureter. In any case, check the size of the tunnel by inserting a mosquito clamp.

B, Pass a clamp holding the stay suture down through the tunnel, grasp the suture with another clamp, and draw the ureter through. Again check the caliber of the tunnel and hiatus. The tunnel should lie within the square outlined on the trigone, depicted in the inset figure.

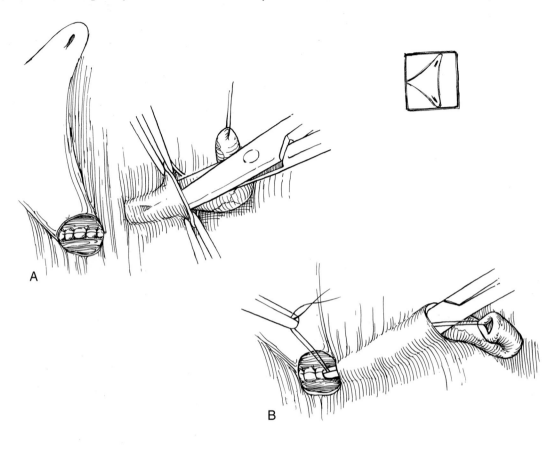

7 **A,** Trim the old meatus from the ureter, and, if it is small, spatulate the end on the medial aspect. Alternatively, if the ureter has a normal configuration, leave the old meatus intact. Anchor the tip with two sutures placed deeply into the trigonal muscle and through the vesical epithelium. Be certain that the ureter is not twisted, takes a straight course, and is under no tension.

B, Complete the anastomosis with carefully placed 4-0 or 5-0 SAS for an epithelium-to-epithelium coaptation. Close the upper incision vertically with the same suture material. Pass a 3.5 F or 5 F infant feeding tube up the ureter to make sure that no ureteral kinks are present.

Stent the ureter with an infant feeding tube to align it and prevent kinks or adhesions and, in the case of dilated ureters, to allow them to regain tone. An 8 F Dow Corning cystocatheter with extra holes can be inserted with a self-contained trocar for insertion of the stent through the skin and into the bladder and connected to a leg bag. The KISS catheter (Cook Urological, Inc.) has a longitudinally open slit to prevent clotting and obstruction.

Fix the stent to the opposite side of the bladder near the neck with a 4-0 PCG suture, and bring it out through a stab wound, or transurethrally if a 1- to 2-day intubation is planned. If the intubation will need to be prolonged, use an indwelling double-J stent.

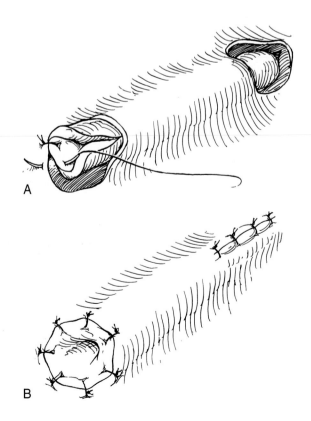

8 **A,** *Additional tunnel length:* Dissect distally under the epithelium to form a second hiatus.

B and **C,** Draw the ureter through to the new hiatus, and suture it in place. Close the two epithelial defects longitudinally.

D, Alternatively, rather than actually tunneling further, advance the meatus by incising the more distal epithelium and closing it over the ureter (see Step 9).

To drain the bladder in males, insert a 14 F or 16 F Malecot catheter in the bladder dome. A small transurethral silicone balloon catheter can also be used effectively. Bring the stenting catheter through a stab wound in the bladder to the surface just above the abdominal incision. In females, the ureteral stents can easily be brought out through the urethra alongside a small balloon catheter. In many cases, it is easier to insert an 8 F to 12 F red rubber catheter in the urethra, put a 2-0 silk stitch through its tip, and bring both ends of the suture through the bladder

and abdominal walls so that it may be tied over a gauze roll (see page 429).

Close the bladder in layers with a running 4-0 subepithelial PCG suture, followed by interrupted 3-0 chromic catgut (CCG) or SAS to the muscle. Place a small Penrose or suction drain in the space of Retzius, and bring it out through a stab wound below the incision. Reapproximate the rectus muscles and fascia with 3-0 or 4-0 SAS. Close the subcutaneous tissue with fine PCG sutures and the skin with a subcuticular 4-0 or 5-0 SAS.

Postoperatively, continue with prophylactic antibiotics. Perform intravenous urography or sonography at 6 weeks and voiding cystography at 12 weeks. Monitor the urine by culture. If reflux has ceased, stop the suppressive antibiotics, but continue checking the urine for infection. At 1 and 3 years postoperatively, perform renal ultrasonography to assess renal growth and rule out hydronephrosis.

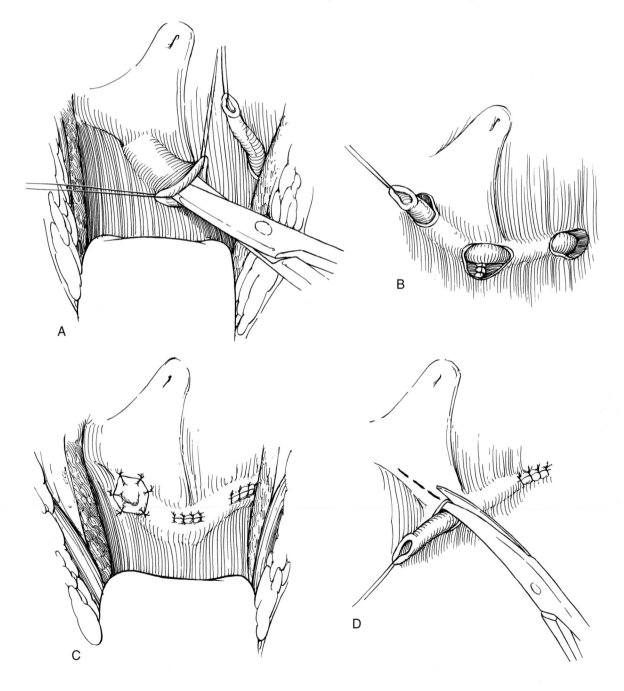

Ureteral Advancement Technique (Glenn-Anderson)

This technique is done under direct vision without blind extravesical dissection. It fixes the ureteral orifice well down on the trigone, providing for maximal closure and prevention of reflux and an orifice that is readily catheterized.

9 **A,** Free the ureter as described in Steps 1 to 4. Create a subepithelial tunnel distally to form a new hiatus.

B, Incise the entire thickness of the vesical wall above the original hiatus. Do not deviate laterally.

C, Close the defect behind the ureter with interrupted 4-0 SAS.

D, Draw the ureter through the tunnel with a right-angle clamp. Trim, fix, and anastomose it to the vesical epithelium. Close the original epithelial defect.

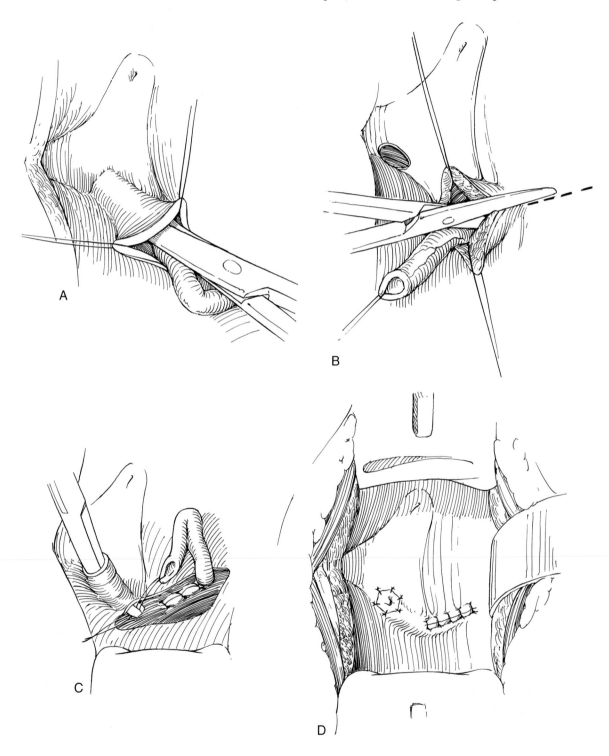

Transtrigonal Technique (Cohen)

Free the ureter as described in Steps 1 to 4. Assess the size of the hiatus; if it is too large, narrow it with one or two fine SAS, but take care not to constrict the ureter. Be sure the ureter is freely mobile. If more exposure is needed, incise the superolateral margin of the hiatus with the cutting current, and lift the edge with small vein retractors. This maneuver also allows a higher and, consequently, longer tunnel.

10 **A,** Incise the epithelium vertically just above and slightly lateral to the opposite ureteral orifice, depending on the size of the trigone. Pull up on that edge of the bladder with Allis clamps to tent and flatten the bladder wall. Insert Lahey scissors, and gently open and close them to advance across the bladder just above the trigone to a point about 1 cm above the opposite orifice. Of course, much depends on the size of the ureter and the trigone. When crossing the midline with the scissors, be careful not to let the tips go too deeply into the muscle and, especially, not to let them curve too much anteriorly and perforate the epithelium. Pulling the orifices laterally and stretching the supratrigonal area causes this surface to become flatter and makes the dissection easier. Remove the tube from the ureter. Insert a curved clamp, and draw the ureter through the tunnel by its traction suture until it lies free of tension.

B, Trim the end of the ureter while the traction suture is relaxed, spatulate it if small, anchor it with a 4-0 CCG suture through all layers of ureter and bladder, and approximate the edges with interrupted fine sutures. Alternatively, if the original epithelial cuff is adequate, suture the ureter in place epithelium to epithelium with 5-0 SAS without trimming. Close the original hiatus with the same material. Check the course of the ureter with an infant feeding tube.

11 **A,** For bilateral reimplantation, make a separate tunnel for the second ureter that extends from the hiatus of the first ureter. Alternatively, lead this ureter through the original tunnel.

B, Bring the second ureter to the hiatus of the first ureter, and suture it in place. Insert a 3.5 F or 5 F infant feeding tube to be sure that the ureter has a smoothly curving course. If there is concern about the quality of the anastomosis, tack the tube laterally to the epithelium with a 3-0 PCG suture and leave it as a stent. In males, place a Malecot catheter for 48 hours. It should exit from a stab wound. In females, a Robinson catheter suffices, held by a silk suture through the bladder dome and skin. Insert a Penrose drain in the retropubic space. Close the bladder in two layers and the wound in layers. Leave the stent in place for 48 hours.

For dilated ureters, resect the obstructing segment to allow the ureter to contract. If it remains large, turn to a technique designed for megaureters (see page 803).

An *alternative* to actually tunneling under the mucosa across the trigone, sometimes difficult to do in a trabeculated bladder, is to incise the epithelium and subepithelium and suture the ureter into the trough (Keramidas, 1993).

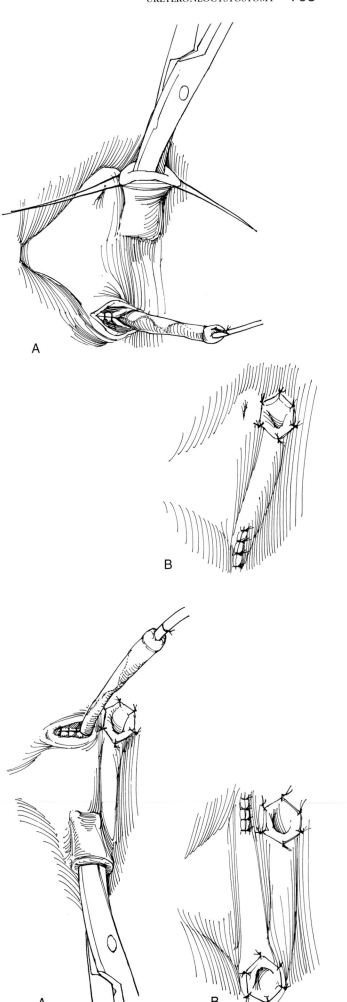

Sheath Approximation Technique
(Gil Vernet)

Make a transverse incision between the two laterally placed orifices to expose the underlying trigonal muscle. Catch the periureteral sheath at the inferior margin of first one ureter and then the other ureter with a single nonabsorbable mattress suture. Tie the suture to draw the ureters together in the midline.

Spatulated Nipple Technique

The spatulated nipple technique, a method for direct anastomosis, is preferable to the older fish-mouth method. It may be the last resort if the ureter cannot be extended without tension and forming a psoas hitch or bladder flap is not practical. It is also a simple technique for adults requiring ureteral implantation.

12 **A,** Pass the ureter directly through the bladder wall near the hiatus, and incise the lateral border for a distance of 2 to 2.5 cm.
B, Turn the ureteral wall back on itself, and tack it in place with 4-0 CCG or SAS. Anastomose the collar to the bladder epithelium.

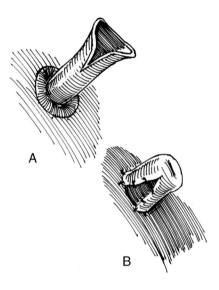

Commentary by Mark F. Bellinger

A transvesical approach is acceptable for most ureters, and I generally have a low threshold to reimplant the contralateral ureter, based upon a history of reflux or an abnormal ureterovesical junction upon gross inspection. Cystoscopy is used prior to incision to rule out cystitis. This can be easily accomplished in females using the frogleg position, obviating movement of the patient down into the lithotomy position. The bladder is left partially full after cystoscopy, and a Foley catheter with the balloon deflated is passed all the way into the bladder and connected to a drainage bag with the tubing clamped. When the bladder is opened, the catheter is easily pulled up out of the way and replaced at the end of the procedure, at which time the balloon is inflated.

A skin crease incision is very cosmetic, and when the fascia is opened in the midline, good exposure of the entire pelvis can be obtained. After dissecting out the ureter and closing the muscular hiatus, leave the muscular sutures long, held laterally as retraction to stretch the trigone and facilitate dissection of the submucosal tunnel. Optical magnification allows precise placement of ureteral sutures, and leaving the mucosal collar of the distal ureter intact lessens worry about meatal stricture.

A urethral catheter removed the following morning works fine in most uncomplicated cases, and a small perivesical suction drain is easier to manage than a Penrose drain. In infant girls, no bladder catheter may be necessary. We generally prefer a combination of adjunctive caudal anesthesia and belladonna and opium suppositories for 12 to 24 hours postoperatively. If postoperative flank pain and prolonged ileus occur, early placement of an indwelling stent is warranted, and this should be left for a few weeks. If anuria secondary to ureteral edema occurs soon after bilateral reimplantation in an infant, overhydration and dilutional hyponatremia can occur quickly, so serum electrolytes should be closely monitored.

EXTRAVESICAL TECHNIQUES

Reimplanting the ureter extravesically has the advantage of reducing postoperative bladder spasms and overall hospital stay. The ureters are subsequently easy to catheterize, and complications are minimal.

Extravesical Tunnel, Open Technique (Lich-Gregoir)

Place an indwelling balloon catheter with a Y adaptor so that the volume can be regulated during the dissection. Fill the bladder to one-third capacity.

13 *Incision:* Make a lower midline incision (see page 487) or, better, a transverse incision (see page 490). Incise the transversalis fascia superficially over the bladder, and draw it cephalad with a finger on either side to expose the obliterated umbilical arteries.

Insert a ring retractor. Dissect the obliterated umbilical artery on one side to its crossing of the ureter. Undermine the artery with a right-angle clamp, and divide it between the ligatures. Avoid dissecting toward the origin of the artery and thus entering the pelvic venous plexus there. Expose the ureter, and encircle it with a Penrose drain or surgical loop. Ligate the several perforating vessels behind the ureter, but dissect laterally to preserve all the adventitial vasculature possible. Dissect toward the bladder, ligating uterine vessels as necessary.

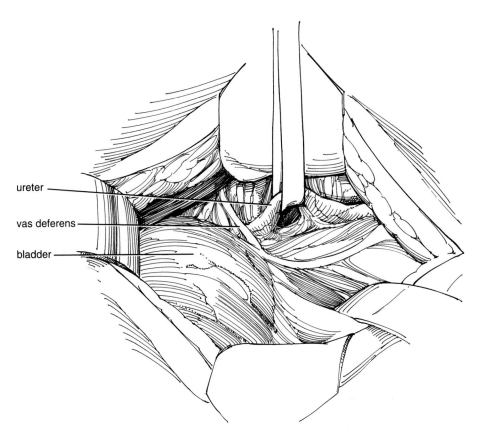

ureter

vas deferens

bladder

14 Lift the ureter in the Penrose drain sling. Separate the intramural portion of the ureter from the detrusor muscle circumferentially, using a Schnidt clamp in order to reach the vesical subepithelium, which may be identified more readily if dilute methylene blue has been instilled in the bladder.

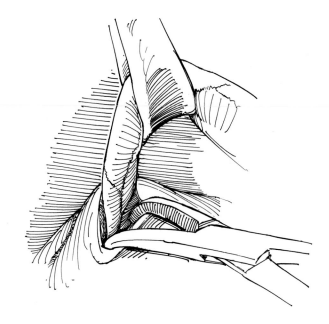

15 **A,** Divide the detrusor muscle down to the subepithelium with a #15 blade, cutting a groove for a distance of 2.5 to 3 cm in an almost vertical direction. Because this cut is made with the bladder elevated and rotated, the direction it should take may not be immediately apparent. Let the bladder drop back to be sure that the incision follows the natural course of the ureter.

B, Undermine the bladder muscle against the subepithelium to provide lateral flaps for coverage. Make a T-shaped incision proximally if necessary to release the flaps. Replace the ureter in the groove. *Alternatively,* divide the ureter at its junction with the bladder, and make a small opening at that site. Place a 3-0 absorbable mattress suture in the ureteral tip, and cut the needle off. Rethread both ends on a larger needle, and pass them through the opening and then through the seromuscular layer of the bladder. Tie them on the surface. This fixes the distal end of the ureter in the subepithelial tunnel.

C, Close the detrusor loosely over the ureter with interrupted 3-0 SAS. If an extravesical diverticulum is present, invert it into the bladder. If it is very large, excise it, close the defect, and implant the ureter through a new incision in the detrusor. Avoid constriction of the ureter at the point of exit. Allow the bladder to fall back, insert a Penrose drain, and close the wound in layers.

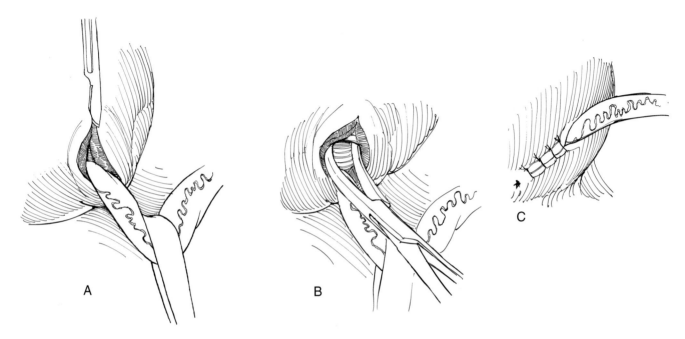

A   B   C

External Tunnel Technique

Single Ureter
(Barry)

The external tunnel method of implantation is especially suitable for the ureter in kidney transplantation (see pages 964 to 965).

Insert a urethral balloon catheter connected by a Y tube to a saline reservoir and a drainage bag. After exposure of the bladder, clamp the outflow and fill the bladder with 100 to 200 ml of water. Roll the bladder medially with a stay suture in the bladder wall, or use a shallow padded retractor.

16 Score the seromuscular layer with the electrocautery for two parallel incision 3 cm apart. Make two incisions 2 cm long through the adventitia and muscularis with the scalpel, down to the subepithelium. With a curved clamp, make a tunnel between the incisions; spread the clamp to make the tunnel 2 cm wide. If a small tear is accidentally made in the epithelium, lift it with fine forceps and ligate it with a fine absorbable suture. Close large tears with a fine running absorbable suture.

17 Grasp the epithelium through the distal incision with vascular forceps. Have the circulating nurse release the urethral clamp, and drain the bladder. Excise a button of uroepithelium.

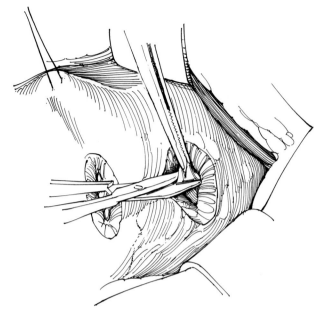

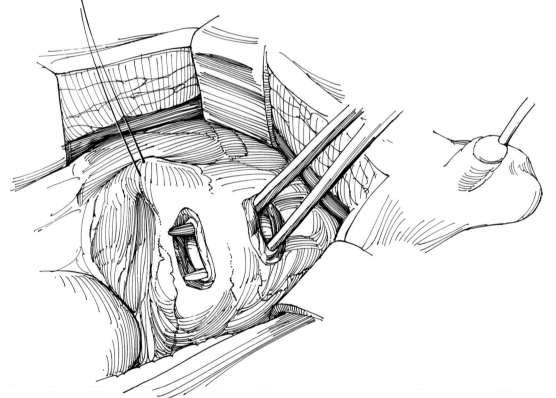

18 **A** and **B,** Draw the ureter through the subepithelial tunnel, spatulate it, and suture it to the opening in the bladder with three 4-0 SAS, one at the apex of the spatulation and the others at the 9-o'clock and 3-o'clock positions. Place a fourth suture through the full thickness of the tip of the ureter, cut the suture long, and thread each end on a curved needle. Pass one end out through the full thickness of the bladder wall to exit 1 cm distally, and pass the other end only through the seromuscular layer. Tie the two ends together. Close the distal bladder opening with 4-0 SAS to all layers but the epithelium. Stents are not needed. Place a suction drain, and remove it when drainage is less than 30 ml/day. Leave the balloon catheter in place for 5 days.

Double Ureter
(Barry)

Trim the ends of adventitia, and spatulate them along the medial edges. Suture the dorsal edges together with a fine running stitch. Bring the double-barreled ureter through the submucosal tunnel as described above, and suture it around the opening in the vesical epithelium, adding a mattress suture through the full thickness of the conjoined ureters and through the seromuscular layer of the bladder distal to the implantation.

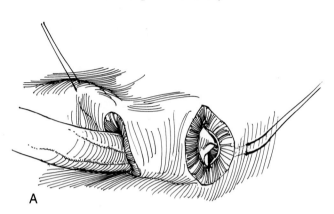

A

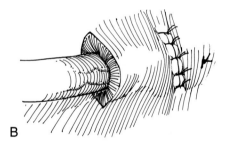

B

Megaureters. This technique may also be used for large ureters, especially in newborns and infants (Perovic-Sremcevic, 1994). Because the ureter folds in the tunnel, tailoring is not required as long as sufficient ureter is resected to avoid kinking.

Commentary by John M. Barry

We have used the parallel-incision extravesical ureteroneocystostomy in more than 1000 kidney transplant recipients, including children. The reoperation rate has been less than 2 percent because of urinary leakage, obstruction, or bleeding. The reflux rate has been 0.4 percent. The mattress anchoring suture through the tip of the ureter and the bladder wall is very significant because it prevents the ureter from sliding in the tunnel. I usually place this anchoring mattress suture 1 cm distal to the mucosal opening because if it is placed too far distally, it can pull the ureter into the bladder and cause one of the apical or dog-ear sutures to pull out. Sometimes the proximal horizontal incision in the detrusor is too large. When that occurs, simply place an extra stitch or two to prevent a periureteral diverticulum. Indwelling ureteral stents are recommended when the bladder is very thin or very thick or when several premature bladder mucosal entries have been made. A suction drain is commonly used following renal transplantation because extensive lymphatic dissection is necessary for vascular reconstruction, because the patients receive anticoagulants in the perioperative period, and because wound healing is impaired with immunosuppressant therapy.

The technique has been used successfully in nontransplant patients, including those in whom the urinary tract reconstruction required a psoas hitch. It has also been adapted to ureteral reimplantation into continent intestinal pouches, and the principles have been applied to a modification of the Mitrofanoff procedure.

Detrusorrhaphy
(Hodgson-Firlit-Zaontz)

Through a Pfannenstiel incision, insert a ring retractor and rotate the bladder to follow the obliterated hypogastric vessel and thus expose the ureter extravesically. Place a vessel loop around it to use for traction to allow dissection to its junction with the bladder. Preserve as much of the periureteral vasculature as possible, but free the terminal ureter of its perivesical and muscular attachments. Distend the bladder moderately.

19 Place traction on the ureter to define its course so that a limited, laterally oriented incision can be made with the cutting current in the line of the ureter. Carry it through the detrusor to the subepithelium proximal to the attachment of the ureter. Continue the incision distal to the ureter. Starting laterally, place multiple traction sutures (not shown) to allow elevation of the muscle from the epithelium. Dissect first distally toward the bladder neck and then proximally for a distance of 5 to 6 cm. Include the fibers from Waldeyer's sheath to form detrusor flaps. Take care not to perforate the bladder epithelium. (If it is breached, empty the bladder and close the defect with a fine figure-eight suture before proceeding.) The degree of pouching of the epithelium may be regulated by filling and emptying the bladder.

Use 3-0 or 4-0 long-acting SAS material (not catgut, which is absorbed too quickly). Place the suture first through the muscle of the bladder wall at the lower edge of the opening from outside in to exit at the edge of the epithelial-muscularis dissection; then pass it through the ureteral serosa and muscularis at the level of the former ureterovesical junction at the 5-o'clock position. Finally, pass it distally to exit inside out near the point of entry. This is a vertical mattress suture that forms a Vest-type stitch. Place a second suture in the same way at the 7-o'clock position of the ureter.

20 A and B, Tie the sutures to telescope the ureter into the bladder, thus forming a long subepithelial tunnel. For duplex ureters, place an extra suture between them. Close the hiatus loosely with running or interrupted 4-0 SAS to back up the tunnel. Check for ureteral torsion, and test for possible constriction with a right-angle clamp. Neither a stent nor a drain is needed. Drain the bladder, and leave the balloon catheter in place overnight to cope with the effects of atropinization; remove it the next day. Check for incomplete emptying, especially in bilateral cases (which might be better repaired transvesically to avoid perivesical denervation), and be prepared to start clean intermittent catheterization.

A similar technique may be followed for megaureters, except that the ureter must be disconnected for tapering. Intubate it with a stent passing out through the bladder. After reanastomosing it with fine catgut sutures, insert the detrusorrhaphy sutures at the 5-o'clock and 7-o'clock positions, and close the defect in the detrusor.

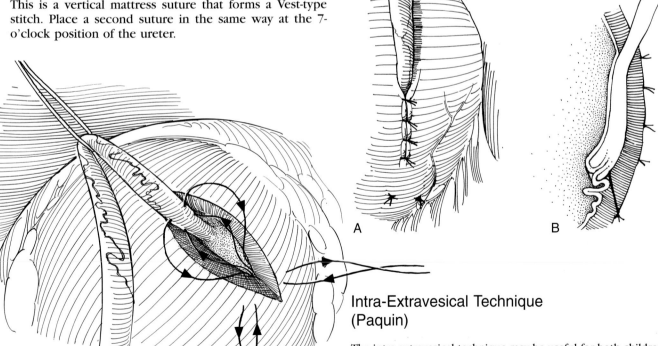

A   B

Intra-Extravesical Technique
(Paquin)

The intra-extravesical technique may be useful for both children and adolescents.

Mobilize the ureter extravesically as previously described. In adolescents, divide the superior vesical pedicle for access. Open the bladder, and make an epithelial incision medial to the original hiatus. Create a subepithelial tunnel beginning outside the bladder, and draw the ureter through it with a catheter passed in retrograde fashion. Alternatively in adults, consider a psoas hitch with direct subepithelial implantation (see page 818).

LAPAROSCOPIC TECHNIQUES

Extravesical Tunnel (Lich-Gregoir Adaptation)

Cystoscopically insert a ureteral catheter into the ureter. Fasten it to an 8 F balloon catheter draped into the field. Create a pneumoperitoneum, and insert two 11-mm trocars, one in the left midclavicular line 5 cm above the umbilicus for the camera and one in the midline below it for various instruments, and insert two 5-mm trocars in the left and right midclavicular line at the level of the anterior superior iliac spine for the dissecting instruments (see page 21). Identify the obliterated umbilical artery. Open the peritoneum over the iliac vessels, and identify the ureter.

21 A and B, Grasp the ureter with Babcock-type forceps to put tension on the periureteral tissue and allow blunt dissection of the terminal 2 or 3 cm. Cauterize the serosa along the line of the proposed incision, and incise into the muscle layer of the bladder wall electrosurgically or with the laser for a distance of 3 cm proximal to the ureterovesical junction. Complete the trough by cutting with scissors and bluntly dissecting to expose the subepithelium.

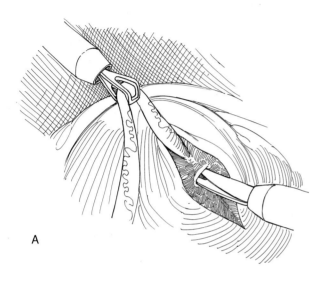

A

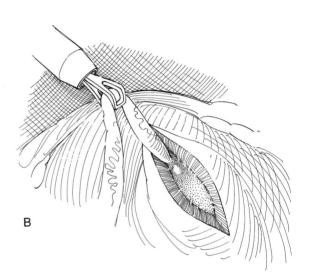

B

22 A, Place the ureter in the trough, and hold it there with a retractor while approximating the edges over the ureter distally with a pair of grasping instruments. Place a staple with the hernia stapler through the edges at the distal end to contain the ureter.

B, Staple the rest of the incision together. *Alternately,* close the trough with four SAS tied with extracorporal or intracorporal knots.

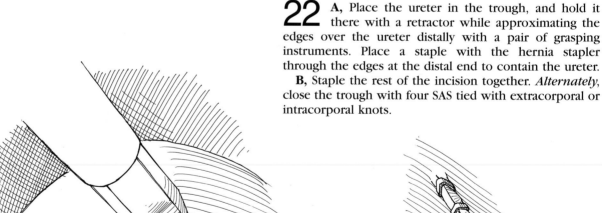

A

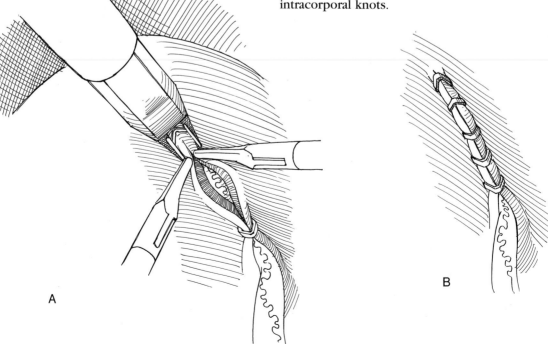

B

Percutaneous Endoscopic Trigonoplasty
(PET Procedure)
(Cartwright, Snow)

This is a laparoscopic adaptation of the sheath approximation technique (Gil Vernet) (see page 794) that can be accomplished as an outpatient procedure in 1 to 1.5 hours.

Place two laparoscopic ports through the prevesical space into the bladder under cystoscopic control. With small laparoscopic scissors or harmonic scalpel, cauterize the mucosa between the two orifices; then incise and dissect a trough along the trigonal ridge between them. Place one or two horizontal mattress sutures just medial to each orifice with the aid of a laparoscopic needle holder. Tie the knot(s) to advance the ureters across the incised trough.

POSTOPERATIVE PROBLEMS

Previously unrecognized *bladder dysfunction* is the most common cause of problems with ureteral reimplantation. Perivesical dissection can itself cause bladder dysfunction. The *non-neurogenic neurogenic bladder syndrome,* if not recognized preoperatively, can lead to failure to correct the reflux or to secondary obstruction at the new orifice.

Early ipsilateral reflux is usually of low grade and resolves spontaneously. *Persistent reflux* (for more than 2 months) may be due to technical failure such as insufficient ureteral mobilization, too short a tunnel, or inappropriate placement of the orifice; to ureterovesical fistulization; or to inadequate closure of the trigonal muscular hiatus. More often it is due to continued abnormal bladder function, often on a non-neurogenic basis. Look first for day and night wetting, frequency, urgency, and bowel soiling. If the failure is on this basis, dysfunction must be corrected by retraining before reoperation is attempted. For neurogenic dysfunction, augmentation cystoplasty may be required.

Contralateral reflux may occur postoperatively, but it usually corrects itself. Usually, both ureters are implanted whenever the other side shows any evidence of abnormality, but implantation of the minimally affected side may be done by simple advancement (Step 9).

Ureteral obstruction may occur early, after removal of the stent, causing flank pain, nausea, vomiting, ileus, and even sepsis. Treat the condition conservatively; rarely is retrograde or antegrade placement of a ureteral stent or percutaneous nephrostomy required. The obstruction is the result of edema or contraction of the thickened bladder wall during spasm. It is especially troublesome in infants under 3 months of age and in those with dilated ureters preoperatively. In such patients, stenting should be routine.

Persistent ureteral obstruction, evidenced by increased dilation of the upper tract, may be detected on routine urography or ultrasonography. Confirm obstruction with diuretic renography. For severe obstruction, perform percutaneous nephrostomy as a temporizing method and as a means to allow evaluation after repair. Obstruction is of concern if it is present for longer than a few weeks and may require endoscopic manipulation or reoperation. It is the result of ureteral ischemia, angulation, or a narrow tunnel. If it occurs when the bladder is full, it may be the result of extravesical ureteral angulation. Too large a hiatus may allow compression of the ureter by a paraureteral diverticulum. An ischemic ureter due to too much dissection may contract and obstruct. In every case of continued hydronephrosis, look first for persistent bladder dysfunction, as well as residual valves and high urine output. The unrecognized dysfunctional bladder is the most common cause of failure of ureteroneocystostomy. With neurogenic dysfunction, bladder augmentation may be required.

Delayed obstruction may occur within the first 5 years; thus, regular imaging is needed. If the obstruction is at the meatus,

pass a stent or balloon catheter, or make a limited meatotomy. Otherwise, approach the ureter extravesically and reimplant it, ignoring the initial implantation. Resort to ureteroureterostomy if the ureter is still too short. If both ureters are involved, implant one ureter into a psoas hitch and perform transureterostomy (see pages 838 to 839).

Extravasation, especially after tailoring, indicates early obstruction from edema, angulation, or constriction at the hiatus unless the catheter has been kinked. Prolonged stenting is indicated. *Gross hematuria* is not unusual. Clots indicate inadequate operative hemostasis, but they rarely require transurethral fulguration or re-exploration. *Anuria* should respond to furosemide and adequate fluid support. Infants should be closely monitored for dehydration, which can severely alter electrolytes. Check the ureteral catheters for patency. If stents are not used, perform intravenous pyelography, and, perhaps, place retrograde catheters or install a percutaneous nephrostomy tube. *Fever* may occur postoperatively if the urinary tract has not been cleared of infection. Antibiotic administration continued for 4 to 6 weeks reduces the chance of chronic infection. *Sepsis* means obstruction and must be handled by drainage. Later recurrent infections are limited to the lower tract and are usually related to bladder dysfunction.

Bladder dysfunction, evidenced by incomplete emptying, is a minor problem whether the procedure is done intravesically or extravesically. However, emptying is less complete after bilateral extravesical reimplantation, but with time all patients empty normally.

Life-long surveillance is needed after ureteroneocystostomy. Start with voiding cystography at 3 months, and then perform yearly ultrasonographic studies for the first 5 years. Further study is needed if infection occurs.

REOPERATION

A second operation may be required because reflux persists or obstruction occurs.

Persistent Reflux

For persistent reflux associated with neurogenic dysfunction and a poorly compliant bladder, augmentation cystoplasty may be needed. Observe the patient for 2 or 3 years before proceeding to correction, meanwhile maintaining low-dose antibiotic prophylaxis. If the kidney has less than 15 percent function and the other kidney is normal, consider nephrectomy rather than reimplantation, especially if tailoring would be required.

Technique for Reimplantation. Approach a persistently refluxing ureter transvesically through a midline incision. Insert an infant feeding tube, and stitch it in place to use it for traction. Circumscribe the meatus, and open the entire subepithelial tunnel to allow removal of the ureter intact with its blood supply. Mobilize the ureter above the hiatus into normal territory to avoid angulation and to get more than enough length. Create a new hiatus by inserting a right-angle clamp into the old hiatus, and dissect in a superolateral direction along the posterior wall of the bladder under direct vision by placing small retractors in the hiatus. Clear enough of the retrovesical tissue to prevent kinking. Cut down through the muscularis and uroepithelium onto the tip of the clamp, and stretch the opening so that it does not constrict the ureter. At this point, the ureter may be tapered by a folding technique (see page 807) if necessary to create a 5:1 ratio of length to diameter. Bring the ureter through the new hiatus as with the Politano-Leadbetter technique (Steps 5 to 8). To reduce tension, reduce the chance for angulation, and allow a longer tunnel for large ureters, provide a psoas hitch as an adjunct (see page 818).

With bilateral reflux, it may not be possible to implant both ureters properly. Consider implanting the better ureter with an adequate tunnel and trimming the other ureter and performing transureteroureterostomy with a running 5-0 SAS (see pages 838 to 839).

Obstruction

Obstruction at site of implantation results from mishandling the ureter and damaging the blood supply with ischemia; from angulating it, usually just outside the hiatus; or from providing an abnormally narrow tunnel. It also may be the result of implantation into a poorly compliant bladder. It is detected on routine urography or ultrasonography that shows dilation of the upper tract greater than that found preoperatively. Confirm obstruction by diuretic renography. For severe obstruction, a ureteral stent or percutaneous nephrostomy with a stent may be a temporizing measure that allows pressure-flow studies through the anastomosis before it is removed. Delayed obstruction may occur within the first 5 years and requires regular imaging to be detected.

Technique to Correct Ureteral Obstruction. For obstruction limited to the meatus, apply endoscopic methods such as passage of a stent, balloon dilation, or a limited meatotomy. For a more extensive obstructive lesion, approach the ureter extravesically to obtain an unoperated portion for reimplantation, ignoring the original intravesical portion. If that leaves the ureter too short, proceed with a psoas hitch. If both ureters are involved, one solution is to reinsert one ureter into the bladder with a psoas hitch and anastomose the other to the implanted ureter (transureteroureterostomy, see page 838).

VENTRICULOURETERAL SHUNT
(Smith, Lee, and Middleton)

This technique does not require nephrectomy and, in contrast to transureteroureterostomy (see page 838), interferes with only one renoureteral unit. Be certain that the bladder operates at low pressure and can be kept free of infection.

23 Divide the ureter 3 cm above the bladder. Reanastomose the ureter to the bladder by an extravesical technique. Insert the shunt tube into the remaining stump to leave the tip 1 cm proximal to the ureteral orifice. Fix both tube and ureter to the bladder wall externally. Perform a psoas hitch (see page 818).

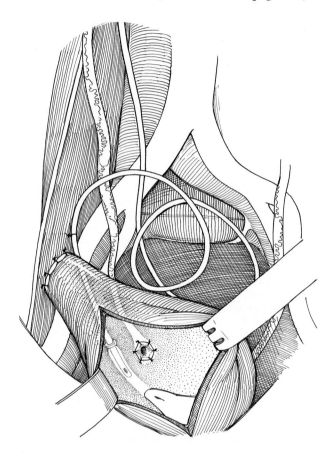

Postoperative problems include *kinking* or *migration* of the tubing. *Infection* may intervene and must be treated and subsequently suppressed. *Metabolic complications* are possible, especially with dehydration. The *increased voiding volumes* may tax the neurogenic bladder.

Ureteroneocystostomy with Tailoring

Megaureters may be either refluxing or obstructive and can have either primary or secondary causes. Intravenous urography shows a dilated ureter with a distal funnel shape. In obstructed megaureter, voiding cystourethrography shows no reflux or outlet obstruction. In refluxing megaureter, it reveals the reflux. Obtain an isotope scan to assess renal function and drainage; added furosemide can help differentiate hydronephrosis with or without obstruction. If there is reflux, the bladder should have an indwelling catheter for drainage during a renal scan study. Perfusion pressure studies can be helpful in equivocal cases. If the narrowed distal segment causes functionally significant obstruction, excise, taper, and reimplant it.

If bilateral megaureter repair and reimplantation are required into a bladder with a small or reduced capacity, reimplantation of the better ureter combined with transureteroureterostomy should be considered (see page 838) because it may be impossible to fashion two good ureteral reimplants in a poor bladder.

1 Identify the type of megaureter: **(A)** obstructive megaureter; **(B)** refluxing megaureter; and **(C)** paraureteral diverticulum with megaureter, a condition usually associated with massive reflux. With obstructive megaureter, the hypertrophied, helically oriented muscular coats become circular at the site of obstruction, just proximal to the longitudinal bundles of the intramural segment.

Perform cystoscopy of the bladder, in particular to assess the contralateral ureteral orifice.

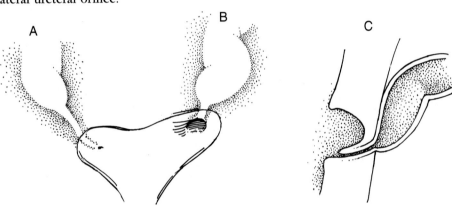

2 **A,** *Incision:* Lower transverse (see page 490). A midline incision gives better exposure if ureteral tortuosity is so great that the upper ureter also needs narrowing or if this is a reoperation.

B, Insert a ring retractor and open the bladder, holding its edges with stay sutures. Insert an infant feeding tube into the ureter, and suture it to the ureteral orifice. Dissect as much ureter as possible intravesically, as described for the ureteroneocystostomy (see pages 787 to 789). If the ureter is only moderately dilated, it may occasionally be reimplanted intravesically through a new tunnel (see pages 790 to 791). For dilated, tortuous ureters, it is better to dissect extravesically to obtain a straight length of ureter to trim and reimplant.

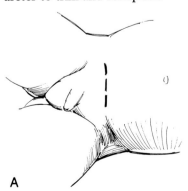

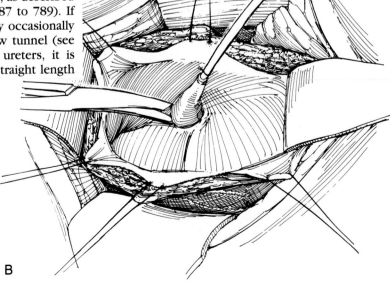

3 From outside the bladder, dissect along the internal iliac vein until the medial umbilical ligament (the obliterated hypogastric artery) is reached. This route causes the least damage to the vesical nerve supply. Divide the ligament, exposing the ureter. Retract the peritoneum upward. Pull the end of the ureter that had been previously freed intravesically out of the bladder, and rotate it into the paravesical field. Distending the ureter with saline may help in the dissection. Free the ureter from the adjacent peritoneum, saving all the periureteral tissue by sweeping the peritoneal attachments toward the ureter, thus skeletonizing the peritoneum, not the ureter. This mobilization seldom needs to extend higher than the common iliac vessels unless the ureter is very tortuous and so must be considerably shortened, such as that found with the prune-belly syndrome.

4 Open the periureteral sheath longitudinally on the lateral aspect of the ureter, and dissect beneath it just deeply enough to allow insertion of straight scissors. Keeping on the lateral aspect, open the sheath to uncover the entire segment to be narrowed, usually up to the level of the iliac vessels. Turn the sheath back on either side for about half the circumference of the ureter, preserving the contained collateral vessels.

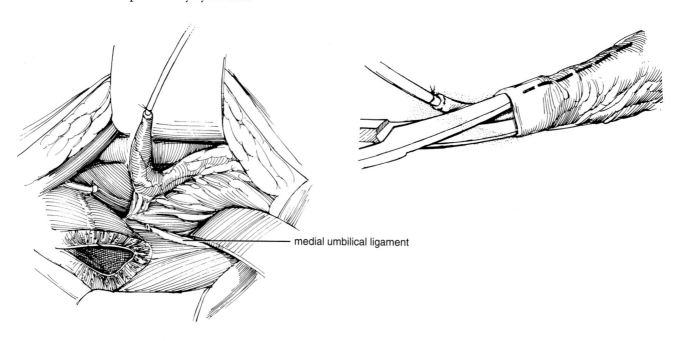

medial umbilical ligament

5 **A,** Distend the ureter with saline, and mark the portion to be excised with a marking pen. Usually make the strip for excision about one third of the ureteral circumference because some of the remaining wall is used up in closure. Taper only enough of the ureter to have the end of the taper several centimeters outside the bladder wall after reimplantation. Excise the longitudinal strip of ureteral wall freehand with scissors. Excising too much jeopardizes the blood supply and can cause stenosis. Leave the terminal segment attached as a handle.

B, Close the proximal two thirds with a running locking everting stitch of 5-0 SAS to form the tapered segment of the ureter. Complete the closure of the distal third with interrupted sutures of the same material because the length needed is uncertain at this stage. Take care not to constrict the lumen. Check the suture line by refilling the ureter with saline.

6 Approximate the flaps of preserved periureteral tissue with a loose running 4-0 or 5-0 SAS.

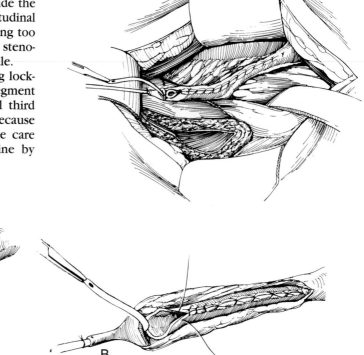

A

B

7 Return intravesically and close the original hiatus with several 4-0 SAS. Incise the epithelium on the back wall of the bladder with a knife 1 to 2 cm distally and 3 to 4 cm proximally in order to prepare a long bed in which to lay the tapered ureter. Fold back the vesical epithelial flaps. Insert a right-angle clamp to make a new hiatus through the muscle from inside the bladder at the proximal end of the bed, making sure that it is large enough. It is vital that the new hiatus be in the back wall of the bladder; if it is misplaced to the side wall, bladder filling angulates and obstructs the ureter. Guide the clamp to enter the paravesical space, avoiding the overlying peritoneum. Alternatively, create a tunnel by dissecting subepithelially as in the Politano-Leadbetter technique (see pages 789 to 791).

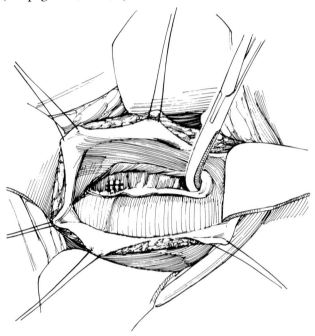

8 Remove the catheter, and draw the ureter through the new hiatus. The taper should end at about the level of the common iliac vessels.

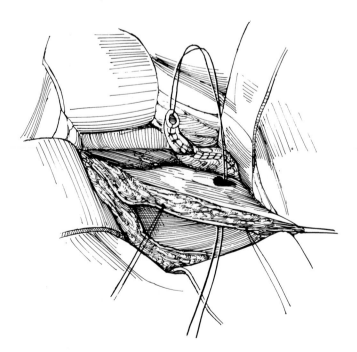

9 **A,** Place the ureter in the trough with the suture line posterolaterally to reduce the possibility for fistula formation. Cut the end of the ureter to an appropriate length. Anchor the ureter in place by placing two 4-0 or 5-0 SAS through the tip into the bladder wall at the end of the tunnel, each stitch to include muscle and epithelium.

B, Complete an epithelium-to-epithelium anastomosis of the ureteral tip, and close the epithelial flaps with interrupted fine stitches of 5-0 SAS. The ureter can also be implanted by the cross-trigonal technique (see page 793). Insert a fenestrated 5 F plastic catheter to drain the kidney.

When the bladder is small relative to the size of the ureter, and especially in reoperative cases, perform a psoas hitch (see page 818).

Close the bladder in two layers. Provide a Penrose drain to the area. If a stent was placed, leave it in place for 10 days. Drain the bladder with a straight catheter anchored to the anterior abdominal wall. Remove it 1 day after the ureteral stent is withdrawn.

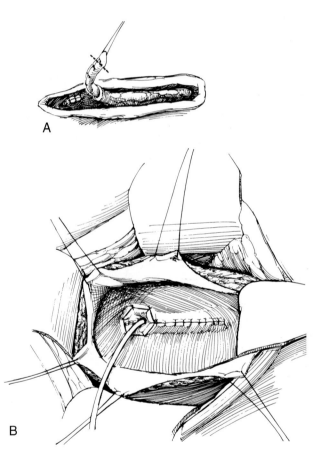

A

B

Important Factors. The tunnel should be long enough (five times the diameter of the revised ureter), the hiatus should not be situated laterally in the bladder, the tapering should not go higher than the level of the iliac vessels, the ureteral suture line should lie posterolaterally, and the ureter should not be angulated.

Duplex Systems. It is not uncommon to see one dilated ureter next to a nondilated one. If the renal segment to the very dilated ureter is nonfunctional, it is best removed together with almost all of the dilated ureter. If both renal segments function, the ureter can be managed in two ways. One is to remove the dilated ureter, reimplant the smaller one and do a transureterostomy, or anastomose one renal pelvis to the other. Alternatively, taper the large ureter and perform a double-tunneled reimplantation.

ALTERNATIVE IMPLANTATION TECHNIQUE (Hodgson-Zaontz)

An extravesical implantation by the Hodgson modification of the Lich-Gregoir technique, as illustrated on pages 795 to 796, may be faster than a intravesical or extravesical method and as effective. This is not a practical solution for a very dilated ureter or for bilateral megaloureters.

Working extravesically, dissect the detrusor from the bladder epithelium before detaching the ureter in order to make a space for the inversion. Tailor the ureter over a 10 F catheter. Excise the distal end, and reanastomose it to the bladder epithelium over a stent that is brought out above the incision. Insert two vertical mattress sutures, and draw the ureter beneath the epithelium. Close the hiatus. Bring the stent through the urethra in females or through a stab wound in males. Drain the bladder through the urethra in females or suprapubically in males.

ALTERNATIVE TAILORING TECHNIQUES

Folding techniques are less complicated than excisional ones and work well. Folding may have the advantage of preserving more of the intrinsic ureteral blood supply, which would be transected during excision, and it also interferes less with the extrinsic supply. It does leave a bulky mass of ureter to be implanted, so for wide, thick ureters and for those in infants, excision is better.

Incision-Excision Technique (Hodgson)

This alternative approximates the ureter over a stent and excises the redundancy.

10 **A,** Insert an infant feeding tube, and place a row of 5-0 SAS in the ureter beside it. Incise the lumen of the free portion of the ureter.
B, Trim the free edges.
C, Approximate the edges with a continuous suture, completing it distally with interrupted sutures to allow for trimming to length.

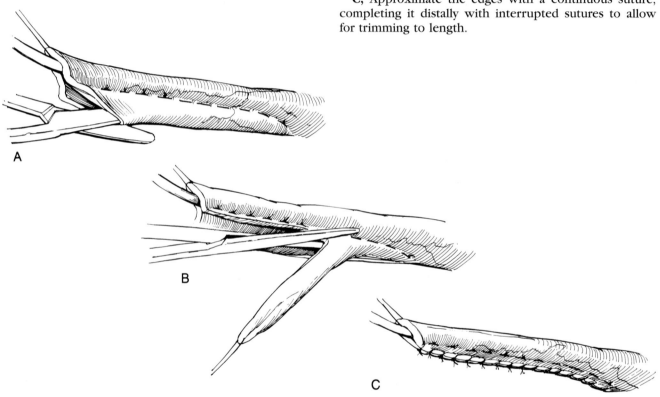

Ureteral Folding
(Kalicinski)

11 **A,** After dissection extravesically, pull the ureter into the bladder. Place a 10 F infant feeding tube in it and, with the fingers around the tube, pinch the walls to displace the tube medially. Run a 3-0 SAS down the ureter on the lateral side, away from the catheter. Tie it several centimeters from the end, and continue suturing with interrupted mattress sutures to allow trimming.

B, Fold the free margin around the stented portion, and fasten it with multiple interrupted 4-0 SAS. Trim the ureter to proper length, and proceed with implantation by a standard technique. Stent the ureter for 4 or 5 days.

C, Alternately, fold the lateral margins of the deflated ureter inward, and hold them with imbricating sutures.

Psoas Hitch. To obtain an adequate submucosal tunnel length, perform a psoas hitch (see page 818) and form the tunnel in the back wall of the extended bladder.

POSTOPERATIVE PROBLEMS

Complications after tailoring procedures are more common than after simple ureteroneocystostomy but of a similar nature.

Bladder spasms are common. Use epidural continuous infusion of bupivacaine to greatly reduce the problem. Oral diazepam and oxybutynin are also useful.

Obstruction results from angulation or from ureteral stricture. *Reflux* is secondary to too short a tunnel. Perform intravenous urography or ultrasonography 4 to 6 weeks postoperatively to assess obstruction and radionuclide cystography to check for persistent reflux. Do not hurry to reoperate because high-grade reflux may resolve as long as 2 years after implantation. In addition, these patients often have decreased renal function with high urine output that places an added load on the ureterovesical transport mechanism. Provide adjunctive measures postoperatively, such as intermittent catheterization if the bladder empties poorly, anticholinergic medication if compliance is poor, and bladder augmentation if the bladder is small, scarred, and noncompliant. Careful follow-up for at least 5 years to detect silent malfunction is mandatory.

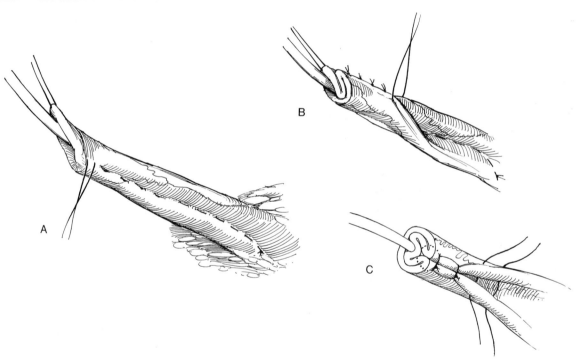

Commentary by W. Hardy Hendren, III

Megaureter is a descriptive term for a ureter that is wide and sometimes very tortuous; it is not a diagnosis. A megaureter can be obstructive or refluxing. In primary obstructive megaureter, the ureteral orifice looks normal endoscopically. A terminal segment 1 to 3 cm long contains excess fibrous tissue and lacks muscle. Biopsy of the dilated ureter above that segment shows muscle hypertrophy. The kidney in obstructive megaureter is often better preserved than in refluxing megaureter. In megaureter secondary to massive reflux, the ureteral orifice is usually dilated and often laterally placed. Some have a paraureteral diverticulum just above the orifice. In a case with massive reflux, the kidney frequently is badly damaged from a combination of backpressure from the bladder during voiding and infection. Paradoxically, a few megaureters can have both obstruction and reflux when the ureter ends ectopically in the bladder neck or urethra. In the resting state, the ureter is obstructed, but during micturition it can show reflux.

Not all wide ureters need to be corrected surgically. For example, in boys, endoscopic ablation of urethral valves can reduce intravesical pressures, allowing secondary megaureter to improve spontaneously. Similarly, megaureters in association with myelodysplasia can resolve when the bladder is emptied by intermittent catheterization.

When a large ureter must be corrected surgically, dissecting the ureter free from the bladder and shortening, tapering, and reimplanting it to provide normal drainage without reflux are involved. The tunnel length should be about five times the diameter of the ureter to be reimplanted, just as in ordinary ureteral reimplantation. Thus, tapering the terminal ureter makes it feasible to reimplant a dilated ureter and achieve a satisfactory ratio of tunnel length to ureter diameter. Ureteral peristalsis cannot be effective when the ureter is dilated because the walls do not coapt. Tapering the lower ureter to improve peristaltic efficiency allows the ureter to empty actively. This effect results in improvement in dilation of the upper tract.

When the ureter is not tortuous, the operative approach can be made through a transverse lower abdominal incision. This approach affords adequate exposure of the lower ureter, as would be customary for a usual ureteral reimplantation. However, when ureteral tortuosity is great, as is often the case in the prune-belly syndrome, dissection higher into the gutters may be necessary to shorten excessive length of the ureter. Here it is better to use a vertical transabdominal approach to provide greater operative exposure. The Denis Browne ring retractor is very useful. After a catheter is sewed into its orifice, the ureter is mobilized intravesically; the ureter is then freed using that approach, as long as it proceeds easily. Then exposure is shifted paravesically to continue its mobilization upward. To locate the ureter with minimal paravesical dissection, which can cause nerve damage to the bladder, dissect along the hypogastric vein to the obliterated umbilical artery-ligament and divide it. This allows retraction of the peritoneum cephalad. The ureter lies immediately beneath the ligament. Mobilizing the ureter and bringing it upward into the paravesical field are facilitated by dissecting along the anterior wall of the ureter from below, penetrating the paravesical tissue at the level of the ligament, and then pulling the ureter through to that point. When the attachments of the ureter are divided during its mobilization, it is important that they be divided as far as feasible from the ureter. This retains as much as possible of the attached periureteral tissue for collateral blood supply. Unless the ureter is extremely elongated and tortuous, we generally mobilize it only as far as the point where it crosses the common iliac vessels.

Tapering the ureter is performed on its lateral aspect because the main collateral blood supply runs along its medial wall. Further, when the suture line for tapering is closed, it should be placed posteriorly next to the detrusor muscle when the ureter is reimplanted into the bladder. This reduces the likelihood of a fistula forming into the bladder. We formerly used special ureteral clamps, but in recent years we have generally not used them. The ureter is distended via the catheter used in its mobilization. A ligature around the tip of the ureter retains the saline within it. The periureteral sheath is opened by dissecting between the sheath and the wall of the ureter on its posterolateral aspect. The sheath is incised and laid back about half the circumference of the ureter to expose the segment to be removed; this area is identified with a skin-marking pencil. Sharp, straight scissors are used to remove the strip of ureter, which must not be too wide. Trimming the ureter excessively makes it too narrow and jeopardizes its blood supply. Some added width is taken up in the closure, which is done with a running, locking suture to avoid reefing the closure. The ureter is filled again with saline to make certain that it is watertight. The periureteral tissue is then closed over the ureteral suture line.

It is important that the new hiatus through which the ureter will be brought be in the back wall of the bladder. It is a common error to bring the ureter through the side wall, which causes it to be angulated when the bladder fills. After closing the original ureteral hiatus, a bed is prepared for the ureter. This bed starts at the new hiatus, which is more cranial and more medial than the original hiatus. The bed extends downward to just above the bladder neck. Instead of making a submucosal tunnel, which is often used in ordinary ureteral reimplantation surgery, it is easier to lay back mucosal flaps before implanting the ureter. Bring the ureter through the new hiatus, taking care to avoid angulation and tension. The ureter is laid in the bed prepared for it, with the ureteral suture line posteriorly against the bladder muscle. The ureter is trimmed to appropriate length. The two most distal sutures are placed in bladder mucosa and muscle to the 6-o'clock position of the ureter; this anchors it firmly. Remaining sutures close the mucosa of the bladder to the open end of the ureter, and mucosa-to-mucosa closure covers the ureter. A small plastic drainage catheter is passed up the ureter to the kidney for 8 to 10 days while the repair heals. Contrast medium is injected before removing the catheter to make certain that no extravasation occurs. After bilateral megaureter repair, catheters are removed on successive days, not simultaneously. Lower megaureter repair, when done as described, should have a complication rate almost as favorable as reimplantation of nondilated ureters— that is, less than 5 percent.

In some highly abnormal bladders, such as in boys with urethral valves or the prune-belly syndrome or in patients with multiple previous operations, it may be impossible to get two good ureteral reimplants into the bladder. In many such instances we have found it best to reimplant the better ureter, together with psoas hitch fixation of the bladder, with transureteroureterostomy of the contralateral ureter.

In the majority of cases, successful repair of the lower ureter results in straightening of the tortuosity of the upper ureter and gradual reduction in its caliber. In some cases, however, the upper ureter needs to be repaired. This is technically easier than repair of the lower ureter. The kinked ureteropelvic junction is resected just as in any dismembered pyeloplasty. This may be all that is required. If the upper ureter is also quite dilated, it can be trimmed in the same fashion as the lower ureter. A temporary nephrostomy is placed when the upper tract is dilated. Contrast medium is injected through the nephrostomy tube 1 week later to be certain that there is free passage to the bladder and no extravasation. The tube is removed.

Kalicinski et al (1977) have described an infolding technique to narrow the functional lumen of the lower ureter, as illustrated. This technique was developed to lessen the risk of devascularizing the ureter while trimming it. This infolding has also been successfully used by other surgeons. It should be stated, however, that the likelihood of devascularizing the ureter by trimming should be minimal if it is performed in the manner we have described. In 425 megaureter repairs in the past 34 years, ureteral fibrosis from devascularization has rarely been a problem. Somehow it seems more appealing to place a trimmed ureter into a tunnel, rather than one with excessive bulk. Infolding the dilated ureter in experimental animals has been shown to result in spontaneous disappearance of the infolded segment in some cases, presumably from its devascularization from being infolded. Thus, it may be that both methods achieve a similar outcome after healing is complete. Like many problems in surgery, more than one way is often available to get the desired end result!

Operations for Ureteral Duplication

Start the diagnostic steps with ultrasonography, followed by intravenous urography if sufficient functioning parenchyma remains. If function is minimal, a delayed renal scan may demonstrate a poorly secreting upper-pole system. Even with nonfunction, lateral and downward displacement of the lower-pole segment is strongly suggestive of duplication. A delayed film may show contrast medium in the upper-pole segment when the ectopic orifice lies within the sphincter, and voiding cystography may show reflux in these cases. In difficult cases, CT scanning with delayed imaging after intravenous contrast administration can be helpful.

Continued leakage of clear urine after the bladder is filled with indigo carmine points to an orifice distal to the internal sphincter. To locate it, perform cystourethroscopy and vaginoscopy.

Approach the operation knowing the degree of damage to the involved segment and the presence or absence of reflux in the lower segment. Removal of the nonfunctioning or infected upper pole with subtotal excision of the ureter in the absence of reflux is usually the best solution (Step 8). However, even with minimal function in the upper pole, ureteral reimplantation, ureteroureterostomy, ureteropyelostomy, and pyelopyelostomy are alternatives, selection among these depending on the length of the duplicated ureter.

URETERONEOCYSTOSTOMY FOR REFLUXING DUPLICATED URETERS

1 **A,** *Incision:* Use a lower transverse incision (see page 490).

B, After opening the bladder, place a 5 F infant feeding tube into each ureter, and suture them in place with a 4-0 purse-string SAS. With traction on the catheters, incise the epithelium around the orifices with a hooked knife; then develop a periureteral plane inside the sheath with Lahey scissors, and free up the ureters well outside the bladder. Do not attempt to separate them.

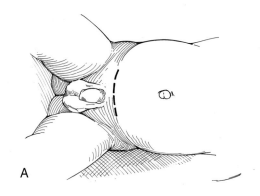

A

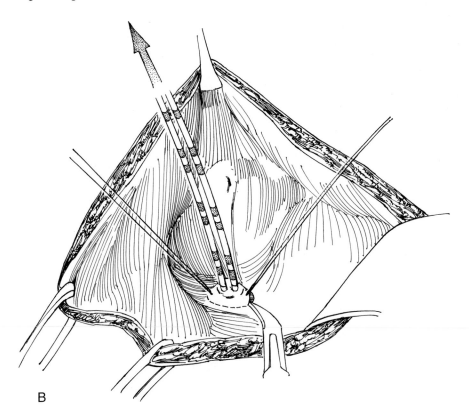

B

2 **A,** Usually trim and discard the distal end of the ureters. If the duplication is incomplete, trim the terminal segment of the ureter to expose two lumens.

B, Suture both to the vesical epithelium as described for ureteroneocystostomy by the Politano-Leadbetter (see pages 789 to 791) or Glenn-Anderson (see page 792) technique, suturing the luminal edges to each other if

necessary and to the vesical epithelium. The ureters may then lie side by side, or the lower segment may be located closer to the vesical neck.

C, *Alternative:* Tunnel the ureters across above the trigone by the Cohen transtrigonal technique (see page 793).

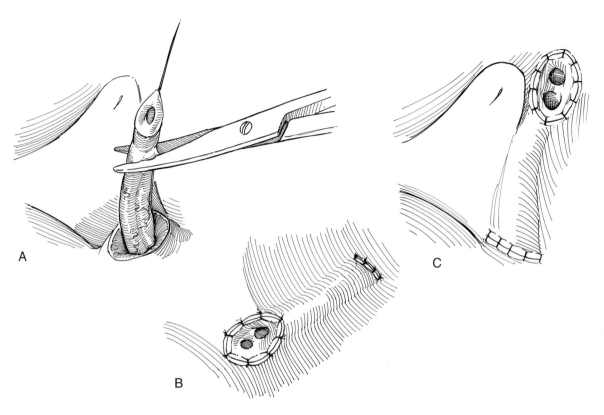

URETEROURETEROSTOMY FOR DUPLICATED URETERS

Anastomosis of the diseased ureter to the normal mate is used for ureteral dilation and reflux of one part of a duplicated system.

If the age and sex of the child permit, with the aid of a cystoscope transurethrally place a 5 F infant feeding tube in the recipient ureter.

3 Through a lower transverse incision (see page 490), dissect the terminal portion of the double ureters extraperitoneally nearly to the bladder. By sharp and blunt dissection, separate the ureters where they are readily accessible above their common sheath, preserving the adventitia, and loop each of them with a small Penrose drain.

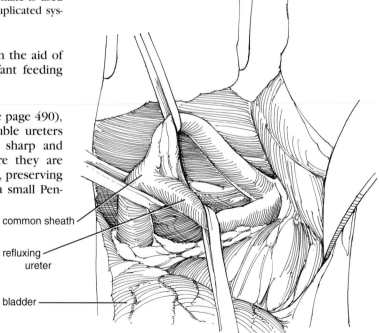

common sheath

refluxing ureter

bladder

4 After placing a stay suture in the refluxing donor ureter, clamp and divide it obliquely below the suture. Ligate the stump as low as possible with a 3-0 SAS.

5 Place two stay sutures in the recipient ureter 1 to 2 cm apart, depending on its size, and incise between them with a hooked blade.

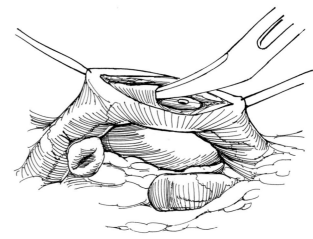

6 **A,** Withdraw the catheter from the recipient ureter, and pass it up the donor ureter. Insert a 4-0 or 5-0 SAS through the proximal end of the ureterotomy, then through the posterior rim of the donor ureter. Place a second suture through the distal end of the ureterotomy and through the anterior rim of the donor ureter.

B, Tie them, then run each suture down the respective side, with an occasional lock stitch. Tie each to the origin of the other. Drain accurately with a Penrose drain (see page 917).

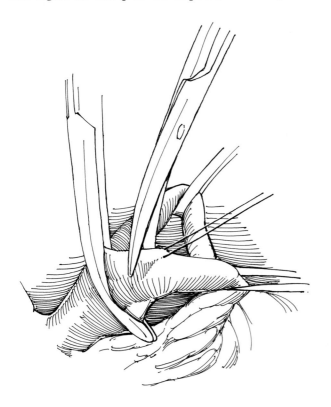

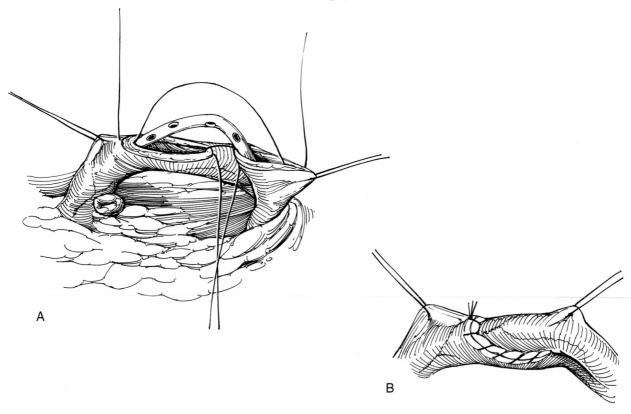

A

B

URETEROPYELOSTOMY

Anastomosing the upper portion of the diseased duplicated ureter to the ipsilateral renal pelvis eliminates ureteroureteral reflux but requires a recipient ureter of adequate caliber. Make an extraperitoneal incision.

7 **A,** Resect as much of the defunctionalized lower-pole ureter as feasible to prevent it from acting as a blind sump.

B, Anastomose the pelvis directly to the upper-pole ureter.

C and D, For a short duplication, make a U-shaped incision and connect the limbs.

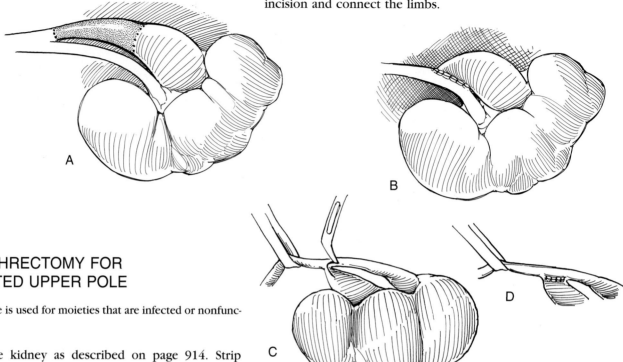

HEMINEPHRECTOMY FOR DUPLICATED UPPER POLE

This procedure is used for moieties that are infected or nonfunctioning.

Expose the kidney as described on page 914. Strip back the small amount of perirenal fat from the capsule to expose the vessels entering the hilum.

8 **A,** Identify the branches of the renal artery and vein supplying the segment (they are small), and loop them with sutures. Tightening the suture loops shows the ischemic areas. If they are limited to the upper pole, tie the sutures. Control of the entire pedicle is seldom necessary. Locate the groove between the firm normal kidney and the soft upper pole. Incise the renal capsule 1 to 2 cm distal to the groove, and strip it back if possible. Enter the cleavage plane slightly distal to the groove, and separate the tissue with the back of a knife. Continue the dissection transversely. Suture-ligate any vessels that are encountered with figure-eight 4-0 SAS. Avoid entering the upper-pole calyces (indicating that the dissection is too peripheral), and avoid the lower-pole calyces (the dissection is too proximal). If an upper-pole calyx is divided,

resect the adherent portion from the main kidney. Conversely, if a lower-pole calyx is entered, close it with a fine running absorbable suture. Dissect between the two pelves. Identify the vessels that supply the upper pole (they are usually small). Clamp, divide, and ligate them. Resect as much of the upper-pole ureter as is feasible from this incision. Total ureterectomy can be done later in the uncommon event that the stump becomes symptomatic. Control any ooze with fine figure-eight sutures. If the correct plane was followed and vessels were ligated as they were encountered, bleeding is minimal.

B, Cover the exposed area with the capsule, held in place with interrupted 3-0 SAS. Mattress sutures in the parenchyma should not be needed. Fix the kidney to the posterior body wall (see page 922).

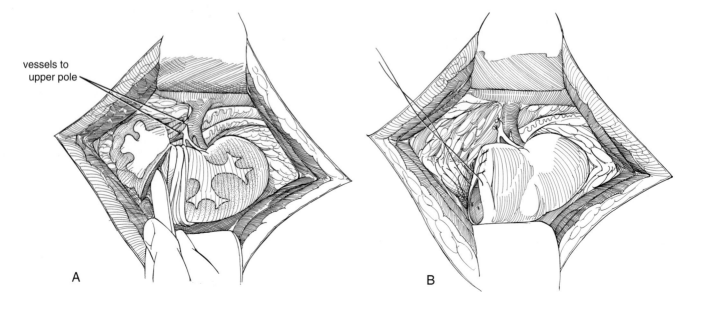

vessels to upper pole

URETERECTOMY

Heminephrectomy alone with partial ureterectomy is adequate if reflux is not present. Refluxing ureters require ureterectomy, best done at the time of partial nephrectomy, rather than waiting for symptoms to prove that the procedure is necessary.

9 If ureterectomy is required, it is hazardous to resect the entire ureter of a nonfunctional kidney in a duplicated system because it has a common wall and blood supply with its normal mate.

Dissect the extra ureter within 1 or 2 inches of the bladder, divide it, and incise it with scissors down its anterior wall to approach the bladder wall. Close the short stump adjacent to the bladder with 4-0 SAS, or merely trim the edges. Drain the area for a few days.

If reflux and infection persist in the residual ureteral stump, excise it. The transvesical approach similar to that shown on page 834 for excision of a utricular cyst allows access to the stump, an approach less formidable than a dissection from above.

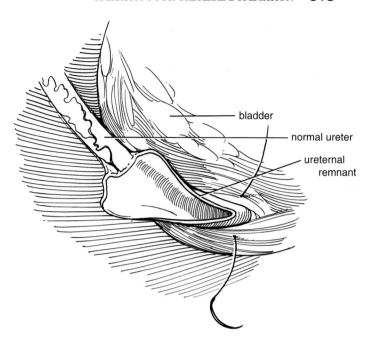

POSTOPERATIVE PROBLEMS

Complications are similar to those after ureteroneocystostomy (see page 801) and include extravasation, gross hematuria, ureteral obstruction and anuria, persistent reflux, and sepsis.

Commentary by Ricardo Gonzalez

Duplication anomalies of the collecting system may require surgical treatment for reflux, obstruction, or urinary incontinence when the upper-pole ureter is ectopic in an extrasphincteric position in a female. In deciding what operation to perform, consider what needs to be accomplished and the risk to the normal system of the proposed procedure. For example, ureteropyelostomy for an obstructed upper system may risk the normal lower moiety more than a partial nephrectomy.

Reimplantation. The indications for operation on a refluxing duplicated ureter are the same as for single systems. To do a reimplantation of duplicated ureters for reflux, I almost always preserve a cuff of bladder mucosa around the orifices. I dissect the ureters without catheterizing them after tagging them with a 4-0 monofilament suture that provides traction and helps later with orientation without traumatizing the distalmost portion of the ureter I prefer to preserve. The method of reimplantation is almost invariably the Cohen technnique. Although the Cohen technique is frequently referred to as the "transtrigonal technique," tunneling in the trigone is cumbersome, and enough room for a tunnel of adequate length is seldom available. It is more realistic to make the tunnel more cephalad in the posterior bladder wall. There the dissection of the mucosa is easy, and the potential length of the tunnel is limited only by the size of the bladder. I do not separate bifid ureters, and in incomplete duplications I treat both ureters as a unit.

Ureteroureterostomy. The key with this technique is the proper identification of the ureter to be divided (i.e., the refluxing one) and the ureter that receives the proximal end of the refluxing ureter (the recipient ureter). Repeated preoperative cystography to exclude reflux to the upper-pole ureter and endoscopic placement of a catheter into the refluxing ureter for unequivocal identification are essential. I prefer not to dissect the recipient ureter circumferentially but rather to leave it in situ to avoid angulation and devascularization. I prefer running sutures of 6-0 or 7-0 polydioxanone in a watertight fashion. No ureteral catheters are used unless the distal recipient ureter has been reimplanted at the same time, as may be the case in some operations for ureterocele with good function of the upper pole. In those cases I leave two fine feeding tubes that pass through the common segment of the ureter, then split at

the level of the anastomosis to the respective ureters. A Penrose drain should be left in the vicinity of the anastomosis. This operation has the advantage over a reimplantation of being performed through a small McBurney-type incision and of avoiding postoperative bladder spasms. Despite this, I seldom use it for lower-pole reflux and prefer a modified Cohen ureteroneocystostomy.

Ureteropyelostomy. This procedure can be useful for reflux to the lower pole or for obstruction or ectopia of the upper-pole moiety when its function is deemed to be worth preserving. In each case, of course, the procedure is reversed, anastomosing the diseased (dilated) ureter to the normal renal pelvis. I never do this procedure for reflux. For obstruction, one must recognize that it may be difficult to perform owing to the discrepancy of diameters between dilated upper ureter and normal lower pelvis. Is the preservation of function of the upper pole worth risking an obstructive complication that would jeopardize the normal lower moiety? In my experience, this is seldom the case. Considerations of stenting and drainage are as for lower anastomosis.

Heminephrectomy. Two extremes are possible in the surgical findings when performing a heminephrectomy for duplication. At one end of the spectrum is the very small, atrophic or dysplastic upper-pole moiety that may be difficult to detect even with the most sophisticated imaging modalities. At the other end is the markedly hydronephrotic upper pole with very thin cortex. I usually approach the partial nephrectomy through a 12th-rib supracostal approach, keeping the incision small and very posterior. My philosophy is to not isolate the vessels that supply the upper pole at the beginning of the operation because this often requires much dissection in the hilum and the vessels that we think go to the upper pole may go elsewhere. Instead I approach the partial nephrectomy from lateral to medial sides and come to the vessels at the end. If the upper moiety is hydronephrotic, I open it in the coronal plane (from lateral to medial) with the electrocautery, exposing the dilated collecting system. Bleeding is not a problem and is controlled with the electrocautery or with an occasional suture. Now we can incise, also from lateral to medial, the two halves of the opened upper pole, as one would do when unroofing a cyst.

When I come to the medial aspect, I suture-ligate every vessel that enters the upper pole; sometimes I ligate them as a bundle. The two halves of parenchyma remain attached solely to the ureter. A catheter is introduced into the ureter, the lateral and caudal attachment of the ureter to the remaining upper-pole collecting system epithelium is divided, the ureter is transected, and the catheter is sutured to the ureter. The remaining epithelium of the upper-pole moiety is peeled off or fulgurated. The two lips of the lower moiety can be sutured with CCG or Monocryl sutures, but usually this is not necessary. The catheter in the upper-moiety ureter is then identified by palpation below the renal hilum, and with gentle traction and blunt dissection the ureter is brought entirely infrahilarly, dissected caudally, and excised as low as deemed necessary. Care is taken not to injure the lower-moiety ureter. This technique has several advantages: (1) the lower-moiety collecting system is never entered, avoiding fistulas; (2) only diseased parenchyma is excised; (3) only the vessels reaching the upper moiety are ligated; and (4) no dissection of the hilum is necessary. When the upper-pole collecting system is not dilated, the external demarcation between the two moieties is clear. Cut with the cautery in the plane of demarcation from lateral to medial until the upper pole is attached only by the ureter and vessels, which are handled in a similar fashion. I treat the distal ureter by excising it as far down as is comfortable and suture-ligating. I have used this technique exclusively for 15 years without fistulas, injury to the lower-pole vessels, or bleeding.

Repair of Ureterocele

Ultrasonography is the first diagnostic procedure. It is usually adequate to delineate the relationships of the ureterocele and assess the degree of ureteral dilation. Intravenous urography demonstrates most of the characteristics of an ectopic ureterocele, such as obstruction of the upper segment and the typical off-center bladder deformity of variable size, but this study may not be necessary. Supplement ultrasonography with voiding cystourethrography to assess the bladder and to detect reflux into the ipsilateral (lower pole) ureter or into the contralateral ureter, which then must be concomitantly reimplanted. It not only may demonstrate the ureterocele but also may provide information on the size, urethral extension, and support behind the ureterocele, and an oblique voiding film may supplement that information. Finally, assess the function of the two renal moieties by radionuclide scan to confirm that heminephrectomy is the more practical course. Cystoscopy, at low pressure so as not to flatten the ureterocele, is done as part of the operation.

The management of ureteroceles depends on several factors (Table 1). Endoscopic transverse incision of the ureterocele at the distal inferior edge initially is a valuable procedure; not only is it a temporizing measure to avoid sepsis but it may also be corrective because more than half of selected cases, especially if the ureterocele is not ectopic, require no further treatment.

For management of the child who is *septic*, if incision proves inadequate (particularly in a neonate), as shown by ultrasonography and persistence of symptoms, percutaneously decompress the kidney, drain the lower tract by catheter, or do both. Formal pyelostomy or ureterostomy may have to be considered.

For a ureterocele associated with little or *no upper-pole function*, incise it endoscopically immediately to relieve obstruction and sepsis. However, incision is not the recommended treat-

Table 1. Surgery for Ureteroceles in Duplex Systems

Upper pole function
Little or no function
  Endoscopic incision
  Upper pole nephrectomy; drainage of distal segment
  No treatment
Useful function with grossly dilated ureter
  Endoscopic incision
  Pyelopyelostomy; drainage of distal segment if needed
Good function, more normal ureter
  Ureterocele excision, ureteral reimplantation, with or
    without tailoring

ment for most cases with a functioning upper pole because it risks making the ureterocele reflux and requires a second procedure. In these cases, operate to remove the upper pole, and drain the distal segment (Table 1). Usually when the ureterocele is not too large or prolapsing, it collapses spontaneously after removal of the upper pole. If the upper pole is functional, perform ipsilateral ureteropyelostomy or ureteroureterostomy (see page 834), and reimplant the orthotopic ureter if necessary because of reflux. If the function is good, proceed with excision of the ureterocele and reimplantation of both ureters together (see page 810).

INTRAVESICAL REPAIR

If function of the upper-pole segments warrants its salvage, excise the ureterocele and reimplant both ureters together after clearing infection with appropriate antibiotics.

1 **A,** *Position:* Supine. Before draping, endoscopically visualize the ureterocele. Avoid distending the bladder, which may cause the ureterocele to flatten or prolapse extravesically, making assessment difficult. *Incision:* Use a transverse lower abdominal incision (see page 490). Alternatively, make an oblique lower-quadrant Gibson incision (see page 495).

B, Open the bladder through a Y incision, with the extension toward the bladder neck. Intubate the orifice of the ureterocele with an infant feeding tube. Identify the orifice to the lower pole, and intubate it as well as the contralateral orifice. Hold the tubes in place with fine sutures (not shown for clarity). Place five traction sutures around the orifice of the ureterocele, and gather them together in one clamp. With a hooked blade or needle electrode, incise the epithelium and subepithelium at the border of the ureterocele. Include the orifice to the lower pole inside the incision.

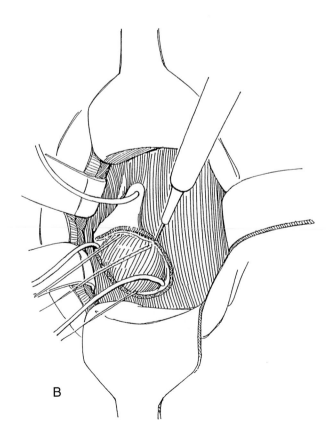

B

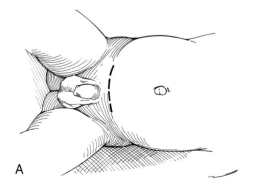

A

2 Elevate the lateral border with stay sutures, and separate the subepithelium from the underlying bladder muscle with scissors.

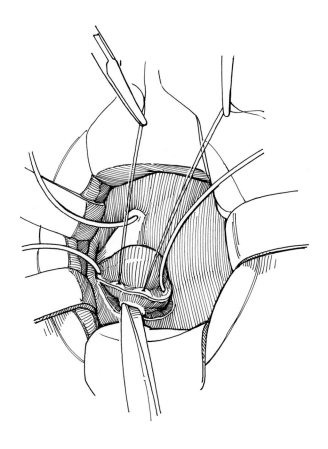

3 Dissect the combined ureteral complex through the ureteral hiatus as for ureteroneocystostomy (see pages 787 to 788). If the ureterocele extends into the urethra, the dissection requires great patience because the wall of the ureterocele blends with that of the trigone. If more exposure is needed, extend the limb of the Y incision by incising the anterior bladder wall to the level of the bladder neck; do not go beyond. Continue the dissection of both ureters proximally through the ureteral hiatus. Extravesical dissection is usually not necessary. Close the defect in the detrusor distal to the hiatus with 5-0 SAS. If the ureterocele is large, the weakened detrusor should be reinforced with transverse sutures.

4 Close the vesical epithelium and subepithelium over the trigone. Remove the tubes from the double ureters. Place a stay suture through the epithelium-subepithelium above the contralateral orifice. Elevate the epithelial edge, and insinuate scissors beneath it to create a transverse tunnel that exits at the stay suture (Cohen technique, see page 793).

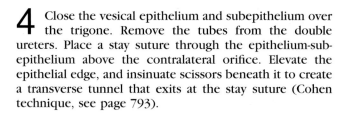

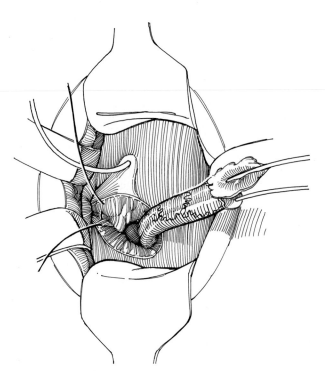

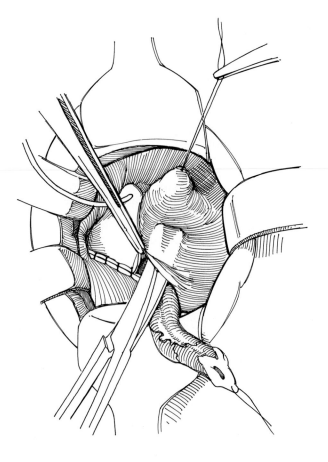

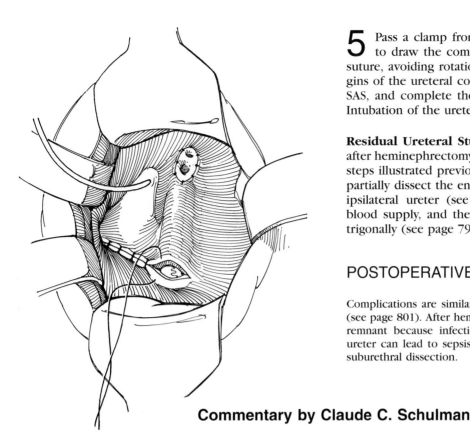

5 Pass a clamp from right to left through the tunnel to draw the combined ureters through on the stay suture, avoiding rotation and angulation. Suture the margins of the ureteral complex to the vesical wall with 5-0 SAS, and complete the closure over the original hiatus. Intubation of the ureters is not necessary.

Residual Ureteral Stump. A ureteral stump remaining after heminephrectomy may be removed by following the steps illustrated previously, except that it is necessary to partially dissect the end of the accessory ureter from the ipsilateral ureter (see page 813), preserving the joint blood supply, and then implant the single ureter crosstrigonally (see page 793).

POSTOPERATIVE PROBLEMS

Complications are similar to those after ureteroneocystostomy (see page 801). After heminephrectomy, do not ligate the distal remnant because infection confined in a closed segment of ureter can lead to sepsis. *Incontinence* results from extensive suburethral dissection.

Commentary by Claude C. Schulman

Each large extravesical ureterocele is managed differently, depending on the child's age and clinical condition, the presence of renal failure or sepsis, the presence of associated lesions of the lower pole and contralateral kidney, the presence of bilateral ureteroceles, and the expertise of the surgeon. For an ectopic ureterocele, no general agreement on the optimal treatment exists. The extravesical extension of the ureterocele, which causes bladder outlet obstruction, is important in management, as well as the relative strength of the underlying detrusor muscle backing, which might appear as an extensive defect after excision of the ureterocele.

A conservative approach cannot be justified except in special cases because dysplastic lesions and severe damage to the upper-pole parenchyma are associated with the ureterocele. Such procedures as ureteropyelostomy should be considered only when a solitary kidney is present or both kidneys are damaged. Thus, in most patients, heminephrectomy is the procedure of choice. It is accomplished easily through a retroperitoneal flank incision with resection of the proximal portion of the involved ureter. In a child with a nonfunctioning or very poorly functioning upper pole, I do not recommend transurethral incision because it carries a risk of causing the ureterocele to reflux. A second operation would then be needed. These ureteroceles should be left untouched in most cases, and only the upper-pole heminephrectomy should be performed. Usually, if the ureterocele is not prolapsing and not too large, it spontaneously collapses after the upper pole is removed, and a second stage is not needed.

The controversial question is whether excision of a ureterocele itself is necessary after the upper pole has been removed. Complete excision with extensive reconstruction of the floor of the bladder and reimplantation of the ipsilateral and sometimes contralateral ureter is advocated as the standard procedure by several pediatric urologists. This approach is advocated when the ureterocele is large, when detrusor backing is weak, when ipsilateral and even contralateral reflux is present, and when the ureterocele extends down into the urethra. Complete dissection of the ureterocele may be difficult, particularly at the lower end, where it may adhere closely to the bladder neck and urethra. There, a combination of an intravesical and an extravesical approach is useful for complete distal dissection of the ureterocele with mobilization of the entire bladder. During dissection, care should be taken not to injure the external sphincter area. When the ureterocele is unroofed, it is important to remove the entire wall of the ballooning portion,

particularly near the bladder neck and in the posterior urethra, to prevent a retained lip of incised ureterocele from acting as a valvular fold and causing obstructive problems. After the ureterocele has been excised completely, the urethra and trigone should be reconstructed with reimplantation of the lower-pole ureter, and sometimes the contralateral lower-pole ureter, following the Politano-Leadbetter technique or Cohen's crossed-advancement procedure.

An essentially extravesical dissection has been advocated to avoid potential damage to the urethra or vagina. Individual skill and experience determine the choice of approach.

In the last decade, an increasing number of authors have advocated a more conservative approach, consisting of heminephrectomy with removal of the upper-pole ureter to the level of iliac vessels, if excision of the ureterocele is not considered mandatory. Complete decompression of the ureterocele, as well as disappearance of mild to moderate reflux in the ipsilateral lower-pole ureter, can be anticipated in a significant number of cases. This approach avoids the risk and potential complications of extensive surgical reconstruction at the bladder level because the bladder is never entered. The procedure is completed entirely through a single retroperitoneal flank incision. The ureteric stump is left open and drained so that urine remaining in the ureterocele and distal ureter empties in a retrograde fashion when the child voids and intravesical pressure rises. If reflux was noted in the obstructed system or if the ureterocele was incised, causing reflux, the distal stump is ligated. This more conservative approach gives satisfactory results in about two thirds of cases. If the ureterocele fails to collapse and remains obstructive or if reflux persists in the lower-pole ureter, it is likely to result in recurrent infection, bladder outlet obstruction, bladder diverticulum, or reflux, all of which necessitate an additional operation through a suprapubic incision in a second stage some time later in one third of cases. This expectant approach, however, allows total reconstruction at a separate time, usually in easier and safer conditions, in the naturally selected cases that really need it. With the advent of prenatal ultrasonography, an increasing number of uropathies are discovered before they become manifest clinically.

In neonates and young infants, there is also a place for cystoscopic incision of asymptomatic ureteroceles discovered by ultrasonography. A small horizontal incision is carefully made at the base of the ureterocele; this approach does not seem to lead to reflux and allows good drainage of the obstructed but otherwise salvageable kidney with a single or duplex system.

Psoas Hitch Procedure

When the ureter is too short for reimplantation without tension, the bladder may be brought to the ureter and anchored to the psoas muscle. The technique is suitable for cases requiring reimplantation for persistent reflux or obstruction after failed ureteroneocystostomy and for those with loss of the distal ureter from other causes. After previous diversion, this operation is useful in conjunction with reimplantation because the ureters are short. In some cases a psoas hitch combined with transureteroureterostomy allows urinary tract reconstruction.

Estimate the capacity of the bladder to be sure that the bladder is sufficiently large and compliant. Provide antibiotic coverage.

Position: Supine. Place children in the frogleg position, but do not use that position for adolescents and adults because it may cause anteromedial thigh pain and paresthesia from stretching of the lumbosacral plexus. Examine the bladder cystoscopically. Place a balloon catheter transurethrally, and half fill the bladder.

Incision: Either place a lower transverse incision (see page 490), or, for greater exposure, make a long midline incision (see page 487), depending in part on previous incisions. If a transverse incision is made, it may be extended on the involved side.

1 Mobilize the peritoneum medially to expose the ureter. Dissect it free, taking care to preserve as many as possible of the medial segmental vascular attachments to the mid and upper portions. Trim the distal end obliquely, and insert a traction suture. Ligate the stump with a 2-0 SAS. Then determine the length of the defect.

Free the vas in males; the round ligament may be divided in females. Circumcise the peritoneal reflection on the dome of the bladder, and close the peritoneal defect with a running PCG or CCG suture. Take care when freeing the peritoneum over the dome that the bladder wall is not overly thinned; saline instillation in the subperitoneal connective tissue helps this dissection. Follow the obliterated hypogastric artery down to the superior vesical pedicle. Divide the pedicle, ligating the vascular stump with a 2-0 SAS.

Alternatively, especially in secondary cases, open the peritoneum and mobilize the ureter transabdominally, taking care to preserve its blood supply.

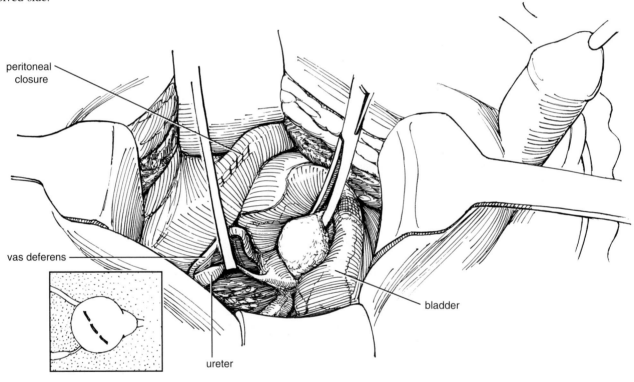

peritoneal closure

vas deferens

ureter

bladder

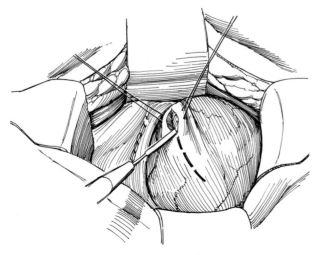

2 Place stay sutures just above the midpoint of the anterior bladder wall. Open the bladder with a semi-oblique incision near its equator (see inset in Step 1) between the stay sutures using the cutting current. This incision should cut across the middle of the anterior wall at the level of its maximum diameter and should extend a little more than halfway around the bladder. When it is closed vertically, the anterior wall of the bladder becomes elongated for a distance somewhat more than half of the maximum circumference of the bladder. The apex of the bladder can then be lifted above the iliac vessels as high as with a Boari bladder flap (see page 822). In a few cases, it may be necessary to make a Z-plasty bladder incision (Cormio et al, 1993) to obtain sufficient length.

3 **A,** Insert two fingers into the fundus of the bladder, and elevate it to the psoas tendon to meet the ureteral stump, thus converting the transverse incision into a vertical one.

B, If necessary to obtain additional length, incise the margins of the opening laterally with the cutting current (*dashed line*).

Except with very large bladders, further mobilization of the bladder is needed to allow this extension. Expose the contralateral side of the bladder, dissect the peritoneum and connective tissue from the pelvic wall, and divide the endopelvic fascia.

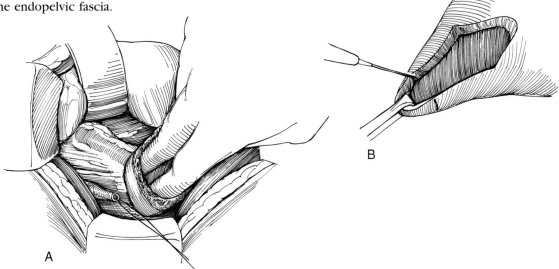

4 If, after the edges of the incision are incised, the bladder still does not reach the end of the ureter and provide a 3-cm overlap for the anastomosis, proceed with ligation of the superior vesical pedicle. The pedicle carries the superior vesical artery, a branch of the internal iliac artery. It may be single but usually has two or three branches that supply the dome and posterior aspect of the bladder. Dissect and divide the superior vesical pedicle; then ligate it with a 2-0 SAS.

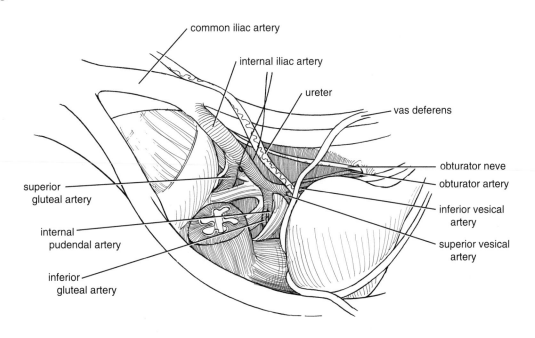

5 Clear the psoas minor muscle and tendon. Insert two fingers into the bladder, and hold it without tension against the tendinous portion of the psoas minor muscle to determine where the ureter will enter. Place two or three heavy nonabsorbable traction sutures into the detrusor (do not let them enter the lumen), extending from the bladder wall to the tendon, for stabilization during ureteral implantation. Tie the sutures, and place more if necessary to support the bladder.

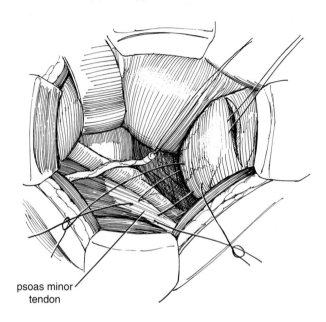

psoas minor
tendon

7 Place one 4-0 SAS through the tip of the ureter, then deeply into the bladder wall. Complete the anastomosis with four or five interrupted sutures to include the vesical urothelium and half the thickness of the ureteral wall. If the bladder cannot be elevated high enough to allow an adequate tunnel, resort to a direct (refluxing) anastomosis (see page 794).

Insert an 8 F infant feeding tube to the renal pelvis as a stent, and bring the end of the stent through the bladder and body walls in a stab wound. Suture the tube to the skin with 1-0 silk. (Alternatively, insert a double-J stent.) Tack the ureteral adventitia to the bladder wall at the exit site with two or three interrupted 4-0 sutures.

6 Perform a ureteroneocystostomy as described for the Politano-Leadbetter procedure on pages 789 to 791. From within the bladder, incise the urothelium transversely at the proposed site of the meatus. Tunnel distally under the urothelium for 3 cm with Lahey scissors. Invert the scissors, and pass the tips obliquely through the bladder wall. Substitute a curved clamp, grasp the stay suture, and draw the ureter into the bladder. Alternatively, leave the scissors in place through the bladder wall, and push the connector end of an 8 F infant feeding tube over the blades to draw the tube into the bladder. Tie the ureteral traction suture to the other end of the catheter, and draw the ureter into the bladder.

An *alternative method* to create the hiatus is to insert a peanut dissector into the bladder against the wall where the new hiatus is to be created. Incise the wall against the dissector with the cutting current. Pass a clamp through the defect, and draw the ureter into the bladder to check its position. Withdraw the ureter, and create a suburothelial tunnel with Lahey scissors.

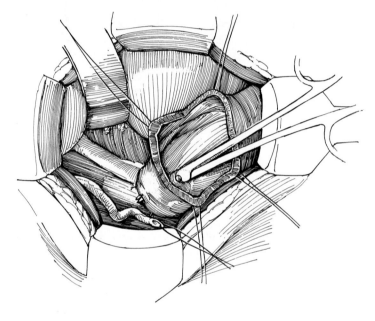

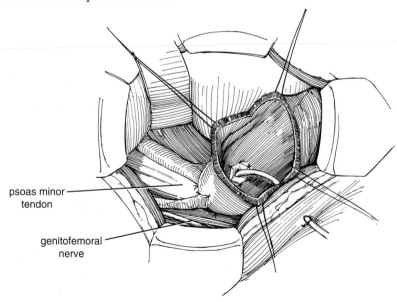

psoas minor
tendon

genitofemoral
nerve

8 Hold the bladder wall against the psoas minor tendon 2 cm above the site where the ureter exits by elevating it with two fingers from within. Place five or six 1-0 or 2-0 SAS to fasten the bladder to the psoas tendon and to the psoas major muscle above and lateral to the iliac vessels. If the tendon is not developed, take deep bites in the muscle itself to anchor it so that it cannot be distracted by detrusor contraction. Take care not to include the genitofemoral nerve trunk. Tie the sutures loosely to avoid devitalization of the bladder wall.

Insert a suitable Malecot or balloon catheter into the bladder through a stab wound. This is especially important if there is concern over the quality of the anastomosis. Check the closure of the peritoneum over the dome of the bladder if it was opened. Close the bladder opening with a layer of running 3-0 PCG suture in the subepithelium and an interrupted layer of 2-0 SAS in the muscularis and adventitia. Place a Penrose drain in the adjacent retrovesical area, and close the wound in layers. Remove the drains 2 or 3 days after drainage stops. Remove the stent in 1 week, and perform cystography. If that shows no extravasation, remove the suprapubic tube.

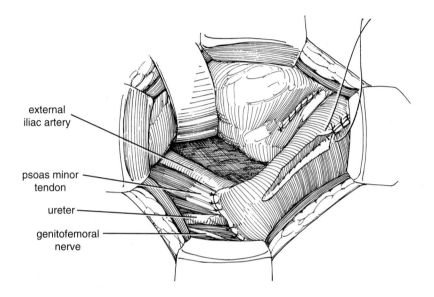

external
iliac artery

psoas minor
tendon

ureter

genitofemoral
nerve

POSTOPERATIVE PROBLEMS

Prolonged urinary drainage is an indication for retrograde cystography to ascertain whether the leak is at the ureterovesical anastomosis. If it is, insertion of a double-J stent and a urethral catheter may allow the fistula to heal. *Obstruction* may be the result of constriction in the tunnel and/or the ureteral orifice or of angulation of the ureter during fixation of the bladder extension. Endoscopic catheterization with insertion of a stent may correct the problem.

Commentary by Michael J. Droller

The importance of the psoas hitch is based on the opportunity it provides to compensate for problems that have compromised the lower ureter. It provides an effective alternative for situations that might otherwise have required other, more complex types of urinary bypass surgery, or even removal of a normal kidney, solely because of a defective ureter. A well-performed psoas hitch can provide surprising length of the extended bladder, often reaching as high as the middle portion of the ureter.

The most important aspects of the psoas hitch are to obtain sufficient flexibility of the bladder, so that it can be brought up to the normal portion of the ureter, and to provide fixation of the posterior wall of the bladder above the level of the iliac vessels, to permit nonrefluxing ureteral reimplantation without undue tension. Although it may be possible to accomplish these through the intrinsic pliability of the bladder, it is often necessary to divide the contralateral bladder pedicle down to the level of the inferior vesical artery to permit the bladder to reach the contralateral normal ureteral segment comfortably. A wider incision of the bladder wall is also occasionally needed to permit extension of the bladder toward the ureter.

If a Boari flap is needed to compensate for a longer ureteral defect, a rhomboid flap can be created from the anterior portion of the bladder wall cephalad to but incorporating the initial bladder incision. The flap can then be extended toward the ureter and the defect in the bladder wall closed with a vertical suture. Sufficient length should be provided in creating the bladder flap so that it can be fixed to the psoas muscle above the common iliac vessels, using absorbable interrupted sutures.

Care should be taken not to incorporate too much of the psoas muscle into the sutures to avoid potential pain, limitation of lower extremity mobility, and tissue necrosis with consequent loosening of the tacking sutures. Care should also be taken to avoid incorporating any branches of the genitofemoral nerve into the sutures. After ureteral reimplantation (using either a refluxing end-on or a tunneled nonrefluxing approach), a ureteral stent should be placed and left indwelling. It should be brought out through a separate stab wound in the bladder wall and the skin. This technique minimizes the amount of potential urinary extravasation, which could compromise the rapidity of healing and the flexibility of the operative site. The bladder wall defect (remaining either from the cystotomy incision or from the flap used to further extend the bladder wall to the mid or upper portion of the ureter) should be closed in as watertight a fashion as possible, using a continuous musculoepithelial absorbable suture followed by an interrupted seromuscular imbricating absorbable suture. Drainage should be provided both above the bladder incision and in the fossa of the ureteral reimplant, with care taken to avoid direct contact of the drain with the suture line. Urethral catheter drainage of the bladder should also be provided to minimize any tension that might be created through bladder distention. A suprapubic catheter is generally not necessary.

The psoas hitch is easily performed safely and satisfactorily. Its generic applicability in a broad range of clinical situations allows the urologist to maintain the continuity of the urinary tract without resorting to urinary diversion. It provides an effective treatment option in situations that might otherwise require far more complex solutions and, in some instances, loss of kidney function.

Bladder Flap Repair

(Boari)

A psoas hitch procedure (see page 818) is preferable to a bladder flap. Only rarely is the ureteral deficit so great that a hitch is not sufficient. Other alternatives are ureteroureterostomy (see page 838), renal displacement (see page 830), and renal autotransplantation (see pages 831 and 956). A relative contraindication to bladder flap repair is a small bladder, especially one involved in neurogenic disease.

For bilateral injury, consider combining a transureteroureterostomy (see page 838) with a psoas hitch or a bladder flap procedure. The appendix can be used to bridge a gap. Rarely is ileal substitution (see page 842) needed.

1 **A,** *Position:* Supine. Insert a balloon catheter connected to a gravity bottle and draped to be accessible during the operation. *Incision:* The site may be predetermined by the scars from the previous operations, which caused the destruction of the distal ureter. Either a midline incision (see page 487) or a transverse lower abdominal incision (see page 490) is suitable.

B, Mobilize the peritoneum medially, along with the vas or round ligament, to expose the normal ureter above the defect, usually best identified at or above the level of the bifurcation of the common iliac artery. Encircle it with a Penrose drain, and dissect it toward the bladder as far as practical.

At reoperation for a very scarred ureter, to avoid dissection in the retroperitoneum with the accompanying risk of injury to the iliac vein while mobilizing the peritoneum laterally, the ureter can be approached transperitoneally through a midline incision. Reflect the cecum or sigmoid colon medially to open the posterior peritoneum along the lateral gutter, and dissect the ureter distally over the iliac vessels as far as the bladder.

To prepare the bladder flap, infiltrate the subperitoneal tissue with saline to help dissect the peritoneum from the posterolateral surfaces of the bladder. Isolate and divide the urachal remnant.

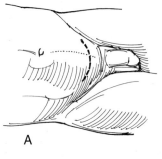

A

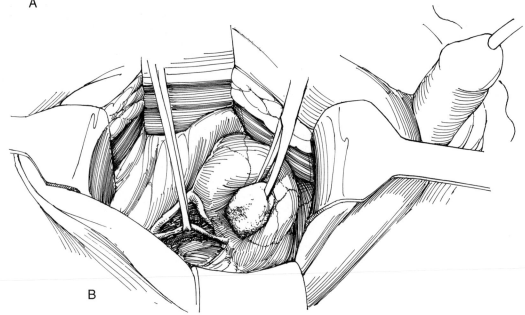

B

2 Excise the diseased portion of the ureter if practicable, and place a fine stay suture in the proximal, normal end for traction. Ligate the distal end.

Fully mobilize the bladder, including division of the superior and, if necessary, the inferior vesical pedicles on the opposite side (see page 818). Try pulling the unopened bladder as a tube onto the psoas muscle to see if a psoas hitch is all that is needed. If the bladder does not reach the ureter, proceed with formation of a flap. Fill the bladder from the gravity bottle and measure, on an umbilical tape, the length of flap needed to bridge the defect, extending from the posterior wall of the bladder to the proximal cut end of the ureter. In general, the width of the flap should be 2 cm at the tip or three times the diameter of the ureter to avoid constriction after tubulation, and at least 4 cm wide at the base. The flap is a random flap and should be two to three times as wide as it is long. Site the flap transversely, or, if greater length is required, make an oblique or S-shaped incision. Mark the outline of the flap with a marking pen.

Place two stay sutures 4 cm apart in the fixed portion of the bladder at the proposed base of the flap. The longer the flap, the wider the base must be. Avoid scarred regions of the bladder. Place two more stay sutures at the distance measured by the umbilical tape at the distal end of the flap. Then re-outline the flap very superficially with the weak coagulating current, which can also serve to fulgurate surface vessels. Recheck the dimensions of the flap. Empty the bladder.

With the cutting current, cut through the bladder wall across the distal end of the flap inside the stay sutures. Place two more stay sutures in the corners of the proposed flap, and cut the rest with the cutting current as outlined. Fulgurate bleeders when they are encountered; ligate larger vessels with fine PCG. Inspect the flap for vascularity, and trim ischemic areas accordingly. Insert a 5 F infant feeding tube in the contralateral ureter. Hitch the bladder distal to the base of the flap to the psoas tendon with 3-0 SAS.

3 The flap should overlap the ureter by at least 3 cm to allow for a proper tunnel. If not, mobilize the ureter but leave its adventitia undisturbed because it derives most of its blood supply from the renal pedicle. Trim any compromised ureter. Omission of a tunnel may be necessary if the ureter is too short; in that case, directly anastomose the ureter to the edge of the bladder flap. If the ureter is still too short, free the kidney inside Gerota's fascia and move it down to gain 4 or 5 cm in ureteral length (see page 830). Avoid tension at all costs.

Dissect a subepithelial tunnel with Lahey scissors for a distance of 3 cm; then bring the tip of the scissors through the epithelium. Injection of saline subepithelially helps in the formation of the tunnel. Install the broad end of an 8 F infant feeding tube (with the cap removed) on the tip of the scissors, and draw the tube up through the tunnel.

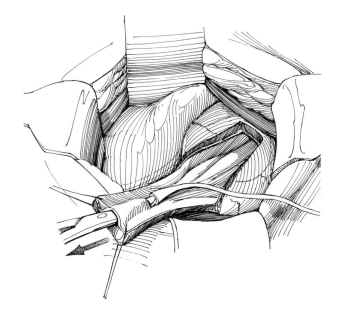

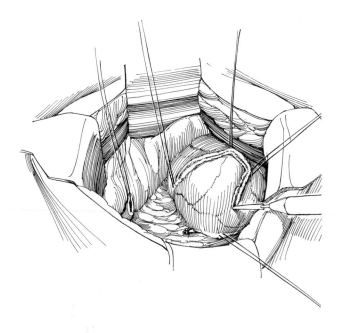

4 Attach the ureteral stay suture to the tube, and draw the ureter down through the tunnel. Spatulate the ureter after trimming it obliquely.

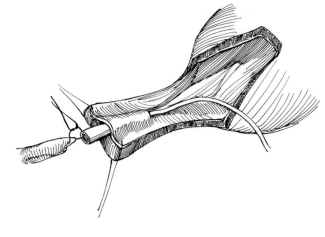

5 **A,** Fix the end of the flap to the psoas minor muscle and its tendon with 3-0 SAS, avoiding the ilioinguinal and genitofemoral nerves.

B, Anchor the apex of the ureter to the bladder wall with a 4-0 SAS that includes the vesical subepithelium and muscularis. Complete the anastomosis with three or four more interrupted sutures to the epithelium.

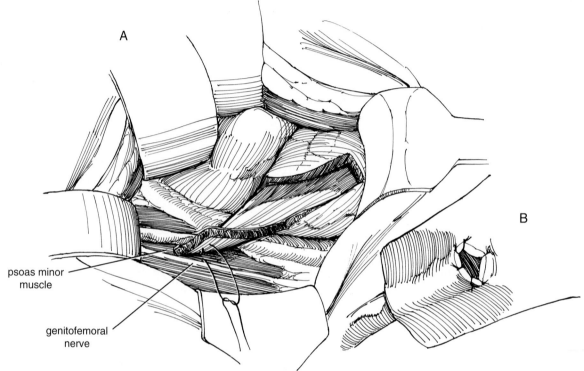

A

B

psoas minor muscle

genitofemoral nerve

6 Insert an infant feeding tube in the ureter as far as the renal pelvis, and tack it to the epithelium of the flap just distal to the anastomosis with 3-0 PCG. Bring the free end through a stab wound in the bladder and body wall, and fix it at once to the skin with a 2-0 silk suture. Place a Malecot or silicone balloon catheter through the opposite bladder wall, to exit through a stab wound. Suture it to the skin.

Close the bladder tube and bladder with a running 4-0 PCG suture in the subepithelial layer. Place a second row of interrupted 4-0 SAS through the adventitia and muscularis, excluding the epithelium. Place a few additional sutures to approximate the end of the flap to the adventitia of the ureter. Check that the bladder at the base of the tube is well secured to the psoas tendon. Place a Penrose drain retroperitoneally, to exit through a stab wound. If a transperitoneal approach was necessary, close the peritoneum but drain the area extraperitoneally. Remove the stent on the eighth postoperative day, and, if no drainage occurs, remove the bladder catheter 2 days later.

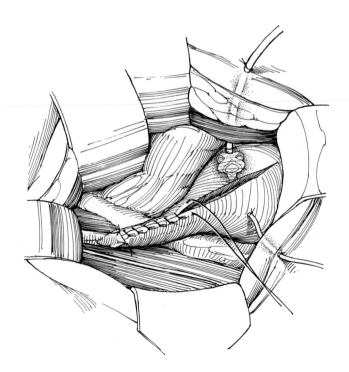

POSTOPERATIVE PROBLEMS

Injury to the opposite ureter should be considered if the patient has pain or low-grade fever. Perform intravenous urography or sonography and bulb ureterography.

Urinary infection with a febrile reaction may occur on removal of the stent; treat it with antibiotics. If it is severe and prolonged, ultrasonography followed by percutaneous nephrostomy is indicated to bypass obstruction at the anastomosis.

Leakage usually arises from the area of the bladder closure, not from the anastomosis. Leave the suprapubic catheter indwelling until it stops. If it continues, perform cystography and intravenous urography to localize the site of leakage. If the anastomosis is at fault, intubate it endoscopically and leave the stent in place 5 to 10 days. In a few difficult cases, a nephrectomy may be required. *Late stenosis* from scarring can occur and requires revision or, if detected too late, nephrectomy.

Commentary by J. Dermot O'Flynn

The psoas hitch has effectively superseded the Boari flap, which is now very rarely indicated. Avoid ureteroureterostomy because it can compromise both ureters. The Rutherford Morison muscle-cutting iliac fossa incision should always be considered; it is easily extended to give excellent access to the whole ureter and kidney.

Leave some fluid in the bladder to make it easier to handle. It is remarkable, with the division of the superior pedicle and dissection, how much bladder can be made available. It is probably never necessary to divide the inferior pedicle on the opposite side. When vesical mobilization is satisfactory, the bladder should be fixed with two or three sutures to the psoas muscle. This gives stability and makes the anastomosis technically easier.

Direct end-to-side anastomosis of ureter to bladder can be done. I suspect that reflux may be demonstrated, but renal deterioration does not seem to occur. If one is dealing with a hyperreflexic neuropathic bladder, the possibility of upper urinary tract deterioration exists following any form of implantation.

Ureteral Stricture Repair and Ureterolysis

URETERAL STRICTURE REPAIR

For most post-traumatic or postoperative strictures, the first intervention is endourologic. If open surgery is required because of failed endourologic attempts or because of the extent or density of the obstruction, the approach is determined by the location of the stricture. Proximal strictures may be managed like failed pyeloplasties (see page 923). Distal strictures may be resected and the system reunited by a psoas hitch (see page 818) or a bladder flap (see page 822). If the stricture is short, ureteroureterostomy is feasible (see page 834). Rarely, renal displacement (see page 830) or interposition of an ileal segment (see page 842) is required. Inform the patient about these options.

Preoperatively, perform retrograde, and if necessary, antegrade ureteropyelography (the patient may have a nephrostomy tube in place) to delineate the site and length of the stricture. If the stricture is secondary to previous surgery, prepare the bowel, and provide antibiotic coverage, especially in the presence of a tube in the kidney, and enough blood. Insert a ureteral catheter retrogradely to allow intraoperative identification of the distal ureter and of the level of the obstruction. Choose an incision to approach the defect from a route different from that taken previously, even choosing a transperitoneal route. After repair by whatever method, stent the area for 1 to 2 weeks while maintaining nephrostomy drainage. Perform antegrade pyelography before removing the stent and tube.

URETEROLYSIS FOR RETROPERITONEAL FIBROSIS

Ultrasonography can be a useful screening test for retroperitoneal fibrosis, and intravenous urography shows poor visualization but only moderate hydronephrosis. Bulb ureterography, rarely needed, demonstrates medially deviated and constricted ureters. CT scanning can identify the typical distribution and confluent configuration of the fibrosis. Perform a thin-needle biopsy if you suspect a neoplasm. Venography may help if evidence of venous obstruction is present. In high-risk patients, consider corticosteroid therapy alone.

If obstruction is severe, perform bilateral percutaneous nephrostomies to allow return of chemical balance and to await possible resolution of the process after the offending drugs are stopped and corticosteroids are given.

Instruments: Provide a basic pack, a GU long set, a Schnidt clamp, a right-angle clamp, and vascular sutures.

Limited Fibrosis (Aortoiliac Involvement)

Hydrate the patient and consider giving antibiotics. Insert a balloon catheter in the bladder, and place a nasogastric tube.

1 **A,** *Position:* Supine. After induction of anesthesia, consider performing cystoscopy of the patient and inserting ureteral catheters for identification of the ureters and localization of the lower level of obstruction. *Incision:* Make a long midline transperitoneal incision extending from xiphoid to symphysis. Pack the intestines superiorly, and place a self-retaining ring retractor. Identify the junction of the dilated ureter with the fibrosis above and the normal ureter below.

B, Incise the posterior peritoneum over the dilated upper portion of the ureter first (*dashed line*), put a Penrose drain around it, and dissect it from its bed caudally, stopping at the plaque. Then find the lower end of the ureter below the plaque, encircle it, and trace it upward. Dissect from the normal lower ureter because the dilated upper ureter can be more easily damaged. Palpate for malignancy (found in one case in 12), and take multiple deep biopsies of any suspicious areas for frozen-section diagnosis.

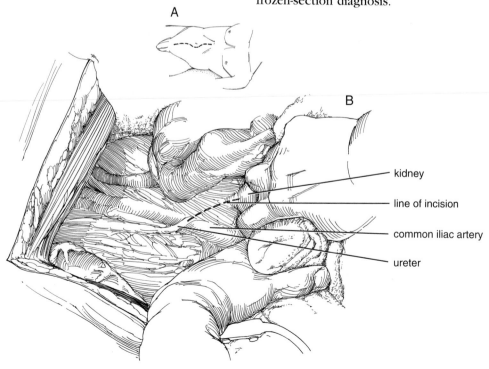

A

B

kidney

line of incision

common iliac artery

ureter

2 **A,** To free the ureter from the plaque, insinuate a curved clamp or a right-angle Schnidt clamp under the fibrosis against the adventitia of the ureter inside the onion skin–like layer; then cut onto the clamp. Apply blunt dissection with the finger tip under the coating to try to peel out the ureter.

B, Once the anterior surface is breached, dissect bluntly around the ureter to free it posteriorly. Loop it with a vessel loop.

Note: If the ureter does not fill as it is freed, further dissection is needed by peeling off additional layers of fibrous tissue. The underlying vessels are protected by the fibrosis, but remember that the aorta, on the medial side of the left ureter, and the vena cava, on the medial side of the right ureter, are closer to the ureter than normal. Do not stop the dissection until entirely normal tissue is reached.

Dissect the opposite ureter, even though it shows no obstruction radiographically (Baker et al, 1988). If the ureter is opened, do not try to suture it, but leave a J stent in place. If the defect is large, cover it with adjacent fat or with a tongue of omentum.

C, If possible, dissect a layer of retroperitoneal fat, interpose it between the ureter and its bed, and tack it as shown to the medial peritoneal edge with 3-0 CCG sutures. Alternatively, place the ureter intraperitoneally (Step 4). Consider excision and reanastomosis (see page 834) if only a short segment of ureter is involved. Alternatives include a bladder flap (see page 822), interposition of an ileal segment (see page 842), renal displacement, and autotransplantation (see page 830). Nephrectomy should be avoided because of the bilaterality of the disease.

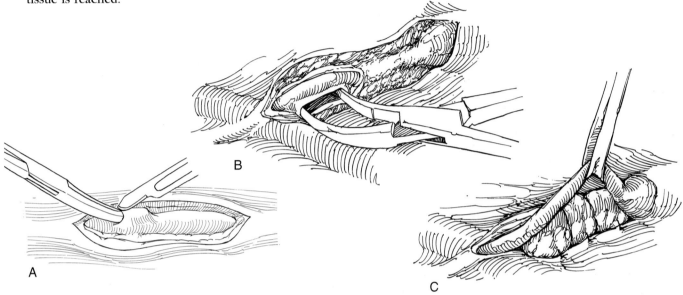

A

B

C

Extensive Fibrosis with Involvement of Most of the Ureter

Have the patient predeposit blood in the blood bank or match 4 units of packed cells in case the aorta or vena cava is entered. Prepare the bowel. Consider parenteral nutritional support.

Incise the parietal peritoneum lateral to the colon from the hepatic flexure or flexure on the left to the iliac vessels, and reflect the colon medially to the fibrotic process. Do the same on the other side.

3 Identify the ureter over the common iliac artery where it is usually less involved, dissect it free, and encircle it with a Penrose drain. Free the ureter from within its onion skin–like coat starting from below. Use a small curved clamp, a right-angle clamp, and, if possible, your fingernail for blunt dissection, and use sharp dissection where necessary. If the ureter does not strip out easily, suspect neoplasm and obtain a biopsy specimen for frozen section examination. Continue the dissection to the renal pelvis, leaving the fibrosis in place posteriorly. Watch out for the gonadal vessels; they are easily inadvertently divided. Remember that the great vessels cannot always be felt and that they lie closer to the ureter than normal. Place the ureter intraperitoneally as described in Step 4. If the ureter is perforated, repair the tear, complete the operation, and then insert a nephrostomy, proximal ureterostomy, or J stent.

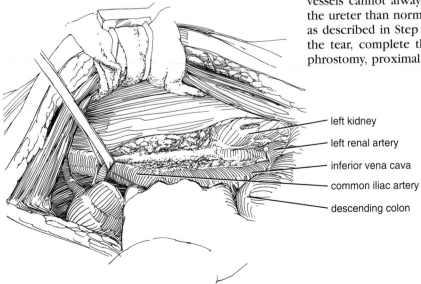

— left kidney

— left renal artery

— inferior vena cava

— common iliac artery

— descending colon

Intraperitoneal Displacement of the Ureter

4 Close the peritoneum behind the ureter with 3-0 CCG sutures, displacing the entire ureter anteriorly and laterally. Avoid making the sites of entry and exit too tight, resulting in obstruction. If you test for patency with a pressure-flow study through a proximal needle, you need subsequently to install a nephrostomy tube or stent because of the risk of extravasation.

As an alternative, mobilize a flap of peritoneum with some subperitoneal tissue from the lateral abdominal wall, swing it under the colon and the mobilized ureter, and tack it in place.

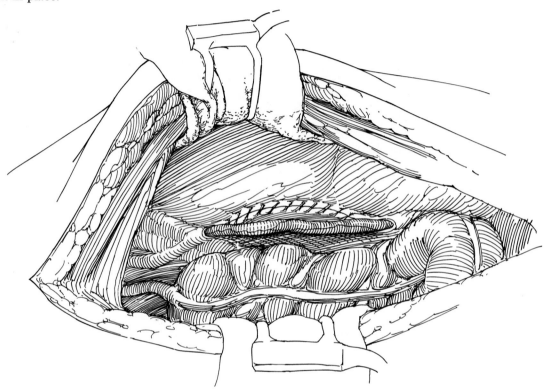

Extraperitoneal Placement for Extensive Fibrosis or Intraperitoneal Involvement

5 **A** and **B,** Dissect the peritoneum laterally to expose normal retroperitoneal fat, and move the ureter laterally into this uninvolved area. Hold it in place with four or five mattress sutures of 3-0 CCG that attach a more medial area of the parietal peritoneum to the psoas or quadratus lumborum muscle along a plane medial to the ureter. Close the peritoneal defect. If the fibrosis is extensive and the ureter poorly vascularized, wrap the ureter in an omental sleeve before displacing it (Step 6). Close the wound with retention sutures in the expectation of delayed wound healing.

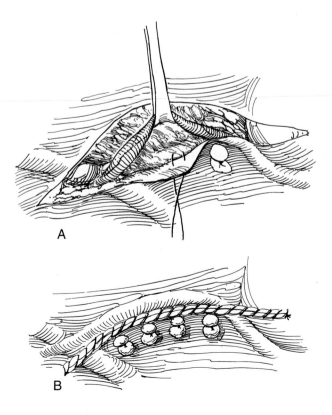

A

B

Omental Sleeve for Extensive Fibrosis

This technique provides the greatest protection against recurrence.

6 Separate the omentum from the transverse colon (see page 71). Divide the apron in half, ligating the vascular connections and the gastroepiploic arch in the center. Divide the short gastroepiploic arteries. Bring the omental apron lateral to the colon, insinuate it under the ureter, and wrap it around the ureter for the entire length of the involvement. Tack it in place with fine PCG sutures.

At the end of the procedure, remove the ureteral catheters if they were placed.

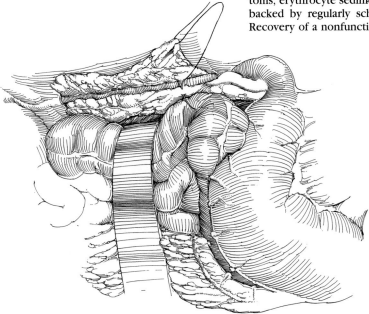

Excision and Reanastomosis

If the fibrosis involves the muscular coat of the ureter over a distance of less than 4 cm, resect that segment and reanastomose the ureter (see page 834). Place it in a fresh bed.

POSTOPERATIVE PROBLEMS

Ureteral injury is possible and should be detected intraoperatively; if it is not, urinary extravasation results in urinary ascites. Immediate retrograde stenting is required, with or without nephrostomy drainage. Watch for *salt-losing diuresis. Recurrent obstruction,* the result of ureteral ischemia or further retroperitoneal fibrosis, should be thwarted by routine administration of corticosteroids. Long-term follow-up is mandatory, using symptoms, erythrocyte sedimentation rate, and renal function studies backed by regularly scheduled screening by ultrasonography. Recovery of a nonfunctioning kidney should not be expected.

Commentary by Euan J. G. Milroy

Although idiopathic retroperitoneal fibrosis is usually bilateral, occasional cases may be encountered in which a short segment of a single ureter is obstructed. For those cases, an extraperitoneal approach to the ureter is very satisfactory, with fixation of the ureter laterally well out of the way of the obstructing fibrosis as described.

More commonly, both ureters are involved, even when the obstruction is more obvious on one side and the other appears virtually normal. In such patients bilateral intraperitoneal exploration is mandatory. I always use omentum, carefully mobilizing it from the greater curvature of the stomach, dividing it in the midline as described, and swinging it laterally down each paracolic gutter in order both to wrap each ureter carefully and, by suturing the omentum to the psoas muscle, to fix the ureters laterally.

Rather surprisingly, difficulties in mobilizing the ureter are not often encountered in idiopathic retroperitoneal fibrosis. Care is certainly needed in following the ureter through a dense plaque of fibrous tissue. The rare, worrisome cases are those in which the fibrosis involves the wall of the ureter; usually an obvious and well-defined plane is seen between the fibrosis and the ureter itself. In these cases it is essential to peel off all the fibrous tissue, even into the ureteric wall itself. Only rarely does ischemic damage occur, although a short area of very severely

affected ureter may be excised with an end-to-end anastomosis. In these, and certainly with any perforation, I leave a ureteric stent in addition to nephrostomy drainage. In the straightforward case, no drainage is necessary.

If preoperative decompression has been used, the sooner the nephrostomy tube is clamped and urine passes down the previously obstructed ureters, the better. An adequate biopsy of the fibrosis is important, but one must guard against taking biopsy samples of the walls of great vessels in the area!

We have found that ultrasonography and CT scanning are effective ways of monitoring the plaque of fibrosis, both preoperatively and postoperatively. It is also important to note the value of renography preoperatively and postoperatively to assess renal function and degree of obstruction and to monitor postoperative improvement. Many internists are enthusiastic about the value of corticosteroids for this condition. Although steroids certainly can be effective and may have a place in mild cases of obstruction and in patients genuinely unfit for surgery, in my experience a surgical approach, although it requires meticulous and careful dissection, is not a difficult procedure and usually results in immediate and complete resolution of the obstruction without the need for long-term steroids with all their complications. Provided that adequate mobilization, repositioning, and protection of the affected ureters are carried out, recurrent obstruction is rare.

Renal Displacement and Autotransplantation

RENAL DISPLACEMENT

Caudal displacement of the kidney without transplantation of the renal artery is an alternative to ileal interposition or auto-transplantation for defects in the mid or upper ureter when a bladder flap or psoas hitch is not feasible. The kidney can be moved down a significant distance by transecting the renal vein and reanastomosing it at a lower site on the vena cava. Because of the greater length of the right renal artery, the right kidney can be moved farther than the left.

1 *Incision:* Use a midline or anterior subcostal incision, depending on whether the projected site for ureteral anastomosis is high or vesical implantation is necessary. Dissect the renal vessels and adjacent vena cava. Heparinize the patient systemically. Occlude the renal artery close to the aorta with a vascular clamp, preferably a Rumel or bulldog clamp (not shown). Consider cooling the kidney with slush.

Place two Satinsky clamps on the side of the vena cava proximal to the entrance of the renal vein. Use different-sized clamps to allow transection of the renal vein flush with the cava for maximum length and to provide an edge to facilitate closure of the cava. Transect the vein on the renal side of the outer clamp.

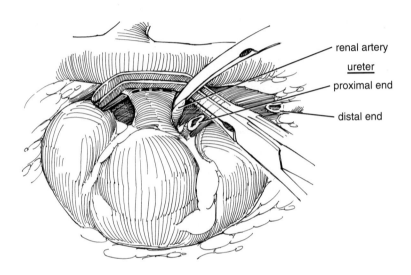

renal artery
ureter
proximal end
distal end

2 Remove the distal clamp, and close the cavotomy with a running 5-0 nonabsorbable suture (NAS). Remove the remaining clamp.

3 Reapply the Satinsky clamp to the vena cava at a lower level, at a site selected to achieve a tension-free ureteral anastomosis. On the right side, greater length can be obtained by ligation and transection of the lumbar vein that tethers the renal artery. Incise the vena cava for a distance equal to the diameter of the renal vein. Anastomose the vein to the vena cava by an end-to-side technique. Begin suturing posteriorly, working from inside the vein, because the kidney cannot be flipped over as in renal transplantation.

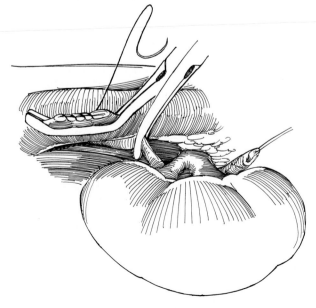

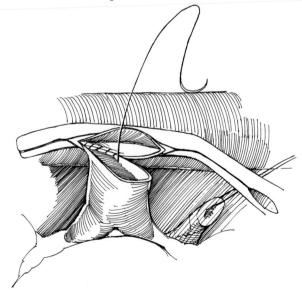

4 Fix the kidney to the psoas muscle and proceed with the ureteroureteral (shown), ureterovesical, or other anastomosis.

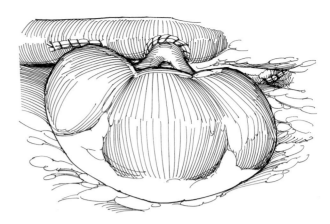

AUTOTRANSPLANTATION

Autotransplantation is used in cases of extensive ureteral loss and also for severe renal trauma and complicated renovascular disease. For *extensive ureteral disease,* autotransplantation can be a good alternative to ureteroileocystostomy. However, if inflammation involves the kidney and hilum, the kidney may not tolerate temporary ischemia. For *renal lithiasis,* extracorporeal reconstructive surgery has been used for cases of recurrent stones and pelvic stenoses and for a few cases of recurrent staghorn calculi, especially in solitary kidneys. Infection of the vascular anastomosis is a possible complication. For *renal trauma* it is possible in a patient with severe, multiple system injury to remove the kidney and repair it extracorporeally. Perfuse the kidney with hypothermic pulsatile perfusion, and perform autotransplantation 1 or 2 days later when the patient's condition is stable (or if the patient does not survive, use the kidney for homotransplantation). For *neoplasms,* even those involving the central portion of the kidney, bench surgery with transplantation (see page 1027) is rarely needed. For the loin pain–hematuria syndrome, autotransplantation is probably not effective.

Incision: Make an anterior subcostal incision (see page 856) for freeing the kidney and a lower oblique extraperitoneal incision to expose the iliac artery and vein to implant the kidney.

Proceed as for live donor nephrectomy (see page 974). Dissect between the vena cava and aorta in order to move the artery out from under the vena cava. To obtain as much length as possible, divide the renal artery as close to the aorta as possible. Similarly, divide the renal vein very close to the vena cava. Dissect the adrenal gland carefully from the kidney. Preserve pelvic and ureteral blood supply by avoiding the adventitia of the pelvis and ureter. Flush the kidney with cold Collins 2 solution, and cool it in iced slush before transfer to the iliac fossa. Anastomose the renal to the iliac vein, and then anastomose the artery to the internal iliac artery (see page 959). Restore ureteral continuity with stented ureteroureterostomy. Alternatives are ureteroneocystostomy and pyelovesicostomy with or without a bladder flap.

Replacement of blood, fluids, and electrolytes must be carefully monitored because the patient was without renal function during part of the procedure.

Commentary by Marc S. Cohen

The preoperative assessment of patients should include an accurate evaluation of the length of the ureteral defect (when surgery is performed for ureteral stricture disease) by either antegrade or retrograde studies or both. A preoperative evaluation of bladder distensibility can also be of benefit when distal ureteral loss is apparent and bladder mobilization by either psoas hitch or Boari flap is a consideration. The preoperative assessment of patients is also aided by arteriography or digital subtraction angiography. Such evaluation may reveal renal artery disease or generalized atherosclerotic change, which may impact the potential success of either procedure. Although the principles of dissection and vascular management are founded on the techniques of living related donor nephrectomy and renal transplantation, associated disorders related to previous surgery, infection, or retroperitoneal change (fibrosis) may be encountered. Both the surgeon and patient should be prepared for other surgical alternatives, including nephrectomy.

At the time of surgery, the patient should be well hydrated. During dissection of the vascular pedicle, care is taken to avoid vigorous traction on the renal artery or overdissection of the renal hilum to prevent renal and ureteral vascular compromise. Papaverine is used in a topical application when vascular spasm occurs. Renal perfusion is enhanced by adequate hydration and the use of intravenous mannitol during and following the dissection of the vascular pedicle.

Renal Displacement. The choice of incision may be impacted by several factors noted previously (previous surgery, anticipated ureteral repair, concurrent pathology) as well as the patient's body habitus. Certainly a midline or anterior approach affords the best options; however, in selected instances a flank approach may give adequate access when displacement is certain and an extraperitoneal approach is preferred.

The principles of hydration and the technique suggested previously are followed. The use of a Rumel tourniquet or a bulldog clamp on the proximal renal artery is the preferred method of arterial occlusion. Prior to occlusion, thorough dissection of the renal vein (and appropriate portions of the renal vein and vena cava), with ligation of renal venous and lumbar tributaries, facilitates renal mobilization. Although systemic heparinization is employed, protamine is rarely used as a reversal agent unless troublesome bleeding is encountered. In the case of ureteral repair, because prolonged or delayed urinary drainage is a frequent complication, a ureteral stent is almost always used, and the area of repair is drained via a Penrose or closed drainage (Jackson-Pratt) system. Many patients enter into such surgery with existing percutaneous nephrostomy tubes, and in such instances this drainage is usually maintained as part of the early postoperative management. Placement of a nephrostomy tube at the time of surgery is not usually necessary.

Autotransplantation. In addition to the previous preoperative suggestions, it should be re-emphasized that autotransplantation is a technically demanding procedure that may be contraindicated in atherosclerotic disease. Autotransplantation may, however, afford the opportunity to manage well-defined renovascular disease surgically. One should be prepared to manage a variety of potential vascular situations at the time of autotransplantation (end-to-end or end-to-side anastomosis, multiple renal arteries). The most frequently recognized complication of such surgery is urinary leakage, which can be managed initially via ureteral stenting (if not already present) or percutaneous nephrostomy. Prolonged drainage not responsive to such therapy suggests ureteral ischemia and requires operative intervention. Bleeding requires immediate intervention. Renal artery thrombosis occurs infrequently but must be considered. Definitive diagnosis can be made by nuclear scan. Late arterial stenosis can occur but is frequently manageable by percutaneous technology. Ureteral strictures can frequently be managed by endourologic/percutaneous routes.

Repair of Ureterovaginal Fistula

During work-up for vaginal urinary leakage (see page 587), if the ureter appears involved on intravenous urography and preliminary tests for vesicovaginal fistula are negative, suspect a ureteral source for the leakage. Perform retrograde ureterography with a cone-tipped catheter to demonstrate the fistula. If this fails, perform antegrade pyelography. Pass a double-J stent, and leave it in place for 6 to 8 weeks. If that is not possible or the ureter is completely divided or frankly obstructed, proceed at once with ureteroneocystostomy (see page 797) with or without a psoas hitch (see page 818), or perform ureteroureterostomy (see page 834) because the defect is easier to repair while the tissues are fresh. Provide prophylactic antibiotics.

Mobilization of the Ureter

Position: Supine. Insert an 18 F 5-ml balloon catheter, and instill 200 to 300 ml of water from a suspended bag with a Y tube.

Incision: Make a transverse lower abdominal (see page 490) or lower midline extraperitoneal (see page 487) incision.

1 Dissect the lateral wall of the bladder, and then empty the bladder through the catheter. Expose and dissect the ureter from above as for a ureteral calculus (see page 847), following the obliterated hypogastric artery. Divide the artery, and then progress caudally under successive bridges of connective tissue and vessels. These usually must be divided because of scarring from the original operation. If the ureter is not found retrovesically, look for it at the pelvic rim where it crosses the bifurcation of the common iliac artery, or open the peritoneum and follow it down intraperitoneally and extraperitoneally. Keep the dissection lateral to the ureter to preserve its blood supply.

Divide the ureter just above the fistula. Place a traction suture, and mobilize the ureter carefully to limit devascularization. It is not necessary to close the vaginal defect, but if the bladder is involved (ureterovesicovaginal fistula), close the vagina with 2-0 SAS and the bladder with two layers of sutures.

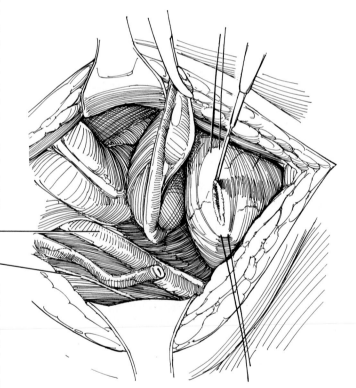

iliac nerve

genitofemoral nerve

Review the options for implanting the ureter. If minimal reaction and little ureteral loss occurs, ureteroneocystostomy (see page 797) is a good choice. If the defect is relatively high, do a ureteroureterostomy (see page 834). Usually there is moderate ureteral loss (or possibly the fistula is complex, such as a ureterovesicovaginal fistula) so that ureteroneocystostomy combined with the psoas hitch procedure (see page 818) is the best choice. Consider nephrectomy in ill or elderly patients with complicated fistulas. A permanent nephrostomy should be accompanied by ureteral ligation.

URETERONEOCYSTOSTOMY COMBINED WITH A PSOAS HITCH

2 Open the bladder near its equator with a semi-oblique incision between stay sutures using the cutting current. From within the bladder, incise the urothelium transversely at the proposed site of the new meatus. Tunnel distally under the urothelium for 3 cm with Lahey scissors. Invert the scissors, and pass the tips obliquely through the bladder wall. Substitute a curved clamp for the scissors, grasp the stay suture, and draw the ureter into the bladder. Place one 4-0 SAS through the tip of the ureter, then deeply into the bladder wall. Complete the anastomosis with four or five interrupted sutures to include the vesical urothelium and half the thickness of the ureteral wall.

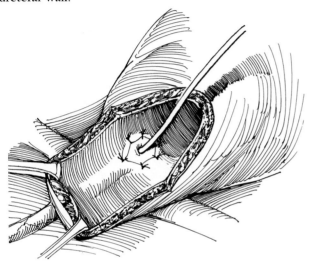

Alternative for Short Ureters. Cut a Boari flap (see page 822), and make the tunnel by inserting the Lahey scissors beneath the subepithelium at the edge of the defect. Have the tips emerge 3 cm distally, and draw the ureter through. Close the anterior bladder wall.

3 Hold the bladder wall against the psoas tendon 2 cm above the site where the ureter enters by elevating it with two fingers from within. Place five or six 1-0 or 2-0 SAS to fasten the bladder to the psoas minor tendon and to the psoas muscle above and lateral to the iliac vessels. Close the bladder opening vertically with a layer of running 3-0 PCG suture in the submucosa and an interrupted layer of 2-0 SAS in the muscularis and adventitia.

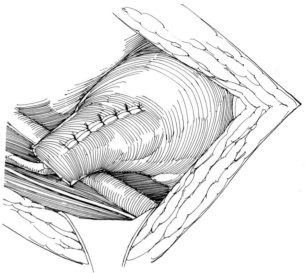

Laparoscopic reimplantation (see page 800) is possible in selected cases, particularly if the patient is seen early before reactive fibrosis or infection sets in.

POSTOPERATIVE PROBLEMS

Leakage at the ureteral entry site usually stops if drainage is adequate, although retrograde stenting may be necessary. *Stenosis* of the anastomosis, usually secondary to attenuated ureteral blood supply or tension, may require revision if instrumental attempts to open it fail.

Commentary by M. J. Vernon Smith

Cystography is helpful prior to surgery for two reasons: It rules out a vesicovaginal fistula, and it allows some idea of vesical capacity and gives one an abbreviated urodynamic study. The crux of all the procedures in managing ureterovaginal fistula is aggressive mobilization of the bladder. The contralateral as well as the ipsilateral ligaments and the superior vesicle artery should be ligated because the aim of a psoas hitch is to take the dome of the bladder to the psoas minor. The vertical closure of the transverse incision gives one even more length with little or no loss of bladder function.

A conscious effort should be made to identify the genitofemoral nerve, which lies on the anterior surface of the psoas major. While the tendon of psoas minor is on the anteromedial surface, some surgeons advocate deep bites of suture material into the psoas. I advise against this procedure because it can lead to hematomas in the psoas muscle and can compromise the posterior related branches of the femoral nerve, which are in intimate contact with the posterior surface of the psoas major.

I believe that the psoas hitch should be done before the reimplantation in order to decrease the likelihood of kinking of the ureteral implant at the bladder or pelvic brim.

On the basis of some earlier studies of the influence of suture material on the hitch, I always use CCG because the inflammatory response to this suture keeps the hitch intact. Although the NAS appears to interfere with the neoureteral tunnel (50 percent reflux), in adults this is probably of no significance. The ureteral anastomosis should be carried out with interrupted CCG sutures. The posterior stitches should be placed deep into the detrusor muscle, whereas the superior stitches should be mucosa to mucosa, thus allowing for ureteral mobility at the new hiatus.

Handle the bladder and ureter with sutures or skin hooks; otherwise edema becomes an unwelcome complication. It is important to place the suture in the ureter in either the anterior or posterior wall, rather than in the medial or lateral wall, where the blood supply is found in the majority of ureters. Finally, it is remarkable how often a stent can be passed in an antegrade manner; this neglected maneuver should be routine. It has been reported that ligation or partial obstruction of the ureter can be managed in this manner. In my experience, the success rate is less than 30 percent, but nevertheless it should be tried.

Ureteroureterostomy and Transureteroureterostomy

URETEROURETEROSTOMY

Resection and reanastomosis of the ureter may be required for ureteral stricture, low-grade ureteral tumor, high-velocity projectile blast injury, intraoperative injury, or retrocaval ureter. In surgical injuries, stenting for 1 or 2 weeks may be all that is necessary.

For ureteral stricture, determine the site of obstruction by a combination of antegrade and retrograde urography. Try passing a stent through the stricture or attempt direct-vision ureterotomy. For tumor, obtain brush biopsies. High-velocity injuries require extensive débridement because of the blast effect. With operative injury, the site must be identified, repaired, and stented from below. A retrocaval ureter is usually elongated, making partial resection and reanastomosis possible.

Retroperitoneal Approach

1 A, *Position and incision:* Make an incision appropriate to the level of the lesion. A Gibson incision (see page 495) shown here may be adequate, but for lesions in the lower ureter, a midline extraperitoneal incision (see page 487) gives better exposure because the ureters in the pelvis lie not far from the midline. Such an incision also allows cephalad extension if the kidney must be mobilized (see Step 6). For upper ureteral lesions in children, the anterolateral approach is suitable (see page 863).

B, Mobilize the peritoneal sac medially. Locate the ureter extraperitoneally, realizing that it is displaced anteriorly during exposure because it adheres to the peritoneum. It crosses the bifurcation of the iliac artery and lies just under the obliterated hypogastric artery. If in doubt, pinch it with forceps to elicit peristalsis. A dilated ureter may be so large as to be deceptive; aspiration of urine with a fine needle distinguishes it from bowel. In difficult cases, transperitoneal exposure with subsequent extraperitoneal drainage is easier.

Isolate the ureter by sharp and blunt dissection, carefully preserving the adventitia that contains the ureteral blood supply. Place a Penrose drain or vessel loop around it. Identify the site of obstruction; a previously placed ureteral catheter, on a stilet to keep it in place, may be of help.

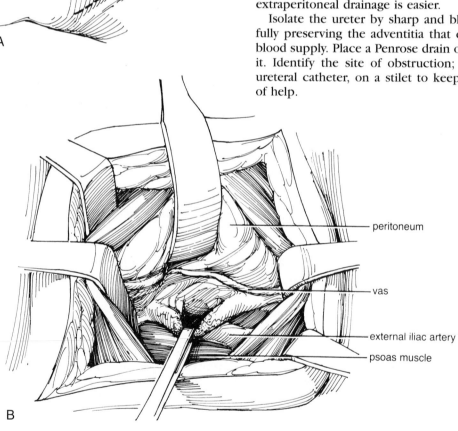

A

B

peritoneum

vas

external iliac artery

psoas muscle

2 Place stay sutures in the ureter above and below the lesion, and excise the defective portion, being sure to leave only healthy ureter. This débridement to normal ureter is important, especially in the presence of infection, after radiation, and after trauma. Replace the stay sutures with a fine traction suture on the medial aspect in each end of the ureter, and carefully dissect sufficient length for the anastomosis while avoiding the vessels in the adventitia.

Intubated ureterotomy is an alternative in long strictures with minimal periureteral involvement. Incise the stricture throughout its length, and insert a double-J stent of suitable size that extends into the pelvis and bladder. Pad the area with fat or omentum (see page 71). Leave the stent in place 6 weeks or more.

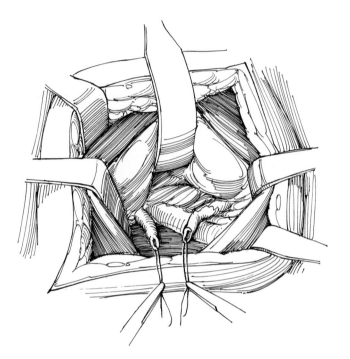

Transperitoneal Approach

Either ureter may be approached through a vertical incision in the left leaf of the small bowel mesentery, extending from over the sacral promontory to the ligament of Treitz. Divide the inferior mesenteric artery if necessary for exposure. For an approach to the lower left ureter, a better alternative is to mobilize the sigmoid colon medially.

To identify a distal end of the ureter transected during pelvic surgery, elevate the patient's knees, and place a ureteral catheter through a flexible cystoscope. Leave the catheter as a stent after repair.

Technique of Ureteroureteral Anastomosis

3 Transect the ureteral ends obliquely. Resect any abnormal tissue. Place fine stay sutures, and spatulate each end for a distance of 2 to 3 mm. If the distal lumen is very small, gently dilate it to 8 F. Do not use forceps on the ureter; manipulate it with the stay sutures.

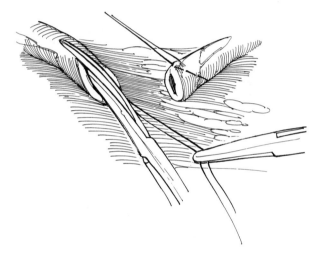

4 **A,** Insert two running 5-0 or 6-0 SAS in through the tip of the spatulated portion and out through the notch of the opposite ureteral wall. It helps to use a binocular loupe, especially in children. Place a double-J stent if the vitality of the ureteral wall is in doubt, but be sure its upper end lies within the renal pelvis and its lower end in the bladder. Tie the two sutures. Do not continue suturing if the ureter is under tension, but apply an adjunctive method, such as renal displacement.

B, Run one of the apical sutures down one side of the defect with bites 2 mm apart, working from inside the ureter and catching more serosa and muscularis than epithelium. Lock the suture every third or fourth stitch. Run the other suture from the outside. Tie each suture to the free end of the other suture. Alternately, insert interrupted sutures. Place a Penrose drain to exit extraperitoneally by the long-suture technique (see page 917), taking care not to let the drain lie against the anastomosis. Fasten the drain to the skin with a suture. Replace the retroperitoneal fat around the repair, and close the wound. An omental wrap (see page 74) may aid healing by decreasing periureteral scarring and providing neovascularity.

If urinary drainage occurs postoperatively, leave the drain in place until leakage has ceased for 2 or 3 days, and then remove it gradually. The timing of stent removal depends on the degree of ureteral injury.

SIMPLE RENAL MOBILIZATION

When the ureter is too short for safe anastomosis during ureteroureterostomy, even with a psoas hitch (see page 818) or Boari flap (see page 822), release the kidney from its bed. For greater mobilization, divide the renal vein (see page 830).

5 Reflect the colon medially, and continue the retroperitoneal dissection of the ureter cephalad, staying inside Gerota's fascia. The peritoneum may need to be opened in some cases. Bluntly free the renal capsule from the perirenal fat. If it is very adherent, extend the incision in the gutter so that Gerota's fascia may be opened and the dissection carried out under vision, as for simple nephrectomy (see page 987). The kidney rotates downward on its pedicle, adding 3 to 5 cm of ureteral length. Fix it to the psoas muscle with two 2-0 mattress SAS, incorporating fat pads (see page 922).

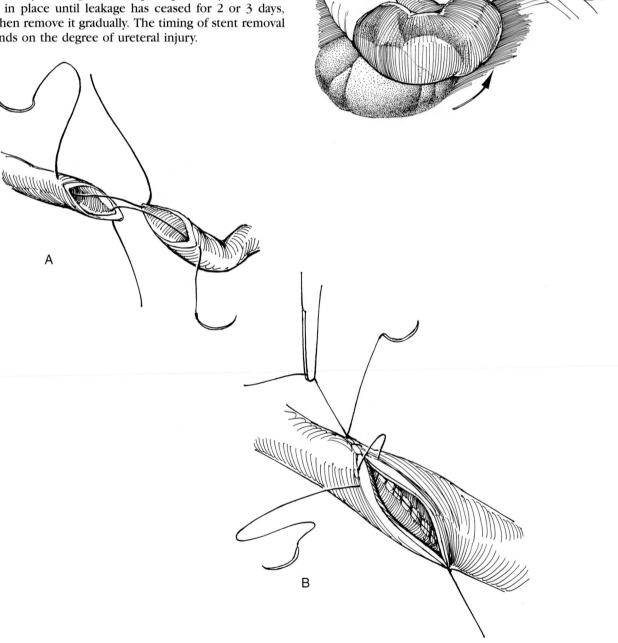

A

B

RETROCAVAL URETER

If the diagnosis of retrocaval ureter is in doubt, perform venaca-vography simultaneously with retrograde pyelography. Note on intravenous urography whether the ureter crosses behind the inferior vena cava at the level of the third lumbar vertebra (Type I), in which case a ureteroureterostomy should be done, or at the level of the renal pelvis (the less common and less obstructive Type II), in which case a pyeloureterostomy is appropriate.

6 Approach the ureter through an anterior subcostal incision (see page 856). First look for a persistent postcardinal vein instead of the vena cava itself as the obstructing vessel, in which case the vessel can simply be ligated and divided to free the ureter. Do not bother to dissect the ureteral segment from behind the vena cava because it probably is secondarily stenotic, and the ureter is always elongated.

A, Expose the ureter below its emergence from behind the medial side of the vena cava, and place a Penrose drain around it. Dissect it to the border of the vena cava, transfix it with a stay suture, and divide it. The proximal stump need not be ligated.

B, Moving laterally to the vena cava, identify the dilated pelvis and upper ureter. Dissect the ureter similarly to the lateral margin of the vena cava. Fix it with a stay suture, and divide it distally with an oblique cut. This end of the ureteral stump does not need to be ligated either because the formerly obstructive segment is now isolated. Anastomose the ureter to the pelvis by the Anderson-Hynes technique (see pages 914 to 918), as shown. Alternatively, anastomose it directly to the dilated upper ureteral segment by ureteroureterostomy, with or without placing a double-J stent. Drain the area with an accurately placed Penrose drain exiting extraperitoneally. Remove the stent after a week or two if the anastomosis was firm, and remove the drain several days after drainage has stopped.

INTRAOPERATIVE INJURY TO THE LOWER URETER

To repair an intraoperative injury to the lower ureter, immediately extend the existing incision to gain exposure, lack of which probably led to the injury. (If the patient's condition does not allow repair, place a silicone tube or double-J stent up the ureter to the renal pelvis, and bring it out extraperitoneally for interim drainage.)

Stenting the Repair. Place a double-J stent by inserting one end of a guide wire to the cephalad end through a hole in the middle of the stent and inserting the other end of the guide wire through an adjacent hole to the caudal end, leaving a loop of wire between. Insert the stent in both directions until the wire loop exits at the site of proposed repair. Withdraw the wire. Check the intravesical position of the stent by filling the bladder with dilute indigo carmine and observing its efflux from the intra-abdominal end of the ureter (Barone et al, 1993). Alternatively, first place a guide wire into the renal pelvis and pass the stent over it, insert the guide wire into the other end of the stent through a hole in the middle to straighten it, and then pass it into the bladder.

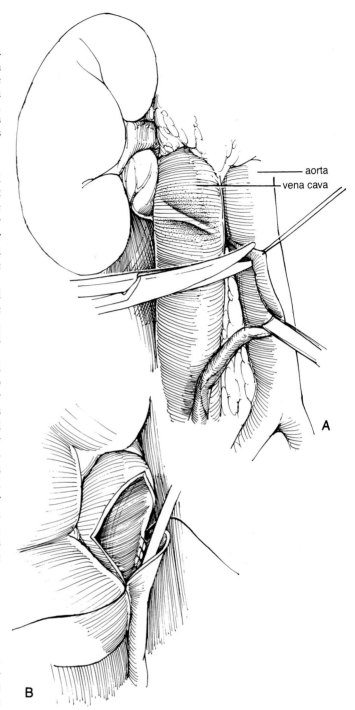

aorta
vena cava

A

B

TRANSURETEROURETEROSTOMY

If the recipient ureter does not appear entirely normal on intravenous urography, check it by voiding cystography to be sure it does not allow reflux and is not even minimally obstructed because the single distal ureter now carries double the load. If the patient has had pelvic radiation, plan a high anastomosis away from the field, although usually both ureters are damaged. The procedure is impractical in infants because of the small size of the recipient ureter. Provide antibiotic coverage.

7 **A,** *Position:* Supine. *Incision:* Use a midline transperitoneal incision (see page 867) unless the patient has had extensive abdominal surgery, in which case an extraperitoneal approach may be easier.

B, *Left-to-right ureteroureterostomy.* Hold the descending and sigmoid colon to the right, and pack the small bowel into the upper abdomen. Incise the parietal peritoneum lateral to the colon, and expose the damaged ureter, preserving all the adventitial tissue with its vasculature. Clamp the ureter just above the diseased portion. Place a 3-0 synthetic absorbable stay suture proximal to the clamp, divide the ureter, and ligate the distal stump with the same suture material. Free the donor ureter for a distance of 9 to 12 cm while preserving the adventitial vessels.

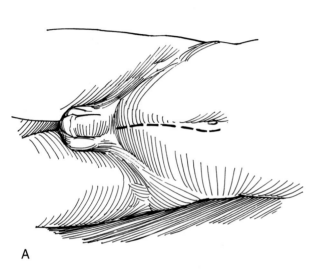

A

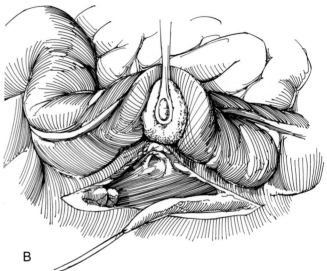

B

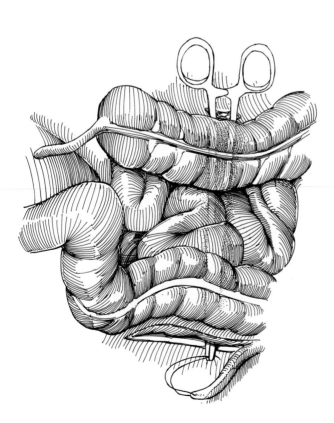

8 Free the cecum, and mobilize it with the terminal ileum into the upper abdomen. Incise the posterior peritoneum transversely just above the pelvic brim. This should be at a level 4 to 6 cm above the level of transection of the donor ureter to allow enough length to bring that ureter over. Realize that the ureters lie only about 5 cm apart at this level. Expose the recipient ureter. Start laterally to dissect it from its bed, freeing it only enough to provide space for the anastomosis, a few centimeters at most. The exception is a short left ureter. In that case, mobilize 6 to 8 cm to allow the ureter to be drawn medially with two Penrose drains.

Mobilizing the cecum is the preferable technique, but if this is not done, make a wide retroperitoneal tunnel under the sigmoid between the ureters digitally. Pass a large clamp from the recipient side, and draw the left ureter through by its stay suture. The ureter may pass over (preferably) or under the inferior mesenteric artery, depending on the available length of ureter, but it must not be wedged under it where it may become trapped between artery and aorta and obstructed from fibrosis. Be sure the ureter is not angulated and is under no tension at all. However, realize that tunneling, as shown here, carries the risk of angulating or constricting the ureter; mobilizing the cecum may be preferable.

9 **A,** Trim the ureter obliquely to provide a 1.5-cm opening. Spatulation is rarely needed. Manipulate it with a stay suture. Incise the wall of the recipient ureter on its medial surface with a hooked blade for a distance slightly longer than the opening in the donor ureter. Avoid placing the incision on the anterior wall because of the risk of angulation of the donor ureter.

B, Place a 4-0 or 5-0 SAS from outside in at each end of the incision in the recipient ureter, then through each extremity of the end of the donor ureter from inside out. Tie both sutures.

C, Run the upper suture down the back wall from the inside, occasionally locking a stitch. Tie it to the lower suture; then run that suture up the front wall from the outside. Prior to closure, consider inserting a double-J stenting catheter into the recipient ureter distally and into the donor ureter proximally. It is usually not practical to place a second stent in the recipient ureter because of its small size. Place an omental wrap (see page 71) if the quality of either ureter is questionable. This can usually be done without mobilizing the omentum by merely bringing it through the peritoneal defect. Tunnel a Penrose drain extraperitoneally from the site of the anastomosis through the body wall and skin of the flank. Close the peritoneal defects with 3-0 SAS. Drain the bladder with a suprapubic tube or urethral catheter. Close the wound.

Instill contrast medium into the stents 10 days postoperatively; if you see no extravasation, remove the stents. Then remove the cystostomy tube or urethral catheter.

TRANSURETEROURETEROSTOMY WITH CUTANEOUS STOMA

Transureterostomy in conjunction with cutaneous ureterostomy can be a useful procedure in a patient with one dilated ureter. It has more recently been applied in salvage of failed reimplantations and in undiversion procedures, often with implantation of the better ureter in the bladder accompanied by a psoas hitch or implantation of one ureter into an augmented bladder or a pouch. For a description of the procedure, see page 642.

POSTOPERATIVE PROBLEMS

Leakage almost always stops spontaneously. If it is prolonged, suspect that the drain is in contact with the repair and shorten it. Distal obstruction may be responsible. Pass a double-J stent to the renal pelvis, and leave it in place 2 to 3 weeks. *Intraperitoneal leakage* can result from tension on the anastomosis and manifests itself as ileus from urinary ascites. Stenting or diversion by percutaneous nephrostomy may be needed. A *urinoma* may form if the drain is removed before drainage has ceased. *Obstruction* at the site of anastomosis can be diagnosed by ultrasonography and by retrograde ureterography through the cutaneous stoma. Late *stenosis* at the stoma must be watched for; follow-up intravenous pyelography or sonography at regular intervals is important to detect silent obstruction.

Stricture of the normal ureter is rare and usually can be treated by ureteroscopic techniques. *Pelvic abscess* has been reported.

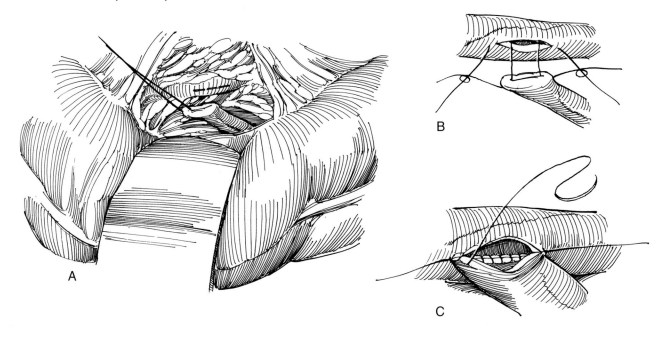

Commentary by Joseph C. Smith

The techniques described in this chapter should be part of every urologist's armamentarium.

Surgical injuries of the ureter, if recognized at the time, can usually be repaired as described, unless a segment of ureter has been excised. In that case, a transureteroureterostomy is probably the best option, but the normality of the recipient ureter should be assessed by on-table retrograde ureterography.

Delayed recognition of surgical injury is not uncommon, and the presentation may be an extravasation of urine with urinoma formation or a cutaneous or (after hysterectomy) vaginal fistula. Diagnosis is confirmed by retrograde ureterography, and an initial attempt to correct the injury by stenting is worthwhile. If stenting is successful, the double-J stent should be left in for 3 months to allow the healing of the local tissue to stabilize. The possibility of future stricture formation remains, and follow-up by ultrasonography is necessary.

Transureteroureterostomy is usually an easy operation to perform, and it is important to remember that even when the opposite kidney has been removed, a viable lower ureter may be present. I have personally used a ureter 60 years after nephrectomy (for trauma) when the patient developed a tumor of the lower ureter draining his solitary kidney.

Calicoureterostomy

Anastomosis of the ureter to a lower calyx ensures dependent drainage from a large hydronephrotic kidney. When, after failed pyeloplasty with consequent fibrosis in the hilum, the ureter proves to be too short to reach the renal pelvis, anastomosis to a lower pole calyx is an appealing solution. The renal cortex over the markedly dilated calyx must have become thin; otherwise the parenchyma would contract around the ureter with resultant obstruction.

Consider other procedures for bridging a defect because of the risk of stricture. Alternatives include the Davis intubated ureterotomy (see page 920), renal displacement or autotransplantation (see page 830), ileal ureter (see page 842), and nephrectomy (see page 987). It is well to have the bowel prepared in case a segment of ileum is needed.

Incision: An anterior subcostal incision (see page 856) is usually adequate, but an anterior transperitoneal incision (see page 867) allows intestinal interposition if that proves necessary. Place a ureteral catheter cystoscopically if you suspect that identification of the ureter may be difficult. Proceed to expose the renal pelvis as for a pyeloureteroplasty (see page 914). In addition to adequately mobilizing the kidney, it is important to expose the renal artery to be able to control it if the need arises. Identify the normal ureter distally, and place a small Penrose drain or vessel loop around it. Continue the dissection up to the scarred ureteropelvic junction. (After the diseased portion is resected, you may find that the ureter is long enough to allow repair by ureteropyeloplasty.) Place a fine traction suture in the ureter and a clamp just above it. Divide the ureter obliquely below the clamp, and ligate the stump on the pelvic side with a 2-0 SAS.

1 Incise the capsule over the lower pole of the kidney in the frontal plane instead of circumferentially. This provides more membrane for cover. Carefully peel the capsule back. It is likely to be quite adherent but is worth preserving intact. Estimate the level of the lower pole infundibulum from the pyelogram. It is helpful to place a curved sound through the pelvis into the target calyx. Bluntly divide the renal parenchyma with the knife handle, cutting the arcuate vessels with scissors. Remove more parenchyma than appears necessary so that the infundibulum of the lower calyx protrudes from the surface. Free the calyx itself enough to provide an edge for sutures, or mobilize the infundibulum and cut it tangentially. If excess parenchyma remains, it contracts around the ureter and constricts it. Control the bleeding by placing a hand around the lower half of the kidney and figure-eight 4-0 SAS, tied by your assistant, to control the arteries. Hemostasis must be complete.

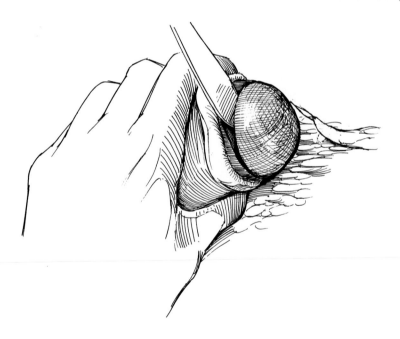

2 Spatulate the ureter on its lateral side for a distance equal to the length of the caliceal or infundibular defect, which should be between 1.5 and 2 cm. The anastomosis is similar to that for a pyeloureteroplasty (see pages 916 to 917). Place two 4-0 SAS side by side through the capsule and medial end of the calyx or infundibulum, and then out through the ureter at the notch of the spatulation. Tie them. Run one suture along the posterior edge to the opposite end, with each bite catching the capsule, ureter, and calyx. Lock an occasional stitch. Do the same with the anterior suture, here including in order the capsule, ureter, and calyx.

Alternative: Before anastomosing the ureter, run a 4-0 SAS circumferentially to appose the capsule to the edge of the calyx or infundibulum.

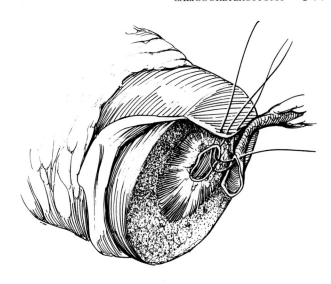

Before the defect is completely closed, insert a double-J stent that extends into both the bladder and the renal pelvis. Additionally, with a curved clamp, draw a small Malecot catheter through the cortex into a middle calyx, and fix it to the capsule with a 2-0 SAS (see pages 928 to 929). Complete the ureterocaliceal anastomosis, and tie the two sutures together. Irrigate through the nephrostomy tube to be sure that the closure is watertight.

If the kidney has been extensively mobilized, place a nephropexy stitch (see page 922). Drain the area well with a Penrose drain that exits retroperitoneally. Replace the perirenal fat, and tack it in Gerota's fascia to encase the repair. If coverage of the repair appears inadequate, bring the omentum into the retroperitoneum and fasten it around the anastomosis.

Remove the stent after 3 to 6 weeks, and test for leakage and pressure flow through the anastomosis. Clamp the tube to see if the patient tolerates the clamping before removing the nephrostomy tube.

Pyelocaliceal Anastomosis

3 Extend the caliceal-infundibular incision toward the renal pelvis, as is done for pyelonephrolithotomy (see page 1050). The pelvis may not require complete transection.

POSTOPERATIVE PROBLEMS

Leakage is the most frequently occurring problem but usually ceases spontaneously, although stenting may be required if the anastomosis is relatively stenotic. *Stricture* of the anastomosis is not uncommon; it usually results from constriction by residual parenchyma. *Pyelonephritis* is treated with antibiotics, to which it responds if drainage is free.

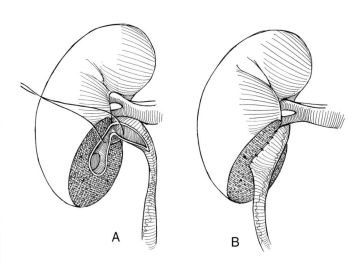

A   B

Commentary by Robert M. Weiss

The use of a calicoureterostomy is appropriate only with severe hydronephrosis and significant thinning of the renal parenchyma. Although the procedure has been used in instances of marked hydronephrosis secondary to a primary ureteropelvic junction obstruction, its greatest use follows failed pyeloplasty, in which scar tissue prevents reanastomosis of the ureter to the renal pelvis.

A running suture through the renal capsule and parenchyma to the divided calyx or infundibulum is important in preventing obstruction. The edges of the calyx or infundibulum need to be everted. If the defect is too long for a tension-free primary anastomosis, interposition of a short tapered segment of ileum is indicated. The ileum is tapered on its antimesenteric border, and an end-to-end calicoileoureterostomy is performed. The segment of ileum may be quite short, and, at least in children and thin adults, the peritoneal opening may be small.

Ileal Ureteral Replacement

Explore all alternatives that use tissue from the urinary tract before electing to use ileum. Determine that the bladder neck is widely open and that the bladder is easily emptied. If not, consider a YV-plasty as part of the procedure. In males, resection of the prostate transurethrally may be adequate. Be certain that the patient has adequate renal function; serum creatinine level should be 2.2 mg/100 ml or less. Nephrostomy drainage should already be in place.

Prepare the patient as for an ileal conduit (see page 647). Do not place a urethral catheter, but allow the bladder to fill. If the ureter is to be excised, insert a ureteral catheter cystoscopically.

1 *Position:* Place the patient in a lateral position with the table flexed and the shoulder and chest held at right angles to the table. Allow the hip to fall back as far as reasonable, and place a sandbag under it.

Incision: Palpate the 12th rib, and begin the skin incision over its posterior portion. Continue semiobliquely to the midline, then vertically to the pubis. Cut through the anterior part of the latissimus dorsi muscle onto the surface of the 12th rib. Place the index finger in an opening in the lumbodorsal fascia at the tip of the rib, and work posteriorly, cutting the serratus inferior posterior muscle and intercostal muscles if encountered. Divide the external and internal oblique and transversus muscles, and enter the peritoneum. Divide the rectus muscle, and retract it laterally while continuing the incision down the midline, opening the peritoneum farther at the same time.

Alternatively, use a thoracoabdominal incision (see page 890) for better exposure for the renal anastomosis. For bilateral cases, a long midline incision is best.

Incise the peritoneal attachment of the terminal ileum to the sacral promontory, and divide the lateral attachments of the ascending colon in the white line of Toldt to mobilize it to the region of the duodenum and as far medially as the great vessels, as done for retroperitoneal lymph node dissection (see pages 387 to 390). Let the bowel fall back. Open the peritoneum, and continue anteriorly in the line of the incision.

2 Select a 20- to 30-cm segment of ileum near the ileocecal junction; the length depends on the size of the patient and on how much ureter must be replaced. Choose sites of transection to allow for total mobilization of the segment of ileum by allowing for the cuts in the mesentery deep enough for the upper end to reach the renal area (this can be difficult) and for the distal end of the loop to reach the bladder. Special care must be taken to get a good arterial supply and make certain that two major branches of the superior mesenteric artery enter the loop. On the left side, a segment of descending colon can be used instead of the ileum. Mark the bowel at each end with a stay suture; throw a loose tie onto the suture at the distal end as a marker to be sure that the segment is placed isoperistaltically.

Divide the mesentery deeply between the ileocolic artery and the terminal branches of the superior mesenteric artery. Divide it also at the proximal end deeply enough to allow that end to reach the kidney. Apply Kocher clamps and divide the bowel. Restore bowel continuity by one of the techniques described for ileal conduit (see pages 650 to 654). Irrigate the loop with a catheter and a 50-ml syringe containing saline solution, followed by 1 percent neomycin-bacitracin solution, and finally by air. Close the mesenteric defect with 4-0 silk sutures.

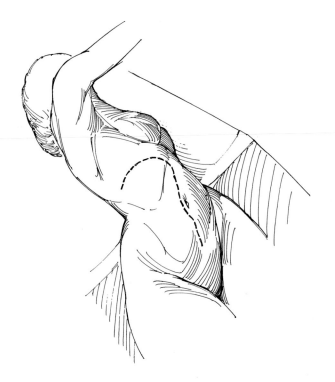

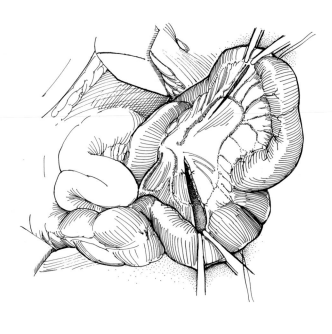

3 For replacement of the *right* ureter, place the ileal segment extraperitoneally by lifting the cecum forward and exposing the retroperitoneal space. Make a small opening in the mesentery of the ascending colon near the cecum, and bring the ileum through it. For *left* ureteral replacement, mobilize the descending colon medially by incising along the white line. Make a window in the colonic mesentery, and push the isolated segment of ileum out through it so that it lies in an isoperistaltic manner in the left retroperitoneal space. Because the anastomoses to the pelvis and the bladder are retroperitoneal, the ileum lies behind the descending colon. Rotate the ileum 180 degrees counterclockwise to place the

knotted stay suture marking the distal end near the bladder, ensuring isoperistaltic orientation. Carefully close the opening through the mesentery to prevent internal herniation, but at the same time avoid constriction.

Grasp the end of the loop again with the Kocher clamp. For unilateral ureteral substitution, close the proximal end of the loop, spatulate the ureter, and anastomose it to the ileum as described for ureteroileostomy (see pages 658 to 659). Connect the ureter end to side if it is dilated, even if tailoring (see page 803) is necessary. At this time, consider placement of a nephrostomy (see page 928).

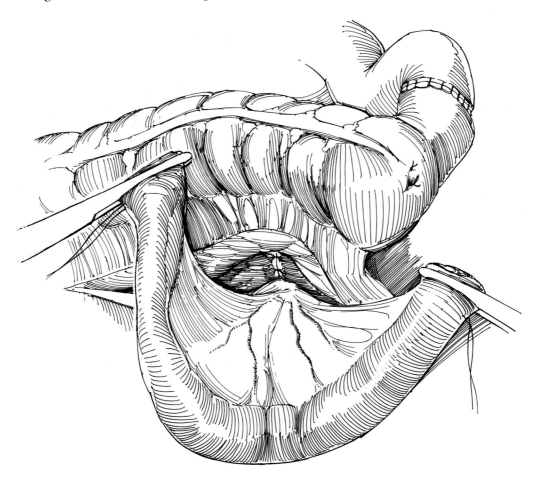

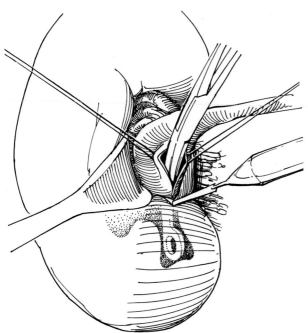

4 Direct pyeloileal anastomosis may be advisable for children with recurrent xanthine stone formation. The renal pelvis must be mobilized, often a difficult undertaking after previous stone procedures. If the pelvis is obscured by scar, insert curved Randall forceps through the nephrostomy site and cut upon its tip, staying away from the vascular pedicle. Leave the ureter in situ. If small calculi are present, consider instillation of coagulum (see pages 1042 to 1043).

Open the renal pelvis widely vertically. Pass Randall stone forceps through the pyelotomy into the lower pole calyx, and cut down on the forceps with the cutting current to open up the entire lower collecting system. Place 3-0 CCG sutures from the capsule to the calyx to control parenchymal bleeding. Remove persisting calculi with the aid of a nephroscope. Insert a small Malecot nephrostomy tube with two wings removed through the parenchyma via a middle calyx.

5 Spatulate the ileum to form an ellipse by opening its antimesenteric border and incising it until the opening is the same size as the pelvic defect. Place a 3-0 or 4-0 CCG suture through all layers of the tip of the bowel, then through the upper margin of the pelvic defect, and tie it. Run the suture down the back wall, occasionally locking a stitch. Continue the suture up the anterior wall, and tie it to the end of the original suture. Alternatively, use interrupted 3-0 or 4-0 CCG sutures, placing the posterior row with the knots outside. Either suture line may be reinforced with serosa-to-adventitia sutures. Fill the pelvis through the nephrostomy tube, and reinforce the anastomosis at sites of leakage.

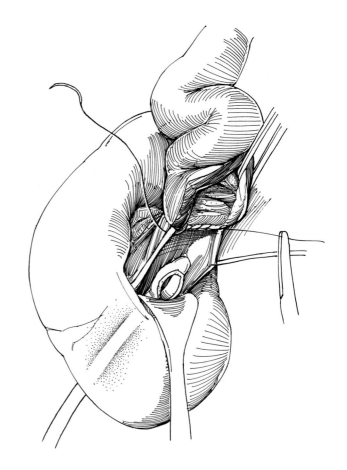

6 Mobilize the peritoneum from the upper and lateral margins of the bladder, and make a short incision in the dome extraperitoneally. Insert the index finger and move the posterolateral wall of the bladder toward the psoas muscle. If the ileal loop is short, so that it is necessary to get greater vesical mobilization, carry the dissection down to include the superior vesical pedicle by incising the peritoneum in the cul-de-sac. Grasp the bladder with an Allis clamp at the site of the finger tip over the psoas muscle, and excise a small circle of bladder wall. Suture the posterior wall of the bladder to the psoas muscle with several 3-0 CCG sutures.

Move the ileal segment alongside to determine the needed length. Keep the loop as short as feasible, but allow enough redundancy to permit formation of a nipple. If the operation is done for stone disease, omit the nipple. Excise the redundant portion of the ileum, first dividing its vessels close to the bowel to avoid interference with the major blood supply.

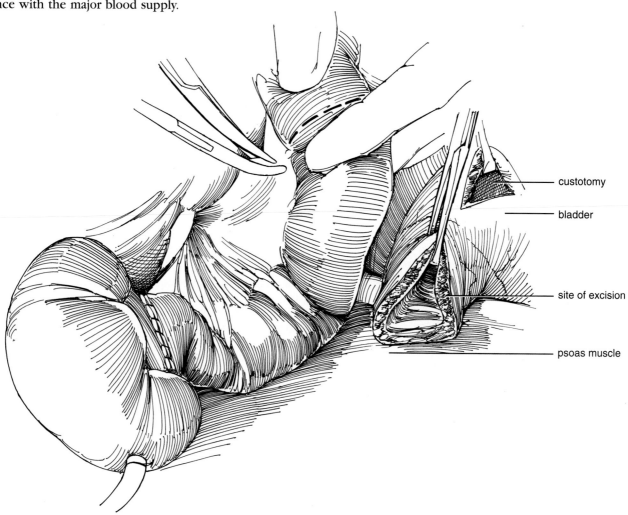

custotomy

bladder

site of excision

psoas muscle

7 **A,** Suture the bowel to the bladder wall with interrupted 3-0 CCG sutures. It is often easier to open the bladder wide and anastomose the ileum by suturing from inside the bladder. Prevention of reflux is important for preservation of renal function. Arrange for an antireflux mechanism, although none has proved entirely satisfactory (Shokeir and Ghoneim, 1995).

B, Antireflux valve: Turn the bowel back on itself as a cuff, and suture the mucosa to the vesical epithelium as an ileovesical intussusception. *Alternative 1:* Taper (tailor) the ileum, and insert it in a subepithelial tunnel as done for large ureters (see page 803). *Alternative 2:* Perform an ileoileal intussusception (see pages 688 to 689).

Place a Malecot cystostomy tube through a stab wound, and close the bladder defect in two layers. Insert a small silicone balloon catheter transurethrally. A stent in the ileum is probably unnecessary. Place a medium-size Penrose drain near the pyeloileal anastomosis, and bring it out retroperitoneally through a stab wound in the posterior axillary line. Place a second Penrose drain by the long-suture technique (see page 917) near the vesical anastomosis, and bring it out anterolaterally. Adequate drainage is essential. Tack the colon laterally to the peritoneal edge to extraperitonealize the entire segment. Close the peritoneum and the wound. Finally, suture the nephrostomy and cystostomy tubes to the skin with heavy silk, and tape them in place.

Remove the urethral catheter on the fifth postoperative day. The cystostomy tube may be clamped on the seventh day for a trial of voiding, but there is no hurry about this. Perform gravity nephrostography and cystography subsequently to check for leaks; if no leaks are detected, remove the cystostomy and nephrostomy tubes. Remove the drains 24 hours later. Check the functional result by following the level of the serum creatinine and the anatomic result by intravenous urography at 6 weeks.

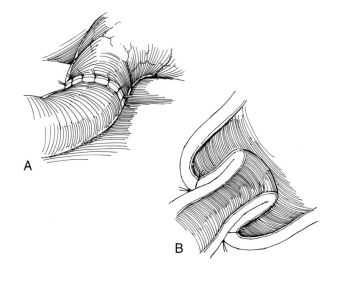

A

B

Bilateral Total and Subtotal Ureteral Replacement

8 **A,** If a portion of the ureters may be preserved, perform ureteroileal anastomoses. Bring the ureters through the posterior peritoneum near the midline, anastomose the ureters to the loop (see pages 658 to 659), and fasten the loop to the bladder extraperitoneally.

B, When the ureters are not salvageable, by working anteriorly and intraperitoneally, anastomose the ileal loop to the left pelvis end to end, and connect it to the right pelvis end to side.

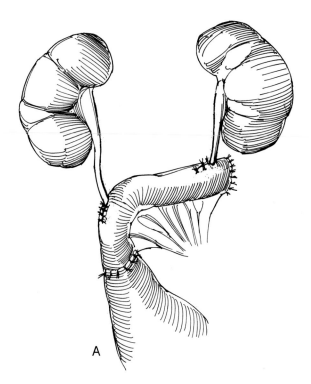

A

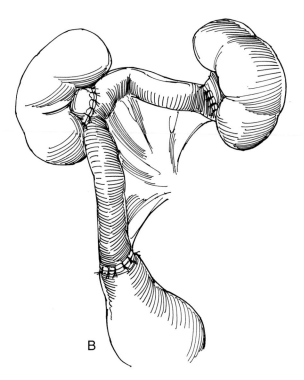

B

POSTOPERATIVE PROBLEMS

Anastomotic leakage with consequent urinoma or fistula can be picked up on a nephrostogram, in which case the nephrostomy tube is left for a longer time. *Obstruction* is usually due to edema or excessive production of mucus. A kink in the ileum must also be suspected. Leaving the nephrostomy tube in place may allow resolution of these factors. *Ischemic necrosis* of the segment requires immediate reoperation.

Electrolyte imbalance is rare if preoperative renal function is adequate and the segment is short and drains well. Preventing reflux by construction of an ileovesical valve may help preserve renal function. Long-term follow-up is needed to detect incipient outlet obstruction.

Commentary by John A. Libertino

The admonition to use tissue from the urinary tract before using bowel and making certain that the bladder neck is widely patent, especially in males, is very much on target.

We use a transabdominal incision and reserve the thoracoabdominal incision for reoperative procedures in the region of the renal pelvis, such as after failed pyeloplasty or ureterocalicostomy.

I usually measure the distance from the renal pelvis to the bladder with an umbilical tape to determine the length of the ileal segment that is required. It is extremely important to have an isoperistaltic ileal segment, which is more tedious to achieve on the right side for right ureteral replacement than on the left. The ureter is brought to the posterior wall of the bladder, and a Paquin type of intra-extravesical implantation (see page 799) is created at the ileovesical anastomosis. In a redo procedure, we usually protect the anastomosis with a percutaneous or open nephrostomy tube. Nephrostography determines when the nephrostomy and suprapubic tubes are removed. We perform nephrostography on the 10th postoperative day; if no leakage occurs, the tube is clamped and then removed sequentially. Attention to details has provided good long-term results in a large series of ileal substitutions.

Ureterolithotomy

Ureterolithotomy is now rarely performed unless it is combined with a reparative procedure because endoscopic and ultrasonic techniques are usually applicable, including laparoscopic removal. Because of the length of the ureter, a different incision is required for each level of involvement. Consequently, care must be taken to prevent the stone from moving out of the area exposed by that incision.

Radiography the morning of operation or on the way to the operating room is mandatory.

APPROACHES

To the Upper Third. Use a lumbotomy incision (see page 887) for high stones and a subcostal or supracostal incision (see pages 871 and 879) for a stone approaching the middle third or one located in a dilated ureter such that it might fall back into the renal pelvis. A pyeloplasty, if indicated, may be done through either incision. A Foley muscle-splitting incision (see page 885) is useful if the stone is impacted just below the ureteropelvic junction, usually in line with the lower margin of the kidney. A midline incision (see page 867) is used if much

of the ureter must be exposed or if it needs to be approached transperitoneally because of previous extensive extraperitoneal procedures (but expect more intra-abdominal adhesions subsequently).

To the Middle Third. Usually a midline extraperitoneal incision (see page 487) is best, but a Foley incision (see page 885) or a dorsal lumbotomy incision (see page 896) may be suitable.

To the Lower Third. Use a midline extraperitoneal incision (see page 487), a midline transperitoneal incision for reoperation (see page 867), or a Gibson incision (see page 495). A transvesical approach may be useful for a large stone in the terminal ureter. A vaginal approach may be suitable for a larger palpable stone.

Approach the ureter extraperitoneally above the level of the stone. If it has been exposed before and lies in scar tissue, a transperitoneal approach may be preferable. Sweep the peritoneum medially. The ureter adheres to its posterior surface so that as it is mobilized, the ureter no longer lies against the posterior body wall. Identify the ureter; it shows peristalsis if pinched with forceps.

URETEROLITHOTOMY, LOWER THIRD

1 **A,** Make a midline extraperitoneal incision (see page 487). Extending the incision around the umbilicus (as shown) adds little to the exposure of this section of the ureter.

B, Mobilize the peritoneum medially. After exposing the lower ureter, pass a Penrose drain around it near its crossing of the iliac vessels to aid in mobilization.

Technique for Mobilization of the Distal Ureter. Dissect toward the bladder until the first vascular arcade of the superior vesical pedicle crosses over it. Open the

tissue lying over the ureter distal to this restricting band but proximal to the next arcade, and reapply the Penrose drain at this level. Continue this process until the ureter is free enough for ureterolithotomy (or for repair or reimplantation).

To reach the midureter, cut the crescent of transversalis fascia that holds the peritoneum to the lateral body wall with Lahey scissors. In females, this portion of the ureter passes beneath the vessels to the uterus, and care must be taken during the exposure to preserve them. Occasionally, as in approaches to the ureter after previous surgery, opening into the peritoneal cavity facilitates exposure and allows dissection of the ureter transperitoneally.

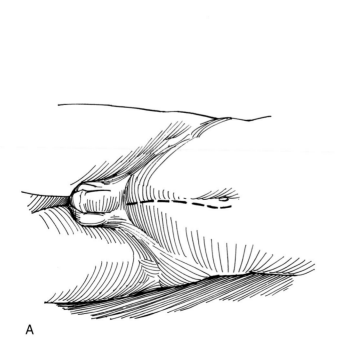

A

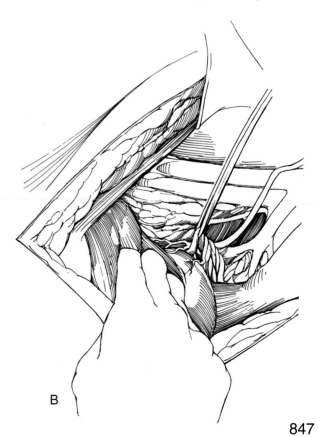

B

2 Place a Babcock clamp or a Penrose drain or vessel loop around the ureter above the anticipated site of the stone. The stone can be seen as a bulge or can be felt by gentle finger-tip palpation. Avoid manipulation. A second Babcock clamp below the stone may help deliver the ureter and prevents downward migration. Dissect the ureter as little as possible. Do not open the ureter until you can identify the stone. Place two 4-0 SAS vertically in the wall, and incise vertically directly on the upper end of the stone with a hooked blade. Feel the grating of the knife on the stone, and do not open above it. Enlarge the incision with the knife or Potts scissors (the muscle is readily divided, but the epithelium can easily be shredded and lost). Be sure to make the opening larger than the stone.

With upper ureteral stones, avoid cutting across the ureteropelvic junction, where subsequent scarring could interfere with its peristaltic function.

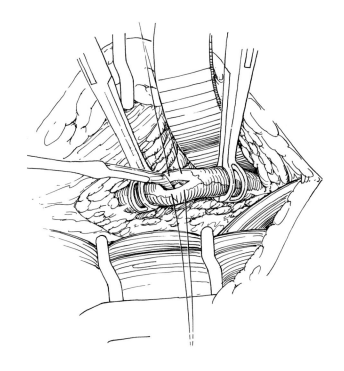

3 Loosen the stone from the epithelium, into which its irregularities are often embedded, by running the tip of a Mixter clamp around it. Gingerly extract the stone with a Mixter clamp or dissector. Avoid fragmentation. Release the upper Babcock clamp; the resultant urine flow from the proximal ureter can wash out residual fragments. Release the lower clamp and pass a 5 F or 8 F infant feeding tube through the ureterotomy down to the bladder to be certain no obstruction remains. If it does not pass into the bladder, suspect a second stone or a stricture. Irrigate if fragmentation has occurred. If the ureter has been extensively traumatized, place a double-J stent to the pelvis and bladder before closure.

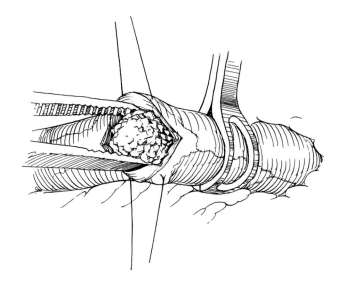

4 Close the ureter to make it watertight either by loosely tying the stay sutures or by putting one or two 4-0 SAS through the adventitia only. Do not constrict the ureter because some edema is to be expected. Replace the ureter inside Gerota's fascia, and suture a Penrose drain in the immediate vicinity (see page 917), bringing it out of the wound. Replace the periureteral fat between the ureter and the psoas muscle, tacking it in place with 3-0 PCG sutures. Close the incision.

Contact of the drain with the ureteral defect may promote leakage; shorten the drain slightly. In any case, shorten the drain on the fourth postoperative day, and remove it the following day unless leakage persists.

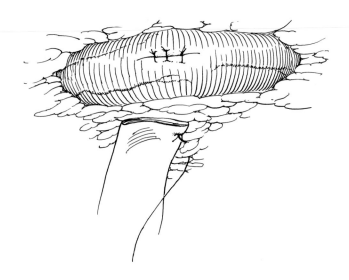

Nonpalpable Stone

If the stone cannot be felt, several alternatives are possible: (1) Perform radiography on the table (often very difficult, requiring loss of operative position). (2) Pass a ureteral catheter gently to locate the stone; then make a counter-incision in the ureter at the site of obstruction. Sometimes a basket or a ureteroscope can be helpful. (3) Pass a stone basket distally (especially useful for stones near the ureterovesical junction). (4) If the stone has retreated to the renal pelvis, pass Randall stone forceps into the pelvis, open them, and (if you are lucky) gently shake the stone into the instrument and remove it. If this fails, expose the kidney and perform radiography. (5) If the stone cannot be recovered, place a J stent because an obstructing stone distal to a ureterotomy is an abomination, especially if infection supervenes.

TRANSVESICAL URETEROLITHOTOMY

Expose the bladder through a transverse lower abdominal incision (see page 490), and make a vertical incision in the bladder. Place a stay suture 1 cm medial and distal to the orifice. With traction on the suture, incise the uroepithelium transversely 3 cm above the orifice. Expose the ureter by splitting the detrusor fibers, and grasp it in a Babcock clamp. Locate the stone by inspection or palpation, and make a longitudinal incision directly over it. Lever the stone out with a probe. Irrigate the ureter proximally and distally. Insert a stent through the ureteral orifice, and close the defect with interrupted fine CCG sutures. Bring the stent and a Malecot catheter through a stab wound in the anterior bladder wall. Close the bladder with a running 4-0 plain suture in the subepithelial layer and interrupted 3-0 CCG sutures in the muscularis. Keep the stent in place for 5 days, and remove the suprapubic catheter the next day.

Alternatively, transurethrally resect the bladder wall over the intramural ureter, and loop the stone out. Leave a J stent if you are concerned about stricture. Reflux follows.

VAGINAL URETEROLITHOTOMY

When a large stone is impacted at the ureterovesical junction and can be felt vaginally, it may be readily approached vaginally, especially in a parous woman with some degree of prolapse.

5 Place a weighted speculum, and suture the labia laterally. Pull the cervix down with a tenaculum. Insert stay sutures on either side of the palpable stone in the vaginal vault.

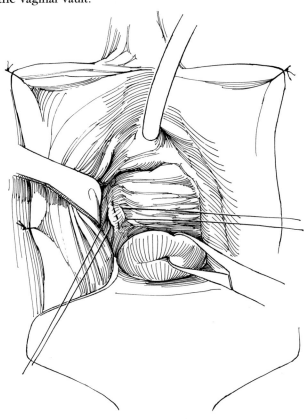

6 **A,** With a #15 blade, incise through the full thickness of vaginal wall, and expose the ureter above and below the stone. Grasp the ureter in a Babcock clamp if necessary to expose it. Make a longitudinal incision in the ureter, and gingerly extract the stone.

B, Close the ureter transversely with interrupted 4-0 CCG sutures.

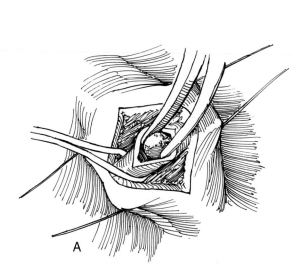

A

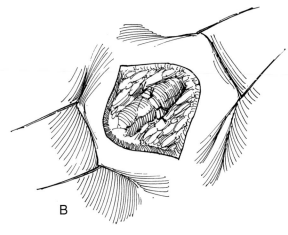

B

7 For oozing, insert a small Penrose drain; if the wound is dry, close the vaginal wall with everting sutures of 3-0 CCG.

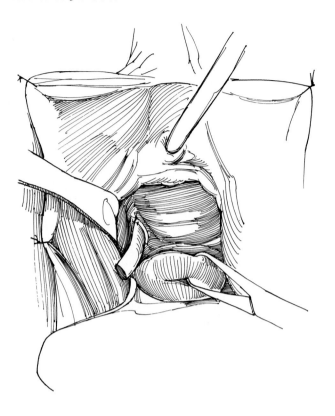

SECONDARY URETEROLITHOTOMY

Start with the patient on an x-ray table. Look in the bladder to see whether the stone can be extracted or destroyed endoscopically. If that cannot be done, pass a catheter to the stone and leave the catheter indwelling.

Proceed with transperitoneal exposure of the ureter. Incise the white line, and mobilize the appropriate segment of the colon. Dissect the ureter above the site of the stone. Remove the stone and insert a double-J stent, run a Penrose drain out extraperitoneally through the flank, and close the peritoneal defect. For low-lying stones, the parietal peritoneum can be opened directly over the ureter on the appropriate side of the sigmoid colon. Remember, the stone lies lower than expected.

For stones too low to reach by this approach, divide the obliterated hypogastric ligament and the superior vesical pedicle to free the bladder. Open it and run one finger down inside and another finger outside the bladder to feel the stone between them. Insert a needle into the stone to be sure that it is calcareous; then incise down upon it from inside the bladder. Be aware of the arterial branch running transversely there. Insert a double-J stent.

POSTOPERATIVE PROBLEMS

Persistent drainage suggests distal obstruction (perhaps an overlooked fragment) or local devascularization. After 12 days, obtain a plain film to check for the presence of a residual stone in the ureter. A drain placed too close to the ureteral incision can also cause persistent leakage and needs to be prudently shortened. If drainage persists longer than 2 to 3 weeks, ischemia is usually the cause; pass a J stent and leave it for at least 1 week after the wound is dry.

Strictures may form if the ureter has been made ischemic by extensive adventitial dissection. Intubation, balloon dilation, or transureteral incision may correct the problem, but construction of a psoas hitch or formation of a bladder flap may be required. Transureteroureterostomy is contraindicated in patients with stone disease. A *urinoma* may develop if the drain is removed too soon. Try to probe and reopen the tract, and protect the patient with antibiotics. A J stent may be required because a urinoma is the result of extravasation.

Commentary by Ken Koshiba

Identification of the ureter is still one of the time-consuming steps, even with a ureteral stent indwelling. Placement of a fiberoptic ureteroscope up to the stone site helps locate the ureter because the light at its tip can be visualized at laparoscopy (Ao et al, 1993).

Commentary by William W. Bohnert

Open ureterolithotomy is required infrequently today with the technologic advances of in situ shock wave lithotripsy and endoscopic and percutaneous approaches to ureteral stones. However, for longstanding, impacted larger stones, it should still be a part of every urologist's armamentarium.

Most importantly, one must approach the ureteral stone above its location and secure it with a Babcock clamp, or encircle the ureter above and below the stone with a Penrose drain or vessel loop to prevent stone migration. Careful dissection for exposure rather than gross manipulation yields fewer migration events.

Meticulous closure with 4-0 absorbable suture shortens the period of urinary drainage; make sure not to make large purchases of ureteral wall with each suture, as such stitches could compromise the ureteral lumen.

One should attempt to use a lumbotomy or muscle-splitting approach, if possible, to minimize morbidity and shorten inpatient days. Dissection and salvage of the 12th intercostal nerve are preferable to prevent flank muscle denervation and eventration when using a subcostal approach.

Drain placement at the ureterotomy site is critical. I prefer a suction drain to a Penrose drain. It seems to decrease morbidity and the inconvenience of frequent dressing changes, allowing the patient to leave the hospital in a relatively short time if adynamic ileus is not a problem.

Devascularization of a ureteral segment is the most devastating complication of ureterolithotomy. Dissection and open exposure of long segments of the ureter should be avoided. Locating the stone exactly with preoperative radiography, choosing the best incisional approach to allow the surgeon access to the ureter above the stone, and securing the stone in the ureter to prevent migration ensure a successful outcome with minimal chance of ureteral devascularization.

LAPAROSCOPIC APPROACHES

Transperitoneal Laparoscopic Ureterolithotomy

Insert a guide wire and a ureteral stent cystoscopically to the level of the stone, taking care not to displace it. While the patient is still supine, induce pneumoperitoneum and insert five trocars: one subumbilical observation trocar and three contralateral trocars and one ipsilateral trocar in the midclavicular line. Place the patient in the lateral position.

After freeing any interfering adhesions, incise the posterior peritoneum along the white line of Toldt with scissors. Reach the hepatic flexure for stones on the right and the splenic flexure for those on the left. Put traction on the medial peritoneal edge, and use blunt and sharp dissection to free the colon from the retroperitoneal tissues. Retract the spermatic vessels laterally. The ureter may remain adherent to the peritoneum but stands out because of the contained stent.

Place a vessel loop around the ureter above the stone to prevent proximal migration, but dissect the ureter as little as possible. An endoscopic Babcock clamp may be placed. Incise the ureter vertically over and just above the stone, making the incision slightly larger than the stone. Loosen the stone from the ureteral epithelium and gingerly extract it. Release the vessel loop to allow urine to flood the site. Close the ureterotomy with a single suture of 4-0 CCG tied either intracorporally or extracorporally. Alternatively, leave the ureterotomy open.

Cystoscopically advance the stent over the guide wire into the kidney. Place a Penrose drain by pressing the grasping forceps against the flank to make a short incision, and draw the drain retroperitoneally. Grasp both peritoneal edges, and clip them together with hernia staples to attach the colon.

Proceed to withdraw the trocars.

Retroperitoneal Laparoscopic Ureterolithotomy

Proceed as described on page 994 to insert a balloon in the retroperitoneal space. Identify the ureter by its contained stent and the bulge of the stone. Incise it and extract the stone. Provide extraperitoneal drainage.

SECTION
20
Surgical Approaches to the Kidney

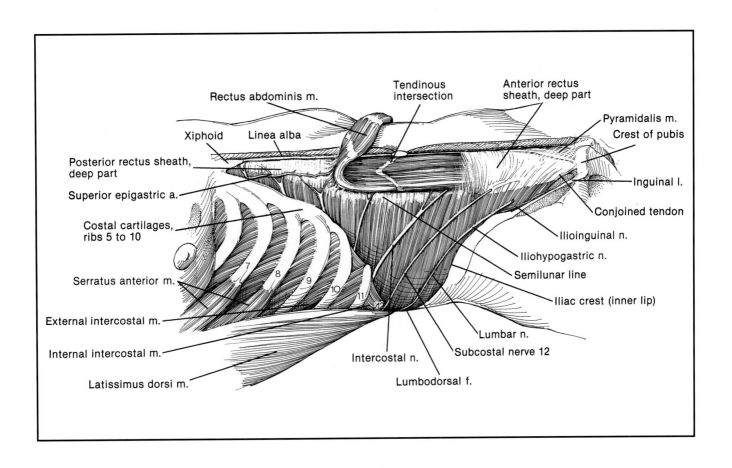

Anatomic Basis for Renal Incisions

BLOOD SUPPLY TO THE UPPER ABDOMEN

Refer to Step 1 (see page 486) in the first article of Section 12. The superior epigastric artery, which supplies the upper portion of the rectus abdominis, originates from the inferior mammary artery (internal thoracic artery) that runs anterior to the upper margin of the transversus abdominis to pass through the rectus sheath behind the rectus abdominis near its lateral border. As it runs caudad on the anterior surface of the posterior rectus sheath, it penetrates and supplies the rectus muscle and then passes through the anterior rectus sheath to supply the overlying skin. The falciform ligament supporting the liver contains vessels from a branch of the superior epigastric artery that are destined to enter the hepatic artery; the ligament therefore requires ligation after division.

RETROPERITONEAL FASCIAS AND SPACES IN TRANSVERSE OBLIQUE VIEW

1 Three layers of the retroperitoneal fascia differentiate as the inner, intermediate, and outer strata. The inner stratum envelops the intestinal tract. The intermediate stratum is associated with the urinary tract. The outer stratum, as the transversalis fascia, covers the muscle surfaces within the body cavity. This thin fascia is intimately associated with the actual investing layer, or epimesium, of the internal surface of the muscles of the abdominal wall. It is continuous with the iliac and pelvic fascias inferiorly and the anterior lamella of the lumbodorsal fascia posteriorly.

The *retroperitoneal fascias* form the boundaries for the retroperitoneal spaces.

Gerota's fascia (renal fascia) is derived from the intermediate stratum of the retroperitoneal connective tissue, the stratum related to the urinary organs. The kidney and adjacent structures lie in the perirenal space between its anterior and posterior lamina. The *anterior lamina* of the renal fascia, a layer that includes the attached perirenal fat, covers the anterior surface of the kidney and adrenal. The *posterior lamina*, also derived from the intermediate stratum, covers the posterior aspects and is thicker than the anterior one.

Over the psoas major and quadratus lumborum, the posterior lamina becomes fused with the fascia of the outer stratum, represented by the transversalis fascia. In the midline, the posterior lamina is attached to the ventral surfaces of the vertebral bodies and to the anterior lamina of Gerota's fascia as the two lamina fuse and blend with the connective tissue around the aorta, the vena cava, and the renal artery and vein, as well as the tissue surrounding the autonomic nerves of the superior mesenteric plexus.

Laterally, behind the ascending and descending colon, the anterior and posterior laminas of Gerota's fascia fuse to make a single layer, the *lateroconal fascia*. It joins the properitoneal fascia (from the inner stratum) at the white line of Toldt.

The peritoneum on each side of the colonic mesentery fuses with the single layer of the primary retroperitoneum behind them to form a single layer, the colonic-peritoneal fusion-fascia. This fused layer meets the lateral parietal peritoneum and the fused lamina of the renal fascia (lateroconal fascia) at the white line of Toldt.

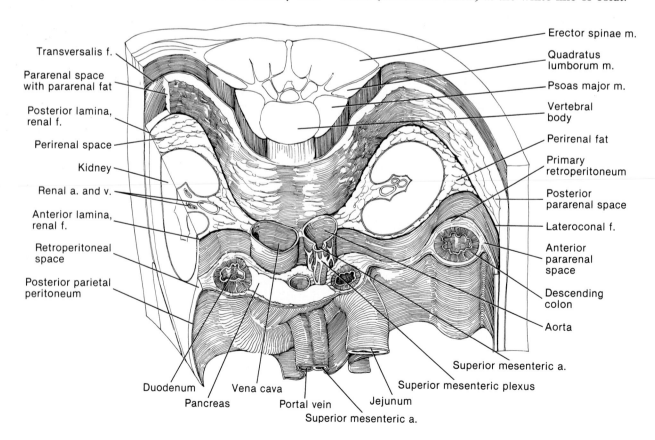

Labels (left side, top to bottom): Transversalis f.; Pararenal space with pararenal fat; Posterior lamina, renal f.; Perirenal space; Kidney; Renal a. and v.; Anterior lamina, renal f.; Retroperitoneal space; Posterior parietal peritoneum

Labels (bottom): Duodenum; Pancreas; Vena cava; Portal vein; Superior mesenteric a.; Jejunum; Superior mesenteric plexus; Superior mesenteric a.

Labels (right side, top to bottom): Erector spinae m.; Quadratus lumborum m.; Psoas major m.; Vertebral body; Perirenal fat; Primary retroperitoneum; Posterior pararenal space; Lateroconal f.; Anterior pararenal space; Descending colon; Aorta

Surgically, the single layer from the three-ply colonic-peritoneal fusion-fascia may be separated from the underlying anterior lamina of the renal fascia by blunt dissection to allow medial mobilization of the ascending or descending colon.

The fascias enclose the three *retroperitoneal spaces*: an anterior pararenal space, a perirenal space, and a posterior pararenal space.

The *anterior pararenal space* lies between the inner stratum, the layer associated with the posterior parietal peritoneum, and the anterior lamina of the renal fascia. It is limited superiorly by the adherence of the renal fascia to the inner stratum in the colic gutters but is continuous laterally with the properitoneal compartment. During surgery, this location is important because the plane of this space is followed medially from the white line of Toldt during mobilization of the colon to expose the kidney.

The *perirenal space* lies between the anterior and posterior laminas of the renal fascia and contains a kidney, adrenal, and ureter encased in fine areolar tissue and perirenal fat. The compartment is limited medially, laterally, and superiorly by fusion of the laminas of the renal fascia.

The *posterior pararenal space* separates the posterior lamina of the renal fascia from the transversalis fascia (from the outer stratum of the abdominal fascia). It is continuous with the properitoneal space in the flank and contains coarse fatty-areolar tissue, the pararenal fat.

Medially the posterior lamina of Gerota's fascia fuses with the transversalis fascia to close the pararenal space over the psoas major and quadratus lumborum. The line of fusion is encountered surgically as a dense band that usually must be divided sharply.

Table 1. Approaches to the Kidney

Anterior routes
　Anterior subcostal
　Pediatric extended anterior
　Anterior transverse
　Midline transperitoneal
　Paramedian
Lateral routes
　Subcostal
　Transcostal
　Supracostal
　Foley muscle-splitting
　Dorsal flap
　Thoracoabdominal
Posterior route
　Dorsal lumbotomy

APPROACHES TO THE KIDNEY (Table 1)

An *anterior transperitoneal route* is an excellent approach for major procedures on the kidney, ureter, and adrenal, especially in infants and young children with protuberant bellies. It provides maximal exposure and an opportunity to evaluate other intra-abdominal organs; it gives superior access to the renal vessels and better control of the great vessels should they be injured. The disadvantages are the limited access that is obtained in obese patients and the risk of generating intestinal adhesions. A wider access is gained from an *anterior subcostal incision* (for localized lesions) and even wider access from an *anterior transverse* (chevron) *incision* (ideal for excision of bilateral Wilms tumors and for neuroblastoma and pheochromocytoma). A *midline* (vertical) *incision* is useful for gastric augmentation procedures. In children, the costal margin is high, so it does not limit a direct approach to the kidneys through the midline as much as in an adult. For difficult upper abdominal urologic cases, a *bilateral subcostal incision with a cephalad T extension*, such as used for liver transplantation, can give maximal exposure, especially if a mechanical retraction system is used.

An *anterolateral extraperitoneal approach* through an *anterior subcostal incision* provides greater exposure in infants than it does in adults because of the wide costal flare and the more relaxed abdominal musculature. In debilitated children, a firm closure is assured because stress is distributed among the three fascial layers of the anterior abdominal wall. This approach induces fewer problems with ventilation than the standard flank incision, reduces postoperative pain, and allows earlier mobilization. The *pediatric extended anterior incision* benefits from its extension onto the anterior abdominal wall. It is a valuable incision for the removal of Wilms tumors.

An *extraperitoneal lateral subcostal approach* through a *subcostal* or *supracostal incision* has the advantage of reaching the kidney where it lies closest to the surface and is especially valuable in obese adolescents. If necessary for wider exposure for extensive surgery on the kidney, a lateral incision can be extended into a *thoracoabdominal incision* or converted into a *dorsal rib flap*. The disadvantages of these lateral incisions are the need to divide large muscles, the risk of injuring nerves, the need to make a relatively large incision, and the fact that the vascular pedicle lies on the opposite side of the kidney from the one exposed. In spite of these limitations, a lateral incision may be safer in neonates, even for bilateral pyeloplasties that require two flank incisions, in order to avoid the intestinal adhesions with resultant intestinal obstruction that are associated with a transabdominal transperitoneal approach.

A *lumbar approach* is ideal for more limited reconstructive operations. A *dorsal lumbotomy* avoids division of muscles and nerves and heals quickly with minimal pain. Although the exposure is limited, it provides the most direct approach to the ureteropelvic junction, and, because it avoids crossing muscles and nerves, it is followed by minimal postoperative discomfort and a quicker recovery.

Anterior Subcostal Incision

EXTRAPERITONEAL APPROACH

1 *Position:* Place the patient in the supine oblique position, with the buttocks flat and the shoulders turned up 30 to 40 degrees. For infants, place a folded towel under the sacroiliac joint; for adults, flex the table in addition to placing a sandbag behind the shoulders.

Incision: Start the incision in the midline anteriorly, one third of the distance from the xiphoid to the umbilicus (*dashed line*). End the incision on the left at the tip of the 11th rib, near the anterior axillary line. Curve it to avoid the costal margin.

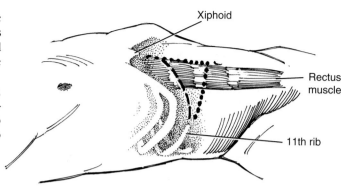

2 Divide the left side of the anterior rectus sheath and the external oblique muscles in the line of the incision for a short distance. If the rectus muscle must be divided, clamp, divide, and ligate the superior epigastric artery behind it.

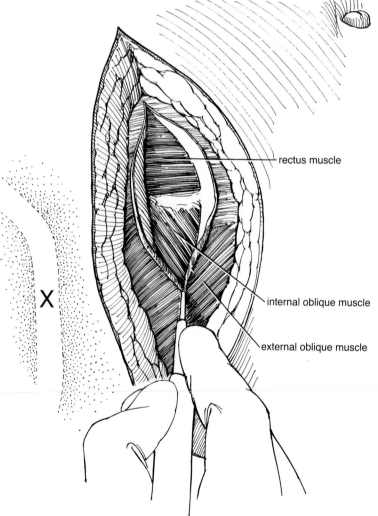

3 Divide or bluntly split the internal oblique, and digitally separate the fibers of the transversus abdominis, starting as far laterally as possible, where the peritoneum is less adherent. Incise the transversalis fascia and also its condensation at the lateral margin of the rectus muscle as the peritoneum is bluntly stripped down from the transversalis fascia covering the inferior portion of the anterior abdominal wall. Free the peritoneum superiorly as well.

For more exposure, divide some of the contralateral rectus sheath. Further exposure can be gained by extending the incision posteriorly as a flank incision or by cutting across both rectus muscles to open the peritoneum as a chevron incision (see page 865).

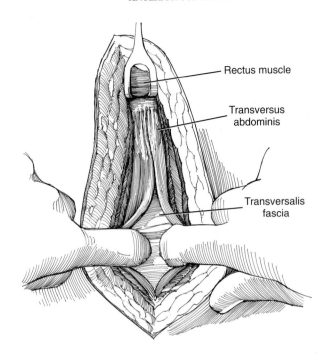

Rectus muscle

Transversus abdominis

Transversalis fascia

4 Use one hand to sweep far posteriorly to the lateral edge of the psoas muscle in the extraperitoneal space; then bluntly strip the peritoneum from the overlying muscle layer. The peritoneum is quite adherent there; use a peanut dissector or a sponge stick to avoid tearing it. Some sharp dissection with the scissors may be required. Make a transverse incision through the transversalis fascia as it passes behind and condenses with the posterior rectus sheath and a sagittal incision through it as it descends into the pelvis beneath the lower musculature, after separating the peritoneum from it medially. The limitations in exposure with the anterior incision are not primarily of muscular origin but originate with the transversalis fascia enveloping the peritoneum.

Free the peritoneum from the transversalis fascia for a distance of at least a few centimeters above and below the wound so that it may be mobilized anteriorly to expose the posterior lamina of Gerota's fascia.

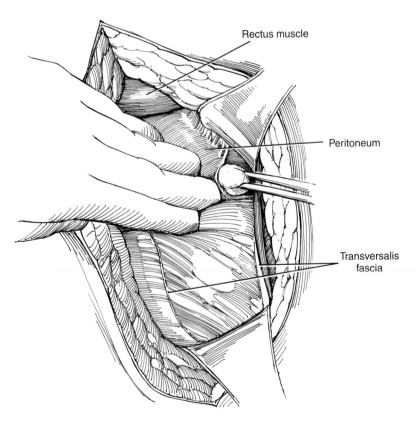

Rectus muscle

Peritoneum

Transversalis fascia

5 Enter Gerota's fascia over the lateral aspect of the kidney; reflect the fascia anteriorly.

6 **A,** Carry the peritoneum anteriorly with Gerota's fascia. Dissect the perirenal fat from the kidney so that the posterior portion remains behind the kidney to isolate it from the posterior body wall after repair. Expose the renal pelvis.

B, Dissect the anterior surface of the kidney and the renal pedicle. Proceed with the definitive operation.

Close the wound in layers after inserting a Penrose drain, which may be allowed to exit through the wound to permit escape of trapped air.

Intraoperative problems may arise with this incision if the upper pole is large or adherent, but initial control of the pedicle reduces the risks. Bleeding from an accessory vessel may require extension of the incision across the midline. Pressure of the retractor on the 10th and 11th intercostal nerves may produce temporary hypesthesia postoperatively.

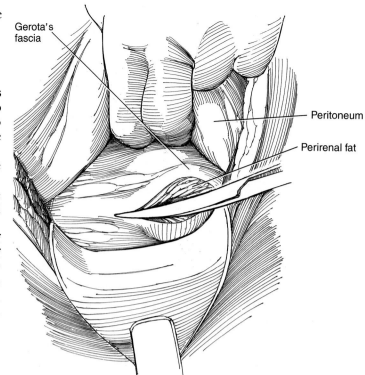

Gerota's fascia

Peritoneum

Perirenal fat

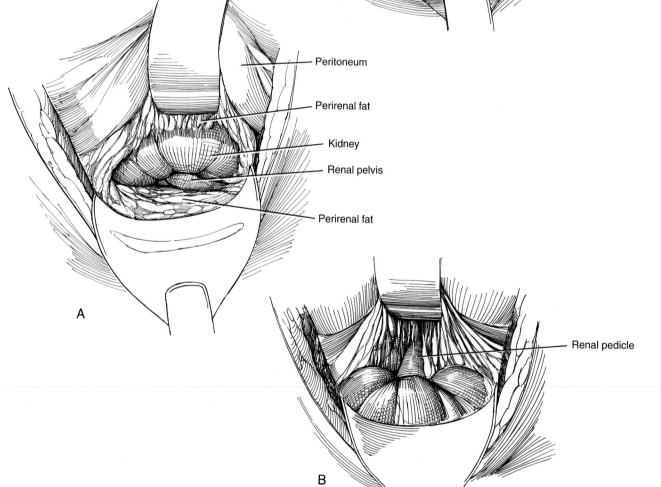

Peritoneum

Perirenal fat

Kidney

Renal pelvis

Perirenal fat

A

Renal pedicle

B

TRANSPERITONEAL APPROACH

7 Make the same subcostal incision described in Step 1 (*dashed line*); alternatively, form a flap as shown there by the dotted line. Bluntly separate the fibers of the internal oblique and transversus muscles, and expose the outer surface of the peritoneum. Divide the peritoneum in the line of the incision to expose the liver, the ascending colon, and the greater omentum covering the transverse colon.

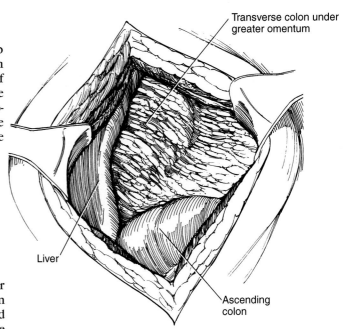

8 *Right kidney:* **A,** Use the *Kocher maneuver* for direct approach to the right renal hilum: Make an incision in the posterior peritoneum lateral to the second portion of the duodenum (*dashed line*). (Also see page 986.) This exposes the anterior surface of the vena cava, posterior to the portal vein and anterior to the renal vein.

B, Identify the right gonadal vein emptying anterolaterally into the vena cava, any accessory polar veins, and the large adrenal vein that enters posterolaterally 4 to 6 cm cephalad of the renal vein.

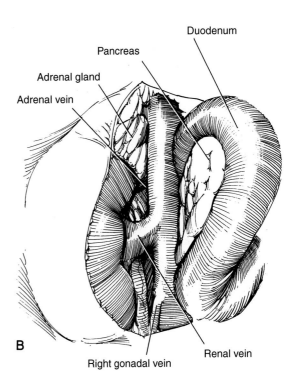

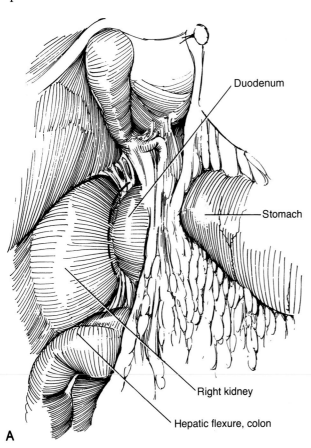

9 *Left kidney:* **A,** For approach to the left renal hilum, make a vertical incision in the posterior peritoneum just caudad to the ligament of Treitz beside the fourth portion of the duodenum, and expose the anterior surface of the aorta.

B, Identify the left renal vein as it crosses the aorta and the anterior-lying left gonadal artery, as well as the inferior mesenteric vein and artery.

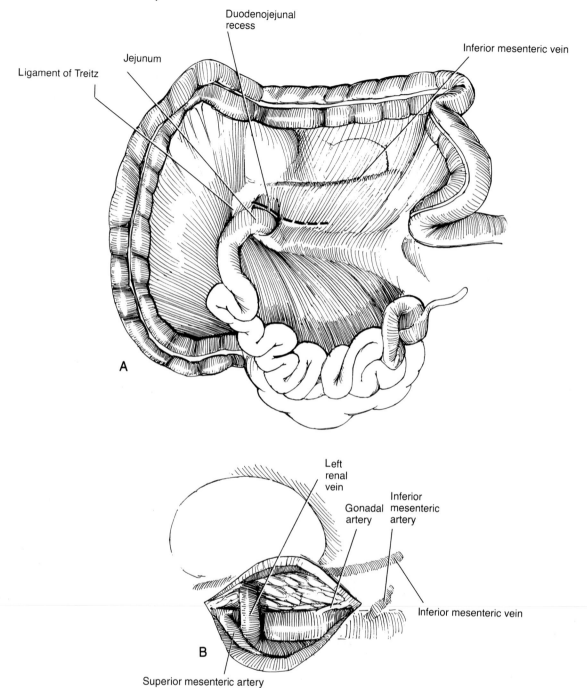

ANTERIOR APPROACH TO THE ADRENAL GLAND

10 **A,** *Position:* Semioblique. *Incision:* Anterior subcostal (Steps 1 to 6).

B, Divide the gastrocolic portion of the omentum to enter the sac anterior to the pancreas and behind the stomach.

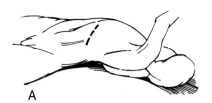

A

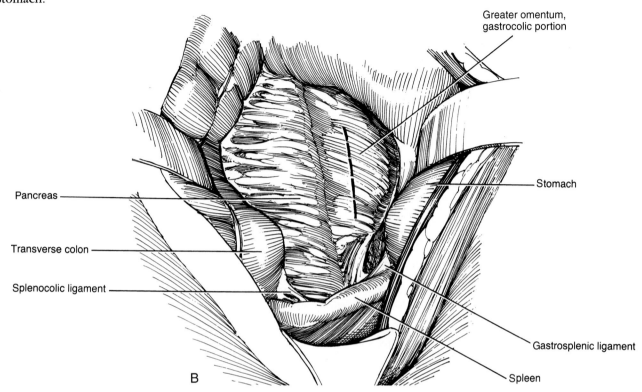

Greater omentum, gastrocolic portion

Stomach

Pancreas

Transverse colon

Splenocolic ligament

Gastrosplenic ligament

Spleen

B

11 Retract the transverse colon inferiorly, incise the retroperitoneum just below the pancreas, and continue to expose the left renal hilum by dividing the splenocolic and renocolic ligaments.

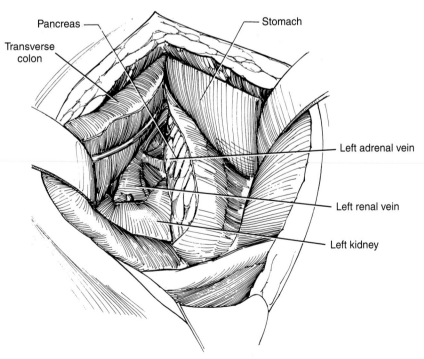

Pancreas

Stomach

Transverse colon

Left adrenal vein

Left renal vein

Left kidney

CLOSURE

Before closure, insert a drain if it is needed (it helps to drain trapped air and serum), and bring it out extraperitoneally through the wound or through a separate stab wound. With transperitoneal incisions, it is not essential that the peritoneum be reattached behind the colon. Place a running synthetic absorbable suture (SAS) to join the edges of the peritoneum and posterior rectus sheath. Approximate the transversalis and internal oblique muscles with interrupted SAS. Close the external oblique fascia and anterior rectus sheath similarly. Complete the closure of the subcutaneous layer and the skin.

Commentary by Michele Pavone-Macaluso

The anterior subcostal approach, widely used in general surgery (somewhat less so now since the advent of laparoscopic cholecystectomy), is relatively less familiar for the urologist. In my personal experience, the curvilinear anterior subcostal incision, as depicted in Figure 1, is generally used for an anterior extraperitoneal approach. For the anterior transperitoneal route to the kidney, I prefer a right-angle subcostal flap (dotted line in Figure 1).

The anterior extraperitoneal incision gives a relatively limited exposure, so it is best suited for pyeloplasty, pyelolithotomy, marsupialization of cysts, and simple nephrectomies. The indications for surgery for renal cysts and stones have drastically decreased in recent years, so the number of urologic operations using the anterior extraperitoneal approach has also decreased. The approach still offers some advantages in selected cases because the sacrifice of muscles and nerves is relatively small. The rectus can be spared and retracted medially in most cases, and the transverse muscle is separated along the direction of the fibers. This is often possible also for a portion of the internal oblique. Postoperative pain is usually less than after a lumbar approach.

Whenever a transperitoneal approach is to be selected, my technique differs. A right-angle flap is obtained by incising the linea alba vertically from the xiphoid to 1 cm above the umbilicus, with the addition of a transverse horizontal incision that starts medially from 0.5 to 1 cm lateral to the umbilicus and extends laterally almost to the tip of the 12th rib (dotted line in Figure 1). The rectus muscle is divided, and fibers of both oblique muscles and of the transversus abdominis must be sacrificed to a greater extent than with the curvilinear subcostal approach. However, the exposure is much greater, the flap is self-retracting, and reconstruction is easy. If the exposure is meticulously done, no postoperative hernias should occur.

The main indication for this wider approach is radical nephrectomy for renal cell carcinoma, with or without regional lymphadenectomy. It is very useful also in other conditions for which a primary approach to the vessels of the renal hilus is needed, such as a difficult nephrectomy in a previously operated kidney.

For a better visualization of the left hilar vessels, I prefer to divide the ligament of Treitz. The inferior mesenteric vein may also be divided if necessary. The transmesocolic approach, with opening of the lesser sac, is seldom required unless the left renal artery is located too high or it is double, with a branch to the upper pole. This approach can also be used to reach the left adrenal gland, but this is seldom necessary. Many authors encourage a wider use of either a laparoscopic or a mini-invasive retroperitoneal approach for adrenal surgery.

Whenever the transperitoneal route, particularly the transmesocolic approach, to the left kidney is adopted, great care must be taken to avoid injury to the tail of the pancreas. *Caution:* Check the position of the retractors, pad them with moist sponges, and avoid forceful traction.

Ligate the renal artery before the vein whenever possible, on either side. The right renal artery can be ligated in the aortocaval space. This is especially useful when regional lymphadenectomy is performed because access to this space must be obtained anyway. In this way, excessive manipulation of the short right renal vein can be avoided during the preliminary isolation of the artery (which lies posterior to the vein), carrying the risk of tears or laceration in the renal vein itself or in the vena cava.

TRANSVERSE "S" LAPAROTOMY
(Srougi)

With the patient semioblique and hyperextended, make a transverse (chevron) incision, and inspect the abdomen before proceeding. Continue the incision along the 11th costal interspace to the posterior axillary line as for a 12th-rib supracostal incision (see page 879), mobilizing the diaphragm and pleura as needed in the posterior aspect. Close the peritoneum with a running SAS, and approximate the external surface of the internal and external oblique muscles, as well as the rectus sheath, with interrupted 1-0 nylon.

BILATERAL SUBCOSTAL INCISION WITH T EXTENSION
(Marsh-Lange)

For adrenal malignancies and large renal cell carcinomas, adaptation of the incision developed for liver transplantation and organ procurement provides an expanded exposure.

Position: Place the patient supine with arms extended. Attach the bar of an Oliver retractor 4 inches above the level of the patient's chin.

Incision: Make a bilateral subcostal incision two fingerbreadths below the costal margin and extended to the midaxillary line on the involed side. Extend the incision up the xiphoid. Enter the abdomen in the midline, and extend the incision with the electrocautery. Insert the blades of the Oliver retractor, and fasten the chains to the previously placed bar to elevate the thoracic cage. In addition, attach the upper arm of an Iron Interne retractor system to the table below the arm board, and fasten the lower arm to the table above the level of the groin.

Pediatric Extended Anterior Incision

This incision allows early access to the renal pedicle and retroperitoneal nodes and provides excellent exposure for excision of Wilms tumor. It can also be used for simultaneous bilateral pyeloplasty, although two subcostal incisions may be just as easy to make and offer fewer complications. Moreover, dividing the rectus muscle results in a long-term abdominal deformity and scar.

1 *Position:* Place the child in a 30-degree oblique position with the lumbar spine over the break in the table. Place small wedges or bolsters (rolled towels, padded sandbags, or gel pads) under the left thorax at the shoulder and under the buttock, and place a larger pad under the loin. The loin pad should be accessible to the circulating nurse for removal at the time of closure. Bend the elbow approximately 90 degrees, and suspend the forearm from the anesthesia screen to avoid stretch injury to the brachial plexus. Hyperextend the table if necessary to accentuate the renal area; raising the kidney rest may improve the position.

For bilateral tumors or for concurrent pyeloplasty, place the child flat and hyperextended at the loin.

Incision: Make a long transverse incision above the umbilicus, ending at the tip of the 12th rib on the involved side. For large tumors, make the incision higher so that it extends through the 11th or 10th intercostal space, or consider a thoracoabdominal approach (see page 890).

2 Divide the anterior rectus sheath and both rectus abdominis muscles. (In neonates and infants, each muscle layer can be separated bluntly, as in the Foley incision; see page 885.) Divide and ligate the superior epigastric vessels. After opening the posterior rectus sheath, insert two fingers under the body wall, and divide all layers with the cutting current as far back as the tip of the 12th rib and extending forward beyond the linea semicircularis of the rectus sheath. If the pleura is entered during posterior extension of the incision, aspirate the air from the pleural cavity with a small catheter at the time of closure, and suture the pleura closed (see page 902). Open the peritoneum, and contain the bowel with packs. Divide the falciform ligament above.

Assess operability by palpating and visualizing the para-aortic nodes, the liver, and the spleen and by looking for any direct tumor invasion into adjacent structures.

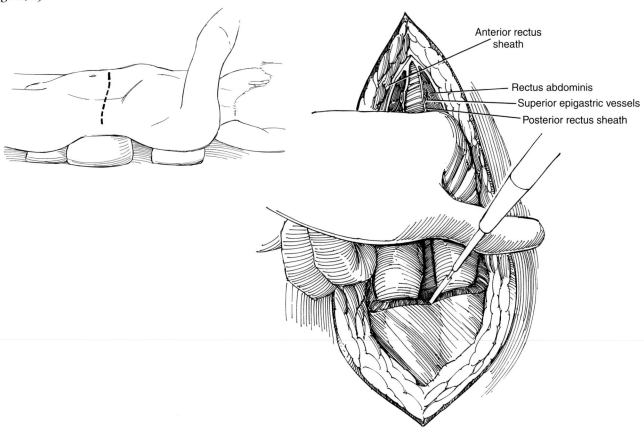

Anterior rectus sheath

Rectus abdominis
Superior epigastric vessels
Posterior rectus sheath

3 To gain access to the aorta through an incision in the retroperitoneum, displace the small bowel toward the opposite side, and have your assistant hold the descending colon medially. Incise along the white line of Toldt to free the colon; then divide its attachments to the spleen on the left (or to the liver and gallbladder on the right). Gingerly dissect the colonic mesentery from the surface of Gerota's fascia over the tumor, taking care to preserve the colonic blood supply within it. For tumors on the right side, a Kocher maneuver permits dissection of the duodenum and pancreas from the anterior aspect of the kidney (see page 986).

Identify the aorta and vena cava. Right-sided tumors may compress and displace the inferior vena cava, and in its collapsed state it is very easily divided and removed with the specimen. On the left side, avoid injury to the pancreas and superior mesenteric artery when dissecting the mesentery medially to gain reach to the renal pedicle. In addition, because the renal vessels may be displaced and distorted with large tumors, make positive identification of the artery and vein to the *opposite* kidney. If in doubt, place vascular tapes around the respective vessels.

It is good practice before closing to open Gerota's fascia on the opposite side and expose the kidney to look for tumor involvement.

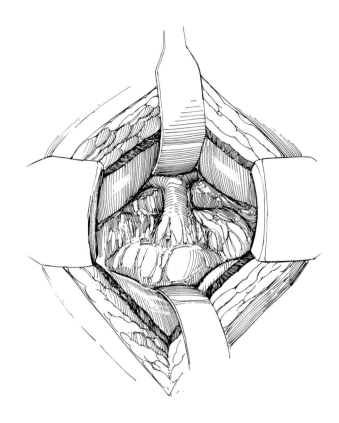

Commentary by Alan D. Perlmutter

When you are planning an extended anterior incision, the most important consideration is hyperextension of the loin area in all cases. This maneuver elevates the renal area to maximize exposure of and access to the hilar structures. The decision to place the trunk in an oblique position and the degree of obliquity (not more than 30 degrees of elevation, and generally less or flat) should be part of the surgical strategy. For known bilateral tumors, the trunk should be flat or minimally oblique, with the larger tumor on the elevated side. Hyperextension can be achieved more conveniently and precisely with the use of a bolster under the loin, such as a rolled towel, padded sandbag, or gel pad, than with hyperextension of the table top. When obliquity of the trunk is also required, place narrower pads under the ipsilateral chest and shoulder above and buttock below. In the oblique position, the ipsilateral upper extremity should not be abducted but should be elevated with the elbow bent and suspended by the forearm from the anesthesia screen. This protects the brachial plexus from stretch injury.

In infants and younger children it is unnecessary to use a chevron incision; a straight, transverse incision curving slightly cephalad laterally to above the tip of the 12th rib generally provides excellent exposure and can be readily extended into the 11th interspace for additional room. For a small tumor, particularly in the younger child, the incision can be directed slightly caudad as it is brought medially. In this circumstance, only the ipsilateral rectus need be divided. If the exposure proves to be inadequate, the incision can be enlarged by dividing the contralateral rectus muscle partially or completely, with or without division of the contralateral parietal muscle layers as needed.

It is not uncommon to encounter a large Wilms tumor crossing the midline and obscuring access to the great vessels and hilar structures. In this instance, an oblique positioning of the patient may actually make exposure of these structures more difficult. An early approach to the aorta, vena cava, and hilar vessels in the presence of limited exposure is contraindicated because of the risk of a tear or avulsion, particularly to the venous system. The dissection should begin peripherally to achieve sufficient renal mobility to help expose the hilum. If exposure is still not adequate, a lateral extension of the incision into the 11th or 10th interspace with splitting of the diaphragm should allow gentle lateral displacement of the tumor sufficient to expose the hilum. Generally, I have not found it necessary to place vascular tapes around the aorta or vena cava even in difficult cases; they increase the risk of vascular perforation or tear, particularly to the dorsum of the cava.

The extended anterior incision with its transverse axis provides excellent exposure of the epigastric structures and should be the procedure of choice for major renal surgery in infants and children. The vertical midline laparotomy incision is more limiting.

For bilateral, concurrent pyeloplasty, I do not favor an extended anterior incision with wide transperitoneal exposure of the pelves. Small bilateral subcostal incisions allow excellent exposure for pyeloplasties, usually accomplished without opening the peritoneum or, if needed, with only a small lateral opening to improve exposure. The peritoneum should not be violated unnecessarily, particularly in infancy, because of the risk of later symptomatic intestinal adhesions.

Anterior Transverse (Chevron) Incision

As an extension of an anterior subcostal incision across the midline, the anterior transverse (chevron) incision provides excellent bilateral exposure of the upper portion of the retroperitoneum. For removal of a large renal or adrenal mass on the left side, the incision provides more exposure for dividing the splenocolic ligament to avoid injury to the spleen. Avulsion of the right adrenal vein from the vena cava is avoided by the improved access. The exposure allows the caudate lobe of the liver to be lifted from the vena cava to allow safe division of the small hepatic veins. The incision is most valuable when access to both sides of the retroperitoneum is required for left renal neoplasms invading the vena cava, for bilateral renal or adrenal tumors, and for large residual abdominal masses remaining after chemotherapy for metastatic testis tumor.

Convert the incision to a thoracoabdominal approach by extending either limb upward below the 11th rib and dividing the diaphragm to expose intrathoracic extension of neoplasms. Or form a wide V incision by splitting the sternum at the apex; this approach allows pursuit of renal cancer with caval involvement extending to the suprahepatic level.

1 *Position:* Place the patient in a supine position, hyperextended over a folded towel or a break in the table.

Incision: From the tip of the 11th rib, incise the skin toward the midline below the costal margin to just below the xiphoid process. Continue down the opposite side to the tip of the opposite 11th rib (*dashed line*). If you are uncertain about operability or the need for such an extensive incision, make only half of it first. The dotted line shows the equivalent pararectus incision.

2 After incising the subcutaneous tissue, divide both sides of the anterior rectus sheath. Insinuate a finger under the rectus muscle (not shown), and divide it with the cutting current. Ligate the superior epigastric artery as it is encountered.

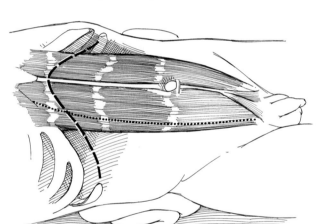

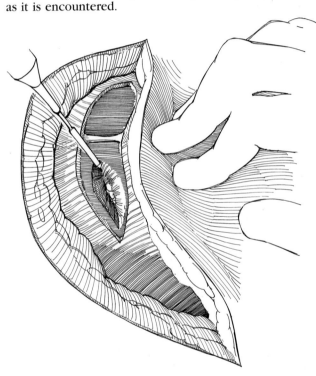

3 Divide the investing fascia and muscles of the external and internal oblique muscles and split the fibers of the transversus abdominis muscle. Incise the transversalis fascia and peritoneum, and enter the peritoneal cavity just lateral to the posterior rectus sheath.

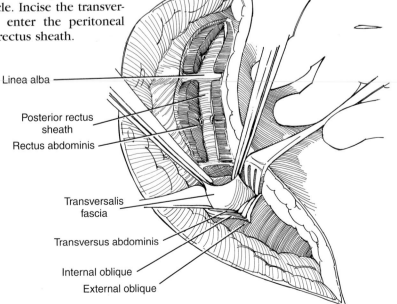

Linea alba

Posterior rectus sheath

Rectus abdominis

Transversalis fascia

Transversus abdominis

Internal oblique

External oblique

865

4 Complete the incision with cutting current or scissors against one or two fingers inside the abdomen. Divide the round ligament of the liver between clamps, and ligate each end.

5 *Closure:* Remove the towel from under the back, and straighten the table if flexed. Reapproximate the round ligament of the liver. Place three heavy sutures through the skin and linea alba at the apex of the incision to secure the linea alba in the midline; tie them when the rest of the closure is completed. Close the peritoneum, transversalis fascia, posterior rectus sheath, and linea alba in one layer with a running suture. Approximate the internal and external oblique muscles and the anterior rectus sheath individually with interrupted stitches of the same material. Alternatively, all fascial and muscular layers may be quickly closed with a Prolene running suture. Close the subcutaneous tissue and skin, and tie the three midline retention sutures over bolsters.

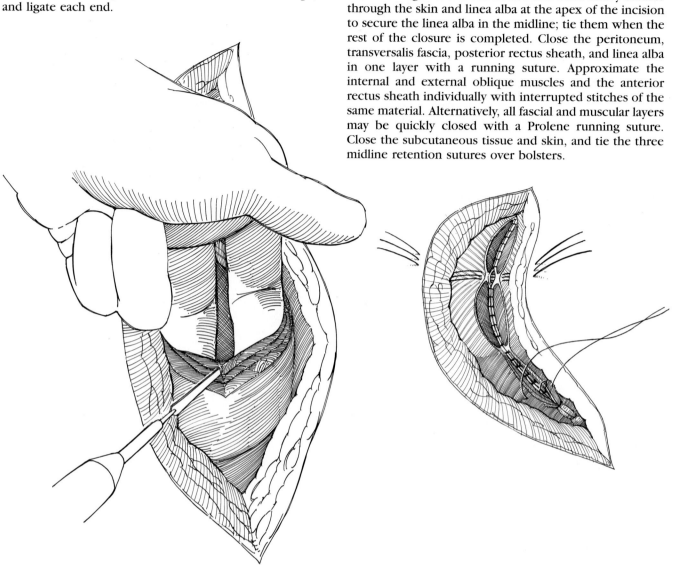

Commentary by Thomas P. Ball, Jr.

The subcostal incision, particularly with hyperextension, is one of my favorites. It provides excellent exposure for most retroperitoneal tumors and adrenal masses with less postoperative discomfort than is usually experienced with a thoracoabdominal incision. I still prefer to cut the subcutaneous fat, rectus, and oblique muscles sharply, using the cautery selectively on bleeders rather than cutting with the cautery because I believe that cleanly cut tissues heal better than burned tissues—certainly better than when the coagulating current is used for cutting. We have seen seroma formation and muscle separation when heavy cautery has been used, presumably because muscle burns respond like any other third-degree burn and the suture line sloughs to some degree.

The closure described is excellent. My preference for approximation of the muscles and rectus sheath is to use figure-eight interrupted sutures because they are less likely to tear through the muscle and fascia than are simple interrupted sutures. Placing the midline "retention" sutures at the initiation of the closure is a good technique, particularly for the fat or very muscular individual.

Midline Transperitoneal Incision

1 *Position:* Place the patient supine with a rolled towel under the side of the lesion.

Incision: Make an incision in the midline from the xiphoid to just below the umbilicus (*dashed line*). For greater exposure, continue the incision to the symphysis (*dotted line*).

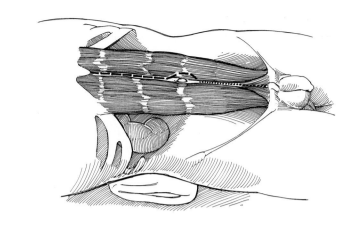

2 Divide the subcutaneous tissue with the cutting current, and identify the fine decussations of the fused aponeuroses of the muscles of the anterior abdominal wall that form the linea alba. The rectus sheath is covered with a delicate investment that may be opened to be certain of the position of the midline.

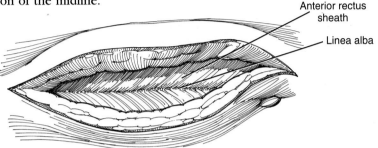

Anterior rectus sheath

Linea alba

3 **A** and **B,** Incise through the linea alba into the loose properitoneal fat covering the peritoneum. Successively elevate the areolar tissue and fat with forceps in one hand, and have your assistant tent the peritoneum with a second forceps. Incise the properitoneal tissue carefully between them, taking care with each grasp not to include any bowel.

C, After three or four such maneuvers, the peritoneum itself is tented up. As it is penetrated with the knife, air enters and the bowel falls away.

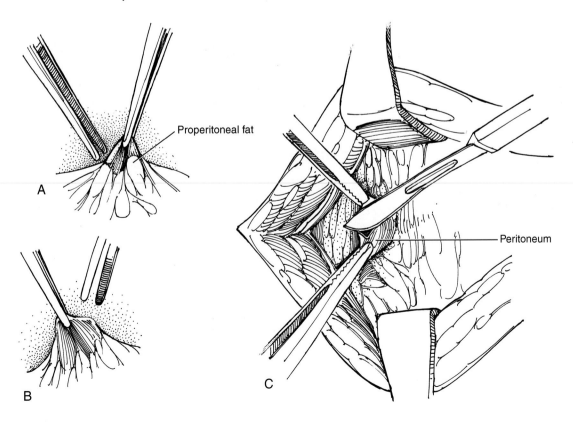

Properitoneal fat

Peritoneum

A

B

C

4 Hold each edge of the peritoneum in a curved clamp, and open it in both directions with curved scissors while protecting the abdominal contents with two fingers of the left hand. Divide and ligate the ligamentum teres.

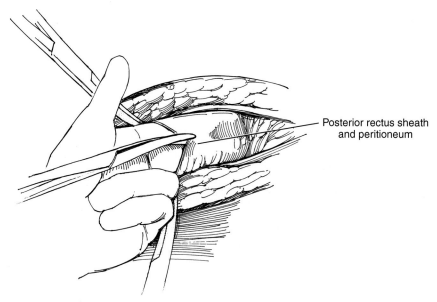

Posterior rectus sheath
and peritoneum

CLOSURE

Tie a length of #2 monofilament suture (Prolene, Novafil, or nylon) with six or seven knots at the xiphoid end of the incision. In thin patients, be sure to bury the knot under the subcutaneous tissue to avoid a chronic sinus. Run the suture continuously to the other end of the wound, catching only the fascia and ignoring the peritoneum. Tie that end securely. For greater safety, use three such sutures, each closing one third of the wound. *Alternatively*, close the peritoneum with a running SAS; then close the fascia with interrupted SAS, either as simple sutures or as figure-eight sutures. Sutures are spaced by the standard rule of 1 cm apart and 1 cm back from the edge.

Approximate the subcutaneous tissue with fine SAS, and close the skin with a fine absorbable subcuticular suture, with fine skin clips, or with removable sutures placed as end-on mattress stitches to elevate the skin edges.

Patients susceptible to wound disruption require special attention. Place figure-eight interrupted nonabsorbable stitches (Prolene) incorporating all layers, including the peritoneum where it can be grasped. These sutures must be tied square with multiple knots to prevent slipping, and the knots must be placed so that they do not protrude under the skin.

POSTOPERATIVE PROBLEMS

Abdominal dehiscence may be a complication of any major abdominal operation; it is heralded by (pink) discharge from the wound, an indication that intestines are lying subcutaneously. Hold the wound with tape, or, if bowel is apparent, cover it with a sterile towel. Place a nasogastric tube, and start intravenous fluids. In the operating room, with anesthesia, rinse each intestinal loop with saline solution and replace it in the abdominal cavity. Wash the omentum and cover the replaced bowel with it. Place through-and-through sutures of braided nylon, and thread a length of red rubber catheter on each before tying. Start antibiotics.

Commentary by John P. Hopewell

This is a clear and satisfactory account of a standard incision. When tissues are thin and when postoperative distension is a possibility, I have been more confident with a paramedian vertical transrectal incision. This incision is made about 1 cm lateral to the medial border of the rectus muscle and affords some reliable tissue to hold the sutures during repair. It appears to have no deleterious effect on the later strength of the rectus muscle. One more point was made to me by the late Sir Denis Browne at the Hospital for Sick Children in London. On opening the peritoneum, leave only one forceps to pick it up: If bowel is unfortunately included in its grasp, it falls away from the knife. This incision was most valuable when more laparotomies were exploratory in nature, but it still has much to commend it today.

Paramedian Incision

Access may be obtained to all four quadrants of the abdomen through either this or the midline incision, allowing major vascular and post-trauma reconstruction. It may be used for bilateral retroperitoneal lymphadenectomy and for major undiversion procedures. It is easy to open and close, but special precautions are need to prevent dehiscence. Any transperitoneal incision may be associated with a high incidence of postoperative bowel adhesions.

Whether the paramedian incision is stronger than one made in the midline is questionable because the midline incision may be closed in one layer with heavy sutures. The rectus-retracting incision described here aims to keep the rectus abdominis muscle intact, but it does disturb the blood supply where it enters the muscle at the tendinous intersections. An alternative is to split the rectus and retract the halves.

1 *Position:* Supine. *Incision:* The incision extends from the xiphoid to below the umbilicus for nephrectomy or to the symphysis pubis for renovascular operations. Place the skin incision 3 cm from the midline.

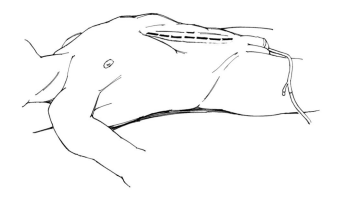

2 Incise the rectus sheath 3 cm to the right of the midline. Free the anterior surface of the rectus muscle from the sheath by retracting with clamps. Cut sharply at the tendinous insertions.

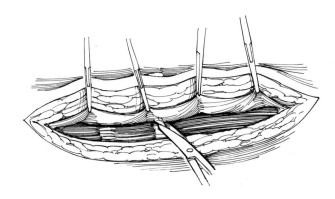

3 Insert U.S. Army retractors, and free the medial and lower surfaces of the muscle, taking care to preserve the intrinsic blood vessels and nerves.

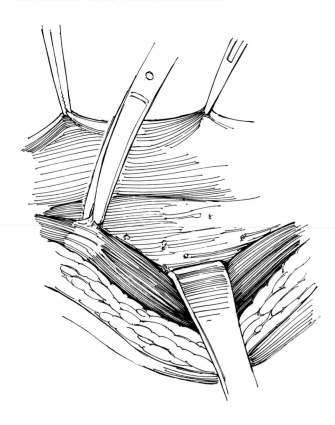

4 Divide the posterior rectus sheath; then open the peritoneum by carefully lifting it with two pairs of smooth forceps on either side and cutting into the tented area.

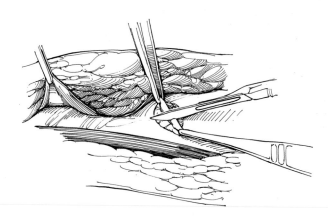

5 Insert two fingers, and divide both structures to both ends of the incision. Proceed with the intra-abdominal operation.

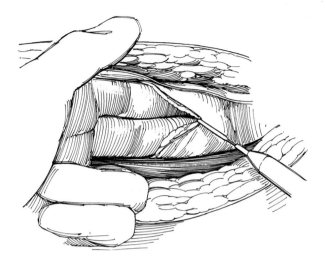

6 Close the peritoneum and posterior sheath in one layer with a heavy running absorbable or nonabsorbable suture. Close the anterior sheath with interrupted sutures of the same material. Retention sutures may be needed in poor-risk patients.

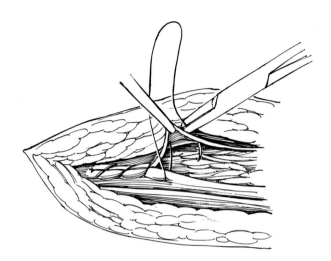

Commentary by J. Warwick F. Macky

Both the paramedian and abdominal incisions give adequate access to the four quadrants of the abdomen for most radical resections and for renovascular and urinary diversion/undiversion procedures. The midline abdominal incision may be used to extend a thoracic sternum-splitting incision. In general, the midline incision is probably most used by urologists, whereas the paramedian may be favored by general surgeons. There is no place for the pararectal incision—the "baleful battle" described by Sir Heneage Ogilvie. The midline incision offers speedy opening and closing, which may be significant in prolonged operations. In principle, the paramedian incision offers minimal interference with tissue planes and with the rectus abdominis and increased security of closure. Muscle splitting should be avoided as much as possible.

Subcostal Incision

A subcostal incision provides limited access and requires almost as much effort to make as a supracostal incision. It may be used for placement of a permanent nephrostomy, for drainage of a perinephric abscess, or for a pyeloplasty in the presence of an extrarenal pelvis. It may be useful for removal of stones from the upper ureter, although the Foley incision (see page 885) or the lumbotomy approach (see page 896) may be better. Other incisions are more suitable for access to the renal pedicle. The availability of percutaneous methods has decreased the use of open approaches to the kidney.

1 **A,** By drawing a horizontal line on the urogram from the lateral border of the rib cage, access can be evaluated because only structures below that line can be adequately exposed. Note the angle of the rib to the xiphisternum; if it is sharp, access may be limited. Kyphosis also may make renal access impossible by this route; a rib resection or supracostal incision is then required.

B, *Position:* Place the patient in the classical flank position (as shown), with the dependent 12th rib directly over the kidney lift. For children, use a rolled towel instead. Elevate the kidney lift in conjunction with table flexion to place tension on the muscles of the flank. Watch for hypotension from poor venous return, mediastinal shift, and displacement of the liver. Fix the patient in position with broad tape extending from the table top anteriorly, over the hip, and to the table top posteriorly, placed after the table has been flexed.

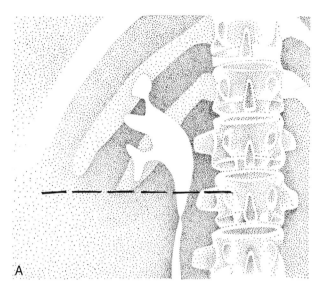

A

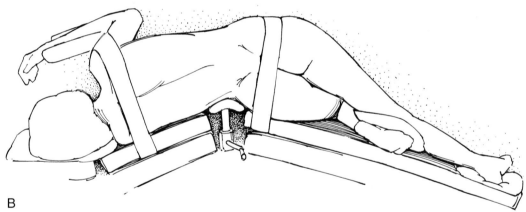

B

2 *Incision:* Start the incision at the lateral border of the sacrospinalis muscle, 1 cm below the lower edge of the 12th rib. Follow the lower border of the rib anteriorly, curving the incision caudally as it crosses the anterior abdominal wall to avoid the subcostal nerve. Avoid extending it very far caudally until you are sure that access to the pedicle is not needed. End it no farther than the lateral border of the rectus sheath. With a rudimentary 12th rib, place the incision well below the 11th rib.

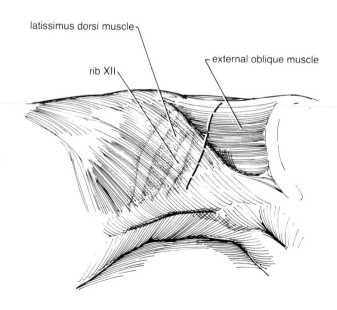

3 Incise the latissimus dorsi and serratus posterior inferior muscles, cutting back from their anterior free borders. Use the cutting current to minimize blood loss and trauma to the tissue secondary to application of multiple clamps and ligatures.

4 Incise the external and internal oblique muscles starting at their posterior free border, and incise the serratus posterior inferior muscle. Watch for the 12th intercostal neurovascular bundle that lies between the internal oblique and transversus abdominis muscles. It is necessary to free it and push it upward. Divide and ligate the small intercostal veins accompanying it.

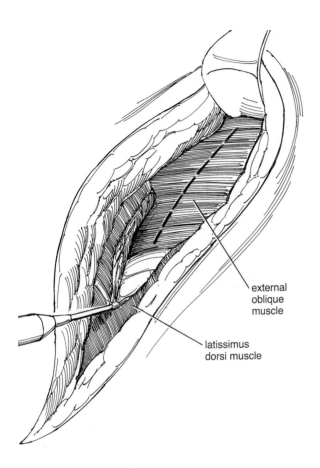

external oblique muscle

latissimus dorsi muscle

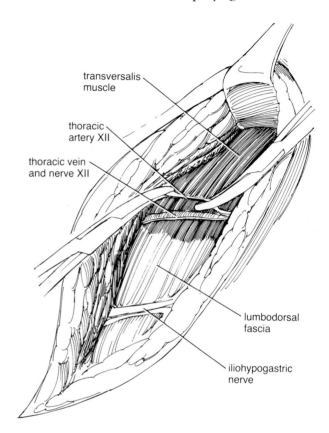

transversalis muscle

thoracic artery XII

thoracic vein and nerve XII

lumbodorsal fascia

iliohypogastric nerve

5 Identify the firm white lumbodorsal fascia, and incise it in the middle of the incision. This allows insertion of two fingers to push the peritoneum forward before completing the incision through the muscle and thus avoids cutting into it. The fingers also aid hemostasis. Sharply cut the fascia to its junction with the anterior musculature. Incise and digitally split the transversus abdominis to expose the retroperitoneal fat and peritoneum, which can be bluntly dissected and pushed anteriorly.

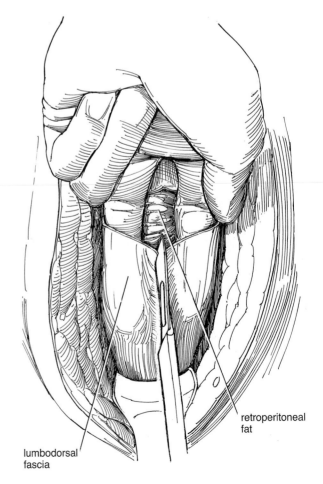

lumbodorsal fascia

retroperitoneal fat

6 Incise the posterior layer of the lumbodorsal fascia, working back from the anterior border of the sacrospinalis muscle, along with a few fibers of the serratus posterior inferior muscle. Divide the sacrospinalis muscle with the cutting current so that the costotransverse ligament is exposed.

7 Elevate the rib, and cut the costotransverse (costovertebral) ligament with partially opened Mayo scissors, advanced curved side down to avoid cutting the intercostal artery or entering the pleura, which lies beyond the tip of the transverse process. Free the subcostal nerve further, and move it superiorly. Insert a self-retaining retractor, and proceed with entry into Gerota's fascia.

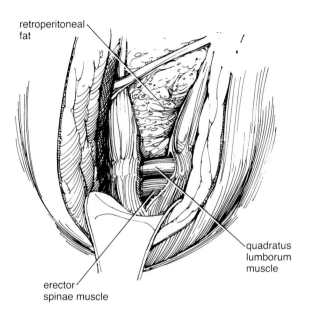

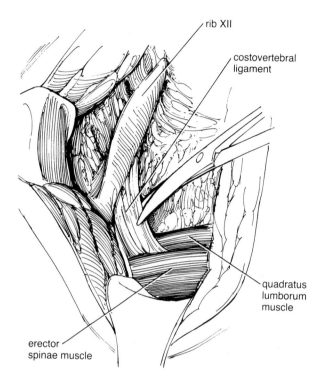

Extension of the Incision. If, after reaching the kidney, exposure is insufficient because the kidney lesion lies higher than anticipated, make a costal extension to allow surgical control, as is done for a dorsal flap procedure (see page 887). Do this by lifting the deep margin of the intercostal muscle at the angle of the rib. Elevate the serratus posterior inferior fibers attached to the lower edge of the 12th rib. Bluntly and sharply expose the periosteum of the rib. Incise the periosteum, and scrape and strip it from the rib for a short distance. Resect 2 cm of the rib. Divide the diaphragm close to the body wall with Metzenbaum scissors. Swing the anterior rib segment over the upper rib, and hold it there with a retractor.

Wound Closure

8 Lower the kidney rest, and partially flatten the table top. Completely flatten it after the first layers of sutures have been placed and tied. Have the assistant pull the shoulder back if it has fallen forward. (Note that rotation of hips and shoulders in opposite directions opens or closes flank incisions.) Insert a Penrose or suction drain to exit through a stab wound, and place an infant feeding tube to supply bupivacaine analgesia postoperatively. Start anteriorly to close the transversus abdominis and internal oblique muscles in one layer with interrupted 2-0 SAS. Alternatively, close the flimsy transversus muscle first. Work posteriorly, and close the lumbodorsal fascia by approximating the aponeurotic portion of the transversus abdominis muscle and the posterior layer of the lumbodorsal fascia. Approximate the external oblique muscle, beginning anteriorly, and the serratus posterior inferior and latissimus dorsi muscles, beginning posteriorly, with interrupted 2-0 SAS. Close the skin.

Alternative: To allow observation of the kidney bed for any oozing during closure and to make suture placement easier, insert figure-eight sutures through all layers and clamp the ends. Then lower the lift and tie the sutures in sequence.

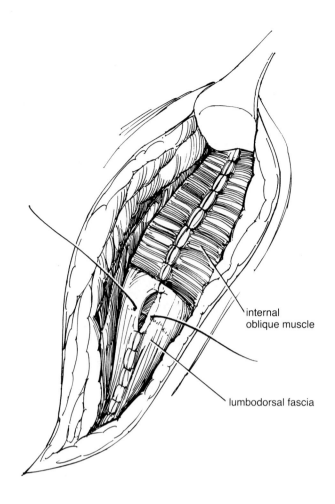

internal
oblique muscle

lumbodorsal fascia

POSTOPERATIVE PROBLEMS

In addition to the problems common to all approaches to the kidney, *hernia* may be encountered. Usually the appearance of hernia is musculofascial sagging from denervation.

Commentary by Peter A. Harbison

The subcostal approach to the kidney is rarely used nowadays because removal of calculi, for which it was very satisfactory, is usually performed by percutaneous or shock-wave therapy. In renal surgery, one can never be sure that access to the renal pedicle will not be required; this uncertainty, in my view, is its chief disadvantage. Even in stone surgery, exposure may be inadequate, especially if the stone slips into the renal pelvis or, worse still, into a calyx and requires extensive mobilization or radiography of the exposed kidney.

The technique of exposure is well described, but I have found that many of the fibers of the internal oblique muscle can be separated longitudinally without extensive incision, as can be done with the tranversalis muscle. In all cases, preserva-

tion of the subcostal nerve is essential because damage often results in areas of skin anesthesia, unsightly asymmetric bulging of the flank, and occasional hernia. Care must also be taken in closing the wound to see that the nerve is not included in sutures.

Closure must be meticulous in layers; layered closure is preferable to all-layer sutures. For drainage, I prefer a closed-tube system through a stab incision placed sufficiently anterior to avoid both kinking of the tube when the patient lies back and the pain associated with lying on the tube.

Most of my problems over many years of renal surgery have been due to inadequate exposure, and thus I believe that this approach has limited indications.

Transcostal Incision

When functioning renal tissue is to be retained and drainage or infection is anticipated, a lateral retroperitoneal incision may be appropriate. The choice of a subcostal, transcostal, or supracostal incision depends on the position of the kidney, the location of the lesion in the kidney, previous surgical incisions in the flank, and the experience and preferences of the surgeon.

The transcostal incision approaches the upper retroperitoneum through the bed of the 12th rib. It may be used for simple or partial nephrectomy and for simple adrenalectomy, although an 11th- or 12th-rib supracostal incision is easier to make and gives equal or better exposure.

Instruments: The special rib instruments used by thoracic surgeons are necessary: Snyder and Alexander periosteal elevators, Matson and Doyen rib strippers, guillotine rib cutter, and rongeurs, as well as a self-retaining retractor.

1 *Position:* Place the patient in the flank position (see page 871) over the break in the table and the kidney rest. Palpate the 12th (and 11th) ribs, and scratch the skin vertically in several places along the course of the 12th rib to guide the incision and to help align the skin at the time of closure.

A, Incise the skin starting at the margin of the erector spinae muscles, running obliquely forward following the line of the 12th rib, and ending at the lateral border of the rectus abdominis. If the rib cannot be felt through a thick body wall, estimate its site, and cut through enough of the subcutaneous tissue that it can be palpated before you divide fascia and muscle.

B, Once the rib can be felt, divide the external oblique muscle and the latissimus dorsi muscle directly over its center line with the electrosurgical blade to expose its periosteal surface. Incise the periosteum sharply with a knife blade.

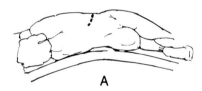

A

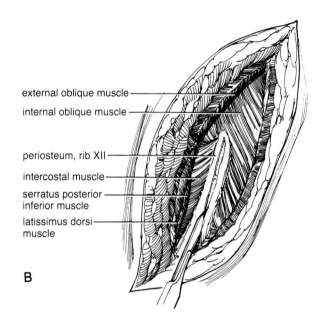

external oblique muscle
internal oblique muscle
periosteum, rib XII
intercostal muscle
serratus posterior inferior muscle
latissimus dorsi muscle

B

2 **A,** Scrape the periosteum from the rib with the chisel end of the Alexander periosteal elevator, beginning at the junction with the neck. Use small strokes to free it from the convex surface of the rib, and then free the upper and lower edges. A dry sponge may also be used to strip back muscle and periosteum. Finally, run the elevator along both edges at an angle to free the periosteum under them.

B, The curved blades on the other end of the Alexander elevator are useful here to free the periosteum from the edges of the rib.

C, Because of the angle of attachment of the intercostal muscles, push the Matson rib stripper anteriorly on the upper edge of the rib and posteriorly on the lower.

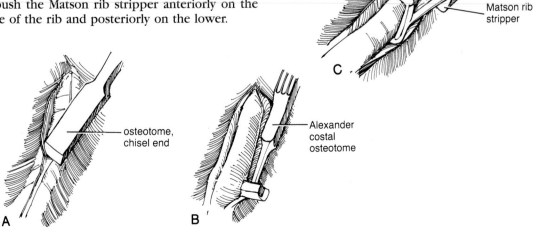

osteotome, chisel end

Alexander costal osteotome

Matson rib stripper

A   B   C

3 Insinuate the Doyen rib stripper under the rib inside the periosteum. Lift up on the shaft, and pull back along the undersurface to the angle of the rib. Depress the handle and push forward to the tip of the rib, thus using each of the cutting edges effectively.

Alternative: The rib may be excised extraperiosteally, not by incising and freeing the periosteum but by proceeding directly to inserting the Doyen rib stripper superficial to the transversalis fascia and forcibly separating the rib from the muscles and fascia that insert in the rib. This cannot be done as cleanly and easily as removing the rib subperiosteally.

4 Grasp the rib with a Kocher clamp to steady it. Insert the rib cutter with the blade on the medial side, and pull it well posteriorly to divide the rib as far back as possible. Cut the rib. After division, use rongeurs to trim more of the rib if needed and to round the edges. Press bone wax into the cut end if it is bleeding (rare with the 12th rib). After lifting up the posterior end, cut the anterior fibrous attachment of the rib with Mayo scissors, and remove it.

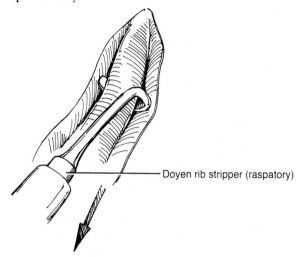

Doyen rib stripper (raspatory)

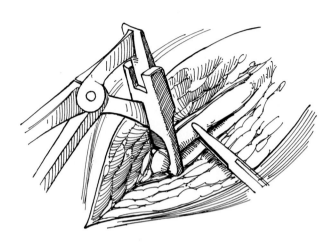

5 Incise the posterior layer of periosteum at the anterior end under the site of the rib tip to enter the retroperitoneal space. Insert a finger to depress the pleura and peritoneum; then extend the incision both ways with scissors. Spare the branches of the 12th intercostal neurovascular bundle by palpating them and letting them move caudally. Watch out for a vessel joining the 12th and 11th bundles anteriorly.

6 Divide the internal oblique muscle electrosurgically. Incise the thin epimesium over the transversus abdominis, and then digitally split the muscle to the anterior end of the wound.

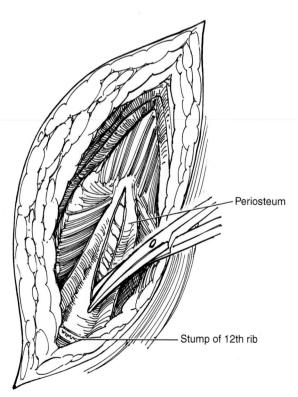

Periosteum

Stump of 12th rib

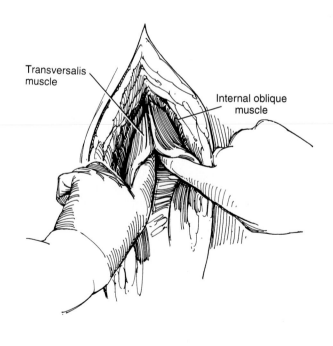

Transversalis muscle

Internal oblique muscle

7 Identify the pleura posteriorly, and have the anesthetist inflate the lung for easy visualization. Gently dissect the pleura from the endothoracic fascia beneath the 11th rib. (For the repair of pleural tears, see page 902.) At the same time, cut the attachments of the diaphragm against the body wall with Metzenbaum scissors. Separate the diaphragm from the retroperitoneal connective tissue to allow its displacement superiorly.

Free the peritoneum thoroughly by blunt dissection from the transversalis fascia on the undersurface of the abdominal wall, not only medially but superiorly and inferiorly as well. This facilitates placement of retractors and achieves optimal exposure.

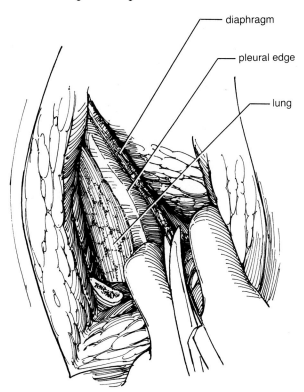

diaphragm

pleural edge

lung

8 Insert a self-retaining retractor. Enter Gerota's fascia bluntly to displace part of the perirenal fat posteriorly (to be used later to protect the repair), and expose the kidney.

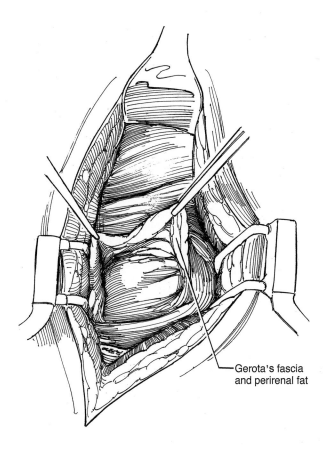

Gerota's fascia and perirenal fat

CLOSURE

9 Insert a Penrose drain through a separate stab wound. Approximate the anterior layer of the cut periosteum beginning dorsally at the superior margin, catching it superficially to avoid the intercostal bundle. Then close the combined transversus and internal oblique muscles; begin anteriorly using interrupted SAS. Before tying the sutures, ask the anesthetist to lower the kidney rest and flatten the table. The tapes holding the patient in position become loose, so have the assistant pull the shoulder back into alignment. (As noted, rotation of hips and shoulders in opposite directions opens or closes flank incisions.) Close the external oblique along with the posterior inferior serratus muscles, and approximate the latissimus muscles with the same suture material. Do not cinch the sutures too tightly. Approximate the subcutaneous tissue obliquely so that the caudal part of the wound does not sag posteriorly. Close the skin by aligning the scratches made initially. Suture the drain to the skin, and insert a safety pin.

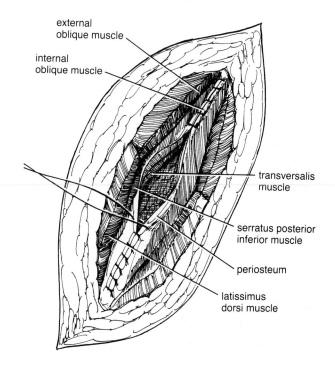

external oblique muscle

internal oblique muscle

transversalis muscle

serratus posterior inferior muscle

periosteum

latissimus dorsi muscle

Commentary by T. E. D. McDermott

I consider indications for the 12th rib approach to be a low-lying 12th rib when attempting lower-pole access and a low-lying kidney. As stated previously—and this must be emphasized—this approach is not generally suitable for radical renal pelvic or adrenal surgery because it usually compromises renal artery access.

Identifying correct access can be difficult. Use contrast intravenous pyelography to help you decide the height of the incision. Place your thumb on the iliac crest on the radiograph, and with the palm of your hand measure the height of the renal pelvis above the iliac bone. When the patient is in the lateral position, use the same measurements, but with the thumb on the iliac crest and the hand on the flank skin. This marks the approximate skin approach required to access the renal pelvis and vessels easily. The level of this access usually requires an 11th- or even 10th-interspace approach for ease of operative access.

When using the 12th rib approach, watch the stump of the rib after rib removal. A sharp edge often persists which can tear gloves peroperatively. Waxing and sometimes covering it with a swab are required.

The peritoneum and pleura can be extremely difficult to mobilize without causing tearing. Blunt swab dissection should be used to retract the peritoneum from the lower abdomen, mobilizing it upward toward the upper abdomen. The peritoneum in the upper abdomen is significantly thinner.

Pleural retraction can also be difficult and usually leads to a small perforation of this tissue. Pleural holes per se do not cause any peroperative difficulty. The anesthetist should be made aware of the problem. Closure at operation should not be attempted because further tearing normally occurs. When one is closing the perforation, (1) be quite clear that any clots have been removed from the chest cavity; (2) for a small hole, simply close the pleura once the lung is held in full inspiration to remove any air from the pleural space without the need for a chest tube; (3) if a chest tube is required, insert it in front of the anterior axillary line to facilitate the patient's comfort in the recovery phase. Any chest tubes should generally be removed within 24 hours once full expansion of the lung has been achieved. There is no benefit to leaving them for a longer period of time when the lung is expanded.

Closure of renal access wounds can be extremely difficult. I personally use an interrupted full-thickness closure with absorbable suture in order to achieve (1) correct approximation of the muscle layers, (2) approximation of all muscle layers, and (3) adequate approximation to achieve good muscle closure for long-term healing. The patient should be warned about the likelihood that desensitization below the wound will last an extended period of time.

Open surgical access to one or the other kidney usually results in an incision that is too low rather than too high. When approaching a difficult upper-pole renal resection, be sure that the incision you make gives suitable access to this area. A high flank approach, whether it be transcostal or intercostal, provides excellent access.

Supracostal Incision

A flank incision immediately above the 12th or, better, above the 11th rib can be made more easily than a transcostal incision and gives equal exposure.

1 *Anatomic description:* Review the kidney-ureter-bladder film to ascertain the length of the 11th and 12th ribs, and decide above which one an incision will give the appropriate exposure. If the 12th rib is long, an incision between it and the 11th rib gives excellent exposure. Entering above the 11th rib is advantageous in patients with short 12th ribs and for those requiring greater exposure, as for radical nephrectomy or adrenalectomy. Extra exposure is gained through the 11th rib incision with little increase in technical difficulty or risk.

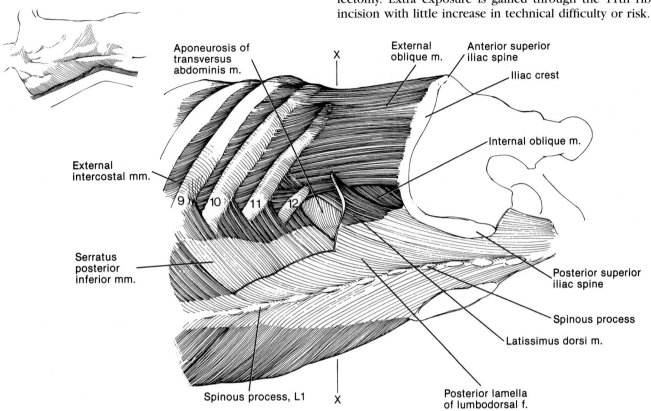

Aponeurosis of transversus abdominis m.

External oblique m.

Anterior superior iliac spine

Iliac crest

Internal oblique m.

External intercostal mm.

9 10 11 12

Serratus posterior inferior mm.

Posterior superior iliac spine

Spinous process

Latissimus dorsi m.

Spinous process, L1

X

Posterior lamella of lumbodorsal f.

2 Place the patient in the flank position (see page 871). If the incision is to be extended to or across the midline, a folded towel is placed under the chest to angle the patient 30 degrees posteriorly.

A, Expose the muscle layers in order in making the incision: latissimus dorsi, serratus posterior inferior, external and internal intercostal muscles, extrapleural fascia, and diaphragm.

B, The route of the incision is through the skin, dividing the latissimus dorsi, the serratus posterior inferior, and the external and internal intercostal muscles.

C, The innermost intercostals are cut to enter the retrocostal space. The attachment of the extrapleural fascia to the posterior surface of the rib is divided; this leaves the intercostal nerve against the rib in its own compartment of investing fascia.

D, The extrapleural fascia is cut and the diaphragm divided along the posterior body wall.

The supracostal 11th-rib incision is not shown, but it differs from the supracostal 12th only in that the pleura extends lower and is more exposed to possible entry during its dissection from the inner aspect of the 12th rib, to which it is somewhat adherent.

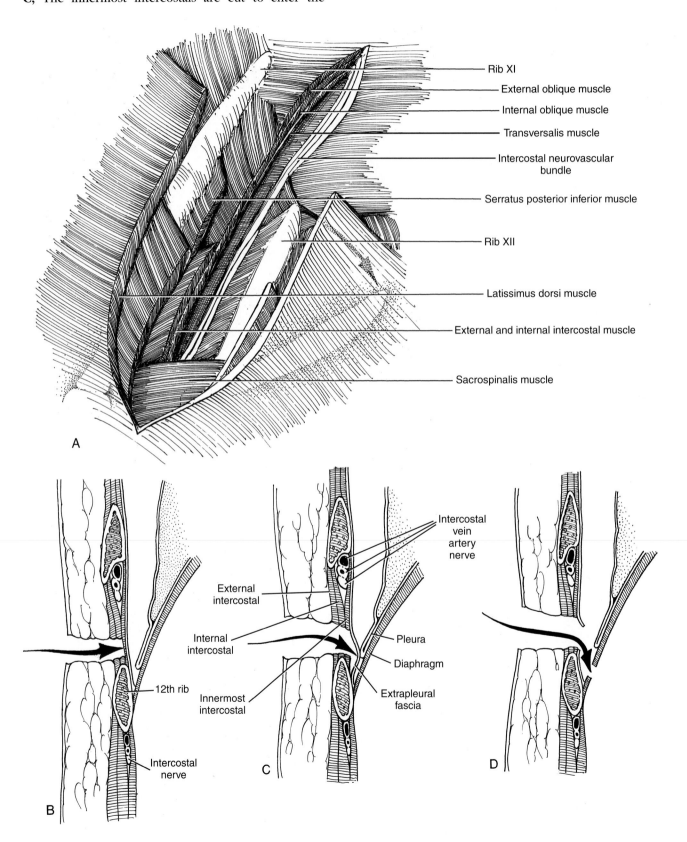

3 *Incision:* Palpate the line of the selected rib, and mark the skin with vertical scratches to facilitate its alignment at the time of closure. Start the skin incision obliquely over the selected rib (here the 12th rib), and extend it anteriorly to its tip. Posteriorly, carry the incision to the margin of the erector spinae muscle group and expose the external oblique and latissimus dorsi muscles.

4 Cut directly down onto the rib through the overlying muscles with the cutting current. Make the cut right down *into* the periosteum. This neatly divides the external and internal oblique muscles and the latissimus dorsi, as well as the serratus posterior inferior. Just anterior to the tip of the rib, incise the thickened layer of the abdominal wall fascia where its layers coalesce.

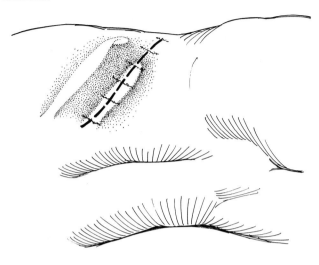

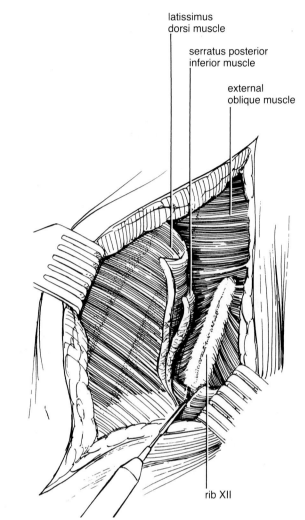

latissimus dorsi muscle

serratus posterior inferior muscle

external oblique muscle

rib XII

5 **A,** Reduce the setting for the cutting current, and use it to divide carefully the external intercostal muscle along the upper margin of the rib. Start at the tip of the rib, which is away from the pleura, and divide the muscles for an inch or so.

B, Insinuate the index finger to displace both the extrapleural fascia and the pleura. Progressively divide the inner intercostal muscle against the finger tip, separating it from the rib throughout its length. This leaves the intercostal nerve lying against the lower border of the rib.

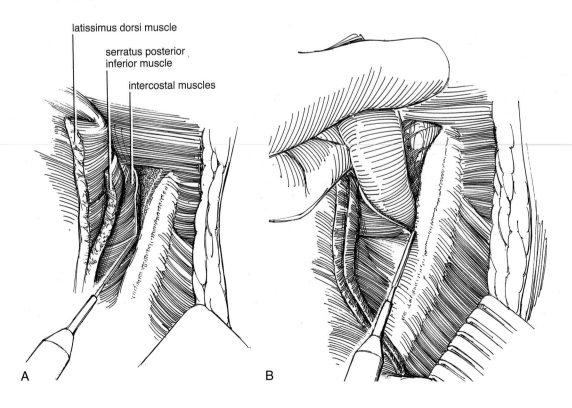

latissimus dorsi muscle

serratus posterior inferior muscle

intercostal muscles

A   B

6 Using a finger, separate the thin extrapleural fascia from the undersurface of the rib. This fascia splits into two layers to form a tunnel that contains the intercostal nerve (see Step 2C). Carefully divide the external layer. As the posterior part of the wound is reached, the pleura can be pushed down by the index finger, away from the intercostal muscle and rib.

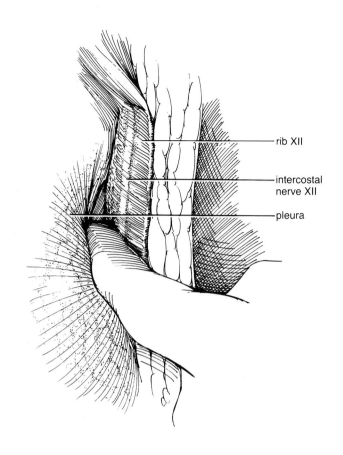

rib XII

intercostal nerve XII

pleura

7 Run the pad of the left index finger back along the top edge of the rib until it meets the sharp edge of the costovertebral ligament. Insert slightly opened heavy curved scissors, curve down, over the rib and under the finger. Hug the top of the rib with the blades to divide the ligament sharply and at the same time avoid the intercostal bundle that lies below the upper (11th) rib. The lower rib can pivot on its costovertebral joint (both the 11th and 12th ribs have a single attachment to the vertebra) and be retracted inferiorly to be held out of the way with a self-retaining retractor. To prevent the retractor from being levered out of the wound, support the handle with rolled towels stabilized with towel clips.

Complete the anterior part of the incision by dividing the external and internal oblique muscles and splitting the transversus abdominis sufficiently to allow the lower rib to be fully retracted downward until it lies alongside the lateral border of the quadratus lumborum muscle. Incising the anterior layers earlier would risk tearing the pleura before it was freed from the 12th rib. Insert a laminectomy (Sheldon) retractor, and support its arm on a rolled towel.

8 Push the diaphragm away from the undersurface of the rib and from the lateral arcuate ligament over the quadratus lumborum muscle.

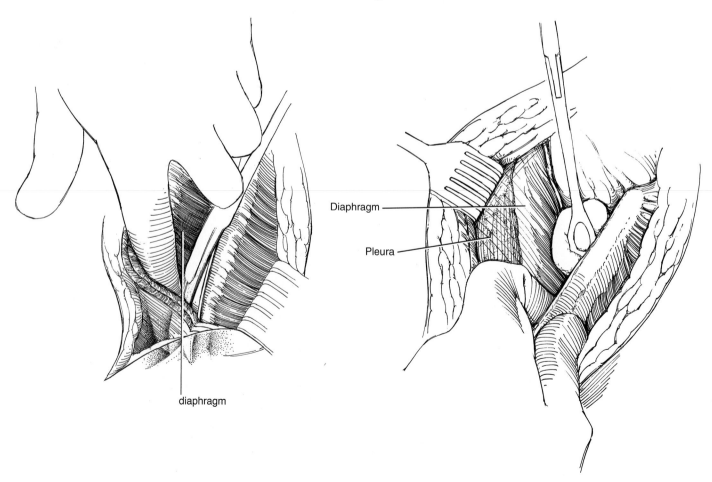

diaphragm

Diaphragm

Pleura

9 Divide the diaphragm close to its origin with scissors. Coagulate those vessels encountered. Stay well away from the pleura, especially when starting the division anteriorly. As the diaphragm is freed, the pleura rises out of the way.

For exposure of the renal pedicle, peel the peritoneum from the transversalis fascia with a cherry sponge in one hand while depressing the peritoneum with a laparotomy tape with the other. This should be done even if the incision is to be extended across the midline by division of one or both rectus muscles because it is difficult to retract the peritoneum from the body wall once it has been opened.

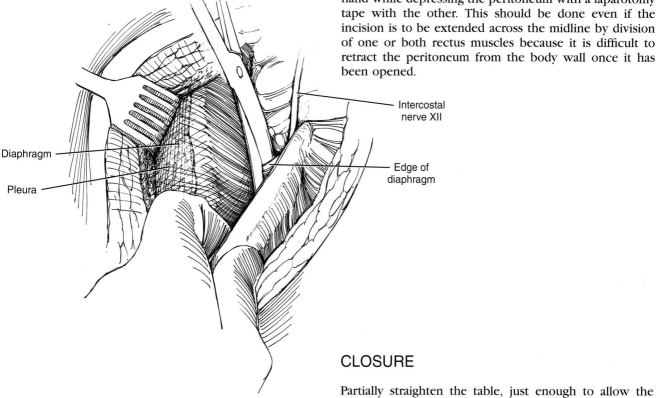

Diaphragm

Pleura

Intercostal
nerve XII

Edge of
diaphragm

CLOSURE

Partially straighten the table, just enough to allow the edges of the wound to come together but not enough to impede the insertion of sutures.

10 Open Gerota's fascia laterally, and expose the kidney through the perirenal fat.

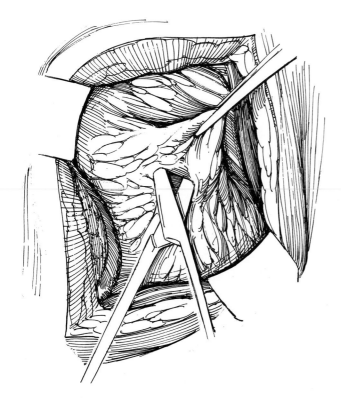

11 Place a figure-eight heavy SAS into the condensed musculofascial tissue at the tip of the 12th rib, bring it through similar tissue below the 11th rib, and tie it. The rib pivots upward into its original position.

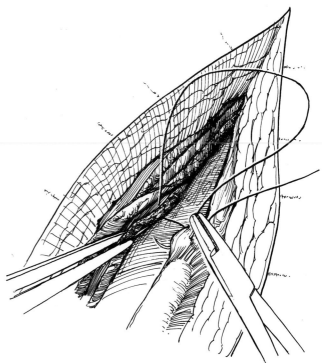

12 A and B, Starting posteriorly, pull the detached diaphragm and intercostal muscles out through the intercostal space, and stitch them progressively to the edges of the muscles below the incision external to the inferior rib (serratus posterior inferior posteriorly and latissimus dorsi anteriorly) with interrupted SAS. Because this maneuver also closes the pleura if it was inadvertently opened, the anesthetist must expand the lung before the final sutures are tied. Never encircle the lower rib with a closure suture; this risks damage to the intercostal vessels in the notch on its inferior surface.

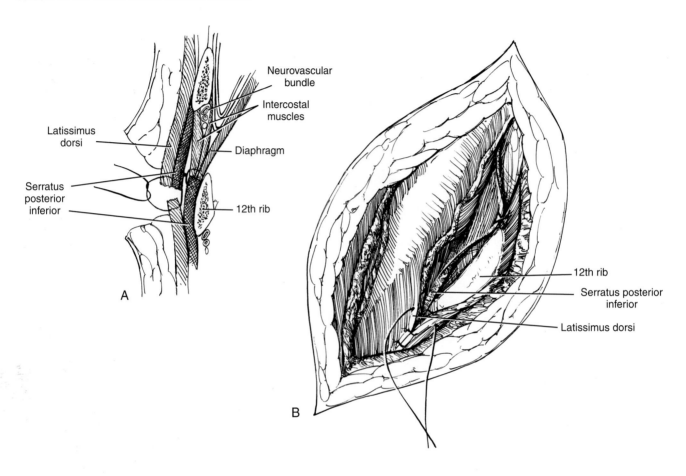

13 Stitch the upper margin of the incised latissimus dorsi to the external surface of the serratus, then to the lower margin of the latissimus dorsi. Place a Penrose drain through a stab wound below the 12th rib to allow the escape of trapped air and exudate. Close the subcutaneous tissue and skin. If the pleura has been entered, leave a small catheter in the pleural space, and put the end under water as a seal.

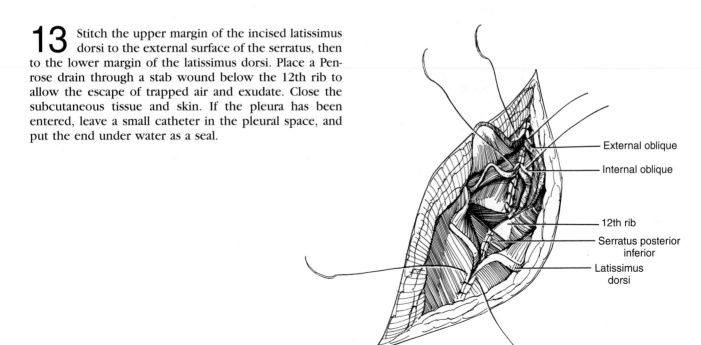

Foley Muscle-Splitting Incision

The muscle-splitting incision of Foley is ideal when an open operation is required for a stone impacted in the ureteropelvic junction opposite the lower pole of the kidney. Because it does not divide the muscles of the lateral abdominal wall, the abdominal wall is not weakened, nor is recovery delayed. It may be adapted for a minilaparoscopic approach, which it resembles. Two assistants are needed.

Instruments: Provide three Deaver retractors, and DeBakey forceps. An intraoperative ultrasound instrument may be helpful. A portable x-ray machine should be available. Good assistance is essential.

1 *Position:* Place the patient in flank position (see page 871) with minimal flexion of the table.

Incision: Palpate three landmarks: the lower border of the 12th rib, the erector muscles, and the iliac crest. Make the incision obliquely toward the iliac crest, starting at the angle where the rib and back muscles meet.

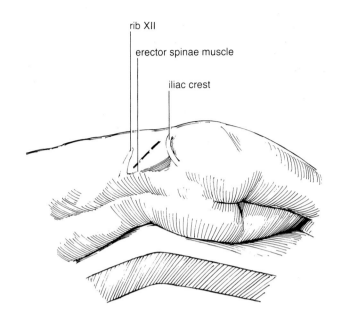

2 The latissimus dorsi is the superficial muscle posteriorly. The external oblique muscle has a free posterior border and may be reflected anteriorly to expose the internal oblique muscle and the lumbodorsal fascia.

Push the latissimus dorsi muscle posteriorly. Dissect the fascia from the external oblique muscle. Use the fingers along with further sharp dissection to free the muscle well anteriorly.

3 Repeat this fascial dissection for the internal oblique muscle; then pull the latissimus posteriorly and the obliques forward. Incise the lumbodorsal fascia in the line of its fibers.

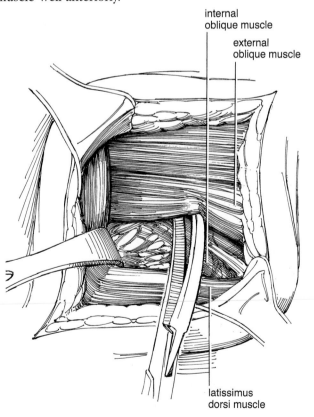

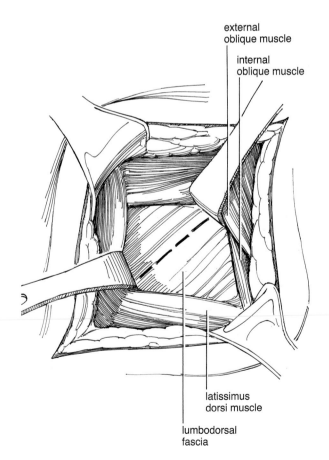

4 Expose the ureter by moving the peritoneum, to which it is attached, medially. Several narrow Deaver retractors, well handled by assistants, are a necessity. Look for periureteral edema. Open Gerota's fascia. If there is trouble with exposure, the incision can always be enlarged by dividing the muscles subcostally to convert to a regular flank incision.

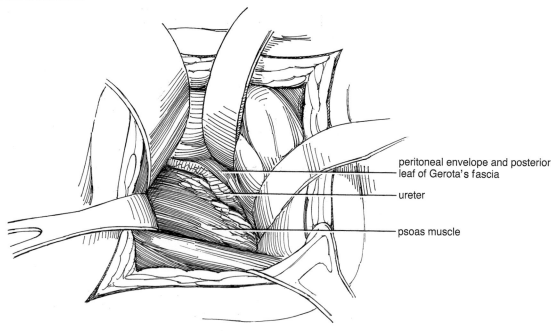

peritoneal envelope and posterior leaf of Gerota's fascia

ureter

psoas muscle

5 The stone may be seen through the ureteral wall. If not, grasp the ureter with a Babcock clamp above the expected site of the stone. Locate the stone with DeBakey forceps; the incision is too narrow to admit a hand for palpation. Open the ureter over the upper end of the stone, and remove it as described on page 848.

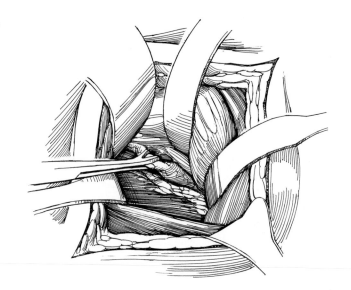

Commentary by Roberto Rocha Brito

The Foley muscle-splitting incision was described by Frederic E. B. Foley in 1935 as being an anatomic route, incising only the lumbodorsal and Gerota's fascias, preserving the musculature, and allowing access to the renal pelvis and the upper ureter. This small incision provides a quicker and less painful recovery with minimal intestinal distention. Long retractors are needed; the surgical field is not wide, but the incision may be extended further if necessary.

The incision is suitable for pelvic and upper ureteral calculi, as well as ureteropelvic junction obstructions, when we are dealing with an "in situ" operation. It is not suitable for very obese patients, renal anomalies, reoperations, or situations in which the kidney needs to be fully mobilized.

The advances of modern endourologic interventions by means of ureteroscopes, nephroscopes, laser, electrohydraulic or ultrasound probes, and extracorporeal shock wave lithotripsy have made the use of this incision quite rare.

Dorsal Flap Incision

(Nagamatsu)

The dorsal flap incision can give exposure well above the kidney and is an alternative to the thoracoabdominal incision (see page 890). A subcostal or 12th-rib incision can be extended with this technique if it proves inadequate. Instruments are the same as those used for a transcostal incision (see page 875).

1 *Position:* Lateral, rotated 15 degrees anteriorly over the kidney rest with the table flexed. Support the upper arm. After the patient has been taped in position, the table may be rotated anteriorly or posteriorly to facilitate making the lumbar or the dorsal parts of the incision.

Incision: Start the skin incision at the level of the 9th interspace, run it vertically down the edge of the sacrospinalis muscle, and then curve it anteriorly along the upper edge of the 12th rib to meet the lateral rectus sheath. If you are uncertain about the operability of lesion, make only the abdominal portion of the incision to allow preliminary palpation and visualization.

Divide the latissimus dorsi and the posterior inferior serratus muscles over the three lower ribs medial to their angles. Avoid the intercostal bundle.

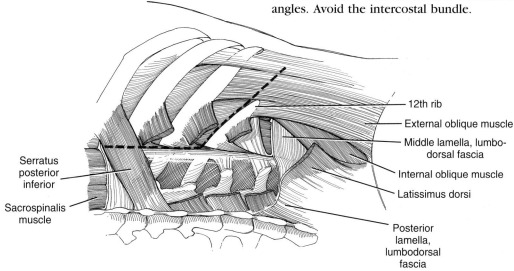

Serratus posterior inferior

Sacrospinalis muscle

12th rib

External oblique muscle

Middle lamella, lumbo-dorsal fascia

Internal oblique muscle

Latissimus dorsi

Posterior lamella, lumbodorsal fascia

2 Divide the lumbocostal ligament and the tendinous slips of the sacrospinalis muscle before they insert into the two lower ribs. Tag each end of the lumbocostal ligament to aid in approximation at closure.

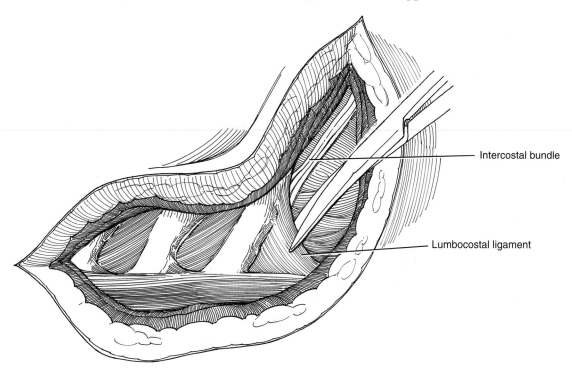

Intercostal bundle

Lumbocostal ligament

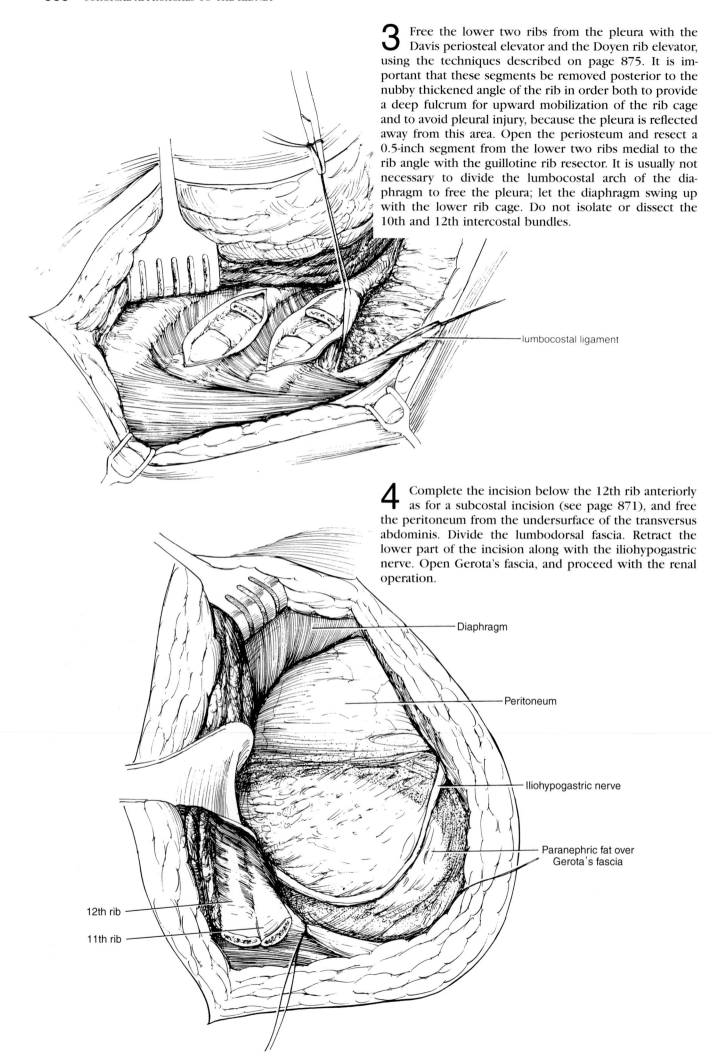

3 Free the lower two ribs from the pleura with the Davis periosteal elevator and the Doyen rib elevator, using the techniques described on page 875. It is important that these segments be removed posterior to the nubby thickened angle of the rib in order both to provide a deep fulcrum for upward mobilization of the rib cage and to avoid pleural injury, because the pleura is reflected away from this area. Open the periosteum and resect a 0.5-inch segment from the lower two ribs medial to the rib angle with the guillotine rib resector. It is usually not necessary to divide the lumbocostal arch of the diaphragm to free the pleura; let the diaphragm swing up with the lower rib cage. Do not isolate or dissect the 10th and 12th intercostal bundles.

lumbocostal ligament

4 Complete the incision below the 12th rib anteriorly as for a subcostal incision (see page 871), and free the peritoneum from the undersurface of the transversus abdominis. Divide the lumbodorsal fascia. Retract the lower part of the incision along with the iliohypogastric nerve. Open Gerota's fascia, and proceed with the renal operation.

Diaphragm

Peritoneum

Iliohypogastric nerve

Paranephric fat over Gerota's fascia

12th rib

11th rib

CLOSURE

5 Lower the kidney rest. Replace the osteoplastic flap by reapproximating the lumbocostal ligament with interrupted 2-0 or 3-0 SAS or NAS. Be certain that the ribs do not override. Close the anterior portion as for a subcostal incision. Place Penrose drains through the superior lumbar triangle. Suture the posterior inferior serratus and latissimus dorsi muscles, followed by the subcutaneous tissue and skin.

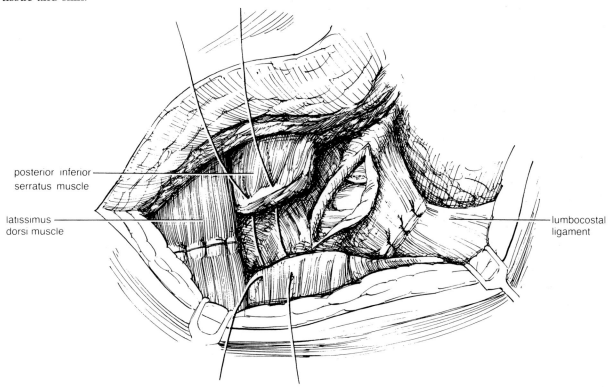

posterior inferior serratus muscle

latissimus dorsi muscle

lumbocostal ligament

Commentary by George R. Nagamatsu

Before taking this procedure to the operating room, we developed it by making detailed sequential anatomic maneuvers on the warm cadaver. The initial operative cases were fully detailed in the original descriptions. Clinical experience through the years has demonstrated the applicability of this operation and has allowed for simplification of the steps, which has greatly reduced the operative time without compromising its aim of adequate exposure of the upper retroperitoneum, in the majority of cases without entering the pleural cavity. The versatility of this exposure has been extended as a modification of the Young bilateral simultaneous lumbar exposure and as an optional extraperitoneal approach for bilateral retroperitoneal lymph node dissection in testis tumor in combination with a Cherney type of incision.

The key is to divide the lumbocostal ligaments anchoring the lower two ribs. Often the fixed overhanging rib cage springs upward together with the attached pleura and the lateral crus of the diaphragm, thus demonstrating the mobility attained by this division. Conversely, accurate reapproximation of this ligament is the first step in the closure. Prior to dividing the ligament, both ends of the ligament must be marked with sutures to ensure correct realignment of the ribs without overriding.

With only the abdominal limb made initially, as for a subcostal incision, it is possible in most cases to assess the removability of large renal tumors and gain early access to the renal pedicle, often anteriorly. Initial clamping of the renal artery under direct vision is often feasible because of the double advantage afforded by the unroofed costal overhang and the abdominal exposure. If it is necessary to open the peritoneum, especially in the right-sided cases, this may be done freely without compromising the final result. The artery can be secured, and further toilet as indicated can proceed visually in the wide-open field.

With increased familiarity with the technique and the avoidance of surgical manipulation after division of the lumbocostal ligaments as described, pleural injury is rare. If it does occur, notify the anesthetist, protect the area with a pad, and proceed with the operation. Attempts to suture the pleura at the time of injury are to be avoided. At the conclusion of the operation, close the rent around a small catheter buttressed with overlying muscle and fascia, and remove the catheter at the last suture, with the lung expanded by the anesthetist. Small Penrose drains are ordinarily placed at the superior lumbar triangle. However, in cases of pleural injury, place these drains at the anterior portion of the incision. Chest films at the conclusion of the operation and the following morning are desirable. Postoperative management and ambulation do not differ from those of routine incisions. With experience, the simplified bony mobilization requires only 5 to 10 minutes.

Several decades of long-term follow-up of patients managed with this type of incision have disclosed no restriction of lumbodorsal mobility. Cartilaginous or bony reunion at resected rib sites with normal realignment is the rule, owing to the accurate reapproximation of the lumbocostal ligament.

Thoracoabdominal Incision

A thoracoabdominal approach is definitely needed if the size of the tumor in the anteroposterior dimension is great in relation to the space between the abdominal wall posteriorly and the undersurface of the ribs anteriorly because of the difficulty in moving the tumor enough to reach the upper pole through lower incisions.

TRANSTHORACIC APPROACH

The transthoracic approach gives superior exposure for radical nephrectomy (see page 1016) and large retroperitoneal tumors. If you are in doubt about operability, make the anterior segment first, as done in the extrathoracic approach described in Steps 6 to 12.

Enter through rib 10, 9, or 8, depending on the height of the renal pedicle; the 10th rib is shown in this description. For major surgery, provide overnight hydration with lactated Ringer's solution.

1 Insert a nasogastric tube. *Position:* Place the patient flush with the ipsilateral (in this case, the right) side of the table, with the flank directly over the break in the table. Place the pelvis almost flat by bending the opposite knee. Rotate the upper torso 30 degrees, and support it with a rolled towel or sandbag. Place the upper arm across the chest onto a padded Krause armboard that is affixed to the table top. Alternatively, place it on a padded Mayo stand or suspend it on an anesthesia screen. Protect the left axilla with a pad. Hyperextend the table, and hold the patient in position with wide strips of adhesive tape from shoulder to table top posteriorly and from hip to table top both anteriorly and posteriorly. Pad all exposed areas.

Incision: Identify the 10th rib, and mark the overlying skin with needle scratches or marking pen ink (*heavy dashed line*). For large renal tumors, place the incision above the 9th rib. Incise the skin and subcutaneous tissue directly over the rib, extending the incision anteriorly across the rectus muscle high in the epigastrium and well above the umbilicus. Curve the incision inferiorly to avoid injury to the intercostal nerve and its branches as they emerge from under the rib above. The incision can be extended across the midline to the contralateral costochondral junction (*short-dashed line*). For retroperitoneal dissection, a midline or paramedian extension is useful (*dotted line*).

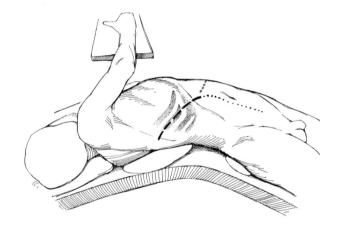

2 Incise the latissimus dorsi, posterior inferior serratus, and external oblique muscles with the cutting current; then divide the internal oblique muscle by cutting directly on the convex surface of the 10th rib. Carry the incision well posteriorly to allow the costovertebral ligament to be divided.

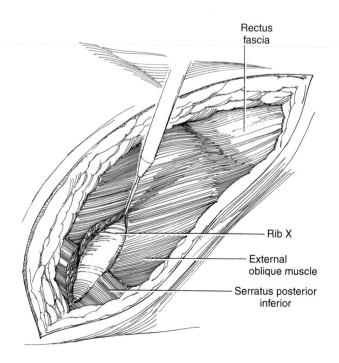

Rectus fascia

Rib X

External oblique muscle

Serratus posterior inferior

890

3 For a supracostal approach (shown), divide the intercostal muscles sharply just above the rib (see page 881). Alternatively, resect the rib (see page 875). Carefully enter the pleura above the costal sinus by opening it with curved scissors after the lung comes into view during inspiration. Place a laparotomy pad under a retractor to protect the lung.

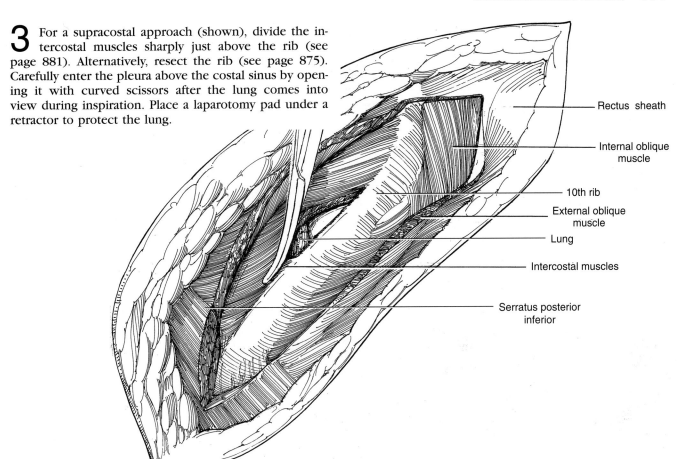

Rectus sheath

Internal oblique muscle

10th rib

External oblique muscle

Lung

Intercostal muscles

Serratus posterior inferior

4 Open the diaphragm where it is covered with pleura, and extend that incision anteriorly to divide its extrapleural portion. By keeping the incision near the attachment of the diaphragm to the chest wall, one can avoid damage to the phrenic nerve. Insinuate curved scissors under the costochondral junction, and divide the costal cartilage. Proceed to divide the internal oblique and transversalis muscles anteriorly, as well as the rectus muscle with its sheath.

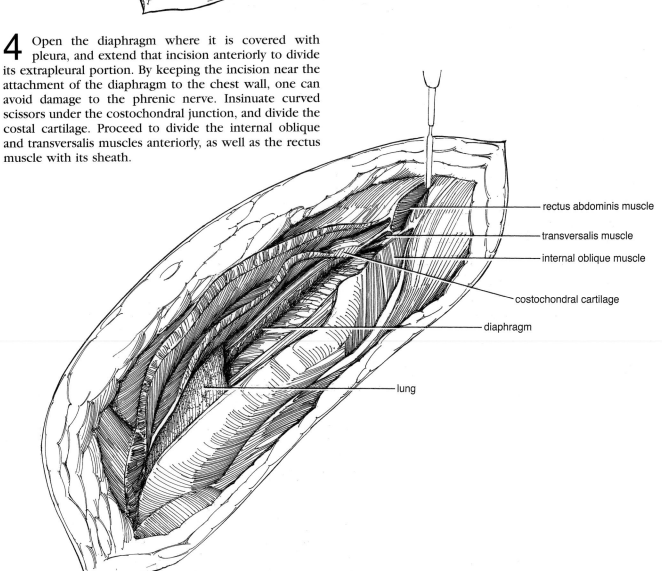

rectus abdominis muscle

transversalis muscle

internal oblique muscle

costochondral cartilage

diaphragm

lung

5 Open the peritoneum. Insert a self-retaining (Finochietto) retractor at the tip of the 10th rib, catching the ends of cartilage in its slots. Displace the liver on the right (and the spleen on the left) upward to expose the posterior peritoneum. Grasp the lateral edge of peritoneum near the diaphragm, and dissect the avascular plane between Gerota's fascia and the peritoneum. Continue the dissection medially to identify the superior mesenteric artery, which in turn allows location of the right renal vein.

Proceed with radical nephrectomy (see page 1016) or adrenalectomy (see page 1061). At the end of the procedure before closure, place a finger inside the chest wall, and inject 5 ml of 0.75 percent solution of bupivacaine hydrochloride into the incisional intercostal space and into the interspaces above and below.

If more exposure is needed, continue the incision across the midline (small-dashed line in Step 1). For retroperitoneal node dissection, extend the incision inferiorly in the midline (dotted line in Step 1) or as a paramedian incision. For adrenalectomy, provide two incisions in the diaphragm. Make the first one laterally between the lumbocostal arch and the left leaf of the central tendon. This allows access to the adrenal area. Proceed with adrenalectomy. Before closure, place a second incision in the diaphragm more anteriorly, running parallel to the muscle fibers between the left leaflet and the site of attachment of the costal cartilages. Incise the peritoneum beneath, and proceed with abdominal exploration and palpation of the other adrenal. For even better exposure, make a single incision that extends medially from the lateral margin of the diaphragm.

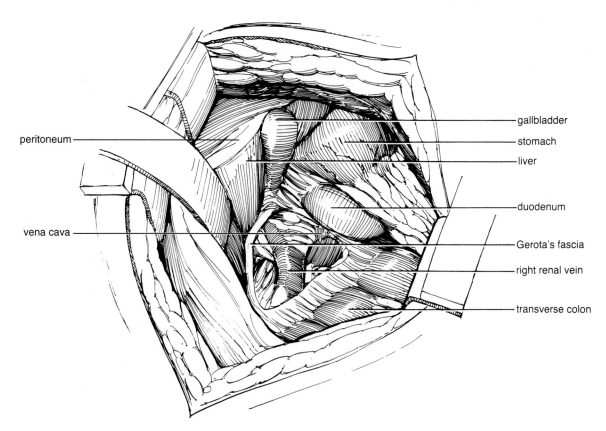

peritoneum

vena cava

gallbladder

stomach

liver

duodenum

Gerota's fascia

right renal vein

transverse colon

EXTRATHORACIC 11TH RIB APPROACH

The extrathoracic approach may be useful if you have doubt about operability, as it allows preliminary abdominal exploration. In some cases, the lesion is more accessible than expected and can be removed without entering the chest.

6 Mark and incise the skin over the 10th rib from its angle to the midline anteriorly. Divide the anterior rectus sheath and the external oblique, latissimus dorsi, and serratus posterior inferior muscles with the cutting current. Transect the rectus abdominis muscle; then divide the internal oblique and transversus muscles right up to the tip of the 10th rib. Open the peritoneum, and explore the peritoneal cavity.

7 Protect the liver with the fingers of the left hand (not shown), and divide the cartilaginous arch between the 9th and 10th ribs.

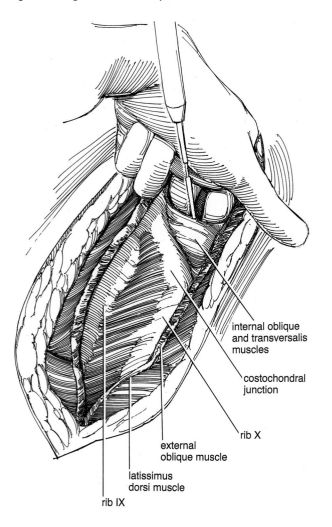

internal oblique and transversalis muscles

costochondral junction

rib X

external oblique muscle

latissimus dorsi muscle

rib IX

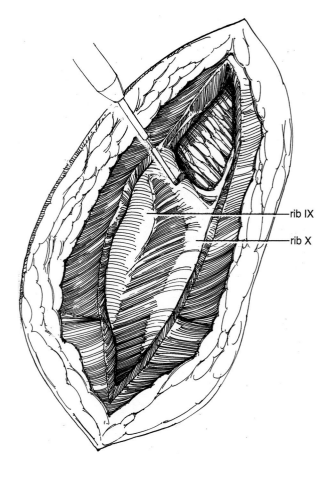

rib IX

rib X

8 Cautiously divide the intercostal muscles against the upper edge of the 10th rib with scissors or electrode, exposing the diaphragm first and then the pleura, as is done for the supracostal incision (see pages 881 to 882, Steps 5 to 7). Ask the anesthetist to expand the lung. Carefully dissect the pleura from the undersurface of the 10th rib, and reflect it upward with the diaphragm. This maneuver is facilitated by dividing attachments of the diaphragm first and then reflecting the pleura cephalad. Alternatively, enter the pleura as described in Step 3. Divide the costovertebral ligament, and hinge the 10th rib downward.

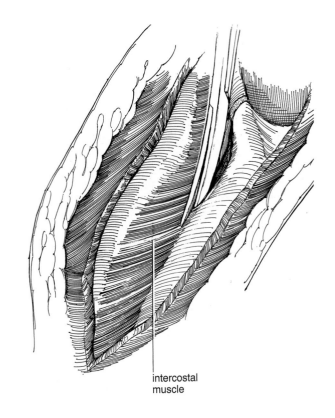

intercostal
muscle

9 Incise the diaphragm about 2 cm below the pleural reflection, behind the rib. By staying near the insertion of the diaphragm into the chest wall, one can avoid damaging the phrenic nerve.

10 Tack the upper edge of the diaphragm to the serratus posterior inferior and latissimus dorsi muscles to protect the pleura. Open the peritoneum completely, and divide the posterior rectus sheath. Insert a self-retaining retractor to separate the ribs, and place an abdominal retractor as well. Proceed with radical nephrectomy or other procedure.

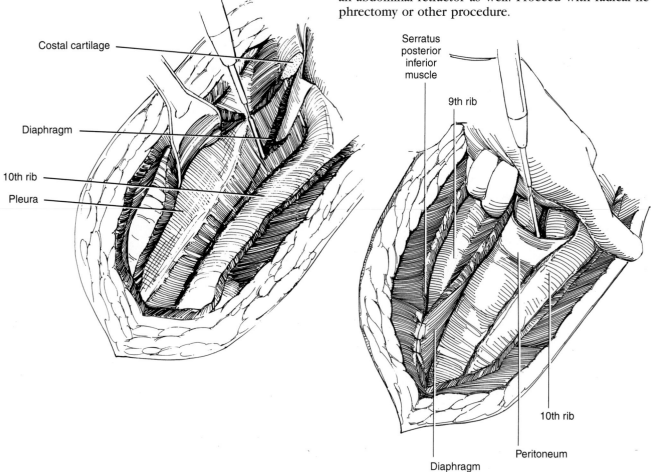

Costal cartilage

Diaphragm

10th rib

Pleura

Serratus
posterior
inferior
muscle

9th rib

Diaphragm

Peritoneum

10th rib

CLOSURE

11 Close the posterior peritoneum with a running 3-0 or 4-0 SAS. A retroperitoneal drain (optional) is placed to exit through a stab wound. Approximate the diaphragm with horizontal mattress sutures of 4-0 NAS (Maxon) with the knots buried. Inject 5 ml of 0.75 percent bupivacaine into the area of the 9th and 10th intercostal nerves percutaneously at the posterior end of the incision, or place a catheter into this area for postoperative infusion of bupivacaine.

Protect the lung with a finger in the pleural space beneath, and avoid entering the costal veins. Place a 3-0 monofilament nylon suture through the cut edges of the costal arch, but do not tie it. Install a 20 F chest tube, bring it out through a stab wound in the posterior axillary line, suture it to the skin with heavy silk, and close the pleura and intercostal muscles with a running fine SAS. Alternatively, insert a 14 F Robinson catheter in the pleural cavity. Preplace several interrupted sutures near the costophrenic sinus. Tie the sutures in the costal arch and then the sutures over the costophrenic sinus.

12 Close the thoracic part of the incision by first placing figure-eight 2-0 or 3-0 SAS through all the muscular layers of the chest wall; include the anterior pleural edge and the diaphragm in the last few sutures. Tie these sutures successively, beginning posteriorly. Reapproximate the costal cartilage with a single figure-eight 1-0 Prolene suture. Suture the peritoneum with a running 4-0 absorbable suture; approximate the posterior and anterior rectus sheaths and the muscle layers with 2-0 or 3-0 SAS. Close the subcutaneous tissue and skin.

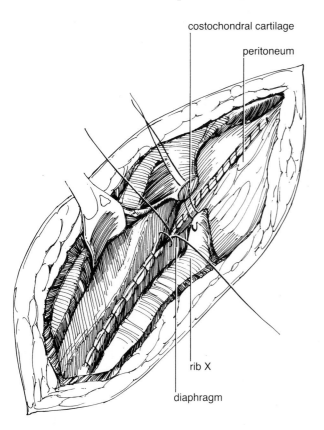

costochondral cartilage

peritoneum

rib X

diaphragm

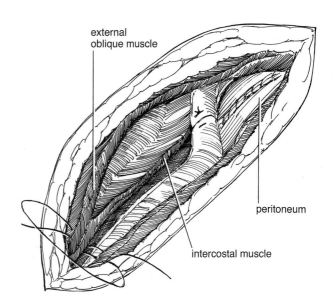

external oblique muscle

peritoneum

intercostal muscle

Commentary by Jerome P. Richie

The thoracoabdominal incision is an exceedingly useful incision for patients with large renal tumors and for retroperitoneal lymph node dissection. The advantage for large renal tumors is the ease of exposure, especially around the upper pole in the region of the adrenal. Incidental splenectomy on the left side should be less frequent with the use of this incision. Even though it involves a pleurotomy and generally requires a chest tube for 24 hours, the improved exposure actually reduces the operating time. Median time for radical nephrectomies is approximately 80 to 90 minutes, including placement of a chest tube. Most patients are discharged from the hospital on postoperative day four or five.

The left thoracoabdominal dissection, with the patient in the torque position, is exceedingly useful for a retroperitoneal lymph node dissection. Especially in postchemotherapy retroperitoneal lymph node dissection, this incision provides excellent exposure at the level of the renal hilum. In patients with bulk disease, a higher thoracoabdominal incision is preferred, either an 8th- or 7th-rib incision, as opposed to a 9th- or 10th-rib incision. As a general rule, I prefer to resect the rib rather than enter between the ribs.

Adequate reapproximation of the costal cartilage is imperative. Because cartilage does not grow or remodel, I use a single figure-eight suture of 1-0 Prolene to fix the costal cartilage. I prefer to close the anterior chest wall in a single layer of interrupted figure-eight 1-0 polydioxanone sutures, catching both muscle and pleura. Toward the medial surface, the diaphragm is also included to close off the pleural space and allow an effective seal. All sutures are placed and then tied down sequentially to prevent sewing oneself into a corner. This incision is one of the most versatile and useful for major urologic cancer procedures.

Dorsal Lumbotomy

UNILATERAL POSTERIOR LUMBOTOMY

Although this incision provides a more limited access to the kidney than do flank approaches, it has many uses: pyeloplasty especially in children, open renal biopsies, removal of small kidneys, large pelvic stones, and stones fixed in the upper or mid ureter. It can be combined with coagulum and/or nephroscopy for free stones, although it is often difficult to perform nephroscopy of all calyces even with a flexible nephroscope. It is not suitable for malignant lesions nor for malpositioned kidneys. If the skin incision is made somewhat transversely, the disadvantage of a scar that results from crossing Langer's lines is eliminated without sacrifice of exposure.

Instruments: Provide Gil-Vernet retractors and long curved retractors. For stone cases, include a flexible nephroscope and coagulum.

1 **A,** *Position:* After tracheal intubation, place the patient in a dorsolateral position, with the shoulders placed forward at a greater angle than the pelvis. Draw the knees in flexion to reduce lordosis. Flex the table minimally to avoid putting tension on the muscles of the back; a pad in the loin is usually not needed. (For renal biopsy, the lateral position without knee flexion keeps the kidney from falling away from the surgeon and is less limiting on respiration.)

Incision: Make a semioblique *skin incision (short dashes)* that extends from the angle of the 12th rib where the lateral border of the sacrospinalis muscle crosses the lower margin of the rib (about 5 to 6 cm from the spinal processes) to a point between the tip of the 12th rib and the crest of the ilium. Make the *fascial incision (long dashes)* more vertically.

B and **C,** Approach is made anterior to the sacrospinalis and quadratus lumborum muscles via the lumbodorsal fascia (*dotted line* and *arrow*). Dividing the latissumus dorsi exposes the posterior lamella of the lumbar fascia and its continuation over the sacrospinalis. Division of this lamella exposes the lateral projection of the sacrospinalis muscle. Divide the muscular attachments of the sacrospinalis to the 12th and 11th ribs, and retract the muscle medially to allow division of the middle lamella over the quadratus lumborum. Retraction of this muscle medially also permits division of the anterior lamella and entry into the paranephric space.

After making the semioblique skin incision, free the subcutaneous tissue to allow sufficient space for the more vertical incision in the posterior projection of the latissimus dorsi and posterior inferior serratus muscles.

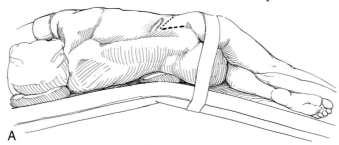

A

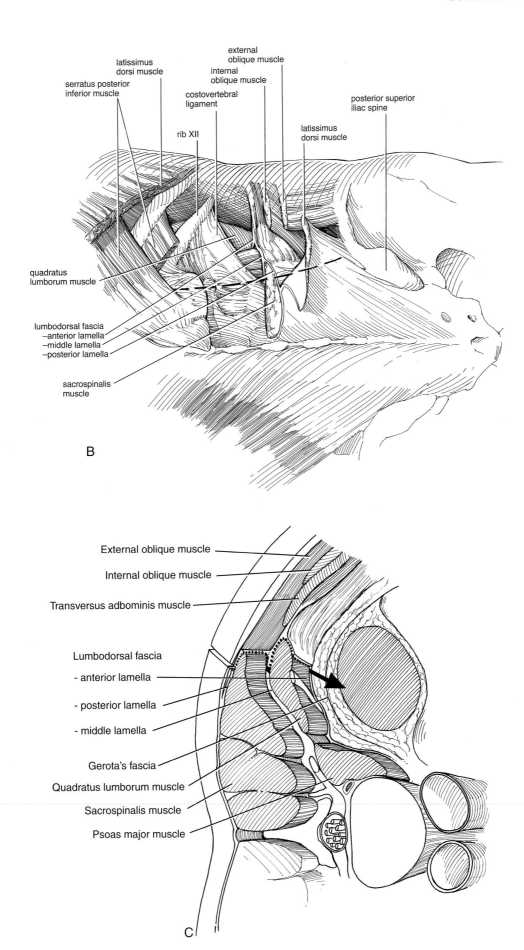

latissimus
dorsi muscle

serratus posterior
inferior muscle

external
oblique muscle

internal
oblique muscle

costovertebral
ligament

posterior superior
iliac spine

rib XII

latissimus
dorsi muscle

quadratus
lumborum muscle

lumbodorsal fascia
–anterior lamella
–middle lamella
–posterior lamella

sacrospinalis
muscle

B

External oblique muscle

Internal oblique muscle

Transversus adbominis muscle

Lumbodorsal fascia

- anterior lamella

- posterior lamella

- middle lamella

Gerota's fascia

Quadratus lumborum muscle

Sacrospinalis muscle

Psoas major muscle

C

2 If necessary, divide the posterior projections of the latissimus dorsi and posterior inferior serratus muscles.

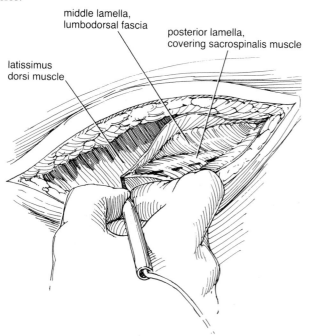

middle lamella, lumbodorsal fascia

posterior lamella, covering sacrospinalis muscle

latissimus dorsi muscle

3 Divide the posterior lamella of the lumbodorsal fascia vertically over the belly of the sacrospinalis muscle, not along its lateral border.

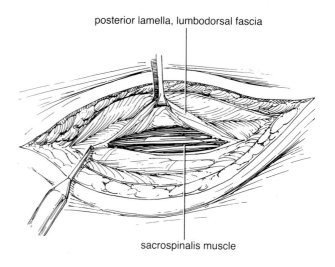

posterior lamella, lumbodorsal fascia

sacrospinalis muscle

4 Elevate the lateral edge of the cut lumbodorsal fascia with Allis clamps to retract the lateral edge of the sacrospinalis muscle medially.

5 Bluntly dissect the lateral margin of the sacrospinalis muscle to expose the subcostal vessels and the costovertebral ligament. Under vision, divide the ligament with scissors. Incise the exposed fused middle and anterior lamellae of the lumbar fascia about 1 cm under the edge of the quadratus lumborum muscle, down to the iliac crest. This fascia surrounds the quadratus lumborum muscle and is the origin of the internal oblique and transversus abdominis muscles. Watch out for the iliohypogastric nerve under the fascia during exposure and closure. Extend the incision in the lumbodorsal fascia cephalad to divide the costovertebral ligament and allow upward rotation of the 12th rib.

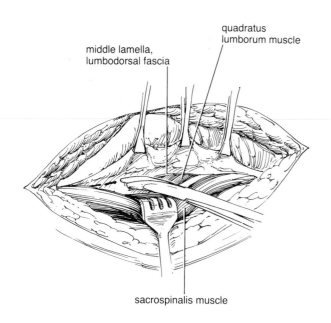

middle lamella, lumbodorsal fascia

quadratus lumborum muscle

sacrospinalis muscle

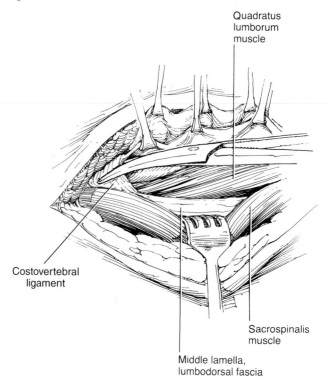

Quadratus lumborum muscle

Costovertebral ligament

Middle lamella, lumbodorsal fascia

Sacrospinalis muscle

6 Retract the quadratus lumborum muscle medially, exposing the anterior lamella of the lumbodorsal fascia. Incise this lamella, and incise the transversalis fascia between the subcostal and iliohypogastric nerves that course obliquely across, exposing the paranephric fat.

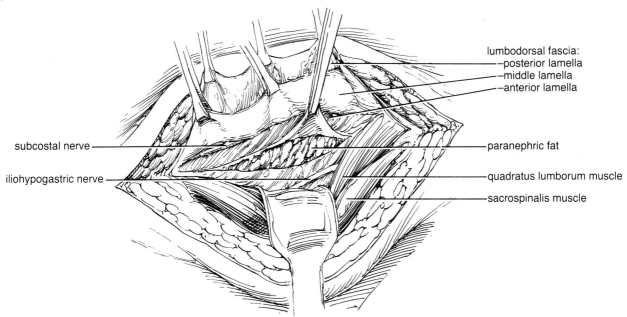

lumbodorsal fascia:
—posterior lamella
—middle lamella
—anterior lamella

subcostal nerve

iliohypogastric nerve

paranephric fat

quadratus lumborum muscle

sacrospinalis muscle

7 Pick up Gerota's fascia with two forceps at the cranial end of the wound and incise it. Extend the opening caudad with two fingers. Insert a laminectomy retractor.

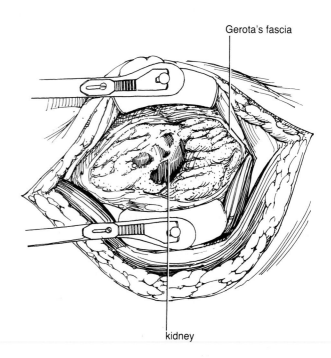

Gerota's fascia

kidney

8 Pick up the ureter and begin renal dissection at the hilus.

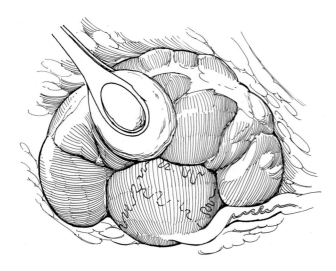

9 For pyelolithotomy, develop the renal sinus first. Insert Gil-Vernet retractors to control the kidney position and assist in removal of the stone. Have coagulum and a flexible nephroscope available.

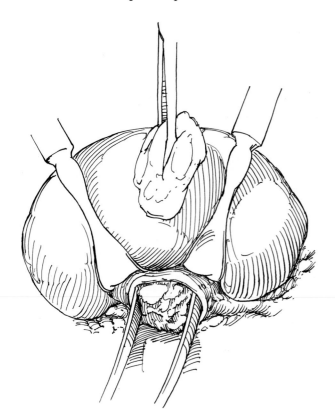

10 Insert a Penrose drain upon completion of the procedure. Close the incision with six to eight 2-0 or 3-0 SAS in the lumbodorsal fascia. It is not necessary to put stitches in the tenuous middle lamella of the lumbar fascia, a maneuver fraught with the danger of catching the iliohypogastric nerve that runs close by. The strong vertically disposed and overlapping sacrospinalis and quadratus lumborum, as well as the thick posterior lamella of the lumbar fascia, provide adequate strength to the closed wound.

Tie the second layer after the kidney rest has been lowered. If the latissimus dorsi and posterior inferior serratus muscles were divided, reunite them. Approximate the subcutaneous tissue and skin.

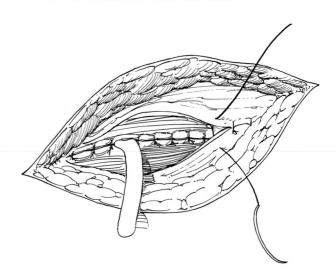

EXTENDED DORSAL LUMBOTOMY

If the exposure is limited by the presence of the 12th rib above and the iliac crest below, especially if a radiograph is needed, mobilize the 12th rib by dividing the costovertebral ligament and resect a 2-cm segment from it posterior to the angle. Incise the diaphragm up to the level of the 11th rib, keeping close to the 12th rib to avoid the pleura. The subcostal (12th thoracic) nerve and the iliohypogastric nerve cross the incision and should be freed; preserve at least the latter nerve. Insert a self-retaining retractor, and open Gerota's fascia vertically. For more exposure, extend the incision anteriorly as a T.

BILATERAL POSTERIOR LUMBOTOMY

Bilateral posterior lumbotomy is used for simultaneous nephrectomy in transplant patients and for simultaneous exposure for adrenalectomy.

11 *Instruments:* Provide a Burford retractor or a ring or a Finochietto retractor with the blades reversed.

Position: Place the patient prone with bolster support under shoulders and pelvis to avoid compression of chest and abdomen and allow diaphragmatic breathing. Flex the table slightly.

Place one surgeon and one assistant on each side of the table to allow simultaneous exposure.

Incisions: Make oblique skin incisions (*dashed lines*) more or less along the skin lines, each of which extends from the angle of the 12th rib where the lateral border of the sacrospinalis muscle crosses the lower margin of the rib (about 5 to 6 cm from the spinal processes) down to the iliac crest at a point one third of the distance from the anterior superior iliac spine to the spinal processes. Proceed as for unilateral dorsal lumbotomy. A self-retaining retractor can be placed to compress the muscles medially, but Deaver retractors in the hands of the assistant provide more adaptable retraction. Keep to the anatomic plane because the peritoneum is displaced dorsally by the prone position and is easily entered.

For bilateral simultaneous exposure of the adrenal glands (see page 1079), make two 12th-rib incisions (*dotted lines*).

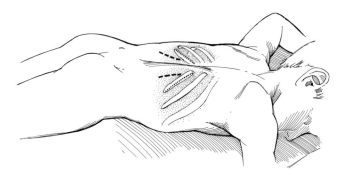

Commentary by Mani Menon

This incision is excellent for exposing the kidney and can be used for almost any non-oncologic procedure. When used properly, "it can offer excellent exposure while making for very comfortable and grateful patients."

I use some minor variations in technique. I do not flex the table, and I do allow the patient to fall forward slightly.

I make a vertical incision, more medial than the figure shows, directly over the belly of the sacrospinalis muscle. The fascia enclosing the sacrospinalis muscle is the strongest fascia in the body. I approach the kidney through this fascia and use a single layer of closure of this fascia on the way out. Superiorly, the fascia thins out over the 12th and 11th ribs, and a few fibers of the latissimus dorsi, the serratus posterior inferior, and the trapezius may be incorporated into the fascia.

After opening the fascia over the sacrospinalis, I dissect away the fleshy mass of the muscle from beneath the fascia. The muscle does not adhere to the fascia and can easily be swept away. I then incise the fused middle and anterior layers of the dorsolumbar fascia, lateral to the sacrospinalis.

When mobilization of the upper pole of the kidney or the adrenals is required, I extend the incision above the 12th rib. I then cut the costovertebral ligament, which may also have a few muscle bundles in it. I then resect a 1- to 2-cm segment of rib posterior to the costal angle, taking care to avoid injury to the subcostal vessels during this maneuver. Once the segment of the rib is removed, I incise the diaphragm close to its origin. The pleura can be dissected away or opened in the line of the incision. These maneuvers effectively double the exposure obtained. I usually use a Finochietto retractor with deep blades for the exposure.

Repair of Pleural Tear

1 **A,** If the pleura has been mobilized and the possibility exists that it is torn, have the anesthetist inflate the lung to identify the leak before closing the wound. Then have the lung deflated to draw the lung margin away from the site of the tear. Insert a small red Robinson catheter into the pleural space through the tear. Tie a running 4-0 plain catgut suture beyond the anterior end of the pleural defect, continue it as a running suture around the catheter, and tie it beyond the end of the defect. Alternatively, include the diaphragm on one side and the intercostal muscles on the other (avoid the intercostal vessels and nerve). For small defects, have the anesthetist inflate the lung while you aspirate pleural air through the catheter with a large syringe; then tie the suture as the catheter is withdrawn.

B, If the defect is larger, leave the catheter in the pleura until the entire wound is closed, taking care not to position a Penrose drain near it. Place the end of the catheter under water, and have the anesthetist fully inflate the lung. Remove the catheter when no more bubbles appear. Expose a portable chest film in the recovery room.

C, If there is any possibility that the lung itself has been perforated, guide the catheter from the wound and place it under water in a sterile vacuum system (Pleur-Evac).

A pleural tear that involves injury to both the underlying lung and the intercostal vessels in the chest wall usually results in hemopneumothorax. Insert a large right-angle tube with all the holes within the chest. The tube must be fastened to the chest wall with a silk suture that closes the skin firmly around the tube and also grasps the catheter so that it is not inadvertently withdrawn. Add a seal of petroleum jelly gauze around the tube, and connect it to continuous drainage using a three-bottle suction apparatus. Make a portable upright chest radiograph to make sure that the lung is expanded and all fluid has been evacuated from the pleura. When no air has been aspirated for 8 hours, remove the tube.

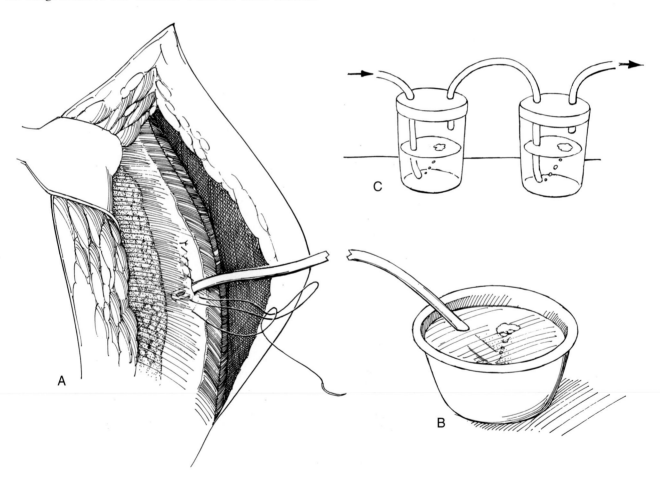

Commentary by Rolf Ackermann

The risk for a pneumothorax is low for surgery of the kidney or the adrenal. Patients with prior renal surgery and patients with a history of pyelonephritis, however, are at higher risk for sustaining a pneumothorax. In these patients, the upper pole of the kidney frequently adheres to the diaphragm and the pleura. Entry to the pleura is also more frequent when an incision is chosen in the 11th or 12th interspace. As described above, a small pleural tear can be closed with a running suture. It is important to instruct the anesthesiologist to fully inflate the lung prior to completing the closure of the pleura. This maneuver ensures that no air remains in the pleural space. One must also ensure that no significant amount of blood remains in the pleural space, in which case a fibrothorax occasionally develops and the lung becomes "trapped." In addition to its restrictive effect on ventilation, a fibrothorax may result in a mild scoliosis of the thoracic region of the spine. As already mentioned, it is of paramount importance that a postoperative radiograph is taken whenever the pleura has been opened during an operation.

Splenorrhaphy and Splenectomy

SPLENORRHAPHY AFTER INTRAOPERATIVE INJURY

Injury of the spleen during an operation, especially during left transperitoneal nephrectomy, usually results from avulsion of the capsule by forcible retraction of the spleen away from the retroperitoneal surface. It is held in place by the splenomental fold that runs between the greater omentum and the medial aspect of the lower pole of the spleen. The splenic capsule may also be torn by traction against the splenocolic and splenorenal ligaments. For a difficult left nephrectomy, take down these ligaments first. In any case, use padded retractors, place them carefully yourself, and instruct your assistant to use care in retraction. Removal of the spleen results in a life-long susceptibility to infection.

Segmental splenectomy may be feasible because of the segmental distribution of the blood supply. It is the preferable alternative if the laceration itself cannot be repaired by splenorrhaphy.

Initial Control

Start by covering the avulsed area with hemostatic gauze (microfibrillar collagen, Avitene) that has been immersed in thrombin and firmly holding it in place with a dry laparotomy pad. Avoid holding it with a retractor, which usually makes the tear worse or starts a new one. Remove the pad and trim any excess gauze. If the area is still bleeding, add more gauze, cover it again, and proceed with the intended operation. If necessary, place a row of 4-0 synthetic absorbable mattress sutures over it. Small bolsters of hemostatic gauze can be inserted under the longitudinal loops of the suture to decrease cutting into the capsule. Take great care not to tear the capsule further.

Compression of Splenic Vessels

If the bleeding is brisk and time is needed for repair, open the lesser sac and compress the tail of the pancreas over the splenic vessels. Mobilize the spleen by incising the lienorenal ligament to allow delivery of the spleen and tail of the pancreas into the wound (see Step 4). The splenic vessels are then readily compressed, and the splenic wound itself can be tamponaded and repaired under direct vision.

SPLENORRHAPHY

Place a running 3-0 SAS in the capsule 1 cm from the edge over hemostatic gauze bolsters. If the laceration is deep, separate the edges and ligate the torn vessels or remove the involved segment as described for repair of renal injuries (see pages 934 to 935).

1 **A,** Bring the omentum over to cover the tear. Fix it in place with mattress sutures held by figure-eight sutures with fat bolsters.

B, For gross injury, stretch polyglycolic acid knitted mesh over the spleen and sew the edges of the mesh together, either to encase the entire spleen or to cover one pole as a cap.

Accessory spleens may be encountered, usually with independent blood supplies, and should be preserved.

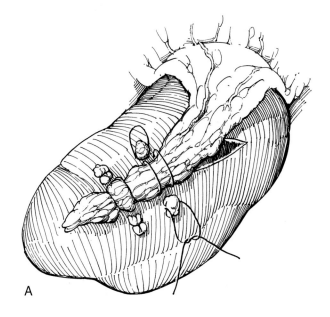

A

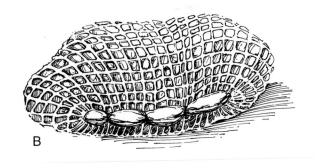

B

PARTIAL SPLENECTOMY

The vasculature to the spleen, being somewhat like that of the kidney, allows segmental splenectomy. Selective ligation is possible because the splenic artery, before it reaches the spleen, gives off a superior polar artery supplying the upper segment of the spleen. Near the hilus it divides again into two branches to the middle and lower polar segments. By preliminary ligation of one of these vessels, a segment of the spleen may be removed along a relatively avascular plane.

Tip the spleen down and work on the posterior portion. Isolate the main splenic artery, and encircle it with a vessel loop. Follow the artery to its main branch (to the upper pole) and into its two inferior divisions. Compress the appropriate vessel to find which one supplies the injured portion by observing immediate blanching there. Ligate and divide the selected artery.

Incise the capsule, and divide the parenchyma with sharp and blunt dissection. Use a Frazier neurosurgical suction tip to help identify and clip the intrasplenic vessels. For dissection of the parenchyma, apply an argon-beam coagulator, although blunt dissection with hemostasis by pressure alone is usually adequate. Clip or ligate vessels as they are encountered. The arteries are obvious as they protrude from the parenchyma, where they can be clamped and ligated. The veins lie flush with the surface and require figure-eight sutures. Control residual ooze with microfibrillar collagen. Place long mattress sutures in the edges of the capsule to occlude the parenchyma even if the capsule itself cannot be approximated. Drainage is not necessary.

SPLENECTOMY

Removal of the spleen should be the last resort because the result is life-long susceptibility to infection. Because patients undergoing left transperitoneal radical nephrectomy have an increased risk of splenic injury with resulting splenectomy and consequent increased susceptibility to infection, administer pneumococcal vaccine preoperatively to those older than 65 years.

2 The blood supply to the spleen is from the celiac artery through the terminal branches of the splenic artery that runs in the leinorenal ligament.

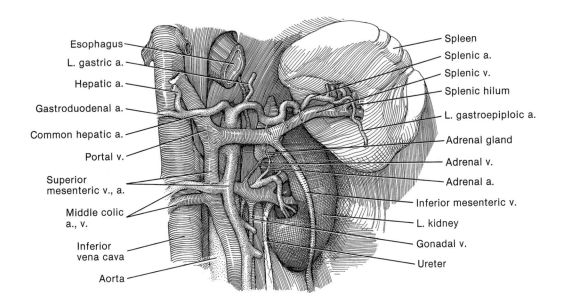

Esophagus — L. gastric a. — Hepatic a. — Gastroduodenal a. — Common hepatic a. — Portal v. — Superior mesenteric v., a. — Middle colic a., v. — Inferior vena cava — Aorta

Spleen — Splenic a. — Splenic v. — Splenic hilum — L. gastroepiploic a. — Adrenal gland — Adrenal v. — Adrenal a. — Inferior mesenteric v. — L. kidney — Gonadal v. — Ureter

3 With the right hand, gently retract the greater omentum and transverse colon inferiorly.

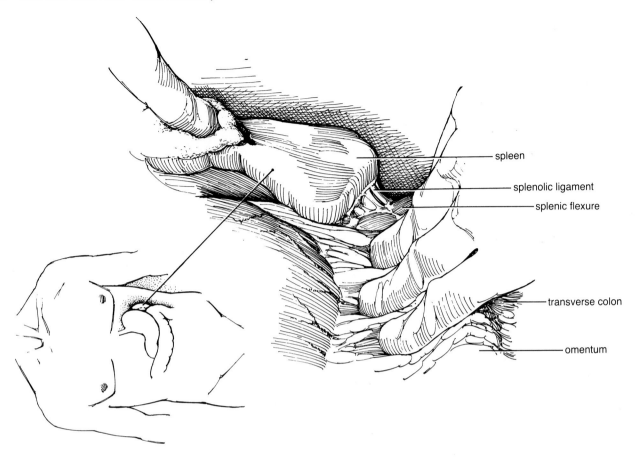

spleen

splenolic ligament

splenic flexure

transverse colon

omentum

4 With the left hand, reach over the top of the spleen and rotate it anteriorly and medially. First incise the attachments to the peritoneum, then those to the kidney (lienorenal ligament), diaphragm, and colon (splenocolic ligament).

Lienorenal ligament

Spleen

Splenic flexure of the colon

Splenocolic ligament

5 Slide the left hand more laterally to hook the finger tips under the medial edge of the peritoneum that was just divided. Avoid traction injury to the splenic capsule or vessels. Incise the posterior parietal peritoneum superiorly and inferiorly to the pancreas, and release the final attachments of the splenocolic and splenodiaphragmatic ligaments. Place one or two laparotomy tapes into the bed to ensure hemostasis and to keep the spleen from dropping back into the wound. Identify the gastrosplenic ligament and the short gastric vessels where the spleen abuts the stomach. Be sure to work high on the greater curvature of the stomach in a caudad to cephalad direction to expose and avoid tearing the most cephalad short gastric vessels.

Splenic flexure

Splenocolic ligament

Omentum

Spleen

6 Lift the spleen with the left hand. Hold the tail of the pancreas out of the way with the left thumb and index finger during dissection of the vessels under direct vision and during clamping. Dissect the artery from the vein before it divides into its branches. Clamp and ligate the artery first; contraction of the spleen gives the patient a transfusion. Clamp each vessel with three clamps. Be sure not to clamp or ligate any part of the stomach. Divide the vessels, and have your assistant tie them beneath the clamps. The *splenic vein* pursues a tortuous course above the pancreas that allows it to be ligated at one of its anterior bends. If the pedicle is small, it may be clamped in toto, but with some risk of an arteriovenous fistula.

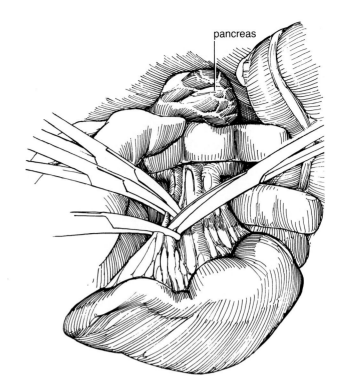

pancreas

7 Cut between the distal clamps. Tie beneath the first clamp with a 2-0 or 3-0 SAS, and remove the clamp. Repeat for the second clamp. Remove the packs from the bed. If any bleeders are seen, oversew them with 4-0 SAS. Drainage is not necessary.

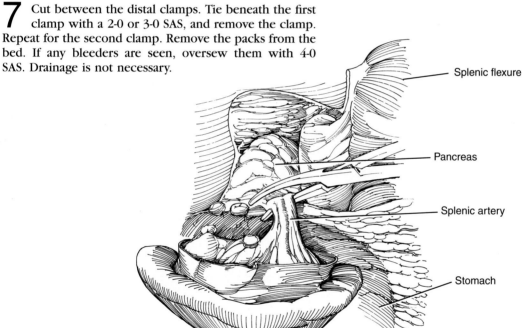

Splenic flexure

Pancreas

Splenic artery

Stomach

POSTOPERATIVE PROBLEMS

Because of the risk of overwhelming infection, administer 14-valent pneumococcal polysaccharide vaccine and penicillin.

Commentary by George F. Sheldon

The details of splenectomy and management of operations in the region of the spleen are well illustrated in the text. To emphasize several of the essential ingredients: On entering the abdomen, if the spleen is to be in the operative area, it is well to see if any adhesions are present from the capsule of the spleen to the anterior or lateral abdominal wall. Occasionally a few of these are present and can easily be divided at that point; preclude avulsion of part of the splenic capsule by using a retractor. A second maneuver that is useful to avoid injury to the spleen is, immediately upon entering the abdomen, to grasp the splenic flexure of the colon and the greater curvature of the stomach in one hand as one begins to mobilize. Such a maneuver avoids putting a torque on the spleen.

If the capsule of the spleen has been injured, the magnitude of injury needs to be ascertained. If the injury is on the edge of the spleen, prior to using thrombostatic agents it is useful to set the cautery on high levels and coagulate the areas in a circular fashion; begin at the edge where the capsule was first avulsed and move to the center. The cautery can actually be inserted into the substance of the spleen a small distance and allowed to induce coagulation in that position. Following that, it is withdrawn, leaving a char on the site. Thrombostatic agents can then be used.

If the posterior edge of the spleen is injured or if control of the bleeding does not occur easily, it is mandatory to divide the splenocolic, splenorenal, and splenodiaphragmatic attachments to allow mobilization of the spleen into its embryonic position, which is midline. The capsular attachments of the spleen to the posterior parietes and diaphragm are variable. Sometimes they are flimsy and can almost be avulsed with finger dissection. More often it is better to incise them sharply or with a cautery in order to get the proper plane. The spleen is then mobilized anteriorly, making it possible to (1) control directly the site of bleeding, (2) do a partial splenectomy or hemisplenectomy, or (3) place the spleen in a Dexon mesh bag.

It is my practice when mobilizing the spleen not to be committed either to mobilization from a posterior approach to the midline or to control of the splenic vasculature through the gastrosplenic omentum. It is more useful to incise the gastrosplenic omentum and identify the splenic artery and vein coursing over the superior surface of the pancreas. One can begin then to encircle the spleen by dissecting the various capsular attachments. The difficult part of the dissection is usually at the most superior attachment, where the top of the spleen abuts against the stomach. Often the ligamentous attachment is firmest there, but if one dissects it with a right-angle clamp that is then cut over, one can easily find the top of the short gastric vessels, divide them between clamps, and mobilize the spleen readily without further injury. It is usually practical to place a large hemoclip on the splenic side and do a standard 4-0 suture tie on the stomach side. My practice has been to do a suture ligature as well to ensure that the short gastric blood vessels remain ligated if gastric distention occurs. The operation, then, is to dissect where dissection is easiest.

Several postoperative issues are important. The patient should receive immunization with a polyvalent pneumococcal vaccine and also immunization against other capsulated organisms, such as *Hemophilus*, which is now available. Re-immunization is now being recommended by some workers in the field. Because the risk of overwhelming post-splenectomy sepsis syndrome is small, I do not recommend that prophylactic penicillin therapy be instituted in adults. Patients are instructed to carry penicillin with them and, if they are away from medical attention at the time a respiratory infection occurs, to take the medicine on a 2- or 3-day cycle.

A practice I have found useful over the years is to sit with the patient and family and assist them in filling out a Medic Alert identification bracelet or tag. It is important to help the patient do this, as other bits of useful information can be placed on this identification, such as blood type, medications, and the like. The fact of doing this is prima-facie evidence that the surgeon has informed the patient of the dangers of splenectomy and presumably serves as some warning in case of litigation.

Repair of Incisional Hernia

Debility, perioperative deficiency of protein and vitamin C, previous wound infection, postoperative sepsis, vertical rather than transverse incisions, failure to use nonabsorbable or retention sutures when indicated, and excessive postoperative coughing are factors responsible for most postoperative incisional hernias.

Bulging of the flank after lateral incisions is more often denervation atrophy of the muscles of the ipsilateral body wall secondary to division of the subcostal nerve and rarely is an actual hernia in which the skin is lined only by peritoneum. For these denervation "hernias," repair may be done for cosmetic reasons or for local discomfort; the risk of intestinal incarceration is small.

Provide prophylactic antibiotics before and after the operation.

IMBRICATED REPAIR

1 *Position:* Lateral or oblique, depending on the site of the hernia. Place a nasogastric tube if the hernia involves the peritoneum.

A, *Incision:* Make an elliptical incision, and excise the scar and excess skin.

B, Extend the incision through the subcutaneous layer circumferentially, exposing normal fascia and muscle layers around the defect. Have your assistant elevate the wound edges with large rake retractors. Mobilize the fasciomuscular flaps, and define the margins of the defect. Do not open the hernia sac prematurely. Meticulous hemostasis is important.

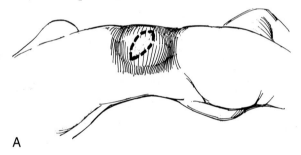

A

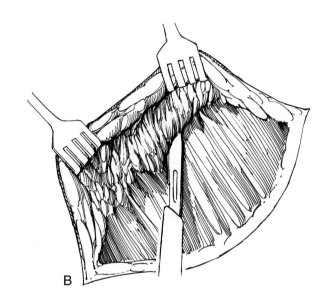

B

2 Deliberately open the peritoneal sac, which comprises attenuated subcutaneous tissue and peritoneum. Free the peritoneum from the intestinal contents if it is adherent. Trim the edges of the hernia sac until sound fascia and muscle layers are reached.

3 Imbricate the fascia in a vest-over-pants technique with heavy SAS placed as interrupted mattress stitches. Do this by entering the upper fascia 2 or 3 cm from its edge and then passing the suture through the lower fascia 1 cm from its edge. Exit from the lower flap 1 cm lateral to the site of entry; then exit from the upper flap 1 cm lateral to the original site of entry. Clamp the ends of the suture. Repeat these stitches 1 cm apart for the length of the defect. Tie them sequentially while your assistant keeps tension on the remainder.

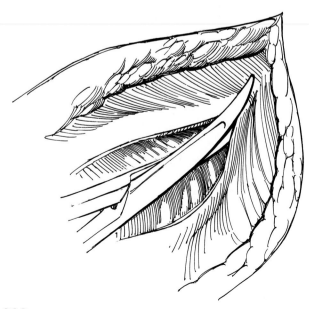

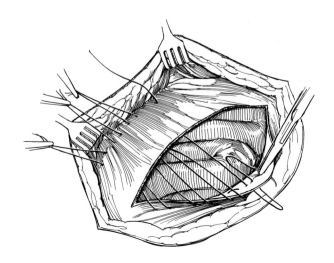

4 Run a heavy SAS under the flap just below the first row of sutures. Take care not to go through the fascia and involve the underlying bowel in the stitch.

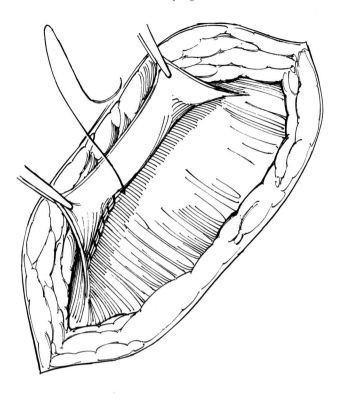

5 Place a row of interrupted figure-eight sutures of heavy synthetic absorbable material between the upper flap and the adjacent lower (posterior) flap. Insert two suction drains in the subcutaneous space, but do not place sutures there in an attempt to close another layer. Close the skin with interrupted or subcuticular sutures. An abdominal binder over the dressing is usually not necessary. Nasogastric suction may not be necessary if all fluids by mouth are withheld until good propulsive peristalsis is heard.

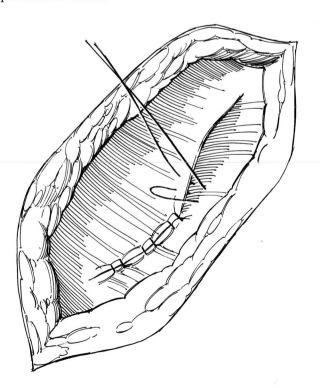

DARNING METHOD

Close the defect edge to edge with interrupted sutures, and strengthen the closure by running a firmly placed monofilament nylon suture back and forth both vertically and horizontally to "darn" the defect. This technique, however, encourages closure under tension, which is associated with recurrence. If this technique is to be used, relaxing fascial incisions placed well lateral to the defect are necessary to reduce the tension.

INVERSION REPAIR

Free the sac and expose the surrounding fascia. Invert the sac into the abdomen, and approximate the fascial edges with heavy figure-eight sutures that include the full thickness of the fascial wall and an edge of infolded peritoneum. If the hernia is anterior, close with muscle and fascia in layers, if possible.

AUGMENTED REPAIR OF LARGE DEFECTS USING SYNTHETIC MATERIALS

Proceed as previously described, clearing the fascial surfaces of fat. If possible, close the peritoneum separately with 3-0 or 4-0 SAS. Cut to the necessary shape a piece of polypropylene mesh large enough to overlap the edges of the defect by 2 to 3 cm. Suture the mesh to the aponeurosis with interrupted 2-0 or 3-0 NAS. A stronger repair can be obtained by placing the mesh under the fascial layer rather than on top of it. Additional support for the mesh inferiorly may be obtained by drilling holes in the iliac crest for insertion of polypropylene sutures (Sutherland and Gerow, 1995). If asepsis or hemostasis is questionable, do not use polypropylene mesh because the mesh must be removed if the wound becomes infected. Substitute tantalum mesh if asepsis is in doubt. Close the subcutaneous tissues and skin over suction drains.

POSTOPERATIVE PROBLEMS

Infection is the greatest concern, especially if synthetic materials have been placed. It must be treated aggressively, although removal of the mesh is usually necessary. *Recurrence* of the hernia is not as common as persistent bulging of the area.

Commentary by Andrew W. Bruce

Imbricated repair: It is essential to delineate clearly the different fascial and muscle layers. If the hernia is situated posteriorly, the repair may involve the tendinous aponeuroses of the muscle layers (lumbodorsal fascia). If the hernia is in the anterior end of the wound, actual muscle with intervening fascial layers may be involved. It is essential, in the latter situation, to repair the hernia using both muscle and fascial sheaths. I use interrupted sutures for at least one layer. (I prefer all layers to be closed with interrupted sutures.) Excise adequate amounts of excess skin and subcutaneous fat.

Treat the underlying bowel with respect. It may be possible to avoid opening the peritoneum; nevertheless, take care to avoid bowel injury when inserting repair sutures. Use tissue forceps to identify the different fascial muscle layers; using forceps is more effective than using a rake retractor. A self-retaining retractor may be helpful after the individual muscles are cleared and allows layer-by-layer closure. If the peritoneum is opened, excise the excess; then close the peritoneum as a single layer with a continuous absorbable suture. I agree with the vest-over-pants technique.

In the illustrations, only one layer of closure is shown with the vest-over-pants technique. It is better to identify the different muscles and close them separately, particularly in anteriorly located hernias. A supporting dressing is useful, with interrupted cotton ties if necessary. An abdominal binder is seldom needed.

I do not use the darning repair. The inversion repair is the best technique for dealing with the peritoneum. The rest of the repair should be in layers. As for the use of synthetic materials, I agree with the comments in general, but I have needed to use those materials very infrequently.

SECTION
21
Kidney: Reconstruction

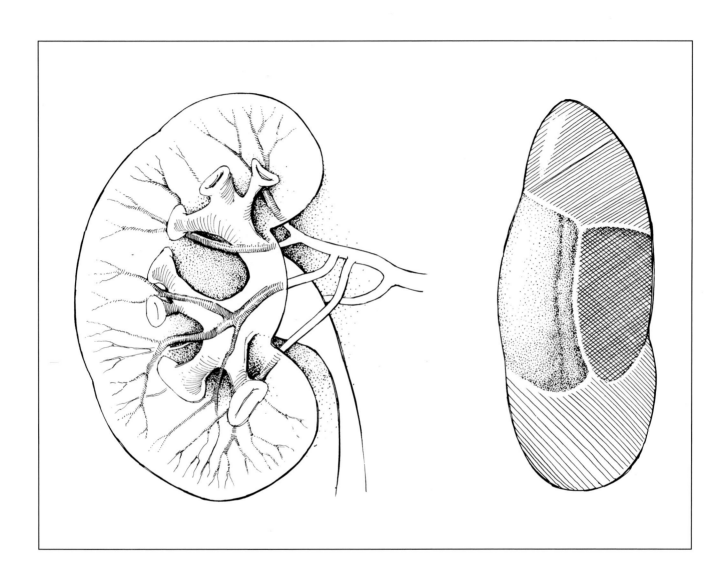

Principles of Renal Reconstruction

RENAL BLOOD SUPPLY

Knowledge of the blood supply to the kidney, especially to the pelvis and calyces, should precede reconstructive procedures.

1 The main renal arteries arise from the abdominal aorta and almost always lie between the upper edges of the first and third lumbar vertebrae. In one fourth of cases, additional small vessels may go directly from the abdominal aorta to the poles of the kidney.

The *renal artery* forms an anterior division that typically supplies three quarters of the blood and a posterior division that carries the rest. The "avascular plane" between these divisions lies in the axis of the posterior calyces (see pages 911 and 1049).

Five important branches originate as segmental arteries—apical or suprahilar, upper, middle, lower, and posterior segmental arteries—and supply the five corresponding segments of the kidney.

Pelvic arterial plexuses lie in the peripelvic connective tissue sheath of the wall of the pelvis and the major and minor calyces, supplied by branches from an interlobar artery that pass to the wall of a nearby calyx, where the branch becomes very tortuous, forming a spiral artery. The pelvis also receives blood directly from the renal artery through a ureteral branch and from arteries in the perirenal fat.

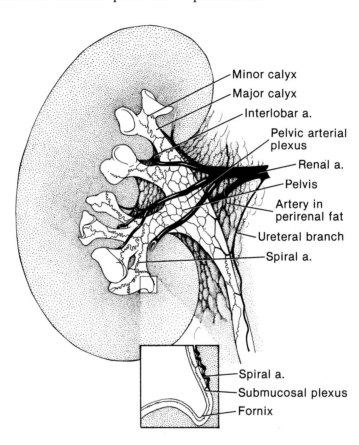

- Minor calyx
- Major calyx
- Interlobar a.
- Pelvic arterial plexus
- Renal a.
- Pelvis
- Artery in perirenal fat
- Ureteral branch
- Spiral a.

- Spiral a.
- Submucosal plexus
- Fornix

INDICATIONS FOR REPAIR

Indications for repair of hydronephrosis and estimation of the potential for recovery are among the recurrent controversies in urology. Now that fetal ultrasonography is routine, more cases are detected that require a decision for management soon after birth.

Imaging techniques applied to renal trauma similarly offer the opportunity for early treatment but require judgment so that unnecessary procedures are avoided. Vascular surgeons have developed procedures that experienced urologists with some special training are able to apply to the vessels supplying the kidney. The harvesting of kidneys for renal transplantation and the implantation itself are simple extensions of those techniques.

Pyeloureteroplasty

Endoscopic incision is an alternative, by either an antegrade or a retrograde technique, to open and laparoscopic procedures; its use is increasing, and success rates appear to be comparable to those for open repair. Among open procedures, the Anderson-Hynes dismembered pyeloplasty is the most adaptable technique because it not only uniformly provides a funnel but also allows resection of diseased portions of the pelvis and ureter. For selected cases, the YV-plasty and pelvic flap operations are elegant, the latter being especially useful for long ureteral defects. Intubation techniques are reserved for cases not suitable for a more anatomic repair.

Clear the urinary tract of infection if possible. Ascertain the presence and degree of obstruction as well as the function of the affected renal unit by radioisotope and pressure-flow studies. It is seldom necessary to perform ureterography to visualize the ureter when a preoperative superhydrated ultrasound study does not show a large ureter behind the bladder or dilation of the upper ureter below the ureteropelvic junction (UPJ). If there is doubt, perform a Whitaker test during surgery. Rule out reflux by voiding cystourethrography.

In a newborn infant, perform ultrasonography to evaluate the extent of the renal pelvic dilation, but delay further evaluation for 4 to 6 weeks if the problem is unilateral. Obtain voiding cystourethrography and a diethylenetriaminepentaacetic acid (DTPA) renal scan at that time. If obstruction is present and function is less than 35 percent, it is reasonable to repair the lesion within the following 6 weeks. Retrograde and antegrade studies are not needed in most instances. Pyeloplasty rather than nephrectomy should almost always be done in infants, even with renal function in the affected kidney as low as 10 percent of total, especially if the contralateral kidney does not show compensatory hypertrophy. Every nephron may be needed in later life when single-nephron hyperperfusion supervenes.

In bilateral cases, both sides may be corrected at the same session through anterior subcostal or posterior lumbotomy incisions. Use magnification, together with fine instruments and sutures.

Instruments: Provide a Basic pack, a GU fine set, Lahey and Potts scissors, Gil-Vernet retractors, 3× binocular loupes, 5 F and 8 F infant feeding tubes, Lahey and vascular forceps, a #11 hooked blade, a skin-marking pen, and swaged 4-0 to 6-0 synthetic absorbable sutures (SAS). In contrast to multifilament sutures, monofilament sutures do not drag nearby areolar tissue into the suture tract, tissue that may become necrotic and lead to leakage. Provide an internal stent. Drain the bladder with a catheter.

Place an anterior subcostal incision (see page 856), taking care to stay out of the peritoneal cavity, or use a flank incision (supracostal, see page 879, or subcostal, see page 871), as shown in the steps that follow. In infants, approach the renal pelvis through a dorsal lumbotomy incision (see page 896).

1 A, P*osition:* Flank position. Alternatively, for a more anterior approach to the renal pelvis, place the patient in a semioblique position, flexed over a rolled towel, air-filled intravenous bag, or sandbag.

Incision: Make an incision from the tip of the 12th rib to a point lateral to the rectus muscle and above the umbilicus, curving the anterior portion downward. Mobilize the colon medially. For bilateral cases, separate subcostal incisions are better than a single transperitoneal incision. If this is a secondary operation, make the new incision one rib higher and work from normal tissue to that involved previously. Place a self-retaining retractor.

B, Open Gerota's fascia laterally to preserve its dorsal layer with its contained perinephric fat, which is used later to cover the repair. Avoid entering the peritoneum. Dissect sharply and bluntly while rotating the kidney clockwise on the right and counterclockwise on the left to expose the posterior aspect of the pelvis. Free as little as possible of the kidney itself (unless some ureter must be resected and the kidney moved down), and leave some fat attached for traction and manipulation. Have your assistant hold the lower pole up and anteriorly with a sponge stick to expose the UPJ posteriorly.

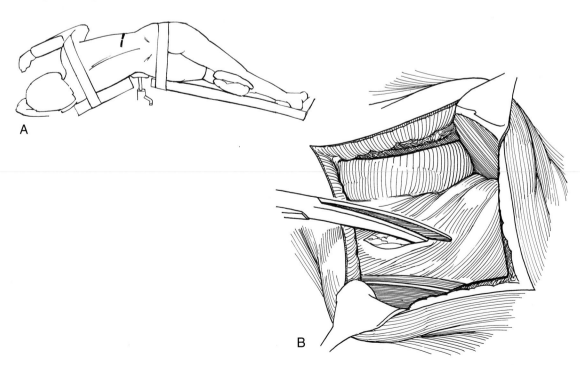

A

B

2 **A,** Expose the ureter below the UPJ, taking care not to interfere with the segmental blood supply to this area that enters the ureter from the medial side. Placing a small Penrose drain or vessel loop around the ureter may help mobilization but risks interfering with the ureteral blood supply. For secondary operations, locate the normal part of the ureter distally, and dissect proximally from normal to abnormal. Dissect as short a length of the ureter as possible, and preserve all its adventitial vessels. It is better to mobilize the kidney than the ureter.

B, Palpate and look for an aberrant lower-pole vessel, which is common with this anomaly. It can usually be moved out of the way after the ureter is divided because sacrificing it could result in segmental renal ischemia and systemic hypertension.

Selection of Technique. After exposure of the UPJ, make a decision about what type of operation to use. Obstructions are located (1) at the UPJ from a high insertion anomaly with or without stricture, the most common finding; (2) just below the UPJ owing to stricture; or (3) in the upper segment of the ureter as a stricture or ureteral valve. It is necessary to ask whether the ureter is long enough to allow dismemberment and excision of the UPJ. If it is, a modified Anderson-Hynes dismembered pyeloplasty is most often suitable, although a Foley Y-plasty works well with high insertions of the ureter. For a long, dependent obstruction of the UPJ, the Culp or Scardino technique may solve the problem of insufficient ureter for approximation. If the site of the obstruction is in doubt, fill the pelvis with saline through a scalp vein needle and observe the site of hold-up.

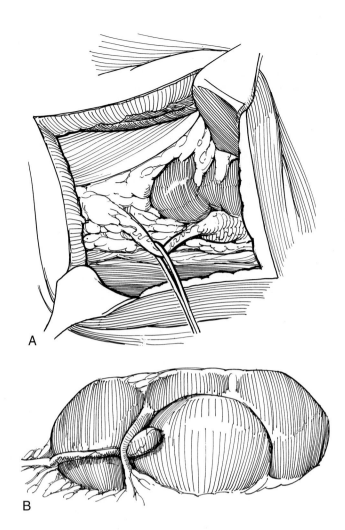

A

B

DISMEMBERED PYELOPLASTY
(Anderson-Hynes)

3 Place a stay suture in the ureter at its junction with the pelvis. Divide the ureter obliquely, and spatulate its less vascularized lateral surface for a distance equal to the length of the proposed V-shaped flap, a step often more accurately done after the pelvic flap is formed.

Alternatively, divide the ureter transversely, insert a traction suture, and spatulate the end; excise the pelvis and form a V-flap at the caudal rim; insert the V-flap into the spatulated ureter to provide a tapered junction.

If distal ureteral obstruction was not ruled out by preoperative sonography, checking for narrowing of the upper ureter by passing a 5 F infant feeding tube distally may not be wise because it could instigate a stricture. Instead, insert an infant feeding tube attached to an open syringe filled with saline into the ureter for a short distance. Flow at an elevation of 10 cm indicates adequate ureteral patency.

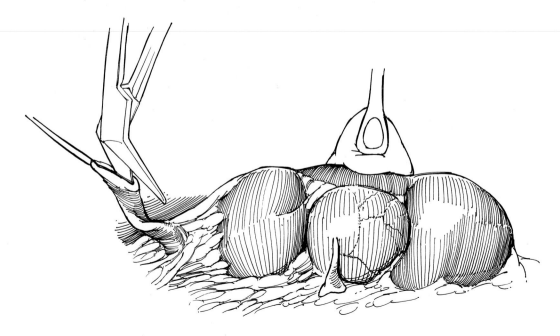

4 With the pelvis full, dissect it free and map out the proposed diamond-shaped incision with a skin-marking pen, angling the caudal triangle medially to form a V-flap. The kidney can be brought up into the wound with vein or Gil-Vernet retractors or rotated with a sponge stick. Place stay sutures of 5-0 silk at the angles of the diamond. Because considerable pyelectasis is the rule, the diamond should include a portion of the pelvis for reduction pyeloplasty as part of the repair.

Caution: Do not place the stay sutures too far apart and thus remove too much pelvis, especially in a bifid system. Keep the incision well away from the caliceal necks, which can be surprisingly close to its edge after pelvic excision; otherwise, closure is difficult and infundibular stenosis may result.

Start dismemberment by incising for a short distance along one of the planned lines with a #11 hooked blade.

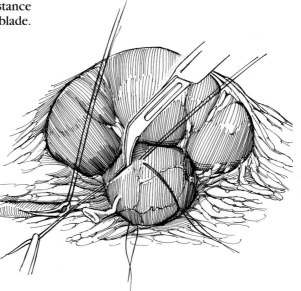

5 Complete the resection with Lahey or Potts scissors, cutting from inside one stay suture to inside the next. Remove the specimen.

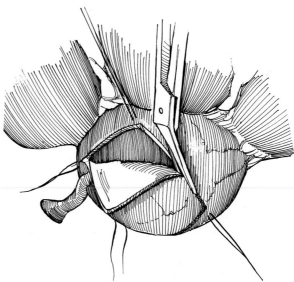

6 **A,** Insert an infant feeding tube of suitable size into the ureter to prevent catching the far wall in a suture. Using binocular loupes, place one 6-0 or 7-0 SAS adjacent to the apex of the V-shaped flap from outside in, then out through the apex of the ureteral slit. Place a second suture 2 mm away from the first. Tie both sutures with four knots, and cut the short ends. Use the ureteral stay suture for manipulation; do not use forceps. Alternatively, place a mattress stitch with a double-armed suture, and run one end up the back wall from inside the lumen and the other up the front wall.

B, Catch minimal epithelium; include more muscularis and adventitia in the stitch.

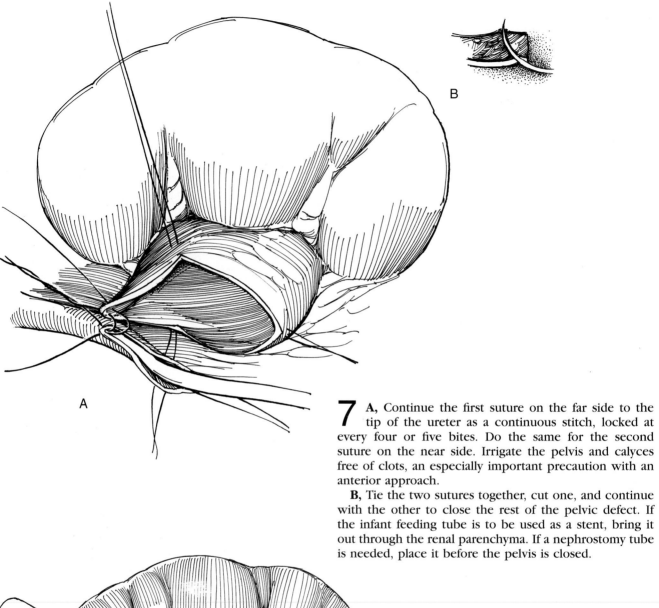

A

B

7 **A,** Continue the first suture on the far side to the tip of the ureter as a continuous stitch, locked at every four or five bites. Do the same for the second suture on the near side. Irrigate the pelvis and calyces free of clots, an especially important precaution with an anterior approach.

B, Tie the two sutures together, cut one, and continue with the other to close the rest of the pelvic defect. If the infant feeding tube is to be used as a stent, bring it out through the renal parenchyma. If a nephrostomy tube is needed, place it before the pelvis is closed.

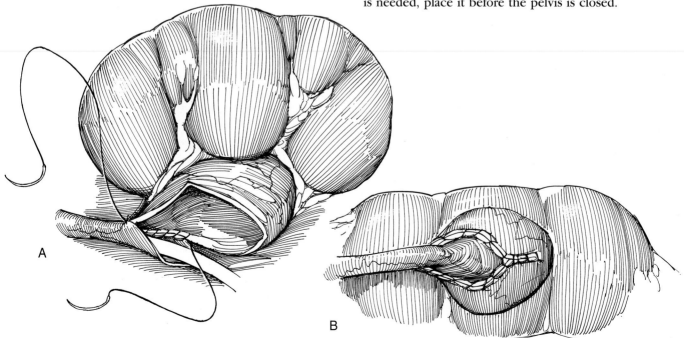

A

B

8 Alternatively, form a purse-string opening around the central defect by starting a third suture from the upper end.

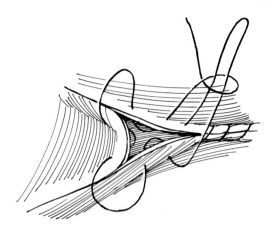

9 Inject saline with a fine needle through the pelvic wall to test for watertightness and for patency of the anastomosis. Alternatively, if the infant feeding tube was left in place, withdraw it until the tip lies in the renal pelvis, and allow saline to flow through it by gravity at an elevation of 10 cm. Add a suture or two if needed to close a leak. Use an omental wrap (see page 74) if the tissues appear poorly vascularized or if the operation is a second one.

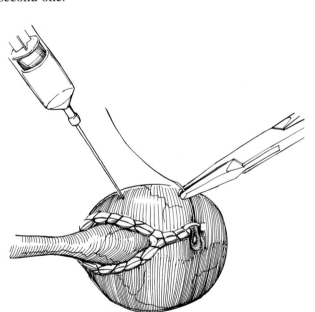

10 Insert a Penrose drain, and fasten it near but not touching the anastomosis or the ureter below it. Use the *long suture technique* (see page 12) to ensure that contact is not made. Alternatively, use a suction drain. Accurate drainage is important. If the kidney has been mobilized, hold it up into normal position with nephropexy stitches (Step 19); otherwise the lower pole falls forward against the ureter. Such fixation is more often needed with a flank approach. Tack the preserved posterior edge of Gerota's fascia to the anterior edge with fine plain catgut (PCG) to hold the perirenal fat around the kidney and isolate the repair from the body wall. Close the wound in layers, leading the drain laterally so that the patient does not lie on it.

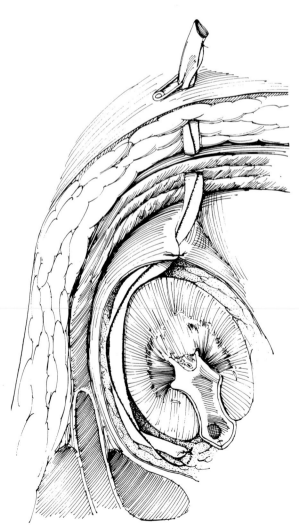

11 *Stenting:* In general, avoid placing a stent, although it may prevent kinking by a large floppy pelvis. A good compromise may be to place a nephrostomy tube in an infant and to use both a tube and a double-J stent in any difficult repair.

A, If the repair has been difficult, as after previous pyeloplasty, and appears tenuous or if the kidney is infected, insert a nephrostomy tube (see page 928) before closing the pelvis. Alternatively, insert a nephrostomy tube along with a double-J stent, or use a grooved KISS catheter that stents and exits through the pelvic wall or a perforated length of soft silicone tubing.

B, A Cummings tube, combining nephrostomy and stent, is an alternative. If such a stent is too long, it may enter the bladder and siphon off the bladder contents, an event that can be very disturbing.

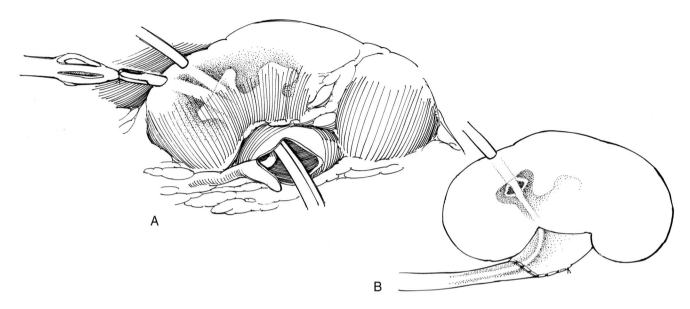

Unless a stent or nephrostomy tube has been placed, insert a balloon catheter into the bladder to prevent back pressure on the repair, and remove it in 24 to 48 hours. This is especially important in infants, who may not void for 12 to 24 hours. Consider giving suppressive antibiotic therapy. Avoid irrigating a nephrostomy tube. Discharge the patient with the drain in place. Shorten the drain 2 days after drainage stops, and then remove it. If a stent has been placed, take it out in 10 to 12 days unless the repair was tenuous. Remove the nephrostomy tube when nephrostography shows no extravasation and ready drainage of the contrast medium when the pelvis is filled. Little residual urine should remain after a trial of intermittent clamping. Perform intravenous urography after 3 months, 1 year, and 5 years.

LAPAROSCOPIC DISMEMBERED PYELOPLASTY (Schuessler)

Caution the patient about the limited data on the results of the procedure. Insert a 6 F or 7 F double-J stent in the affected ureter at operation or, preferably, 2 to 3 weeks before, with fluoroscopic guidance if necessary.

Insert a 16 F balloon catheter in the bladder. *Position:* Place the patient in the lateral decubitus position at a 75-degree angle, held with a vacuum bean bag. Induce a pneumoperitoneum. Place one 10-mm trocar two fingerbreadths below the costal margin in the midclavicular line. Place a second trocar caudad to the first and a third in the anteroaxillary line. Remember that veins injured by trocar insertion do not bleed during pneumoperitoneum but do so copiously at the end of the procedure.

Mobilize the appropriate part of the colon, and reflect it medially. Place one or two more 10-mm trocars more laterally in the midaxillary line if needed for renal traction. Two or three stay sutures in the pelvis, either supported transabdominally or exiting transcutaneously and manipulated outside the body, expand and support the pelvis during the dissection and anastomosis and reduce the need for extra ports (Recker et al, 1995).

Identify the proximal ureter as far as the UPJ, and dissect it free. Look for crossing vessels; if any are found, clip and divide them. Dissect the entire renal pelvis free on both aspects.

Mark the proposed incision with the electrocautery. To excise the anterior part of the pelvis, make diverging incisions with the rotating endoscopic scissors, starting from the superior medial aspect of the pelvis. As the incisions progress, close the opening left behind them with a running 4-0 SAS on a straight or ski needle. Before either spatulating the UPJ or detaching the ureter, insert a suture between the apex of the ureter and the lowest part of the pelvis and leave it untied. Cut the ureter 1.5 cm above the apex of the spatulation, and cut the pelvis through the posterior layer, excising the UPJ. Insert a second suture anteriorly near the first, and tie the two sutures. Place one additional interrupted suture anteriorly; then close the posterior wall with a running suture, held at the end with a resorbable clip. Alternatively, spatulate the ureter and start two 4-0 SAS at the apex. Run two sutures lines in opposite directions to close the UPJ. In some cases, rather than excision of the defect, the simpler Heinecke-Mikulicz incision and closure can be applied.

Insert a 7-mm suction drain retroperitoneally through a trocar site with grasping forceps using two trocars. Replace the colon and hold it with hernia staples. Leave the stent in place for at least 6 weeks. The procedure may also be done extraperitoneally by inflating a balloon in the retroperitoneum (see page 994).

YV-PLASTY
(Foley)

The Foley Y-plasty can be used for a high insertion of the ureter, especially when the pelvis has a box shape. It requires more ability to visualize the rearrangement than does the dismembered operation.

12 **A,** Free the ureter but preserve the adventitia. **B,** Draw the ureter cephalad with a Penrose drain. Mark a long Y-shaped incision between stay sutures. Incise the pelvis between the stays with a #11 hooked blade, and open it with Potts scissors, forming a V with arms equal to the length of the ureteral incision. At this point, consider placing a nephrostomy tube with or without a ureteral stent.

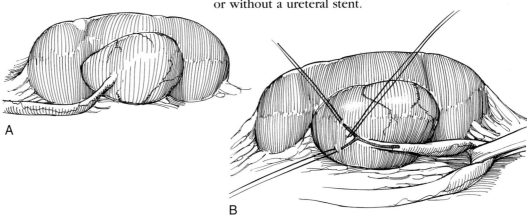

A

B

13 Suture the apex of the flap to the apex of the ureteric incision by placing a 7-0 SAS in through the apex of the V and out through the apex of the ureteral incision, and tie it. Include a minimal amount of epithelium.

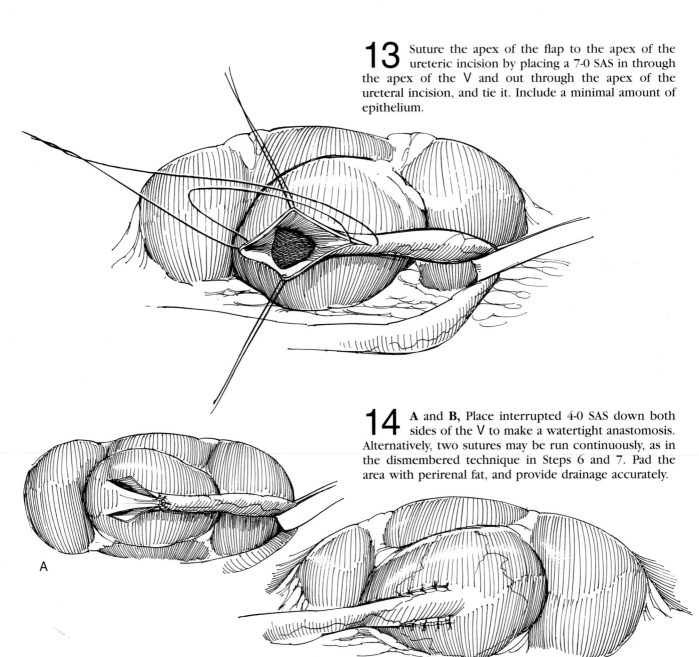

A

B

14 **A and B,** Place interrupted 4-0 SAS down both sides of the V to make a watertight anastomosis. Alternatively, two sutures may be run continuously, as in the dismembered technique in Steps 6 and 7. Pad the area with perirenal fat, and provide drainage accurately.

PELVIC FLAP PYELOPLASTY
(Culp-DeWeerd)

Use the Culp-DeWeerd procedure for long, low defects with a dilated pelvis, for which a dismembered procedure would result in tension. The Scardino-Prince variation (not shown) uses a vertical instead of a spiral flap; it is more suitable for cases with higher insertion of the ureter. Alternatives are dismembering the spiral flap and performing calicoureterostomy (see page 841).

15 **A,** Mark a spiral (Culp) flap running obliquely around the enlarged pelvis, and extend the incision down the ureter for a distance equal to the length of the flap.

B, Incise the flap, and deflect it down with a stay suture.

C, Approximate the posterior edge of the flap to the lateral ureteral edge with a running 4-0 or 5-0 SAS.

D, Close the anterior edge of the flap and pelvis with similar sutures. It helps to place the sutures over a small infant feeding tube (not shown).

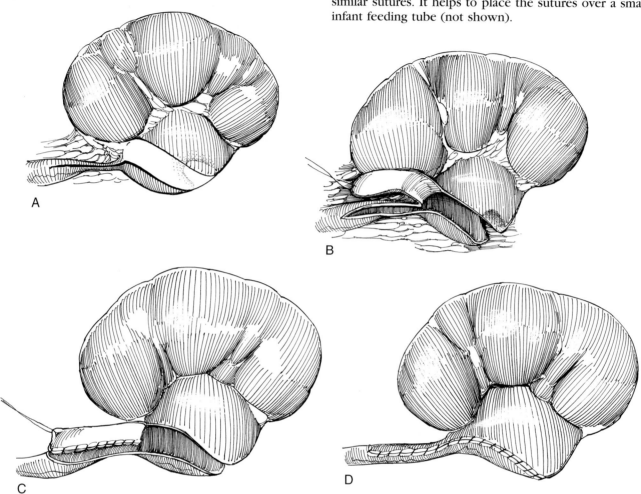

INTUBATED URETEROTOMY
(Davis)

Intubated ureterotomy is used for scarred defects near the UPJ, but endoscopic incision is usually preferred unless the defects are very long.

16 With a #11 knife blade, incise the pelvis just above the UPJ between two stay sutures. Open the ureter with Potts scissors until normal caliber is reached.

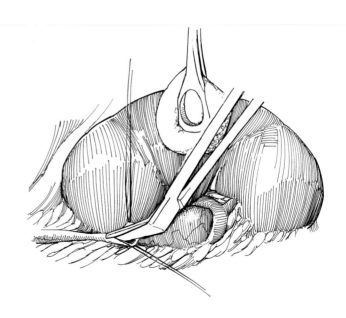

17 Insert an 8 F silicone double-J stent and a nephrostomy tube. Tack the edges of the defect together loosely with 5-0 SAS.

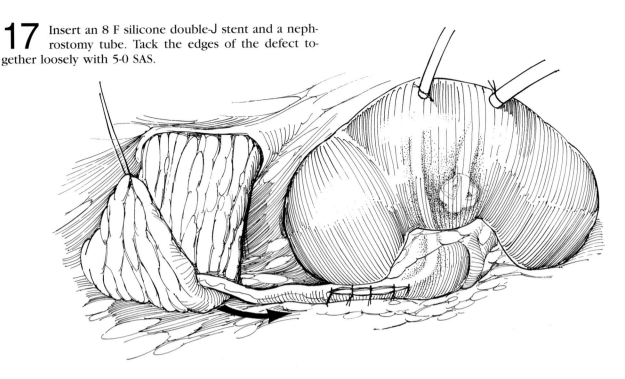

18 For a lower defect, incise it laterally over a small-caliber double-J stent. Place a few fine sutures to hold the ureter loosely against the stent, being sure not to constrict it.

Close the pelvic defect after placing a nephrostomy tube. Tack retroperitoneal fat around the defect, or bring the omentum through the posterior peritoneum and wrap it around the ureter (see page 74) (not shown). Perform a nephropexy (see Step 19).

Drain the area of the repair very accurately with the long suture technique (see page 917), taking care that the end of the drain neither touches the repair nor is so far away that urine can accumulate in a pocket. Leave the stent in place at least 6 weeks, testing for sealing with nephrostography before and after removing it.

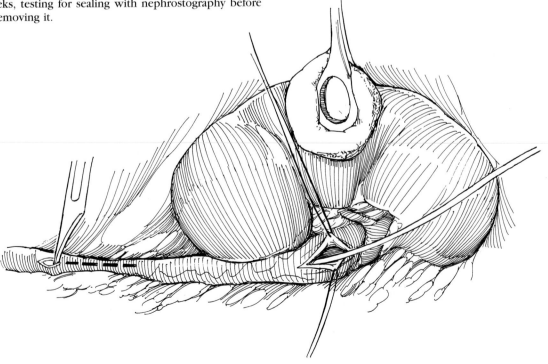

NEPHROPEXY

19 To prevent the lower pole of a kidney that has been extensively mobilized from sliding medially and making contact with or angulating the repair, fix it to the posterior body wall.

Place two mattress sutures in the renal capsule on the posterolateral aspect of the lower portion of the kidney, and tie them over bolsters of fat or absorbable sponge so that they do not cut through the capsule. Adherence is greater if a square of renal capsule is removed between the stay sutures.

Insert the sutures with mattress stitches into an appropriate area on the quadratus lumborum. Rotate the kidney into proper orientation, and tie the sutures.

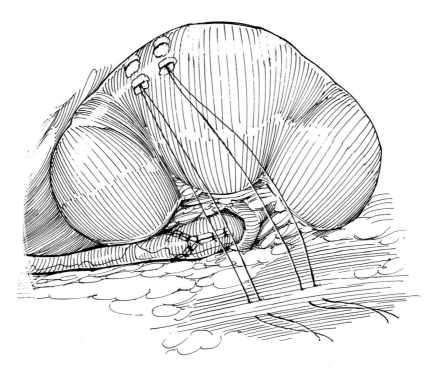

POSTOPERATIVE CARE

Test for patency of the anastomosis if a nephrostomy tube has been left in place by taping the tube to patient's chest and observing the filling level. When urine cannot be seen in the tube, the anastomosis is patent and the tube can be removed. It is also possible to perform a pressure-flow test (Whitaker). Remove the tube when the pressure at a flow of 10 ml/min is 15 cm H$_2$O or below.

At 3 months, obtain a diuretic nuclear renal scan. Repeat the scan in 6 months, and obtain a baseline sonogram. Follow with sonography at intervals. Further improvement in pelviocaliectasis is not to be expected after 24 months, although children exhibit good growth of the parenchyma after repair ("catch-up" growth). Do not expect complete resolution of caliectasis.

POSTOPERATIVE PROBLEMS

Bleeding can jeopardize the repair by the formation of clots that obstruct the outlet. The source of bleeding is usually the nephrostomy tract. If bleeding cannot be tamponaded, immediate re-exploration may be required. In general, avoid irrigation of the nephrostomy tube because irrigation introduces infection and can disrupt the suture line. *Acute pyelonephritis* indicates infection behind obstruction. If a nephrostomy tube was not inserted at operation, place one percutaneously.

Urinary leakage may occur within the first 24 hours as a result of an overfilled bladder (an argument for leaving a balloon catheter indwelling for the first day). Drainage lasting more than 1 week should be investigated because subsequent peripelvic and periureteral fibrosis harms the anastomosis and results in secondary procedures. First be sure that the drain is not in contact with the anastomosis or with the ureter below it. Shorten it and subsequently remove it, substituting a piece of red rubber catheter to keep the fascia open if drainage continues. Intravenous urography may identify the site of the leak and detect obstruction distal to it. Leakage may be managed expectantly by applying an adhesive stomal bag. It is usually necessary to insert a double-J stent from below or to place a percutaneous nephrostomy tube and a stent from above. Do this as soon as obstruction is suspected, the exception being in a small child. A *urinoma* may form if the drain is removed too soon, but passing a curved clamp down the drainage tract can usually relieve this problem. If the drain has fallen out prematurely, replace it with a cut-off small Robinson catheter with extra holes that is passed through the fascia. Transfix the catheter with a safety pin to prevent its loss in the wound and to aid in fixation to the skin. Before removing a stent, fill the system with contrast medium to test for leakage, removing the drain only after making sure the ureter is intact.

Obstruction at the UPJ after the stent is removed can be managed by leaving the nephrostomy tube in place, by placing one percutaneously until nephrostography shows an open tract, or by passing a double-J stent from below. To detect silent obstruction, check the renal status by sonography at 4 to 6 weeks, by a DTPA scan at 3 months, and by an intravenous pyelography at 6 months.

For *persistent obstruction,* attempt intubation from below. Perform antegrade ureterography to visualize the defect under fluoroscopy. Negotiate the stricture with a guide wire, and dilate it with a balloon catheter to 5 F to 8 F. If this fails, allow the area to heal; then traverse the stricture with a guide wire and proceed with direct-vision cold-knife *endopyelotomy* by either a retrograde, or more often, a percutaneous route. Incise the stricture on the posterolateral wall with a single incision into the perirenal fat to achieve a funnel appearance of the ureter. Place a 16 F Malecot nephrostomy tube percutaneously, with or without a ureteral extender, for access and diversion. A ureteral stent made from an infant feeding tube with extra side holes to allow drainage from the pelvis and bladder may also be placed. For strictures but not for fistulas, cap the stent when the antegrade drainage is satisfactory and the initial hematuria has resolved. Remove the stent in 4 to 6 weeks by exchanging it for a nephrostomy tube over a guide wire, followed by antegrade pyelography to be sure that the ureter is intact. Clamp the tube if it is intact; remove the tube in 2 or 3 days if the patient does well. If the ureter appears narrow, perform a perfusion pressure test. A few cases need formal reoperation (see later), but the explanation may lie in the initial involvement of the pelvis in extensive fibrosis. Pathologic examination of the resected portion of the pelvis, instead of showing muscular hypertrophy, may show fibrosis, explaining the poor function after a technically adequate repair. Other alternatives are transplanting the kidney to the true pelvis (see page 956) and constructing an ileal ureter (see page 842).

Other postoperative problems include granuloma formation around catgut sutures, wound infection, incisional hernia (see page 908), and complications associated with broken stents (see page 70).

REOPERATIVE PYELOPLASTY

Excessive urinary drainage in the immediate postoperative period signals eventual recurrence of the obstruction. An endourologic approach by placement of a percutaneous nephrostomy tube for immediate drainage and subsequent antegrade dilation or incision of the obstructed section, as is achieved in the intubated ureterotomy, may be done. Alternatively, the obstructed area may be approached and incised retrogradely.

For an open operation, approach the area from a different direction, if feasible, to start the dissection in previously unoperated territory. Avoid approaching the major vessels. Free the ureter first, keeping as much periureteral tissue adherent to it as possible. It is necessary to dissect the pelvis completely so that enough tissue is available for the repair.

Commentary by Terry W. Hensle

Pyeloureteroplasty or pyeloplasty is frequently—perhaps too frequently—done for the correction of UPJ obstruction. I do not share Dr. Hinman's optimism for the endopyelotomy as a primary therapy for UPJ obstruction, particularly in children. I do agree that the best procedure to obtain uniformly acceptable results is the Anderson-Hynes dismembered pyeloplasty. This procedure can be done at almost any age and is adaptable to almost any anatomic variant, except perhaps the extremely long upper ureteral stricture.

Several important technical points must be considered to ensure uniform success for a dismembered pyeloplasty. Exposure and visualization must be adequate. Excise enough redundant renal pelvis. Excise all the abnormal upper ureter, but do not devascularize the upper ureter. Design a long, spatulated, watertight anastomosis. Use optical magnification and fine long-acting absorbable sutures.

To accomplish each of these technical requirements, I follow several particular steps to ensure success. I find that a relatively short subcostal anterolateral incision provides the best retroperitoneal exposure for a dismembered pyeloplasty. The posterior (dorsal) lumbotomy incision causes less postoperative discomfort, but it does not provide nearly the exposure of the anterolateral subcostal incision. I do not use a kidney bridge, and I rarely flex the operating table except in older adolescents or young adults. Very adequate retroperitoneal exposure can be obtained using a soft rolled towel in infants or a plastic intravenous fluid bag inflated with air via a blood pressure pump in older children.

For retraction I use either a small Balfour retractor with an adjustable third blade or a curved Denis Browne ring retractor. The use of self-retaining retractors greatly enhances one's ability to manipulate the lower pole of the kidney and the UPJ without having too many hands or instruments in the operating field. Mobilization, exposure, and manipulation of the UPJ are best done with fine silk traction sutures. The use of traction sutures helps the surgeon avoid squeezing the tissue and causing trauma to the upper ureter and the area of anastomosis.

One should take care to outline a very adequate segment of renal pelvis for excision. Leaving excess pelvis causes stasis of urine behind a newly created anastomosis. One must also take great pains to completely excise all of the abnormal upper ureter. The abnormal segment should be discarded prior to spatulating the upper ureter for anastomosis. If at all possible, avoid using abnormal ureter as part of the anastomosis.

In most instances, spatulating the ureter on the ventral surface and the renal pelvis on the dorsal surface enables one easily to create a triangulated, funnel-shaped anastomosis. The initial suture of the anastomosis should be made at the most proximal portion of the ureteral spatulation, bringing the renal pelvis to the spatulated ureter and using that suture as a handle for manipulation. Following the initial suture, a second suture can be used in a running fashion up either side of the ureteropelvic anastomosis to create a watertight closure. I do not routinely use either an indwelling ureteral stent or a nephrostomy tube. If there is a particular reason for concern, as in a reoperation, a nephrostomy tube can be used to protect the anastomosis.

Postoperatively I use a Penrose drain and bladder catheter just as Dr. Hinman describes. It is unusual for a child to need more than 72 hours of hospitalization following a dismembered pyeloplasty. Follow-up is done with an ultrasound study at 1 month and a diuretic-augmented renal scan at 3 months.

Surgery for the Horseshoe Kidney

The horseshoe kidney retains parts of its developmental blood supply from the pelvic vessels. The isthmus and lower poles frequently receive blood from the common iliac arteries. The gonadal vessels pass over the lower renal vessels. Also, the ureters lie closer to the midline than normal. Realize that the isthmus itself is rarely obstructive; consequently, symphysiotomy is seldom indicated.

1 The approach to the horseshoe kidney depends on the objective of the operation. For correction of unilateral ureteropelvic junction (UPJ) obstruction or for nephrectomy, an anterior subcostal extraperitoneal incision provides good access (see page 871). In order to operate on both pelves and divide the isthmus as well, make a longer supraumbilical transverse incision, going transperitoneally and then reflecting the ascending and descending colon to reach the retroperitoneum. This gives excellent exposure and is recommended for a child. In an adult, a long midline incision is required.

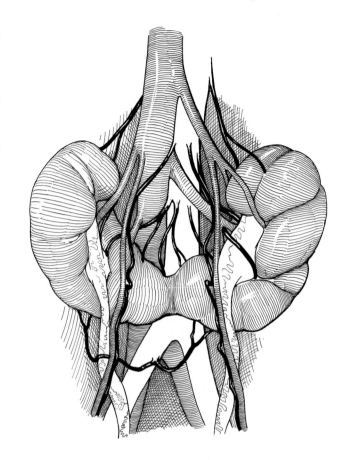

PYELOPLASTY

2 Approach the pelvis through an anterior subcostal incision. Mobilize the colon, and move Gerota's fascia and perirenal fat medially to provide cover for the repair later.

A modified Anderson-Hynes pyeloplasty is usually suitable (see page 914), although a Foley YV-plasty (see page 919) may occasionally be easier to perform.

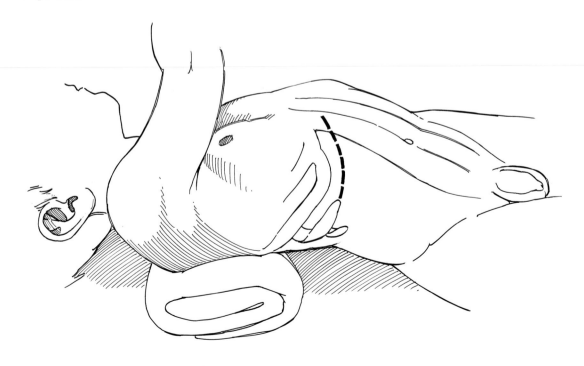

3 **A,** Place a stay suture in the ureter at its junction with the pelvis.

B, Divide and spatulate the ureter. Position the flap high on the pelvis so that when it is turned down its apex does not reach the isthmus; contact could compromise the repair. Mark it with three stay sutures.

C and **D,** Suture the ureter to the flap, starting at the apex of the flap and using two running 4-0 or 5-0 SAS with an occasional locked stitch. Install a Penrose drain fixed by the long-suture technique (see page 917), and bring it out extraperitoneally. Replace Gerota's fascia and perirenal fat around the drain.

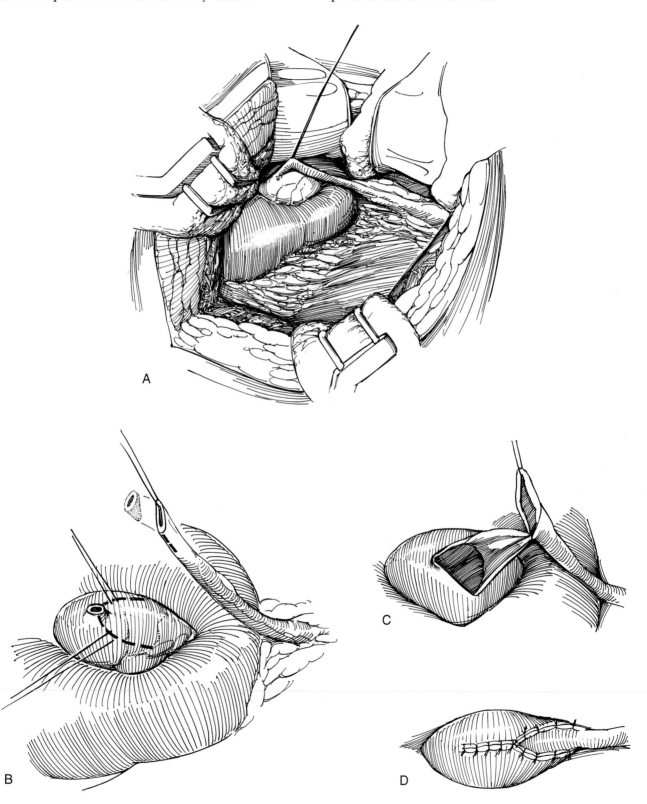

A

B

C

D

4 **A,** The Foley Y-plasty (see page 919) can be used in some situations. Hold the ureter cephalad with a Penrose drain. Incise the ureter vertically to its insertion into the pelvis. From this point, form a V with arms equal to the length of the ureteral incision. Consider placing a nephrostomy tube with or without a stent.

B, Place a 4-0 SAS in through the apex of the V and out through the apex of the ureteral incision, and tie it.

C, Place interrupted 4-0 SAS down both sides of the V to make a watertight anastomosis. Pad the area with perirenal fat, and provide drainage accurately. Use a similar incision and approach for pyelolithotomy.

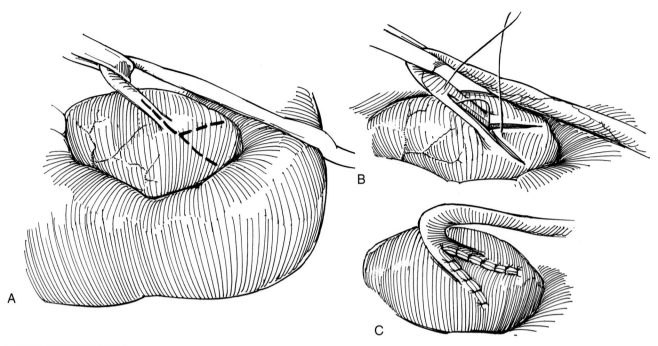

NEPHRECTOMY

5 **A and B,** Obtain wide exposure through a transperitoneal incision, long transverse in children or long midline in adults. Incise the peritoneum over the aorta and vena cava to get exposure of the vascular pedicles as for radical nephrectomy (see page 1016). Anterior-lying veins can be sacrificed. Free the upper pole of the affected kidney, and divide the ureter. Proceed to expose

the remainder of the anomalous vascular supply, and individually clamp, ligate, and divide each artery and then each vein supplying that kidney. Divide the isthmus last by making a V-shaped incision that leaves a notch in the remaining portion of the isthmus to aid in closure. The fixation of the kidney to pelvic blood vessels usually allows only minimal rotation of the lower poles.

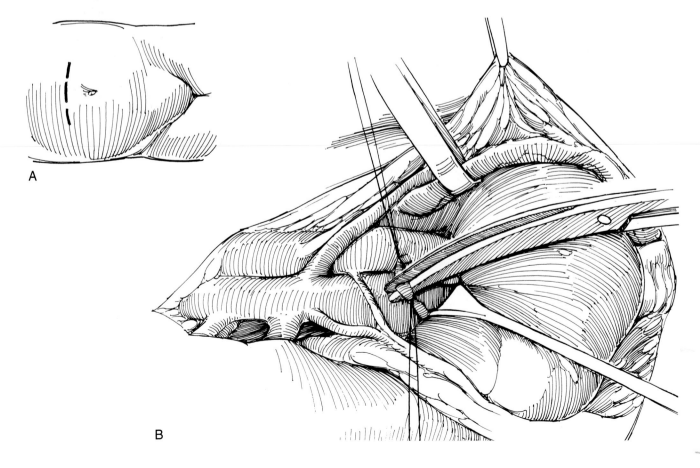

DIVISION OF THE ISTHMUS

Division of the isthmus is rarely indicated alone because ureteral obstruction usually results from high insertion rather than impingement by the isthmus. Division does allow the kidneys to be rotated into a somewhat more normal position for improved drainage from the pelves after pyeloplasty or to undergo radiography after removal of a staghorn calculus.

Mobilize the ascending colon and cecum along the white line, and move it across the great vessels. Enter Gerota's fascia laterally; take care to preserve it to cover the repair. Expose the isthmus by blunt dissection, and dissect the vessels entering it from the aorta and vena cava. Other vessels may come from the iliac arteries.

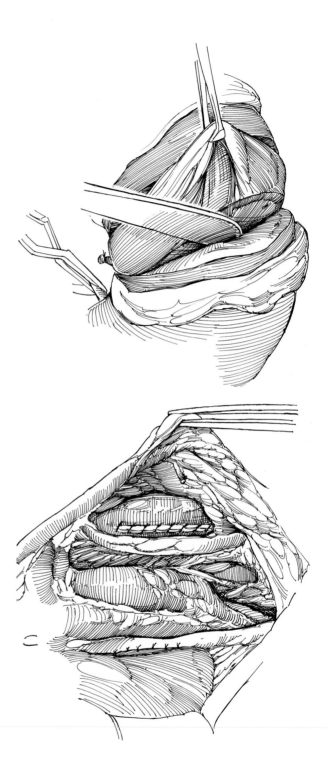

6 Identify the center of the isthmus by observing lobulation, palpating the thinnest portion, and inspecting the radiographs to avoid entering a calyx. Lift up the isthmus and loop the posterior vessels. Place a padded bulldog clamp on any vessel that supplies the isthmus, and observe for ischemia. Ligate and cut only those vessels that prevent division of the isthmus; spare every vessel possible. If the isthmus is thin, place a Satinsky clamp on either side and divide between them. For a thick isthmus, apply padded clamps (not shown); then incise and peel back the capsule. Divide the parenchyma bluntly with the back of the knife (see page 1001). Avoid entering a calyx, but if a calyx is transected, close it meticulously. Resect any devascularized tissue. Place figure-eight 4-0 SAS to transfix the arcuate vessels. Digital compression is useful to reduce blood loss during suturing. When lateral rotation of the lower pole is sought, divide one or more arteries to the isthmus and resect any ischemic tissue that results.

7 Close as much of each of the capsules as possible, using running or interrupted 4-0 SAS. Mattress sutures with hemostatic gauze bolsters that incorporate capsule and parenchyma may be used if necessary. Lift the lower pole of each kidney, and place a mattress 3-0 SAS over fat bolsters. Pass the suture superiorly and laterally into the psoas muscle. Have your assistant push the kidney cephalad with a sponge stick, holding the stump away from the ureter while you tie the suture.

Commentary by William J. Cromie

Any surgical procedure involving horeshoe kidneys requires thoughtful preparation. The approach in children is straightforward and varies little from the standard approach to the kidney. In bilateral lesions, or in cases involving multiple fused collecting systems near or crossing the midline, I would suggest a chevron incision in adults to both the hilum and the isthmus.

Whenever an extirpative procedure is considered, I have always felt more comfortable obtaining an angiogram to delineate the multiplicity of vascular variations. Wilms tumors, hypernephroma, giant segmental hydronephrosis, and the management of coexistent aortic disease represent situations in which this approach is particularly appropriate.

Improved diagnostic imaging encouraged the use of endoscopic surgery for the horseshoe kidney. Endopyelotomy, percutaneous calculus extraction, and management of complex calculi, as well as laparoscopic partial nephrectomy, have been successfully accomplished. Regardless of the procedure or technique, the major hazard of surgery on horseshoe kidneys is the potential for inaccessible bleeding directly from the aorta, posterior to the kidney. Appropriate radiographic projections and meticulous dissection will minimize such problems or surprises.

Nephrostomy and Ureterostomy

A nephrostomy is used to divert urine after a difficult pyeloplasty or other renal operation. For ureteral obstruction, percutaneous nephrostomy is usually better than open placement of a nephrostomy tube for temporary drainage, although the quality of drainage is inferior. It is not a good solution for long-term drainage.

Subcutaneous diversion is an alternative (Lingam). Place a pigtail stent in the pelvis percutaneously. Lead it down subcutaneously by making two more small incisions in the skin of the flank and forming a tunnel between them with a special introducer and sheath. Insert the end into the bladder through a peel-away suprapubic puncture kit.

If diversion is needed during an operation, arranging a *ureterostomy in situ* by intubating the ureter and bringing the tube out retroperitoneally is a simple, quick, temporary procedure compared with nephrostomy, and the catheter can emerge in a more comfortable position for the patient.

NEPHROSTOMY

1 **A,** *Position:* Flank position with the table flexed. *Incision:* Make a subcostal incision (see page 871).

B, Expose the renal pelvis as described for pyelolithotomy (see page 1041). Hold the edge of the hilum with vein or Gil-Vernet retractors to expose the renal pelvis. Alternatively, if the pelvis is large, approach it from its anterior surface.

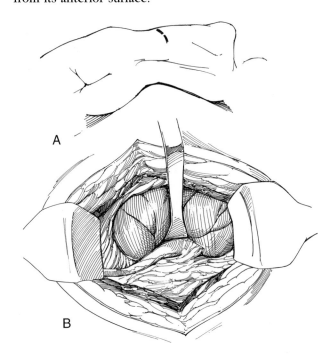

2 **A,** Place two 5-0 SAS in the pelvis well away from the ureteropelvic junction (UPJ), and make a 1- to 2-cm incision parallel to the border of the hilum with a hooked knife blade. Prepare a small Malecot catheter by transfixing the tip with a 1-0 silk suture. (A whistle-tip plastic Foley catheter has the advantage that it may be replaced by merely passing a guide wire through it down the ureter, although it does not provide equal drainage.) Insert a long curved clamp or Randall stone forceps with a suitable curvature into a lower calyx. An alternative is a pediatric right-angle Muynon clamp with fine tips to grasp the Malecot catheter directly, without the need for the suture. Press it firmly into the parenchyma while palpating for the tip. Cut the capsule in a radial direction over the clamp to allow it to exit. Open the clamp slightly to dilate the tract. Grasp the suture on the catheter in the clamp.

B, Have the assistant steady the kidney. Stretch the wings on the tip of the catheter by pulling on the clamp with one hand and the catheter with the other. The spread of the wings can also be reduced by inserting a curved clamp into the hollow tip between them. Gradually move both hands in concert to draw the catheter through the tract and out of the pelvis. Because the parenchyma is usually thin, little force is needed. Cut the suture; then draw the catheter back until it fits in or near the lower calyx.

Alternative: Insert a curved sound with a hole at the distal end through the pelvis and into a lower calyx. Cut down on the tip. Pass a suture through the hole of the sound and the holes on the catheter, and tie it. Slightly dilate the parenchymal opening and draw the catheter into the pelvis.

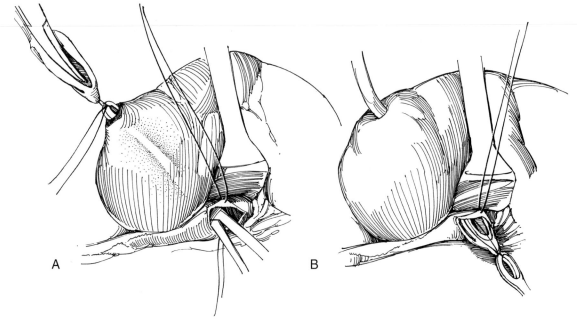

3 Suture the catheter to the capsule with a figure-eight 3-0 SAS over fat bolsters. Bring the tube out with a straight run through a separate stab wound in the flank placed well anteriorly so that the patient does not lie on it. Fix it to the skin with a 1-0 silk suture. Close the pyelotomy incision with a running 5-0 SAS. Place a Penrose drain, and replace the perirenal fat and Gerota's fascia.

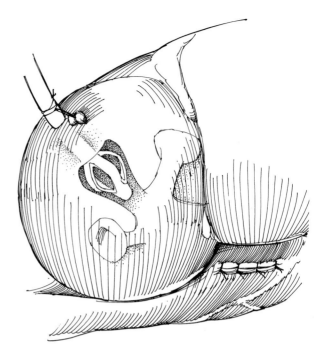

Alternative Technique

4 Prepare a Malecot catheter by cutting the distal end obliquely and making a vertical slit in it to create an eye. After inserting the clamp through the parenchyma as described above, grasp a length of moistened umbilical tape and draw the end out through the pelvis. Pass a mosquito clamp through the eye of the catheter, bring the tape through, and tie it. Draw the tape and catheter out through the cortex, and position the catheter as described. Take care not to saw the parenchyma.

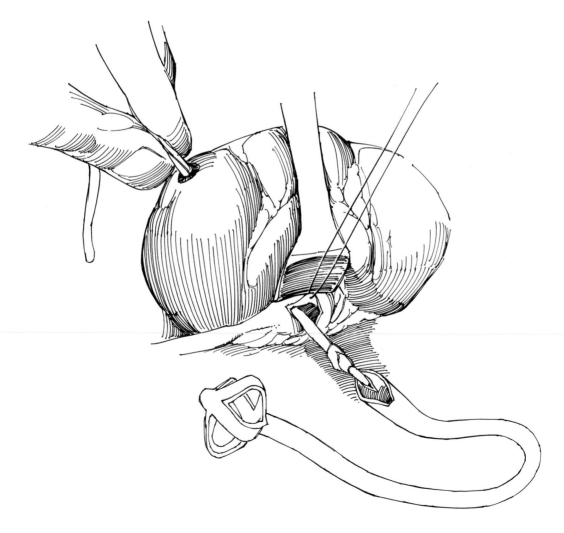

URETEROSTOMY IN SITU

5 For temporary diversion, expose the upper ureter through the retroperitoneum. Make a short ureterotomy, and insert an infant feeding tube into the renal pelvis. Fix it in place with a suture in the ureteral wall. Make a stab wound in the anterior axillary line, draw the tube out, and stitch it to the skin with a heavy silk suture. A similar procedure can provide temporary diversion if the ureter is injured during difficult pelvic surgery

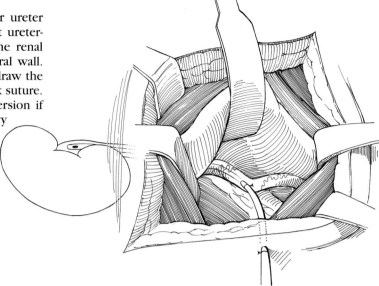

END URETEROSTOMY

If both ureters are dilated, after bringing the less dilated ureter across the midline, either bring them both through the body wall side by side or form an end-to-side anastomosis of the smaller to the larger one, which is brought to the skin in the lower quadrant (preferable to a midline subumbilical stoma). Form a stoma by everting the ureter to form a nipple.

POSTOPERATIVE PROBLEMS

For *excessive hematuria,* clamp the tube and allow a clot to form unless this will disrupt a repair. *Inadvertent removal* of the tube is due to inadequate suturing and taping to the skin.

These fastenings must be checked daily and replaced immediately if loose. After a week or two, the nephrostomy tube probably can be replaced with a small silicone balloon catheter on a stilet. Insert it to the same depth indicated by the color change on the catheter that was removed. Inflate the balloon with 3 ml of water, and check its position with gravity nephrostography.

Obstruction to drainage requires gentle irrigation. Give an intravenous push of mannitol to be certain dehydration is not the cause. If this fails to produce drainage, perform gravity nephrostography to be sure that the end of the tube is in the right position. If it is displaced, reposition it percutaneously. If the patient is anuric, treat for acute tubular necrosis secondary to intraoperative ischemia.

Continued drainage after removal of the tube suggests distal obstruction, which must be looked for radiographically and treated with retrograde intubation.

Stones may form in patients with chronically alkaline urine. Use a silicone tube, and change it every 6 weeks.

Commentary by William H. Lakey

Open placement of a nephrostomy tube is unusual today, thanks to the innovation of percutaneous nephrostomy drainage performed by radiologists and the placement of double-J stents by urologists. With a complete obstruction of the ureter or UPJ, percutaneous or open nephrostomy drainage of the kidney can be a life-saving procedure for the obstructed patient.

Several important considerations in the open nephrostomy operation require attention: (1) Be sure that the drainage tip of the Malecot catheter is placed in the lower pole calyx by Randall forceps for maximum drainage. (2) Be sure that the incision in the renal pelvis does not compromise the UPJ when it is closed. (3) Be sure that the skin exit site of the tube is well placed to prevent angulation or kinking. My variations in the technique are minor but include the occasional placement of the Malecot tip in a large dilated pelvis and the fixation of the renal parenchyma exit site to the abdominal wall muscles to ensure a direct approach for insertion of a new tube.

Problems that can occur include laceration of the renal parenchyma and bleeding from a parenchymal vessel injured during the insertion of the tube down the lower-pole infundibulum or through the parenchyma. The use of an umbilical tape to pull the distal end of the tube from the pelvis to the outside of the renal parenchyma may cause injury. Adequate fixation of the tube to the parenchyma is essential, without compromising the caliber of the lumen. Careful closure of the pelvis is also essen-

tial to prevent leakage or necrosis of the pelvis. I have had no experience with the subcutaneous diversion technique of Lingam. Although it would obviate a cutaneous site for the drainage tube, one would have to be careful that the tube is not kinked as it is placed from one subcutaneous site to another. Drainage of urine at the site of entry into the bladder could become a problem when voiding is resumed.

The *ureterostomy in situ* can ensure drainage through a more tolerable location in the loin. I use catgut fixation of the tube to the ureteral wall to allow easy removal but provide adequate fixation in the early postoperative period. The removal of such a tube is simple; if no distal obstruction is present, the site seems to close quickly. I have used this technique on very few occasions. Infant feeding tubes can be a problem if bleeding from the kidney is significant, so adequate fixation is essential.

The end-ureterostomy, in my experience, has been used only with chronically dilated, tortuous ureters. The survival of the ureteral stoma is more likely when the ureteral wall has become thickened with prolonged obstruction. I would be concerned with the use of this technique in acute obstruction with a thin wall of the acutely dilated ureter. The eversion of the larger ureter into a stoma is helpful to prevent stenosis. I have usually left fine feeding tubes through the stoma, draining both ureters until healing and viability have been ensured.

Open Renal Biopsy

Open biopsy is preferable to percutaneous biopsy in adults who have solitary or small contracted kidneys and very poor renal function, who are very obese, or who have some bleeding tendency and in children, who frequently are uncooperative. Laparoscopic biopsy is an option. Avoid biopsies in patients with severe hypertension and uncorrected coagulopathies. Use general anesthesia.

1 **A,** *Position:* Place the patient in the lateral position. *Incision:* Approach the kidney through a dorsal lumbotomy incision (see page 896). An alternative is the subcostal incision (see page 871).

B, Enter Gerota's fascia over the lower pole of the kidney, and mobilize the perirenal fat caudad to expose the renal capsule. Insert a narrow Deaver retractor between the kidney and the fat to draw the kidney down. Insert two fine stay sutures on either side of the proposed incision. Insert a third suture in the parenchyma, and make a deep elliptical incision into the cortex around it. Lift the specimen out on the suture, and place it on saline-moistened, coated gauze, not in formalin.

Obtain a needle biopsy specimen under direct vision from the deep cortical and juxtamedullary levels. If that site bleeds, close it with a fine figure-eight suture.

Close the capsule by tying each of the stay sutures first to itself and then to each other across the incision. If bleeding continues, carefully rotate a taper-cut needle swaged with 5-0 or 4-0 chromic catgut (CCG) through the renal cortex to cross at the depth of the incision as a horizontal mattress suture. Tie it carefully over pieces of fat with two-handed square knots to avoid tearing the suture from the tissue. Place a second suture if necessary.

Approximate Gerota's fascia, then the muscles, fascia, and skin in layers. Close the skin with subcuticular SAS. If skin clips are used in immunosuppressed patients, leave them for 10 or 12 days. Divide the biopsy tissue into three portions directly on the gauze, and place the portions into formalin, into 2 percent glutaraldehyde, and into a container for quick freezing.

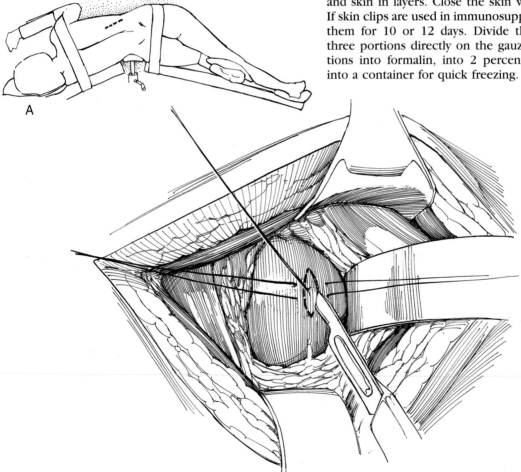

A

POSTOPERATIVE PROBLEMS

Bleeding occurs, especially in hypertensive patients or those with minor coagulation problems. *Gross hematuria* usually stops after 24 hours of bed rest. A *retroperitoneal hematoma* may form, but a *wound infection* is uncommon.

Commentary by Hugh N. Whitfield

There has been an historical reluctance on the part of nephrologists to subject patients with a solitary kidney to a closed renal biopsy. This stems from the recognized risks of severe complications requiring nephrectomy. Early series quoted figures of 1 percent, but with the use of ultrasound-guided biopsy and fine-needle biopsy techniques this risk has become significantly less. Nevertheless, the medicolegal position remains uncertain, and it might be argued that the risks of an open biopsy in a patient with a solitary kidney are less than with a closed biopsy because active steps can be taken to stop bleeding.

The biopsy must contain both cortex and medulla. However, because the kidneys from which biopsy specimens are taken often have a thin parenchyma, it may be helpful to perform preoperative ultrasonography to assess renal parenchymal thickness. A urinary fistula is a risk if the biopsy is too deep.

LAPAROSCOPIC RENAL BIOPSY

Transperitoneal
(Squadrito-Coletta)

Expose the lower pole of the kidney as described for laparoscopic nephrectomy (see page 993), preferably inducing the pneumoperitoneum with the Hasson sheath for safety. Select a site on the skin overlying the lower pole, and percutaneously insert a Biopty gun or Tru-Cut biopsy needle into the identified site on the kidney. Take one or more biopsy specimens. Observe the area for a few minutes, expecting spontaneous cessation of bleeding. If bleeding continues, compress the site or treat it with a laser-beam coagulator.

Retroperitoneal
(Gaur)

Place the patient in the flank position (see page 871), and make a 2-cm subcostal incision in the posterior axillary line. Pick up and enter Gerota's fascia. Insert a prepared balloon (see page 994), and inflate it for 5 minutes with 8 to 10 pumps of a sphygmomanometer bulb. Insert a 10-mm trocar sheath, and place a mattress suture to close the opening. Insufflate with nitrous oxide at a pressure between 10 and 20 mm Hg. Insert a 0-degree telescope and a 5-mm trocar under vision at the angle of the 12th rib and the sacrospinalis muscle to aid in exposing the renal capsule. Obtain a wedge-shaped biopsy specimen with laparoscopy cup biopsy forceps, and coagulate the site. Deflate the space, and close the wound with a few interrupted SAS without a drain. If bleeding is a problem, open the incision and close the defect under direct vision.

Repair of Renal Injuries

Obtain urine for microscopic analysis, either by having the patient void or by catheterization, collecting the urine in either case after the first 30 ml has passed. More than five red blood cells per high-power field signifies injury. With vascular avulsion, the kidney becomes nonfunctional and no red cells enter the bladder.

Staging. To stage the injury, perform one- or two-shot intravenous urography in the emergency room by inserting a large-bore intravenous catheter and rapidly injecting up to 2 mg/kg

of contrast medium. Nephrotomography can be done during the same injection. If the urogram is normal, observe the patient. If it is somewhat abnormal and if the condition of the patient allows, obtain a computed tomographic (CT) scan, which stages the injury accurately and allows a decision on whether observation, aortography, or operation is appropriate. When the urogram is markedly abnormal or if major renal bleeding is occurring, operate. Be certain that the contralateral kidney is present and normal. Do not neglect to assess the effects of other injuries.

1 *Incision:* Make a midline transperitoneal incision (see page 867). First explore the abdomen for associated injury. Repair injuries to the liver, spleen, and bowel first unless renal bleeding is more rapid than can be replaced. In the meantime, apply pressure on laparotomy sponges in the kidney area to help control the renal bleeding.

Lift the transverse colon superiorly, and place the large and small bowel in a plastic bag on the chest. Palpate the aorta, and incise the peritoneum over its exposed length *(dashed line)*. Extend the opening cephalad to 10 cm from the ligament of Treitz. If the aorta cannot be felt because of hematoma, identify the inferior mesenteric vein, and incise the posterior parietal peritoneum medial to it.

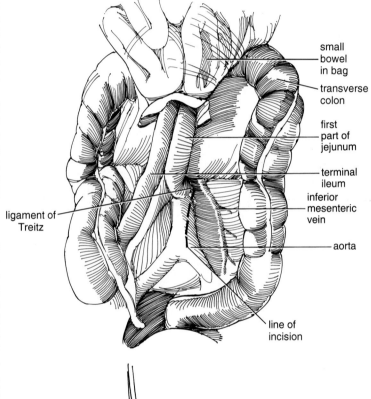

2 Dissect superiorly along the aorta to reach the left renal vein, which crosses it anteriorly. Avoid disturbing the perirenal hematoma by keeping the dissection medial, away from the kidney. Note that the left renal artery lies not only behind the vein but superior to it, and the right renal artery is also superior but medial to the vein. Place a vessel loop around the vein, and retract it superiorly to expose first the left renal artery and then the right one. Beware of tearing the left posterior lumbar vein that comes directly off the renal vein. Place vessel loops around the renal artery of the injured side to make it ready for placement of vascular clamps, but unless bleeding is heavy, do not apply the clamps at this time. For control on the right side, pass a loop around the right renal artery.

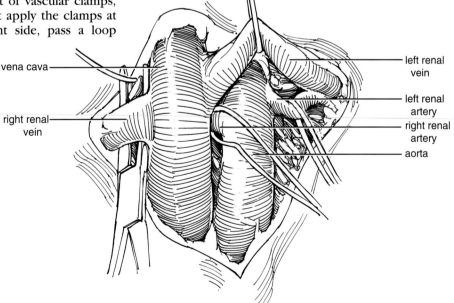

3 For left renal injury, as shown, incise the parietal peritoneum in the white line of Toldt lateral to the descending colon, and reflect the colon medially to expose the hematoma inside Gerota's fascia. Dissect directly into the hematoma through Gerota's fascia and the perirenal fat to reach the kidney. Quickly free the kidney because the tamponade is now released. Expose all aspects, and carefully look over the entire kidney. Stay outside the capsule, and leave the adrenal behind superiorly. Keep

away from the tail of the pancreas. If the bleeding warrants, lift up on the appropriate vessel loop, and clamp the left renal artery with a bulldog vascular clamp or a Rumel tourniquet before proceeding with definitive repair of the renal defect(s). In most cases, however, compression with the fingers is sufficient. For extensive injuries requiring reconstruction, consider cooling with iced slush.

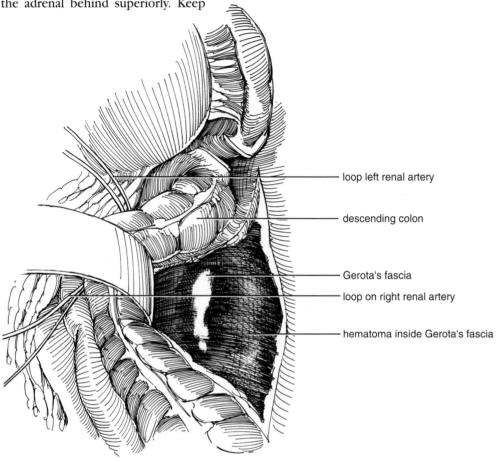

loop left renal artery

descending colon

Gerota's fascia

loop on right renal artery

hematoma inside Gerota's fascia

4 Remove the intrarenal hematoma residing in the laceration, and ligate the contributing intrarenal arteries and veins. Resect any necrotic tissue, and secure hemostasis by placing fine figure-eight 4-0 CCG sutures on the interlobar, arcuate, or interlobular arteries; catgut sutures slide through tissue better than do woven ones. Injured segmental veins can be ligated without concern for renal infarction because of the generous intrarenal collateral circulation. Ligate a segmental artery if it supplies less than 15 percent of the kidney; if the resulting infarction is greater than 15 percent, remove that portion of the kidney. If the injury is near the pelvis, look for pelvic laceration and repair it with a fine absorbable running 4-0 chromic suture. Check for leaks, as described in Step 5.

If there is a major injury of the upper or lower pole, perform partial nephrectomy (see page 1001). If the damage is restricted to the midportion of the kidney, excise the devitalized tissue, down to the collecting system if necessary, and close the calyx. Perform renorrhaphy by approximating the parenchymal margins with interrupted 3-0 SAS placed through the capsule and tied over absorbable gelatin sponge bolsters to prevent them from cutting through and to provide some hemostasis. If you expect reconstruction to take more than 30 minutes, cool the kidney with slush (see page 1048).

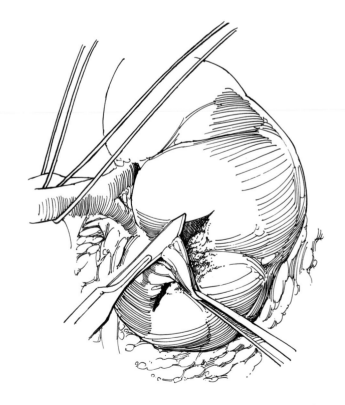

5 Make a watertight closure of any open calyces or infundibula with running 4-0 CCG sutures. To be certain that no leakage is present, give indigo carmine intravenously, and pinch the upper ureter closed. Alternatively, inject a small amount of dilute methylene blue directly into the renal pelvis through a fine needle. Close any remaining openings.

6 **A,** Apply a patch of gelatin sponge or microfibrillar collagen to persistently oozing areas before approximating the parenchymal surfaces. Cover the defect with any available capsule, and hold it in place with CCG mattress sutures over bolsters of fat or absorbable sponge. A patch of synthetic fabric may be applied if the defect is large. It is easier to close the capsule before releasing the arterial clamp, but this may allow delayed bleeding. In any case, do not reclamp a kidney that has been cooled.

B, Alternatively, apply a long bolster of gelatin sponge impregnated with Avitene or thrombin, and hold it with mattress sutures in the capsule. The capsule is often lost; in that case, bring a pedicle flap of omentum through a window in the mesocolon without dividing the short gastric vessels, and tack it in place with interrupted 4-0 CCG sutures. If the capsule is extensively destroyed, as from a blast injury, apply synthetic mesh (NU-KNIT), or even enclose the kidney in an absorbable synthetic mesh bag.

Because the calyces usually have been opened and there is risk of urinary leakage, insert a closed-system (Jackson-Pratt) drain that exits through a stab wound retroperitoneally from the flank. This is preferred over Penrose drainage because it reduces the chance for infecting the retroperitoneal hematoma. Do not close Gerota's fascia.

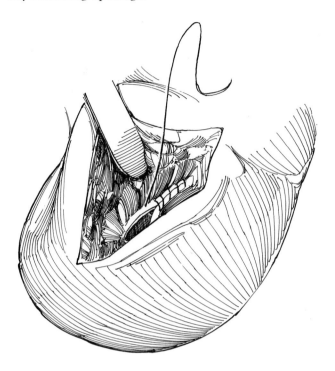

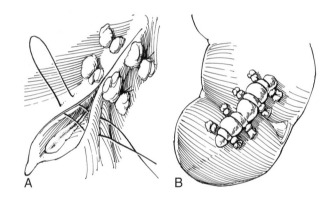

7 Repair *traumatic renal artery thrombosis*, especially if the kidney is solitary. Remove the obstructed segment of the artery, and replace it with a vascular graft obtained from the saphenous vein or hypogastric artery. Close lacerations of the main renal vein with fine vascular sutures, but ligate a lacerated venous branch and depend on internal collateral circulation. With deceleration injury to the renal artery, the defect is usually at the origin of the artery from the aorta, leaving the artery suitable for autotransplantation (see page 830).

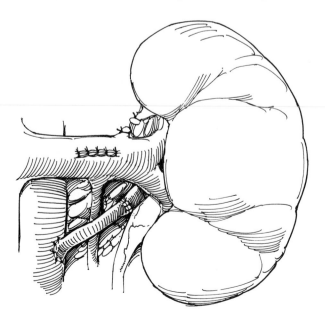

POSTOPERATIVE MANAGEMENT

Provide antibiotic coverage. Continue gastric suction for 3 or 4 days; then ambulate the patient. Follow the blood pressure and hematocrit data closely, and provide intravenous fluids to achieve a high urine output. Test drainage for creatinine to detect leakage of urine. Remove the drain within 3 days if no leakage is present, to prevent infection. If fever persists or hematocrit falls, obtain a CT scan.

Study renal function 2 weeks and 2 months after injury, and follow the blood pressure for at least 1 year.

POSTOPERATIVE PROBLEMS

Watch for *delayed bleeding* and *infection*, with possible perirenal abscess formation. Open *urinary drainage* may continue, or closed urinary leakage (suspected by prolonged ileus) may lead to the formation of a *urinoma* or *abscess*. Percutaneous drainage techniques may be effective and prevent reoperation. *Arteriovenous fistula* and later *hypertension* may occur. Renal scans are useful for follow-up monitoring. Obtain follow-up intravenous pyelography (IVP) 3 months after injury.

Commentary by Mitchell Edson

Penetrating renal trauma, especially gunshot injuries, should be explored surgically. A significant number of patients have associated injuries involving the liver, colon, small bowel, spleen, and great vessels, and these should be managed aggressively. In the absence of a hematoma within Gerota's fascia, control of the renal vessels is recommended. However, one can choose to explore and repair the kidney, approaching it laterally using finger pressure to control bleeding.

The argon-beam coagulator, if available, is helpful for resection of injured renal parenchyma and control of bleeding from the wound edges. In the absence of renal capsule to close the defect, the omental flap technique is extremely useful. We have routinely used fibrin glue instilled beneath the omental flap to control troublesome oozing effectively. The control of vascular supply, evacuation of hematoma, débridement and watertight repair of the collecting system, and adequate drainage should ensure a good result. The use of nephrostomy tubes is controversial, and we have rarely used them in our renal repair cases.

One word of caution is that even in the presence of normal IVP in penetrating injuries and in the presence of nonexpanding perirenal hematoma, renal exploration must be performed. Preoperatively, IVP is a must; if it is not performed, an intraoperative study must be done prior to a nephrectomy to ensure the presence and function of a contralateral kidney.

Open surgery in both early and late complications can often be avoided with the use of percutaneous drainage techniques, stenting maneuvers, and vascular embolization methods.

Renal Artery Reconstruction

For fibrous dysplasia, percutaneous transluminal angioplasty (PTA) is a good procedure. For arteriosclerotic obstruction, the first choice is aortorenal bypass. The patient with an aorta that is surgically difficult to treat, as after a previous operation or with severe arteriosclerosis, warrants alternate surgical procedures, such as autotransplantation; splenorenal, ileorenal, or hepatorenal bypass; and, in selected cases, aortic replacement. Branch disease can sometimes be repaired in situ but may require extracorporeal microvascular reconstruction and autotransplantation (see page 830). With severe renal atrophy (that is, renal length less than 8 cm) or total infarction, perform nephrectomy.

Preoperative evaluation can be minimal in the young patient with fibromuscular disease, but the older patient with arteriosclerotic lesions often has serious disease in the coronary or carotid vessels that must be identified before operation by an exercise stress thallium study and carotid duplex sonography. It may be well to correct these other atheromatous vessels before tackling the renal vessels. The renal arterial lesion is assessed by angiography, including oblique views.

Correct hypokalemia before surgery, and monitor the patient by determining central venous pressure, arterial pressure, and, in some cases, pulmonary wedge pressure.

Thorough hydration intravenously is needed during the 12 hours before operation, and 12.5 g of mannitol given intravenously not only at the start of the procedure but also at the time of clamping the renal artery is necessary. Add furosemide and more mannitol as indicated.

Instruments: Provide a Basic set, a GU fine set, DeBakey clamps, Metzenbaum and Strully scissors, vein and vena cava retractors, an endarterectomy knife, one straight and two curved aorta clamps, tonsil forceps, Potts scissors, a GU vascular pan, chilled perfusate, a flowmeter, pressure transducers, materials for cooling the kidney (see page 1048), and heparin solution.

1 *Position:* Place the patient supine with the lumbar spine hyperextended over a rolled towel. The legs may be placed in a modified frog-leg position. Prepare and drape the skin over the thighs in case a saphenous vein graft must be harvested. The lower legs may be placed in bowel bags so that their circulation may be observed during the procedure.

Incision: Although a midline incision may be adequate in thin individuals, it is better to make a transverse upper abdominal incision (see page 865) that extends from the lateral border of the contralateral rectus muscle to the costal margin between the 11th and 12th ribs. The incision should cross 2.5 to 4 cm above the umbilicus. For more exposure, convert it to a thoracoabdominal or chevron-shaped incision. Divide both rectus abdominis muscles and the internal and external oblique muscles with their attached peritoneum. Divide the ligamentum teres between clamps.

Explore the abdomen, lyse adhesions, and move the small intestine aside in a bowel bag.

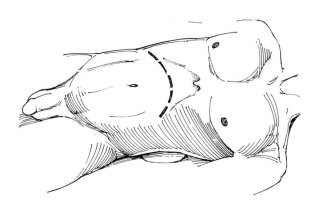

EXPOSURE FOR LEFT RENAL ARTERY STENOSIS

2 Standing on the left side, mobilize the splenic flexure and descending colon downward and medially by cutting along the white line of Toldt. Divide the

gastrocolic ligament; then free the lienocolic ligament to protect the spleen. For splenorenal bypass (Steps 19 to 23), dissect the splenic artery at this stage. Identify the tail of the pancreas in the upper margin of the incision, and incise the peritoneum behind it. Develop a plane between Gerota's fascia and the pancreas, and retract the spleen and pancreas medially. Insert a self-retaining retractor.

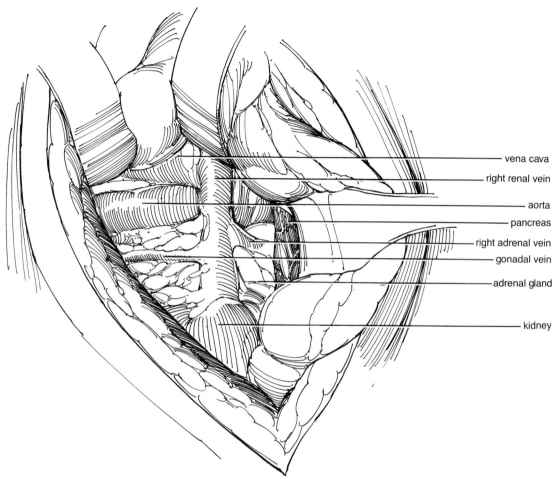

3 Open Gerota's fascia over the renal hilum. Protect the spleen under a laparotomy pad (splenectomy would create hypercoagulability). Do not mobilize the kidney from its bed, which would reduce the possibility for developing collateral circulation. Widely dissect the renal vein from the surrounding structures. A lumbar vein is usually found behind the renal vein that requires dissection, ligation, and division. Clamp and divide the left adrenal and gonadal veins, and ligate them with 3-0 silk ligatures. Pass a tape around the renal vein and elevate it.

4 Open a window in Gerota's fascia laterally over the lower pole of the kidney to allow monitoring of the condition of its circulation, but do not open Gerota's fascia farther, thus avoiding interference with collateral capsular circulation.

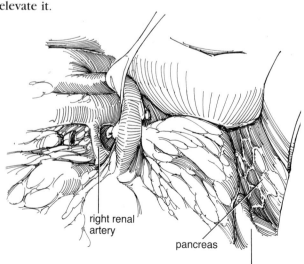

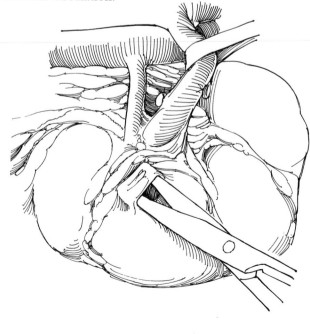

EXPOSURE FOR RIGHT RENAL ARTERY STENOSIS

5 Stand on the right side of the table. Reflect the hepatic flexure and ascending colon downward and medially by incising the white line of Toldt. Elevate the liver and gallbladder. Perform the Kocher maneuver on the duodenum (see page 986), and expose the vena cava and aorta. Watch out for the hepatic ligament, which contains vessels, and the common bile duct. Insert a self-retaining retractor.

Dissect the tissue from the anterior surface of the vena cava above the renal vein to the entrance of the right renal vein. Take special care not to injure the lumbar veins entering the vena cava. Some of these veins may have to be doubly ligated and divided to provide enough mobility of the vena cava.

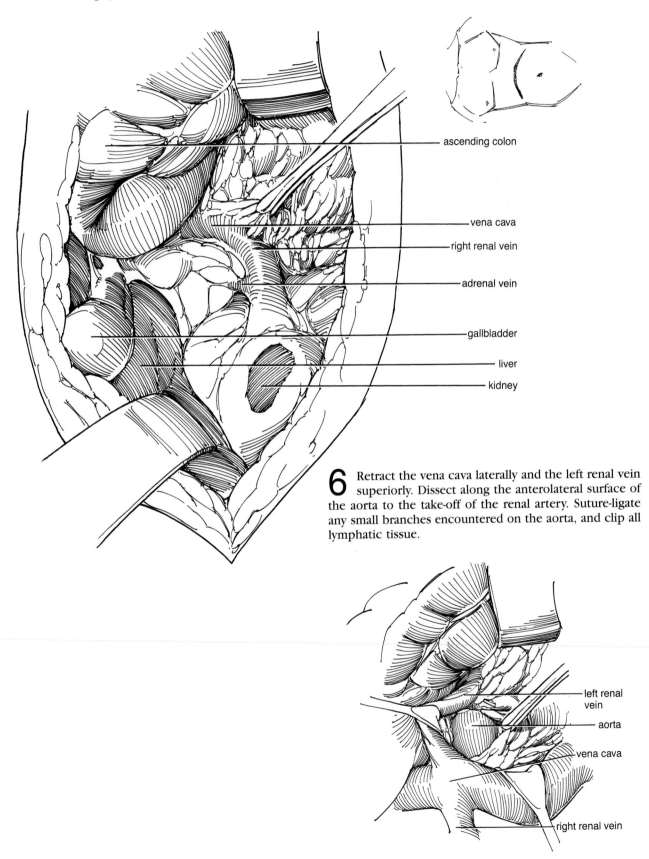

ascending colon

vena cava

right renal vein

adrenal vein

gallbladder

liver

kidney

6 Retract the vena cava laterally and the left renal vein superiorly. Dissect along the anterolateral surface of the aorta to the take-off of the renal artery. Suture-ligate any small branches encountered on the aorta, and clip all lymphatic tissue.

left renal vein

aorta

vena cava

right renal vein

7 Retract the vena cava medially and the right renal vein superiorly. Dissect the underlying renal artery free. It often is involved in inflammatory fibrosis, making dissection tedious. Avoid manipulation of the arterial wall that could release arteriosclerotic plaques. Arterial spasm can be mitigated by application of papaverine with lidocaine.

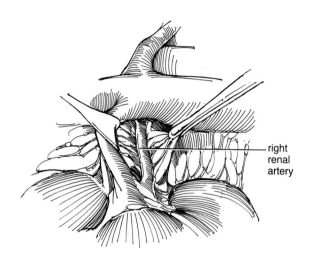

right renal artery

AORTORENAL BYPASS GRAFT, RIGHT

A graft is used for lesions involving major sections of the renal artery (medial fibroplasia and long atherosclerotic lesions). The procedure on the left is similar to that on the right.

8 Stand on the right side. Be certain that the aorta and vena cava are widely exposed, as described above. Dissect the aorta from the level of the renal vessels down to the inferior mesenteric artery. Carefully clamp, ligate, and divide interfering lumbar arteries.

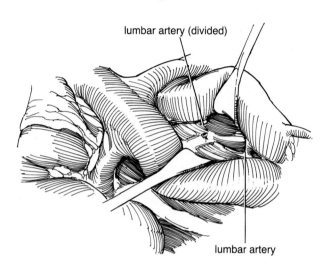

lumbar artery (divided)

lumbar artery

9 Free the right renal vein, but defer dissecting the artery to avoid vasospasm with consequent renal ischemia. Obtain an autogenous graft from the ipsilateral hypogastric artery (see page 1029). If that artery is too short or too sclerotic (as shown by preoperative radiography), a graft from the saphenous vein is satisfactory (see Step 43 for harvesting the graft).

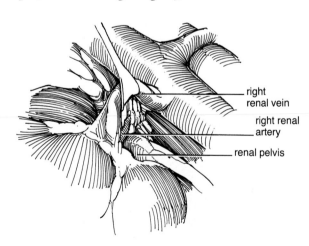

right renal vein

right renal artery

renal pelvis

10 Consider systemic heparinization before clamping the aorta. Place a DeBakey clamp on the anterolateral surface of the aorta in such a way as to allow distal flow and avoid interference with the mesenteric and contralateral renal arteries.

Remove an oval of aorta larger than the diameter of the hypogastric artery or saphenous vein graft. If arteriosclerotic plaques are found in the hypogastric artery graft, perform endarterectomy (see Steps 30 to 38).

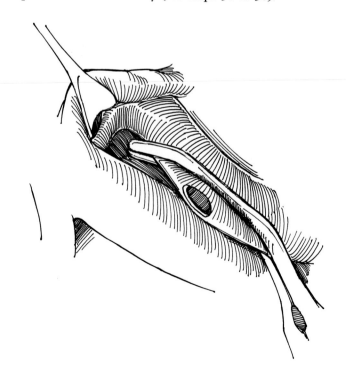

11 Cut the graft obliquely or spatulate it. If the graft is long enough, place the apex of the spatulation caudad to allow a smooth take-off; if it is too short, reverse it. Rotate the aorta anteriorly and run a 6-0 arterial silk suture down the posterior wall. If the aorta resists rotation, place this posterior layer of sutures from inside the graft. Alternatively, use interrupted sutures. It is important that the graft take an anterolateral course from the aorta and not have a lateral or an anterior take-off.

12 Rotate the aorta back. Look at the posterior suture line from the inside to make sure that the intima has been included in the stitches. Finish the anterior row with a second running 6-0 arterial silk suture, or use an interrupted suture technique. Check for leaks by placing a bulldog clamp on the graft and momentarily releasing the DeBakey clamp on the aorta. Place additional 6-0 silk sutures as needed. Flush the graft by temporarily releasing the bulldog clamp; reclamp and flush the distal end with heparin solution.

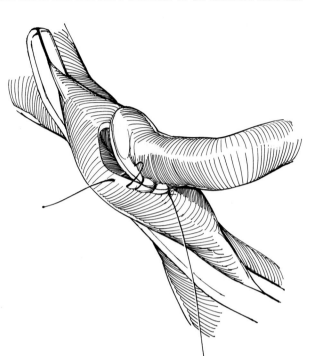

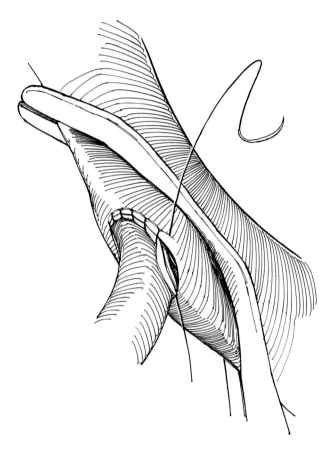

13 Dissect the right renal artery, beginning at the aorta and continuing into its branches. Clamp it proximally, divide it, and doubly ligate the stump. Resect the diseased portion. Pass the graft over the vena cava unless it is a synthetic graft (see Step 18). Trim it to the appropriate length. Relax pressure on the retractors to allow the aorta to return to its normal position before trimming the graft because proper length is important. Dilate both the arterial graft (or saphenous vein) and the renal artery with sounds or hemostats, and irrigate them with heparin. Clamp the renal artery distally near its branches with a bulldog clamp.

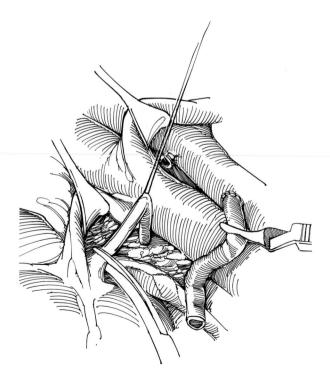

14 A and B, For large vessels (those greater than 1 cm), either use an interrupted suture technique or begin a running suture posteriorly from inside the vessel with a 5-0 double-armed vascular suture. Run it first to the right to the anterior quadrant.

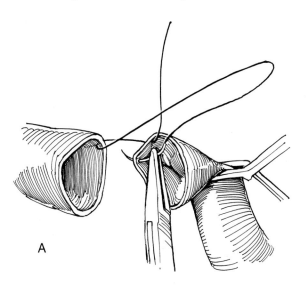

A

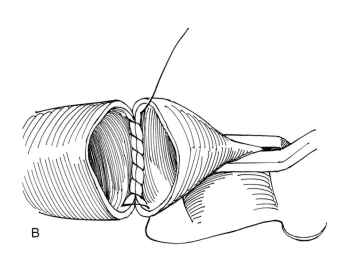

B

15 A and B, Pick up the other needle and run the suture to the left and across the anterior portion; then tie the sutures together. *Note:* It is not necessary to be consistent in entering and leaving the lumen in the same direction with each stitch; place these stitches in whichever direction is convenient.

16 For smaller vessels (less than 1 cm), transect the vessel obliquely with an S-shaped cut.

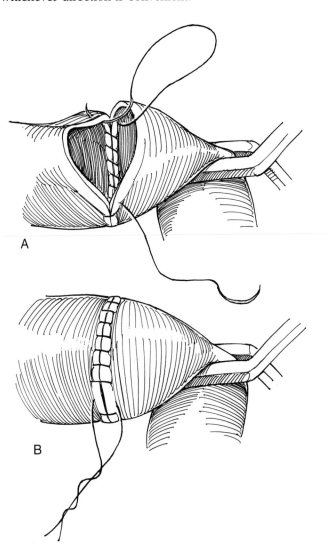

A

B

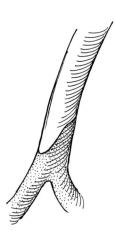

17 **A,** Start a 6-0 double-armed vascular suture posteriorly from inside the vessel.

B, Continue to the right side.

C, With the other end of the suture, run up the left side and across the anterior section. Before completing the anastomosis, release the occluding clamp to flush the vessel. Tie the sutures together. Again, the sutures may be placed from outside in or from inside out, as convenient. Release the distal clamp, and control the bleeding with

additional sutures, or apply absorbable hemostatic material. Release the proximal clamp, and check the perfusion of the kidney through the window. For disease extending into the bifurcation of the renal artery, suture the arteries together before anastomosis, as described on pages 960 to 961. Alternatives include use of a saphenous graft to which a side arm of vein has been anastomosed and use of the hypogastric artery with its branches (up to five).

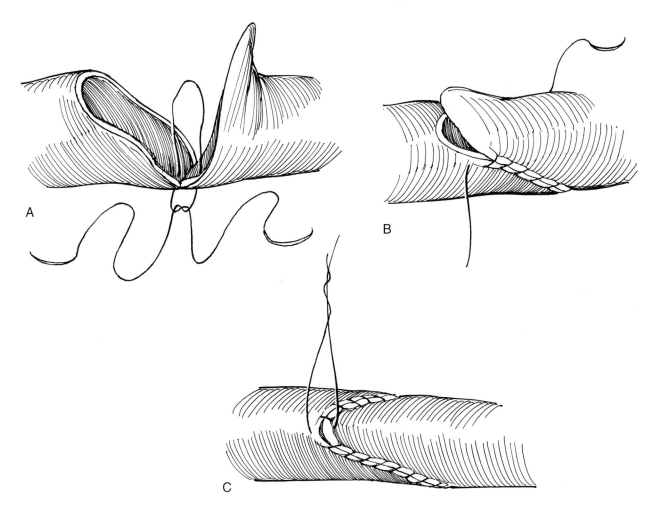

18 Alternatively, a synthetic prosthesis may be substituted, but do not expect comparable long-term results. If a prosthesis is used, place it behind the vena cava to avoid erosion of the duodenum.

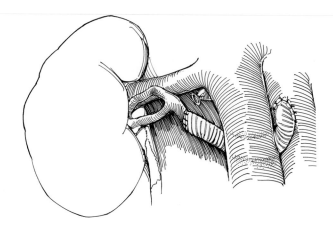

ALTERNATIVES TO AORTORENAL BYPASS

Two alternatives are available if aortorenal bypass is not feasible, splenorenal bypass and hepatorenal bypass.

Splenorenal Bypass

Splenorenal bypass is a practical alternative for a patient requiring left renal artery reconstruction in whom aortorenal bypass has failed or is not feasible because of severe, diffuse atherosclerosis, aneurysmal disease, or dense fibrosis after a prior operation.

Anterior Approach

Perform selective celiac angiography to rule out regional stenosis. It is important to obtain a lateral view of the origin of the celiac artery from the aorta to be sure that no stenosis is present at that site.

19 **A,** *Position:* Supine. Stand on the left. Insert a balloon catheter. Drape the legs into the field in case the saphenous vein is needed. *Incision:* Make a chevron incision (see page 865).

B, Incise the peritoneum in the gutter, and reflect the left colon and duodenum medially. Develop a plane just anterior to Gerota's fascia, and bluntly dissect the pancreas and spleen superiorly. Open Gerota's fascia over the renal vessels. Dissect the left renal vein free, and clamp, divide, and ligate the gonadal and adrenal tributaries. Make a window in Gerota's fascia over the lower pole to monitor renal oxygenation.

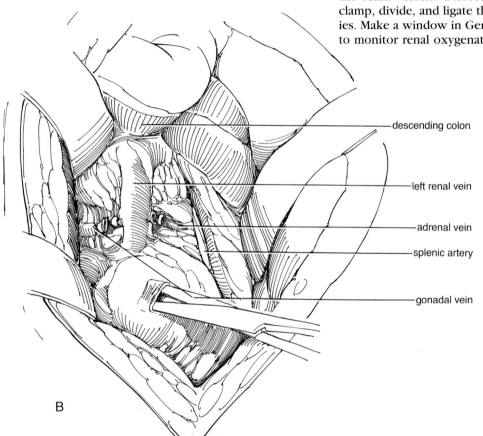

descending colon

left renal vein

adrenal vein

splenic artery

gonadal vein

A

B

20 Mobilize the left renal vein, and free the entire length of the main renal artery with the aid of vascular tapes. This may be done better after dissecting out the splenic artery to avoid producing vasospasm. Lift the pancreas, and palpate the splenic artery, which lies above and behind the splenic vein, to be certain that it is not involved with arteriosclerotic changes. Check the flow with the Doppler gauge; the flow should be more than 125 ml/minute. Place a self-retaining retractor. Select that section of the artery closest to the renal artery, which is an area least likely to have arterial disease. Encircle it with a vascular tape, and dissect it as far as the celiac axis, carefully clipping the small branches to the pancreas and the left gastroepiploic artery at its origin.

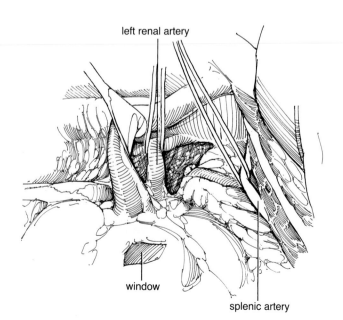

left renal artery

window

splenic artery

21 Place a bulldog clamp proximally on the splenic artery. Tie two 3-0 silk sutures around the artery distally, and divide it just proximal to the ties. Leave the spleen in position; it receives sufficient collateral blood supply from the gastroepiploic and short gastric vessels. Gently dilate the proximal end of the splenic artery with coronary artery dilators, or, preferably, spatulate it for a distance of 1 cm to match the size of the renal artery.

22 Clamp the renal artery distally with a bulldog clamp. Doubly ligate it with 2-0 silk, and divide it proximally. Trim the diseased segment from the proximal end for pathologic examination. Dilate the renal artery distally with coronary artery dilators if it is in spasm; then insert a catheter and flush the kidney with 250 ml of chilled perfusate.

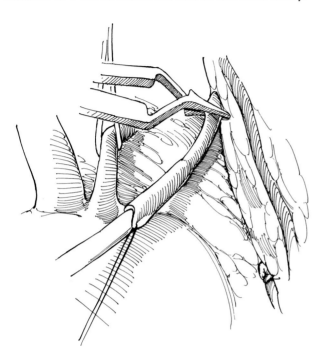

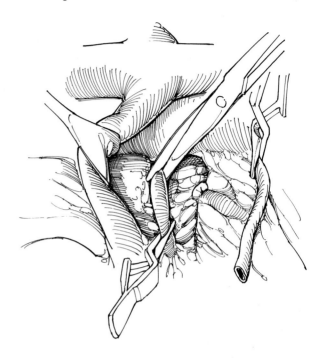

23 **A,** Anastomose the two arteries end to end. An end-to-side anastomosis is an alternative, especially for repeat procedures. A saphenous graft may be interposed. Use interrupted sutures, or place a posterior row with a running 5-0 arterial suture, tying both ends.

B, Run an anterior row. Before tying this suture, release the clamp on the renal artery first and then the one on the splenic artery to flush the vessels. Check the kidney through the window for adequate perfusion. Fix the kidney in position. Inspect and replace the pancreas after making sure its artery has not been kinked.

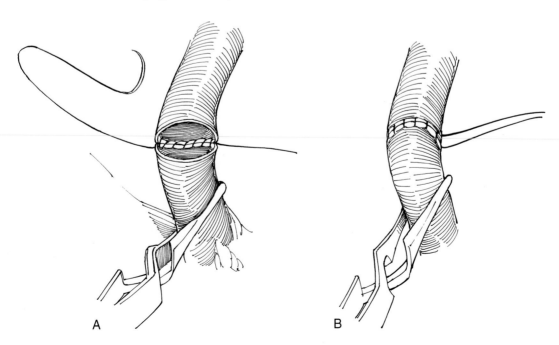

A

B

Thoracoabdominal Approach to the Left Kidney

24 **A,** *Position:* Semioblique, with the left side elevated 75 degrees. Raise the kidney rest below the lower rib. Stand on the left. *Incision:* Make a thoracoabdominal incision (see page 890) in the ninth interspace, extending posteriorly to the angle of the rib.

B, Incise the diaphragm in the direction of its fibers.

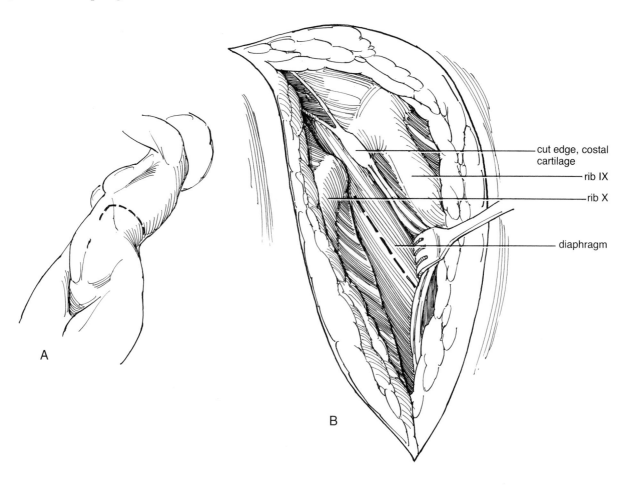

cut edge, costal cartilage

rib IX

rib X

diaphragm

A

B

25 Divide the lienocolic ligament. Move the splenic flexure of the colon anteriorly and the stomach anteriorly and superiorly.

26 Lift the spleen, and free the hilum to expose the splenic vessels. (For additional illustrations, see page 903.)

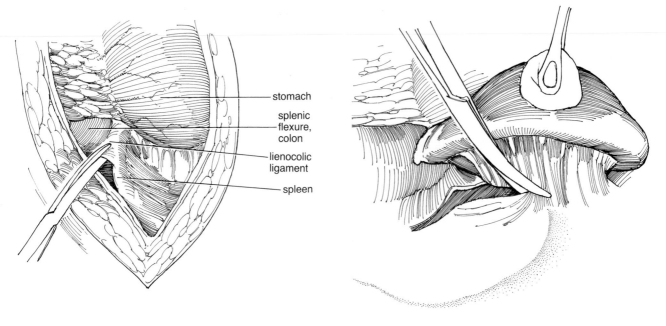

stomach

splenic flexure, colon

lienocolic ligament

spleen

27 Open the posterior peritoneum medially, and elevate the inferior margin of the tail of the pancreas.

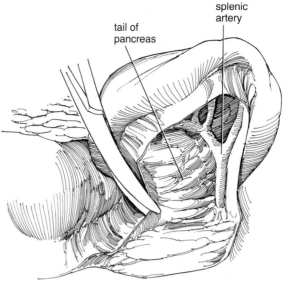

tail of pancreas

splenic artery

28 Expose the renal artery and vein through Gerota's fascia. Divide the adrenal vein at its take-off from the renal vein. Place a vascular tape around the artery. Continue the dissection of the artery peripherally beyond its first bifurcation, and encircle these branches with vascular tapes. Palpate the distal portion of the renal artery; if it is involved with arteriosclerosis, its use for reconstruction is not advisable.

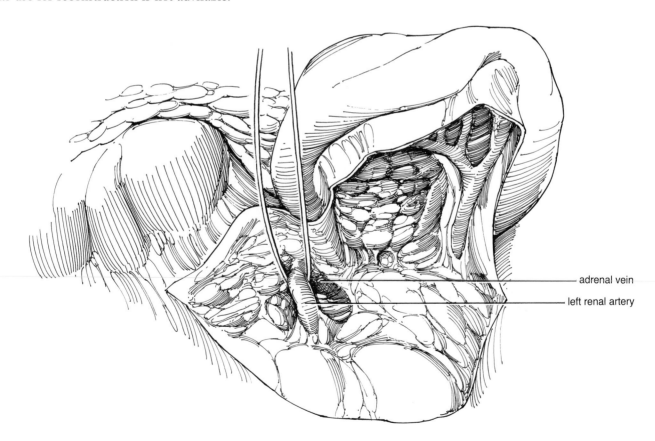

adrenal vein

left renal artery

29 Dissect the splenic artery along the upper border of the pancreas; divide and ligate its branches to the pancreas, as well as those to the left gastroepiploic artery. Continue the dissection all the way to the take-off of the splenic artery from the celiac axis. Occlude the splenic artery both proximally and distally with bulldog clamps. Divide the artery near the distal clamp. Proceed as described for the anterior approach for splenorenal bypass in Steps 22 and 23.

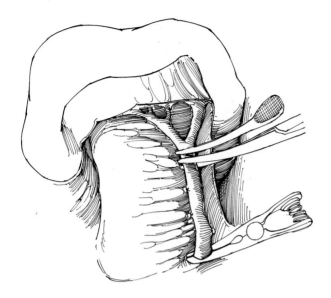

For the right kidney, if an aortorenal bypass graft is impossible to perform, an hepatorenal bypass can be substituted by a technique similar to that for the splenic artery for left renal revascularization. Depending on the anatomic configuration, use the common hepatic artery alone accompanied by cholecystectomy or use a saphenous graft. If the hepatic arteries bifurcate soon after take-off, use the right hepatic artery, leaving sufficient vascularization of the gallbladder.

Hepatorenal Bypass

The hepatic artery may be used for right bypass when the aortorenal bypass has failed or when use of the aorta is precluded and the celiac and hepatic arteries are found to be clear, as seen in a lateral film by angiography. Mobilize the common hepatic artery to its bifurcation into a gastroduodenal branch and the main hepatic artery. (Division of the hepatic artery results in ischemia of the gallbladder.) Interpose a section of saphenous vein end to side immediately before the bifurcation. Anastomose the venous interpositional graft end to end to the spatulated renal artery.

Other Vessels for Bypass

Certain other arteries are suitable donors for a bypass operation: The iliac artery may substitute for the aorta for an interposition graft when the aorta is diseased. Similarly, the graft may be connected with the superior mesenteric artery. For the left kidney, the distal thoracic aorta (supraceliac aorta) is often free of arteriosclerotic involvement and may be exposed by a thoracoabdominal incision (see Step 24 and following).

ENDARTERECTOMY

Aortorenal Endarterectomy (Wylie)

30 *Incision:* Midline transperitoneal (see page 867). A flank incision is usually not adequate because both renal arteries should be exposed. Stand on the left side. Cut the fibers attaching the crura of the diaphragm to the vertebral bodies over the aorta.

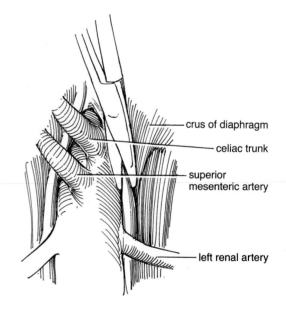

crus of diaphragm

celiac trunk

superior mesenteric artery

left renal artery

31 Divide and ligate the small adrenal arteries arising from each side of the aorta. With the index finger, bluntly dissect laterally and behind the aorta against the crus of the diaphragm to provide an opening for an occluding clamp between the superior mesenteric artery and the celiac arteries.

32 Insert a long, straight aortic clamp behind the aorta from below to occlude the two pairs of lumbar arteries along with all the retroaortic tissue.

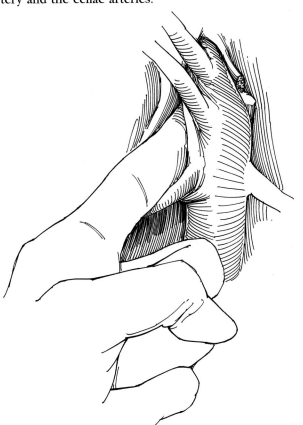

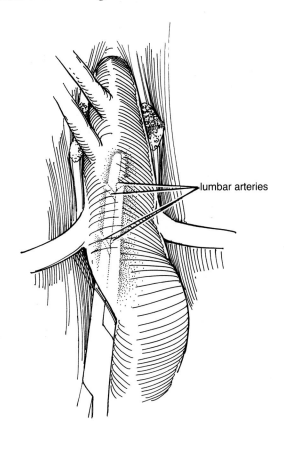

lumbar arteries

33 Place vascular clamps on the superior mesenteric artery and on the renal arteries beyond the plaques. Also place one on the aorta proximal and distal to the site of the aortotomy after palpating the aorta to select areas of minimal thickening for their application. Make an 8- to 10-cm incision in the aorta between the renal arteries, and extend it just to the left of the take-off of the superior mesenteric artery. Bluntly free the sleeve of aortic intima with an endarterectomy probe, and transect it circumferentially at the distal end in an area where the thickening is minimal. Continue cephalad with the endarterectomy to free the entire aortic portion, leaving the regions around the renal orifices until last. Divide the proximal end of the sleeve just distal to the orifice of the superior mesenteric artery.

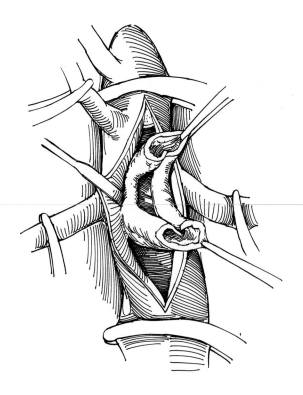

34 **A,** As the assistant moves the kidney medially, grasp the loose intima with vascular forceps, and with the probe push the media of the renal artery away to evert the artery into the aorta.

B, Continue until the attenuated plaque breaks free. Extract residual fragments, and flush the artery. Provide flushing by alternate release of the proximal and distal aortic clamps. Close the arteriotomy with a continuous 4-0 silk suture. Palpate the renal arteries for residual plaques, and obtain an arteriogram by injecting contrast medium into the aorta while it is occluded. If plaques are detected, clamp the take-off and remove them through a transverse arteriotomy.

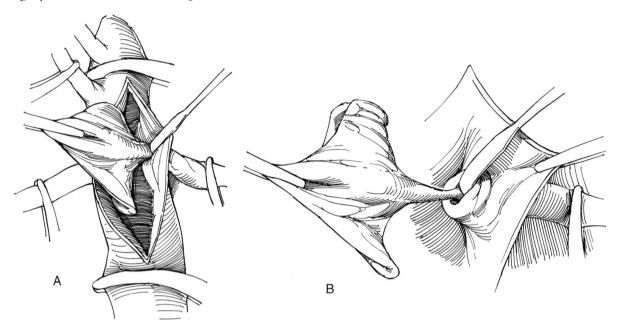

Endarterectomy with Patch-Graft Angioplasty

A patch graft can be used for atherosclerotic lesions of the left renal artery. Those on the right are more easily managed by bypass grafts. Obtain a segment of saphenous vein (Step 43) and keep it moist.

35 **A,** *Position:* Supine.
Incision: Chevron (see page 865). Stand on the left.

B, Expose the left renal artery, and divide the adrenal vein as described previously (Steps 2 and 3). Remove a wedge from the crus of the diaphragm behind the origin of the renal artery to relieve possible posterior compression of the repair.

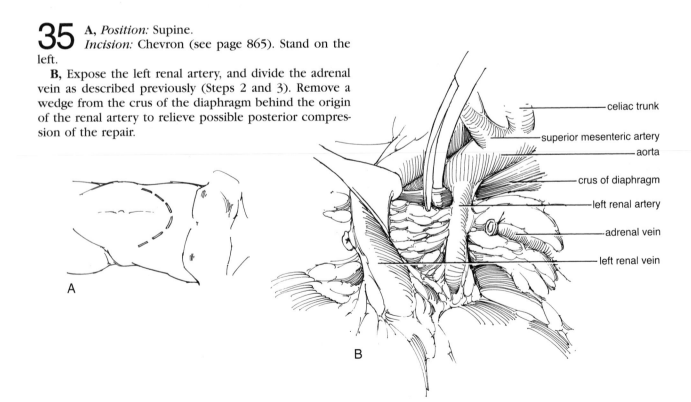

36 Free the left side of the aorta to allow application of a DeBakey vascular clamp. Keep the tip of the clamp well below the superior mesenteric artery, and apply it so that enough blood passes alongside it to preserve a pulse in the aorta below it. Palpate the renal artery, and incise it over the plaque. Extend the incision in the artery beyond the plaque into the aorta for a distance of 1 cm. Irrigate the artery with 10 ml of heparin solution, and clamp it distally with a bulldog clamp.

37 Establish a plane between the plaque and the media of the artery with an endarterectomy knife, and dissect around the plaque proximally and distally. Use Potts scissors to transect the intra-aortic end. Try to remove the plaque intact; if it does break up, remove the pieces with tonsil forceps. Be sure to break off the distal end cleanly at its attachment to the media so that no intimal flaps are raised. If they are, tack them down with a few transmural stitches of 6-0 arterial suture, tying the knots on the outside of the artery.

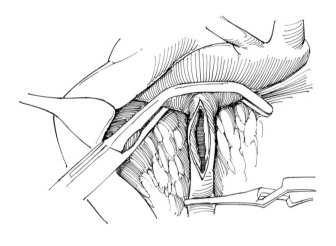

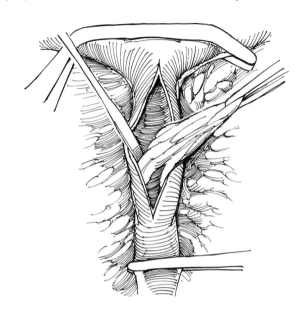

38 **A,** Open the saphenous vein, and cut a patch of suitable size and shape. Stitch the graft in place with 6-0 arterial sutures, beginning at the aortic apex and running down the upper side and then around the apex on the renal artery. Insert the suture from inside to outside to catch the intima, especially distally.

B, Start a second suture at the aortic apex, run it out

the lower side, and tie it to the end of the first suture. Temporarily release the distal bulldog clamp, and repair any leaks with 6-0 vascular sutures. Remove the DeBakey clamp, and check the color of the kidney. Palpate the renal artery, expecting good pulsation without a thrill. Close the wound without drainage.

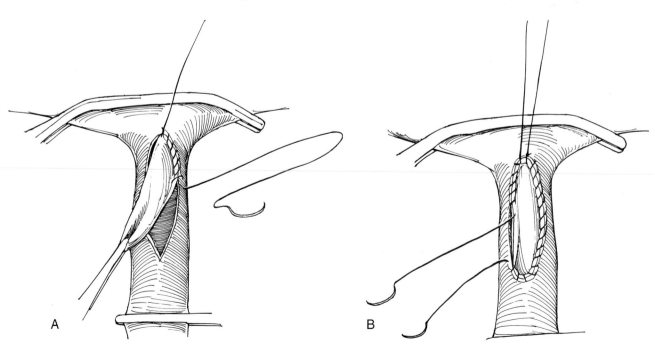

A

B

AORTORENAL REIMPLANTATION, RIGHT

Right aortorenal reimplantation is suitable for short fibrous lesions in the proximal part of the renal artery.

39 **A,** *Position:* Supine. Stand on the right. *Incision:* Chevron (see page 865).

B, Expose the aorta and vena cava as described above. Ligate and divide enough arteries and veins to provide exposure of the right renal artery and the medial aspect of the aorta.

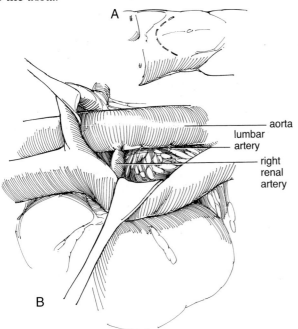

aorta

lumbar artery

right renal artery

40 Place a DeBakey vascular clamp on the lateral aspect of the aorta below the renal artery, and rotate the aorta forward. Excise an oval of aortic wall. When atherosclerotic plaques lie beneath, remove them locally. Mobilize the right renal artery from the aorta, extending out to its hilar bifurcation. Clamp the artery just distal to the obstructing lesion, divide it, and ligate the stump doubly with 2-0 silk suture. Place a bulldog clamp on the artery distally. Spatulate the end on the cephalad aspect.

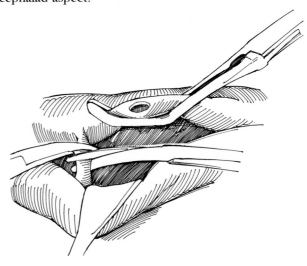

41 **A,** Fix the apex of the spatulation to the cephalad end of the aortotomy with a 5-0 arterial suture. Place interrupted sutures or run the suture down the back wall, working from inside the vessels to include the intima of the renal artery in each stitch.

B, Start a second suture at the apex; run it to meet the first and tie it. In children, use interrupted sutures for the anterior row.

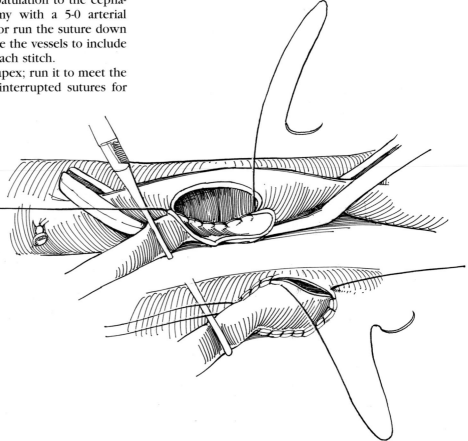

42 Release the distal bulldog clamp, and check for leakage. Apply absorbable hemostatic agents if necessary. Slowly release the DeBakey clamp to allow the kidney to fill, and then check renal color. Close the wound without drainage.

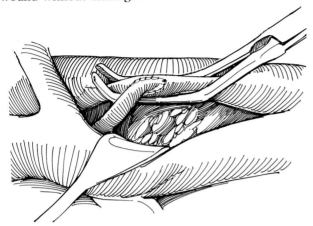

HARVESTING A SAPHENOUS VEIN GRAFT

43 **A,** The long saphenous vein drains into the femoral vein just below the inguinal ligament. Tributaries include the superficial inferior epigastric vein, the superficial external pudendal vein, and, often, an accessory saphenous vein.

B, Standing to the patient's right, make a 12-cm longitudinal incision on the anteromedial surface of the leg, beginning 4 cm below and 4 cm lateral to the pubic tubercle. Insert two self-retaining rack retractors.

C, Expose the vein for the length of the incision. Divide each branch as it is exposed. Suture-ligate the stumps of the tributaries on the vein segment one by one (they will be subjected to arterial pressure). Clear the adventitia from the surface of the proposed graft. Clamp the vein just outside the fossa ovale where it joins the femoral vein below the tributaries; divide it and ligate the stump with 2-0 silk. Free 1.5 times the length considered necessary. Ligate the vein with 2-0 silk before dividing the distal end. Place a fine suture in this distal end of the graft to mark it for anastomosis to the aorta so that the valves conform to the direction of flow. Also mark it longitudinally with a marking pen along the anterior surface to prevent later rotation.

D, Place a bulldog clamp on the proximal end, and distend the vein with heparinized saline solution through a Titus needle to relax it and check for leaks and constrictions. Keep the graft moist until it is needed by storing it in a pan of cold heparinized Ringer's solution.

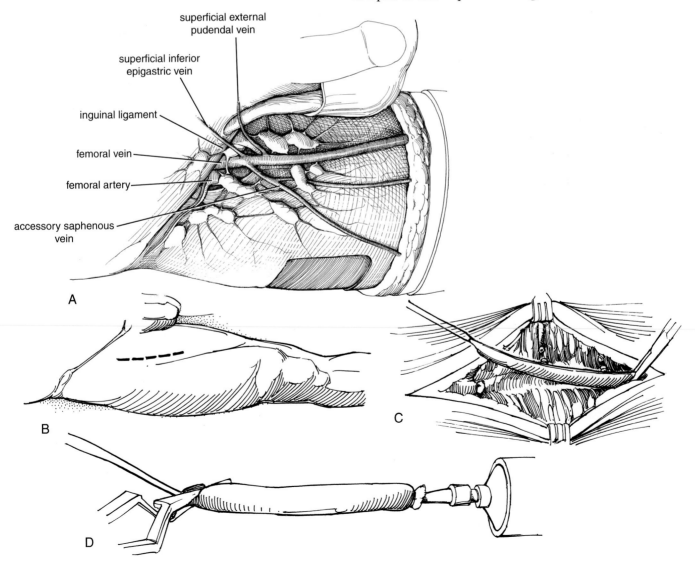

RENAL ARTERY EMBOLECTOMY, RIGHT

Realize that partial renal perfusion continues even with an embolus lodged in the main branches of the renal artery. Perform renal angiography, injecting vasodilators into the artery at the same time. Proceed with embolectomy.

44 From the right side, expose the renal vasculature as described in Steps 5 to 7. Control the artery proximally with a bulldog clamp. Perform a longitudinal arteriotomy, and extract the embolus. Perfuse the kidney with heparin solution. Postoperatively, provide systemic anticoagulant therapy. Search for the source of the embolus. Follow renal function.

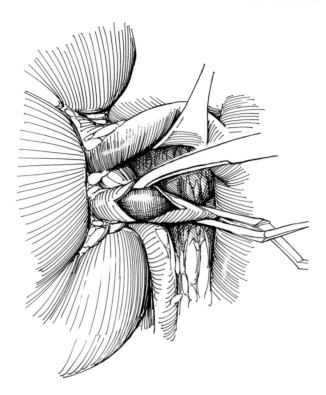

RENAL ARTERY ANEURYSM

After exposure by rotating the kidney so that the lower pole faces anteriorly and local control of the artery is obtained, excise the aneurysm but leave some of its wall on the vessel. Close the defect by overlapping the residual wall in a pants-over-vest fashion.

RENAL AUTOTRANSPLANTATION

Transplantation of the kidney to another site allows extracorporeal microvascular manipulation of the vessels. For a description of renal displacement with or without transplantation, see page 830, and for extracorporeal renal surgery, see page 1027. The kidney is protected from ischemic injury by cooling and occasional perfusion, exposure is excellent in a bloodless field, and the anastomoses can be tested before replacement in the body. Extracorporeal renal surgery should be limited to vascular disease that is not correctable with in situ techniques, to patients in whom in situ repair has not given good results, and to adults in whom microscopic techniques are needed with fibrous disease or aneurysms in multiple branches. Reoperation for renovascular disease may be easier on the workbench.

POSTOPERATIVE PROBLEMS

General complications include atelectasis and pneumonia; bowel obstruction, either mechanical or paralytic; wound infection; pulmonary embolism; and myocardial or cerebrovascular infarction.

Hemorrhage probably means that tension was placed on an anastomosis, that the artery was too diseased for use, or that the sutures either were too widely spaced or everted the intima.

Another cause is neglecting to secure the collateral renal hilar vessels, the parenchyma of the adrenal gland, or the lumbar arteries. When using a saphenous graft, be sure that all the branches are suture-ligated to be able to withstand arterial pressure. If coagulation is abnormal or if an episode of hypertension intervenes, bleeding may begin. When bleeding is not severe and symptomatic, observe it even though the hematoma may eventually contract around the artery; when it is severe and persistent, repair the defect at once.

Late major hemorrhage requires emergency management. Causes may be suture-line infection, rupture of a false aneurysm, and erosion of a synthetic bypass graft into the duodenum. The last can be avoided by routing the graft behind the vena cava and by interposing omentum or peritoneum.

Renal artery thrombosis appears soon after operation, fostered by hypotension, hypovolemia, or hypercoagulability. Reduced flow may be a factor if appreciable intrarenal arteriolar nephrosclerosis exists. The basic cause of thrombosis is a defect in technique, such as anastomosis of diseased vessels, intimal injury or intrusion where the intima was not tacked down, inadequate endarterectomy, anastomosis of vessels of greatly disparate size, and rotation or angulation of a graft. Atheromatous embolization or arterial compression from a hematoma or seroma may be factors. Late thrombosis is usually the result of progressive aortic atherosclerosis. Watch for the sudden onset of hypertension and a rise in serum creatinine level. Routinely do a technetium scan 24 hours after operation. If results are not normal, perform arteriography. Treatment with intra-arterial streptokinase may be effective, and percutaneous extraction of the thrombus can be done. The graft may be revised, but more often nephrectomy for a nonviable kidney is required.

Acute renal failure usually results from prolonged ischemia. Longer than 30 minutes is acceptable time only if a good collateral blood supply is present. Hydration, mannitol, limited surgical manipulation, and maintenance of adequate blood pressure are mandatory to avoid ischemia. Occlude the artery only as long as necessary; plan the steps of the procedure to minimize occlusion time. Look for reduced urinary output and increasing serum creatinine levels; control fluids and electrolytes by using central venous pressure or, preferably, pulmonary artery wedge pressure to monitor therapy.

Renal artery stenosis is a late phenomenon; thus, regular follow-up is necessary. The causes are similar to those for thrombosis. The best treatment is PTA. *Renal artery aneurysm* is also a late complication of vein grafts, or it may result from local infection. *Emboli* to the distal extremities come from aortic atherosclerotic plaques that may be dislodged during clamping. Look for poor peripheral pulses. Heparinization helps, along with the administration of papaverine. Fasciotomy

may even be required, but perform aortography at once followed by thromboembolectomy.

Hypertension is not uncommon immediately after operation and must be controlled to avoid stress on the anastomoses. Give sodium nitroprusside intravenously while carefully monitoring the patient's vital signs. Substitute other agents after a day or two; the hypertension should resolve in a few weeks. If it does not, look for a defect in the anastomotic site.

Laceration of the spleen by a retractor may occur, but the defect can usually be repaired (see page 903). If the splenic vein is torn as the artery is mobilized, repair it with fine vascular sutures. Injury to viscera is usually the result of a difficult secondary dissection, as from mobilization of the intestine, pancreas, spleen, and duodenum from the surface of the kidney.

Commentary by Silas Pettersson

Surgical correction of renovascular abnormalities, including both renovascular disease, with and without impaired renal function, and renovascular hypertension, is an activity in decline. PTA has today replaced most surgical procedures in both categories. Thus, in my hospital, the Sahlgrenska University Hospital in Göteborg, only about 2 percent of cases are corrected surgically; the remaining 98 percent are treated by PTA. The role of the surgeon in the latter group is mainly to be available if a complication occurs. Complications, however, are very rare. The introduction of PTA has also widened the indica-

tion for treatment, and the number of patients treated for renal artery disease by PTA is twice the number treated when surgery was the only technique available.

This change from surgical to minimally invasive therapy, however, does not depreciate the importance of this chapter. I would say the opposite: If a procedure is now rare, most surgeons need to review the technique occasionally. The surgical approaches and techniques described in this chapter are excellent and constitute all the information necessary.

Renal Transplant Recipient

ADULT TRANSPLANTATION

Assess peptic ulcer disease, and obtain cardiology consultations. Avoid pretransplant nephrectomy unless hypertension cannot be controlled or reflux or infection is present. Check bladder function by voiding cystourethrography.

Preparation. If possible, dialyze the patient the day before operation to ensure metabolic and electrolyte balance.

Instruments. Provide a general laparotomy set with vascular instruments, Gemini Mixter forceps, a bent-handled curved De-Bakey aortic clamp, an angled DeBakey clamp, three pediatric vascular clamps, curved DeBakey endarterectomy scissors, an 8 F Robinson catheter, heparinized saline solution, bacitracin-neomycin irrigant, 3-0 SAS; 4-0 PCG sutures; 1-0 SAS; 1-0 or 2-0 braided nylon; 5-0, 6-0, and 7-0 cardiovascular sutures; and 4-0 nylon skin sutures.

1 *Position:* Supine; break the table slightly to hyperextend the abdomen. The kidney is most commonly placed in the right side of the pelvis. Shave and prepare the abdomen. Insert an 18 F 5-ml silicone balloon catheter. Instill 100 ml or more of sterile saline that contains 1 ampule of bacitracin-neomycin solution to partially fill the bladder. Immediately before preparing the abdomen, place a 20 F 5-ml balloon catheter into the bladder, which is drained. Fill the bladder with antibiotic solution to facilitate an extravesical ureteroneocystostomy. This is best done by gravity using the barrel of a Toomey syringe, attached to the balloon catheter. Once the bladder is filled, clamp the catheter and attach it to sterile drainage. Clamp the tubing at an accessible site to allow release at the time of the cystostomy.

Incision: Make a curved right lower quadrant (Gibson) incision (see page 495) beginning below the lower thoracic cage, running 2 cm medial to the anterior superior iliac spine, and staying at least 2 cm above the iliac crest, to reach a point just above the symphysis pubis. Incise the external and internal oblique muscles and the transversus abdominis. If necessary for more exposure, divide part of the rectus sheath and muscle for access to the bladder, and extend the incision up to the tip of the 12th rib.

2 Free the inferior epigastric vessels; divide and ligate them. Divide the thin inner layer of the transversalis fascia and enter the extraperitoneal space. Sweep the peritoneum medially from the iliac vessels.

In the female, transect and ligate the round ligament. In the male, identify the spermatic cord and free it to its entry into the inguinal canal. It can then be surrounded by a Penrose drain and pulled medially, to be retracted with the medial portion of the incision. Division of vessels or vas deferens is not usually required.

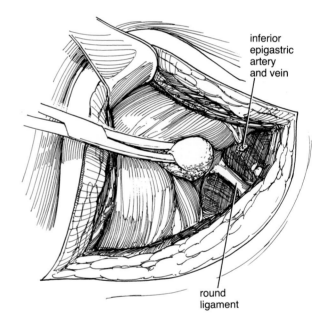

inferior
epigastric
artery
and vein

round
ligament

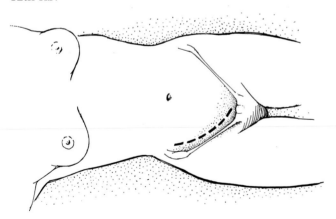

3 Insert a self-retaining Buchwalter retractor. A ring retractor with fixation to the operating table via a post permits many different exposures using a variety of fixed and adjustable blades. Be certain that a blade does not compress the femoral nerve.

Develop the extraperitoneal space over the iliac fossa to expose the distal common and external iliac artery. Start the dissection over the distal iliac artery, elevating the tissue anteriorly with right-angle forceps. Post-transplant lymphocele formation is often due to leakage from donor kidney lymphatics, but it is well to avoid large visible lymphatic trunks from the femoral canal by staying 2 to 3 cm proximal to the canal. Ligate overlying lymphatics before they are divided. Ties are better than clips to prevent lymphoceles. Continue up onto the common iliac artery. Skeletonize and elevate the iliac artery with sharp dissection. Iliac preparation should extend several centimeters proximal to the bifurcation of the hypogastric artery. Try to place the renal artery, especially from the right kidney, on the anterior wall of the common iliac artery.

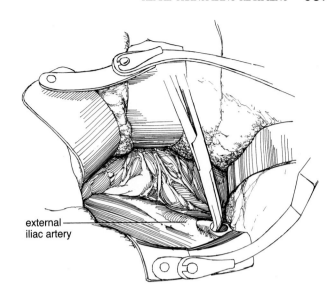

external iliac artery

4 **A,** Palpate the vessel walls at the bifurcation of the common iliac artery and internal iliac artery. Evidence of arteriosclerosis here makes end-to-side anastomosis of the renal artery with the external iliac artery preferable; the internal iliac artery then is not dissected. If little atheromatous involvement is found or if an endarterectomy is feasible, carefully tie the lymphatics over the medial side of the bifurcation, and divide them to allow skeletonization of the internal iliac artery.

B, Expose the internal iliac artery.

C, Clamp the internal iliac artery proximally and distally with artery clamps. Divide it, and ligate the distal stump.

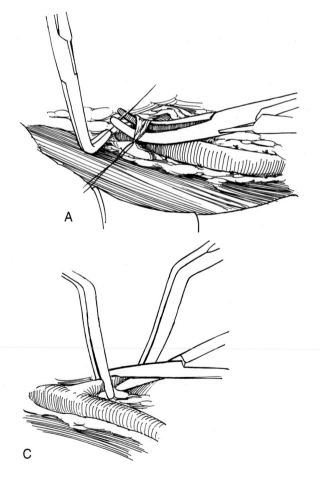

A

C

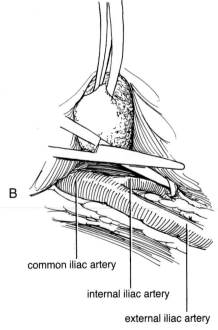

B

common iliac artery

internal iliac artery

external iliac artery

End-to-Side Anastomosis to External Iliac Vein

5 Skeletonize the iliac vein, taking care to tie and divide all the overlying lymphatics and connective tissue. Look for tributaries posteriorly; when they are found, doubly ligate and divide them. Avoid double clamping, which may avulse these delicate vessels. Place a bent-handled DeBakey curved aortic clamp on the vein proximally and an angled DeBakey clamp distally. Cut a smooth ellipse from the vein with the curved DeBakey endarterectomy scissors. Irrigate the lumen with heparinized saline.

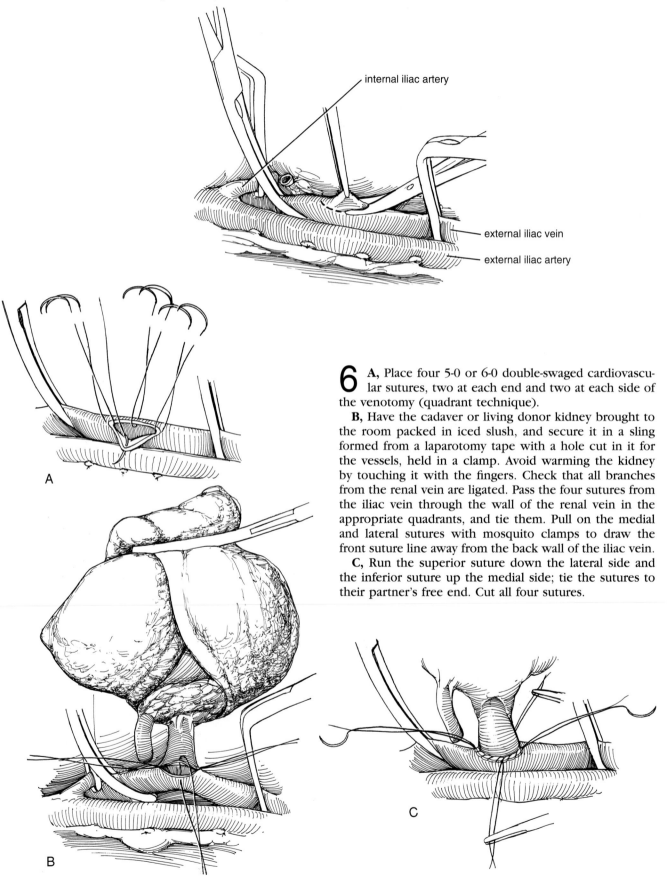

6 **A,** Place four 5-0 or 6-0 double-swaged cardiovascular sutures, two at each end and two at each side of the venotomy (quadrant technique).

B, Have the cadaver or living donor kidney brought to the room packed in iced slush, and secure it in a sling formed from a laparotomy tape with a hole cut in it for the vessels, held in a clamp. Avoid warming the kidney by touching it with the fingers. Check that all branches from the renal vein are ligated. Pass the four sutures from the iliac vein through the wall of the renal vein in the appropriate quadrants, and tie them. Pull on the medial and lateral sutures with mosquito clamps to draw the front suture line away from the back wall of the iliac vein.

C, Run the superior suture down the lateral side and the inferior suture up the medial side; tie the sutures to their partner's free end. Cut all four sutures.

End-to-End Anastomosis to Internal Iliac Artery

7 Place a bulldog clamp on the renal vein, and remove the vascular clamps from the iliac vein.

A, Bring the renal and internal iliac arteries together in a gentle curve. Place a 5-0 or 6-0 cardiovascular suture in the opposite walls of both vessels and tie them, leaving the ends long.

B, Continue closure with interrupted sutures by putting the first one at the midpoint between the apical sutures anteriorly, then approximating each of the two quadrants. Cut these sutures.

C, Rotate the vessels by traction on the apical sutures. Place the posterior sutures in the same manner as the anterior. Avoid a continuous suture. Even if it is placed by the quadrant method described for the venous anastomosis, it may act as a purse-string and partially occlude the vessel.

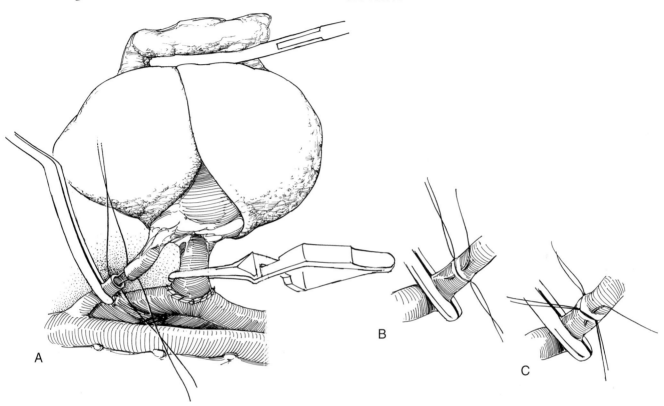

Alternative: End-to-Side Anastomosis

If arteriosclerosis is extensive, an end-to-side anastomosis is a safer alternative.

8 **A,** Occlude the iliac artery above the level of the renal vein anastomosis with a bent-handled DeBakey curved aortic clamp. Place an angled DeBakey clamp below, avoiding discernible atheromatous plaques. Make a longitudinal incision on the anterior or anterolateral surface of the artery with a #11 knife blade. Instill 80 ml of heparinized saline (1000 units/100 ml) into the distal limb of the artery.

B, Remove half an ellipse from the arterial wall on each side of the incision with the curved DeBakey endarterectomy scissors to produce a smooth oval arteriotomy.

Alternatively, use a 4- or 5-mm aortic punch to make the opening in the iliac artery.

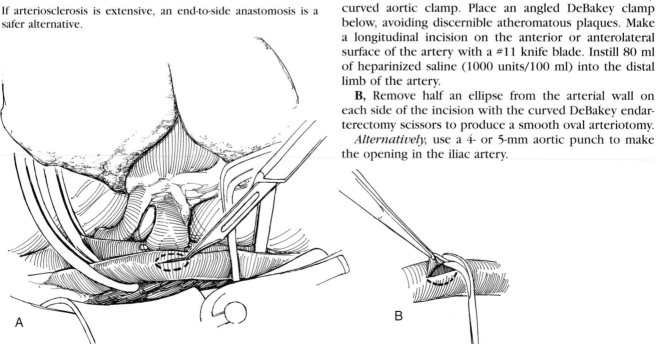

9 **A,** Insert a superior and an inferior suture of 5-0 or 6-0 cardiovascular silk through the iliac and renal arteries and tie them.

B, Close the remaining defect with interrupted sutures, first on the posterior surface and then anteriorly. *Alternatively,* place running double-armed sutures of 6-0 Prolene, taking care not to create a purse-string effect.

Remove the sling from the kidney. Release the vascular clamps, venous side first. If cold agglutinin titers were moderate to high preoperatively, warm the kidney in situ by applying warm saline solution over its surface before re-establishing circulation. Failure of the kidney to become pink and firm immediately suggests a technical occlusion of the renal vein or artery that requires review of the anastomoses. Check for perfect hemostasis. Be certain that the circulation is good in the ipsilateral leg.

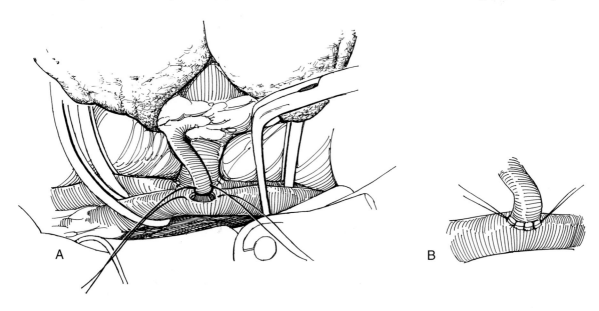

Multiple Renal Arteries

10 For cadaver kidneys harvested with a Carrel patch, make an oval arteriotomy the width and length of the patch with a knife and DeBakey endarterectomy scissors. Err on the small side because the patch can be trimmed slightly. Pass the vein back through the arterial cleft, if necessary, before making the venous anastomosis. Fix the patch in place with one 5-0 cardiovascular suture at each apex. Run the suture from the superior end down the lateral side, and tie it to the free end of the inferior suture. Run the inferior suture up the medial side and tie it.

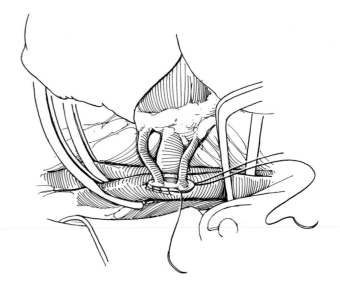

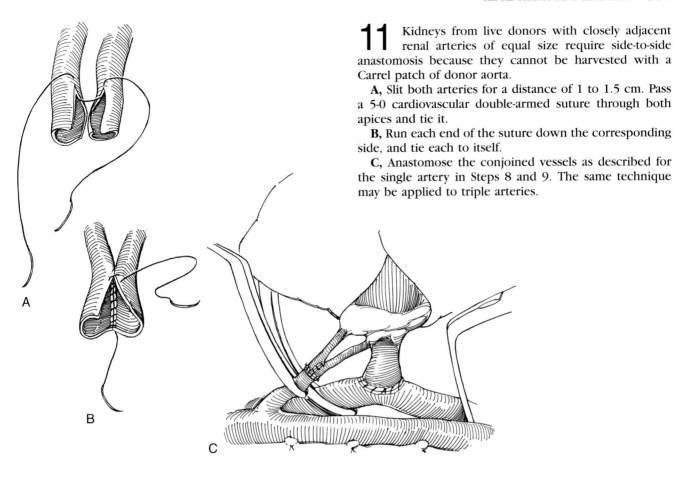

11 Kidneys from live donors with closely adjacent renal arteries of equal size require side-to-side anastomosis because they cannot be harvested with a Carrel patch of donor aorta.

A, Slit both arteries for a distance of 1 to 1.5 cm. Pass a 5-0 cardiovascular double-armed suture through both apices and tie it.

B, Run each end of the suture down the corresponding side, and tie each to itself.

C, Anastomose the conjoined vessels as described for the single artery in Steps 8 and 9. The same technique may be applied to triple arteries.

12 **A,** Alternatively, anastomose the superior renal artery end to end to the internal iliac artery and the inferior renal artery end to side to the external iliac artery.

B and **C,** Another alternative: Before implanting the kidney, perform an ex vivo anastomosis in iced slush of the small polar vessel to the larger main renal artery with interrupted 6-0 or 7-0 cardiovascular sutures, using a

loupe. It is important to preserve circulation in the polar vessels because they often supply the pelvis.

Short Right Renal Vein. Kidneys recovered during *excision of the liver* may suffer from a short right renal vein when the inferior vena cava is transected through the cephalic portion of the renal vein to provide a wide inferior vena cava cuff for caudal inferior vena caval anastomosis. To fill the defect, use a patch graft from the vena cava distally to patch the superior defect, and use a portion of the cava to extend the lower margin of the renal vein. Alternatively, create a rotation flap from the inferior vena cava, discarding the excess cava (Barry and Lemmers, 1995). The right renal vein of a *cadaver kidney* may be unduly short. When harvesting it, split the attached length of vena cava longitudinally into halves, and fold the proximal and distal ends together, thus converting the caval segment to a clam-shell configuration. Alternatively, excise a segment of donor external iliac vein and interpose it (Barry and Lemmers, 1995).

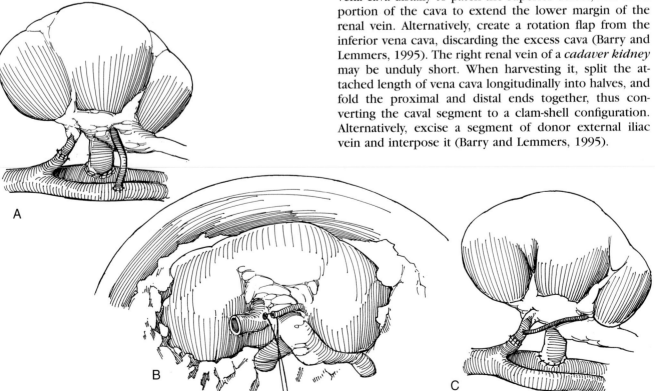

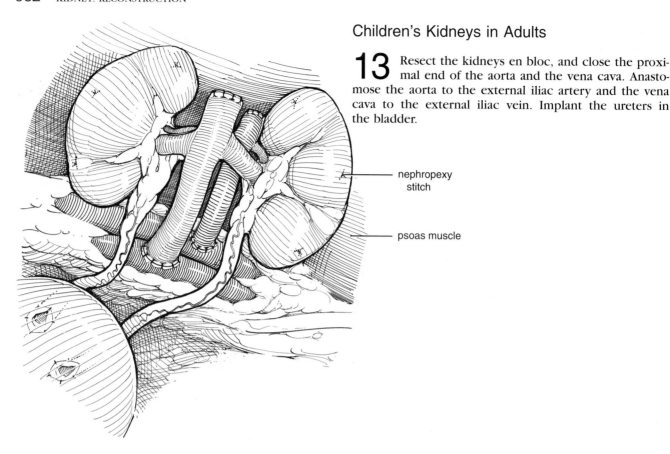

Children's Kidneys in Adults

13 Resect the kidneys en bloc, and close the proximal end of the aorta and the vena cava. Anastomose the aorta to the external iliac artery and the vena cava to the external iliac vein. Implant the ureters in the bladder.

nephropexy
stitch

psoas muscle

RENAL TRANSPLANTATION IN CHILDREN

Voiding cystourethrography provides adequate information on bladder dynamics. In children with voiding dysfunction or prior urinary diversion, formal urodynamic studies and cystourethroscopy are necessary. Cycling the defunctionalized bladder for a week or two through a suprapubic trocar catheter allows assessment of its potential. Do any necessary bladder augmentation at least 3 months before transplantation; then check to make sure the storage and evacuation system works because the bladder should have adequate capacity, empty without residual urine, and have a functional continence mechanism. In children with prior urinary diversion, intermittent catheterization may be necessary if emptying is incomplete. Reflux may be an indication for pretransplant nephrectomy.

Because an adult kidney is usually used for renal transplantation in small children weighing 20 kg or less, use a transperitoneal approach and position the kidney behind (lateral to) the cecum. Older children who require transplantation into a conduit also need a transperitoneal approach. Otherwise the retroperitoneal approach has fewer technical problems and avoids leakage of peritoneal dialysate. Choose the site for the vascular anastomoses that provides adequate arterial supply and venous drainage. In a small child, anastomosis to the vena cava and the aorta or common iliac artery is necessary. Ureteral implantation may be difficult because of multiple previous procedures. If all else is impossible, make a direct ureteral (or even pelvic) anastomosis to the bladder, or anastomose the renal pelvis or ureter to the native ureter.

14 *Position:* Supine.
Incision: Midline, from the xiphoid to the symphysis pubis.

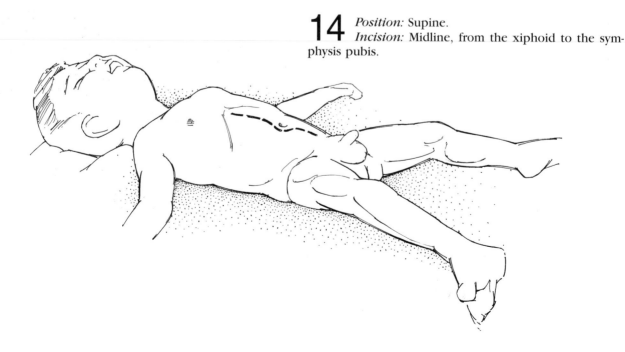

15 Reflect the right colon medially by incising the lateral posterior parietal peritoneum, and develop the retroperitoneal space down to the lateral aspect of the bladder.

Remove the right kidney if necessary. Free the vena cava from the level of the right renal vein to its bifurcation; sometimes it is necessary to mobilize both proximal iliac veins. Identify, doubly ligate, and divide the lumbar veins in the area of the proposed renal vein anastomosis. Mobilize the aorta distally from just below the renal arteries to and including both common iliac arteries. Initiate blood transfusion to compensate for the relatively large volume of blood required to fill the adult kidney.

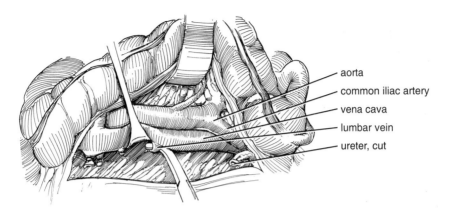

- aorta
- common iliac artery
- vena cava
- lumbar vein
- ureter, cut

16 **A,** Mark the site for the end-to-side anastomosis of the shortened renal vein to the vena cava and the sites for arterial anastomosis to the aorta or common iliac artery. Place vascular clamps above and below the anastomotic site on the vena cava, and isolate a segment of aorta by placing a pediatric vascular clamp inferiorly on each common iliac artery and one superiorly on the aorta.

B, Perform end-to-side anastomosis of the shortened renal vein, using 5-0 or 6-0 cardiovascular sutures as for adult transplantation (see Steps 5 and 6). Perform end-to-side anastomosis of the spatulated renal artery to the lower aorta (as shown) with running or interrupted 5-0 or 6-0 cardiovascular sutures. Remove the superior clamp on the inferior vena cava first, then all three inferior clamps. Finally, release the superior aortic clamp very slowly, but keep it in place in case reclamping becomes necessary.

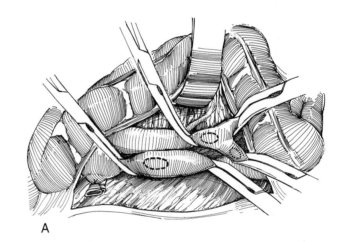

A

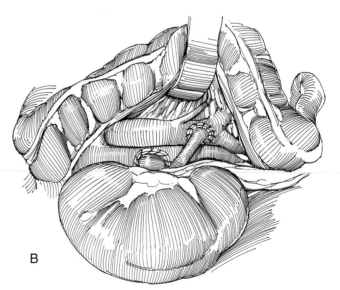

B

URETERAL IMPLANTATION

An *extravesical* ureteroneocystostomy (Lich-Gregoir, see pages 795 to 796, and Barry, see pages 797 to 798) is associated with fewer leaks and is preferable in most cases to a *transvesical* technique. When the donor ureter is short or its circulation is compromised, anastomose the recipient ureter to the donor renal pelvis as an alternative to performing ureteroneocystostomy under tension.

Transvesical Technique

17 Open the partially filled bladder on the anterior aspect. Select a site on the floor of the bladder as near and as lateral to the ureteral orifice as possible, and make a short transverse incision through the mucosa. Make a second transverse incision proximally, and dissect a tunnel between them with curved scissors. The length of the tunnel should be proportional to the size of the child, with a maximum of 2.5 cm in adolescents. Draw an 8 F Robinson catheter through the tunnel retrogradely.

18 Pass a right-angle clamp obliquely through the bladder wall from outside just above the upper end of the tunnel. The tract must provide a smooth oblique exit for the ureter, which with transplantation has a more anterior course than the normal ureter. Stretch the hiatus, making it large enough that it cannot obstruct the ureter. Draw the catheter (below the spermatic cord in males) through the hiatus with a clamp, and fasten it to the tip of the ureter with a 2-0 SAS. Pull the ureter gently into the bladder, leaving a little redundancy outside the bladder.

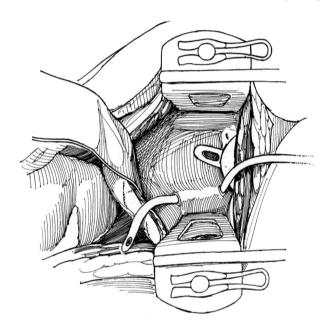

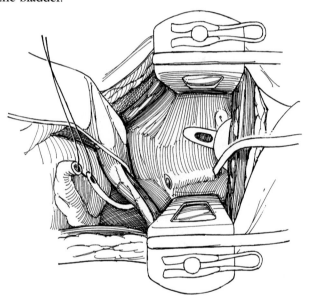

19 Trim and spatulate the end of the ureter, leaving 1 cm protruding. Anchor the apex with a 5-0 SAS to the trigonal muscle and mucosa. Place several mucosal sutures on either side and at the apex. Test for absence of constriction with an infant feeding tube. Close the mucosa over the hiatus. A stent should not be needed, but if one is placed, use a double-J silicone stent.

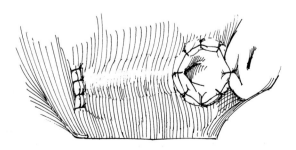

20 Close the cystotomy in one layer with a running full-thickness 3-0 or 4-0 SAS. Catch just the edge of the epithelium, and take a good bite of the muscularis and adventitia. Alternatively, close the bladder in the standard fashion with a running fine suture to the epithelial layer, as shown, and interrupted sutures to the wall itself. Carry the closure beyond the ends of the incision to avoid leakage. Close the peritoneal incision lateral and inferior to the right colon to extraperitonealize the ureter and graft. To prevent lymphoceles, some surgeons make a 12- to 15-cm incision in the peritoneum below and medial to the kidney, pull a tongue of omentum through it, and drape the omentum over the graft. Flood the wound with bacitracin-neomycin solution, and aspirate it. Obtain perfect hemostasis; these patients may bleed from azotemic coagulopathy if a spastic vessel opens. Consider a retroperitoneal suction drain. Close the abdomen appropriately. Place a balloon catheter through the urethra into the bladder.

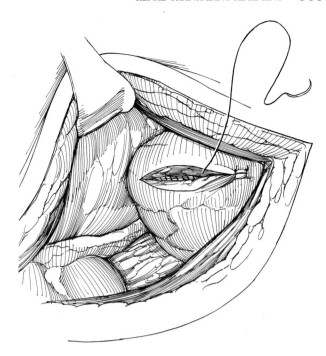

OPERATIVE AND POSTOPERATIVE SUPPORT

It is important that the graft be supplied with adequate fluids and electrolytes and that the patient be supported with packed cells and colloids. Give mannitol at the end of the procedure. Because the patient has been cooled by the iced slush, neuromuscular function may return slowly. Delay extubation until the patient is stable.

POSTOPERATIVE PROBLEMS FROM RENAL TRANSPLANTATION

Bleeding is the most frequent cause for re-exploration of the graft. Although a small hematoma in the iliac fossa is to be expected, bleeding is heralded by pain and the signs of blood loss, followed by a distended wound, an unstable blood pressure, and usually anuria. Reopen the wound, dissect the peritoneum from the surface of the kidney, and evacuate the hematoma. Expose the arterial and venous anastomoses, the area of the hilum, and the surface of the kidney. The bleeding may come from the arterial anastomosis because of inadequate technique, from atherosclerosis, or from hypertension; place additional sutures. Look for small vessels in the hilum that were not tied during procurement. Often no source for the bleeding is found.

Allograft rupture due to acute rejection is suggested by acute, severe pain over the graft. Nephrectomy is usually necessary. *Hyperacute rejection* is heralded by swelling and discoloration of the kidney soon after it is revascularized. It must be differentiated from renal vein obstruction or thrombosis. Take a biopsy specimen to confirm the diagnosis of hyperacute rejection. If the finding is positive, removing the kidney may be advisable; if the situation is doubtful, leave the kidney in place and hope for reversal.

Try not to confuse the signs and symptoms of *rejection* with those of *urologic complications*. Use ultrasonography and renal scintigraphy to differentiate among acute tubular necrosis, rejection, and urinary obstruction. One can resort to intravenous urography, cystography, and even retrograde or antegrade pyelography. Percutaneous nephrostomy is the diagnostic test for total or partial obstruction and moreover is therapeutic.

Ureterocutaneous fistulas are heralded by bulging of the wound, decreased urine output, weight gain, and rising serum creatinine. Fistulas are the result of devascularization during harvesting and implantation, especially with kidneys from live donors and in children who are of small size, may have congenital abnormalities, and usually have experienced multiple preceding operations. Fewer leaks occur after external methods of ureteral reimplantation. Rejection may play a role.

Leakage may occur at the ureterovesical anastomosis or from the bladder closure, or, later, directly from the ureter. Evaluate the patient with ultrasonography and a mercaptoacetylglycine (MAG 3) renal scan. Determine a vesical source by cystography if the leakage is at the cystostomy site or the ureteral anastomosis. Because urine is irritating and conducive to infection and disruption of the vascular anastomoses, intervene within 72 hours of the appearance of a fistula to avoid wound and systemic infections that may be fatal. Place a balloon catheter. If cystography does not show extravasation and the source is the ureter itself, insert a nephrostomy tube percutaneously and perform antegrade pyelography. Place a ureteral stent if the defect appears limited. It is easier to insert the stent antegradely because inserting it endoscopically through the bladder after ureteral reimplantation is difficult. If the extravasation is in the proximal ureter without communication with the bladder, if it is in a child, or if it appears late from extensive ureteral necrosis, do not use the percutaneous approach. If leakage continues, maintain renal drainage, and later do a ureterovesical or pyelovesical anastomosis with a psoas hitch or a Boari flap; alternatively, consider an anastomosis of the ureter or pelvis to one or the other residual terminal ureter. A nephrostomy tube or silicone stent may be needed in complicated situations. Fistulas can occur from a calyx if a renal pole is devascularized. In that case, partial nephrectomy or an omental patch may be effective.

Vesicocutaneous fistulas are not common when the bladder has been opened through a normal wall and has been closed carefully. When a cystostomy is necessary in an infant because of the small urethra, it may not close spontaneously. Delay treatment of fistulas by inserting a balloon catheter and using suction drainage and antibiotics, but do not be afraid of surgical excision and closure of the tract with an omental or muscle wrap. For *calicocutaneous fistulas* secondary to segmental infarction of one of the vessels, insert a nephrostomy tube percutaneously. If that fails, first be sure that the fistula is not secondary to obstruction; then débride and close the defect by open operation.

Ureteral obstruction in the first week or so is usually from edema, but hematoma, lymphocele, or technical error may be the cause. A common cause, with later subtle onset of obstruction, is periureteral fibrosis or contraction of the ureter from partial ischemia. The immediate treatment is percutaneous diversion or occasionally transurethral insertion of a silicone stent. Some cases may respond to percutaneous transluminal ureteroplasty. If these measures are inapplicable or if they fail, reoperate and reimplant the ureter. Alternatively, use the patient's own structures: Anastomose the native ureter to the grafted pelvis (pyeloureterostomy); anastomose the grafted ureter to the native ureter ipsilaterally or contralaterally (ureteroureterostomy or crossed ureteroureterostomy); bring the severed pelvis down for anastomosis to the grafted pelvis (pyelopyelostomy); or even perform calicocystostomy combined with a psoas hitch.

Lymphoceles, although often confused with extravasation, appear several weeks after surgery rather than at once. Look for reduced renal function due to compression of the ureter, local swelling, genital edema, increased blood pressure and body weight, and edema of the ipsilateral leg from compression of the iliac vein. Ipsilateral iliofemoral venous thrombosis may occur. Aspirate the lymphocele with the aid of ultrasonography. Identify the fluid as lymph by finding lower levels of creatinine and potassium than in urine. If the lymphocele recurs, consider inserting a tube for drainage, a process that may take 4 to 6 weeks. Alternatively, for large accumulations, marsupialize the lymphocele into the peritoneal cavity with a laparoscope (see page 468).

Renal artery stenosis comes from a defective anastomosis, from chronic rejection, or from kinking or torsion due to excessive length. In children, the cause may be inadequate size of the recipient vessels. Stenosis can occur both early and late. Look for hypertension. Even though this could be due to rejection or renal disease, perform angiography, especially if you find a diastolic bruit or a decrease in renal function. Use selective renin determinations to be sure the kidney is the cause of the hypertension, and locate the lesion with anteroposterior and oblique views on digital subtraction imaging. Delay treatment if renal function is stable and hypertension can be controlled medically. In any case, try transluminal angioplasty before proceeding with a difficult surgical procedure (saphenous vein graft, page 953) that carries a real chance for loss of the graft.

Arterial thrombosis usually comes from tearing of the intima either when the kidney is secured or during perfusion, but rejection and poor anastomotic technique may be factors, as well as hypercoagulability, arteriosclerotic disease in the recipient artery, and embolus. Treatment is usually prompt nephrectomy. *Venous thrombosis* is secondary to such errors as kinking of the graft when the kidney is put in place. Distinguishing the signs of swelling of the graft, oliguria, and proteinuria from those of rejection is difficult. Perform renal venography when suspicion is aroused, and re-explore immediately to do a thrombectomy.

Acute tubular necrosis is a complication in the immediate postoperative period. Follow the patient with nuclear scans to check on blood flow and evidence of rejection and with sonograms to rule out obstruction and extravasation.

Be alert for *wound complications.* Wound infections are uncommon even though patients are immunocompromised, but infections may have serious sequelae. If fever persists, look for a pelvic or retroperitoneal abscess by sonography and CT scans, as well as for urinary leakage and rejection of the graft.

In patients with poorly controlled renin-mediated hypertension, persistent urinary tract infection, renal stones, prior urinary diversion, or severe reflux, the *native kidneys* usually should be removed before transplantation. Use bilateral posterior incisions (see page 896) because of the low morbidity and mortality. Polycystic kidneys may require removal in two stages through the flanks. Bilateral nephroureterectomy is recommended for a patient with existing urinary diversion. Nephrectomy of the native kidney is usually performed weeks before transplantation.

NEPHRECTOMY AFTER FAILED TRANSPLANTATION

Removal of the failed graft is not always necessary, but once the patient requires maintenance dialysis, stopping the immunosuppressive drugs that are no longer needed usually results in fever and painful swelling of the graft, requiring nephrectomy.

Nephrectomy soon after transplantation is straightforward. Resect the artery at the anastomosis; this may require a vein patch if the anastomosis was end to side. The low-pressure renal vein may simply be ligated and divided beyond the anastomosis but as close to the iliac vein as possible to avoid formation of a thrombus. Pull the ureter out of the bladder, close the defect with absorbable sutures, and maintain bladder drainage for 1 or 2 days.

Late nephrectomy can be very difficult because of the rejection reaction and the adherence of the kidney to the recipient artery and vein. If possible, have the original transplant surgeon perform the nephrectomy because he or she knows best how to clear the vessels. Allograft nephrectomy more than 1 or 2 weeks after transplantation is usually best done subcapsularly because of perinephric fibrosis (see page 926).

Reopen the transplant incision, staying lateral to avoid penetrating the peritoneum. In early cases, suture-ligate the renal artery and vein and remove the whole kidney. Otherwise, incise the capsule over the lateral surface, and bluntly dissect the kidney from the capsule. At the hilus, incise the capsule vertically, dissect the branch arteries free, and ligate them. Dissect and ligate the veins. Avoid an approach near the iliac artery or peritoneum, structures that may adhere to the renal capsule and hilus. Ligate and then suture-ligate the vessels, leaving small portions of the donor vessels in place if necessary. Finally, ligate and divide the ureter. Leave a portion of the donor ureter if necessary, although hematuria from rejection may be noted for a few weeks. Coagulate or apply the argon beam to oozing spots within the capsule. Irrigate with antibiotic solution, and spray the capsule with thrombin. Avoid placing drains, or, rarely, insert a suction drain to remain a short time. Provide antibiotic coverage.

RENAL ARTERY STENOSIS AFTER TRANSPLANTATION (Banowsky)

If possible, the original surgeon should conduct the reoperation. Harvest an appropriate length of saphenous vein (see page 953). Approach the kidney through a midline transperitoneal incision. With the patient in Trendelenburg position, pack the intestines away. Incise the posterior peritoneum over the external (or common) iliac artery, and clear it from the vessel. A right-angle clamp is useful to free the posterior aspect. Encircle the artery with a vessel loop. Repeat the procedure for the distal portion of the external iliac artery. With Metzenbaum scissors, carefully dissect the adventitia and scar tissue from the artery at both sites. Expose the area of the anastomosis and a length of renal artery. Occasionally it is necessary to mobilize the entire renal unit. Take care to avoid the renal vein and ureter.

Obtain control of the external iliac vein with a vascular clamp. Open the anterior wall of the artery with a #11 blade. Insert a 4-mm aortic punch to make an elliptical opening. Anastomose the vein to the artery with two double-armed 6-0 Prolene sutures inserted inside out at either end, tied and run down either side. Be sure to incorporate the intima. Clamp the vein near the anastomosis with a bulldog clamp, and release the arterial clamp to check for leaks.

Hold the vein in position and trim it to the proper length. Place a small bulldog clamp on the renal artery, divide the artery, and spatulate it if necessary to match the caliber of the vein. Place a 6-0 silk suture in through the dorsal aspect of the opening in the vein and out through the apex of the arterial spatulation. Place a second suture in the vein and out through the arterial base. Place interrupted sutures under direct vision on the back wall from each end to the middle. Turn the vessel over and repeat the suturing. Remove the bulldog clamp, and

allow back-bleeding for visualization of any leaks that require extra sutures. Remove the clamp on the iliac artery, and again check for patency and leakage. Irrigate the wound with 1 L of saline, and close it in two layers with interrupted 0 nonabsorbable sutures or #28 wire. Close the subcutaneous tissue with 3-0 SAS and the skin with clips or subcuticular stitches.

Postoperatively, control excessive blood pressure with a nitroprusside drip. Replace blood volume. If anuria occurs and it does not respond to furosemide or mannitol, suspect failure of the anastomosis and check by a technetium-99m renal scan.

Commentary by Stuart M. Flechner

Donor kidneys are scarce, so select the recipient carefully. Although physiologic age of the recipient is often more important than chronologic age, carefully evaluate the recipient, taking care to rule out those with uncorrectable cardiopulmonary or peripheral vascular disease, ineradicable infections, malignancy, or vascular compromise. Ultrasound examination of the upper abdomen is useful to rule out native kidney lesions and hepatobiliary problems. Voiding cystography is useful in patients with small-capacity bladders or prior urologic problems. It is not routinely performed on young patients with recent-onset renal failure, especially those undergoing preemptive transplantation.

The techniques used for vascular re-anastomosis should be flexible enough to accommodate the many possible alignments of the renal vessels and the recipient vessels. In principle, it is useful to use a cuff of donor vena cava for the renal vein or aorta for the renal artery. This, of course, can be accomplished only in cadaver donor renal transplantation. This rim of extra tissue obviates suturing of the actual ostia of the renal vessels and is often thicker than the wall of the donor artery and vein. This approach lends itself more favorably to the use of the end-to-side anastomosis rather than an end-to-end anastomosis to the hypogastric artery. Because an increasing number of recipients are older males, it is useful to avoid compromise of the pelvic blood flow from the hypogastric artery that may contribute to the maintenance of potency. Alternatively, many hypogastric blood vessels in diabetics and older patients have extensive atherosclerotic plaques that require endarterectomy and further manipulation.

The wall of the right renal vein is often thin and attenuated, making the use of a vena cava patch especially helpful. Some have advocated extending the length of the right vein by using a tube of vena cava. This tube is created by closing the superior and inferior ends of the vena cava with running suture. This technique is most helpful in recipients who weigh more than 100 kg.

For most vascular anastomoses, the quadrant technique is used, with 5-0 monofilament suture for the vein and 6-0 monofilament for the artery. Each end of the anastomosis is placed with a double-armed suture, and one fourth of the anastomosis is run from the apex to the midpoint. Sutures are then tied at the midpoint. In most cases, the venous anastomosis is done first; a bulldog clamp is placed across the renal vein, and the iliac vein clamps are removed to restore circulation to the leg. Anastomotic integrity of the vein can be tested and repaired if necessary at this time. In a similar fashion, a bulldog clamp is placed on the renal artery, and the occluding vascular clamp is removed from the iliac artery to test the integrity of the arterial anastomosis. This technique provides the best opportunity in a clear operative field to repair any vascular leaks. The bulldog clamps are then removed in sequence from the vein first and then the artery to restore circulation to the kidney.

A helpful tool in creating a smooth arteriotomy on the anterior wall of the iliac artery is the aortic punch. Originally designed to create an aortotomy for aortocoronary bypass, a 4- or 5-mm punch makes a smooth opening for renal artery anastomosis to the iliac vessels.

An extravesical ureteroneocystostomy, a derivative of the Lich-Gregoir technique, has become popular and has replaced the intravesical Leadbetter-Politano technique in the majority of transplant centers. The advantages of this technique include a shorter length of donor ureter required, absence of a complete cystotomy incision, diminished postoperative bleeding, diminished incidence of obstruction as the bladder fills, and shorter operative time. The incidence of ureteral fistula appears to be decreased, and post-transplantation bladder fistula is eliminated. The one disadvantage is the greater difficulty in subsequently identifying and cannulating the transplant ureter, if that becomes necessary. A useful addition to this technique is the placement of a U stitch joining the anterior ureteral wall to the full thickness of the bladder. This anchors the ureter and prevents dislodgment. Both the ureteral anastomosis to the mucosa and the muscular tunnel should be created using absorbable suture, either polyglycolic acid or polydioxanone. It is important not to use electrocautery directly on the ureter. If cautery is necessary, a bipolar rather than a unipolar cautery unit should be used. The extravesical technique also permits earlier removal of the catheter, usually on day four or five. Some have recommended the use of an internal double-J ureteral stent for all cases. It is certainly helpful when the bladder wall is thin and poorly vascularized, a condition often encountered during re-transplantation in patients who have received many years of steroid therapy.

The technique of en bloc transplantation of small pediatric kidneys, usually from children under age 3, is useful. It is essential to place both kidneys in a perpendicular fashion lying directly on the psoas muscle. If not given this support and if placed medial to the iliac vessels, the medial kidney often twists and thromboses. Either the arterial anastomosis can be created end to side to the iliac artery, or a direct end-to-end anastomosis from the hypogastric artery to the lower aorta can be fashioned. It is useful to use a small 4 F internal ureteral stent for these small pediatric kidneys. With stents in place, the two ureters can be conjoined, creating one ostia to be re-implanted into the bladder by an extravesical technique. The stents can then be removed endoscopically at about 6 weeks after transplant. It is also most helpful to leave the perirenal tissues on the surface of these pediatric kidneys. The kidneys can then be anchored to the psoas muscle using interrupted 3-0 CCG sutures. This helps to avoid further mobility and possible kinking of the delicate renal vasculature if the kidney changes position.

BLADDER AUGMENTATION WITH RENAL TRANSPLANTATION

For a patient with a small contracted bladder and end-stage renal failure, perform bladder augmentation (see Section 17) as a first stage prior to transplantation. Left nephrectomy can be

done at the same time. At the second stage, mobilize the right colon, and remove the right kidney. Transplant the donor kidney into the right iliac fossa, and tunnel its ureter retroperitoneally to exit near the augmented bladder. Anastomotic alternatives include ureteroureterostomy and implantation into the bladder or into an ileal nipple, if that has been formed.

VASCULAR ACCESS BY RADIAL ARTERY–CEPHALIC VEIN SHUNT (Barry)

Instruments: Provide a cut-down tray, an electrocautery, two winged-in-line Ramirez shunt tubes, vessel tips (two small, two medium, and two large), a straight connector, neomycin-bacitracin irrigating solution, 100 ml heparinized saline, a 10-ml syringe with a plain tip, and 1 percent lidocaine.

21 Use the nondominant arm, if possible. Prepare and drape it. Palpate the radial artery, and mark its course in the forearm. Apply a tourniquet, and mark the (variable) course of the distal cephalic vein. Mark the skin for a transverse incision four fingerbreadths above the wrist, high enough to keep the shunt clear of the wrist. Infiltrate the area with local anesthesia, and incise the skin. Do not place the shunt higher than necessary in case it must be replaced later, at a high level. Use electrocautery for hemostasis.

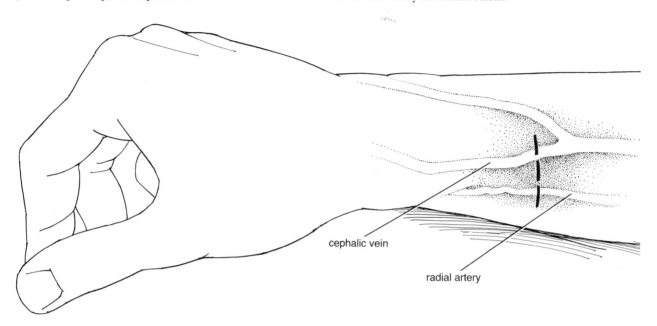

cephalic vein

radial artery

22 Isolate 1.5 to 2 cm of the cephalic vein using a mosquito clamp, and pass two 2-0 silk sutures around it. Palpate the radial artery through the antebrachial fascia, and incise the fascia longitudinally for 1.5 to 2 cm to expose it. Ligate any muscular branches with fine silk. Isolate an arterial segment, and pass two ligatures of 2-0 silk around it.

23 Select the appropriately sized vessel tip for both vein and artery, and insert each into its trimmed wing-in-line shunt until the etched areas are within the tubing. Tie them in place with a 2-0 silk ligature, using three knots, and cut one end of the ligature. Fill the tubing with heparinized saline, and clamp the other end. Skill is needed to have the loop run easily through the incision in the skin and to be sure that the cannulas are not kinked as they enter the vein or artery.

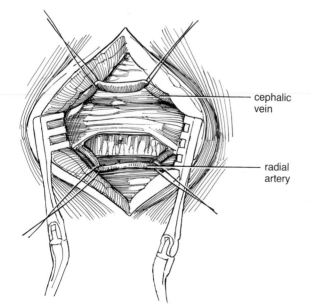

cephalic vein

radial artery

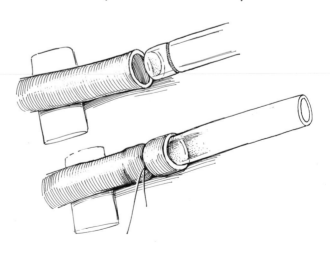

24 **A,** Return to the exposed cephalic vein, and tie the distal ligature, leaving the ends long. Pass a #11 knife blade obliquely, halfway through the vein, keeping the cutting edge up.

B, Lift the edge, dilate the lumen gently with a curved mosquito clamp, and insert the vessel tip.

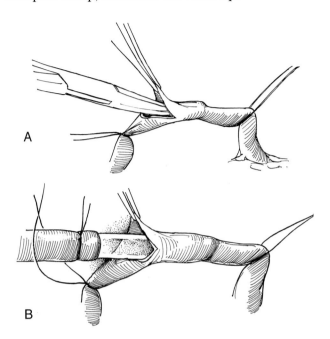

25 Tie the proximal ligature around the vein and vessel tip, and cut one end. Tie the other end to the remaining end of the ligature, holding the tip in the tubing. Pass the ends of the distal ligature around the shunt tubing, tie them, and cut the ends. Make a subcutaneous tunnel distal to the incision to seat the wings of the shunt. Irrigate the tubing with heparinized saline and reclamp it. For the radial artery, tie the distal ligature and leave it long. Put traction on the proximal ligature for hemostasis, and cut the artery as was done for the vein. Dilate the artery gently, and insert the vessel tip with attached shunt. Tie the ligatures as described for the vein.

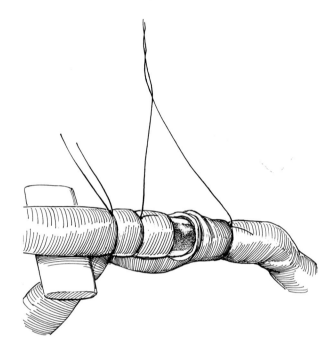

26 Pass the shunt tubing from both artery and vein through stab wounds in the skin. Relax the traction ligature on the artery, and let the tubing fill. Place the shunt connector to join the two assemblies, and fix it with shunt tape. Close the wound in two layers, using a running 4-0 SAS for the skin. Alternatively, other veins and the ulnar artery can be used.

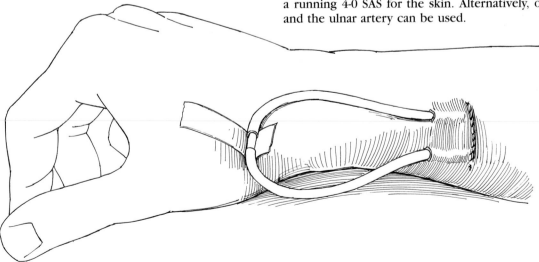

Postoperative Problems

Clotting of the shunt in the early postoperative period can be easily corrected. Prepare the field and then separate the tubing at the connector. Pass a #3 Fogarty embolectomy catheter into the venous side, partially inflate it, and draw it out with the clot. Irrigate the tubing with heparinized saline on a plain-tipped syringe. Repeat the procedure on the arterial side, and reconnect the tubing. Mild anticoagulation helps, but recurrent thrombosis necessitates moving the shunt to other vessels.

Commentary by Stuart M. Flechner

Vascular access for temporary dialysis is often required in tertiary-care hospitals. The use of the surgically implanted Scribner shunt with extracorporeal exposure was used in the early years of hemodialysis. However, frequent episodes of infection, thrombosis, and obliteration of the upper extremity blood vessels needed for later use to create a permanent vascular access have diminished its usefulness. Temporary access is more readily obtained by placing silicone catheters with a double lumen into the superior vena cava. They are generally placed through entry sites in the subclavian vein or internal jugular vein using the Seldinger technique (see page 92). Percutaneous entry is made into the large vein, and a guide wire is passed centrally. A tract is dilated, and then the catheters are passed over the guide wire into the superior vena cava or right atrium. Many of the commercially available percutaneous catheters also have cuffs and extended tubing that can be tunneled subcutaneously several centimeters away from the entry port and have been used successfully for weeks and months. They can be placed under local anesthesia, and sterile technique is essential to long-term maintenance.

CATHETER INSERTION FOR CHRONIC AMBULATORY PERITONEAL DIALYSIS (Tenckhoff)

Catheters for chronic ambulatory peritoneal dialysis may be placed in three ways—blindly, laparoscopically, and surgically.

Blind Insertion

Make a puncture in the abdomen with a needle or trocar and introduce dialysate; make a second puncture and introduce the catheter.

Laparoscopic Insertion

The laparoscopic technique is followed by the fewest complications of infection, outflow failure, and subcutaneous leak.

Puncture the abdomen with a 2-mm trocar with a special sheath covered with a thin plastic guide (Quill guide). Insert a Y-TEC scope through the sheath, and confirm the position of the tip. Infuse 600 ml of CO_2 through the cannula. Reinsert the scope and advance the sheath into position under vision. Remove the sheath, leaving the Quill guide at the proper depth. Dilate the guide to the size of the peritoneal catheter, and insert the catheter until the cuff rests within the abdominal wall. Pass the end through a subcutaneous tunnel, as described in Step 29.

Surgical Insertion

Clear the patient of *Staphylococcus aureus*. (Look for the patient who is a nasal carrier; prescribe special antibiotic nasal creams preoperatively and postoperatively.) Prepare the patient with antiseptic showers, and give prophylactic antibiotics.

Mark the exit site while the patient is standing, as is done for a ureteroileostomy (see page 647).

Catheter: Use a Tenckhoff catheter consisting of a 30- to 35-cm-long Silastic catheter with one or two Dacron felt cuffs attached for fixation. If properly placed, it does not require coils or discs to prevent obstruction by the omentum.

Position: Supine. Local or general anesthesia. Select a site suitable for emergence of the catheter and mark it.

27 **A,** Make a transverse incision at a point lateral to the midline and 3 cm below the umbilicus, usually on the side opposite that of a future renal transplant. Incise the anterior rectus sheath transversely. Split the rectus abdominis muscle in the line of its fibers. Look for the inferior epigastric vessels; ligate them if necessary.

B, Insert self-retaining mastoid retractors. Place a 3-0 purse-string SAS in the peritoneum in a 3-cm circle, leaving the needle attached. Make a 1-cm incision in the

peritoneum (larger if one intends to palpate for adhesions or, in children and thin adults, to resect a portion of a mobile omentum). Mount the catheter on a guide, and direct it into the vesicorectal pouch, leaving the deep margin of the cuff level with the peritoneum, with the cuff remaining in the muscle. If difficulty is met in positioning the catheter, distend the abdomen with 1 to 2 liters of 5 percent dextrose in saline. It is rarely necessary to trim the catheter for length.

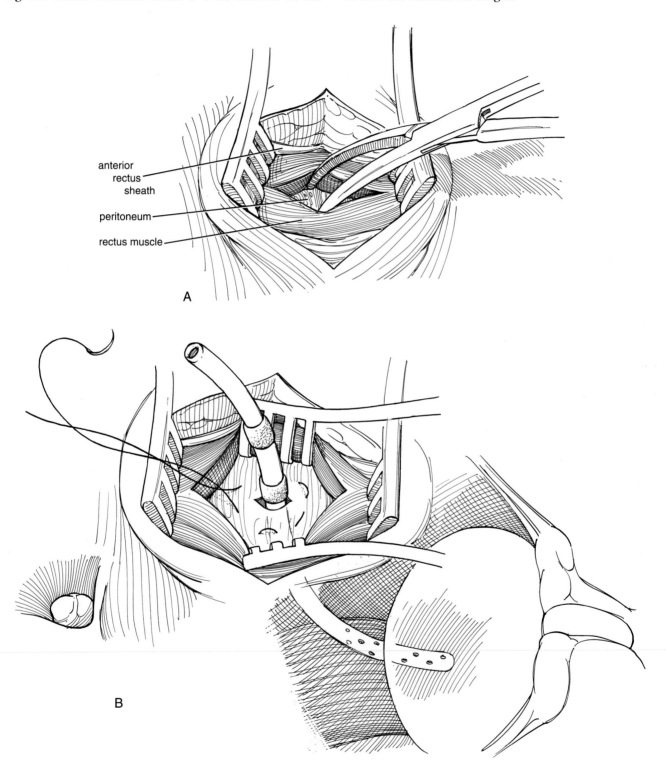

anterior rectus sheath

peritoneum

rectus muscle

A

B

28 Draw the purse-string suture tight and tie it. Pass the attached needle through the cuff, and tie the suture again. Test the closure for watertightness by instilling dialysate containing a high concentration of antibiotics into the peritoneal cavity. If there is leakage from peritoneal needle holes, raise the peritoneum by traction on the catheter, and ligate the tented peritoneal cuff. With the peritoneal cavity full, check drainage through the catheter by aspiration with a syringe.

Close the anterior rectus sheath with interrupted 3-0 SAS, leaving the cuff embedded in the muscle. Have your assistant hold the catheter so that the tip remains caudad to stay in the pouch.

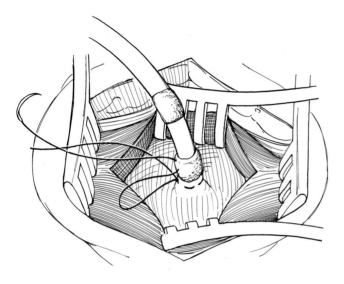

29 Incise the skin 3 cm away at the exit site that was selected preoperatively. Insert a clamp from the implantation site to create a subcutaneous tunnel, and draw an umbilical tape through it. Tie the tape to the catheter, and draw it through the tunnel, leaving the second cuff midway in the tunnel, about 2 cm from the exit site in the skin. Take care not to dilate the exit site to avoid eversion of the subcutaneous tissue and subsequent granulation tissue formation and infection. Instill 1 liter of dialysate, and check for leaks. If any leakage is seen, reinforce the peritoneal suture. Close the subcutaneous tissue with SAS, and approximate the skin with a subcuticular stitch. Insert a titanium adapter in the tube, instill 5 ml of dilute heparin, and cap the tube. Tape the catheter to the skin. Apply separate dressings to the wound and the drain site. Flush the catheter daily with not more than 500 ml of dialysis fluid until intermittent dialysis is begun, usually 5 to 10 days later. Change the dressing at the exit site with strict aseptic technique.

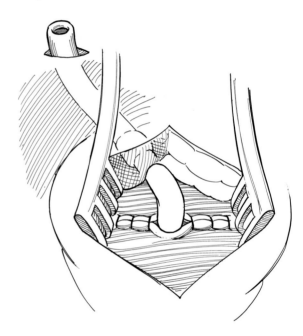

Postoperative Problems from Peritoneal Catheters

Outflow may be impeded if the catheter has shifted into an iliac fossa. External manipulation is seldom successful. Make a vertical midline incision below the entry site, and digitally redirect the catheter. A similar approach can be made for *omental blockage* of the holes. *Leakage* either externally or into the anterior abdominal wall is best managed conservatively by stopping continuous ambulatory peritoneal dialysis for 2 weeks. *Infection* in the body wall around the exit site requires intensive antibiotic therapy; if that fails, the catheter must be removed. *Peritonitis* is usually secondary to contamination of the dialysis system, although it may be hematogenous in origin or arise from bacteria that gain access around the catheter. Look for cloudy dialysate and culture it. Start by adding a first-generation cephalosporin plus heparin to the dialysate; change the antibiotic as necessary. It may occasionally be necessary to remove the catheter.

Commentary by Stuart M. Flechner

The author describes an excellent technique for long-term placement of a double-cuff peritoneal dialysis catheter. It is important to place the catheter through the rectus sheath as outlined. Subumbilical midline placement of the catheter creates an unnecessarily difficult dissection because of the fusion of the peritoneum to the posterior rectus sheath in the midline. Placement of the purse-string suture in the peritoneum is done much more easily in the paramedian position. Placement of the deeper cuff within the substance of the rectus muscle, above the posterior rectus sheath, makes future catheter removal less morbid. The tract of the catheter can then be closed with just a few interrupted sutures on the anterior rectus sheath. Tenckhoff catheters are now available with a single cuff. They can be placed in a similar fashion by anchoring the cuff within the substance of the rectus muscle.

A malleable catheter stilet can be placed through the lumen of the peritoneal dialysis catheter as it is placed into the peritoneal cavity. The temporary rigidity of the tubing facilitates the gentle manipulation of the catheter toward the vesicorectal pouch.

If one is having difficulty in placing the tip of the catheter inferiorly, it is always safer to make a lower midline counterincision above the symphysis pubis. Forcing a catheter through resistance may ultimately result in bowel perforation. The counterincision can be used to pull the catheter tip into the proper position. In most cases, the procedure is safe and can be performed through a small incision. However, bowel perforation is a potentially life-threatening and disastrous complication. It is always safer to make an adequate incision and place the catheter properly even if a general anesthetic and larger laparotomy incision are required.

Migration of the peritoneal dialysis catheter to the upper quadrants of the abdomen and/or ingrowth of omental fat into the catheter can obstruct the flow and make the exchange of the dialysate inadequate. Repositioning of the catheter can sometimes be done by passing a semirigid stilet through the catheter lumen. However, this must be done most carefully. If resistance is encountered, further attempts should not be made. Either the catheter should be replaced or a lower midline incision should be made, as previously described. Some surgeons have recently advocated the use of laparoscopic techniques to manipulate the position of peritoneal dialysis catheters. However, the placement of several laparoscopic entry ports may result in leakage of peritoneal fluid.

Living Donor Nephrectomy

The left kidney is preferred over the right because of its longer vein, unless multiple renal arteries are located on that side. Perform renal arteriography to detect abnormal vasculature. Transfuse 200 ml of whole blood from the donor to the recipient every 2 weeks for three times. Prepare the donor by giving 1000 to 2000 ml of lactated Ringer's solution beginning either the evening before or 2 hours before surgery. Give prophylactic antibiotics with the preoperative medications, and continue for 3 days postoperatively. Do not anesthetize the donor until a good diuresis results from intravenous fluids given in the operating room. Place a 16 F 5-ml balloon catheter into the bladder.

Instruments: Provide Sheldon, Balfour, Harrington, and two Deaver retractors; a Satinsky clamp; 0 silk ties; surgical clips; 5-0 silk arterial sutures; and a basin with cold electrolyte solution.

Two approaches are in use, one extraperitoneal and the other transperitoneal. The former has fewer complications but may be associated with greater difficulty in dissecting the hilar vessels.

SUPRACOSTAL 11TH- OR 12TH-RIB APPROACH

Left Nephrectomy

1 *Incision:* Follow the plan outlined for the supracostal incision (see page 879), but curve the anterior part of the incision toward the symphysis to allow better access to the lower ureter. Open Gerota's fascia over the lateral curvature of the kidney. Fulgurate small capsular branches, but watch for a polar artery that also supplies the renal pelvis. If the artery is inadvertently severed, reanastomose it, using a loupe.

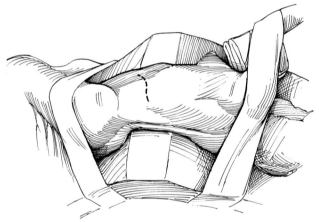

2 Locate the ureter and gonadal vessels as they cross the iliac vessels. Place a 5-0 CCG stay suture in the ureter at the level of the iliac vessels and divide it. Ligate the stump with a 3-0 SAS. Insert an infant feeding tube in the severed ureter to monitor urinary output. Dissect the gonadal vessels, ureter, and intervening areolar tissue en bloc up to the lower pole of the kidney. The periureteral and peripelvic areolar tissues are not shown in order to depict the underlying structures. Divide the gonadal vein where it crosses the ureter.

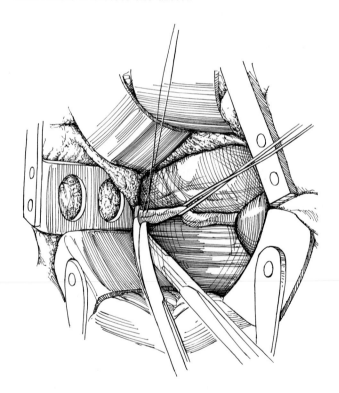

3 At the level of the kidney, dissect as much as possible outside Gerota's fascia. Expose the left renal vein by rotating the kidney posteriorly. Dissect the tissue lying in the angle where the renal vein and artery join the vena cava and aorta. Give mannitol in divided doses during the dissection. Clear the areolar tissue below the vessels as well as above them, mobilizing the tissue toward the hilum and ligating and dividing lymphatics. To reduce vascular spasm, avoid approaching the hilum, and do not pull on the kidney. If the kidney becomes soft from vasospasm, stop dissecting until it is again firm. Ligate and divide the adrenal vein. Locate, ligate, and divide the lumbar vein that enters the left renal vein posteriorly.

4 Shift the kidney anteriorly, and dissect the tissue laterally from the aorta, moving it toward the pelvis and hilum.

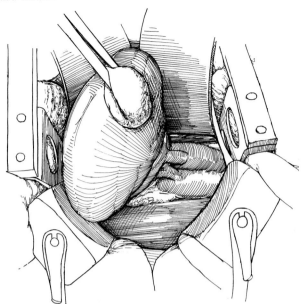

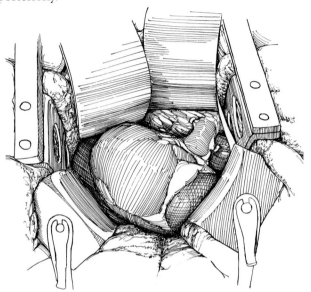

5 When the recipient has been prepared to receive the allograft, give the donor mannitol and furosemide to induce maximal diuresis, as monitored from the ureteral catheter. Clamp the renal artery with a vascular clamp near the aorta, and divide it distal to the clamp. Clamp the renal vein and divide it. Free the remaining areolar and lymphatic tissue. If the renal vein is torn, reclamp it or suture the tear. Remove the specimen and place it in a bowl of chilled electrolyte solution, ready to be perfused and transferred to the operating room of the recipient.

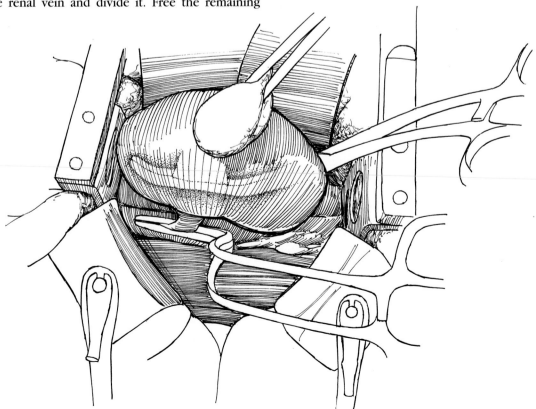

6 **A,** Place a 6-0 silk mattress suture in the renal vein distal to the clamp, and run it as a continuous suture back over the suture line ("baseball stitch"). Remove the clamp from the renal vein.

B, Close the renal artery with a running stitch, beginning at one side and returning to that side. Remove the arterial clamp.

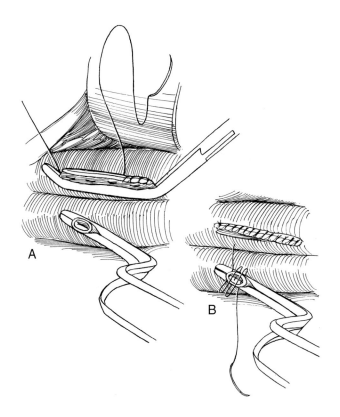

Right Nephrectomy

For right nephrectomy, proceed as described, with a similar incision but in the right flank.

SUBCOSTAL TRANSPERITONEAL APPROACH
(Peters)

The transperitoneal approach has certain advantages over the retroperitoneal route, even though it is associated with slightly greater morbidity and a longer postoperative course because of ileus. Its advantage is excellent anatomic exposure, so that the renal pedicle and the origins of the renal artery and the renal vein are viewed in an anteroposterior position. It also allows exploration of the abdominal cavity for associated disease.

Make a subcostal incision (see page 871), beginning at the tip of the 12th rib on the side of the kidney to be removed, angling about 1.5 inches below the costal margin toward the xiphoid. Cross the rectus sheath on the side of the kidney to be removed, and cut slightly into the rectus sheath at the opposite side, depending on whether the individual is stocky and broadly built or tall with a narrow subcostal arch. Carry the incision down through the external and internal obliques, which are divided perpendicular to their fibers, and through the transversus abdominis muscle and transversalis fascia. Divide the transversus abdominis muscle parallel to its fibers, and open the peritoneal cavity. Extend the incision across the rectus sheath on the side of the kidney to be removed, and continue it into the rectus sheath of the opposite side. If the falciform ligament is encountered, divide it between 2-0 silk suture-ligatures.

Examine the colon and pack the small bowel away. Make an incision lateral to the colon, along the white line of Toldt, and carry it from the splenic flexure of the colon on the left side to a point below the common iliac artery.

Right Transperitoneal Nephrectomy

For nephrectomy on the *right side*, carry the incision from above the upper pole of the kidney near the vena cava around the hepatic flexure of the colon and down to a point over the common iliac artery. Mobilize the colon medially on either side. This exposes Gerota's fascia, the retroperitoneum, and also the ureter as it courses along the psoas muscle. On this side, the ureter may be seen to be adherent to the peritoneum in a major portion of its lower third, but it is easily dissected off. Dissect the ureter to a point 2 or 3 cm below where it crosses the right common iliac artery so that more than the upper two thirds of the ureter is easily removed, this major portion being supplied by collaterals from the renal artery. Clamp the ureter distally, cut it just proximal to the clamp, and tie it with a 2-0 silk ligature.

Dissect the ureter proximally, preserving a lateral triangle of mesenteric and areolar tissue that extends to the lower pole of the kidney from the point where the ureter was cut. Carefully preserve the surrounding areolar tissue and vessels with the ureter as the dissection proceeds superiorly. Open Gerota's fascia, and shell the kidney out from the fascia by a combination of blunt and sharp dissection.

After the cava has been mobilized and the artery beneath it separated as much as possible, direct attention to a space between the aorta and vena cava to expose the arterial exit of the renal artery on the right side. Continue dissection until it is completely separated from the posterior aspect of the cava. Then ligate it at the time of removal of the right kidney.

Make an attempt to place the Satinsky clamp on the vena cava so that a small cuff of cava can be taken in addition to the usually short right renal vein. Ligate the artery with a size 0 or 2-0 silk in its ampullary portion at its point of exit from the aorta, and further close it with a suture ligature of 3-0 silk.

Left Transperitoneal Nephrectomy

Continue the incision made lateral to the colon at the splenic flexure medially to the border of the aorta so that upper-pole adhesions of the kidney to Gerota's fascia may be easily exposed and clipped, or tied if they contain vessels, and divided between clips or ties to free the upper pole of the kidney and separate it from the adrenal gland. Preserve the lienorenal ligament, the reflection of the peritoneum between the spleen and colon, and dissect with the hand beneath it so that a pack may be placed there under a large retractor to give exposure of the upper pole of the kidney. The spleen is protected by the peritoneal reflection, the pack placed posterior to the incision in the parietal peritoneum, and the Harrington retractor placed outside the pack. This usually gives excellent exposure of the upper pole of the kidney on the left side so that upper-pole adhesions may be easily divided.

Carry the dissection around the kidney down to the pedicle. Look for the gonadal and adrenal tributaries, and divide them between 3-0 silk ligatures. Mobilize the vein free from underlying areolar tissue, and then retract it superiorly or inferiorly to expose the renal artery, which is then dissected back to its ampullary portion. Shell the kidney from Gerota's fascia by a combination of blunt and sharp dissection. The gonadal vein usually empties into the vena cava and may be left undisturbed, but occasionally dividing it near its point of entry may be necessary. Mobilize the kidney, expose the renal artery posteriorly, and dissect it beneath the cava.

Make an effort to preserve the fat lying in the hilum of the kidney, as this supplies the collateral circulation for the upper two thirds of the ureter. In addition, preserve the triangular pedicle of areolar tissue and mesentery that extends from the tip of the ureter at its point of transection to the lower pole of the kidney. Otherwise, clear off Gerota's fascia completely, and ligate any small emissary tributaries traversing the renal capsule with 5-0 silk, or fulgurate them with the coagulating current. Check to be sure that the recipient is ready to receive the kidney.

Ligate the artery at its point of exit from the aorta with 2-0 silk, and place a 3-0 silk suture-ligature distal to this tie. Dissect the renal vein to its point of entry into the vena cava on the left side after the gonadal and adrenal tributaries have been divided. Place a Satinsky clamp on the vena cava, divide the renal vein on the left side near its point of entry into the vena cava, and remove the kidney. Have it taken to an adjacent table for perfusion with a cooled heparinized balanced salt solution before being transported to the adjacent room for transplantation.

Multiple Renal Arteries. An aortic patch, such as a Carrel patch, cannot be taken from a living donor as it can from a cadaver donor. When multiple arteries are present, divide them at their point of exit from the aorta in the ampullary portion. If double arteries are nearly the same size, spatulate them and insert them under magnification side to side to form a single ostium. If the vessels are of unequal size, anastomose the spatulated polar branch end to side to the main renal artery after excising a small patch. This makes it essentially a primary branch of the renal artery. With three or more vessels, apply a combination of these two techniques to form a single ostium. The incidence of late thrombosis in a vessel 1 to 2 mm in diameter is much less by making it a primary branch of the renal artery than by attempting to anastomose it separately into a recipient external iliac artery. Ligate accessory veins with impunity.

After removal of the kidney, inspect the wound to make certain that hemostasis is complete. Reperitonealize the posterior parietal peritoneum with a running 2-0 CCG suture, using a continuous suture or short sections of continuous suture as needed. Perform a layered closure of the abdominal wall with slowly absorbed suture material, such as polydioxanone suture (PDS) or Prolene. The latter is preferred because it has no interstices, is associated with minimal blood loss from the wound, and has, because of its homogeneity, a low incidence of infection. Close the internal oblique and transversus muscles together with the peritoneum with a running 2-0 PDS or Prolene suture. Close the rectus sheath with interrupted Prolene sutures anteriorly and posteriorly, along with the linea alba. Make no attempt to reconstitute the falciform ligament. Use no drains in the usual case. If oozing appears from cut edges of a structure, make every effort to control the oozing prior to closure. Close the anterior rectus sheath with interrupted 0 or 2-0 PDS or Prolene suture. Close the subcutaneous fat, including Scarpa's fascia, in a single layer with running 4-0 Vicryl or 4-0 CCG, and close the skin with staples. Because of the small risk of primary peritonitis, appendectomy is not performed in living donors.

POSTOPERATIVE CARE

Transfusion is rarely necessary. Leave the nasogastric tube indwelling, and maintain the patient on intravenous fluids until bowel sounds are active or the patient passes gas.

POSTOPERATIVE PROBLEMS

Complications after extraperitoneal donor nephrectomy are those of simple nephrectomy (see page 987). The most frequent problem is *pneumothorax*, treated by observation or aspiration. Rarely is a chest tube required. Wound infections, aspiration pneumonia, and urinary retention may be seen. Complications after transperitoneal nephrectomy are more frequent and include splenic injury, incisional hernias, and bowel obstruction.

Commentary by Lynn H. Banowsky

Living donor nephrectomy presents the surgeon with unique challenges. This is the only circumstance in which a surgeon knowingly removes a healthy organ from an asymptomatic patient. The old axiom of "do no harm" assumes even more importance. The donor's surgeon must carefully balance the safety of the donor with procurement of an organ that will have maximum utility in the recipient.

A broad-spectrum antibiotic is given intravenously as a single dose at the start of the operation. Little evidence indicates that postoperative prophylactic antibiotics give additional protection against wound infection.

An important aspect of donor management is the vigorous administration of intravenous fluids. Every effort should be made to bring the donor to the operating room with a brisk diuresis underway. To minimize donor discomfort, no intravenous infusion is started the night before surgery; rather, an intravenous line is placed at 6:00 AM on the day of surgery, and 1000 to 1500 ml of fluid are given rapidly with 12.5 g of mannitol. A balloon catheter is inserted at the same time. In the operating room, a central venous pressure line is inserted. During the donor operation, lactated Ringer's solution and 5 percent Albumosol are given liberally to maintain the diuresis. If the urine output decreases, mannitol 12.5 g IV may be repeated (not to exceed a total dose of 50 g), and intravenous furosemide may also be given. It is helpful to divide the donor ureter early to be able to observe that urine output from the kidney being dissected is adequate. Under virtually no circumstances should the kidney be removed in a state of antidiuresis.

Some comments about the anatomy of the renal artery, vein, and ureter make donor nephrectomy more logical. The left kidney is preferred over the right because the left renal vein is both larger and thicker than the right renal vein. The right renal vein is shorter, usually has no extra renal branches, and almost always has a venous valve located where the vein inserts into the vena cava. The presence of the valve is accompanied by a thinning of the vein that makes suturing it almost impossible. For this reason, a cuff of vena cava should always be taken during right donor nephrectomy. The left renal vein is sufficiently long and thick that no caval cuff is necessary. Frequently more than one renal vein is encountered. It is almost always safe to ligate the smaller of the two veins.

Approximately 20 percent of donors have unilateral multiple arteries, and approximately 10 percent of donors have multiple renal arteries bilaterally. When reviewing the renal angiogram, one must first decide if the extra artery is an accessory renal artery or one of the segmental renal arteries. If the extra artery supplies an anatomic vascular segment of the kidney, it must be revascularized by one of a variety of acceptable techniques. Failure to revascularize a renal segment causes a segmental infarct with the possibility of hypertension or a caliceal urinary fistula. An accessory artery that does not supply a renovascular segment can be safely ligated. All renal arteries exit the aorta with an ostial diameter approximately 25 percent larger than

the remainder of the artery. Division of the renal artery to include the larger ostial diameter greatly facilitates the arterial anastomosis in the recipient.

Injury to the ureteral blood supply during donor nephrectomy may create up to a 100 percent possibility of a urinary fistula in the recipient regardless of the technique used by the recipient surgeon. The main blood supply of the pelvis and lumbar ureter comes from a small branch arising from the main renal artery or from a separate artery arising from the basilar segmental artery of the kidney. Injury to this vessel can result in necrosis of the upper ureter and/or renal pelvis. A small interlocking network of arteries in the ureteral wall is also a key to successful ureteral mobilization. Injury to this arterial network by the use of abrasive tapes (umbilical tapes) or unnecessary dissection of the ureteral wall can create necrosis of an isolated area in the ureteral wall.

The choice of incisions for donor nephrectomy is a personal matter. In general, I prefer a flank incision (either 11th or 12th rib) to an anterior subcostal incision. A flank incision provides more than adequate access to the renal vessels, exposure is more easily obtained in heavy or obese patients, and the possibility of subsequent intestinal obstruction from adhesions is eliminated.

In general, any arterial reconstruction of multiple arteries is done by the recipient surgeon. Preferred solutions for flushing and cooling the kidney are EuroCollins solution or UW (University of Wisconsin) solution. An excellent instrument for division of the renal artery and vein is a pair of curved gallbladder scissors.

In summary, the important features to remember in performing donor nephrectomy are (1) adequate donor hydration with crystalloid and colloid solutions and the vigorous use of mannitol; (2) avoidance of injury to segmental renal arteries; (3) acquisition of maximum length in the artery, vein, and ureter to facilitate vascular and urinary reconstruction in the recipient; and (4) avoidance of devascularization of the ureter.

Cadaver Donor Nephrectomy

Nephrectomy from cadaver donors as an isolated procedure is being done less often and must now be coordinated with recovery of other organs. The usual order of harvesting is heart and lung, liver, pancreas, kidney, and spleen.

Donor Selection. Use the "minimum hundreds criteria" (systolic blood pressure greater than 100 torr, Po_2 greater than 100 torr, and hourly urine output greater than 100 ml). If only the kidneys are to be retrieved, consider heparinization with 20,000 units intravenously. At the same time, take a blood sample to confirm the ABO blood type. Serum creatinine level should be normal, but an elevated serum creatinine level as high as three times normal may be acceptable, as long as evidence indicates that it is improving as a consequence of intravenous fluid administration and that the cause of the elevation was a prerenal condition rather than a primary renal parenchymal dysfunction. Some cases may require bilateral renal biopsies, examined by frozen section, after harvesting to determine if the kidneys are suitable for use. Take the donor to the operating room while continuing cardiac monitoring along with intravenous fluids and ventilation, using an ambulatory bag attached to a small oxygen tank. Avoid hypoxia.

Place two intravenous lines for rapid fluid replacement during diuresis. A central venous catheter for volume monitoring is useful. Add mannitol and furosemide to sustain diuresis over the hour before nephrectomy. Some surgeons give 100 mg phenoxybenzamine or phentolamine IV 20 minutes before nephrectomy to reduce intrarenal vasospasm.

For the stable donor, use an in situ dissection. For the unstable donor, cannulate the vessels and remove the organs (Starzl).

In Situ Approach to Kidney Retrieval (Streem and Bretan)

Instruments: Perfusion catheter, 2 L iced (4° to 8° C) Collins 2 or UW-1 solution, cold lactated Ringer's solution, povidone-iodine solution and amphotericin, a GIA stapler, a large Péan clamp, a self-retaining multiple-blade retractor, and a perfusion catheter.

Preparation: Prepare the abdomen and chest while continuing to monitor blood pressure and urine output.

Multiple Organ Retrieval. The techniques for recovering the heart and liver vary considerably from one transplant team to another. Generally, freeing the kidneys en bloc with in situ cooling can precede removal of the heart, lungs, liver, and pancreas. Actual removal of the kidneys occurs last.

1 *Incision:* With the electrocautery set on high coagulation to minimize bleeding, make a sternum-splitting incision in the midline from the sternal notch to the pubis. Add a transverse abdominal incision.

Hold the corners of the flaps back with towel clips. Insert a self-retaining multiple-blade retractor. Systematically examine the abdominal contents for abnormalities that would prevent donation.

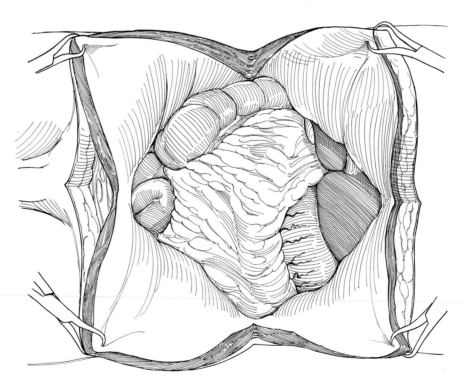

2 Starting on the right side, incise the white line, continuing beyond the hepatic flexure, and Kocherize the duodenum (see page 986). Ligate and divide the inferior mesenteric artery and vein. Free the small bowel on its mesentery as far as the ligament of Treitz. Move both small and large bowel up out of the abdominal cavity.

Give a bolus of fluid intravenously, to include 12.5 g of mannitol to prevent reactive vasoconstriction. Dissect the left common iliac artery, and insert a perfusion catheter that has been cleared of air. Ligate the artery below the insertion site; then ligate the corresponding vein. Ligate and divide the contralateral iliac vessels. Fix the catheter in place with a heavy silk ligature and umbilical tape. Connect the catheter to a 1-L bag of cold Collins or UW-1 solution, and clamp the tubing.

Clip and divide the right ureter near the bladder. Mobilize it from the posterior body wall with all its vessels encased in the periureteral tissue. Stop dissection at the lower pole of the kidney. Mobilize the right kidney superficially without opening Gerota's fascia, leaving the hilar region intact. Do the same for the left kidney. Open a window in the mesentery of the left colon to reach the left kidney.

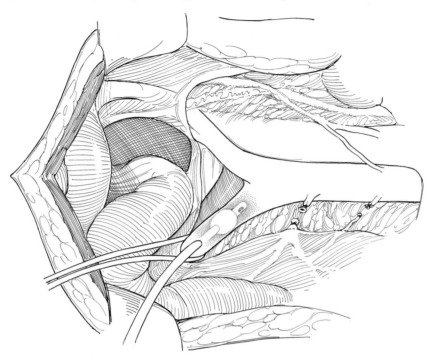

3 Expose, ligate, and divide the superior mesenteric artery by retracting the duodenum and pancreas cephalad. Clear the ganglionic and lymphatic tissue from the base of the celiac artery, and ligate and divide the vessel.

Pass an umbilical tape around the aorta above the kidneys and occlude it. Stop respiratory ventilation. Insert a suction cannula into the inferior vena cava, and flush the aortic segment with cold solution through the iliac catheter. Observe for rapid cooling of the kidneys and for drainage of solution from the venotomy cannula.

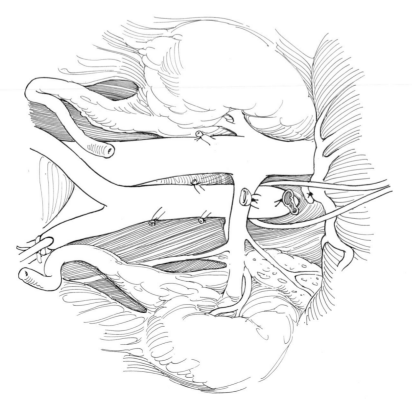

4 Have the assistant hold the kidneys and ureters. Lift the distal aorta and vena cava from the posterior body wall, using the cut iliac vessels for retraction. Dissect progressively cephalad, clipping the lumbar arteries and dividing other attachments with curved scissors. Avoid dissection in the area of the renal hilum.

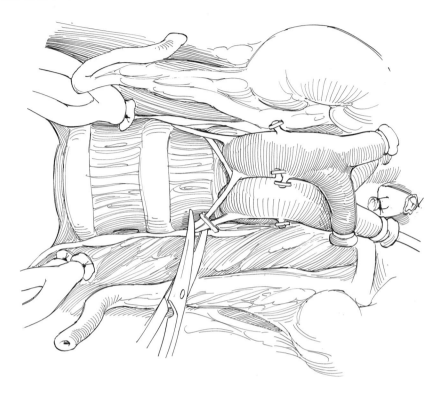

5 The en bloc specimen can be removed while being continuously perfused.

Place the kidneys in cold Ringer's lactate solution on a back table. Open Gerota's fascia, and look for any abnormalities that would preclude transplantation such as congenital anomalies, areas of underperfusion, and petechiae. A small wedge biopsy can be taken from the upper pole of each kidney if systemic or medical renal disease is suspected.

Invert the kidneys, and divide the posterior wall of the aorta between the lumbar arteries. Determine the number and location of the renal arteries leaving the aorta. Turn the kidneys over, and remove the left renal vein from the vena cava with a cuff. Leave the right renal vein attached to the vena cava so that it may be used to make a conduit to extend this usually short vein. Divide the anterior wall of the aorta, and place the kidneys in separate containers of iced Collins or UW-1 solution to be packed in ice for transport.

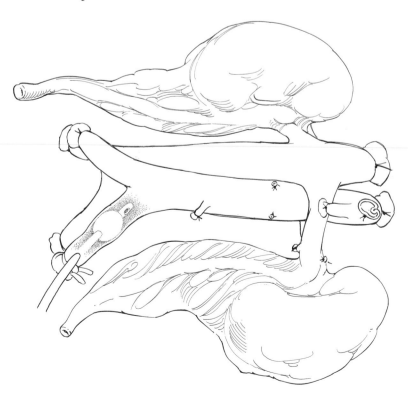

Team Approach for Multiple Organ Retrieval (Starzl)

Preparatory Steps

1. Make a midline incision from the suprasternal notch to the pubis and a transverse extension. Examine the liver for a replaced left or right hepatic artery. Ligate and then divide the falciform ligament.

2. Incise the left triangular ligament of the liver and the diaphragmatic crura between the retrohepatic inferior vena cava and esophagus.

3. Mobilize the ascending and descending colon.

4. Place a tape around the aorta at the diaphragm.

5. Ligate and divide the inferior mesenteric artery.

6. Place a tape around the aorta at that lower level, and cannulate it with a perfusion catheter.

7. Isolate the inferior mesenteric vein, and cannulate it far enough for the tip to reach the portal vein ($\pm$ 5 cm).

8. *Pancreas recovery:* Mobilize the pancreas and spleen and rotate them medially. Ligate and divide the gastroepiploic vessels. Pass a nasogastric tube into the fourth part of the duodenum. Irrigate the area with povidone-iodine and amphotericin solutions. Staple the pylorus and duodenum with a GIA stapler. Isolate the duodenum with the head of the pancreas. Blot all staple lines with povidone-iodine solution.

9. Open and wash the gallbladder. If the pancreas is not harvested, isolate the inferior mesenteric vein and cannulate it. Pass a clamp above this vein to help transect the pancreas.

10. *Heart recovery:* Have the cardiac team remove the heart.

11. Cross-clamp the aorta at the diaphragm.

12. Transect the vena cava at the level of the diaphragm to allow egress of perfusate.

13. Start cold perfusion with UW-1 solution through both the aortic and inferior mesenteric catheters.

14. Place a large Péan clamp across the root of the mesentery before starting the flush.

Liver Recovery

1. Observe blanching of the liver.

2. Remove a patch of diaphragm around the suprahepatic vena cava.

3. Dissect the hepatic hilum, and cut or ligate the gastroduodenal, right gastric, splenic, and left gastric arteries, but stay away from the celiac axis and common hepatic artery. Dissect along the anterior vertebral column while rotating the liver for maximal exposure.

4. Expose the portal vein, and follow it to the junction with the splenic and superior mesenteric veins. Cut these vessels. (Look under them for an anomalous right hepatic artery, which requires inclusion of the superior mesenteric artery in a large Carrel patch.)

5. Remove the origin of the celiac axis from the aorta with a Carrel patch.

6. Place the liver on the back table. Insert a cannula into the portal vein, and cannulate and perfuse it with 1 L of UW-1 solution.

7. Pack the liver in an ice chest for cleaning and placement at the recipient's hospital.

Kidney Recovery (the Final Event)

1. Remove the kidneys en bloc (Steps 1 to 5), and reperfuse them in an ice bath with Collins or UW-1 solution.

2. Harvest iliac vascular grafts for use during liver implantation.

Commentary by Peter N. Bretan, Jr.

The overall technique of cadaver donor nephrectomy is described here, and it has not changed significantly in the past 10 years. What has changed is that the majority (80 to 95 percent) are now multi-organ recoveries. Because of this, isolated cadaver donor nephrectomy is very uncommon. In addition, many centers do not rule out a brain-dead patient as a potential liver donor before attempting a liver recovery initially. Therefore, even if the likelihood of an isolated cadaver donor nephrectomy is high, a midline incision with an open sternotomy is used at the beginning to facilitate the liver procurement if it is feasible. One must also take into account that ruling out a prospective donor of a liver and heart because of significant systemic disease may also preclude cadaver donor nephrectomy. In summary, it is becoming more uncommon to perform cadaver donor nephrectomy (only) procedures. At the rare times that they are done, many centers perform routine upper-pole renal biopsies. The lower pole is not used as a biopsy site because of risk of devascularization of the ureter. In addition, many

centers place kidneys from these high-risk donors routinely on pulsatile perfusion. This requires that the kidneys not be divided because the entire aortic and caval segments are used as conduits for pulsatile perfusion. After an initial observation on pulsatile perfusion, often high pressures are found that preclude the use of these organs because of the significant risk of subsequent nonfunction. Categories of donor patients that are often selected for cadaver donor nephrectomy (only) procedures include hepatitis C antibody–reactive patients with negative (normal) liver biopsies, those with liver cirrhosis (with noninfectious cause, such as alcohol abuse), those with congenital liver disorders, and those with any systemic disease that may affect the liver and heart but spare the kidneys, as determined by biopsies. Finally, the technique for procurement of the liver may be modified somewhat if it is accompanied by whole pancreas retrieval, a procedure that may vary from center to center in the amount of in situ dissection performed.

SECTION

22

Kidney: Excision

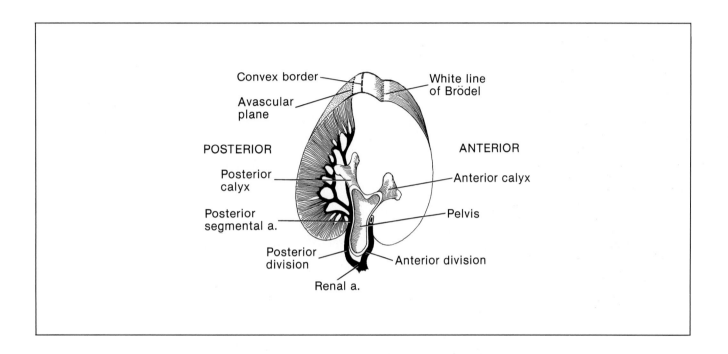

Convex border — Avascular plane — POSTERIOR — Posterior calyx — Posterior segmental a. — Posterior division — Renal a. — White line of Brödel — ANTERIOR — Anterior calyx — Pelvis — Anterior division

Anatomy and Principles of Kidney Excision

RENAL ANATOMY FOR RENAL RESECTION

Arterial Supply

1 **A,** Anterior view. **B,** Lateral view. **C,** Posterior view. The renal artery forms an anterior division that typically carries three quarters of the blood and a posterior division that carries the rest. The "avascular plane" of Brödel between these divisions lies in the axis of the posterior calyces (Brödel, 1901).

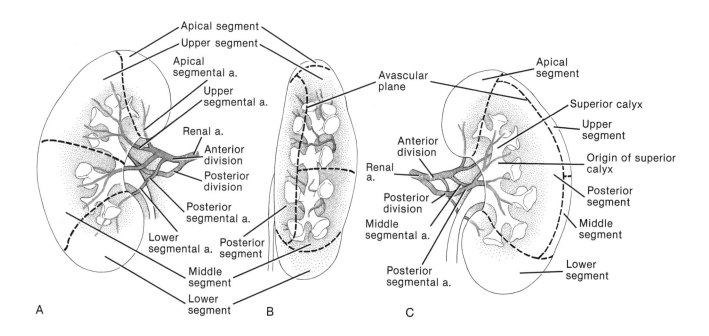

From the major anterior and posterior divisions, five important branches originate as segmental arteries: apical or suprahilar, upper, middle, lower, and posterior segmental arteries that supply the five corresponding segments of the kidney.

Anterior Division. The *apical segmental artery* originates from the anterior division and supplies the apical segment lying on the medial side of the upper pole like a small cap.

An upper and a lateral branch of the *upper segmental artery* supplies the upper segment, restricted to the anterior portion of the kidney, and involves the remainder of the upper pole and the upper portion of the central part of the kidney.

The *middle segmental artery,* also a branch of the anterior division of the renal artery, supplies the middle segment, that part of the anterior portion of the kidney between the upper and the lower segments.

The lower segment involves the entire lower pole and thus is larger than the apical segment. It is supplied by the *lower segmental artery,* which may arise from the renal artery or its anterior division, the upper segmental artery, or it may originate from the main artery at the same point as the other segmental arteries. After the lower segmental artery passes anterior to the pelvis, it divides into an anterior branch supplying the anterior portion of the lower pole and a posterior branch that runs behind the infundibulum of the inferior calyx (a site where it may be entered inadvertently) to supply a small portion posteriorly.

Posterior Division. The *posterior segmental artery* arises from the posterior division of the renal artery and thus provides the entire supply of the posterior segment, involving all of the posterior portion of the kidney except that taken up by the

polar segments. The posterior segmental artery crosses behind the upper portion of the pelvis at a point very close to the origin of the superior calyx and can be injured during surgery. It also may be involved during mid-kidney and lower-pole resection.

Although the kidney is organized into lobes corresponding to papillary drainage, the vascular supply does not follow this embryonic arrangement. The line of incision for resection of a lobe or, more often, for heminephrectomy, follows the midplane of the interlobular septa (columns of Bertin) as far as the arcuate vessels and encounters little vascular interference from interlobular vessels. The arcuate vessel is then ligated on the incisional side of the interlobar artery, causing minimal devascularization.

The size of an artery is a guide to the size of the area supplied. During an operation, injection of indigo carmine into a segmental artery accurately outlines the segment supplied.

Venous Drainage

The *right renal vein* is shorter than the left and drains into the inferior vena cava without gaining tributaries. The *left renal vein* is longer and more complex than the right, being regularly joined by the adrenal and inferior phrenic vein, the gonadal vein, and one of the lumbar veins.

The *lumbar veins* are an important link for collateral circulation. Like those in the intercostal system, they recur typically at each vertebral level, with all five lumbar veins connected by an ascending lumbar vein on each side. On the left side, the trunk of the ascending lumbar veins connects with the lumbar azygos vein more medially. These veins lie against the vertebral bodies covered by the investing fascia of the psoas major, deep to the sympathetic trunk.

Gonadal and adrenal collateral circulation is important after division of the left renal vein because circulation then depends on the integrity of these vessels as well as on supplemental capacity of the pelvic and capsular venous plexuses. Thus, division of the renal vein must be proximal to the entry of these vessels, and the vein cannot be divided after renal mobilization. The gonadal vein provides the principal drainage route, especially in women, anastomosing with the internal iliac veins, but is functional only if the valves are incompetent. The left adrenal vein, by its connection with the inferior phrenic vein, may bypass the renal vein. The reno-azygo-lumbar channel can possibly handle the entire flow.

SURGICAL PLANES

2 The kidney may be approached without entering the renal fascia through two separate planes, one through the posterior pararenal space and one through the anterior pararenal space. The *posterior surface* of the kidney may be approached through the posterior pararenal space by dissecting between the posterior lamina of the renal (Gerota's) fascia and the transversalis

fascia, a dissection aided by an intervening layer of pararenal fat.

Access to the *anterior surface* of the kidney and its vessels is accomplished by opening the anterior pararenal space by medial mobilization of the fusion fascia of the descending or ascending mesocolon (including the parietal peritoneum) from the underlying anterior lamina of the renal fascia, starting at the white line of Toldt.

Partial Nephrectomy. In the last few years, partial nephrectomy has gained advocates who apply it not only to tumors in solitary kidneys but also to tumors diagnosed when they are small by means of widespread use of sonographic and scanning procedures. Radical excision with nodal dissection does not appear to add to the rate of cure. Extracorporeal techniques have proved to be of value in very few cases.

Nephrolithotomy. Shock wave lithotripsy and percutaneous techniques have greatly reduced the number of nephrolithotomies and ureterolithotomies to the point that it is difficult to teach the flank approach to residents. However, staghorn calculi in infants, stones remaining after endoscopic attempts, and stones associated with obstructive lesions still may require open procedures.

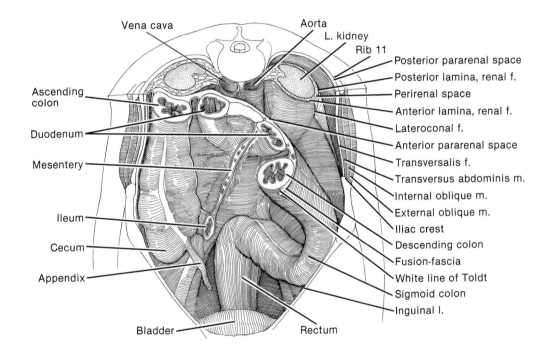

PREOPERATIVE ASSESSMENT

Perform a thorough assessment of the patient's physical condition, with special attention to the status of the lungs. Evaluate the function of the contralateral kidney by serum creatinine determination and by urography. A radionuclide study may be indicated. Assess the characteristics of the involved kidney and the extent of involvement by computed tomography (CT) or

magnetic resonance imaging (MRI) scans. Urography, sonography, and even aortography may have a place in evaluation. Tumor in the renal vein can be visualized by abdominal CT or MRI scanning with intravenous contrast material, perhaps supplemented by inferior venacavography. Be sure to check the serum creatinine level after all these contrast studies. It should rarely be necessary to perform an "exploratory" operation.

Identification of Masses. Subject an adrenal mass detected by sonography to CT scanning to differentiate solid neuroblastomas from cystic adrenal hemorrhage. The CT scan also helps identify retroperitoneal lymphomas and sarcomas. For Wilms tumor, if intravenous pyelography and sonography show a unilateral tumor, proceed with nephrectomy. If nephrectomy is not possible, perform biopsy preparatory to chemotherapy and delayed nephrectomy. If tumors are bilateral, perform unilateral total and contralateral partial nephrectomy or bilateral partial nephrectomy; if that is not possible, obtain a biopsy preparatory to chemotherapy. In a solitary or fused kidney, do a partial nephrectomy or a biopsy if that is not possible. For pyonephrosis, consider percutaneous drainage for 3 months before removing the kidney.

INSTRUMENTS

Provide a Basic set; a GU long set; a GU vascular set; a GU chest set, if taking a rib; Ferguson or Lowsley pedicle clamps, Satinsky clamps, and bulldog clamps, a Major retractor set; a D-tach Balfour retractor; a ring retractor for children; surgical clips; and a Penrose or suction drain.

SELECTION OF INCISION

For infants and children, the anterior subcostal incision usually provides the best exposure. For adolescents and adults, a lateral approach (particularly the 11th- or 12th-rib supracostal incision) is most commonly used. However, the flexion required for the flank position decreases vital capacity and venous return to the heart, and thus it may not be tolerated by obese patients. A further disadvantage is that the kidney is approached before the vessels can be secured. Flank wounds are more prone to subsequent muscular weakness from stretching the intercostal nerves. The advantages are the simplicity of the dissection through the flank, the direct exposure, and the absence of organs or vessels in the retroperitoneum. The pleura and peritoneum, if entered, are readily repaired. If the exposure proves to be limited, it can be increased by segmental resection of the overlying ribs (see page 887). Good visualization of the kidney is obtained, making inspection and repair easy. Even the pelvis is well exposed when the kidney is rotated anteriorly. Closure in layers with dependent drainage makes for a secure wound.

The classic subcostal flank incision is better if reoperation is a possibility, although it has the disadvantage of often proving to be too low (see page 871). The alternatives are resecting the 12th rib (see page 875) or, better, going just above it through a supracostal incision (see page 879). In fact, entering above the 11th rib is not much more difficult than above the 12th rib and gives appreciably better exposure. Of course, the more extensive thoracoabdominal (see page 890) and dorsal flap (see page 887) incisions provide still better access to the renal area for large tumors.

An anterior approach, whether transverse (see page 865), subcostal (see page 856), or midline (see page 867), provides superior exposure to the vascular pedicle of the kidney for renal trauma and neoplasm. An anterior approach is somewhat more difficult than those through the flank and risks both injury to the viscera and later formation of intestinal adhesions. The upper pole is remote, and the renal pelvis lies under the renal pedicle. The peritoneal cavity may become contaminated if the urine is infected. Wound separation is more common than in flank incisions. A posterior approach through a dorsal lumbotomy is quicker and carries less morbidity but provides more limited exposure (see page 896).

KOCHER MANEUVER

For exposure of the right kidney and adrenal from a transabdominal approach, perform a Kocher maneuver to mobilize the duodenum and head of the pancreas to the left (also see page 859).

3 **A,** First have your assistant elevate the second portion of the duodenum to put tension on its retroperitoneal connections. Incise the retroperitoneal surface in a semicircle adjacent to the duodenum. Medially and caudally, continue the incision under the superior mesenteric artery and vein, and have it approach the right gastric artery above the duodenum.

B, Bluntly dissect the duodenum and head of the pancreas from the posterior body wall, and move them to the left, carrying the common bile duct and main pancreatic duct with them.

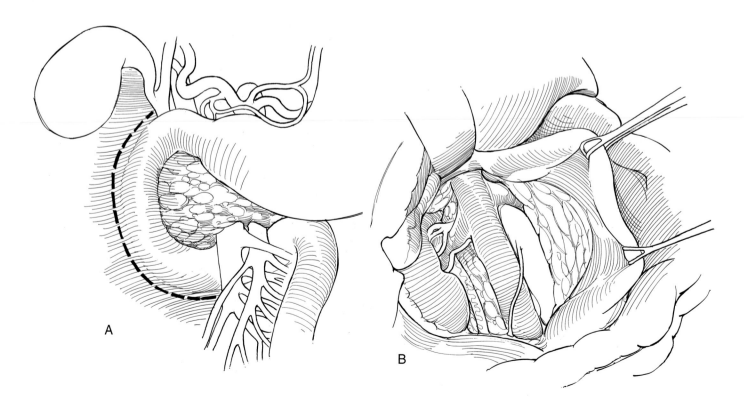

A   B

Simple Nephrectomy

Give intravenous crystalloid fluids preoperatively. Have blood available in case of a vascular accident. Provide endotracheal anesthesia and adequate relaxation.

Position for Flank Operations

1 For the *flank* or *kidney position*, place the patient on the operating table in a true lateral orientation, with the upper leg extended perfectly straight over a pillow, the lower leg fully flexed with the knee near the edge of the table, and the 12th rib centered over the kidney rest and the break in the table. The upper leg acts as a lever to tense the flank. Be certain that the patient's upper foot is not in contact with the table. Have the kidney rest raised, and then have the table extended until the flank muscles become tense. Hold the patient exactly vertical with a hand on the iliac crest, with one sacral dimple lying directly above the other. Apply one end of 4-inch-wide cloth adhesive tape to the slide bar of the table top (not the table itself) in front of the patient just above the flexed knee. Bring it over the hip above the greater trochanter while holding the patient in place; then fasten it to the slide bar of the table top behind the patient. Run another tape from the upper shoulder back to the table top to prevent the upper body from falling forward. Tilt the entire table to position the patient in the Trendelenburg position with the flank parallel to the floor. Place a small pad or pillow under the dependent thorax just caudad to the axilla to take pressure off the axillary neurovascular bundle. Do not fix the upper arm to the anesthesia screen, but support it on pillows. Be sure to support the head and to avoid pressure on the ears.

The patient in the kidney position has physiologic limitations. Vital capacity is decreased 14 percent. The dependent lung may function poorly, resulting in atelectasis. Pneumothorax may be induced with resulting lung collapse, mediastinal flutter, and hypotension. During induction of anesthesia, sudden changes from the supine to the lateral position and then to the kidney position may lead to cardiovascular collapse. Return of blood through the vena cava is impaired, especially in the left lateral position. Consequently, avoid extreme flexion, change the position of the patient gradually, avoid deep anesthesia, and maintain good alveolar exchange and tissue oxygenation with controlled ventilation. If excess fluids are given to correct postural hypotension, be aware that acute cardiac decompensation can occur when the patient is returned to the supine position.

For wound closure, after the table is straightened, the tapes holding the shoulder and hip will become loose. Pull the shoulder back if it has fallen forward. Rotation of hips and shoulders in opposite directions opens or closes flank incisions.

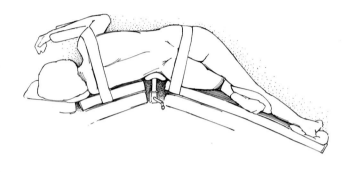

SUBCOSTAL APPROACH

Incision: Make a subcostal incision as described on page 871. Alternatives are the transcostal (see page 875) and (preferably) supracostal (see page 879) incisions.

Dissection of the Kidney

2 Bluntly push Gerota's fascia medially off the psoas muscle, carrying the peritoneal reflection with it. Install a self-retaining retractor.

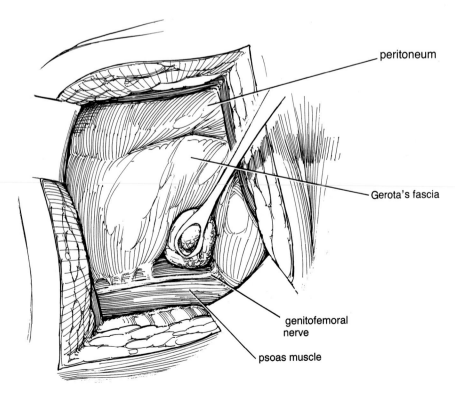

peritoneum

Gerota's fascia

genitofemoral nerve

psoas muscle

3 Insert a Kelly clamp through Gerota's fascia into the pale, lemon yellow–colored perirenal fat. Open Gerota's fascia longitudinally with the scissors through the length of the incision. The index fingers may also be used to separate the thin fascia.

4 Bluntly and sharply dissect the perirenal fat from the lower pole and posterior surface of the kidney. Have the assistant hold Gerota's fascia medially in two curved clamps. Do the easy parts of the renal dissection first, gradually working toward the more adherent areas. Make the greatest effort not to get beneath the capsule, an event that makes the remainder of the dissection more difficult. If the capsule is entered, back out and start a new plane extracapsularly. Take care dissecting ventrally where the peritoneum may be adherent. Use sharp dissection, and, if adherent bowel is suspected, open the peritoneum to aid in dissection. Watch for aberrant blood vessels, especially near the poles. An area resistant to dissection may well contain a vessel that requires clamping and cutting. Adherence to the psoas fascia may be so great as to require inclusion of the psoas fascia with the specimen. If exposure of a large hydronephrotic kidney is difficult, aspirate the contents.

Identify the ureter on the peritoneal side of the wound. Free it with a right-angle clamp, and encircle it with a Penrose drain to allow further dissection. The gonadal vein is easily torn.

Displace the kidney caudally, and develop a plane between the kidney and the adrenal gland. Clip all vessels that are encountered. Finally, dissect sharply under vision near the pedicle. Fulgurate the emissary veins.

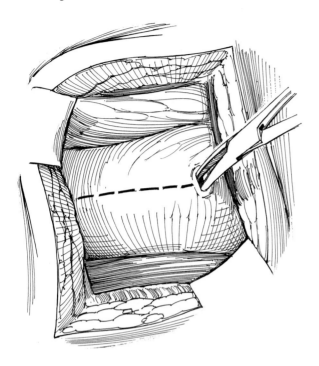

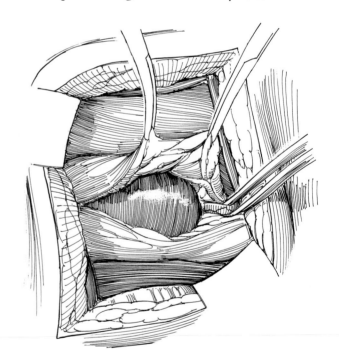

5 Doubly clamp and cut the ureter. Ligate both ends with absorbable suture material, leaving the proximal suture long enough for traction and identification. Dissect proximally along the ureter to free the pelvis.

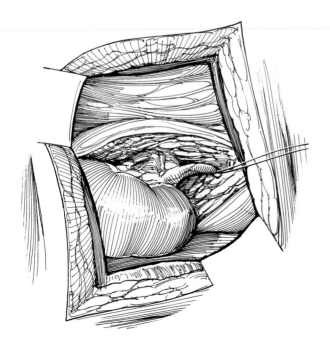

Securing the Pedicle

Retract the peritoneum medially, and complete the dissection of the tissue anterior to the pedicle, trimming it about 1 cm away from the hilum. Identify the renal vein anteriorly, dissect it for a short distance, and encircle it with a vascular loop. Avoid the adrenal veins and the gonadal veins on the left.

With a neoplasm, remove obvious lymph nodes for staging (for radical nephrectomy, see page 1016). Start near the hilum, using sharp and blunt dissection to move the perihilar tissue medially to identify and dissect along the artery.

Clamp Method of Pedicle Ligation

This is a simpler method, especially for those urologic surgeons without experience in handling large vessels, but it does carry some risk of damaging the duodenum or creating an arteriovenous fistula.

6 Bluntly and blindly, if necessary, isolate the pedicle until it has a diameter of 2 or 3 cm. Use heavy curved Ferguson, Lowsley, or similar clamps that have locking male and female blades to prevent the vessels from slipping. Pinch the pedicle between the first and second finger of the left hand, and guide the blades of the lowermost clamp around the pedicle while the fingers keep neighboring tissue away. This finger technique also ensures that sufficient pedicle remains to allow ligation and that the tip of the clamp extends far enough beyond the pedicle to engage the suture. Close the first clamp to the first notch on the ratchet. Place a second clamp above and adjacent to the first.

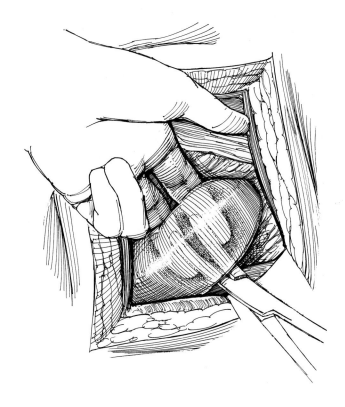

7 Place a third, more curved clamp distal to the second, leaving a few millimeters of pedicle exposed between them. Under direct vision, divide the pedicle in this space between the second and third clamps with a knife.

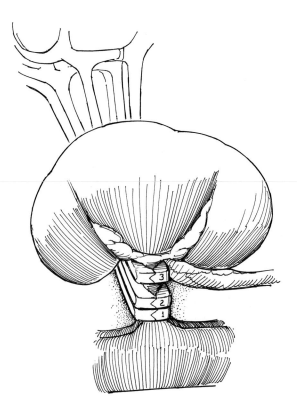

8 **A,** Loop a doubled 2-0 chromic catgut (CCG) suture below the lower clamp, and tie it as the assistant, using two hands, slowly releases the clamp.

B, Insert a doubled 2-0 CCG on a needle below the second clamp as a figure-eight suture.

C, Tie the suture as the clamp is slowly released. Complete the dissection of the upper pole, and remove the kidney. In case of injury to the adrenal, close the defect with a running lock stitch of 4-0 synthetic absorbable suture (SAS) or with large clips or staples.

Clamp and Individual Ligation Method

9 **A,** Doubly clamp the artery, and divide it between clamps; do the same for the vein, and remove the specimen.

B and **C,** Tie the artery with a 1-0 SAS, reinforced with a second 1-0 SAS as a stick tie. Ligate the vein with a 1-0 SAS.

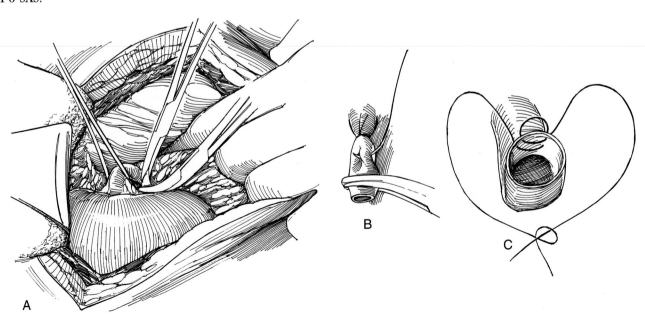

Individual Ligation Method

10 Pass a right-angle clamp under the artery, and successively draw two ligatures around it. Use them to doubly ligate the artery. Do the same for the vein. If the right renal vein is short, use two Satinsky clamps on the vena cava, and oversew the cuff after removing one clamp.

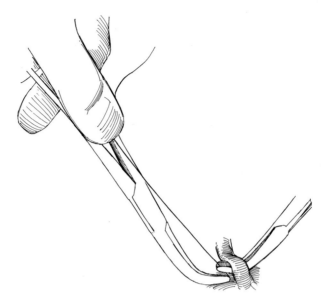

Loss of Control of the Pedicle

Do not get excited. Palpate the spurting blood. Follow it to its source, and compress the vessel digitally for 10 minutes. Alternatively, compress the artery and vein with a stick sponge. Take time to obtain a second suction line, more blood, and some 5-0 vascular sutures and vascular clamps. Inform the anesthetist of the situation. First replace the blood loss. Do not clamp blindly, but get more exposure. Compress the aorta above the renal artery, and clamp the artery with a vascular clamp. Try to visualize one end of the vessel, and put a suture in it. Tie the suture and hold it up as you put a stitch in the part that your assistant exposes next. Run the vascular suture up the defect and down again as your assistant slowly rolls the packs away and you apply suction.

For venous bleeding from the vena cava, hold a finger over the hole, and grasp the wall with the tip of a Kocher clamp. Pulling up on the clamp stops the bleeding, allowing the vessel to be suture-ligated. For the vena cava, Allis clamps are excellent.

On a rare occasion, it may be advisable to close the wound around a clamp. In this case, return the patient to surgery for its removal, and be prepared to manage any further bleeding.

Closure

Fill the wound with saline solution and look for bubbles because the pleura may have been breached. If the pleura does require closure, proceed as described on page 902, and expose an upright chest film in the recovery room. Beware of tension pneumothorax from either a torn pleural adhesion or an actual laceration of the lung. When the pleura is intact, insert a Penrose drain to be left 24 hours to let the air and serum out of the wound and to allow observation for bleeding.

Inject 0.25 to 0.5 percent bupivacaine into the appropriate intercostal nerve, or insert a small feeding tube adjacent to the wound to allow subsequent bupivacaine

administration. Close the wound with 3-0 or 4-0 SAS. If this is a secondary operation, insert the sutures in the muscle first; then tie them successively.

MIDLINE TRANSPERITONEAL APPROACH

To make the incision, follow the description on page 867 through Step 4. Divide the parietal peritoneum on the white line of Toldt lateral to the descending or ascending colon. Enter the plane between the peritoneum and Gerota's fascia, and bluntly separate these structures until the aorta or vena cava is approached. For nonmalignant conditions, enter Gerota's fascia over the medial border of the kidney, and expose the vein and artery. On the left side, secure the renal artery with a heavy silk ligature by retracting the vein caudad; on the right, secure it between the vena cava and aorta. The vein may then be clamped, ligated, and divided. Place a second tie on the artery, divide it, and oversew the end with 4-0 arterial suture. The kidney is then easily removed inside Gerota's fascia. Drain the area through the flank by a stab wound.

PEDIATRIC NEPHRECTOMY (Elder)

For excision of the multicystic and hydronephrotic kidneys in infants as an alternative to laparoscopic removal or nonsurgical management, after inducing general anesthesia, place the child in an extended flank position. Inject a 0.25 percent bupivacaine intercostal block beneath the 10th, 11th, and 12th ribs (the diaphragm lies at a high level in children). Make a 2.5- to 3.0-cm subcostal incision off the tip of the 12th rib, and enter the retroperitoneum. Grasp the kidney with an Allis clamp, bring it into the wound, and puncture the cysts or aspirate the pelvis. Suture-ligate the pedicle as a single entity, divide and ligate the ureter, and remove the kidney. The intercostal nerve block allows the child to go home after the procedure.

SECONDARY NEPHRECTOMY

Have adequate blood available. Prepare the bowel; this is especially important in a patient in whom the bowel may need to be resected.

Choose a new site for the incision if possible (one rib higher or place it anteriorly), and be sure to allow enough exposure. The kidney adheres to the body wall; therefore, it is very easy to cut right into the kidney without realizing it. Open the peritoneum anteriorly to safeguard the duodenum and colon. One can even work transperitoneally.

Palpate the renal artery first, and approach it through the layers of tough fibrofatty tissue. Once you can get a right-angle clamp under the renal artery, draw a suture through and ligate it. The vein, if short, may require a Satinsky clamp, oversewn on the vena cava. Then free the upper pole, keeping close to the capsule to avoid the adrenal gland. (For kidneys that are densely adherent, perform subcapsular nephrectomy; see page 998.)

POSTOPERATIVE PROBLEMS

Hemorrhage can arise from the renal artery, aorta, or vena cava. A vessel in spasm may be overlooked during closure. *Ileus* can be a problem secondary to retroperitoneal dissection around the celiac axis. Because of this reaction even after a flank approach, the patient should not resume oral intake until peristalsis returns.

Commentary by Culley C. Carson, III

One of the most important aspects of simple nephrectomy is preoperative planning. Identification of the location of the kidney and the possible location of its vasculature should guide the surgeon in choosing an appropriate incision. A flank incision that is placed too low makes individual arterial and venous dissection and ligation difficult or impossible. An excessively high incision, while unnecessary, may be complicated by a pleurotomy. Maintenance of the pleura and peritoneal integrity is especially important when simple nephrectomy is carried out for perinephric abscess or pyonephrosis.

It is helpful to open Gerota's fascia as far posteriorly as feasible because a posterior incision permits formation of a "flap" of Gerota's fascia and perinephric fat that can be easily retracted using a Deaver retractor, providing excellent exposure.

The major advance in simple nephrectomy in the past three decades has been the practice of early ligation of the renal artery and separate identification, dissection, and ligation of the vessels rather than pedicle ligation. If early arterial ligation is prevented by scarring, infection, enlarged lymph nodes, or other anatomic abnormalities, pedicle ligation is an excellent

technique to remove a diseased kidney safely and efficiently. Identification of the renal artery, if single, can be performed by palpation over the cephalad border of the renal vein, where the renal artery is most commonly located. Elevating the renal vein using a vessel loop and retracting it inferiorly allows the renal artery to be identified, dissected free, and ligated prior to occlusion of the renal vein. Occasionally, if the renal vessels cannot be isolated satisfactorily from the anterior approach, the kidney can be retracted medially and the renal artery identified beneath the vein by following the retroperitoneum to the spine.

Ligation of the vessels can be carried out effectively with a variety of suture materials. We prefer nonabsorbable sutures for vessel ligation. If perirenal infection or abscess is present, braided sutures should be avoided because they may become a nidus for persistent infection. In this situation, absorbable monofilament suture, whether natural or synthetic, is the best choice. Although many surgeons believe that a single tie in the vessels is adequate, double ligation ensures maintenance of tie position and security. The portion of the artery on the specimen can be single-tied or clipped to decrease back-bleeding and facilitate surgical visualization. An absorbable suture is essential for ligation of the remaining ureteral stump.

Laparoscopic Nephrectomy

TRANSPERITONEAL LAPAROSCOPIC NEPHRECTOMY
(Kavoussi-Clayman)

Prepare the bowel by the balanced lavage method and the administration of three doses of oral antibiotics consisting of 1 g neomycin and 1 g erythromycin base. Give an intravenous dose of a broad-spectrum antibiotic just before surgery.

After induction of general anesthesia, including tracheal intubation to ensure adequate oxygenation and avoid hypercarbia, insert a nasogastric tube. Examine the patient cystoscopically, and, under fluoroscopic guidance, insert an occlusive ureteral balloon catheter into the renal pelvis. Inflate the balloon with 1 ml of dilute contrast solution, and stiffen the catheter with a very rigid guide wire. Place a Councill catheter into the bladder over the ureteral catheter. Move the patient to the operating table. Place the patient supine on an inflated bean bag for later rotation into the lateral position. Apply compression stockings, and pad the contralateral arm (monitor the circulation in that arm with a pulse oximeter). Prepare the entire abdomen and as much of the back as possible.

Induce pneumoperitoneum with a Veress needle or by the Hasson open technique. Insert an 10/11-mm trocar at the umbilicus, and attach the camera to monitor the insertion of the subsequent trocars. Place an 11-mm trocar in the midclavicular line 2 cm below the costal margin and a 5-mm trocar in the midclavicular line 4 cm below the umbilicus. Turn the patient into the full lateral position, and deflate the bean bag to fix the body in position. Place a fourth, 5-mm port in the anterior axillary line at the tip of the 12th rib and another port 4 to 5 cm lower in the same line.

After freeing any interfering adhesions, incise the posterior peritoneum with electrosurgical scissors along the white line of Toldt, including the hepatic flexure on the right or the splenic flexure on the left. Put traction on the medial peritoneal edge, and use blunt and sharp dissection to free the colon from the retroperitoneal tissues. Fully expose Gerota's fascia.

Identify the spermatic cord as it runs under the colon. Locate the ureter by pulling on the ureteral catheter, and bluntly dissect it from its bed in the intermediate stratum of the retroperitoneal fascia by drawing it anteriorly with a tape or a Babcock clamp and dissecting behind it. When the gonadal vessels are encountered crossing the ureter, clip and divide them.

Follow the ureter to the kidney. Clear the perirenal fat from the lower pole of the kidney. Place traction on the ureter, and carefully dissect enough hilar fat to expose the renal vessels outside the hilum, where they are least numerous. Make a window in the connective tissue around each of the vessels. Clip the artery with three 9-mm clips proximally and two clips distally and divide between. Similarly clip the vein(s). If the renal vein is single and thus large, apply multiple clips on opposite sides of the vessel in "staircase" fashion. Alternatively, apply a laparoscopic vascular GIA stapler. If a stapler is used to ligate the pedicle, apply it to one vessel at a time to avoid an arteriovenous fistula. Transect the ureter between two 9-mm clips. With tumors of the upper pole, identify and clip the adrenal arteries and vein, and remove the gland with the kidney.

Insert an impermeable specimen sack (Cook Urological, Inc., Spencer, IN) through the large midclavicular port. Move the laparoscope to the midclavicular port.

Open the sack with three graspers led through the smaller ports. Lead the kidney into the sack, and tighten the drawstring to close the neck.

Move the patient into the supine position. Through the umbilical port, grasp the drawstring and pull the neck of the sack into the sheath as far as it goes easily. Withdraw the sheath to expose the drawstrings on the anterior abdominal wall, and use them to draw the neck of the sack out to the surface.

Open the sac enough to admit an electric tissue morcellator to liquefy and evacuate the contents. Withdraw the sac. Send tissue trapped in the morcellator for pathologic analysis. *Alternative:* Break the tissue into small pieces with a sponge forceps and remove them with the bag. Or extend the trocar incision to 5 to 7 cm and withdraw the bag containing the kidney.

Check the abdomen for injury or bleeding, and remove the ports under vision. Close the fascia of the 11-mm sites with 2-0 absorbable suture and the skin with a subcuticular suture. Remove the catheters in the recovery room, but leave the stockings in place until the patient is fully ambulatory. Start oral intake the following morning. Continue antibiotic coverage for 1 week.

LAPAROSCOPIC NEPHROURETERECTOMY
(Clayman-Kavoussi)

This procedure is used for patients with low-grade transitional cell carcinomas of the renal pelvis. Insert a 0.35-inch Bentson guide wire cytoscopically into the renal pelvis, and place a 6-mm, 10-cm ureteral dilating balloon catheter over it to fit in the distal and intramural ureter. Inflate the balloon to less than 1 atmosphere of pressure. Introduce a 24 F resectoscope, and incise the orifice with an Orandi electrosurgical knife to divide the entire intravesical ureteral wall. Remove the dilating balloon. Insert a 7 F, 12-mm occlusion balloon catheter, and inflate it in the renal pelvis with 1 ml of dilute contrast solution. Exchange the Bentson guide wire for an Amplatz Super Stiff guide wire. To reduce the chance for seeding, reintroduce the resectoscope and, with a roller electrode, coagulate the epithelium of the entire intramural ureter as well as the periureteral area in the bladder. Place a 16 F balloon catheter to drain the bladder.

Continue as described above for laparoscopic nephrectomy, but do not divide the ureter. Insert a 12-mm trocar in the midline halfway between umbilicus and symphysis. Free the ureter to the bladder, and also clear the bladder surface around the ureterovesical junction. Insert the laparoscopic GIA stapler through the large port. Insinuate the bladder cuff into the stapler, being sure that surrounding tissue is not included. Fire the stapler once or twice to transect the cuff and seal the bladder. Check for watertightness by filling the bladder with saline.

Proceed with entrapment and removal. If the specimen is arranged in the sack so that the distal ureter lies in the neck, the ureter can be divided and sent as a separate specimen.

An *alternative* to initially resecting the ureter transvesically is to introduce a ureteral catheter into the renal pelvis. The ureter is divided and the end sutured to the catheter. After removal of the kidney, the ureteral orifice is circumscribed and the ureter invaginated (Janetschek).

LAPAROSCOPIC PARTIAL NEPHRECTOMY

Partial nephrectomy through the laparoscope may still be considered experimental.

Proceed as for laparoscopic nephrectomy to Step 3. In children with duplex systems, dissect the affected ureter, and clip and divide it. Continue the dissection to the hydronephrotic pole. Identify, clip, and divide the vessels supplying it. Apply a bulldog clamp to the main renal artery; then transect the thin parenchyma, staying away from the adjacent normal cortex. Control bleeding with an argon-beam coagulator.

In adults, after exposure of the affected pole, encircle it with a Rumel-type tourniquet (Winfield, 1995) constructed from a length of umbilical tape threaded through a 5-mm suction-irrigation unit. Divide the parenchyma with an electrocautery blade immediately followed by the argon-beam coagulator. It is not necessary to close the severed infundibulum. Clip perirenal fat to the capsule to cover the defect. Provide for drainage by running an additional trocar posteriorly though the quadratus lumborum muscle to place a Penrose drain. If the procedure was done extraperitoneally, bring the drain through the site of the posterior working port. Close the leaves of Gerota's fascia with staples, and bring the colon over it to help isolate the drainage.

LAPAROSCOPIC UNROOFING OF RENAL CYST
(Winfield and Donovan)

This procedure is an alternative to open excision or percutaneous evacuation and alcohol sclerosis. Consider the risk of malignancy.

Position and proceed as for laparoscopic nephrectomy (Step 1). After peritoneal insufflation, reflect the colon medially. Dissect Gerota's fascia and pararenal areolar tissue from the surface of the cyst (Step 2). Insert an endoscopic needle, aspirate the contents, and send the specimen for pathologic confirmation. Enter the cyst cavity with the electrocautery.

Grasp the cyst wall and trim it, leaving a narrow cuff near the parenchyma to avoid larger vessels. Fulgurate the cuff. Search the walls of the cyst for any evidence of malignancy. Take biopsies of any suspicious areas. The inner surface may be cauterized with the argon-beam coagulator. It is not necessary to fill the cavity or drain the site. Send the specimen of the wall for pathologic analysis. Replace the colon with surgical clips.

EXTRAPERITONEAL LAPAROSCOPIC SURGERY

For a description of the extraperitoneal technique for laparoscopic pelvic lymph node dissection, see page 473. Simple insufflation of the retroperitoneum does not provide adequate exposure because gaseous dissection is not uniform, but by inflating a balloon beneath the peritoneum, the fibrous connections between it and the transversalis fascia can be separated, as is done with open techniques of mobilization, and exposure is increased.

The extraperitoneal approach avoids mobilization of the colon and possible injury to the intra-abdominal organs and allows immediate access to the renal artery. But the working space is smaller and the anatomic landmarks are less clear than with the transperitoneal approach. Although the retroperitoneal approach is adequate for simple nephrectomy, it is not suitable for patients with a bleeding diathesis or previous retroperitoneal surgery, or for kidneys involved with malignancy or chronic infection. These should be approached by an open technique.

Under general anesthesia with tracheal intubation to ensure adequate oxygenation and avoid hypercarbia, which is more of a problem with retroperitoneal insufflation, insert a nasogastric tube. Examine the patient cystoscopically, and, under fluoroscopic guidance, insert an occlusive ureteral balloon catheter into the renal pelvis. Inflate the balloon with dilute contrast solution, and stiffen the catheter with a very rigid guide wire. Place a Councill catheter into the bladder over the ureteral catheter.

Move the patient to the operating table. Place the patient supine on an inflated bean bag for later rotation into the lateral position. Apply compression stockings, and pad the contralateral arm (monitor the circulation in that arm with a pulse oximeter). Prepare the entire abdomen and as much of the back as possible.

A balloon dissector is required. One can be made from materials available in the operating room (Gaur, 1992): Tie an index finger from a size 7 washed surgical glove or from an O'Conor drape over an 8 F red rubber catheter. Attach the tube through a T connector to the pump of a sphygmomanometer and to a manometer to allow inflation and simultaneous observation of pressure. Commercial dilators are also available, as is a trocar-mounted balloon that allows visualization of the space through its transparent walls during inflation.

After the usual preparation, including induction of general anesthesia and insertion of a ureteral catheter cystoscopically, place the patient in the lateral position. Make a 2-cm incision through all layers at the margin of the sacrospinalis and 2 cm above the iliac crest. It should pass through Petit's triangle bounded by the latissimus dorsi, the external oblique, and the iliac crest. With a hemostat, followed by the index finger, pass through the transversalis fascia, and dissect an adequate space retroperitoneally between the pararenal fat and the fascia. Creation of this space not only allows accommodation of the balloon but also reduces the initial pressure required for the dissection (Laplace's law). Grasp the knot at the base of the balloon, and direct the balloon into the retroperitoneal space. If possible, penetrate Gerota's fascia and insert the balloon within the perirenal space. This strips the perinephric and periureteral fat away with little bleeding.

Hasson Port Insertion. Insert a Hasson-type port through the short incision, and place the balloon with the aid of a 28 or 30 F Amplatz sheath passed through it. Direct the balloon toward the area to be exposed: toward the umbilicus for exposure of the ureter, toward McBurney's point for the lower ureter and spermatic vessels, and toward the epigastrium under Gerota's fascia for exposure at the lower pole of the kidney.

Clamp Insertion (Gaur, 1996). Make a 10-mm incision in the subcostal area just posterior to the midaxillary plane. Insert a straight clamp through the subcutaneous tissue, and force it through the lumbodorsal fascia. Free up the retroperitoneal space by moving the clamp back and forth over the psoas muscle. Pull it out with the jaws open. Dilate the tract with a 10-mm blunt obturator; then use the obturator to introduce a 10-mm sheath into the space. Dissect a space for the balloon deep to the transversalis fascia or Gerota's fascia under vision using the telescope as a dissector. Remove the telescope and insert the balloon either through the sheath or directly through the tract by stretching it over a clamp. Proceed with inflation.

Inflate the balloon with CO_2 or use up to 1500 ml of saline (the glove finger holds 4 L). The volume depends on the type of operation, nephrectomy requiring the greatest exposure. Inflate until a bulge on the abdomen can be seen. Expect a transient decrease in cardiac output during inflation, especially for right-sided procedures. The balloon pressure varies from the 110 mm Hg needed to separate the transversalis fascia from the properitoneal fat to 40 or 50 mm Hg as the space is developed. Leave the balloon inflated for 5 minutes for hemostasis; then deflate and remove it. After the space is developed, aspirate the gas (or fluid) from the balloon and remove it through the sheath. Connect the port for high-flow CO_2 insufflation to a pressure of 12 to 15 cm. Close the opening in the fascia and skin around the Hasson port with a mattress suture.

Insert additional working ports under camera guidance. Place a 12-mm trocar at the lateral border of the sacrospinalis muscle, equidistant from the iliac crest and costal margin, and a 12-mm port below the 12th rib in the posterior axillary line. Dissect under the transversalis fascia before inserting a 5-mm port below the 12th rib in the anterior or midclavicular line and a 5-mm port in the same line above the anterior superior iliac crest. Be sure they do not puncture the peritoneum. Work with a pressure of 10 to 12 mm Hg to reduce the tracking of gas in the tissue planes. If the peritoneum is entered, the gas soon equilibrates, creating a tension pneumoperitoneum and greatly reducing exposure. The choices are to open the tear and equilibrate the pressure, insert a cannula to vent the peritoneal cavity, or go to an open procedure.

Retroperitoneal Laparoscopic Nephrectomy

Incise and open Gerota's fascia and dissect the fat, first from the posterior and lateral surfaces of the kidney and then from the upper and anterior surfaces. Push the kidney anteromedially to increase the workspace and hold it with a fan retractor. Identify the ureter at the posterior border of the lower pole, and place an umbilical tape around it, held by a grasper in the 5-mm lower anterior axillary line port.

Dissect the hilar vessels as the ureter is retracted. A pneumodissector using short bursts of CO_2 is ideal for stripping off the loose fat. In contrast, an aquadissector makes the tissue soggy, contributing too much water. Clip the renal artery with five 9-mm clips, and cut the artery between them to leave three clips on the arterial stump. Do the same for the renal vein. (For a broad vein, use the Endo-GIA 30 vascular stapler, which provides six rows of staples.) Free the remaining renal attachments. Remove the ureteral catheter, and divide the ureter between 9-mm clips. Insinuate the kidney into a 5- × 8-inch entrapment bag. Morcellate the kidney, and remove it in the bag. For large kidneys, the trocar incision may need to be extended to provide sufficient room. A drain can be inserted and left overnight.

MINILAPAROTOMY

Operating through a limited incision is a compromise between open and laparoscopic surgery for retroperitoneal nephrectomy. Elevate the body wall of the flank by inserting hooks attached to an overhead bar. Make a short incision posteriorly, place retractors strategically, and use standard operating room equipment. To obtain a better view for the operating team, insert a trocar below the minilaparotomy incision, and attach a video monitor so that the field can be viewed both through the incision and on the screen (laparoscopically assisted retroperitoneal nephrectomy). In addition, a laparoscopy port may be placed in the midclavicular line at the level of the umbilicus and another at the tip of the 12th rib to allow the use of laparoscopic instruments in addition to standard instruments.

POSTOPERATIVE PROBLEMS

The overall complication rate for laparoscopic nephrectomy has been reported as 16 percent (Gill et al, 1995). Several complications can occur during access, such as a *hematoma* in the abdominal wall and trocar injury of the kidney. Intraoperatively, problems include vascular injuries and splenic laceration. Postoperatively, one may see a *hernia* at a trocar site. Other problems occur from the gastrointestinal tract (ileus, bleeding duodenal ulcer, and enterocutaneous fistula), from the cardiovascular system (congestive heart failure, atrial fibrillation, and myocardial infarction), from the genitourinary tract (urinary retention and epididymitis), from the lungs (pneumonitis and embolus), and from the musculoskeletal system (brachial nerve palsy and injury to the lateral cutaneous nerve of the thigh), as well as clotted arteriovenous fistula and acute tubular necrosis. In experienced hands, the incidence of electively resorting to open operation is about 5 percent, and opening for emergency control of hemorrhage 1 percent.

LAPAROSCOPIC URETEROLITHOTOMY

This procedure is perhaps preferable to open ureterolithotomy and to shock wave or endoscopic approaches for large stones in the middle and upper ureter.

Insert a ureteral stent or, if that is not possible, an open-ended catheter with a guide wire. For stones in the upper third, approach the area from the tip of the 12th rib; for midureteral stones, enter above and medial to the anterior iliac spine. Bluntly dissect the ureter, preserving the periureteral tissues. Fix the ureter in position, and prevent stone migration by inserting a 2-0 nylon suture on a Keith needle through the abdominal wall and out again, encompassing the ureter. Incise the ureter with knife or scissors, and manipulate the stone free. Place it in a bag (a finger from a glove is suitable) to draw it through the port. Leave the ureteral stent in place, or, if it could not be placed initially, advance the guide wire to the renal pelvis and exchange a double-J stent for the ureteral catheter. Leave a tube drain in place and close the fascia. Remove the drain in 5 days.

DISMEMBERED PYELOPLASTY

Stent the ureter and proceed with retroperitoneal inflation. Find the ureter at the lower pole of the kidney, and free it toward the hilum. Leave the periureteric and any aberrant vessels intact. Dissect the renal pelvis, and mark the limits of pelvic resection by coagulation. Excise the junction and spatulate the ureter posteromedially for 2 cm. Close the superior portion of the pelvis with a continuous 4-0 SAS on a 20-mm curved needle. Tack the ureter above and below with similar sutures, and continue the closure of the anterior and posterior defects with interrupted sutures. Place a tube drain. Because the sutures do not produce a watertight closure, scarring and strictures may result.

Commentary by Günter Janetschek

Transperitoneal laparoscopic nephrectomy: The key to the success of this procedure lies in the identification of the ureter and the transection of the renal vessels. A ureteral catheter is certainly helpful for the beginner; however, once the gonadal vein is dissected free, it is quite easy to identify the ureter without previous stenting. This vein crosses the ureter ventrally a few centimeters cephalad to its crossing of the common iliac artery; this point may serve as a landmark for identification. It is also helpful to keep in mind the succession of layers: first, the mesocolon; second, the gonadal vein; third, the ureter; and finally, the iliac artery.

Generally, the gonadal vessels can be transected whenever necessary without compromising testicular perfusion. In pediatric nephroureterectomy and in young fertile patients, however, we invariably try to preserve them, particularly because in these patients the dissection of the ureter has not been more complicated.

Approaching the renal artery prior to transection of the renal vein is more difficult by the transperitoneal than by the retroperitoneal route. The dissection of the renal artery, which is located dorsal to the renal vein, is greatly facilitated by pulling the ureter and renal pelvis in a ventrolateral direction and by pushing the already freed lower pole ventrally. As a general rule, it is advisable to transect larger vessels step by step rather than in a single maneuver. In this way, incomplete occlusion secondary to malplacement of clips can be recognized early, and placing further clips is much easier as long as the vessel is not transected completely. Also, one must be aware that clips can easily slip off a transected vessel; therefore, further dissection near the vascular stump should be avoided or, if absolutely necessary, performed with great caution. This is why we transect large vessels as late in the procedure as possible.

For most nephrectomies, no more than four trocars are required; in adults we currently use 10/11-mm trocars in virtually all instances so that all 10-mm instruments (clip applier, fan retractor, surgical sponge held with grasper) can be introduced through the trocar, providing the best access at a given time during the procedure. Nevertheless, when four trocars are used, the specimen sack can be held open with two graspers only.

With nephrectomy for benign disease, Gerota's fascia can be left in place. In case of a malignant tumor, however, Gerota's fascia must be removed, and the dissection is performed in the same layers as in the open surgical counterpart. The decision of whether or not to remove the adrenal should be based on the same criteria as in open surgery. If an electric tissue morcellator is not commercially available, the specimen must be morcellated with strong surgical graspers and surgical scissors as it is retrieved from the sack. Tumor-bearing kidneys are not morcellated but are removed within the sack via the most caudal port after extending the initial stab incision as a gridiron.

Nephroureterectomy: The most frequent indication for nephroureterectomy among our patients is vesicoureteral reflux. In open procedures, access to the distal ureter is commonly gained by an extraperitoneal route, which is rather complex because several layers must be transected before the ureter can finally be exposed. In contrast, the laparoscopic transperitoneal approach to the distal ureter is easy because the ureter travels directly underneath the parietal peritoneum in this region.

Because laparoscopic ureterectomy is easier than laparoscopic nephrectomy, complications are less likely to occur during ureterectomy, which should therefore be performed first. If, owing to a complication during nephrectomy, the procedure must be converted to an open operation, the patient has at least been spared the incision for ureterectomy. We prefer to perform ureteral stripping after circumcising the ureteral orifice down to the perivesical fat with an electrosurgical hook. Initially, retrograde ureteral stripping was done in combination with laparoscopic nephrectomy. More recently, antegrade rather than retrograde ureteral stripping has been adopted as the procedure of choice in our department. Unlike retrograde ureteral stripping, the antegrade technique requires additional dis-

section of part of the distal ureter. However, this technique has the advantage that tedious and complicated manipulation of the ureteral catheter and intracorporeal suturing can be avoided. Tearing of the ureteral suture—a potential complication of retrograde stripping—is not encountered in the antegrade technique. Perforation of the bladder has never been a problem, and perfect healing is achieved after catheter drainage of the bladder for 5 days. It should be noted, however, that ureteral stripping is contraindicated in ureteral tumors. The place of laparoscopic nephroureterectomy in transitional cell tumors is still a matter of controversy. In open surgery, a retroperitoneal approach has traditionally been advocated because of the risk of tumor spread. This strategy should not be changed because of the availability of laparoscopy, particularly in view of the fact that complete nephroureterectomy is also feasible by means of retroperitoneoscopy.

Laparoscopic partial nephrectomy: The main problem with this technique is adequate hemostasis. In children with duplex systems, the situation is favorable, and transection of the vessels to the affected pole makes subsequent transection of the renal parenchyma quite safe. Although we have never encountered severe bleeding in this setting, we strongly recommend the use of a bipolar coagulator, which is clearly superior to the argon-beam coagulator. Furthermore, sealing of the cut surface with fibrin glue to prevent delayed bleeding has become common practice in our department. Partial nephrectomy in adults with a nonduplicated kidney is more difficult, and bleeding cannot be avoided completely during the dissection. Allowing warm ischemia using a tourniquet or bulldog clamp is not feasible because the dissection proceeds too slowly. In our hands, bipolar coagulation has proved to be superior to the tourniquet described by Winfield; alternatively, the argon-beam coagulator or tamponade with a Surgicel sponge stick held by a surgical grasper or with similar substances can be used. As a last step, fibrin glue is applied. If available, laparoscopic Doppler flow ultrasonography is helpful to visualize the border of the dissection as well as the vasculature.

Laparoscopic unroofing of renal cyst: In order to preclude recurrences, it is advisable to suture a flap of Gerota's fascia to the bottom of the resected cyst.

Extraperitoneal laparoscopic surgery: The balloon used to create the space required within the retroperitoneum should not be filled with gas, as first described by Gaur. Saline should be used instead because rupture of a gas-filled balloon results in a sudden expansion of the gas, which can cause damage to adjacent structures. With compressed liquid no expansion effect occurs if the balloon ruptures. For most procedures we use four 10/11-mm trocars.

Retroperitoneal endoscopic nephrectomy: This approach is ideal for small kidneys as long as the dissection can be expected to be straightforward and not complicated by interfering intraperitoneal adhesions. In our department, retroperitoneoscopy has become the preferred approach in nephrectomy for benign disease. When dense perirenal adhesions are encountered, it is generally better to convert the procedure to the transperitoneal approach, but this is rarely necessary. The psoas muscle, which can be readily identified, serves as the main anatomic landmark. When the psoas muscle is followed medially, the ureter can be approached quickly and easily. Subsequently, the ureter can be followed to the renal pelvis and the renal artery.

Postoperative problems: Most reports on complications of laparoscopy mainly reflect the early experience and the influence of the learning curve rather than the true impact of the method. Although various complications may occur, some of which are quite serious, the great majority can be avoided by the experienced surgeon. In fact, recent series reporting on laparoscopic adrenalectomy and retroperitoneal laparoscopic adrenalectomy demonstrated both the postoperative morbidity and the complication rate to be lower than in open surgery.

Laparoscopic ureterolithotomy: Retroperitoneoscopy allows for quick and easy access to the proximal ureter, and the same is true for the transperitoneal approach to the distal ureter.

Therefore, laparoscopy is preferable to open surgery for this indication. Experience will show if laparoscopy is superior to antegrade or retrograde ureteroscopy or extracorporeal shock wave lithotripsy in case of large ureteral stones. Only one or two interrupted sutures are required for closing the incision.

Dismembered pyeloplasty: When comparing laparoscopy to endopyelotomy, the argument for the former being less invasive does not apply. However, in a recent study, endoscopic pyelotomy was reported to yield poor results in patients in whom ureteropelvic junction obstruction is caused by a crossing vessel, and it must be noted that the incidence of crossing vessels is as high as 40 to 60 percent. We use a modified transperitoneal approach in which access is gained through the layer between Gerota's fascia and the lateral and the dorsal abdominal wall. Subsequently, the kidney can be rotated anteromedially to permit direct access to the renal pelvis. For the management of aberrant vessels crossing dorsally, dismembered pyeloplasty is the method of choice. In our experience, the different methods of nondismembered pyeloplasty have proved to be more suitable for laparoscopy. We therefore use the so-called Fenger-plasty (longitudinal incision/transverse closure) for the repair of short stenoses.

Subcapsular Nephrectomy

Although dissecting inside the renal capsule is seldom necessary because tissue planes within Gerota's fascia usually persist, it may be the only choice for removal of the pyonephrotic or previously operated kidney.

1 *Incision:* Approach the kidney at a level different from that of the previous operation (flank, if previously anterior; 12th rib, if previously subcostal). Be careful in making the incision because in secondary operations the kidney capsule lies immediately below the transversalis fascia. Because little pararenal or perirenal fat usually remains in this area, the parenchyma can be inadvertently incised. Work at separating the perirenal fat from the capsule with blunt and sharp dissection in the usual way before concluding that subcapsular nephrectomy is absolutely necessary. Place a Penrose drain around the ureter.

Incise the scarred perirenal tissue, including the capsule of the kidney, along the convex border of the kidney, and grasp the medial edge with Mayo clamps. Insert a finger beneath this layer, and bluntly peel the capsule from the parenchyma, working medially until the hilum is reached. A vertical capsular incision directed toward the hilum (*dashed line*) aids in exposure.

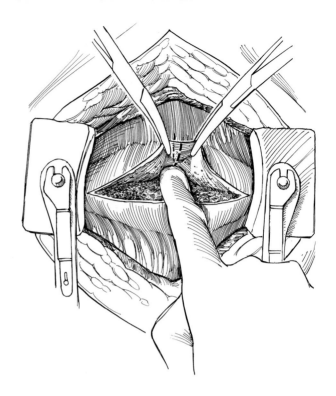

2 Hold the kidney back while retracting the capsule medially. Palpate the renal artery; it is usually small because the kidney is diseased. As the dissection progresses, continue to incise the turned-back capsular flap directly toward the artery.

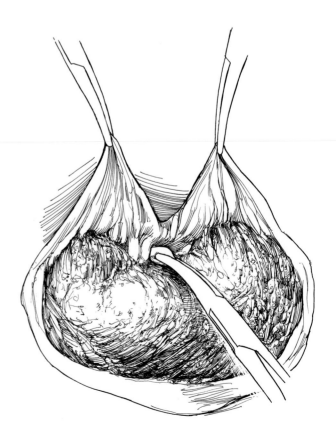

3 If possible, dissect the renal artery first, even though it lies behind the vein. Triply ligate the artery in continuity and divide it. Treat the renal vein similarly. Alternatively, place three heavy clamps and cut between the distal two (see page 988).

Alternative: If visualization is poor and the vessels cannot be separated, place a succession of curved clamps on the bulky tissue, dividing the pedicle between them as they are placed. The ligation of these sections of the pedicle can be delayed until the kidney has been removed.

Rotate the kidney cephalad, and divide and ligate the ureter below the scar tissue. Dissect along the ureter to reach and free the renal pelvis. Trim as much (devascularized) perirenal tissue as feasible. Suture-ligate the renal vessels with 1-0 SAS as the clamps are successively removed.

Close with adequate drainage, to be continued longer than that for an uncomplicated case.

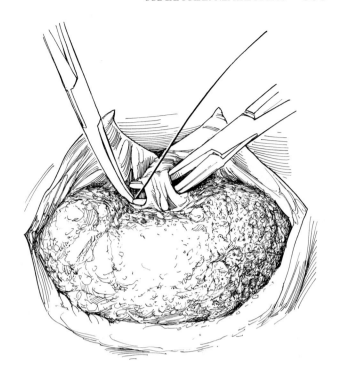

Commentary by Warren W. Koontz, Jr.

At times the renal hilar area is thickened, and the renal artery and especially the renal vein are difficult to identify. Several methods of handling the difficult renal pedicle have been described, such as incising the hilus and securing the vessels as they are cut. An alternative method is to doubly clamp the renal vessels and close the wound around the clamps; then loosen and remove them in 3 to 5 days.

We described a method (Koontz, 1973) in which, after the hilum has been reduced in size as much as possible, the surgeon can apply one vascular noncrushing clamp (or preferably two clamps) to the thickened, indurated mass of tissue containing the renal vessels. (A DeBakey vascular clamp is excellent for this purpose.) The hilum can then be divided close to the kidney, leaving a cuff of tissue distal to the clamp. The vessels become readily apparent and can be oversewn with vascular sutures as one would repair a rent in the side of the vena cava. The clamps are then slowly released. If bleeding occurs, the clamps are reapplied until complete hemostasis is achieved.

Partial Nephrectomy

Partial nephrectomy conserves renal tissue with certain neoplasms and with stone disease.

Neoplasms. Partial nephrectomy is indicated for patients with bilateral tumors or a tumor in a solitary kidney. The limited operation may also be necessary for patients with two kidneys who suffer from chronic renal failure. Partial nephrectomy provides functional renal reserve at the cost of a technically more difficult operation with a greater chance of local recurrence and more manipulation of the tumor. Selective venography is advisable for large or central tumors to detect intrarenal tumor thrombi.

Benign Disease. Removal of the lower pole for stone disease in a thin-walled lower caliceal stump is a reasonable objective of partial nephrectomy. Calicopyelostomy with anastomosis of the opened lower-pole calyx to the incised renal pelvis is an alternative. Other techniques, still experimental, include laser extirpation and ultrasonic aspiration.

Partial Nephrectomy for Neoplasm

A computed tomography (CT) scan precisely delineates the extent of the tumor. For a complicated case with neoplasm, perform renal arteriography. This procedure not only helps in planning the line of excision but also helps detect major arterial disease. Clear infection.

Have the patient well hydrated before surgery; good hydration is a necessity prior to renal arterial occlusion. If the problem may become complex, prepare ice slush for renal cooling (see page 1048). If you suspect that a solitary kidney will be severely stressed by ischemia, arrange for vascular access to be established perioperatively for postoperative dialysis (see page 90).

Extracorporeal surgery (see page 1027) is an alternative for large central tumors to avoid spillage and ensure complete resection, but it is rarely necessary and it carries a higher risk of complications. After removing the entire kidney, cool it and flush the main artery with a cold electrolyte solution until the solution runs clear. Remove the tumor, avoiding injury to the major vessels and ureter. Take special care not to interfere with the vessels supplying the ureter and renal pelvis. Perfusion via artery or vein helps identify vascular branches. After closing the collecting system and parenchyma, transplant the kidney into the iliac fossa.

Bilateral tumors require preliminary node dissection with frozen-section biopsy examination before proceeding. Perform radical nephrectomy on the more involved side and partial nephrectomy on the better kidney. Preserve at least one of the adrenal glands. A more suitable alternative in bilateral cases may be to proceed in two stages, preserving renal tissue on the radiographically better side at the first operation and then preserving as much as feasible, if any, on the other side at a later operation. Note that with asynchronous bilateral tumors, one of them may represent a metastasis.

Make preparations for cooling even though warm ischemia time seldom exceeds 30 minutes. Start intravenous mannitol administration.

1 **A,** *Position:* Lateral, over a kidney bolster or table break. *Incision:* A flank approach usually provides adequate exposure, especially through an 11th-rib supracostal incision (see page 879). If autotransplantation is contemplated, use an anterior approach (see page 865). An anterior approach should be used in children.

B, With a flank approach, open Gerota's fascia in the lateral plane, and insert a Buchwalter ring retractor. Free the entire kidney so that other tumors can be detected if present. Ballottement of the tumor with a finger placed in the hilum against fingers over the parenchyma allows assessment of large tumors and helps determine their suitability for removal by partial nephrectomy.

Be certain to leave the perirenal fat overlying the tumor undisturbed because capsular invasion is a common finding. Dissect the vascular pedicle sufficiently to allow application of vascular clamps. Dissect the vessels entering the hilum, especially those leading to the involved portion of the kidney. Place a vascular tape around the main artery and around the appropriate arterial branch going to the affected portion.

If the operation is for carcinoma, palpate for hilar nodes (left para-aortic for left-sided tumors; right paracaval for those on the right) and send suspicious nodes for frozen-section examination.

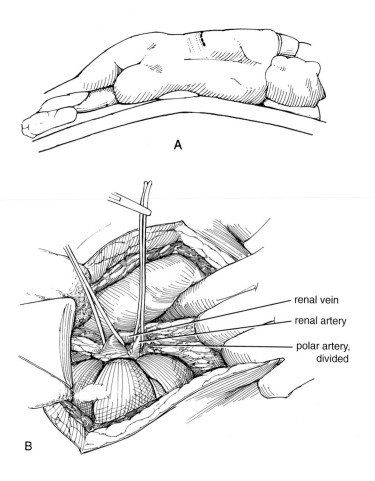

A

B

renal vein

renal artery

polar artery, divided

POLAR PARTIAL NEPHRECTOMY

Inspect the kidney to evaluate the practicality and determine the site of heminephrectomy. Use ultrasonography intraoperatively for this purpose. To identify the line of demarcation for heminephrectomy, place a bulldog clamp temporarily on the artery identified as supplying that portion and observe the kidney for blanching. Indigo carmine injected intravenously may give a line for resection, or a dilute solution of indigo carmine (0.4 percent) may be injected directly into the artery. Place vascular tapes around any accessory vessels. Ligate and divide polar vessels that directly supply the segment to be removed. The plane of excision must follow the radial direction of the pyramids. The assistant may be able to compress the renal pole between thumb and finger, obviating vascular occlusion. Alternatively, a kidney tourniquet (Goldwasser et al, 1987) or clamp (Storm et al, 1975) can be applied.

2 Dissect the arteries in the hilum to identify the artery supplying the involved portion of the kidney. Place a rubber-shod bulldog clamp on it, and leave it in place until the renal incision is closed, at which time it is released to check hemostasis. In some cases, finger compression of the parenchyma may substitute for vascular clamping. It is not necessary or desirable to clamp the renal vein.

If ischemia time is estimated to be more than 30 minutes, ask the anesthetist to inject furosemide or give 20 percent mannitol intravenously. Install a rubber dam or bowel bag with a hole in it under the kidney, and insulate it from the body wall with a laparotomy pad. Then clamp the renal artery in a vascular clamp, and distribute ice slush to cool the kidney for 15 minutes (see page 1048).

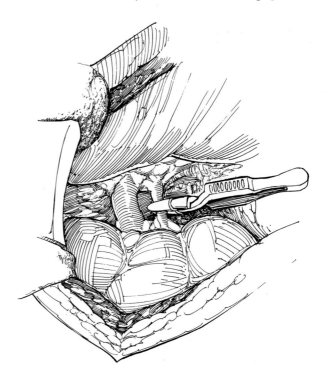

3 Incise the capsule 1 to 2 cm distal to the site of the proposed resection. If this ends up over tumor, move the incision proximally. Reflect the capsule from the normal parenchyma with the back of the knife.

4 Bluntly incise the parenchyma using the knife blade or handle, and leave 1 cm of normal tissue on the side of the tumor. Follow the normal plane between the renal lobules, using neither guillotine nor wedge incisions. Progressive slices may be removed if the disease process extends more proximally, unless you are dealing with carcinoma, in which case nephrectomy is required. Brain retractors may be helpful.

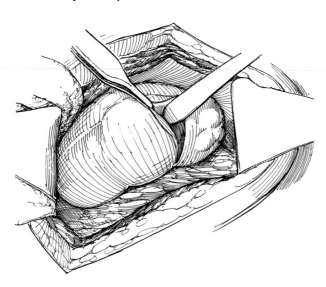

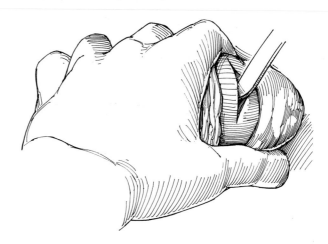

5 For blunt dissection between the nephrons, use the thumbnail, if desired.

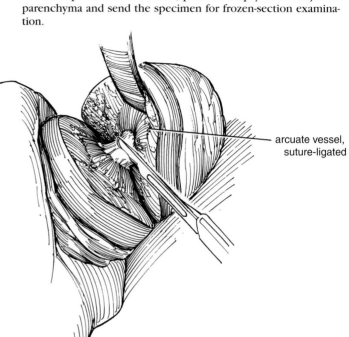

6 Sharply divide the arcuate vessels with Lahey scissors and suture-ligate them with figure-eight 4-0 or 5-0 CCG sutures. Cut each caliceal infundibulum with knife or scissors. In stone cases, excise them as distally as possible.

If the operation is for tumor, perform biopsy of the adjacent parenchyma and send the specimen for frozen-section examination.

arcuate vessel, suture-ligated

7 Suture-ligate all remaining arcuate vessels, paying special attention to the large venous collectors near the hilum. Work rapidly but accurately. Electrocoagulation cannot be used, but argon-beam laser coagulation, if available, is effective. Ligate the interlobar vessels with sutures that include the adjacent infundibulum. Remove the specimen to another table so that the pathologist may check the margins by frozen-section examination. Release the bulldog clamp momentarily to allow identification and ligation of remaining open vessels. Place a self-retaining ureteral stent in the ureter, if desired. Close the infundibulum with a 4-0 or 5-0 continuous SAS to make the suture line watertight. Obstruct the ureter, allow the pelvis to fill, and check for leaks.

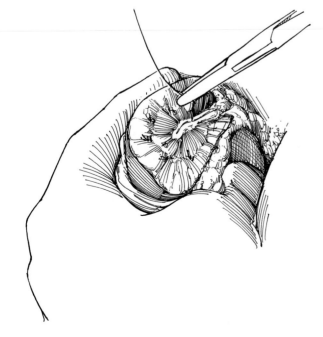

8 Absorbable collagen may be applied to the parenchymal surface for hemostasis. Release the bulldog clamp while compressing the kidney at the suture line for several minutes to assist hemostasis. If this does not stop the bleeding, an arterial branch was not controlled and the kidney must be reclamped and cooled, then reopened to secure the vessel in a suture. If urinary output decreases after release of the clamp, give furosemide intravenously. Close the capsule, including the edges of the parenchyma, using 3-0 or 4-0 CCG vertical mattress sutures. Obtain fat pads from the properitoneal fat, and catch them between the loops as bolsters. A free strip of peritoneum or synthetic mesh can substitute for an inadequate capsule. The omentum may be pulled through into the retroperitoneum and applied as a wrap (see page 71). Perform nephropexy (see page 922) to keep the lower pole away from the ureteropelvic junction and ureter.

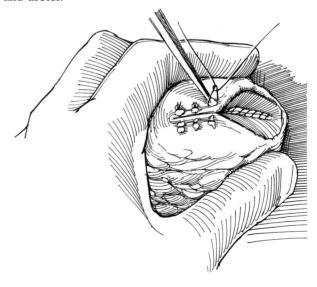

Place a stent only if major reconstruction has been done. Suture a Penrose drain adjacent to the repair by the long suture technique (see page 917), or (less desirable) place a closed suction drain to exit through a stab wound. Close Gerota's fascia so that it cushions the repair inside the perirenal fat. Complete the wound closure. Drain for at least 7 days. If leakage continues, perform retrograde ureterography and consider placing a J stent.

Within the first postoperative month, obtain a CT scan of the kidney as a baseline, and follow with scans every 6 months for the first 2 years. For patients with a solitary kidney, follow the patient's urinary protein excretion because of concern for hyperfiltration nephropathy.

WEDGE RESECTION FOR TUMORS IN THE MIDPORTION

9 Evaluate the extent of malignant tumors with color Doppler intraoperative ultrasonography to determine if renal salvage is possible. Incise the capsule 2 cm away from the tumor margin. Consider clamping the renal artery if the resection will be extensive (Step 2).

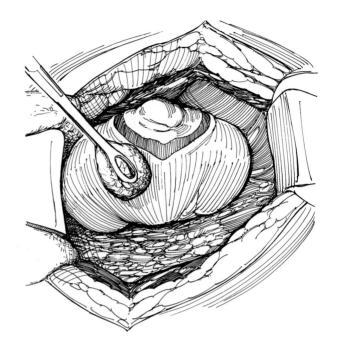

10 Remove a wedge to include normal parenchyma beyond the tumor by following the direction of the nephrons. Secure hemostasis by figure-eight suture ligation.

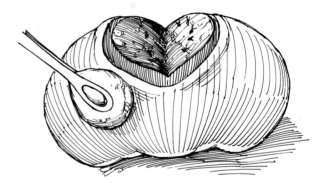

11 Before closing the collecting system, insert an internal stent down the ureter.

A, Close the defect with mattress sutures and fat bolsters to the capsule.

B, If the defect is large, apply absorbable collagen or omentum.

C, A free peritoneal graft may be applied.

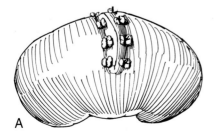 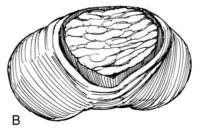 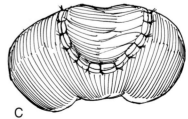

POSTOPERATIVE PROBLEMS

For continued *leakage*, look for distal obstruction. *Fistulas* are not common but occur with central tumors and large tumors and after collecting system reconstruction. They also occur with wedge resections that are closed with large mattress sutures. They usually resolve spontaneously or after stent placement (or removal). *Urinomas* are secondary to poor drainage. Placement of a ureteral catheter or stent is rarely necessary.

Wound infections can occur and often follow operations for infected stones. *Renal artery thrombosis* from *traction damage to the intima* is a rare complication. *Secondary nephrectomy* is reported in less than 3 percent of cases. *Acute renal failure* may follow partial nephrectomy in a solitary kidney, related to large size of the tumor, excessive removal of parenchyma, and prolonged ischemia time. A gradual decrease in renal function may occur in children as a result of hyperperfusion in reduced renal parenchyma.

Commentary by Andrew C. Novick

Partial nephrectomy has become a successful treatment for patients with localized renal cell carcinoma (RCC) who need functioning renal parenchyma preserved—patients with bilateral RCC, RCC involving a solitary functioning kidney, chronic renal failure, or unilateral RCC and a functioning opposite kidney that is at risk for future impairment due to an intercurrent disorder. Some centers have extended the indications for partial nephrectomy to patients with small unilateral RCC and a normal contralateral kidney. The technical success rate with partial nephrectomy is excellent, and long-term cancer-free survival is comparable to that obtained after radical nephrectomy, particularly for early-stage RCC. The major disadvantage of partial nephrectomy for RCC is the risk (4 to 10 percent) of postoperative local tumor recurrence in the operated kidney. Some local "recurrences" may be manifestations of undetected multifocal RCC in the renal remnant.

For most patients, preoperative renal arteriography to delineate the intrarenal vasculature aids in tumor excision with minimal blood loss and minimal damage to adjacent normal parenchyma. This test can be omitted in patients with small peripheral tumors. Selective renal venography is performed in patients with large or centrally located tumors to evaluate for intrarenal venous thrombosis secondary to malignancy.

Preoperative hydration and mannitol administration are important adjuncts to ensure optimal renal perfusion at operation. It is usually possible to perform partial nephrectomy for RCC in situ by using an operative approach that optimizes exposure of the kidney and by combining meticulous surgical technique with an understanding of the renal vascular anatomy in relation to the tumor. We use an extraperitoneal flank incision through the bed of the 11th or 12th rib for almost all of these operations; we occasionally use a thoracoabdominal incision for very large tumors involving the upper portion of the kidney. These incisions allow the surgeon to operate on the mobilized kidney almost at skin level and provide excellent exposure of the peripheral renal vessels. With an anterior subcostal incision, the kidney is invariably located in the depth of the wound, and the surgical exposure is simply not as good.

The kidney is mobilized along with Gerota's fascia while the perirenal fat around the tumor is left intact. For small peripheral renal tumors, it may not be necessary to control the renal artery. In most cases, however, partial nephrectomy is most effectively performed after temporary renal arterial occlusion. This measure not only limits intraoperative bleeding but, by reducing renal tissue turgor, also improves access to intrarenal structures. In most cases, we believe that it is important to leave the renal vein patent throughout the operation. This measure decreases intraoperative renal ischemia and facilitates hemostasis by allowing venous back-bleeding and enabling identification of small transected renal veins. In patients with centrally located tumors, we do occlude the renal vein temporarily to minimize intraoperative bleeding from transected major venous branches.

When the renal circulation is temporarily interrupted, in situ renal hypothermia is used to protect against postischemic renal injury. Surface cooling of the kidney with ice slush allows up to 3 hours of safe ischemia without permanent renal injury. An important caveat with this method is to keep the entire kidney covered with ice slush for 10 to 15 minutes immediately after occluding the renal artery and before commencing the partial nephrectomy. This amount of time is needed to obtain core renal cooling to a temperature (15 to 20° C) that optimizes in situ renal preservation. During excision of the tumor, large portions of the kidney are invariably no longer covered with ice slush, and, in the absence of adequate prior renal cooling, rapid rewarming and ischemic renal injury can occur.

Several surgical techniques are available for performing in situ nephrectomy in patients with RCC. These include (1) polar segmental nephrectomy, (2) wedge resection, and (3) transverse resection. These techniques all require adherence to basic principles of early vascular control, avoidance of ischemic renal damage, complete tumor excision with free margins, precise closure of the collecting system, careful hemostasis, and closure or coverage of the renal defect with adjacent fat, fascia, peritoneum, or Oxycel. Prior to commencing the renal resection, any enlarged or suspicious regional lymph nodes are excised for staging purposes. The value of partial nephrectomy for RCC with lymph node involvement is not established.

Whichever technique is used, the tumor is removed with at least a 1-cm surrounding margin of grossly normal renal parenchyma. Enucleation is ill advised, even for tumors that appear grossly well encapsulated, and carries the risk of leaving residual malignancy in the renal remnant. Intraoperative ultrasonography is very helpful in localizing the tumor accurately, particularly intrarenal lesions that are not visible or palpable from the external surface of the kidney. Excision of the tumor involves dividing the renal parenchyma by a combination of sharp and blunt dissection. Intrarenal vessels that are identified during the resection are directly suture-ligated at that time while they are most visible. Immediately after the tumor is excised, biopsies of the remaining portion of the kidney are done to verify complete tumor excision. It is unusual for such biopsies to demonstrate residual tumor, but if they do, additional renal tissue must be excised.

If possible, the renal defect created by the excision is closed as an additional hemostatic measure. This is done by approximating the transected cortical margins with interrupted 3-0 chromic sutures, taking care to avoid tension on the suture line or distortion of blood vessels supplying the kidney. A retroperitoneal Penrose drain is always left in place for at least 7 days. An intraoperative ureteral stent is placed only when major reconstruction of the intrarenal collecting system has been performed.

Using the techniques described above, even large, complex, centrally located tumors can be completely excised in situ. We have found that extracorporeal surgery is rarely necessary. Specific disadvantages of extracorporeal partial nephrectomy include a longer operative time and a higher incidence of postoperative complications, particularly renal failure.

Heminephrectomy

This procedure is best for removal of the diseased upper pole in duplicated systems.

1 *Position:* Place the patient supine with the involved side slightly elevated on a towel.

Incision: Make an anterior subcostal extraperitoneal incision (see page 871). Open Gerota's fascia posteriorly, and mobilize the usually scanty fat anteriorly to free the entire kidney. Rotate it anteriorly, and expose the ureter, pelvis, and renal pedicle to the upper pole from behind. The line of demarcation is usually obvious on inspection and palpation.

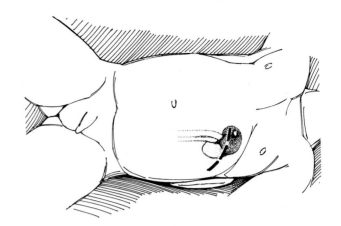

2 Identify both ureters, and trace the dilated one to its entry into the upper pole. Catch it in a vessel loop. Free this ureter from its bed as distally as feasible, at the same time avoiding interference with the blood supply of the normal mate. Insert two traction sutures, and divide the ureter; allow the system to empty. Dissect the distal ureter down to the common sheath. Divide it there, and spatulate it as deeply as possible at this point; it is not necessary to excise the portion within the common sheath, a maneuver that could jeopardize the circulation to the normal ureter. Do not ligate the distal stump, especially if the urine is infected, unless the ureter is known to reflux.

Pass the proximal end of the ureter anterior to the upper pole vessels, taking great care not to pull so hard that the small vascular branches to the upper pole associated with the main blood supply to the upper pole segment are avulsed. Lifting the ureter in its new position while completing the proximal dissection of the ureter and pelvis into the hilum allows the vessels to be readily identified before they are divided. Locate and dissect out the blood supply to the upper segment. If a vessel is not clearly separate from those going to the rest of the kidney, pass a 4-0 SAS around it, occlude it with traction, and note the area of blanching. If it is a part of the upper pole that becomes ischemic, tie the suture and divide the vessel. It is seldom necessary to occlude the main blood supply; if it is, give intravenous mannitol before applying the clamp.

Look for the deep groove between upper and lower moieties and for the difference in thickness and color of the parenchymas. Feel for the pulsation of the arteries to the lower pole. Incise the renal capsule circumferentially 2 cm distal to the obvious line of demarcation, and peel it back with a knife handle.

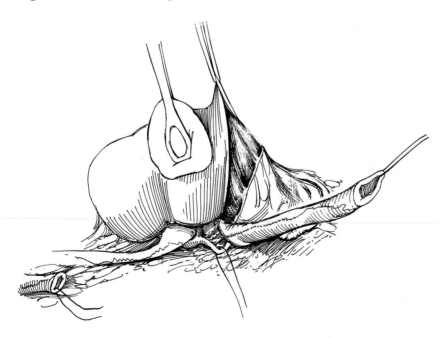

3 Transect the renal parenchyma, which is concave, with knife blade or cutting current, knife handle, and scissors along the plane of demarcation. Sharp dissection is needed because of the fibrous character of the parenchyma. Insert the index finger into the upper-pole renal pelvis; this helps identify the plane between the upper and lower pole. If in doubt, err on the side of leaving a small amount of upper-pole tissue behind. Residual upper-pole tissue and portions of calyces may be trimmed later. As the separation proceeds, place a figure-eight 4-0 transfixion SAS on any major parenchymal vessel, especially on those associated with the calyx and pelvis. Remove remnants of caliceal lining, that is, those not contained in the specimen. Avoid opening into the upper calyx of the lower segment; if it is opened, close the calyx with a running 4-0 SAS.

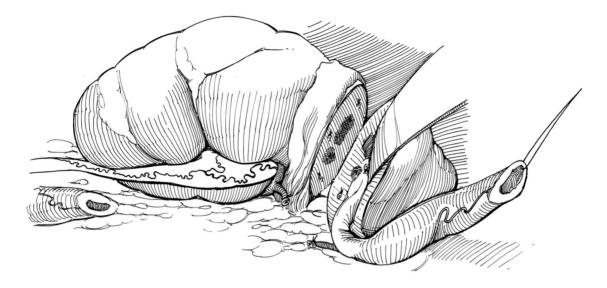

4 Close the capsule over the exposed parenchyma with a running 4-0 SAS. Place a 3-0 mattress SAS over fat bolsters in the capsule of the posterior inferior surface of the kidney to suture the mobile residual kidney to the posterior body wall as a nephropexy (see page 922) to maintain the renal axis and prevent torsion of the vasculature of the remaining segment and kinking of the relatively redundant lower-pole ureter. Tack a Penrose drain adjacent to the area of transection by the long suture technique (see page 917), re-approximate the perirenal fat and Gerota's fascia, and close the wound in layers.

For the rare case requiring lower-pole heminephrectomy, the procedure is similar except that extreme care must be taken to preserve the vascular supply to the upper pole, which is usually a branch from the main vessel that goes to the lower pole.

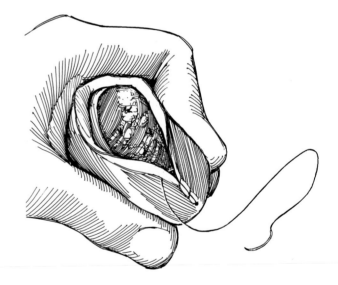

Commentary by Thomas S. Parrott, III

I prefer a more posterior approach in which the patient is placed on his or her side, with a roll under the opposite lumbar area. In larger patients, the kidney rest can be used as in adults. The incision is typically rather small and extends from the tip of the 12th rib transversely across the flank toward the umbilicus. The subcostal (12th) neurovascular bundle rarely presents a problem with exposure, but when it is prominent, the nerve may be retracted inferiorly after the artery and vein are divided. A muscle-splitting approach can be used if desired; however, I have never encountered anything more morbid postoperatively after dividing the flank musculature than a temporary small bulge beneath the incision. Mobilization and exposure of the upper pole are facilitated by this approach. I have at times found myself somewhat confined with the more anterior approach and have thought that less traction on the kidney (for adequate exposure) is needed when the kidney is approached and mobilized posteriorly. This may help to limit spasm of small renal arteries, which often occurs when the kidney is put on prolonged or excessive traction. In addition, a small flank scar is less noticeable than one of similar length presenting anteriorly beneath the rib cage.

I totally agree that it is seldom necessary to occlude the main blood supply. On the other hand, one should consider passing a vessel loop around the main trunk or main renal artery, so that, if occlusion of the lower-pole blood supply is necessary during the course of the operation, the proper vessels can be located promptly and safely. The easiest and safest way to remove the upper pole is to dissect the upper-pole ureter and pelvis proximally, staying in that plane between the pelvis and lower-pole parenchyma referred to as Gil-Vernet's plane (when discussing extended pyelolithotomy). Mobilizing this avascular area usually allows the surgeon to separate the upper pole from the lower, with attachments remaining only at the hilar area. The capsule can be incised as drawn, allowing for a slight excess that can be apposed over the raw top of the upper-pole parenchyma. Nephropexy as described is optional; however, Penrose drainage is mandatory. As with pediatric reconstructive procedures, gentle tissue handling in this operation is essential for uneventful healing. Excessive renal traction causing arterial spasm is to be avoided at all costs. Performed properly, the operation is a fun technical exercise and should give uniformly excellent results.

Nephroureterectomy

Search the entire urinary tract for other transitional cell tumors. Perform intravenous urography to visualize a filling defect; if that is inadequate, resort to retrograde pyelography. Obtain a computed tomography (CT) scan to rule out a nonopaque stone and to evaluate the regional nodes. Cells for cytologic examination can be obtained from voided urine or, better, from a ureteral catheter brush biopsy specimen.

In questionable cases, ureteropyeloscopy can visualize the tumor. If doubt remains, inspect the pelvis or calyx by open or percutaneous methods and perform a biopsy. For carcinoma of the renal pelvis, nephroureterectomy is required, except for the solitary kidney, for which percutaneous endoscopic or ureteroscopic treatment may be applicable. For an upper or mid-ureteral low-grade lesion, excise and reanastomose the ureter. For a low-grade lesion in the lower ureter, resect the ureter and reimplant it in the bladder after taking a frozen-section specimen from the cut end. For a high-grade ureteral tumor, a nephroureterectomy is necessary, although micrometastases probably account for the poor cure rate.

The purpose of nephroureterectomy is removal of the kidney, ureter, and bladder cuff in continuity, along with the regional lymph nodes. Transvesical excision or transurethral resection of the terminal ureter may be needed for its complete removal.

The operation can be done through one or two incisions. If the ureter contains the tumor, reverse the order of the operation and approach the ureter first. Laparoscopic excision is an alternative, but the rapid recovery from the operation must be weighed against the facts that it requires twice the operating time and that it is technically difficult (McDougall et al, 1995). In these cases, the intramural ureter can be resected transurethrally at the start of the nephrectomy to simplify removal of the distal ureter (Palou et al, 1995). Lymphadenectomy helps stage the tumor and may offer therapeutic benefit.

SINGLE-INCISION THORACOABDOMINAL APPROACH WITH NODE DISSECTION

Operation on the Left Kidney

1 *Position:* Elevate the involved flank to a 30- to 45-degree angle on a sandbag, and extend the table to stretch the operative area. Keep the pelvis as flat as possible. It may be helpful to place a bag of intravenous fluid under the contralateral axilla. Insert an 18 F 5-ml silicone balloon catheter in the bladder and attach it to closed drainage, but drape it so that it is accessible for bladder filling.

Incision: Start the incision from the angle of the 11th rib at the posterior axillary line, run it medially to the anterior superior iliac spine, and continue it paramedially to the symphysis in the midline. If the mass is very large, make the incision over the 10th or 9th rib. Cut directly onto the palpable 11th rib through the latissimus dorsi and serratus muscles posteriorly and the external and internal oblique and transversalis muscles anteriorly.

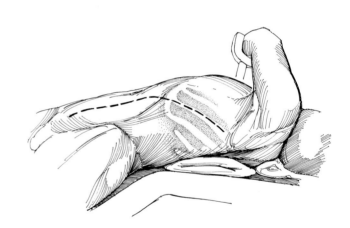

2 Excise the rib as described for the transcostal incision on page 875, or free its superior margin as described for the supracostal incision on page 879.

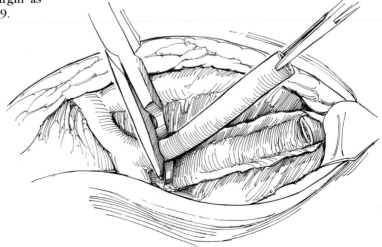

3 Sharply divide the costochondral junction. Incise the bed of the rib, opening the pleura. Alternatively, use an extrapleural approach. Continue the incision anteriorly to the border of the rectus muscle; then carry it to the symphysis.

4 Bluntly dissect under the edge of the diaphragm, and open it in the direction of the incision. This approach should spare injury to the phrenic nerve.

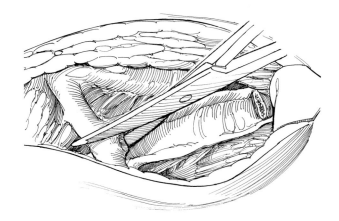

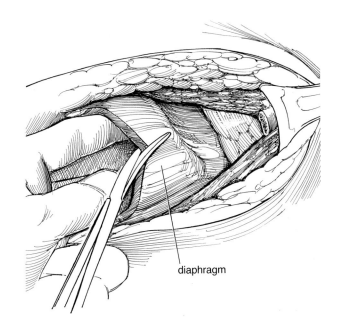

diaphragm

5 Mobilize the peritoneum medially, freeing it first from the transversalis fascia and then from the anterior rectus fascia, where it is quite adherent and must be sharply separated. Also free the peritoneum from the undersurface of the diaphragm to allow the spleen, pancreas, and liver on the right side to be moved medially within the peritoneal envelope, out of the way of the dissection. Enter the avascular plane between the peritoneum and the anterior surface of Gerota's fascia in the thin layer of loose areolar tissue. (For small tumors, open Gerota's fascia and leave behind the fascia around the upper pole and the adrenal gland.) Carry the dissection medially across the great vessels bluntly while the assistant holds up the peritoneal envelope. Ligate and divide the inferior mesenteric vein for left-sided tumors. Trace this vein to its junction with the splenic vein to locate the area of the origin of the superior mesenteric artery (SMA), an important landmark.

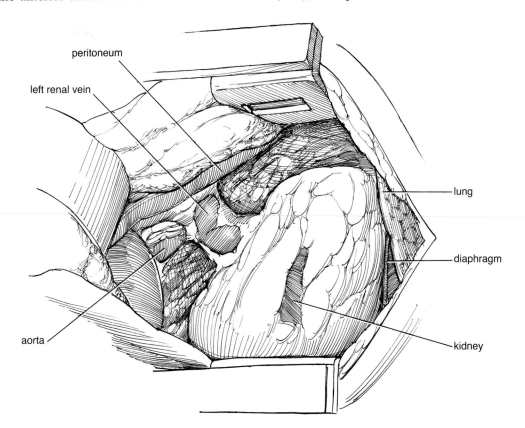

peritoneum

left renal vein

lung

diaphragm

aorta

kidney

6 Dissect the left renal vein lying beneath the SMA. Divide the adrenal, gonadal, and lumbar veins at their origins from the renal vein for left-sided tumors. (This division is not necessary for right-sided tumors.) Expose the renal artery.

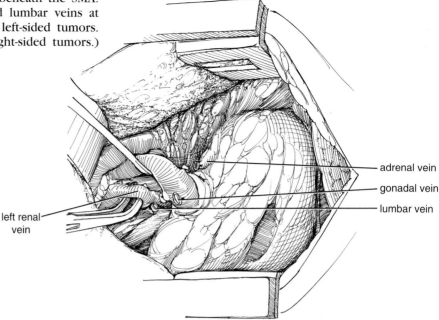

adrenal vein

gonadal vein

lumbar vein

left renal vein

7 Triply ligate the renal artery, including a suture ligature, and divide it. Doubly ligate and divide the renal vein. Mobilize the posterior surface of Gerota's fascia from the lumbar and psoas muscles. Begin dissection of the retroperitoneal areolar and nodal tissue at the diaphragm. Clip the vessels to the adrenal gland. As the dissection proceeds, clip generously to prevent lymphatic leakage.

renal vein

aorta

renal artery

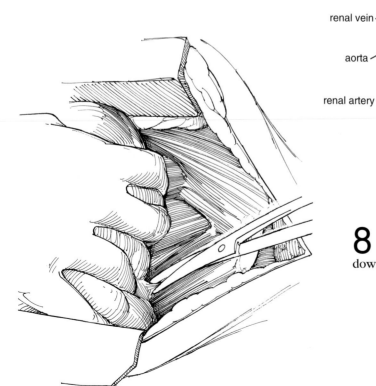

8 Continue the dissection posteriorly outside Gerota's fascia. Clear the tissue from the top of the vena cava down to the level of insertion of the right spermatic vein.

9 Dissect around the vena cava down to the crossing of the right common iliac artery over the left common iliac vein. If necessary, divide each lumbar vein as it is encountered. Ligate the proximal end and clip the distal end.

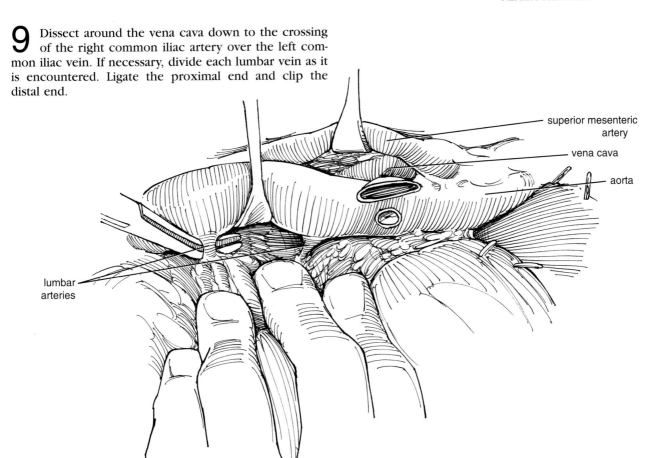

superior mesenteric artery

vena cava

aorta

lumbar arteries

10 Enter the plane superficial to the aortic adventitia, and resect the aortocaval nodal tissue. It may be helpful to ligate the lumbar arteries below the renal pedicle. Protect the right renal artery, and clip the cisterna chyli with a large clip behind the right renal artery where it lies medial to the right crus of the diaphragm.

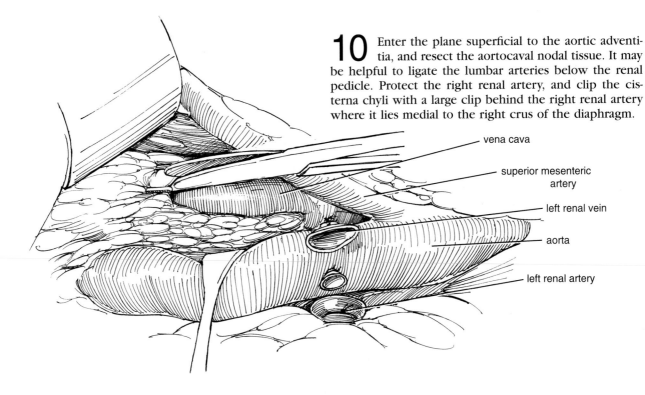

vena cava

superior mesenteric artery

left renal vein

aorta

left renal artery

11 Pass this tissue beneath the vena cava after dissecting it from the intervertebral ligaments.

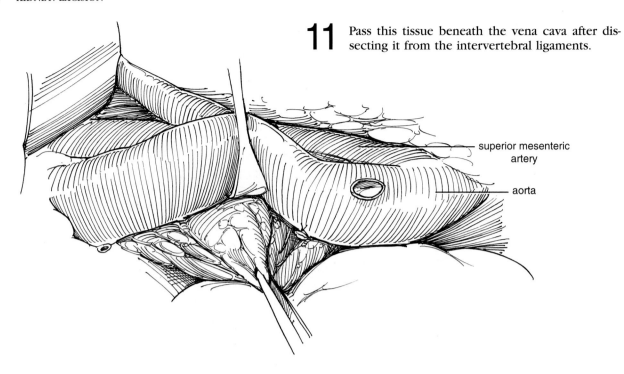

superior mesenteric
artery

aorta

12 Continue the dissection caudally to just above the aortic bifurcation. Clamp, divide, and ligate the remaining tongue of tissue.

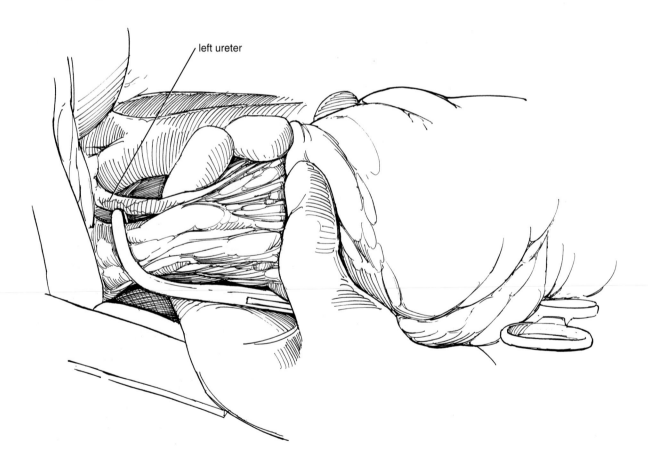

left ureter

13 The undersurfaces of the diaphragm, the psoas muscle, and both great vessels are clear of areolar tissue.

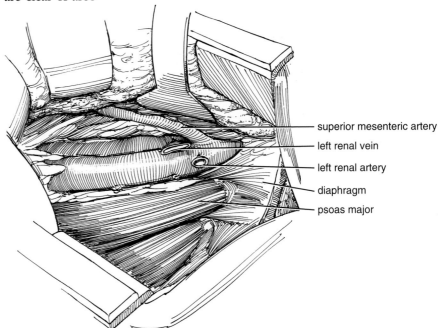

superior mesenteric artery

left renal vein

left renal artery

diaphragm

psoas major

Operation on the Right Kidney

After dividing the tissue over the top of the vena cava and ligating the adrenal vein and lumbar veins down to the bifurcation of the vena cava (Step 6), dissect over the top of the left renal vein, and mobilize the tissue over the aorta down to the origin of the inferior mesenteric artery. If necessary, ligate and divide the lumbar arteries in this area, and sweep the tissue under the aorta and vena cava. Clip the margins on the left side as the vena cava is moved to the right.

Ureterectomy, Left Ureter

14 Draw the ureter aside, and clip and divide its vascular connections. Identify the superior vesical artery (not shown) as it crosses the ureter just above the bladder wall; doubly ligate and divide it. Continue the dissection to expose the bladder wall by dividing the obliterated hypogastric artery. Place a large clip on the ureter at this point to reduce tumor spillage.

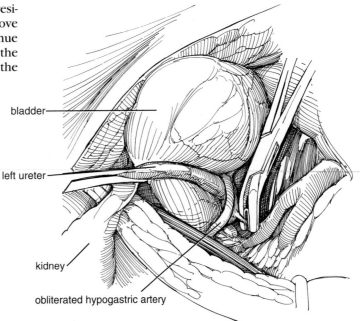

bladder

left ureter

kidney

obliterated hypogastric artery

15 Fill the bladder with saline or an antineoplastic solution, and open it between stay sutures. Suture the ureteral orifice closed with a figure-eight 3-0 SAS, and use the ends for traction. With a hooked blade, incise the mucosa circumferentially; then free the intramural ureter inside Waldeyer's sheath with Lahey scissors. From outside the bladder, draw the ureter out of the hiatus, and remove the specimen. Close the muscle in the hiatus with two or three 3-0 SAS and the epithelium with interrupted 4-0 SAS. To close the cystotomy, run a submucosal 4-0 SAS reinforced with a row of interrupted 3-0 SAS to muscle and adventitia. A tube is not necessary because the urethral catheter remains.

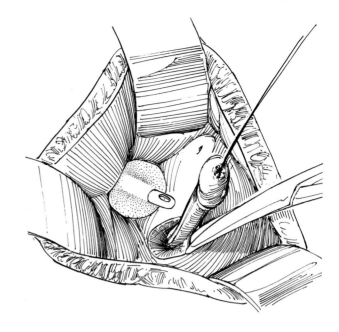

Alternative Treatment of the Intramural Ureter. Opening the bladder and visually excising the orifice and part of the trigone is standard practice, and deviations from it may result in the subsequent development of a tumor in a small segment that is not removed. If the distal ureter is known to be uninvolved, loop the ureter extravesically with a Penrose drain, and insert two stay sutures in the bladder wall adjacent to the orifice. Excise a disk of bladder wall that includes the orifice, and close the defect. To avoid a second incision and pelvic dissection, although with a higher risk of tumor recurrence, use a resectoscope to cut the mucosa around the orifice, and insert a vein stripper from above to free the ureter from the retroperitoneum. Another technique involves transurethrally passing a catheter to the renal pelvis, then incising the orifice. After the kidney is freed, traction on the catheter inverts the ureter into the bladder.

Close the lower part of the wound around a suction drain placed at the base of the bladder and brought out through a stab wound. A second drain may be placed in the renal fossa, exiting from the posterior portion of the wound or from a separate stab wound. Flatten the table. Approximate the diaphragm with interrupted 2-0 or 3-0 SAS. Close the pleura along with the rib bed with a running 2-0 or 3-0 SAS or with 2-0 figure-eight, through-and-through buried sutures around an 18 F Robinson catheter. Close the remainder of the wound after infiltrating the intercostal nerves with 0.5 percent bupivacaine. Remove the upper Penrose drain the next day and the lower one in 4 days unless urinary drainage is present; if drainage is present, leave the lower drain until drainage stops. Remove the chest tube in 2 or 3 days. Take the catheter out in 7 to 10 days.

TWO-INCISION APPROACH

If node dissection is not planned, making two incisions may be a simpler approach. For infants and children, use an anterior subcostal incision for nephrectomy (see page 871) and a lower abdominal midline or transverse incision for ureterectomy. For adults, make a supracostal 11th-rib incision (see page 879) and a midline extraperitoneal incision (see page 487). Place the patient in the semi-oblique position for the anterior subcostal approach and in the lateral position for the flank approach.

Mobilize the colon medially, and bluntly free the area of the renal pedicle. Proceed as previously described for Steps 1 to 13, using a large Deaver retractor for maximal exposure in the lower end of the wound. Take all the perirenal tissue and Gerota's fascia. Resect the regional nodes. Bluntly mobilize the ureter to the level of the iliac crossing, fulgurating or clipping the medial vessels that supply it.

Pack the kidney and nodal tissue retroperitoneally to be retrieved from below. Alternatively, the ureter can be doubly ligated or clipped and divided electrosurgically to prevent spillage of tumor cells. Close the flank incision around a Penrose drain.

Move the instrument table. Place the patient supine. Prepare and drape the patient for a midline incision. (An alternative is an oblique incision extending from the anterior superior iliac spine to the midline two fingerbreadths above the symphysis. Divide the external and internal oblique muscles and the transversalis fascia. Retract the rectus muscle medially.) Bluntly mobilize the peritoneum medially, and identify the ureter 3 or 4 inches above the bladder. Loop the ureter with a vessel tape, and dissect it while clipping its vessels. Bring the kidney into the incision. Proceed as described in Steps 14 and 15.

POSTOPERATIVE PROBLEMS

Pneumothorax can occur if the chest tube fails to function. *Urinary drainage* through the bladder incision is rare.

Commentary by Peter R. Carroll

The treatment of renal pelvic and ureteral cancers is based on tumor grade, stage, position, and multiplicity. Preoperative evaluation should include contrast imaging of the upper urinary tract, cystoscopy, and collection of cytology specimens. Low-grade cancers may be associated with benign-appearing cytology specimens. Patients with indeterminate radiographic findings may benefit from ureteral catheterization, selective ureteral cytology collection, brush biopsy, retrograde pyelography, and, on occasion, ureteroscopy.

Selected patients with accessible low-grade cancers or single systems may be candidates for endoscopic (either retrograde or percutaneous) management. However, the risk of understaging is significant, and a small risk of tumor spillage exists as well. Rare patients with large or multifocal renal pelvic cancers in single systems may be better served by ex vivo excision and renal autotransplantation using a wide pyelocystostomy. The latter allows for easy endoscopic inspection and intravesical chemotherapy or immunotherapy in follow-up. Distal ureterectomy and ureteral reimplantation (often facilitated by a psoas hitch) are adequate treatment for distal ureteral cancers. I prefer an open, end-to-side ureteral anastomosis, which may allow ureteroscopic access to the remaining ureter for follow-up.

Although some adults with small body habitus may have a nephroureterectomy done through a single incision, two incisions are necessary in most adults. I prefer a supracostal approach and make an effort to avoid entry into the pleura. Careful dissection proceeding along the rib medially to laterally, releasing the diaphragm, and exposing the pleural edge may allow one to avoid pleural entry without compromising exposure. Large cancers may be best removed through a thoracoabdominal incision. Renal dissection should proceed outside Gerota's fascia, although the capsule may be entered superiorly in the majority of cases in which the adrenal is preserved. I usually perform a regional lymphadenectomy and do not extend the dissection to the contralateral side in patients without evidence of regional metastases. This dissection extends from the crus of the diaphragm to the level of the inferior mesenteric artery. Fibroareolar and lymphatic tissues over the great vessels are taken, and individual lymphatics are secured with small clips. Lumbar arteries or veins need not be ligated routinely, but only when necessary. The therapeutic benefit of lymphadenectomy is likely to be small.

I attempt to mobilize the ureter with as much periureteral tissue as possible. Lower ureteral dissection is usually performed through a separate midline incision, although it can be performed through an oblique one as well. The ureter is traced to its insertion into the bladder. This is facilitated by dividing the superior vesical artery and obliterated umbilical vein as described. I prefer removing a cuff of bladder and the intravesical portion of the ureter through a cystotomy. A drain is placed at the level of the cystotomy and brought out through a separate incision. I do not drain the renal bed. Suprapubic catheter drainage should be avoided.

All patients with upper-tract transitional cell cancers require endoscopic and cytologic evaluation in follow-up because the risk of transitional cell cancer formation in the bladder is significant.

Radical Nephrectomy

Node dissection for renal carcinoma does not appear to add to the rate of cure from radical excision of the kidney. Nor does simultaneous *adrenalectomy* affect prognosis. However, *removal of tumor thrombus* from the vena cava is beneficial. Ethanol *embolization* may shrink not only the tumor but also its venous extensions.

Partial nephrectomy (see page 1000) has gained advocates who apply it not only to tumors in solitary kidneys but also to those small tumors now diagnosed through the widespread use of sonographic and scanning procedures. *Extracorporeal techniques* for partial nephrectomy have not proved to be advantageous.

Bilateral tumors require preliminary node dissection with frozen-section examination of biopsy specimens before proceeding. Perform radical nephrectomy on the most involved side and a partial nephrectomy on the other kidney, as described on page 1000. Preserve at least one of the adrenal glands. Alternatively, proceed in two stages, preserving tissue on one side at the first operation, then on the other side later. If excision is not possible, obtain a biopsy preparatory to chemotherapy. In a solitary or fused kidney, do a partial nephrectomy or, if that is not possible, a biopsy. Note that with asynchronous bilateral tumors, one of them probably represents a metastasis.

Choice of Incision: The most generally useful incision in adults is the 11th- or 12th-rib supracostal incision (see page 879). For a large tumor, especially if it is at the upper pole, a thoracoabdominal incision is needed (see page 890). In children, the pediatric extended incision (see page 863) is preferred, but an anterior unilateral transverse extraperitoneal incision (see page 865), although it takes longer to make, provides better exposure and obviates entrance into the chest and the abdomen. An anterior approach allows early control of the arterial blood supply and consequently results in the least blood loss. Because of the known risk of splenic injury during transperitoneal removal of the left kidney, administer pneumococcal vaccine preoperatively to patients over age 65, and transect the splenic ligaments before applying traction on the spleen. A vertical transperitoneal incision (see page 867) has certain disadvantages compared with a transverse one (see page 865).

Instruments: Provide GU vascular, GU long, GU chest, and Major retractor sets; Satinsky clamps; a Fish visceral retractor; a Smith ring or large Balfour retractor; an extra-long vascular needle holder; large and medium hemoclips; a 16 F 5-ml balloon catheter; a 14 F Robinson catheter with a 50-ml syringe and a three-way stopcock; a closed suction drain; and, for children, a warming blanket.

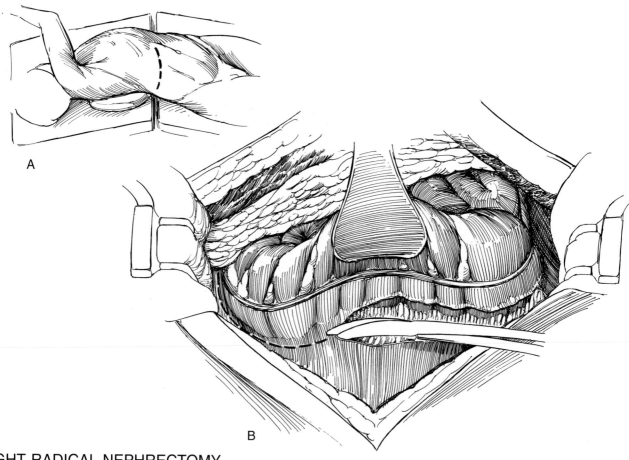

A

B

RIGHT RADICAL NEPHRECTOMY, ANTERIOR TRANSABDOMINAL APPROACH

1 **A,** *Position:* Right semi-oblique. *Incision:* Make an anterior transverse incision (see page 865). Stand on the right.

B, Open the peritoneum fully. Insert a Balfour or Buchwalter retractor while packing the liver and gallbladder superiorly. Palpate the abdominal viscera and nodes. In-

cise the avascular right triangular ligament of the liver to make it easier to shift the liver medially. Pack the liver superiorly, but avoid injury to the underside. Have your assistant retract the ascending colon medially. Pick up the parietal peritoneum and incise it over the kidney near the colon. Extend this incision from the aortic bifurcation to above the renal pedicle in front of the vena cava.

With large tumors, the peritoneum covering the kidney may be infiltrated by the tumor; as a consequence, an incision in it becomes difficult. It may be advisable to begin the incision at the caudal end of the tumor, where the peritoneal layers are intact. Even then, if the tumor has grown in the direction of the colon, detachment may be difficult. Avoid injuring the vessels in the mesocolon. With large tumors obstructing the renal vein, the *collateral circulation* may be widespread not only dorsally in Gerota's fascia and over the psoas and quadratus lumborum muscles but also ventrally between Gerota's fascia and the peritoneum and mesocolon. These thin-walled vessels demand careful individual ligation.

2 Mobilize the hepatic flexure of the colon and "kocherize" the duodenum by blunt dissection (see page 986). The second part of the duodenum may be closely connected to the tumor. Detach it by carefully dividing the connecting fibers by sharp dissection, and only then begin blunt dissection. The duodenum is in danger of injury, with necrosis and perforation as a consequence. In this region, do not coagulate; at the most, use only bipolar coagulation. If a superficial duodenal injury produces an expanding intramural hematoma, incise the serosa over it, clamp and ligate the bleeding vessel, and then close the serosa. If the duodenum is severely damaged, repair it in three layers around a tube brought out through a stab wound, and interpose the omentum.

Hold the bowel medially with retractors over moist laparotomy tapes. Place laparotomy tapes over the inferior edge of the wound, and hold them with a retractor blade. Beware of injury to the liver from inadequately padded retractors; if the liver is lacerated, pressure with warm laparotomy tapes usually controls the bleeding. Repair deep hepatic lacerations with carefully placed and tied interrupted horizontal mattress sutures. Remember to occasionally moisten the bowel and to watch it for compromised circulation.

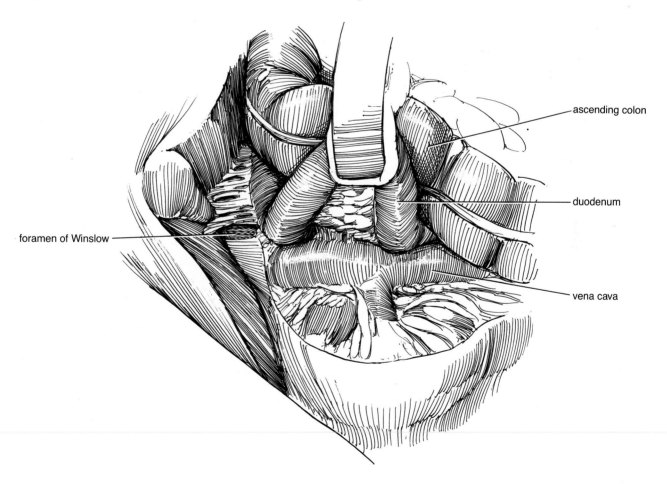

foramen of Winslow

ascending colon

duodenum

vena cava

3 **A,** Open the connective tissue over the vena cava to dissect on the left side. The superior mesenteric artery that runs over the left renal vein marks the upper limit of the operation. Clip or ligate and divide the lymphatics lying over the origin of the superior mesenteric artery, especially the large lacteals. Free the left renal vein. Keep close to the anterior surface of the aorta to avoid the lumbar veins. Palpate the right renal artery, and expose it by elevating the left renal vein and gently retracting the vena cava toward you. For large tumors that overlap the vena cava, it is easier to begin the dissection of the cava caudally, below the lower pole of the kidney, and then slowly work up while applying clips on the aortic side of the vena cava. With large, medially encroaching tumors, the superior mesenteric artery can be mistaken for the renal artery and ligated.

B, Pass a curved clamp beneath the right renal artery, grasp a 2-0 nonabsorbable ligature, pull it through, and tie it close to the aorta. Place a second suture and tie it. Clamp and divide the artery, and place a ligature on the distal end. An additional suture tie may be placed on the proximal stump. A better method may be to put one tie on the artery and proceed to divide the vein (Step 3C) before completing the ligation of the artery.

C, Dissect the right renal vein. Palpate the vein gently for any firmness that suggests a tumor thrombus. (For management of a thrombus, see page 1031.) Be on the lookout for short adrenal veins that empty directly into the side of the vena cava; divide them between ligatures. If the renal vein is large, using a right-angle clamp to dissect the dorsum can be tricky; beware of injury to the vein from excessively aggressive drilling on the hidden dorsal side. Instead, dissect the vein by carefully spreading the clamp. Avoid the entrance of the main adrenal vein into the vena cava. If that area is avulsed, grasp the stump with an Allis clamp and close it with a running 5-0 vascular suture. Or place one Satinsky clamp and then place a larger one beneath it; remove the top one, and oversew the stump. If the adrenal gland is injured, oversew the edge.

Watch for *lumbar veins* that come into the renal vein or vena cava at this level. When you encounter them, do not secure them with clips that may become displaced, but pass a 0 silk ligature on a right-angle clamp and tie it. For any large tumor with infiltration in the region of the hilum, it is advisable to apply a Satinsky clamp to the vena cava and to oversew the cut venous stump secondarily.

Dissect the renal vein distally, and inspect it for blood flow and contained tumor. If it is clear, proceed to clamp, divide, and ligate it. Hold up the stump and look for a lumbar vein entering from behind; such a vein requires ligation. Leave the distal suture on the renal vein long enough to allow identification by the pathologist.

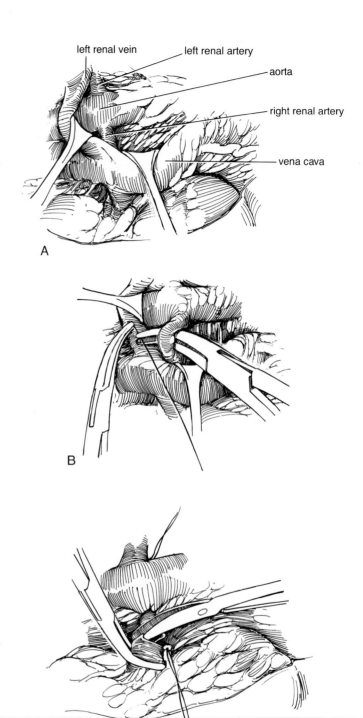

left renal vein   left renal artery

aorta

right renal artery

vena cava

A

B

C

4 Clear the anterior surface of the vena cava, and ligate the gonadal vein. Free the lymphatic tissue from the vena cava, moving toward the right. Clip all lymphatic vessels.

Mobilize the ureter and gonadal vein bluntly to the level of the bifurcation of the aorta. Lift them into the wound; clamp and ligate each of them with 0 silk ligatures, leaving the proximal suture long enough for identification later. Pick up the lateral edge of the peritoneum below the tumor, and incise it vertically up to the liver, then medially to just above the adrenal gland.

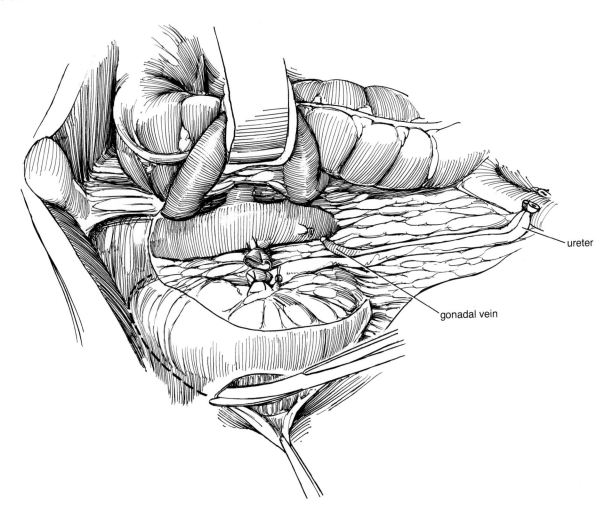

ureter

gonadal vein

5 Lift the lower pole of the kidney with the left hand, and mobilize Gerota's fascia enclosing the kidney from the posterior body wall. Clip small vessels as they are encountered, and doubly clamp and ligate large collateral veins. It may be possible to clip these veins with large clips.

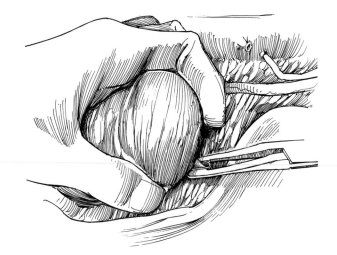

6 Pull down on the upper pole of the kidney to expose the adrenal gland, and progressively divide the connective tissue and vascular and peritoneal attachments. Dissection is easier if one proceeds laterally along the posterior body wall toward the crus of the diaphragm. The cranial connections to the adrenal gland must be divided carefully step by step between clips. Clip the small vessels and especially the lymphatics. In 75 percent of cases, abdominal computed tomography (CT) preoperatively shows that the ipsilateral adrenal gland is not involved (Gill et al, 1994), and ipsilateral adrenalectomy is not required.

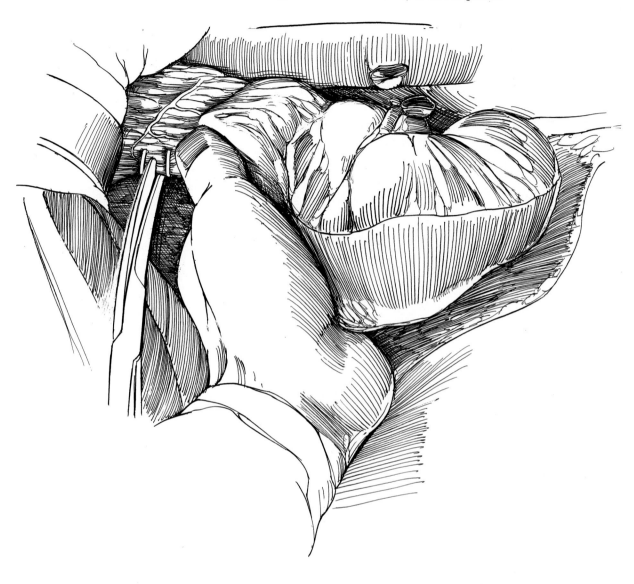

7 Displace the kidney caudally and laterally to visualize the vena cava and expose the right adrenal vein. Divide it between ligatures. Avoid interference with the small veins bridging the space between the liver and vena cava, but clip and divide the lymphatics and small adrenal arteries. Resectable tumors are those with medial extension to the aorta and vena cava; unresectable tumors are those with medial extension to the superior mesenteric vessels and celiac axis. It is of little use to excise part of the tumor; complete removal provides the patient's only chance for cure. If the colon or the spleen is involved, consider removing that organ.

Remove the tumor mass. It may be sensible to oversew the stumps of the renal artery and vein with 5-0 arterial

silk. Close the defects in the mesocolon to prevent internal hernias. Check blood pressure; if it is below normal, anticipate possible later bleeding from small vessels now in spasm.

Hepatic Involvement. Usually the tumor does not actually involve the liver parenchyma, being limited by Glisson's capsule. If the capsule is lacerated, apply hemostatic gauze under a pack, which may have to remain for 24 hours because suture methods of control fail. For invasion of the liver, perform right hepatectomy and right nephrectomy en bloc by controlling the renal vessels and ureter and then resecting the liver by controlling the hilar structures on the right side first. The mass can then be elevated to expose the vena cava to allow control of the hepatic veins.

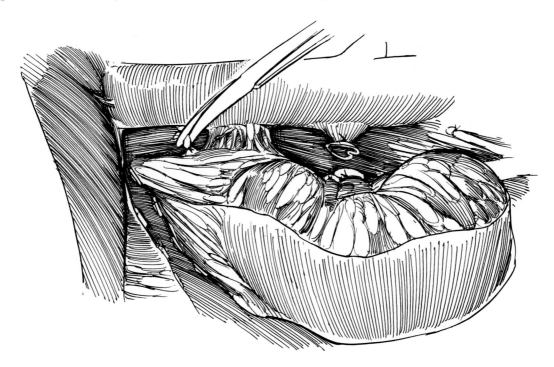

REGIONAL LYMPHADENECTOMY FOR RIGHT RENAL TUMORS

It is generally considered worthwhile to perform limited regional removal of hilar, paracaval, and para-aortic lymph nodes with resection of the corresponding interaortocaval nodes. The lymphadenectomy should extend above as far as the adrenal vein and below to the level of the inferior mesenteric artery.

8 **A,** Draw the vena cava toward you, and lift the left renal vein caudad. Clear the lymphatic tissue from the aorta, and pass it under the stump of the right renal vein. Clip all lymphatic vessels.

B, Continue along the aorta to its bifurcation. The lumbar arteries and veins may or may not require division.

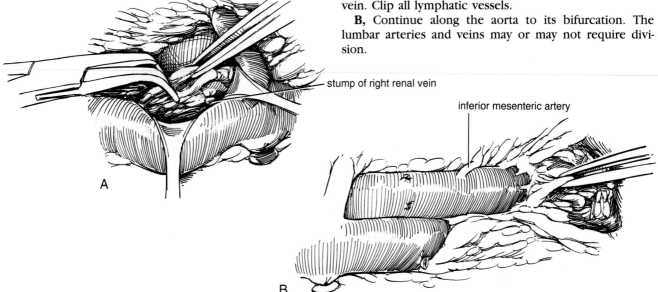

stump of right renal vein

inferior mesenteric artery

A

B

9 **A,** Retract the vena cava to the left, and dissect the tissue from behind it and from the right side of the aorta.

B, Continue to the level of the aortic bifurcation.

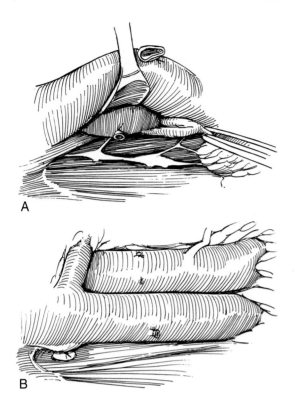

A

B

LEFT RADICAL NEPHRECTOMY, LATERAL APPROACH

A supracostal incision may be preferable to a transverse incision, but for very large tumors the thoracoabdominal approach is best (see page 890). Because a left transperitoneal approach carries an increased risk of splenic injury with splenectomy and consequent increased susceptibility to infection, administer pneumococcal vaccine preoperatively to those older than 65 years.

10 **A,** *Incision:* Make an 11th-rib supracostal incision (see page 879), extending anteriorly, either at an angle as shown or more transversely. Open the peritoneum.

B, Pack the spleen, pancreas, and stomach upward and to the right side. This may not be easy in obese patients. Place a self-retaining retractor, and cover the intestines with a moist pack. Beware of injuring the spleen with a retractor, and be sure to inspect the spleen before closing the abdomen.

Pick up and incise the posterior peritoneum along the white line lateral to the descending colon from the bifurcation of the aorta to a point above the adrenal gland. Divide the anterior lamella of the splenocolic ligament to move the splenic flexure medially. Divide the lienorenal ligaments to mobilize the pancreas and spleen upward and to the right.

Alternative: The pedicle of the left kidney can be exposed by freeing the greater omentum from the transverse colon and splenic flexure and by retracting the colon and the stomach, spleen, and pancreas upward while moving the large intestine downward.

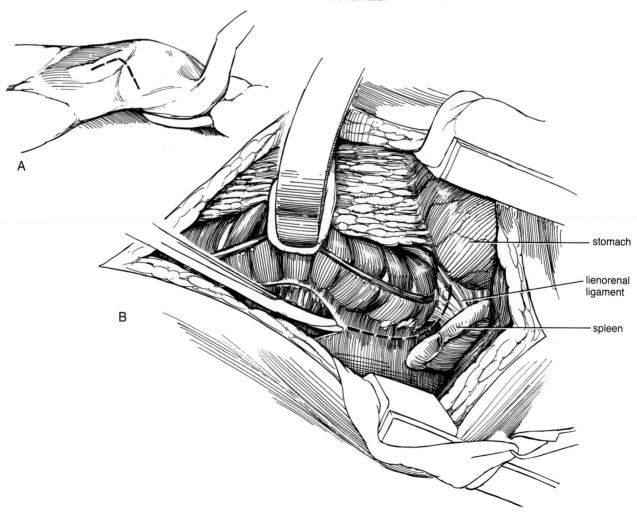

A

B

stomach

lienorenal ligament

spleen

Watch for infiltration and invasion of the mesocolon, the colon itself, and the tail of the pancreas. Preoperative studies often give little evidence of the involvement of these structures.

If the pancreas is injured, obtain a consultation from a general surgeon. Close a simple laceration with synthetic absorbable mattress sutures, and drain the retroperitoneum with a sump drain. If the pancreatic duct is also injured, resect the tail of the pancreas, ligate the duct, close the capsule, and provide free drainage. For repair of splenic injuries, see page 903.

11 Hold the colon up, and dissect between it and Gerota's fascia over a wide area. Dissect medially to first expose the anteromedial aspect of the vena cava and then the aorta. If the tumor is large and extends medially or if the patient is obese, it may be difficult to uncover the aorta. Begin the dissection caudal to the renal hilum, and locate the renal vein where it crosses the aorta. For large tumors with involved lymph nodes, the dissection of the renal artery can be difficult because of its dorsolateral junction with the aorta. Remove the

connective tissue and lymphatics to expose the left renal vein. Apply downward traction on the vein to expose the left renal artery. Be sure to identify the superior mesenteric artery as distinct from the renal artery. Ligate and divide the adrenal vein to prevent tearing it during traction on the renal vein.

In many cases, the mesocolon has attached itself to the anterior surface of the tumor, making this dissection difficult. If such is the case, leave a portion of the mesocolon on the tumor. The colon is adequately supplied by the marginal arcades. In addition, look for connections between the tail of the pancreas and the tumor and, with a cranially situated tumor, for the splenic vessels.

Place and tie a ligature around the renal artery close to its origin. Look for accessory renal arteries and ligate them if present. Generally and theoretically, it is better to ligate the artery first. However, it is sometimes easier, on approaching the pedicle from the front, to ligate and divide the vein first, after which the artery is readily exposed and quickly clamped and ligated.

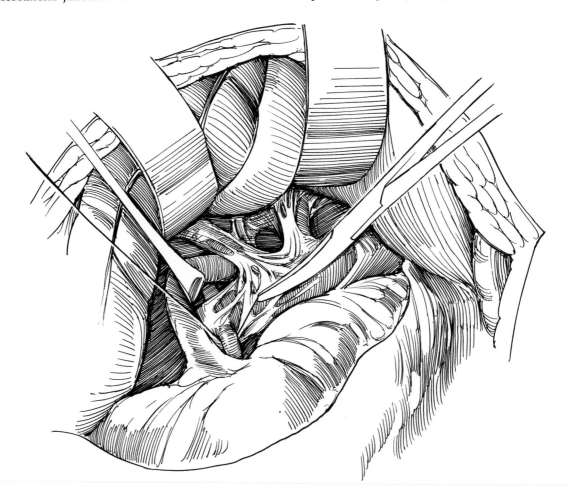

12 Dissect the left renal vein as it crosses the aorta. Palpate it carefully for contained thrombus. Doubly clamp, divide, and ligate it. Dissect it laterally to locate and divide the lumbar vein. Do not expose the adrenal or gonadal veins; they are included in the en bloc dissection. Complete the dissection of the left renal artery and clamp it distally. Divide and ligate the left renal artery both proximally and distally.

Free the ureter and the gonadal veins as low as can be done easily, and divide them between clamps. Ligate the tissue distally and proximally. Leave the sutures long on the side of the specimen.

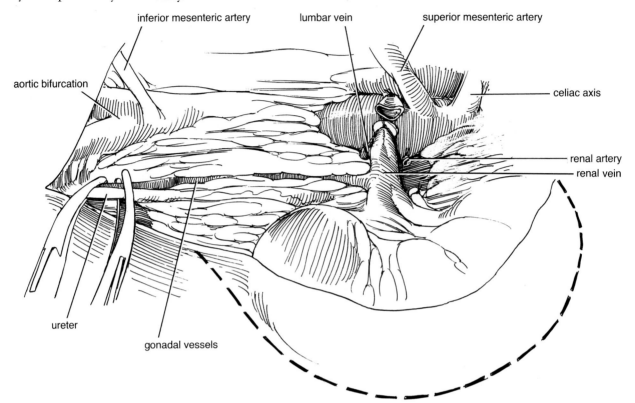

inferior mesenteric artery   lumbar vein   superior mesenteric artery

aortic bifurcation

celiac axis

renal artery
renal vein

ureter

gonadal vessels

13 Divide the peritoneum laterally over the lateral border of the kidney. Free the posterior and lateral surfaces of the specimen by blunt and sharp dissection outside the envelope of Gerota's fascia. Work from the caudal end of the dissection up to the medial border while dividing any additional vessels so that the lower pole of the kidney can be completely freed. Clip each vessel as it is encountered; use large clips on large collateral veins.

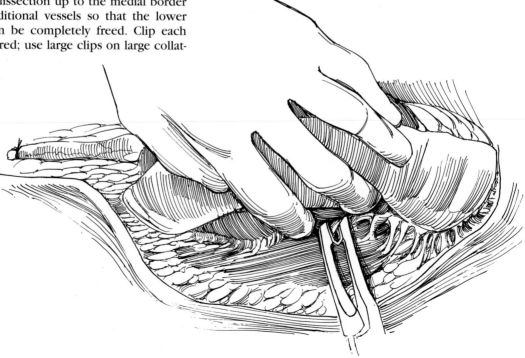

14 Complete the step-by-step dissection on the cranial and medial borders by pressing the kidney downward and laterally to allow dissection along the crus of the diaphragm and to expose the remaining small vessels and the adrenal artery. Remove the specimen.

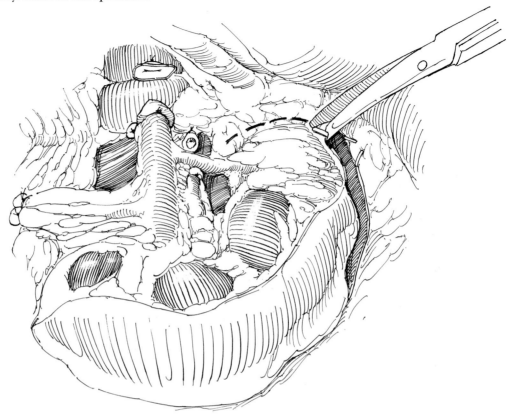

REGIONAL LYMPHADENECTOMY FOR LEFT RENAL TUMORS

15 Retract the vena cava to the right, and dissect the lymphatic tissue from the anterior and lateral surfaces of the aorta. Clip or ligate all the lymphatics at their upper margins.

16 Dissect caudally along the aorta, preserving the superior mesenteric artery as well as the celiac ganglia and splanchnic nerves, which lie on the aorta at its origin. Continue down between the vena cava and aorta and along the lateral surface of the aorta to the inferior mesenteric artery. Lumbar vessels need not be taken. Remove the specimen after appropriately marking it with silk ties for orientation. Check the spleen for injury (see page 903). Close the wound in layers around a Penrose drain.

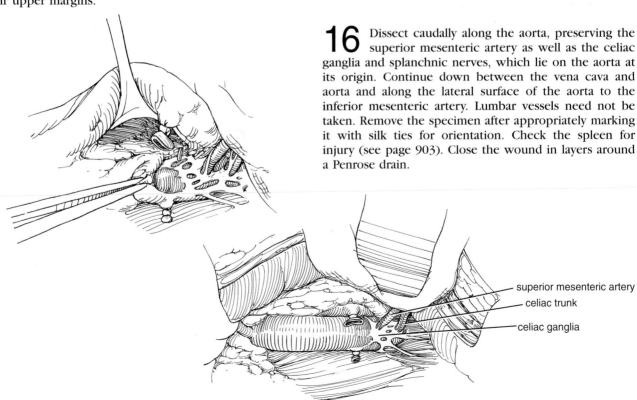

superior mesenteric artery

celiac trunk

celiac ganglia

POSTOPERATIVE PROBLEMS

Postoperative pulmonary care is important because vital capacity has already been reduced by the incision. *Pulmonary complications* of atelectasis and lobar collapse can be prevented by assiduous inflation and suctioning. The diaphragm can be injured as the crus is divided and resutured during retrocrural dissection of nodes that lie above the renal hilum. It is also traversed in the thoracoabdominal approach and, to prevent later herniation, requires reapproximation with interrupted sutures, with a running fine suture on the pleural surface.

For a *collapsed lung* that fails to expand, arrange for bronchoscopy. A *tension pneumothorax* can occur if the lung is inadvertently cut or if an old adhesion separates with a tear. In an emergency, push a needle into the second intercostal space; then insert a pleural drain attached to a water seal (see page 902). *Pleural effusions* should be aspirated.

Pancreatic injury may not be recognized intraoperatively. After operation, an elevation of serum amylase levels, an alkaline drainage from the wound, or a retroperitoneal collection of fluid is highly suggestive. Analyze the fluid for amylase, and obtain a CT scan to identify the pocket; then drain it. Expect spontaneous closure of the fistula, but hyperalimentation is required during that time.

The *spleen* may be injured during left nephrectomy from an anterior approach if the splenocolic and lienophrenic attachments are not divided to allow the spleen to be swung up out of the way. If injury occurs, resort to splenorrhaphy (see page 903) and avoid splenectomy, which increases the susceptibility to septicemia. Pneumococcal vaccine should be given routinely to patients over the age of 65 undergoing left transperitoneal nephrectomy.

Bleeding from the wound is usually from a loose vessel in the muscle layers. Pressure on the area often arrests the bleeding. *Vascular injuries* should be minimal if adequate exposure is obtained through a sufficiently large incision with adequate mobilization of the bowel. On the right side, the adrenal vein is vulnerable to injury where it enters the deep side of the vena cava. If your assistant lifts the right lobe of the liver and retracts the vena cava while you are dissecting, laceration or avulsion may be avoided. The superior mesenteric artery and the celiac vessels are at risk when large tumors create distortion. If one of these vessels is transected, reanastomose it, using a borrowed arterial segment if necessary. *Sagging of the flank* resembling a hernia may result from division of more than the 12th intercostal nerve. *Locally recurrent tumor* may be treated by an aggressive surgical approach, perhaps with neoadjuvant therapy. Here, postoperative complications are common because resection of adjacent organs is usually necessary (Tanguay et al, 1996).

Commentary by Ernst J. Zingg

Radical nephrectomy remains the only effective method of management in renal cell carcinoma. For small tumors, bilateral tumors, and tumors in a solitary kidney, however, partial resection has gained wide acceptance. Radical nephrectomy involves removal of the affected organ, the renal capsule and fatty tissue, Gerota's fascia, and, in tumors of the upper pole of the kidney, usually the ipsilateral adrenal gland. The surgical procedure should include the application of appropriate measures to the renal artery and vein to ensure that no neoplastic cells enter the circulation.

With the exception of the purely lumbar access, which is inadequate for radical nephrectomy, most of the accepted access routes allow tactically correct surgical procedures for nephrectomy as follows: the transverse approach, the midline transabdominal approach, the supracostal approach, and the thoracoabdominal approach. An essential prerequisite is, of course, familiarity with the access routes and with the problems of nephrectomy. We favor a supracostal approach above the 10th or 11th rib, with elongation anteriorly. The pleura can be dissected bluntly, and entering the pleural cavity is not compulsory. In large tumors, especially upper-pole tumors, we use the thoracoabdominal approach. This technique facilitates preparation of the infradiaphragmatic area and also allows simple mobilization of the liver, which can be displaced medially after the triangular ligaments and the coronal ligament are divided.

Invasion of the liver is rather uncommon because the Glisson capsule forms the barrier. Direct infiltration into the duodenum and wall of the colon is rare. Lesions of the duodenum with fistula postoperatively are usually the result of extensive coagulation or excessive retractor pressure. Few cases of renal cell carcinoma of the left kidney were found to have invasion of the tail of the pancreas. Simple resection, oversewing of the pancreatic duct, covering of the resected area with greater omentum, and adequate drainage ensure a subsequent uneventful postoperative course.

We consider the vena cava to be the reference landmark with tumors of the right kidney. This vessel can be followed upward to the point where the left renal vein enters. Before dealing with the renal vessels, we prefer to ligate and dissect the gonadal vein at the point where it enters the vena cava. The right renal artery lies below the renal vein. If preparation is uncomplicated, double ligation and division may follow. If technical difficulties arise, the vessel is ligated but not divided. The blood flow is interrupted and the venous system is no longer under pressure. In the absence of a tumor thrombus in the renal vein or the vena cava, the renal vein may be exposed.

Extracorporeal Renal Surgery

The advantages of extracorporeal repair of the kidney (ECRS) are better exposure and illumination, a bloodless surgical field, the ability to protect the kidney from prolonged ischemia, and the opportunity to use the microscope. For neoplasms, in situ surgery is usually adequate and much easier to perform. However, the procedure is applicable to complex branch renal artery disease and occasionally to renal lithiasis and renal trauma.

Preoperatively, assess renal function with radioisotope renography. Evaluate vascular topography with intravenous urography and selective arteriography to be able to identify the apical, basilar, and anterior and posterior segments. With malignancy, perform computed tomography (CT), magnetic resonance imaging (MRI), or both, and rule out metastases. Assess the internal iliac artery and its branches in anticipation of their use as a graft and the external iliac artery for renal arterial anastomosis.

Instruments: Provide a workbench with a basin, ice slush (see page 1048), cryoprecipitated plasma perfusate, Collins or Sachs solution, 10 percent low molecular weight dextran, a Mox-100 pulsatile perfusion unit, microvascular instruments, and surgical loupes.

The workbench can be a simple table, low enough to allow the surgeons to operate seated. It should hold a flat basin containing slush and can be equipped with an inlet and outlet for constant perfusion with cold dialysate. Except for the most complex procedures, a simple surface hypothermia set-up is adequate and cost effective. However, the advantages of constant pulsatile perfusion are that full vessels are easier to dissect, a nicked artery can be repaired, anastomotic leaks can be detected, core renal temperature is better controlled, and, in cases of partial nephrectomy, transected blood vessels on the surface of the renal parenchyma can be more readily identified.

1 *Incisions:* Select one that allows both nephrectomy and autotransplantation.

A, Anterior subcostal and contralateral oblique lower quadrant incisions are useful in an obese patient, especially when a prolonged extracorporeal operating time is anticipated, because the subcostal incision can be closed and the patient returned to the recovery room for the interval.

B, Midline incision, preferred for most patients.

C, Anterior oblique incision extended into the lower quadrant.

Give 500 ml of 10 percent low molecular weight dextran intravenously during the operation. Expose the kidney and move it outside of Gerota's fascia. Rapidly infuse 12.5 g mannitol intravenously before clamping the renal artery. Preserve as much of the vasculature as possible on the kidney, taking special care not to interfere with the ureteral or pelvic blood supply. If the ureter is not divided, encircle it with a Penrose drain to prevent backbleeding, and perform the dissection of the kidney over the patient's abdomen. In most cases, it is better to divide the ureter and subsequently implant it into the bladder to allow transfer of the kidney to a workbench, where the surgeon can sit and conveniently dissect and anastomose. It also allows a second team to secure a vascular graft, if needed, and to prepare the transplant site in the iliac fossa.

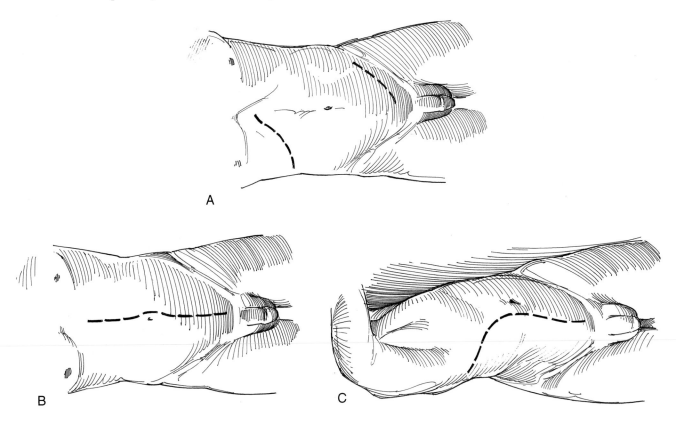

A

B

C

2 Immediately after dividing the renal vessels, place the kidney on the workbench in a pan of ice slush covered with a towel. Flush the kidney intra-arterially by gravity flow with at least 500 ml of Sachs or Collins solution at 6° C; use enough to cool the kidney and to clear it of intrarenal blood. Intermittently reflush the kidney during the repair to maintain low core temperature. Alternatively, after the initial flush, keep the kidney under ice slush in a basin to avoid the need for recurrent flushing.

For renovascular disease, dissect the renal hilum, using loupes or dissecting microscope. For neoplasms, remove Gerota's fascia and the perirenal fat to visualize the extent of the proposed partial nephrectomy (see page 1000). After renovascular repair (see page 937) or partial nephrectomy (see page 1000) (take a biopsy specimen for frozen-section examination to determine clear margins), attach the kidney to the pulsatile perfusion unit and perfuse alternately through the artery and the vein to enable suture ligation of potential bleeding points. Ignore parenchymal oozing. Close a bleeding site if possible.

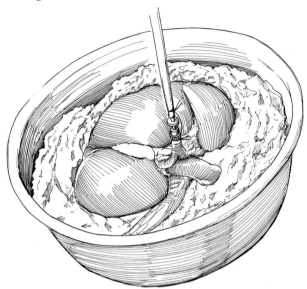

3 Transplant the kidney into either lower quadrant (see page 956). When the ureter is intact, implant the inverted kidney ipsilaterally, or make a retroperitoneal tunnel and move the kidney to the contralateral side. Insert a Penrose drain and close the wound. If the ureter has been transected, consider placing a nephrostomy tube (see page 928). Transfer the kidney to the iliac fossa, and anastomose the renal vein to the external iliac vein and the renal artery either end to end with the hypogastric artery (**A**) or end to side with the external iliac artery (**B**). Implant the ureter into the bladder.

Postoperatively, make baseline radioisotope studies on day 1. If these results are equivocal, perform intravenous digital subtraction angiography. Follow up with tomographic cuts because the bony pelvis interferes with visualization during intravenous urography. If a nephrostomy tube is in place, perform gravity nephrostography before its removal.

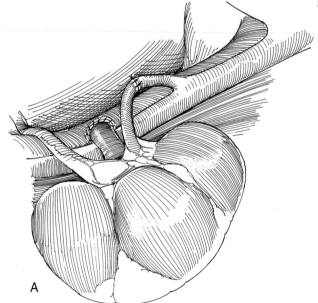

A

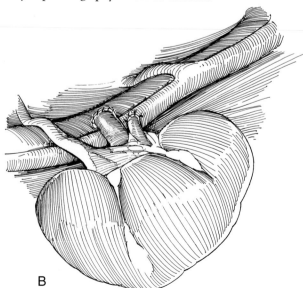

B

RENOVASCULAR DISEASE

Use ECRS for vascular disease not correctable by in situ techniques, such as intrarenal branch arterial diseases causing hypertension and/or impairing renal function. It may be used when in situ repair has not given good results or in an adult with fibrous disease or aneurysms in multiple branches, for which microscopic techniques are needed. Also, reoperation for renovascular disease may be easier on the workbench. For repair, select one of several alternative autogenous vascular grafts, such as the saphenous vein graft (see page 953).

4 **A,** The hypogastric artery, when not involved in atherosclerosis, may be used intact with its branches.

B, Anastomose each branch end to end to a distal branch of the renal artery, using a loupe.

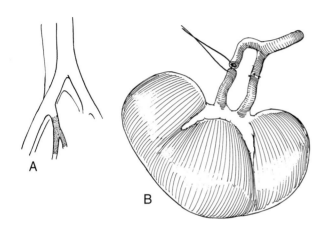

5 If the hypogastric artery is atherosclerotic, select the saphenous vein (see page 953). Construct sequential end-to-side anastomoses to fashion a branched graft.

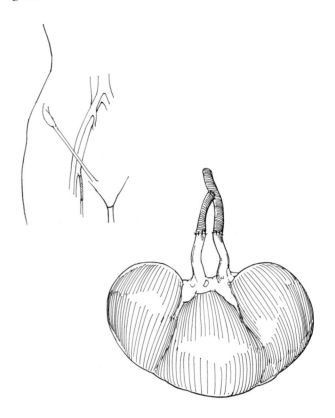

RENAL NEOPLASMS

ECRS has very limited application. It may be used for the solitary kidney or for bilateral disease. It may be appropriate for a large, very vascular, centrally located tumor. Unfortunately, with ECRS, clamping of the vein and artery must be delayed during dissection of the kidney and surrounding tissue, with the possibility for intravascular dislodgment of tumor.

Leave the ureter intact, if possible, to provide collateral circulation after revascularization by performing the procedure on the patient's abdomen, and only (gently) clamping the ureter to prevent back-bleeding.

6 **A,** For partial nephrectomy (see page 1001) of nonpolar neoplasms, clear the fat from the capsule to evaluate the extent of the disease and from the hilum to assess the vascular supply. Begin dissection of the tumor at the hilum and proceed peripherally. Using loupes, dissect, suture-ligate with 4-0 SAS, and divide each artery and vein that supplies the tumor. Leave a 2-cm margin of normal kidney. Insert a nephrostomy tube (not shown). Close the collecting system with running 4-0 SAS. Obtain samples for frozen-section examination to determine if tumor persists. Perform regional lymphadenectomy.

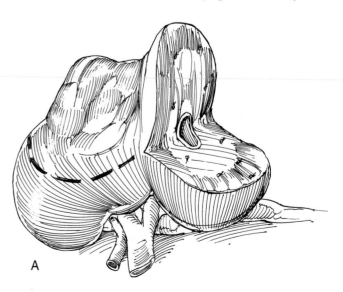

B, Check the security of the vessels by perfusing the kidney on the pulsatile perfusion unit alternately through the artery and the vein. Suture-ligate the transected vessels on the renal surface. Again, ignore parenchymal oozing. If possible, reapproximate the renal parenchyma, or cover the defect with absorbable gauze. Reunite the ureter over a stent (see page 835). Autotransplant the kidney into the iliac fossa and restore urinary continuity by ureteroneocystostomy; ureteropyelostomy is an alternative. If the ureter was not divided, avoid rotation during implantation. Leave a nephrostomy tube in place. Bring

the tube and a Penrose drain extraperitoneally to exit laterally in the lower quadrant.

Blood and fluid losses may be large, requiring careful monitoring and adequate replacement, especially because the patient has been anephric for part of the operation. Hemodialysis may be required for a period of time.

POSTOPERATIVE PROBLEMS

Vascular and ureteral anastomotic problems are similar to those after renal transplantation (see page 965).

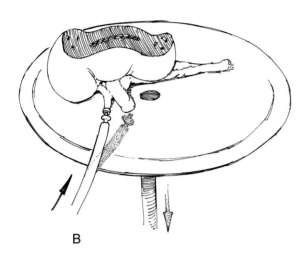

B

Commentary by Michael Marberger

With the use of renal ischemia and hypothermia, ample exposure, and microsurgical techniques with loupe magnification, almost all intricate intrarenal surgery can be performed in situ without division of the vascular pedicle. Bench surgery has become obsolete for removing renal stones. For nephron-sparing excision of renal cell carcinoma, removing only central tumors that invade the renal vein but do not spread systemically appears justified. Reconstruction of the renal vein can be performed more reliably ex vivo. In our experience, tumors of this type are extremely rare.

Lymphadenectomy must be performed before the kidney is removed. If frozen-section examination demonstrates lymphatic spread, neither nephron-sparing excision nor nephrectomy with chronic dialysis can cure the patient. The high morbidity of both approaches renders them unjustified. Bench surgery is therefore today limited mainly to difficult reconstruction of intrarenal arteries, most often after a primary attempt at in situ repair has failed.

Autotransplantation, however, remains an excellent way to bridge extensive defects of the midureter, such as with iatrogenic strictures or after trauma. By bringing the kidney down to the iliac fossa, most or all of the ureter can be removed and urinary drainage accomplished under physiologic conditions. Because extracorporeal manipulation is effective and ureteroneocystostomy is performed with healthy tissues, morbidity is low and the results are excellent. Unless the renal pedicle is scarred from previous surgery, we prefer autotransplantation to ureteral replacement with ileum. We use it to save a good kidney even with a normal contralateral kidney.

Multifocal superficial transitional cell carcinoma of the ureter or pelvis of a solitary kidney can be treated by the same technique. If necessary, the entire upper tract collecting system can be removed. The pelvis is then anastomosed directly to the bladder, anchoring the bladder musculature to the renal capsule around the hilum. The higher bladder pressure seems to have no significant impact on renal function. Follow-up is performed by cystoscopy, and recurrent tumors may even be fulgurated transurethrally.

Vena Caval Thrombectomy

A vena caval thrombus is managed in conjunction with radical nephrectomy (see page 1016).

1 Determine the extent of the thrombus by a coronal cut on magnetic resonance imaging (MRI). Computed tomographic (CT) scanning and ultrasonography identify inferior vena caval involvement but do not indicate the cephalad extent of a thrombus (Goldfarb et al, 1990). Use the more accurate contrast venacavography for a patient with suspected cardiac involvement or one in whom the extent of the thrombus is unclear on MRI. If antegrade cavography does not completely outline the thrombus, perform retrograde cavography to determine the distal limits of the thrombus.

Renal arteriography may show hypervascularity of the thrombus supplied by distinct vessels from the renal artery. This finding is an indication for renal arterial embolization 2 to 3 days before surgery. If the vena caval thrombus lights up on aortography, it probably has acquired an independent blood supply that requires resection of the vena caval wall.

Use ultrasonography or transesophageal echocardiography preoperatively or intraoperatively to determine the extent of the thrombus, especially in patients with conflicting findings on cavography. Ultrasonography can also be of value in detecting venous anomalies and in determining the approach to the vena cava. Echocardiography also gives useful information on venous return and left ventricular function with a thrombus above the level of the hepatic veins.

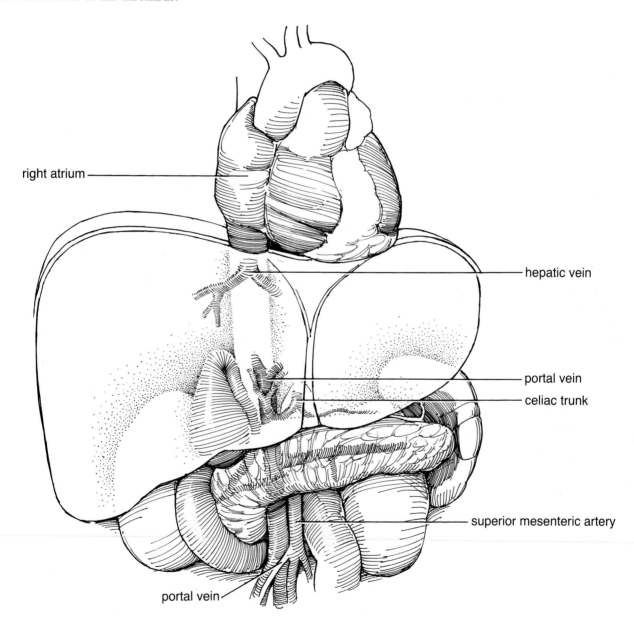

right atrium

hepatic vein

portal vein

celiac trunk

superior mesenteric artery

portal vein

2 Classify the condition into one of three groups: Group I, infradiaphragmatic infrahepatic extension; Group II, supradiaphragmatic intrapericardial or suprahepatic extension; and Group III, supradiaphragmatic intracardiac extension. Consider collaboration with a vascular surgeon. Classification may change after intraoperative ultrasonography more clearly defines the extent of the thrombus.

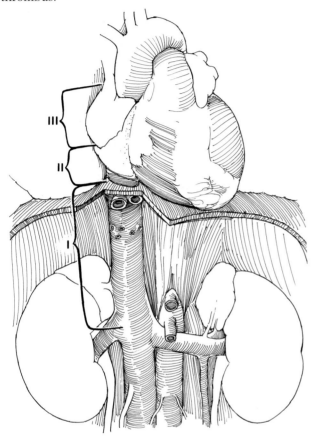

Incisions

A thoracoabdominal incision is appropriate for most cases (see page 890). If supradiaphragmatic extension of the tumor in the vena cava is present and cardiopulmonary bypass is required, a midline incision with a median sternotomy is preferable. The sternotomy can be extended by converting the lower end into a transverse upper abdominal (chevron) incision. If the tumor is very large, a bilateral subcostal incision with T-extension can give needed exposure.

THROMBUS WITH RIGHT RENAL TUMOR

For tumors on the right side, which are more common and in general less difficult to manage than those on the left, a right thoracoabdominal incision may be used, although the liver is in the way. It is necessary to work not only under the liver but also over it, between it and the diaphragm. This is often a difficult maneuver and one that can result in injury to a hepatic vein. It is essential that these patients have normal liver function. Alternatively, use a midline incision with a median sternotomy if more exposure is needed.

If a thoracoabdominal incision is used, open the anterior end first to assess operability (e.g., hepatic metastases, invasion of the mesocolon and hilar nodes, and involvement of the posterior abdominal musculature). Expose and explore the right renal hilum. Perform biopsy on any suspicious nodes for frozen-section examination. Positive findings are usually a contraindication to proceeding. Mobilize the mesenteries of the right and transverse colon, small bowel, and duodenum. Divide the inferior mesenteric vein, and place the bowel in a plastic bag on the chest.

GROUP 1: INFRADIAPHRAGMATIC INFRAHEPATIC EXTENSION

Insert intra-arterial and Swan-Ganz catheters to prepare for large blood losses.

Small Infradiaphragmatic Thrombus

3 Expose the renal vein and retract it gently. It is good practice to control the vena cava above with a Rommel tourniquet or a caval occlusion clamp, to be certain that the thrombus does not become dislodged and embolize. Avoid the lumbar veins. Pass a 2-0 silk suture around the renal artery and ligate it. The dashed line indicates the line of incision in the renal vein and vena cava.

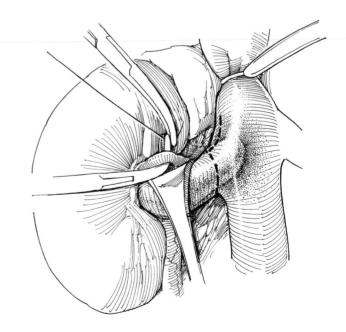

4 Place a Satinsky clamp on the vena cava beyond the thrombus. In a difficult case, consider placing the clamp and dividing the renal vein before clamping the artery, even though that can trap as much as a unit of blood in the kidney. Make a J-shaped incision around the renal vein and up the vena cava to obtain a generous cuff. Take care not to cut into the thrombus.

Alternatively, resect an ellipse of vena cava around the renal vein. Identify the plane between the thrombus and the intima, and gently free the thrombus by using the back of a knife, a finger, or a Küttner dissector to remove all of it from the vena cava. Resection of the wall of the vena cava because of adherence of tumor is rarely necessary. Immediately fasten a 4 × 4 pad of gauze over the thrombus and renal vein and tie it in place to prevent spillage of tumor cells.

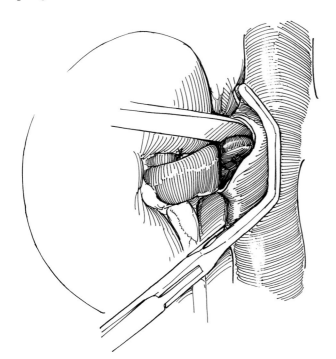

5 Ligate the renal artery again, once it is more exposed, and divide it distal to the ligatures.

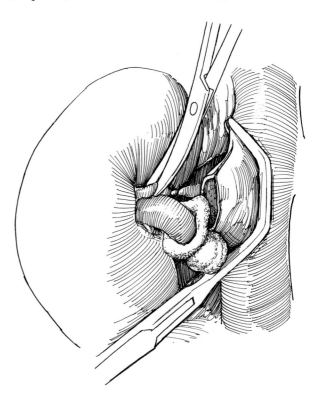

6 Close the vena cava with a running 5-0 vascular silk or Prolene suture; then run it back as a second layer.

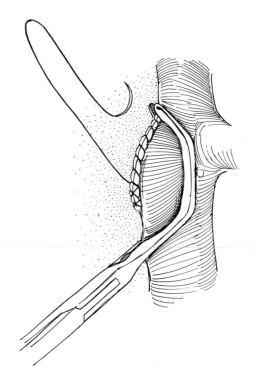

Large Infradiaphragmatic Thrombus

7 Obtain vascular control sequentially as follows: (**1**) right renal artery; (**2**) subhepatic vena cava; (**3**) proximal vena cava, above the bifurcation; (**4**) left renal vein. Control of the porta hepatis (**5**) is not necessary. Expose the vena cava up to the insertion of the hepatic veins, and place an arterial tourniquet around it at this level. Dissect the vena cava below the renal vein, and control bleeding with a tourniquet. Do the same for the left renal vein. If the kidney becomes engorged, control the left renal artery. Ligate the right renal artery.

8 Incise an ellipse of vena cava around the right renal vein, and carefully dissect the thrombus free from the cava. Place a Satinsky clamp in the vena cava. Cover the thrombus with gauze. Ligate the renal artery again and proceed with nephrectomy. Remove the vascular clamps in the following sequence to allow evacuation of air and debris: (**4**) left renal vein tourniquet; (**next**) Satinsky clamp on the cavotomy (hold the edges of the vena cava in forceps to assist the replacement of the clamp and release it momentarily to allow air to escape); (**2**) distal vena caval tourniquet; and (**3**) proximal vena caval tourniquet. Close the defect in the vena cava.

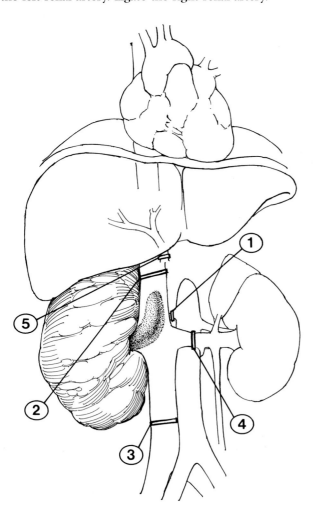

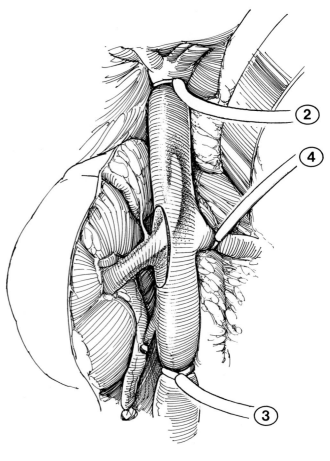

GROUP 2: SUPRADIAPHRAGMATIC INTRAPERICARDIAL OR SUPRAHEPATIC EXTENSION

Use a midline incision with a median sternotomy. A chevron extension may be required. Usually, is a cardiopulmonary bypass via the femoral vessels instituted by the cardiovascular team, even if the thrombus does not extend into the atrium.

Complete the renal dissection except for division of the vein before attachment to the pump.

9 Expose the renal artery as previously (Step 3), and ligate it with 2-0 silk ligatures. Extend the incision cephalad to the sternal notch, and there dissect the plane just beneath the deep periosteum. Insert the sternal saw and divide the sternum in the midline, exposing the pericardium and aortic adventitia. Press bone wax into the cut edges of the sternum. Insert a chest retractor.

Open the pericardium and suture it to the drapes with 2-0 silk sutures. Palpate the inferior vena cava inside the pericardium to locate the apex of the thrombus. Place a cardiac tourniquet loop around the intrapericardial inferior vena cava proximal to the thrombus, and temporarily occlude it while monitoring blood pressure.

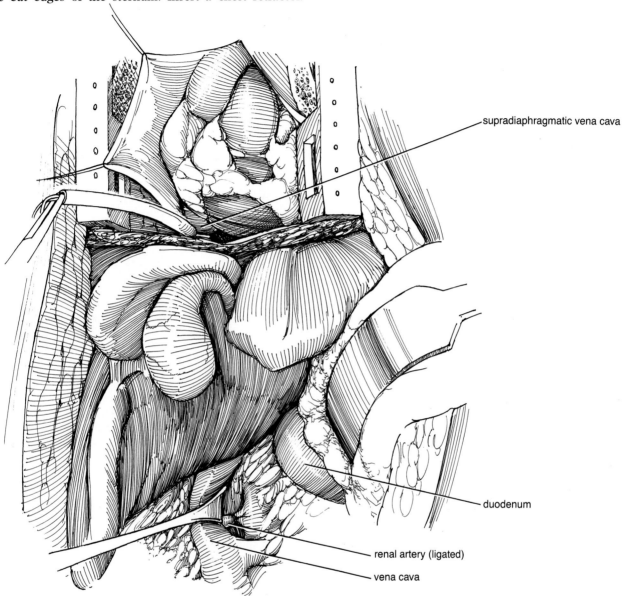

supradiaphragmatic vena cava

duodenum

renal artery (ligated)

vena cava

10 If the blood pressure is not reasonably maintained, an indication of inadequate collaterals, prepare for the possibility of cross-clamping the aorta above the celiac axis in the diaphragmatic hiatus with a vascular clamp. Remember that the right kidney has comparatively little collateral venous drainage.

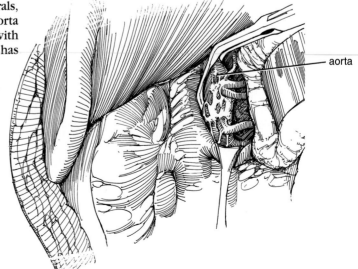

aorta

11 Divide the hepatic, the coronary, and the two triangular ligaments to mobilize the liver from its attachments to the diaphragm.

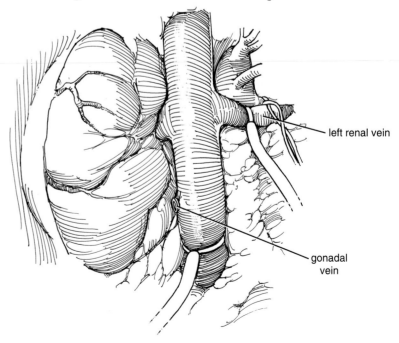

12 Rotate the liver medially to expose the retrohepatic cava. Divide the small inferior hepatic veins that lie caudal to the main hepatic vein. Divide the upper lumbar veins. Give heparin, and give mannitol in a dose of 25 g intravenously.

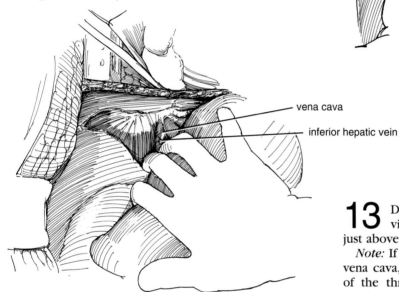

vena cava

inferior hepatic vein

13 Dissect the vena cava below the renal vein. Divide the gonadal vein. Place a Rumel tourniquet just above the bifurcation of the vena cava.

Note: If you feel a thrombus on palpation of the distal vena cava, gain vascular control beyond it. This portion of the thrombus is usually not malignant, but take a specimen for biopsy after extraction. It may be advisable to clip the vena cava to prevent pulmonary emboli. Place a Rumel tourniquet around the left renal vein. Place vascular tape around the left renal artery to reduce blood flow to the left kidney if its venous collateral through the gonadal and adrenal veins is inadequate.

left renal vein

gonadal vein

14 Prepare to clamp the porta hepatis at the foramen of Winslow to reduce back-bleeding from the hepatic veins. Ask the anesthetist to put the patient in a 20-degree Trendelenburg position to prevent air embolization and to facilitate later evacuation of intravascular air.

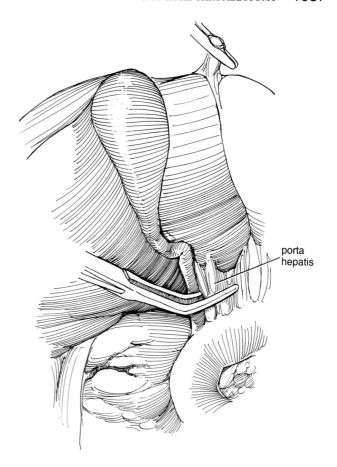

porta hepatis

15 Prepare the several vessels for vascular occlusion; then proceed in the following sequence: (1) cross-clamp the aorta (optional); if it is clamped, limit occlusion to a maximum of 30 minutes to avoid ischemia of the spinal cord, bowel, and left kidney; (2) occlude the vena cava in the pericardial sac after an interval determined by arterial and left ventricular filling pressure, avoiding hypervolemia or hypovolemia of the upper torso; (3) occlude the distal vena cava; (4) atraumatically clamp the porta hepatis; and (5) occlude the left renal vein.

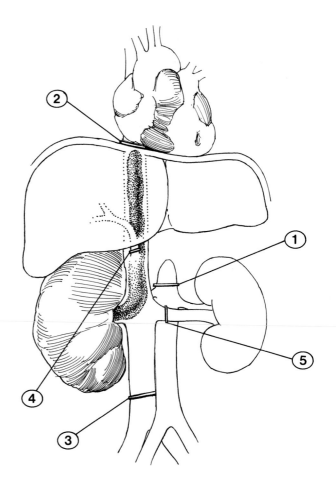

16 Incise the vena cava with a hooked blade, and open it with Potts scissors to about 8 cm below the hepatic veins. If the thrombus extends above the vena caval incision, insert a 20 F 30-ml balloon catheter through the opening until the tip can be felt above the thrombus. Inflate the balloon and gently pull it down while compressing the vena cava beyond it, which is either above or below the diaphragm, with the other hand. If the thrombus is too adherent, sweep it out with an index finger inserted in the vena cava. Occasionally, a Küttner dissector is needed. If the thrombus is solid, it can often be withdrawn intact; if it is friable and adherent to the caval wall, consider cardiopulmonary bypass to allow its resection.

The thrombus can be divided if the upper end is secured; it is not essential that it be removed in continuity. Flush the vena cava copiously with sterile water. Place a Satinsky clamp across the cavotomy. Divide the remaining posterior wall of the renal vein, ligate the distal stump, and cover it with gauze. When the thrombus involves the wall of the vena cava, a segment can be resected, but without much expectation of cure; the ends may simply be closed or a pericardial patch can be used to complete its closure.

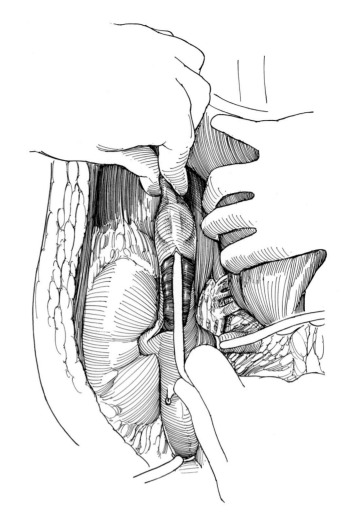

17 Remove the vascular clamps in sequence to allow evacuation of air and debris: (**1**) left renal vein tourniquet; (**2**) clamp on the porta hepatis; (**3**) Satinsky clamp on the cavotomy—hold the edges of the vena cava in forceps to assist the replacement of the clamp and release it momentarily to allow air to escape; (**4**) aortic cross-clamp, if the aorta had been clamped; (**5**) distal vena caval tourniquet; and (**6**) proximal vena caval tourniquet.

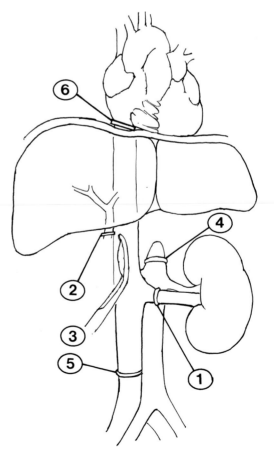

18 Close the cavotomy with a running 5-0 silk suture; then oversew it to provide a two-layer closure. Remove the Satinsky clamp. Drain the chest with two tubes in the mediastinum, and the renal fossa with suction inserted at the time of wound closure. Complete the nephrectomy, and proceed with lymph node dissection.

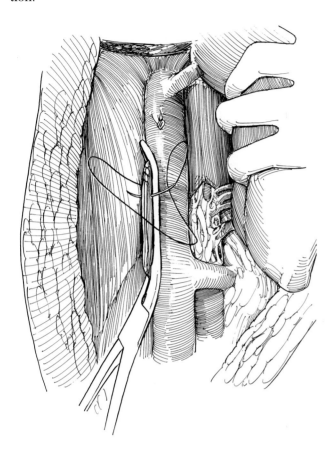

GROUP 3: SUPRADIAPHRAGMATIC INTRACARDIAC EXTENSION

Use cardiopulmonary bypass with deep hypothermic circulatory arrest to reduce the chance for massive hemorrhage or embolization by the thrombus and to allow as much as 1 hour for performing a complicated operation. Extensive retrohepatic or intrapericardial caval dissection is avoided because the distal inferior vena cava does not require formal isolation and control, and such dissection also avoids clamping of the porta hepatis, ligation of multiple lumbar veins, and cross-clamping of the aorta. The entire vena caval lumen can be inspected in a bloodless field, and the atrium can be opened to remove an atrial thrombus and also residual parts of the thrombus in the intrahepatic inferior vena cava.

Institute cardiopulmonary bypass with the cardiac surgery team. To avoid severe restriction in time to complete the operation, do it with deep hypothermic circulatory arrest, using total body hypothermia with exsanguination and circulatory arrest. Pack the patient's head in ice. Use

Left Renal Tumors

In contrast to the right kidney, which has little collateral venous drainage, the left kidney drains into the adrenal, lumbar, and gonadal veins. If the vena cava is resected with the left kidney, insert a section of saphenous vein or a pericardial graft to bridge the gap.

Tumors on the left side are more difficult to treat than those on the right and usually are more advanced. Use an anterior midline incision to allow exposure of both the right and left sides of the abdomen and retroperitoneum. Reflect the left colon.

19 Proceed as described for the right side, but adhere to the following sequence for occlusion: (1) left renal artery; (2) proximal aorta (optional); (3) proximal vena cava intrapericardially; (4) distal vena cava; (5) right renal vein. In addition, the right renal artery should be accessible so that it may be secured with a tourniquet while the right renal vein is occluded. Finally, occlude the porta hepatis (6).

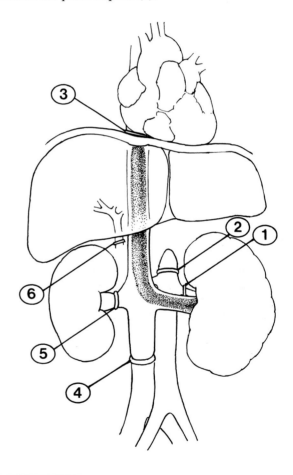

a transverse upper abdominal incision (chevron) combined with a median sternotomy. Mobilize the kidney until it is attached by only the renal vein. Less extensive mobilization of the retrohepatic vena cava is required when using adjunctive circulatory arrest. Heparinize the patient systemically.

Cannulate the heart and the ascending aorta for arterial circulation; cannulate the vena cava and femoral vein for venous circulation. Start the bypass, which allows 45 to 60 minutes for completion of the vascular part of the operation. Open the right atrium, and remove that portion of the thrombus. It may be adherent and require dissection from the wall, as is done with endarterectomy. Remove the infradiaphragmatic portion, as previously described. Sequentially close the atriotomy and the vena cava, and remove the patient from the bypass apparatus. Warm the patient. It is possible to repair coronary disease during cooling or rewarming. Give protamine to neutralize the heparin. Apply elastic stockings.

INTRAOPERATIVE PROBLEMS

For *vena caval wall involvement* with tumor, after resecting the vena cava, send the margin for a frozen-section diagnosis. If the findings are positive, resect more of the vena cava and provide a Gore-Tex graft to repair the defect.

Air embolism is the most serious complication. It can be prevented if the vascular clamps are applied and released in the proper order. Inspect the vena cava for large air bubbles before releasing the proximal clamp. If bubbles are seen, aspirate them with an 18-gauge needle on a syringe, and place a 6-0 silk suture to close the puncture site. *Tumor or clot embolism* occurs when manipulation of the tumor takes place before vascular control or when rough handling occurs during extraction. If respiratory distress is noted during the operation, proceed with thoracotomy, pulmonary arteriotomy, and extraction of the thrombus.

Control *massive hemorrhage* during the operation with laparotomy pad compression while the anesthetist stabilizes the circulation and additional help is mobilized. Release the pad slowly, and aspirate the blood with multiple suction devices until the bleeding site can be located and sutured. Consider placing a pack and removing it the next day. *Splenic rupture* has been reported after clamping of the porta hepatis. For *blood loss,* use the Cell Saver autologous blood recovery system to collect and allow retransfusion of blood lost in operations with estimated blood losses of more than 6 L. The expense of the device is so high, however, that it is not worth the cost for lesser amounts of blood. The device can be useful in patients with bleeding tendencies who are undergoing difficult operations. Whether it increases the risk of tumor seeding in a patient with malignant disease is debatable, but in patients with extensive renal malignancy, it certainly can be used safely before the vena cava is opened.

POSTOPERATIVE PROBLEMS

Pulmonary embolism can occur. Duodenal obstruction and transient encephalopathy have been reported. For *low urinary output,* give furosemide.

Acute renal failure may supervene from renal venous stasis secondary to operative constriction of the vena cava and requires hemodialysis.

To avoid *excessive bleeding* after cardiopulmonary bypass, give adequate platelets and fresh-frozen plasma plus desmopressin acetate, aminocaproic acid, or a combination of these in the immediate postoperative period. High doses of aprotinin can be used to normalize coagulation. Give Factor IX concentrate and cryoprecipitate if needed. Reoperation for massive bleeding may be necessary in a small number of patients

Commentary by Andrew C. Novick

One of the unique features of renal, adrenal, and certain retroperitoneal malignancies is their frequent pattern of growth intraluminally into the venous circulation. In extreme cases, this growth may extend into the inferior vena cava, with cephalad migration as far as the right atrium. The absence of metastases in some children with direct vena caval involvement from a malignancy remains intriguing. In most cases, an aggressive approach is warranted if the tumor is localized and complete surgical removal can be accomplished.

Accurate preoperative information regarding the presence and complete extent of an inferior vena caval (IVC) tumor thrombus is essential to determine the appropriate operative approach. CT scanning and ultrasonography detect gross renal vein and IVC involvement but are unreliable in delineating the cephalad extent of a thrombus. Inferior vena cavography has been the most accurate diagnostic study for assessment of IVC thrombi. However, a single antegrade study may be insufficient in the presence of complete caval occlusion; in such cases a second retrograde injection of the IVC is needed to define the distal limits of the thrombus. Recent data indicate that MRI is an accurate noninvasive method for delineating the full extent of IVC thrombi and is now the preferred caval imaging modality at most centers. Inferior vena cavography is reserved for patients in whom MRI findings are equivocal or MRI is contraindicated.

Renal arteriography remains an important preoperative study in patients with renal malignancy and an IVC thrombus. Large caval thrombi often demonstrate hypervascularity, with a distinct arterial supply from the renal artery. With this finding on arteriography, we perform renal arterial embolization 2 to 3 days before surgery. We have observed several cases of definite shrinkage in the size of a caval thrombus following such embolization, which has facilitated its intraoperative removal.

In performing surgical removal of an IVC thrombus, it is essential to obtain control of the vena cava above the thrombus to prevent intraoperative embolization of a tumor fragment. Temporary occlusion of the infrahepatic IVC can be safely done, but occlusion of the suprahepatic IVC often causes a profound decrease in venous return with hypotension. Additional disadvantages of the latter maneuver when removing a caval thrombus include back-bleeding from hepatic and lumbar veins and occasional swelling of the liver from venous congestion, which interferes with exposure. The adjunctive techniques for minimizing such problems with suprahepatic caval occlusion are outlined in this chapter. An intraoperative vena caval-atrial venous shunt is another available technique for use in this setting.

Cardiopulmonary bypass with deep hypothermic circulatory arrest offers several advantages for removal of a supradiaphragmatic vena caval thrombus. Because formal isolation and control of the distal IVC are not necessary, extensive retrohepatic or intrapericardial vena caval dissection is avoided. Occlusion of the porta hepatis, ligation of multiple lumbar veins, and aortic cross-clamping to prevent hemorrhage are not needed. Cardiopulmonary bypass with deep hypothermic circulatory arrest allows direct visual inspection of the entire vena caval lumen in a completely bloodless field. An atriotomy can be performed easily, which facilitates removal not only of an atrial thrombus but also of friable or adherent pieces of thrombus in the intrahepatic IVC. The risk of sudden massive intraoperative hemorrhage or distal tumor thrombus embolization is lessened. Finally, deep hypothermic circulatory arrest allows up to 60 minutes of safe ischemia in a bloodless field for the performance of vena caval thrombectomy or resection and appropriate vena caval reconstruction. The maximum period of safe ischemia with occlusion of the suprahepatic IVC and porta hepatis is no more than 30 minutes.

We have found that cardiopulmonary bypass with deep hypothermic circulatory arrest is a safe and effective approach. No ischemic or neurologic complications have occurred, and no cases of perioperative tumor embolization have been seen. The most common postoperative complication has been hemorrhage requiring surgical re-exploration, which has occurred in 8 percent of patients. Cardiopulmonary bypass is associated with temporary platelet dysfunction, and this effect may be enhanced with superimposed deep hypothermic circulatory arrest. This problem is generally managed with administration of platelets, fresh-frozen plasma, desmopressin acetate, aminocaproic acid, or a combination of these. Recent data also suggest that high-dose aprotinin has the ability to normalize coagulation dramatically after cardiopulmonary bypass and to reduce transfusion requirements.

Pyelolithotomy

Although the need to remove renal stones by open operation has been greatly reduced with the advent of percutaneous and shock-wave modalities, large stones may be more directly removed by pyelolithotomy or nephrolithotomy, especially if an expert endourologist or a lithotripsy machine is not available. The indications for removing stones surgically are (1) economy and the personal convenience of the patient, (2) associated disorders that require open operation, (3) infected cases needing definitive and expeditious clearance of calculi, (4) cases that have failed lithotripsy and endoscopic removal, and (5) cases that for technical reasons cannot be managed by lithotripsy. An open procedure is still indicated in cases of obstruction of a caliceal infundibulum, the ureteropelvic junction, or the lumbar ureter and when the volume and configuration of the stones contraindicate extracorporeal shock wave lithotripsy (ESWL) or a percutaneous approach, such as with caliceal stones larger than the renal pelvis.

For infected stones, obtain a urine culture while the patient is not taking antibiotics. Treat infection for 24 or 48 hours preoperatively based on sensitivity tests with an agent that achieves high urinary and tissue levels but is not nephrotoxic. Semisynthetic penicillins and cephalosporins are preferable to aminoglycosides. If aminoglycosides are used, check renal function before and after surgery. Obtain a kidney, ureter, and bladder film the morning of surgery, and have it and the pyelograms available for viewing in the operating room.

Instruments: Provide deep blades for the ring retractor; Gil-Vernet retractors; coagulum materials; Randall, Russian, and vascular forceps; a gallbladder set; a grooved sound; a portable x-ray with sterile plastic bag cover; an ultrasonic probe; a flexible nephroscope; an 18 F red rubber catheter or infant feeding tube; a J stent; a Water-Pik; a Küttner dissector; a hooked scalpel blade; angled Potts scissors; Andrews suction; a hand-held electrode; Allis-Adair clamps; and Stevens scissors. Place the latest films on the view box.

1 **A,** *Incision:* Select a flank incision (see page 879) or an anterior subcostal extraperitoneal incision (see page 871). In children, a lumbotomy incision may be effective (see page 896). With a flank incision, raise the kidney rest slowly to allow for circulatory stabilization.

B, Open Gerota's fascia laterally to provide for later fatty enclosure of the pyelotomy. After renal exposure, have the assistant rotate the kidney toward the midline with clamps on Gerota's fascia and the perirenal fat or with a sponge stick. Locate the ureter and encircle it with a small Penrose drain. Continue the dissection sharply and bluntly above the ureteropelvic junction into the hilum, working in the plane found directly on the adventitia of the pelvis. Russian forceps are useful if the fat is matted.

SIMPLE PYELOLITHOTOMY

2 Draw the hilum anteriorly with vein or Gil-Vernet retractors placed in the lip (not shown). Incise the pelvis transversely in the form of a U, starting with a hooked blade and continuing with Potts scissors. Stay well away from the ureteropelvic junction. If small stones are present, pass an 8 F infant feeding tube though the ureteropelvic junction to prevent stone migration. Stay sutures may not be needed; they can tear the tissue.

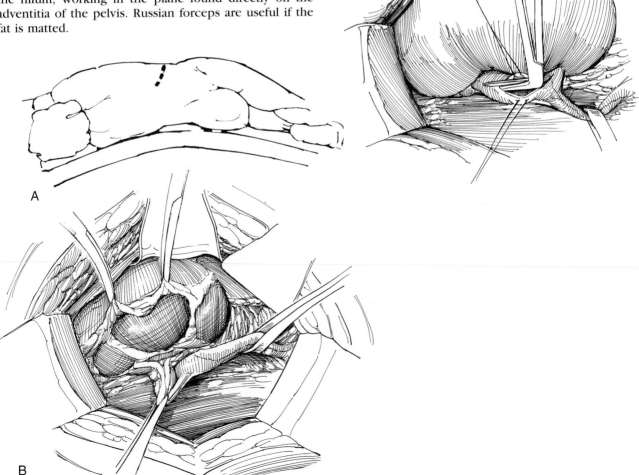

A

B

3 Withdraw the stones with forceps or a Mixter clamp. If a large stone adheres to the pelvic wall, free it by passing a probe around it. Irrigate the interior with water through a cut-off Robinson catheter. Use a Water-Pik. Insert a flexible nephroscope if concern remains about residual adherent stones. Alternatively, close the pelvis and inject coagulum (Step 4). It may be worthwhile before closure to pass a ureteral catheter or infant feeding tube to the bladder to be sure that no fragments are caught in the ureter, which would promote prolonged postoperative drainage. Make a watertight closure of the pelvis with a running 4-0 or 5-0 SAS with an occasional lock stitch. Suture a Penrose drain by the long suture technique near the closure (see page 917), being sure its end does not touch the anastomosis. Tack the edges of Gerota's fascia together, and close the wound.

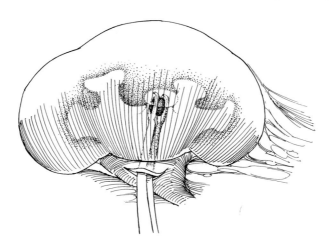

COAGULUM TECHNIQUE

Obtain two bags of thawed cryoprecipitate (about 15 ml each), and keep them at room temperature. Add a few drops of methylene blue to them in a pan. Draw the cryoprecipitate into the 35-ml syringe.

4 **A,** Obstruct the ureter by placing traction on the encircling Penrose drain. Insert an angiocatheter into the renal pelvis, withdraw the stylet, and drain the urine, estimating its volume.

B, Draw 1 ml of 10 percent calcium chloride solution into the syringe containing the cryoprecipitate just before instilling the mixture into the pelvis. Attach the syringe to the angiocatheter, and inject enough of the solution to fill, but not overfill, the pelvis. Remove the angiocatheter.

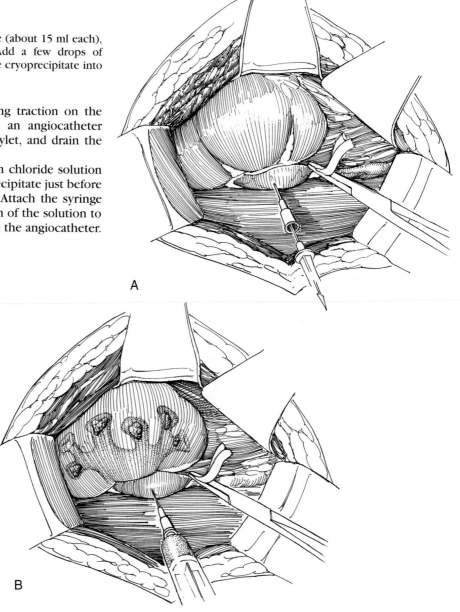

A

B

5 **A,** Wait 5 minutes; then open the pelvis with a U-shaped incision, and gingerly extract the coagulum with the stone. Sometimes pressure on the kidney parenchyma helps extraction. After removing the clot, flush the ureter with saline through the 8 F infant feeding tube.

B, Inspect the coagulum to be certain it is intact. Thoroughly irrigate the pelvis and ureter.

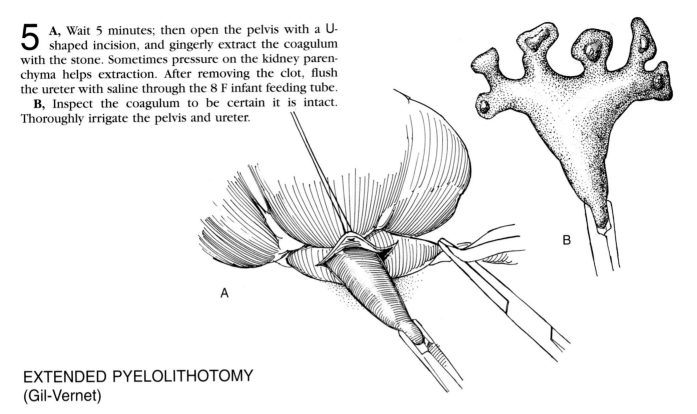

EXTENDED PYELOLITHOTOMY
(Gil-Vernet)

Alternatives are anatrophic nephrolithotomy (see page 1048) and partial nephrectomy (see page 1000).

Contraindications to this intrasinusal approach are a previous extended pyelolithotomy, an extremely intrarenal pelvis, or staghorn calculi in clubbed calyces. Study the radiographs well preoperatively, and have them on display in the operating room.

Expose the kidney as for simple pyelolithotomy. Proceed with complete mobilization of the kidney to allow control of the renal artery and to facilitate roentgenography. Have the assistant rotate the kidney toward the midline. Feel for the arterial pulsation, and expose the renal artery. Draw a sling around it with a right-angle clamp. Try applying a bulldog clamp on it for size and clearance.

6 **A,** Dissect along the posterior surface of the pelvis, entering the renal sinus beneath the sinus fat exactly on the adventitia of the pelvis.

B, Excise excess fatty tissue. It is not necessary to clear out all the fat; the portion remaining cushions the closure line.

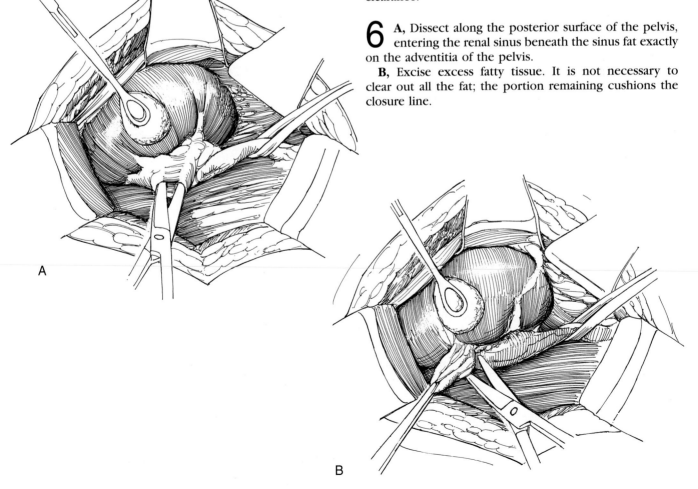

7 Separate the pelvis from the renal hilum and peripelvic fat in the avascular plane by blunt dissection. Avoid the retropelvic artery, which is the posterior branch of the main renal artery. It originates near the superior edge of the pelvis and passes behind it, sometimes outside and sometimes inside the hilum. The scissors must be kept in close contact with the adventitia of the pelvis. Even if there is considerable reaction in the peripelvic fat, this plane remains intact. Insert special Gil-Vernet retractors over the whole mass of peripelvic fat, and insinuate the corner of a moist, opened 4 × 8 gauze pad to expose the bases of the infundibula. Have your assistant lift and rotate the kidney to bring the pelvis into view. If the pelvis is extrarenal, the assistant should relax pressure on the retractors occasionally to allow flow through the retropelvic artery. If exposure is difficult, place a bulldog clamp on the renal artery to reduce parenchymal turgor.

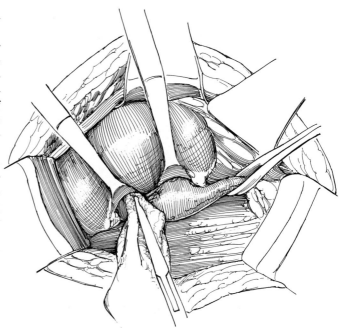

8 Incise the pelvis in an open U shape with a hooked scalpel blade and Potts scissors. Design the cut to fit the configuration of the pelviureteral portion of the stone, keeping well away from the ureteropelvic junction. Usually make the incision from the base of the lowest calyx to the base of the uppermost. Stay sutures are not needed and may tear the pelvic wall.

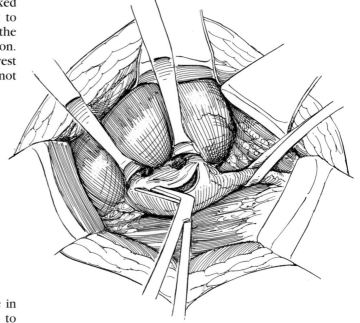

9 **A,** First wipe around the extension of the stone in the ureteropelvic junction with a blunt probe to free it from the pelvic epithelium.
B, Lever the pelviureteral extension out first, thereby exposing as much as 70 percent of the stone.

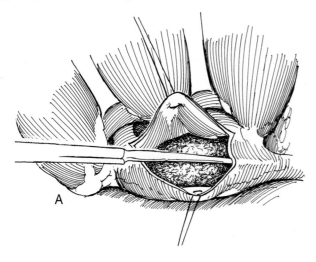
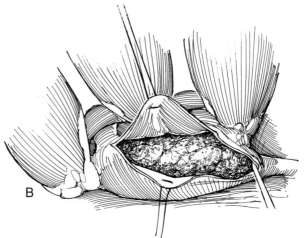

10 Grasp the stone with Randall forceps. Gently rock and rotate it to extract its caliceal extensions. Extricate the shortest branch first. If absolutely necessary, fracture the neck of one or more of the branches and remove the clubbed ends via transverse nephrotomies. Often an infundibulum can be dilated with forceps sufficiently to allow an extension of the main stone to be extracted. If the renal hilum is large enough, a vertical incision along the involved infundibulum (calicotomy) may assist in the removal of large caliceal stones. Remove the stone and fit the pieces together to be sure all were retrieved. Send the stone for culture and analysis.

11 Inspect the interior of the calyces, using a flexible nephroscope if necessary, and remove any remaining calculi, usually with stone forceps or a Mixter clamp. If the stones are too large to pass through an infundibulum, gently dilate the opening with a clamp. Try not to use a finger or high pressure. Irrigate each calyx in turn, using a large syringe and a cut-off 18 F red rubber catheter.

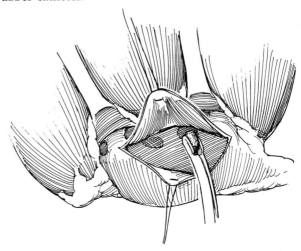

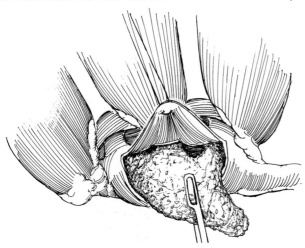

12 **A,** Make a radial nephrotomy over clubbed caliceal stones too large to extract through the infundibulum. Locate the site of the stone by pushing it toward the capsule with a clamp or finger in the infundibulum and palpating it through the cortex. If it cannot be felt, probe for it with a milliner's needle.

B, Sharply incise the capsule circumferentially for a distance equal to the diameter of the stone; then bluntly separate the kidney parenchyma down to the stone, which is supported by a clamp or finger in the infundibulum. Extract the stone with forceps inserted into the nephrotomy. If the cortex is thick, it is helpful to place a bulldog clamp on the renal artery to soften the kidney long enough to locate and remove the stone. If these manipulations are to be prolonged, cool the kidney (see page 1048) and give mannitol intravenously. Irrigate the calyx thoroughly with saline. Avulsion of the ureteropelvic junction is possible. With a segment made ischemic by chronic impaction of a relatively large stone, avulsion can occur during dissection. Repair and intubation are

necessary (Howard and Hinman, 1952), even though the tissue has the quality of wet paper.

C, Close the nephrotomy with 3-0 CCG mattress sutures over fat bolsters.

If the pelvis lies principally inside the sinus, exposure can be improved by inserting a grooved (Gouley) sound along the outside of the inferior pelvis and lowest calyx and out through the lower-pole parenchyma. Cut into the groove and divide the renal cortex. Alternatively, pass successive pairs of sutures, tie them, and cut between them.

Perform radiography (see page 1051). A straight milliner's needle thrust through the cortex can be useful to locate residual stones, and two needles provide a landmark on the roentgenogram. Intraoperative nephroscopy and sonography are the best techniques to detect and clear remaining stones. Coagulum can be used if the pelvis is closed first. Pass an 8 F catheter down the ureter to be sure it is clear.

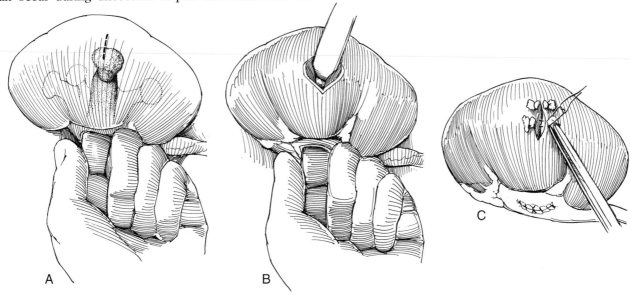

A   B   C

13 A nephrostomy tube made from perforated silicone tubing may be brought out through the lower pole but is necessary only when stone removal is incomplete and irrigation postoperatively with hemiacidrin (Renacidin) must be resorted to.

Close the pelvis with a running 5-0 SAS, occasionally locked. If reaching either end of the incision for suturing is difficult, start and finish the closure at convenient sites because the parenchyma falls over the suture line and prevents leakage. Irrigate the wound copiously. Tack a Penrose drain near the pelvis with the long suture technique (see page 917), although urinary leakage is unusual. Fasten Gerota's fascia over the kidney with 3-0 plain catgut sutures. Close the wound.

At a secondary operation, the kidney is found firmly attached to the transversalis fascia and is readily entered inadvertently. Identify the capsule early, and dissect it carefully from the fibrous bed. Enter the sinus anteriorly and inferiorly, at a site distant from that for the initial pyelolithotomy.

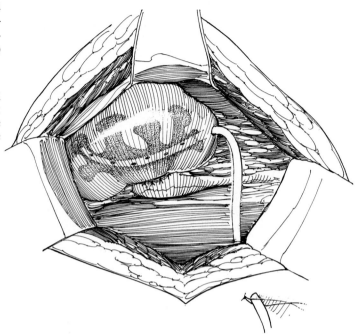

PYELONEPHROLITHOTOMY

This technique is used to recover large stones in a lower-pole caliceal system.

Proceed through Step 7, exposing the renal pelvis and vessels. Make an oblique incision that extends into the infundibulum of the affected calyx but does not approach the ureteropelvic junction. Place a silicone J stent down the ureter to prevent stone migration. Incise the renal capsule over the infundibulum, and, with the knife handle, bluntly separate the parenchyma between the nephrons. Continue the pelvic incision into the infundibulum and into any involved calyces. Extract the stone. Ligate bleeding vessels with figure-eight fine CCG sutures. Irrigate the calyces and explore them for residual stones. If you have any doubt about clearance, obtain a radiograph. If the infundibulum is stenotic, close it transversely or with a sliding pelvic flap (calicoplasty, see page 1051). Leave the stent in place, and close the infundibulum and pelvis with a running suture of 4-0 CCG. Approximate the parenchyma and check for hemostasis. Place a drain by the long suture technique (see page 917), and bring it out through a stab wound. Approximate Gerota's fascia to encase the kidney and close the wound.

LOWER-POLE PARTIAL NEPHRECTOMY

Because stones may reform in a dilated lower calyx, remove that calyx with a portion of the lower pole (see page 1001). Control the main renal artery. Make a transverse incision in the capsule peripheral to the site of resection, and turn the capsule back. Incise the parenchyma with the back of the knife, and divide the interlobar vessels as they are encountered. Divide the infundibulum to the lower-pole calyx, and remove the specimen containing the stone. Transfix the vessels with fine figure-eight sutures, and close the infundibulum with a running 4-0 SAS. Tack the capsule over the defect, as well as any adjacent fat. Do not try to approximate the parenchyma.

ROENTGENOGRAPHIC TECHNIQUE

Wrap a fully opened 4 × 8 gauze pad around the kidney as a sling, and gather the ends in sponge forceps. Insert one or two straight milliner's needles with the threads attached into the parenchyma near the suspected site of the stone.

Place the sterile film (or the film in a sterile plastic bag) behind the kidney. The film may be grasped in the same forceps. Focus the x-ray using an extension tube covered with a plastic bag. Support the kidney with the forceps, and step away from the beam. Expose the film. Leave the needles in place until the film is viewed to orient the site of residual stones.

POSTOPERATIVE PROBLEMS

Bleeding may appear postoperatively, usually from overzealous extraction of caliceal stones. It usually stops spontaneously, but obstructive clots may disrupt the pelvic closure. If hemorrhage continues, reopen the kidney and place sutures appropriately. *Prolonged drainage* may result from such disruption, but suspect obstruction from a stone or stricture and obtain studies needed to rule out such obstruction. *Late stricture* may occur if the pelvic incision crossed the ureteropelvic junction.

Pneumothorax can occur but is usually detected before wound closure. However, pulmonary dysfunction is common and requires careful pulmonary care.

Commentary by Vito Pansadoro

Pyelolithotomy and nephrolithotomy are less often used today because of the extended availability of ESWL and percutaneous procedures. The open operations are, nevertheless, basic surgical procedures for the urologist. Unfortunately, residents are not usually exposed to them because complicated stone cases have become increasingly rare in the Western world. Cases do occur, however, in which these procedures are indicated, and patients must be managed appropriately.

One of the key points to ensure complete stone removal is *accurate localization*. This is best accomplished with preoperative plain tomography or, alternatively, with a CT scan of the kidney to localize the stones in an anteroposterior plane.

Intraoperatively, the best way to localize stones is by sonography, using a 7.5-MHz transducer, which provides information about volume and shape of the stone and is also helpful in defining the size of the calyx and the amount of overlying parenchyma. Once the renal pelvis has been opened, a rigid 90-degree intraoperative nephroscope can be of great help, when combined with sonography, in localizing caliceal stones. It is very important to place a small gauze pad to occlude any calyx from which the stones have been removed, to prevent it from filling with new stones during the remainder of the procedure.

Omental flaps can be of help to cover the pelvis and ureter, but they should be avoided in the presence of infected stones because they may permit bacterial colonization of the peritoneal cavity. In our experience, small precise nephrotomies and the use of an operative nephroscope combined with ultrasonography, lithoclast, and forceps permit complete removal of all stones without the need for extended nephrotomies. Finally, when transnephric surgery is not indicated, a posterior lumbotomy is the ideal approach. This muscle-sparing incision gives good exposure of the renal pelvis and provides the patient with a short, almost painless postoperative course.

Nephrolithotomy

(Smith-Boyce)

Extracorporeal shock wave therapy and endolithotripsy can manage most renal calculi, but for large stones the results from open surgery are as good as, if not better than, those from closed methods and can be done in one operation, at the cost of a longer convalescence. The patient should be referred to a center specializing in renal reconstructive surgery when caliceal stenosis is present and calicoplasty or calirrhaphy is needed to improve intrarenal drainage, when partial nephrectomy is indicated, when the ureteropelvic junction is obstructed, when the stone is very large or does not respond to lithotripsy (cystine), and when the patient's body size, obesity, or other factors contraindicate minimally invasive procedures.

Evaluate the patient's ability to withstand a major procedure. Obtain a basal metabolic evaluation in each case; a more extensive evaluation may be indicated in an active stone former. Intravenous urography with oblique and delayed films allows appreciation of the size and configuration of the stone and shows any obstruction. Retrograde urography may be needed to outline the ureter. Voiding cystography demonstrates the presence or absence of reflux. Renal angiography is very useful for staghorn stones to delineate the vascular supply prior to renal incision. Total renal function is measured by serum creatinine level. Differential function is often important and is obtained by an iodohippurate sodium I-131 or technetium-99 scan, a diethylenetriaminepenta-acetic acid (DTPA) radionuclide scan, and a CT scan for determination of cortical thickness.

Perform urine culture and sensitivity testing, and begin intravenous administration of antibiotics at least 48 hours preoperatively, if indicated. Continue therapy through the postoperative period to attempt eradication of the infection after the stone has been removed.

Obtain culture and sensitivity tests, and give antibiotics preoperatively and intraoperatively. Alternative approaches are the Gil-Vernet pyelolithotomy with nephrotomies or nephrectomy.

Nephrectomy should be the last resort, being acceptable only when the kidney has had an irreversible loss of function to less than 10 percent of normal, even with normal contralateral function.

Instruments: Provide a $4\times$ magnifying loupe; malleable microspatulas; nerve hooks; microretractors; a full set of microsurgical instruments; blunt angular drum elevators; rubber-shod, spring-loaded arterial clamps; Potts scissors; 10 to 20 ml of injectable methylene blue in a syringe; material for coagulum pyelolithotomy (see page 1042); sterile x-ray film; fine 6-0 CCG sutures on taper-pointed, half-circle, double-swaged needles; ice slush; a nephroscope; a marking pen; mannitol; methylprednisolone; and a rubber (dentist's dam) or plastic dam or a large microscope drape. In addition, have available a portable x-ray machine with sterile x-ray film, a high-frequency ultrasonic probe, a Doppler probe, and a small sterile flexible ureteroscope or nephroscope.

RENAL HYPOTHERMIA

The soft ice, formed by freezing, is available as a sterile solution in liter bottles. Slush is formed by placing the bottles of physiologic irrigating fluid as a commercially synthesized ultrafiltrate of plasma in a freezer or refrigerator for 4 hours. During the last 2 hours each bottle is shaken vigorously every 20 to 30 minutes to ensure that the ice forms as small, soft crystals. Alternatively, use a freezer unit (Taylor Freezer Co., Rockton, IL), and dip the slush with a strainer as needed.

Form a dam from an 18×24 inch rectangular latex rubber sheet with a 9-inch slit in the center, stretched around the kidney and clamped closed around the pedicle, over a laparotomy tape for insulation. Alternatively, place a plastic bag over the kidney and make a second opening through which the kidney is delivered. A microscope drape may also be used.

1 **A,** *Incision:* A supracostal 11th- or 12th-rib approach (see page 879) is generally applicable. For young children, use a pediatric extended anterior incision (see page 863).

B, Expose the posterior aspect of the kidney. Open Gerota's fascia over the lateral frontal plane (over the convex surface of the kidney) to provide a fat pad for covering the area at the time of closure. Ligate lower-pole vessels only if necessary. Expose the convex border of the renal capsule, and separate the perirenal fat gently from the capsule anteriorly to the edge of the hilum, superiorly to separate or free the adrenal, and inferiorly to free the lower pole. Posteriorly expose a portion or all of the dorsal pelvis and each renal pole so that the kidney may be suspended by a broad tape or gauze, forming a sling beneath each pole. Continuing posteriorly, palpate the renal vessels and expose the main renal artery at a point between the aorta and its first (posterior segmental) branch. The renal pedicle should be small enough to permit enclosure of the entire kidney within a rubber dam or bag that includes all the parenchyma but excludes most of the ureter.

Dissect the renal pedicle and renal arteries gently, using Potts or similar scissors, applied in line with the long axis of the pedicle. Restrict the dissection to that required to expose the main renal artery and its pertinent branches. Avoid undue traction on the tapes supporting the kidney. Blunt dissection should be done with vascular pledgets. Do not use cauterization around the pedicle. The objective is to not induce arterial vascular spasm, which may invalidate subsequent mapping of the renal arterial segments. Place vascular loops of different colors loosely around each vessel, and note the color so that you may quickly identify the position of each artery during the procedure without removing the slush bath or unnecessarily disturbing the renal pedicle.

Identify the ureter well below the renal pelvis at the most caudal margin of the dissection. Enclose the surrounding plexus of vessels and areolar tissue with the ureter in a Penrose drain for ease of access (which, it is hoped, will not be necessary). Do not attempt to dissect the renal pelvis or ureter. For this procedure, the essential renal vessels are the main renal artery, which has been approached on the posterior (dorsal) side of the dissection, and the first branch to the dorsal segment, which courses posterior to the pelvis, both of which are identified with tapes.

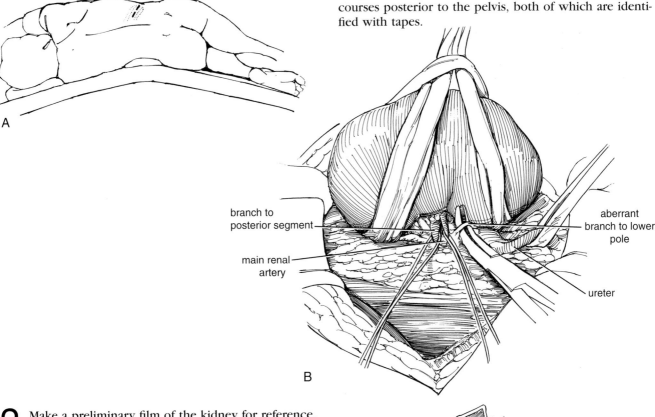

branch to posterior segment

main renal artery

aberrant branch to lower pole

ureter

A

B

2 Make a preliminary film of the kidney for reference. It will be more relevant to the operation than earlier films.

Gently apply a rubber-shod, spring-loaded clamp, and observe blanching of the posterior segment. Have the anesthetist give 10 to 20 ml of methylene blue intravenously to color the remainder of the kidney. Dip an applicator stick in methylene blue (preferable to using the cautery as shown) for marking the intersegmental plane (Brödel's line). If definition is poor, give mannitol and another dose of methylene blue (up to 60 ml total). The injection may be given into the aorta with a long needle, but direct injection into the renal vasculature is inadvisable.

If the blood supply has a less regular separation, the incision in the kidney does not have to be made straight.

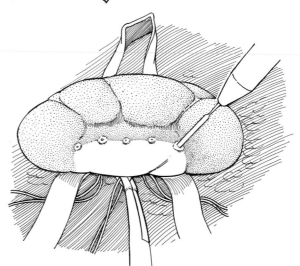

3 Occlude the main renal artery with a Rumel clamp (made of a vascular tape in a section of catheter) or with a rubber-shod bulldog clamp to preserve the methylene blue stain in the kidney. Immediately place a rubber dam or plastic bag under the kidney distal to the clamp, and insulate it from the body wall with dry gauze packs. Cover the kidney with ice slush immediately after occluding the renal artery, and leave it in place for 10 to 15 minutes before incising the kidney. It takes that long to obtain core renal cooling to the effective temperature of 15 to 20° C.

Incise the capsule sharply along the previously marked line, even if it is irregular. Make the incision as short as deemed necessary for exposure of the stone (it can be lengthened later), and be careful to avoid an extension into the upper or lower poles.

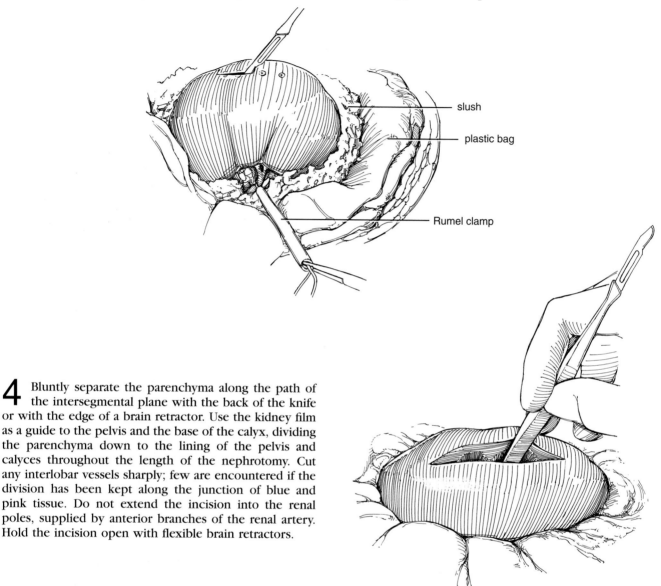

slush

plastic bag

Rumel clamp

4 Bluntly separate the parenchyma along the path of the intersegmental plane with the back of the knife or with the edge of a brain retractor. Use the kidney film as a guide to the pelvis and the base of the calyx, dividing the parenchyma down to the lining of the pelvis and calyces throughout the length of the nephrotomy. Cut any interlobar vessels sharply; few are encountered if the division has been kept along the junction of blue and pink tissue. Do not extend the incision into the renal poles, supplied by anterior branches of the renal artery. Hold the incision open with flexible brain retractors.

5 Incise the pelvis, calyx, or both directly with a knife onto the stone, and open along its surface with Potts scissors. To expose all ramifications of the stone, open adjacent infundibula into the calyces. Review the pyelogram for orientation.

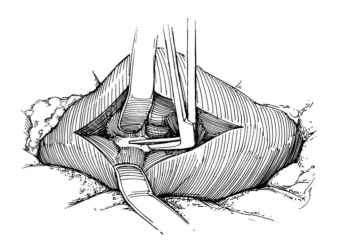

6 After the stone is exposed, gently free it with a blunt elevator. Lift out the main portion of the stone. Insert a silicone stent down the ureter to prevent migration of stones during manipulation, and allow it to remain after closure. Open and inspect each calyx in succession; check with the radiograph to be sure all calyces are opened. Irrigate vigorously and aspirate the irrigant. A Water-Pik may be helpful to free adherent scales but can injure the kidney. Use the nephroscope to check for complete removal. Continually reapply slush.

7 Support the kidney in the sling, and make a radiograph (see page 1045). A straight milliner's needle thrust through the cortex can be useful to locate residual stones, and two needles provide a landmark on the roentgenogram. Intraoperative nephroscopy and sonography are the best techniques to detect and clear remaining stones.

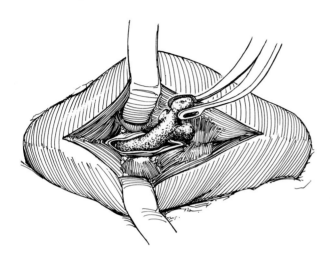

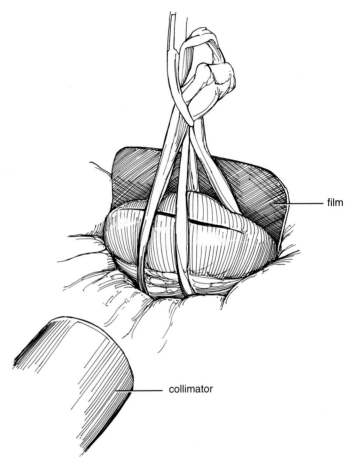

film

collimator

CALICOPLASTY

8 *Calicoplasty on adjacent calyces with stenotic infundibula:* **A,** Approximate the cut edges of adjacent calyces with 6-0 CCG on half-circle taper needles. Use a cross-stitch technique to place the knots outside. Tie the suture while depressing the intervening fat with an angle retractor. The finished suture line is shown in Step 9.

Calicoplasty by YV-plasty technique, combining the infundibula into a single unit: **B,** Incise the adjacent walls of both calyces. **C** and **D,** Suture the edges of both infundibula together to form a single unit.

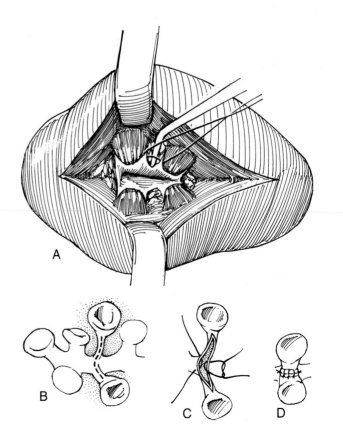

A

B

C

D

9 **A,** Close the pelvis around a Silastic catheter or a double-J stent (not shown), starting with reinforcing pocket stitches.

B, Finish with running stitches.

10 Release the arterial clamp; then reapply the clamp to allow suture of bleeding vessels with figure-eight 4-0 or 5-0 CCG sutures.

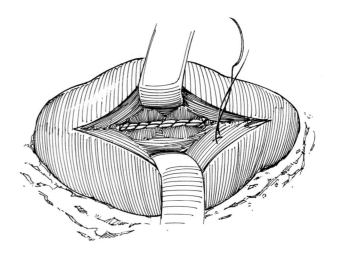

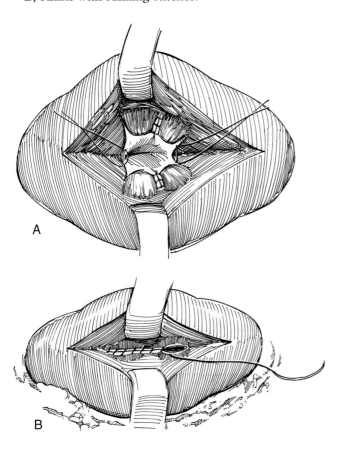

11 **A,** Close the capsule with a running lock stitch of 4-0 CCG.

B, Alternatively, place mattress sutures over fat bolsters.

Insert only a Penrose drain; avoid nephrostomy drainage, if possible, but a large suction drain may be placed through a lower-pole calyx to rest in an upper-pole calyx. Replace Gerota's fascia around the kidney, or consider bringing the omentum through the posterior peritoneum to cover the area (see page 74).

Remove the drains after leakage has ceased. If a nephrostomy tube is in place, check for leaks with nephrostography before removal. Irrigation with a 10 percent hemiacidrin (Renacidin) solution for 2 days may dissolve any inapparent stones; 4 or 5 days of irrigation are needed for fragments seen radiographically. Continue antibiotics for 5 to 7 days. Remove a ureteral stent on the seventh day. Check for persistent urinary tract infection, and treat it if found.

Pyelonephrolithotomy, a technique to remove large stones from a lower-pole caliceal system, is described on pages 1043 to 1046.

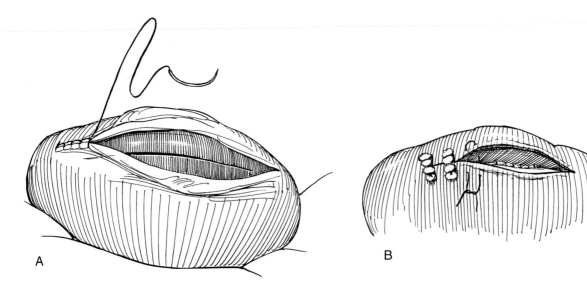

INTRAOPERATIVE PROBLEMS

Arterial injury can be avoided by preserving the adventitia and small vessels of the renal artery, gently clamping the artery with an atraumatic vascular clamp, and avoiding traction on the pedicle during radiographic procedures. Either a small bulldog clamp of disposable plastic or a rubber-shod metal bulldog clamp should be used. Even then, injury to the intima is possible, resulting in a nonvascularized kidney that requires arterial repair (see page 937) if it does not return to normal color after release of the clamp. Segmental arterial injury also requires repair because infarcted segments become infected and injury may also lead to later hypertension.

POSTOPERATIVE PROBLEMS

Pain is a common problem due to the large incision that is required. Risks from transfusion cannot be ignored. *Pulmonary atelectasis* is common, but the incidence can be reduced by vigorous expansion of the lungs before extubation and by coughing, deep breathing, and incentive spirometry along with early ambulation. *Pneumothorax* is a possible complication, especially in patients who have had previous renal surgery and those with a history of pyelonephritis. If the pleura has been entered or if pneumothorax is suspected, obtain portable chest radiography in the recovery room. A pneumothorax may require needle aspiration or, more often, insertion of a chest tube. *Phlebothrombosis* and embolic phenomena are reduced by early ambulation. Full-length stockings may help.

Delayed intrapelvic hemorrhage may occur 4 to 8 days after operation, usually secondary to breakdown of absorbable sutures that were used to ligate intrarenal vessels. Treat hemorrhage expectantly with fluids and blood transfusions. Intraoperative placement of a silicone stent, by reducing the opportunity for obstruction, can reduce the chance of hemorrhage. If there is fibrinolysin activity, epsilon-aminocaproic acid (Amicar) may be given intravenously, followed by oral administration for several days. However, the consequent rubbery clots may be quite obstructive. If significant bleeding persists, suspect develop-

ment of an arteriovenous fistula or false aneurysm. Obtain an arteriogram to define the site, and have an angiographer try to embolize it. If not, reoperation is necessary to suture-ligate the bleeding vessel.

Renal damage from ischemia may follow prolonged arterial occlusion, especially if cooling was not adequate. *Hypertension* may result from ischemia secondary to intimal injury from arterial clamping, with subsequent stenosis. *Persistent infection* means that stones were left behind and requires long-term suppressive therapy.

Residual calculi create problems. A calculus may become obstructive and cause pain and urinary leakage as well as produce serious pyelonephritis in the presence of urinary infection. This condition requires retrograde or percutaneous urinary bypass and removal of the stone. Retained infected stones prevent sterilization of the urine and promote regrowth.

CHEMOLYSIS

Chemical dissolution may be used if stones, especially those composed of struvite, are known to remain at operation. Insert a large nephrostomy tube to exit along a straight path and irrigate postoperatively with large volumes of a solution suitable for the composition of the stone. Sodium bicarbonate and tris-(hydroxymethyl)aminomethane (Tham) with acetylcysteine plus oral alkalis are suitable for cystine and uric acid stones and hemiacidrin for struvite stones. Ethylenediaminetetra-acetic acid (EDTA) may be used for apatite stones, but it produces significant injury to the mucosa and probably should not be used. Exercise great care not to exceed 25 cm H_2O by using an overflow system attached to a central venous pressure manometer. The patient should be provided with antibiotic coverage. Wait 2 or 3 days for intrarenal healing before starting irrigation, and use only saline for the first day to be sure that the solution runs freely down the ureter. Then irrigate at a rate not exceeding 120 ml/hour, and check the progress by means of plain radiographs. Stop treatment if pain, extravasation, and especially fever occur. An alternative is direct removal of the fragments through the nephrostomy tract.

Commentary by William H. Boyce

The fundamental anatomic, physiologic, and serviceable attributes of the kidney plus its conduits are essential to health and to life itself. The human species has been endowed with such reserves of functional renal tissue as to permit survival in health with as little as 15 percent of this total. This largess is no excuse for sacrifice of the system to other considerations, such as financial, technologic, emotional, and questionably scientific factors. Nephrolithotomy is but a small portion of all reconstructive intrarenal surgery, the fundamental knowledge, skills, and technologic and other support systems required for proper execution of which also require ongoing use, research, and education.

At present, no adequate designation has been made of hospitals equipped to support intrarenal surgery. Without question, it is more efficient in every respect to transfer individual patients to centers of expertise than to have them treated in an "occasional" environment. The present sociologic revolution in delivery of medical care is humanitarian, as it has always been; the knowledge, skills, research, and development of medical techniques always reside within the basic tenets of the scientific method. At present we lack the verifiable results required for proper selection from the many available interventional techniques for renal surgery. Our choices are based on "common sense," availability of resources, what payers are willing to pay for, the siren call to self-indulgence, and numerous other rationalizations. The scientific method is our only means to verify outcomes, however slow, cumbersome, expensive, and politically and socially unacceptable the process may be.

Points of technique: A preliminary film is made for reference; such films are far more definitive than conventional kidney-

ureter-bladder films or tomograms. If the pedicle is large enough to obscure aberrant vessels, it may be searched with the Doppler, or the kidney may be scanned with the sonic probe while the films are developed.

For temporary occlusion of the artery, rubber-shod clamps may be used, but a pressure cuff (CR Bard Company) is better. It is a special red rubber 8 F catheter, the lumen of which opens into a latex balloon of 3-ml capacity. An inelastic cuff divided in half is attached so as to surround the catheter and balloon. The artery to be occluded is slipped into the cuff, which is then closed with two ties or a figure-eight ligature passed through four eyelets in the cuff. These blood pressure–type cuffs are not thermal conductors, are soft and not mechanically injurious to the tissue, and once in position are secure. The end of the catheter is brought outside the wound to provide ready access to the balloon during the procedure without disturbing the ice pack.

The segmental distribution of the arterial supply must be mapped because no two kidneys have the same distribution; the variation is of such a magnitude that proper segmental distribution must be mapped and adhered to if the complications of postoperative hemorrhage, poor wound healing, and reduced function are to be avoided. Mattress sutures are a poor substitute for meticulous surgery.

The renal parenchyma is separated down to the renal pelvis with the thin, flat edge of a brain retractor or other microretractor. The kidney film displayed in proper orientation to the patient is a guide to the position at which the pelvis is exposed and the location of the base of the calyx. This makes exploration by separation of parenchyma from pelvis a less traumatic procedure. Some papillae are formed by fusion of anlagen from two segments. The rule is to follow the demarcation and not to attempt to restore the papilla or parenchyma by suturing. The pelvic and infundibular repair is all that is required for healing.

Parenchymal separation should leave a clean cleavage plane without fractures or false passages. The pelvis is incised in line with the parenchyma to the level of the selected infundibulum, where a right-angle extension is made to the base and extended the full length of that structure. The surgeon should resist the urge to remove the stone forcefully or to fragment it. He or she should continue to open all calyces that contain calculi in this manner because all should eventually be inspected for residual fragments. The very best guide to the orifice of unexplored calyces is a comparison of the *preoperative* renal radiographs, pyelograms, and sonograms with the *intraoperative* images viewed in comparable orientation.

The ischemic kidney becomes quite pliable, and the branched calculus can usually be removed intact following these maneuvers, and with minimal trauma to the kidney.

In closing the pelvis, first define the points of anatomic relevance (stress, angled corners, puckering, excess), and fix these positions with reinforcing pocket stitches, which may be oversewn with subsequent continuous closing sutures. This is the final definitive step in the reconstruction of the intrarenal collecting system. Calyces may be enlarged and infundibula elongated by drawing the excess pelvis into their closure. They may be foreshortened to fit the anatomy of the kidney relieved of internal immobile struts (that is, staghorn calculi).

Close the capsule with a running lock stitch or cross stitch. Closure is a very important aspect of the operation because adhesions of the kidney fix it to surrounding structures. The kidney's natural state is semimobile in Gerota's fascia, and it should be returned to that state. We have on occasion resorted to transplanting the omentum when we had no other no alternative to leaving the kidney in contact with striated muscle or fascia of the abdominal wall.

Postoperative care: Infection, hemorrhage, urinary obstruction, and temporary or permanent impairment of renal function are postoperative complications of any open or endoscopic surgery. The incidence should be no greater for reconstructive renal surgery than for any major abdominal urologic or general surgical procedure. The prevention and management of these complications are universal aspects of all such surgery: complete preoperative evaluation, meticulous technique, and intensive postoperative care. Patients who are candidates for such surgery, whatever the disease, should be transferred to medical centers where all services, requisite personnel, and technical support are available and active. Intrarenal reconstructive surgery is not to be performed by occasional operators.

Caliceal Diverticulectomy and Excision of Renal Cyst

CALICEAL DIVERTICULECTOMY

Alternatives: Consider a percutaneous approach directly into the diverticulum; then dilate the caliceal neck endoscopically. A large nephrostomy tube may be left in the diverticulum for 2 weeks, in anticipation of obliteration of the cavity. Laparoscopic excision is an alternative. If stones are present, extracorporeal shock wave lithotripsy may be used, although the fragments are unlikely to pass. Use an open technique when other approaches are not practical.

Incision: Make a short subcostal incision (see page 871) or a lumbotomy incision (see page 896).

1 After exposure of the appropriate area of the kidney, check the location of the diverticulum by palpation or, if it is deep, by aspiration with an 18-gauge needle. Use intraoperative ultrasonography for small fluid-filled diverticula and those containing stones.

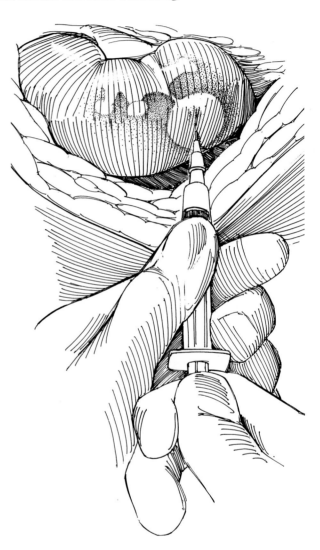

2 **A,** Incise through the parenchyma into the diverticulum, and trim excess cortex and capsule. Marsupialize the edges of the diverticulum with interrupted 3-0 SAS. A wedge excision may be needed (see page 1003). The transitional epithelial lining seldom needs to be removed.

B, If necessary, inject dilute methylene blue into the renal pelvis to identify the narrow neck of the diverticulum. Incise the neck circumferentially, and invert the wall with 3-0 SAS. Pack the cavity with perirenal fat, and place a Penrose drain to the area. Consider partial nephrectomy for deeper, larger, or polar diverticula.

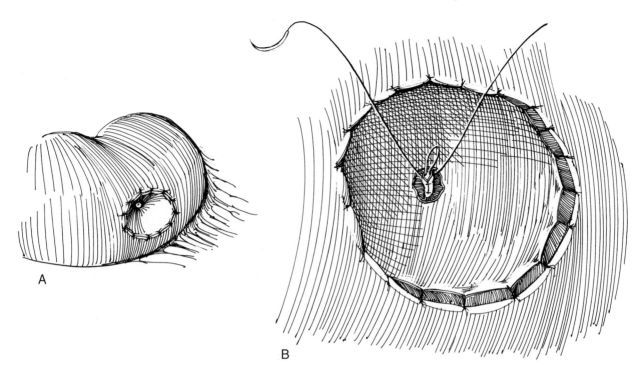

A

B

POSTOPERATIVE PROBLEMS

Prolonged urinary drainage indicates incomplete closure of the diverticular neck. Other problems are similar to those after a partial nephrectomy.

Commentary by Ronald B. Brown

I believe that the most important point during the operation is to incise the neck of the diverticulum circumferentially and then to invert the wall using 3-0 SAS. Failure to completely close the neck of the diverticulum, inadequate hemostasis, and failure to perform a partial nephrectomy rather than an attempted caliceal diverticulotomy are the three main causes of trouble.

EXCISION OF RENAL CYST

Except that the wall is much thinner, cyst excision is similar to excision of a diverticulum. *Position* and *incision* are the same as for diverticulectomy. The blue-walled cyst is usually seen upon opening Gerota's fascia.

Pack the wound with laparotomy tapes in case the cyst contains malignant cells. Using cutting current, open the cyst, aspirate the contents, and send them for cytologic examination. If the contents are bloody, nephrectomy for tumor may be necessary. Grasp the wall with a clamp to steady it, and incise along the juncture of the cyst wall with the renal parenchyma, leaving 1 or 2 mm of the edge of the cyst wall behind. Inspect the lining for tumor.

Fulgurate any small bleeding vessels in the rim. A circumferential running suture is rarely needed. It is not necessary to place filling, such as omentum, into the cavity.

SECTION
23
Adrenal Excision

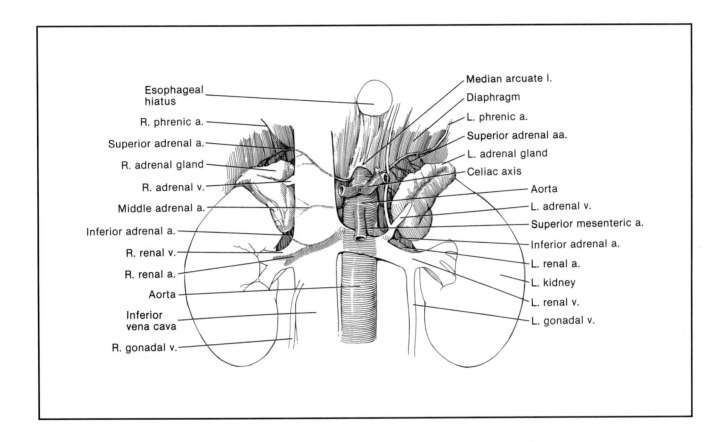

Esophageal hiatus
R. phrenic a.
Superior adrenal a.
R. adrenal gland
R. adrenal v.
Middle adrenal a.
Inferior adrenal a.
R. renal v.
R. renal a.
Aorta
Inferior vena cava
R. gonadal v.

Median arcuate l.
Diaphragm
L. phrenic a.
Superior adrenal aa.
L. adrenal gland
Celiac axis
Aorta
L. adrenal v.
Superior mesenteric a.
Inferior adrenal a.
L. renal a.
L. kidney
L. renal v.
L. gonadal v.

Preparation and Approaches for Adrenal Excision

Preparation for surgery and the surgical approach to an adrenal lesion depend on its type and function. Localization has become so exact that exploration with bilateral exposure is rarely necessary. Endocrine support and supplementation are critical to a successful outcome, requiring a team approach that includes several specialists.

PREPARATION

To prevent adrenal insufficiency, prepare any patient, except those with neuroblastoma and pheochromocytoma, scheduled for adrenal exploration with steroids by giving cortisone acetate in doses of 100 mg orally for 2 days preoperatively. Supplement this with 100 mg given intravenously immediately before and immediately after surgery. Subsequent therapy depends on the amount of adrenal tissue left postoperatively.

Cushing's Disease and Cushing's Syndrome

Excess circulating glucocorticoids produce a symptom complex termed Cushing's syndrome. It is often caused by excess adrenocorticotropic hormone (ACTH) production by the pituitary gland (in 70 percent of patients), producing true Cushing's disease. It may be from the glucocorticoid production of a primary tumor of the adrenal cortex (in 20 to 25 percent) or extra-adrenal tumors such as oat cell carcinomas of the lung or tumors of the thymus (in 5 to 10 percent).

Rule out pituitary tumor. Measure diurnal serum cortisol levels. If they are fixed, suspect the syndrome. Perform a dexamethasone suppression test. If the cortisol level becomes depressed, the diagnosis is bilateral hyperplasia. An autonomous tumor is present if no depression occurs. Measure ACTH levels to detect its ectopic production.

For adrenal-dependent Cushing's syndrome, localize the tumor before exploration with radionuclide studies (65 percent accuracy) or computed tomography (CT) scan (80 percent accuracy). Venous sampling can be very accurate. For pituitary-dependent Cushing's syndrome, consider pharmacologic agents directed at the pituitary (bromocriptine) or the adrenal (o,p′ DDD), pituitary irradiation, transsphenoidal hypophysectomy, or bilateral adrenalectomy. Realize that adenomas, cysts, cortical carcinomas, and myelolipomas may be difficult to differentiate.

For perioperative endocrine control in Cushing's syndrome, give cortisone acetate, 100 to 200 mg IM the evening before and the morning of surgery. Start water-soluble cortisol IV, at a rate of 10 mg/hour. Immediately after the operation, give another 100 mg IM, then give cortisone acetate, 75 mg IM every 8 hours on postoperative days 1 and 2, and every 12 hours on days 3 and 4. Start a maintenance dose of 25 mg orally twice a day, along with fluorocortisone, 0.1 mg/day for a month. Because these patients are susceptible to infection, provide adequate perioperative antibiotics.

Primary Hyperaldosteronism

Suspect hyperaldosteronism if the serum potassium is low. Measure plasma renin; if it is low, give potassium and measure urine aldosterone. If it is high, measure supine and 4-hour ambulatory plasma aldosterone levels. A fall suggests adenoma. Proceed with localization of the tumor by MIBG scintillation scanning (with or without dexamethasone suppression), CT scanning at 0.5-cm intervals, and adrenal vein aldosterone levels. Magnetic resonance imaging (MRI) may be useful. Adrenal venography is rarely indicated. If the tumor cannot be localized, which is a rare occurrence, realize that adenomas are three times more frequent on the left side, so use the bilateral posterior approach described here or the bilateral anterior approach (see pages 865 and 867). Bilateral hyperplasia causing hyperaldosteronism is best treated medically. Exploration and bilateral exposure are now unnecessary; localization has proved to be 100 percent accurate.

Place the patient on 100 to 400 mg of spironolactone (or aminoglutethimide) daily for 2 or 3 weeks before operation, and follow the serum potassium level until it becomes normal and the blood pressure falls. Partial adrenalectomy (so-called enucleation) may be a suitable alternative to total adrenalectomy for aldosterone tumors (Nakada et al, 1995).

Pheochromocytoma

Measure plasma catecholamines, such as epinephrine (adrenal source), norepinephrine (extra-adrenal source), metanephrine, and normetanephrine. An oral clonidine suppression test may be useful in doubtful cases. Localize the tumor (10 percent bilateral, 10 percent multiple, 10 percent extra-adrenal) by CT scan, MRI using both T1 and T2 images (pheochromocytomas light up on T1; adenomas are hypodense compared with metastatic lesions), radionuclide studies with meta-iodobenzyl guanidine (^{131}MIBG scan), or venous sampling.

Prepare an adult patient with 2 units of whole blood a day or two ahead of time, regardless of blood volume studies. Avoid stimulatory diagnostic procedures. Preoperative and intraoperative adrenergic blockade, although it prevents hypertensive crises, makes the detection of small extra-adrenal tumors more difficult by blunting the sudden rise in blood pressure during exploration, which may be the only indication of their presence. If the surgeon and anesthetist desire it, adrenergic blockade can be achieved by a 10-day to 2-week course of prazosin, 2 to 5 mg twice a day, or phenoxybenzamine, starting with 10 mg three to four times daily and increasing the dose as needed to provide freedom from hypertensive attacks and mild postural hypotension. Catecholamine synthesis inhibitors such as alpha-methyltyrosine may be added. If the patient has cardiac dysrhythmia, give a cardiospecific beta$_1$-receptor antagonist (atenolol) orally after the alpha-adrenergic blockade has stabilized. For dysrhythmia during the operation, use IV lidocaine or propranolol. At surgery, to be safe, have two experienced anesthesiologists at the table, with adequate monitoring equipment.

Place one IV catheter to monitor central venous pressure. Insert a second IV catheter for fluid administration. To the connector next to the vein, attach the tubing from the bottle containing the drug for control of excess blood pressure. Keep the connection close to the vein to avoid dead space and resultant delay in getting the drug into the circulation. Monitor intra-arterial pressure with a cannula in the radial or brachial artery. Maintain electrocardiogram tracings continuously. Induce anesthesia with thiopental sodium. For an anesthetic agent, avoid halothane and curare; isoflurane is preferred, along with succinylcholine and nitrous oxide. Use sodium nitroprusside or phentolamine to reverse hypertensive crisis. The hypertensive episodes that occur with intubation or manipulation of the tumor are countered by giving phentolamine IV. In any case, stabilize the patient before beginning the operation. A hypotensive episode during surgery requires the vigorous administration of whole blood and plasma volume expanders to fill the vascular spaces consequent to removal of alpha stimuli. Sympathomimetic amines can be used as back-up. Vasoconstrictors, however, carry the risk of precipitating renal shutdown and cerebral ischemia. For hypotension after removal of the tumor, expand the blood volume with fluids and whole blood.

Postoperatively, continue monitoring the blood pressure because acute hypotension is still a risk, especially if the patient is moved. Correct hypotension with fluids. Check the blood glucose level to detect hypoglycemia before it is fatal. Follow up with metanephrine and vanillylmandelic acid (VMA) levels every 6 months for 3 years and yearly for another 4 years.

IMAGING

Use CT to determine size, calcification, and necrosis as criteria for the diagnosis of adrenal carcinoma. MRI is not necessary except to detect involvement of the inferior vena cava or extension into the liver or to differentiate renal carcinoma of the upper pole (Schlund et al, 1995).

APPROACHES

Surgery of the adrenal glands can be considered in two steps: (1) the approach, requiring selection of an appropriate incision, and (2) the technique of excision of the gland, which concerns its anatomic relationships and vascular supply and requires meticulous hemostasis. The surgical approach depends on the diagnosis, as outlined in Table 1.

A *lateral approach* can provide very adequate exposure for unilateral adrenalectomy for a localized tumor of moderate size if a high flank incision, such as the supracostal 11th-rib incision (see page 879) or a modification of the thoracoabdominal incision (see page 890), is selected. Of course, only one gland can be seen at a time. The lateral approach is not suitable for pheochromocytomas that require abdominal exploration, but a thoracoabdominal incision is excellent for large adrenal tumors, especially on the right side. In children with tumors other than pheochromocytomas, approach the adrenal through one or both flanks; anterior or posterior incisions are less suitable. For a localized aldosterone tumor, a lateral approach may be preferable.

For simultaneous exposure of both glands, a *posterior approach* is direct and quick and carries a low morbidity. It is preferable to the anterior approach for obese patients. It does require the patient to lie in a prone jack-knife position, with concomitant limitations on respiration. It may be ideal for cases of bilateral hyperplasia, because it gives adequate exposure with the least operative disturbance. The exposure is more restricted than that gained by a flank approach and thus may not be suitable for large tumors. However, with the patient prone, by approaching transthoracically through the bed of the 11th rib and continuing through the diaphragm and pleura, excellent exposure is possible. For the rare instance of nonlocalized aldosterone-secreting adenoma, bilateral anterior exposure is required.

An *anterior transabdominal approach* through a high modified chevron-shaped incision (see page 865) is the approach of choice for pheochromocytoma because of the bilaterality of this condition and the high incidence of extra-adrenal sites (15 percent). Remember that in children these tumors are often bilateral and multiple. A "radical" adrenalectomy is required to remove adjacent neural crest tissue. However, current localization techniques make a lateral approach tempting because it results in far fewer complications. A good rule is not to use this approach in patients who have extra-adrenal pheochromocytomas, who are less than 18 years of age, or who are pregnant. An anterior approach is also preferred in infants for excision of neuroblastoma, which is often infiltrating and thus not confined to the adrenal. For the same reason, approaching anteriorly through a modified chevron incision is very suitable for tumors greater than 10 cm in diameter. Also, if a patient must be

Table 1. Surgical Treatment of Adrenal Disease

Disorder	Approach	Comments
Cushing's disease		
Hyperplasia	Bilateral posterior Bilateral 11th-rib (sequential)	Bilateral adrenalectomy as last option
Cushing's syndrome		
Adenoma		
Left	11th-rib supracostal	
	Thoracoabdominal	Especially for large adenoma or secondary operation
	Posterior	Small adenoma
Right	10th-rib transthoracic	Same as left
Children	11th-rib supracostal	Avoid anterior and posterior incisions
Carcinoma	Thoracoabdominal 11th-rib supracostal Transabdominal	
Primary aldosteronism		
Adenoma, localized	Posterior Left 11th-rib supracostal Posterior transthoracic	Protect adrenal vein
Adenoma, nonlocalized	Bilateral anterior	Expose both adrenals, remove the larger (or both if large)
Pheochromocytoma and other functioning tumors		
Adults, localized		
Left	Transabdominal (chevron) 11th-rib supracostal	
Right	10th-rib supracostal Thoracoabdominal	
Children	Anterior transabdominal	
Paraendocrine tumors	Bilateral anterior	
Neuroblastoma		
	Transabdominal 11th-rib supracostal	
Bilateral ablation		
	Bilateral posterior	

reoperated for adrenal disease, exposure is much better through the peritoneum that through the flank. The disadvantages of an anterior incision are several. The exposure takes longer to obtain, and the approach to the adrenal is not as direct. Further, the adrenals are usually found to lie quite deep and quite high. Postoperatively, ileus occurs and intestinal adhesions may become a problem.

In summary, for the right adrenal behind the vena cava, a right transverse incision tends to be too low, but if entry is gained through pleura and diaphragm as in a thoracoabdominal approach, the exposure can be satisfactory. For small lesions in thin patients, a posterior incision with resection of the 12th rib is good if the pleura and diaphragm are traversed and the undersurface of the diaphragm is freed up. By retracting the kidney downward, the avascular superior and lateral surfaces of the adrenal may be freed, and the vessels to the inferior and medial portions are more readily successively clipped. For large, potentially malignant tumors, a chevron incision can be used, although it is less than ideal for tumors on the right side. The best exposure is through an 8th-rib subcostal thoracoabdominal incision, but that takes more time to create. With the adrenal adherent to the undersurface of the liver, the duodenum is reflected to expose the vena cava; this allows early ligation of the adrenal vein. Realize that pheochromocytomas and carcinomas can invade the vena cava. The flank incision is reserved for obese patients, for unilateral disease, and for small tumors.

TECHNIQUE OF EXCISION

The adrenal glands are very well vascularized and require careful hemostasis with both electrocautery and clips. Leave the gland attached to the upper pole of the kidney during dissection. The adrenal capsule is very thin and the gland is very fragile; manipulate it by its attached connective tissue. Free the superior, anterior, posterior, and lateral surfaces first. On the left, complete the dissection of the gland by placing a clamp on the periadrenal tissue, and dissect against the aorta while either ligating or clipping the arteries. Finally, clamp and ligate the adrenal vein at the hilum. Removal of the right adrenal gland can be more troublesome because the adrenal vein is short on that side and it enters the vena cava, in contrast to the longer vein on the left that enters the renal vein. Incidentally, in large functioning adrenal tumors with vena caval obstruction, the veins below are enormous and very friable. After removal, check the vena cava for injury. It may be helpful to pack the fossa with gauze for a few minutes; if oozing persists, add an absorbable sponge. Replace Gerota's fascia before wound closure.

LAPAROSCOPIC ADRENALECTOMY, TRANSPERITONEAL APPROACH

Place the patient in a half-lateral position, establish a pneumoperitoneum, and insert appropriate trocars.

Incise the posterior peritoneum from the hepatic flexure to the duodenum on the right and from the phrenocolic ligament both transversely along the transverse colon and caudally along the descending colon. Expose the renal capsule. Locate the adrenal and tumor in the perirenal fat (a laparoscopic 7.5-MHz ultrasound scanner may be helpful). Identify and clip the main adrenal vein. Do this where it joins the vena cava to make enough room to apply clips, a maneuver not as easily done on the right side. Start the dissection at the upper end between the diaphragm and the gland to establish a plane. Use the argon beam coagulator as needed. Clip and divide the adrenal arteries as they are encountered. Small arteries may be fulgurated. Hemorrhage is of concern with this approach. Remove the gland in an Endobag after morcellization.

Commentary by James F. Glenn

For adrenal surgery, my own preference is the posterior approach with the patient prone and in the jack-knife position. This allows use of a hockey-stick incision, as proposed by Young, or the direct oblique 11th-rib posterior approach, as we have advocated. Such an approach is suitable for unilateral adenomas (Cushing's and aldosteronomas); it may be used in cases of bilateral hyperplasia, including macronodular and micronodular disease. The posterior approach is also useful when it is necessary to explore one adrenal and to be able to turn to the other when the tumor is not found. The simplicity of the posterior approach is augmented by its relatively innocuous postoperative effects because neither the pleural cavity nor the peritoneum needs to be entered. The posterior approach is not suitable for pheochromocytomas or paragangliomas, which should be approached transabdominally, nor is this approach desirable for very large tumors or malignancies of the adrenal because an anterior approach provides the more extensive exposure required. In children, the anterior abdominal approach is preferred for essentially all adrenal tumors.

Lateral Approach to the Adrenal Gland

LEFT ADRENAL GLAND

Instruments: Provide a Basic set, GU vascular and GU chest sets, small and large Satinsky clamps, a GIA stapler, a major retractor set, a D-tach Balfour retractor, a Turner-Warwick retractor, and a fiberoptic suction tip with light source.

Incision: Select one of the flank incisions. A supracostal incision above the 11th rib gives excellent exposure (see page 879). In thin patients, an anterior subcostal incision (see page 871) can be used. For large tumors, make a thoracoabdominal incision (see page 890).

1 A, Place the patient in the lateral position over the kidney rest, and place the left arm on an airplane-type arm board.

B, Through an incision above the 11th rib (supracostal incision, see page 879), mobilize the colon and peritoneum medially. Bluntly dissect the posterior lamina of Gerota's fascia from the posterior body musculature. Sharply divide the splenorenal ligament. Mobilize the peritoneum containing the spleen and pancreas anteriorly to expose the anterior surface of the adrenal gland, seen through a thin layer of Gerota's fascia.

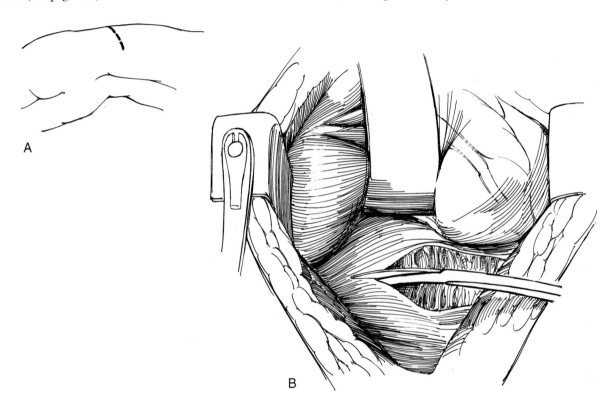

2 Dissect the pale periadrenal fat from the surface of the golden yellow gland. Do not grasp the gland itself; clamp the attached fat as a handle. Start anteriorly with sharp dissection. The connective tissue adheres to hyperplastic glands, less so to those containing a tumor. Clip each small artery with a fine clip as it is exposed and divide it. Continue dissection anteriorly, then laterally and posteriorly, leaving the gland attached inferiorly to the kidney and medially.

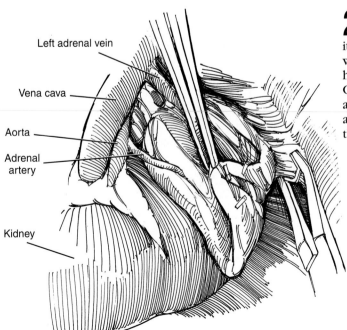

Left adrenal vein

Vena cava

Aorta

Adrenal artery

Kidney

3 For total adrenalectomy, grasp the fat and attached periadrenal tissue with a Babcock clamp and retract the gland laterally, away from the aorta. Free the gland medially by blunt dissection, using a peanut sponge to expose the several small arteries. Clamp and ligate each one with silk ties; clip the smaller vessels. Expose the hilum of the gland, and carefully dissect the large adrenal vein to the vena cava. Clamp, divide, and tie it.

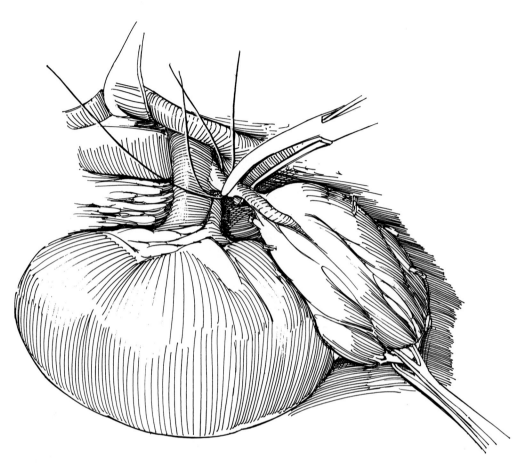

4 For partial adrenalectomy to remove a small localized tumor, place a Satinsky clamp proximal to the mass, cut off the exposed portion, and close the defect with a running suture over the clamp. Alternately, the GIA stapler may be used. Observe the fossa for bleeding. If oozing is seen, pack the site for a few minutes. Absorbable gelatin sponge may be used. Check the adjacent aorta, vena cava, and upper renal pole. Close the wound without drainage.

Large left adrenal tumors: Make the approach anterolaterally through the lesser sac (see page 1066). Carefully divide the omentum on the left above the transverse colon, and lift the stomach to reveal the adrenal through the lesser sac. Divide the inferior mesenteric vein before it joins the splenic vein to enable retraction of the spleen and tail of the pancreas and exposure of the tumor.

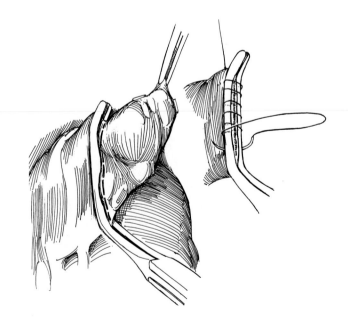

RIGHT ADRENAL GLAND

5 **A** and **B,** Through a right 11th supracostal incision (see page 879), open the peritoneum and incise it again lateral to the ascending colon to the level of the hepatic veins. Retract the colon medially, and lift the liver and gallbladder from the anterior surface of the adrenal gland. Open the exposed Gerota's fascia, and pull the kidney down.

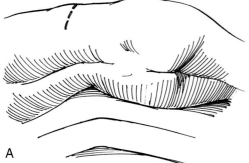

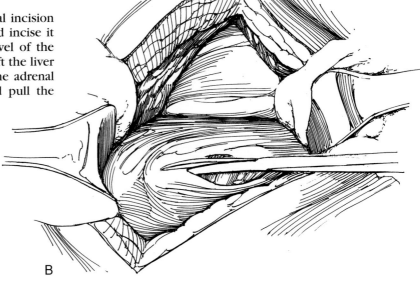

A   B

6 **A,** By downward traction on the kidney with one hand, mobilize the gland along the lateral border by clipping the multiple small arteries.

B, Free the medial border. Watch out for the inferior phrenic vein, which may be large and cause considerable bleeding if not controlled.

C, Dissect the superior margin.

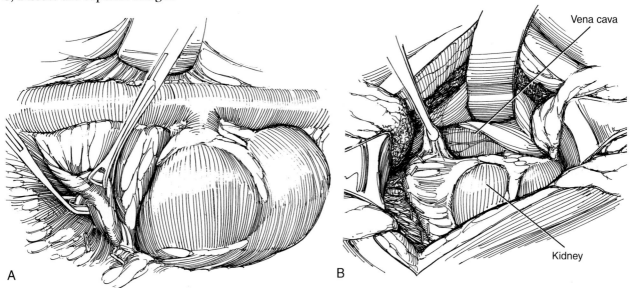

A   B

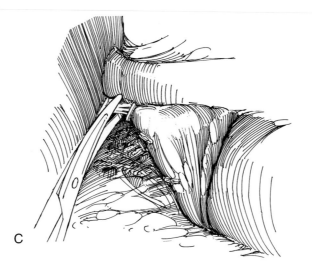

C

7 On the right, the adrenal vein enters the vena cava directly, at a site higher and more posteriorly than expected. To expose it, clip the small medial arteries to allow retraction of the vena cava medially, and displace the kidney with the attached adrenal downward.

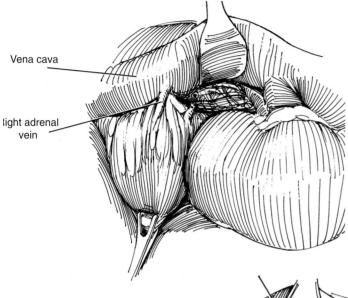

Vena cava

light adrenal
vein

8 Pass two silk ties around the vein, divide it, and remove the gland. If the vein is torn, the tear is close to the vena cava. In that case, apply a small Satinsky clamp to the base, including some of the wall of the vena cava; then place a larger clamp beneath it. Remove the small clamp, and oversew the vein stump and some of the vena caval wall (see page 81).

Large right adrenal tumors: For better exposure of large tumors on the right, extend the incision anteriorly, and continue the mobilization of the hepatic flexure of the colon by freeing the peritoneum across the vena cava and back along the edge of the liver. Bluntly dissect the liver from the front of the vena cava for 3 to 5 cm. As the several lower hepatic veins are encountered, doubly tie and cut them. Retract the vena cava, allowing good exposure of the adrenal vein. Further exposure can be obtained by sharply dividing the triangular and coronary ligaments of the liver, plus the ligamentum teres if needed. Rotate the entire liver to the left to expose the multiple short veins between the tumor and the vena cava, which can then be divided for greater exposure.

Check the area for bleeding, and close the wound in layers.

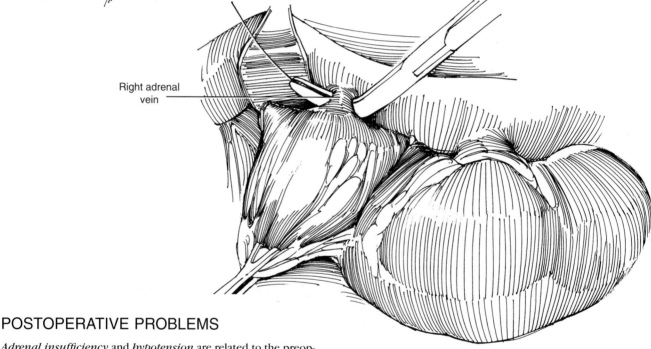

Right adrenal
vein

POSTOPERATIVE PROBLEMS

Adrenal insufficiency and *hypotension* are related to the preoperative diagnosis and the amount of adrenal tissue remaining. Appropriately monitored therapy (see page 1058) replaces the deficits. *Other complications* are similar to those after nephrectomy (see page 1026).

Commentary by John A. Libertino

I find that in the flank the Buchwalter retractor gives excellent exposure through a supracostal 11th-rib incision. I agree completely that a thoracoabdominal approach is best for larger tumors. In general, when mobilizing the adrenal gland, I prefer to approach it by mobilizing the lateral border, which is relatively avascular. Then I mobilize the superior blood supply and the inferior phrenic artery and vein and ligate these vessels. This is facilitated by gentle downward traction on the kidney. At this point, we can take the posterior branches with large Weck clips. Those branches contain the arterial blood supply that comes directly from the aorta. I take the medial blood supply last. This must be done carefully to avoid injury to the main renal artery or the segmental branches.

The major adrenal vein is always ligated in continuity and divided. One should not clip this vessel, as clips are prone to come off and result in significant postoperative hemorrhage. The gland is then sharply divided from the upper pole of the kidney.

The two major complications are hemorrhage and injury to the renal artery or its branches. Complications ca be avoided by very careful dissection of the medial blood supply of the adrenal gland. When one is dealing with a pheochromocytoma, it is imperative to control and ligate the major adrenal vein to prevent excessive catacholamines from getting into the systemic circulation. Such a situation is the only reason to vary the above-outlined approach to mobilizing the gland.

Anterior Approach to the Adrenal Gland

Pheochromocytomas may be bilateral or may occur at sites distant from the adrenal. Choose an anterior transabdominal approach through a modified chevron incision (see page 865). In children, use the pediatric extended anterior incision (see page 863). A thoracoabdominal approach (see page 890) is reserved for a large, well-localized pheochromocytoma in adults or for any large adrenal mass, especially in an obese patient. This approach is safer and avoids traction on the tumor before removal.

LEFT ADRENAL RESECTION

1 **A,** Stand on the left side of the table and place the patient supine. Be certain that the bar is elevated or a rolled blanket is placed under the back to accentuate the lumbar lordotic curve to open the incision. Make a chevron incision (see page 865) that extends from the 10th costal cartilage across the upper abdomen to the opposite 10th costal cartilage. Make it shorter on the contralateral side if the tumor has been localized; if the results of the properative localization studies were questionable, make a full chevron incision. The incision can be amplified by resecting one or both 10th-rib costal cartilages by dissecting them free and breaking them off the ribs.

B, Hold the splenic flexure of the colon medially, and incise the posterior peritoneum vertically just lateral to it. Divide the splenocolic ligament. If necessary to get more exposure, divide the inferior mesenteric vein and incise the ligament of Treitz. Open Gerota's fascia vertically to expose the anterior surface of the left kidney and the left renal vein.

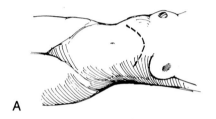

A

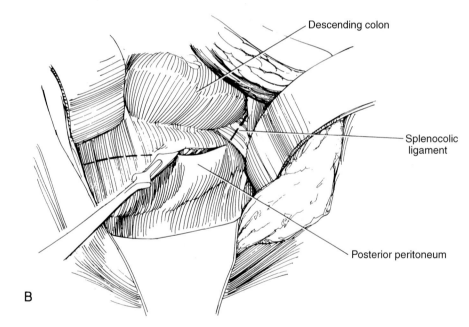

Descending colon

Splenocolic ligament

Posterior peritoneum

B

2 Alternatively and preferably, divide the omentocolic attachment, and enter the retroperitoneum through the lesser sac. Incise the posterior peritoneum just inferior to the pancreas, working medially and leaving the splenocolic ligament above intact.

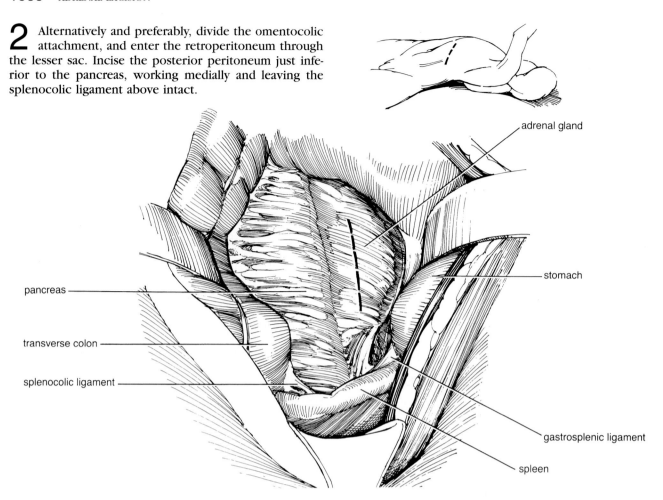

pancreas

transverse colon

splenocolic ligament

adrenal gland

stomach

gastrosplenic ligament

spleen

3 Hold the viscera medially with broad retractors. Draw the kidney down with a stick sponge to bring the adrenal into view. Start dissecting along the lower outer border, leaving some periadrenal connective tissue attached to the gland for traction and rotation. Do not grasp the gland itself. Clip each vessel as it is encountered. Use coagulating current for small potential oozers. Disconnect the superior margin of the gland.

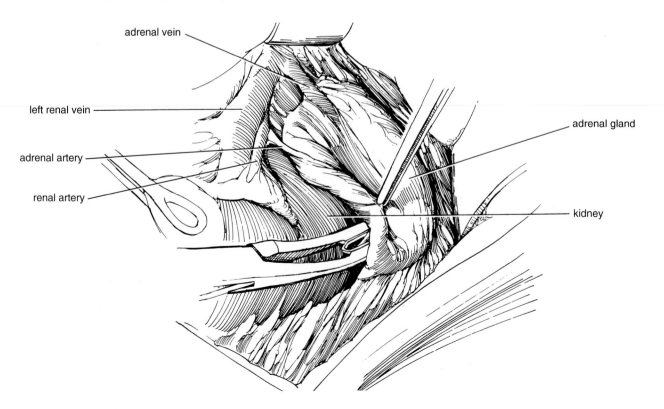

adrenal vein

left renal vein

adrenal artery

renal artery

adrenal gland

kidney

4 Clip the small phrenic branches on the superior margin. Secure the artery or arteries from the aorta with clips.

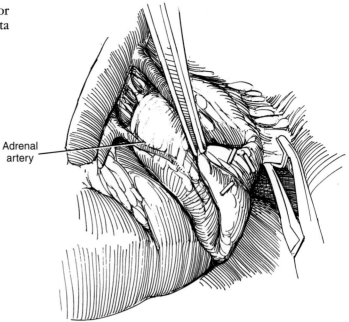

Adrenal
artery

5 Watch for tributaries from the adrenal to the inferior phrenic vein, a structure that may be torn in the dissection. Pass two 2-0 silk sutures around the adrenal vein; ligate, clamp, and divide it.

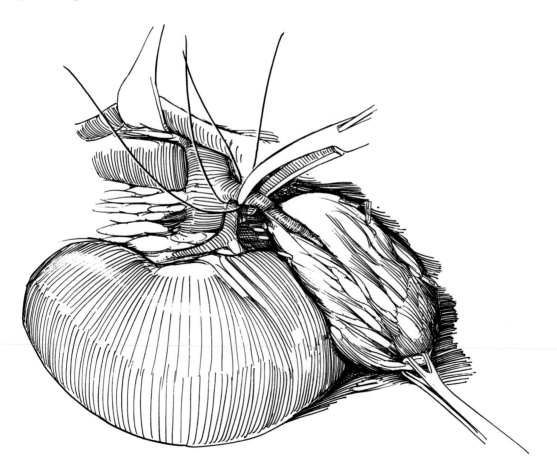

RIGHT ADRENAL RESECTION

6 **A,** Stand on the right side of the table and make a chevron incision.

B, Incise the posterior peritoneum lateral to the duodenum and adrenal. Mobilize the hepatic flexure of the colon, and free the colon down to the cecum. Reflect the duodenum medially.

7 Lift up the liver to visualize the upper pole of the kidney. Pull the kidney down preparatory to dissecting the adrenal. Clear the anterolateral surface of the gland, grasping periadrenal fat but being very careful not to grasp the gland itself. Dissect laterally and posteriorly, dividing each small vessel using clips or ties.

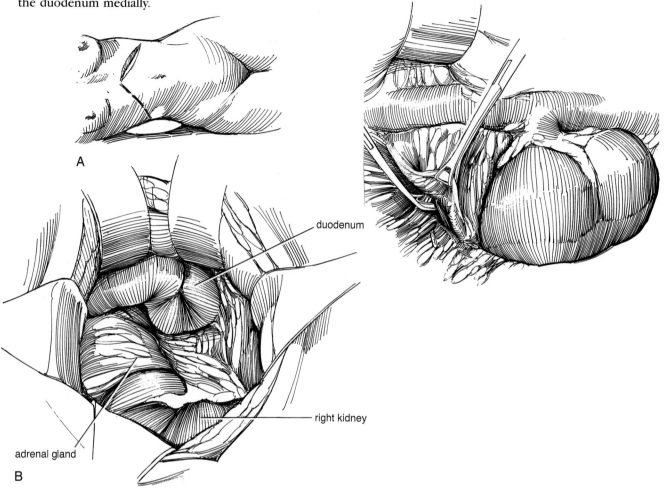

A

duodenum

right kidney

adrenal gland

B

8 Divide the fibrous attachments at the apex. These may reach the lower surface of the liver, which must be protected. Watch for low hepatic veins; these may be easily avulsed from the vena cava and should be ligated and divided.

9 Free the medial surface by clipping the arterial branches. Place two 2-0 silk ties around the vein and ligate it. Clamp the vein distally and divide it. Divide the attachments to the kidney, and remove the specimen.

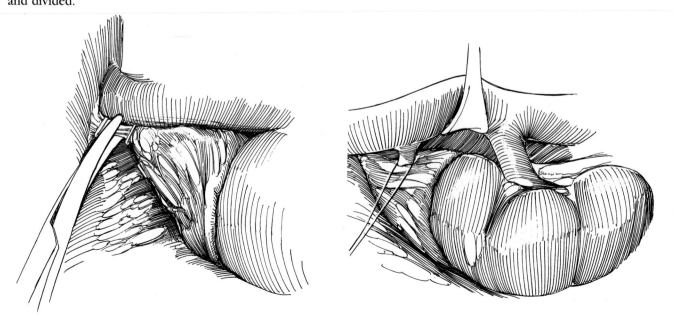

ADRENALECTOMY WITH NEPHRECTOMY

Extracapsular Left Adrenal Tumor

10 **A,** *Position:* Place the patient in the supine position, accentuating the lumbar lordotic curve.

Incision: Make part of a chevron incision (see page 865) that extends laterally over the costal cartilage of the 10th rib, which should be removed or freed supracostally (see page 887).

B, Expose the aorta behind the left renal vein. Dissect the vein to expose the left renal artery beneath it. Clamp the renal artery with a vascular clamp to allow the kidney to become smaller and softer. After clamping the renal artery, ligate the adrenal vein, and dissect enough of the adrenal to be sure that the kidney is not involved. If this is the case, release the arterial clamp and proceed with adrenalectomy. Most adrenal tumors can be dissected off the kidney; in contrast, renal tumors are more likely to invade the adrenal.

If the kidney is involved, ligate the renal artery with a size 0 silk suture passed around it, clamp and divide it, and then ligate both sides with 0 silk. Doubly ligate the left renal vein; then clamp it distally, divide it, and ligate the distal end.

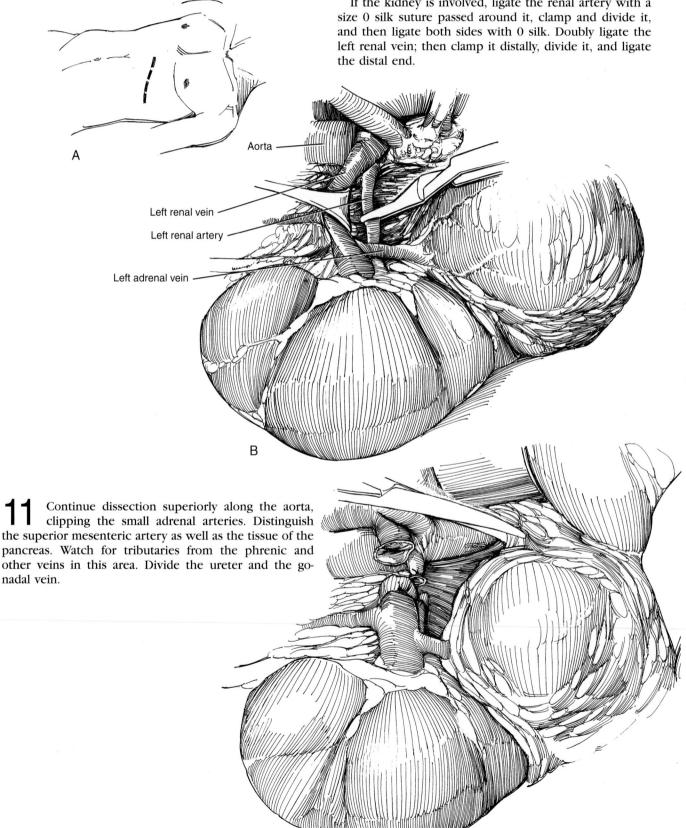

Aorta

Left renal vein

Left renal artery

Left adrenal vein

A

B

11 Continue dissection superiorly along the aorta, clipping the small adrenal arteries. Distinguish the superior mesenteric artery as well as the tissue of the pancreas. Watch for tributaries from the phrenic and other veins in this area. Divide the ureter and the gonadal vein.

12 Have the assistant draw the kidney and tumor medially. Bluntly free both of them from the psoas fascia. The spleen is vulnerable to injury by the retractor and must be protected.

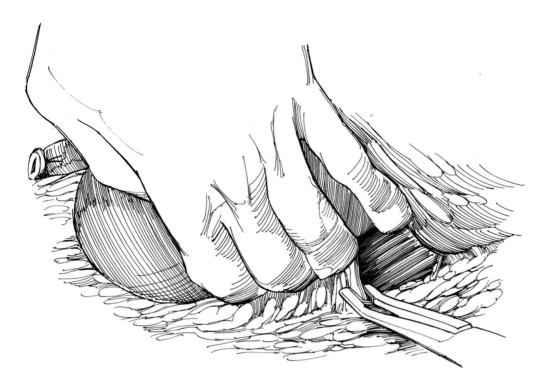

13 Pull the kidney down. Clip and divide the vascular attachments to the upper pole of the adrenal. Remove the specimen.

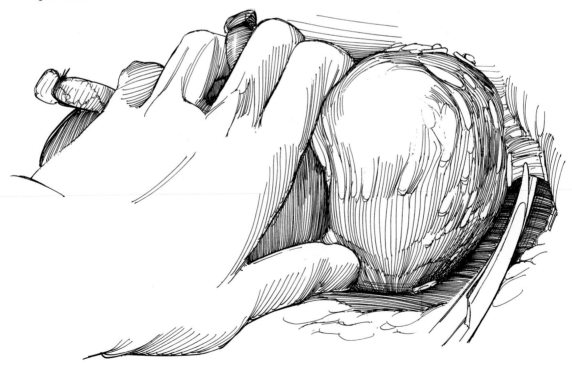

Extracapsular Right Adrenal Tumor

14 **A** and **B,** Proceed as described for the left side, but, because of its inaccessibility, secure the adrenal vein entering the vena cava *after* dividing the renal pedicle. It may be necessary to divide hepatic veins for access. Proceed with regional lymphadenectomy, not necessarily en bloc. Alternatively, if the tumor is a pheochromocytoma and is adherent only to the upper pole of the kidney, dissect beneath the perirenal fat until the upper pole is reached. Resect the upper pole if it is involved (see page 1000); do not try to peel the tumor off the kidney.

POSTOPERATIVE PROBLEMS

Patients with aldosterone tumors may *retain potassium* postoperatively. Patients with glucocorticoid excess have had *suppression of the contralateral adrenal* and require replacement with hydrocortisone. Give it in doses of 100 mg IM every 4 to 6 hours until the patient is able to take oral medications. Because of their defective metabolic state, these patients are subject to wound infection and thromboembolism, as well as cardiovascular and mental problems.

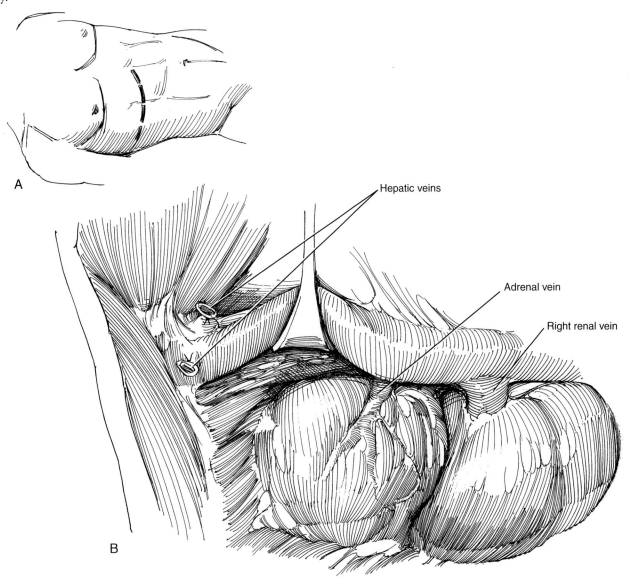

A

B

Hepatic veins

Adrenal vein

Right renal vein

PHEOCHROMOCYTOMA

Approach on Left

Localize the tumor with MRI and perhaps also with [131]MIBG scan. Such localization may make the traditional complete transabdominal exposure unnecessary. In children, however, multiple tumors are more common.

15 **A,** *Position* and *incision* as in Step 1. Make the chevron incision (see page 865), shorter on the contralateral side if the tumor has been localized. After entering the abdomen, gently palpate the adrenal and para-aortic areas while the anesthetist monitors the blood pressure to search for previously undetected tumors.

B, Mobilize the colon medially by incising the splenocolic ligament. For more exposure, ligate the inferior mesenteric vein, and divide the ligament of Treitz. Dissect the pancreas from the surface of the adrenal gland. Incise the retroperitoneum just below the lower border of the pancreas, and open the Gerota's fascia.

An alternative is to approach the adrenals through the lesser sac, rather than reflecting the splenic flexure.

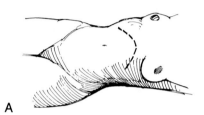

A

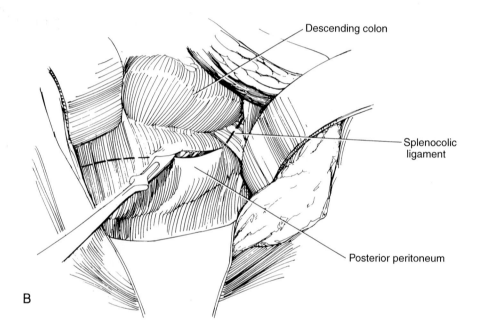

Descending colon

Splenocolic ligament

Posterior peritoneum

B

16 Place retractors; a large ring retractor is best. Realize before starting the dissection that pheochromocytomas, especially large ones, are soft, very friable, and sometimes malignant; thus, any break in the capsule can cause recurrence. Avoid manipulation and engorgement of the gland.

Carefully free the gland from its bed inferiorly. Dissect it laterally to the superior margin of the left renal vein and locate the adrenal vein, which may empty into the inferior phrenic vein or even directly into the vena cava.

Dissect out the vein and notify the anesthesiologist. Pass a 2-0 silk ligature, and be ready to ligate the vein proximally. If the patient is stable, delay venous ligation until the arterial inflow is controlled to avoid venous congestion in the adrenal, which increases friability. Otherwise, clamp and divide the vein and ligate it beneath the clamp. Leave the distal ligature long for traction.

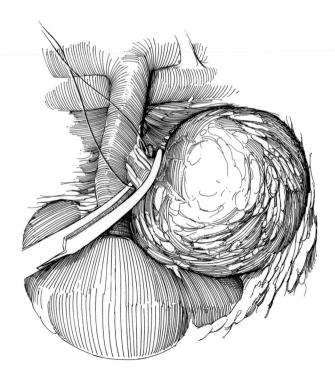

17 Bluntly free the gland posteriorly. Retract the splenic vein with a padded retractor to expose the upper pole. Clip the vascular and fascial attachments. Pull the gland laterally and inferiorly to clip and divide the one or more arteries arising from the aorta and from the inferior phrenic artery. Remove the adrenal gland and tumor.

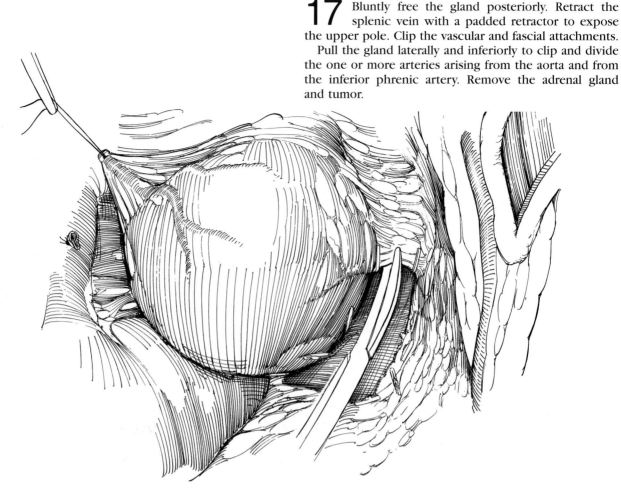

18 If malignancy is suspected for either left or right pheochromocytomas as evidenced by fixation or by invasion of local tissues, proceed with regional lymphadenectomy (see pages 1021 and 1025). Look for other tumors in the para-aortic region by opening the posterior peritoneum over the aorta and palpating the renal pedicle on both sides and the groove between the aorta and vena cava to a point below the bifurcation. Close the retroperitoneal incision. Reapproximate the gastrocolic ligament. Search the retroperitoneal area again thoroughly for additional tumors before closing the retroperitoneum. Close the abdominal wound.

For malignant pheochomocytoma, perform a block dissection that may include the kidney.

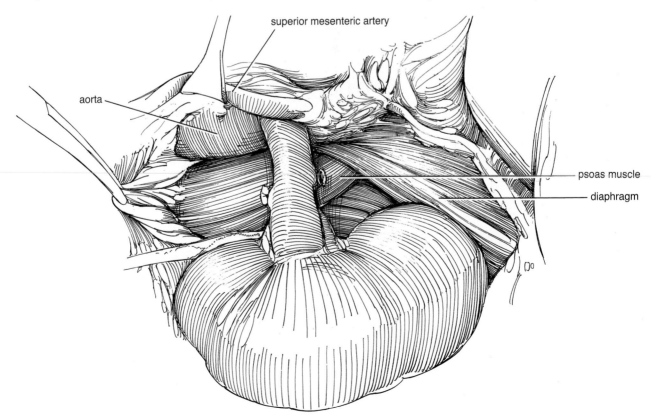

superior mesenteric artery

aorta

psoas muscle

diaphragm

Approach on Right

The general approach is illustrated in Steps 6 to 9.

Incision: The exposure here needs to be wider than on the left side. Make a chevron incision in adults (see page 865) or an extended pediatric anterior incision in children (see page 863). A thoracoabdominal incision is an alternative for large tumors.

Retract the liver. To expose the adrenal area, perform a wide Kocher maneuver (see pages 859 and 986) by making a semicircular incision in the retroperitoneum extending two thirds of the way around the duodenum and mobilizing the first three parts of the duodenum to the left. Free the hepatic flexure of the colon, using clips as needed, to expose the right colic artery. Continue to incise the parietal peritoneum to the level of the cecum.

Pull the kidney down, and gently dissect the mass as described for the left adrenal, exposing the adrenal vein at its entrance to the vena cava by dissecting from above downward. Take great care not to injure the thin-walled vein or tear the vena cava. Gently retract the vena cava with a long vein retractor.

19 Place a 2-0 silk suture around the vein, and notify the anesthesiologist. Ligate the vein near the vena cava with 2-0 silk. If the vein is short and wide, insinuate a Satinsky clamp onto the vena cava and use that for control instead of using a ligature alone. Place a tie or hemoclip distally. Individually clip the small arteries from the aorta; do not try to tie them. Remove the specimen.

Search the retroperitoneal area thoroughly for additional tumors before closing the retroperitoneum and the wound. Place the patient in the intensive care unit for 1 or 2 days.

POSTOPERATIVE PROBLEMS

Cardiovascular lability is reduced by preoperative alpha-adrenergic blockade, with catechol production reduced with alpha-methyltyrosine. During and after operation, management is determined by a team of anesthesiologists, endocrinologists, and urologists. Because acute hypotension remains a risk postoperatively, especially when the patient is moved, continue monitoring the blood pressure. Correct hypotension with fluids. It may take 24 to 48 hours for the effect of the adrenergic blocker to wear off. Check the blood glucose level to detect *hypoglycemia.* Follow up with *metanephrine* and *VMA* levels every 6 months for 3 years and yearly for another 4 years. *Back pain* is not uncommon after long transabdominal operations if the lumbar curve was not maintained.

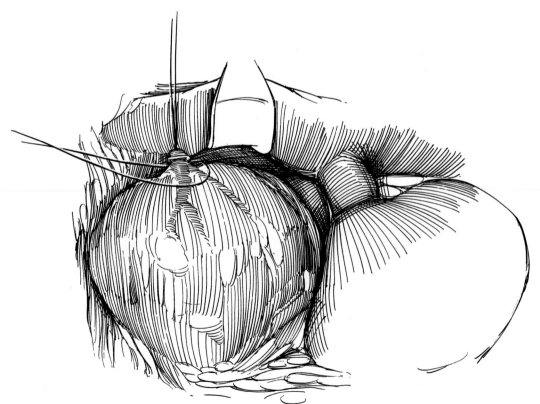

Posterior Approach to the Adrenal Gland

The posterior approach is ideal for small, well-localized benign adrenal tumors, providing adequate access with the lowest morbidity. But it is not suitable for pheochromocytomas in children, for tumors larger than about 6 to 8 cm with their parasitic blood supply, or for malignant tumors with the potential for intra-abdominal extension. For these cases, take advantage of the wider field obtained by a more anterior approach. The posterior approach may also be used for bilateral explora-tion, although there are now few indications for this because of the accuracy of localization techniques. The posterior approach is, of course, suitable for bilateral adrenalectomy.

Instruments are the same as those for dorsal lumbotomy.

For well-localized lesions, a lateral approach through the 11th-rib supracostal incision (see page 879) usually provides adequate exposure, but the transdiaphragmatic exposure described here offers greater access for larger lesions.

POSTERIOR TRANSCOSTAL TRANSDIAPHRAGMATIC INCISION

Left Adrenal Exposure

1 **A,** *Position:* Place the patient in the prone position with the pelvis and shoulders resting on firm pillows to allow the abdomen to sag between them. Flex the table to 35 degrees. Place the incision at the level of the left 11th rib.

B, Start a curved incision three fingerbreadths from the midline at the level of the 10th rib, and pass the incision through the posterior lamella of the lumbodorsal fascia and the associated fibers of the latissimus dorsi muscles. Retract the erector spinae muscle medially and expose the 11th rib. Divide and ligate the several vessels to the erector spinae muscle. Identify the 11th rib (check the radiograph), and free it from the erector spinae muscle with the cutting current.

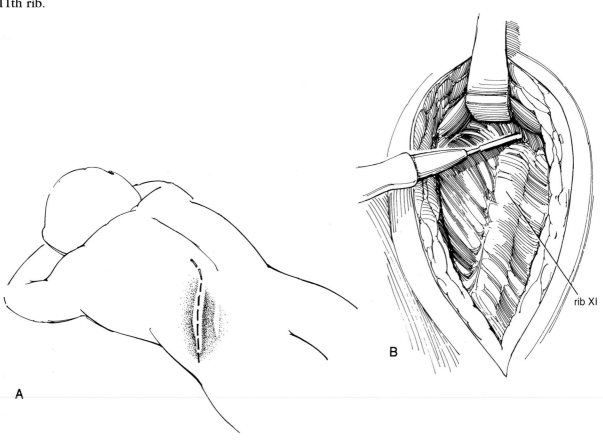

rib XI

A

B

2 Resect the 11th rib subperiosteally (see page 875), exposing Gerota's fascia. Divide the subcostal vessels, but preserve the 11th intercostal nerve.

3 Ask the anesthetist to tilt the table 15 degrees away and to deflate the lung. Incise the pleura in the line of the incision. Insert a self-retaining retractor.

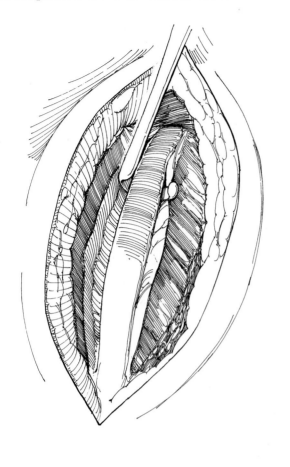

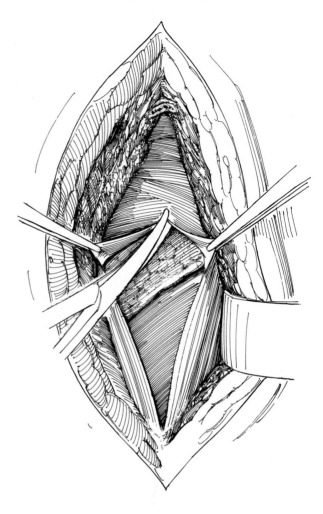

4 With the cutting current, make a small opening in the diaphragm. Insert a finger between it and Gerota's fascia. Bluntly separate these two layers anteriorly and posteriorly, and cut the diaphragm the length of the incision. Or preferably, strip the intact pleura and diaphragm away from the 11th and 12th ribs where they adhere posterior to the midaxillary line and above the back of the L1 spinous process. The adrenal can then be identified beneath the thin layer of Gerota's fascia.

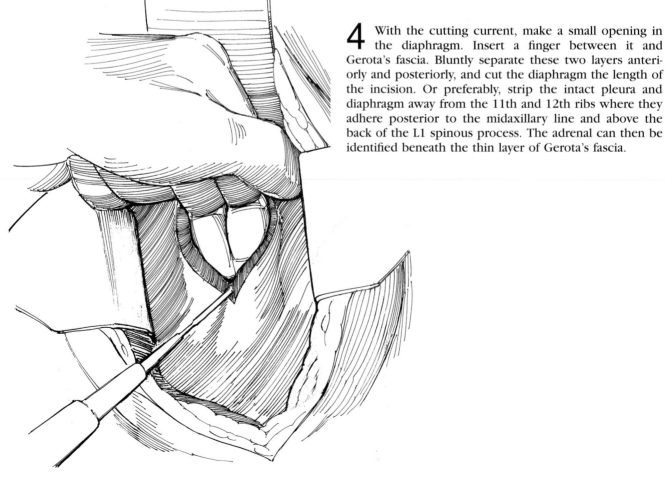

5 Incise Gerota's fascia transversely, and expose the posterior surface of the kidney at the upper pole. Draw the kidney down with a sponge stick or gauze-covered retractor. The adrenal, which lies above it and toward the midline, is brought into the incision. Dissect the pale periadrenal fat to expose an edge of the golden yellow adrenal. After the adrenal is exposed, progressively clip or fulgurate the arterial input arising from the phrenic vessels. Place several silk sutures in the margin of the adrenal; grasping them together in a clamp provides traction without obstruction. Finally, free the attachments to the upper pole of the kidney and renal pedicle, the aorta, and the renal artery.

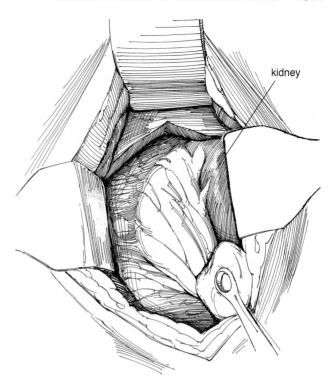

kidney

6 Open a space medially to dissect down to the renal vein. Isolate the adrenal vein. Either clamp it near the renal vein and doubly ligate and divide it or pass two ligatures around it, tie them, and divide the vessel between. If the vein is too short, doubly clip it on either side and cut between the clips. Complete the dissection of the anterior adrenal surface and remove the specimen. Close Gerota's fascia loosely. Check for pleural leaks. Fasten the edges of the diaphragm and the periosteum of the rib to the lumbodorsal fascia, taking care to avoid the intercostal nerve.

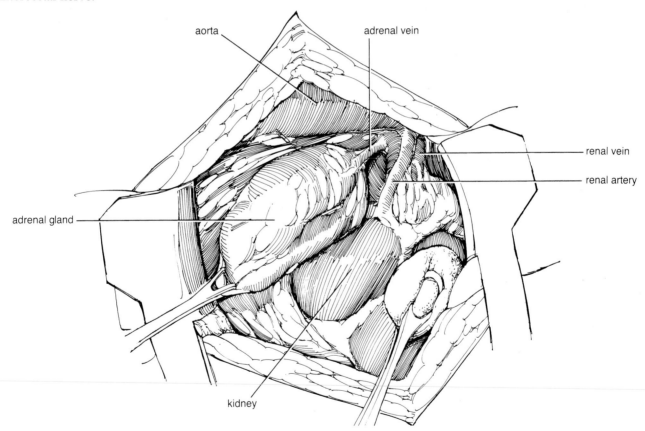

aorta

adrenal vein

renal vein

renal artery

adrenal gland

kidney

Right Adrenal Exposure

The right renal vein is relatively inaccessible from anteriorly or laterally, so a transcostal transdiaphragmatic approach offers the safest exposure.

7 A and **B,** Make a posterior transcostal incision and resect the rib (see page 875). Proceed as previously described for the left side up to Step 6.

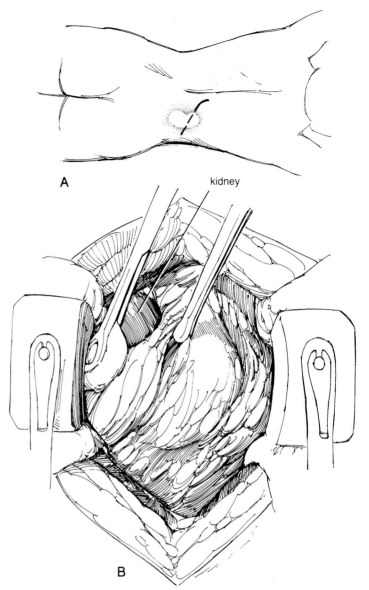

A

kidney

B

8 Start dissecting a few millimeters lateral to the gland to create a "holder" so that it is not necessary to grasp the soft adrenal gland with instruments. Gently retract the adrenal to allow dissection up and down its medial aspect, exposing the surface of the vena cava. (Be aware that large adrenal neoplasms can involve the vena cava. If this is the case, proceed as described for vena caval thrombectomy [see page 1031].) Exposure of a segment of the vena cava is important before dissecting the adrenal vein because a Satinsky clamp must be immediately applied in case of a tear in the adrenal vein or vena cava. Isolate the short adrenal vein with great caution where it approaches the vena cava. Ligate or clip the vein in continuity and divide it. It may be safer to put two clips on the vein at the time that it is first seen. Add a suture tie of fine silk distal to the first tie or clip. Remove the specimen.

If the vena cava or renal vein is lacerated, clamp the vessel with a right-angle vascular clamp, and oversew the clamp with 6-0 arterial silk. Cover the adrenal fossa with perinephric fat; apply absorbable gelatin sponge if oozing is present. Close the diaphragm, checking for pleural leaks. Close the wound in layers without drainage. Obtain a chest film in the recovery room.

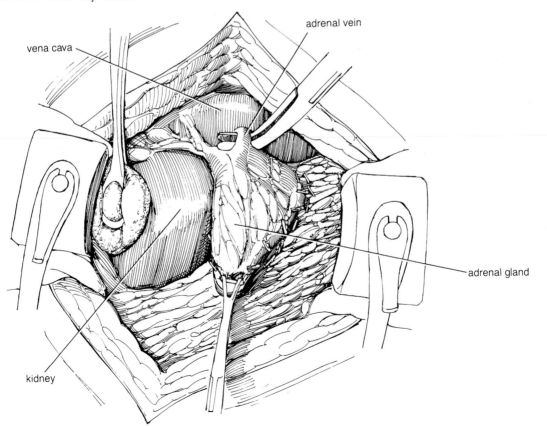

vena cava

adrenal vein

adrenal gland

kidney

MODIFIED POSTERIOR APPROACH
(Vaughan and Carey)

To avoid placing the patient with a small tumor in the stressful jack-knife position, use an obliquely prone position so that the 11th rib is more or less parallel to the table top. Resect the 11th rib, but avoid the pleural reflection (see page 875). Mobilize the peritoneum and liver from the diaphragm. Dissect the peritoneum adjacent to the liver from Gerota's fascia to expose the lateral part of the adrenal gland. Expose the posterior abdominal musculature, and clip and divide the small adrenal arteries behind the gland. Displace the adrenal gland posteriorly to reach the adrenal vein that takes a direct course from the vena cava. Doubly tie or clip it, and divide it.

SIMULTANEOUS BILATERAL EXPOSURE FOR ADRENAL ABLATION

9 **A,** Place the patient prone with pillows under the shoulders and side walls of the chest so that the abdomen is free.

B, Make either bilateral lumbotomy incisions *(long dashes)* (see page 896) or resect the 12th ribs bilaterally *(short dashes)* (see page 875).

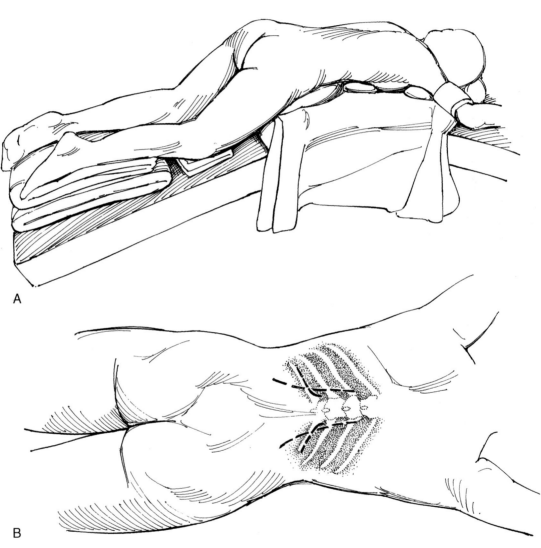

A

B

10 Approach the *left adrenal gland* first, as it is more accessible. Draw the kidney down with a stick sponge to bring it into view. Leave its connective tissue attachments intact. Start dissecting along the lower outer border, leaving some adventitia on the gland for grasping and rotation. Do not grasp the gland itself. Clip or coagulate each vessel as it is encountered. Use coagulating current for small potential oozers. Disconnect the superior margin of the gland.

Rotate the gland medially and expose the anterior surface. Clip the two or three small arteries coming from the aorta, and clamp and divided the adrenal vein arising from the left renal vein.

Approach the *right adrenal gland* by pulling the kidney down preparatory to dissection. Clear the posterior surface of the gland, being careful not to grasp the gland itself. Dissect laterally and anteriorly, dividing each small vessel using clips or ties. Next divide the fibrous attachments at the apex. These may reach the lower surface of the liver, which must be protected. Divide the attachments to the kidney. Secure the aortic branches with clips; then pass two 2-0 synthetic absorbable sutures around the adrenal vein; ligate and divide it.

Close the wounds in layers, without drainage. Carefully monitor serum electrolytes and urinary output.

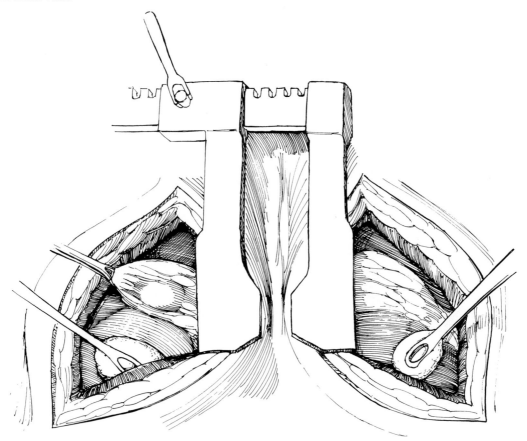

POSTOPERATIVE PROBLEMS

Adrenal insufficiency and *hypotension* are related to the preoperative diagnosis and the amount of adrenal tissue remaining. Appropriately monitored therapy (see page 1058) replaces the deficits. *Other complications* are similar to those after nephrectomy (see page 1026). *Pneumothorax* and *pancreatic* and *splenic injury* are not uncommon, nor are *wound infections,* *retroperitoneal hemorrhage,* and *hematomas* seen less frequently with this approach. *Thrombosis* and *emboli* may result from venous stasis in the legs in the prone position. More special to adrenalectomy are *injuries* to the portal vein, to the vena cava at the entrance of the adrenal vein, and to the hepatic vein—all of which are managed intraoperatively. *Subdiaphragmatic abscess* can be an additional complication.

Commentary by E. Darracott Vaughan, Jr.

For patients with adrenal adenomas, either incidental or causing Cushing's syndrome, smaller adrenal carcinomas, and well-localized pheochromocytomas, I generally use a flank or lateral approach. I limit the anterior approach to patients with multiple pheochromotycomas or bilateral adrenal lesions. Children are in the high-risk group for multiple pheochromocytomas; however, imaging studies—MIBG and MRI—are extremely accurate in identifying multiple tumors. If these tests show only a solitary lesion, I use a flank approach, particularly on the right side, where it is more difficult to isolate the adrenal vein from an anterior approach.

I make it a rule in adrenal surgery to leave the adrenal attached to the kidney and begin the dissection by dividing the most posterior lateral attachments and then the superior attachments. This allows the operator to bring the adrenal gland down into a more accessible area. One exception is in patients with pheochromocytomas, in whom the initial dissection, particularly on the left, should be aimed at early control of the adrenal vein.

If a patient with pheochromocytoma has very high levels of catecholamines or any evidence of cardiomyopathy, we use not only phenoxybenzamine but also alpha-methylparatyrosine to reduce catecholamine production.

SECTION
24

Instruments
GU Cart Contents

DRAWER 1

Medications: Various antibiotics, such as cefazolin (Kefzol), ampicillin, vancomycin, gentamicin, and neomycin (Neosporin); GU irrigant

Papaverine, methylene blue, indigo carmine, flexible collodion [USP], bacitracin ointment, diatrizoate (Hypaque or Renografin 60), lidocaine (Xylocaine, 1%), bupivacaine (Marcaine, 0.25%)

Butterfly infusion sets (19, 21, 23, and 25 gauge), Vacutainer (no additive; used with butterfly needle for penile drainage), and 27- and 30-gauge hypodermic needles

DRAWER 2

Skin stapler clip applier, hemoclip cartridges (large, medium, small), and skin stapler remover

Bovie extensions and cleaners, catheter plugs, urostomy appliance, ureteral catheter adapters, vascular tapes, and umbilical tape

DRAWER 3

Balloon catheters, 5 ml, 8 to 24 F
Silicone balloon catheters, 5 ml, 8 to 18 F
Coudé catheters, 14 to 22 F
Balloon catheters, 30 ml, 16 to 24 F
Malecot catheters, 18 to 24 F
Catheter stilets, pediatric and adult

DRAWER 4

Vasovasostomy supplies

Microscope drape, microsurgical knife, hand-controlled Bovie, needle tip for Bovie, 20-gauge 1¼" angiocath, TB syringe, Weck-cel surgical spears, visibility background material, microinstrument wipe, tongue blade, sterile slides, coverslips for slides, labels, bupivacaine (Marcaine, 0.25%), and lidocaine (Xylocaine, 1%)

Sutures

7-0 Dermalon PRE 20, 5-0 Dermalon D1, 9-0 Dermalon TE 143, 9-0 Dermalon LE-100, 10-0 Dermalon TE 100, and 6-0 Dexon DO-1

DRAWER 5

Suprapubic catheters: Bonanno, Ingram trocar catheters (12 and 16 F)

Feeding tubes (3.5, 5, 8, and 10 F), Jackson-Pratt drains (7 mm and 10 mm), Jackson-Pratt bifurcated extension, Jackson-Pratt reservoirs, bile bags, and Coban dressing (sterile, 1" and 2")

BOTTOM SHELF

Unsterile Ace wraps for legs, Elastoplast tape, urine drainage set, catheterization tray, K-Y lubricant, Montgomery straps, scrotal supporters (medium and large), sanitary belts, sanitary napkins, vaginal prep tray, Chuck absorbent pads, and blue barrier sheets

SUTURES

0 Dexon T12	5-0 Dexon T30
2-0 Dexon CE-10	5-0 Dexon PRE-2
2-0 Dexon TT3	1 Dexon ties (54")
3-0 Dexon TT2	0 Dexon ties (54")
3-0 Dexon T16	3-0 plain ties
3-0 Dexon CE-6	2-0 chromic ties
4-0 Dexon T31	3-0 chromic ties
4-0 Dexon PR-4	1 silk ties (60")
0 silk ties (30")	0 Surgilene T20
2-0 silk ties (30")	2-0 Surgilene T5
3-0 silk ties (30")	3-0 Surgilene T5
2-0 chromic TT3	4-0 Dermalon CE4
2-0 chromic UR5	1 PDS CTX
4-0 chromic C4	0 PDS CT
4-0 chromic RB1	2-0 PDS CT
5-0 chromic RB1	3-0 PDS SH
5-0 chromic CE2	4-0 PDS SH

NEEDLES

Terry Mayo
Fine French eyes
Murphy needles

Standard Instrument Sets

BIOPSY TRAY

Knife handles, (#3)
Metzenbaum scissors
Straight Mayo scissors
Smooth forceps (6″), 2
Tooth forceps (6″), 2
Adson forceps, 2
Providence clamps, 4
Kelly straight clamps, 4
Kelly curved clamps, 4
Mayo clamps, 2
Allis clamps, 2
Kocher clamps, 2
Mixter clamps, 2
Schnidt clamps, 2
Short needle holder
Towel clips (large), 6
Stick sponge
US retractors, 2
Vein retractors, 2
Loop retractors, 2
4-claw retractors (small), 2
4-claw retractors (medium), 2
Mastoid retractor
Dull Weitlaner retractor

BASIC SET

Drape sheet
Mayo tray
Sterile gowns
Large basin set
Towels (pkg)
Laparotomy sponges
Discard-a-Pad
Hand-controlled Bovie
Bulb syringes
Ground pad
Suction tubing
4 × 4 gauze pads
Robinson catheters (8, 10, 12 F)
Balloon catheter (16 F) with 5-ml drainage bag
Medium Penrose drain (½″)
Small Penrose drain (¼″)
Tonsil tip
Catheter adapter (Xmas tree)
Cath-tip syringes (60-ml)
Syringe (6-ml)
Luer-Lok syringe (60-ml)
NaCl solution (1000 ml)
Sterile water (1500 ml)
Prep container

GU LONG INSTRUMENTS

Metzenbaum scissors (9″)
Metzenbaum scissors (11″)
Needle holder, 2
Jones clamp, 4
Allis clamp, 2
Babcock clamp, 2

Mixter clamp, 2
Mayo clamp, 4
Clip appliers (medium and large)
Vascular forceps, 2
Smooth forceps (10″), 2
Toothed forceps (10″), 2
Schnidt clamp (long), 2

GU FINE INSTRUMENTS

Needle holder (5″)
Needle holder (7″)
Andrews suction tip
Knife handle (#7)
Probe
Potts scissors
Lahey scissors
Tenotomy scissors
Cushing forceps (smooth), 2
Cushing forceps (toothed), 2
Adson forceps (smooth), 2

BASIC PLASTIC SET

Scissors
  Tenotomy
  Joseph
  Lahey
  Mayo (straight)
Brown-Adson forceps, 2
Needle holders
  Webster
  GS (general surgical)
Knife handles (#3)
Skin hooks
  Double/fine, 2
  Double/heavy, 4
Ruler

GU VASCULAR PAN

DeBakey forceps, 2
DeBakey angled artery clamp, 2
Satinsky clamp, 3
Potts scissors
Andrew suction with stilet
Bulldog clamp, 5
Metzenbaum scissors (long)
Bent-handled aortic clamp
Curved-handled aortic clamp
Straight aortic clamp
Blunt nerve hook
Vascular needle holder (9″)
Vascular needle holder (10″)
Long tenotomy scissors
Long Weck applier (large)
Long Weck applier (medium)
Weck clips (large)
Weck clips (medium)
Rumel stilet

GU CHEST INSTRUMENTS

Doyen rib stripper
Schneider elevator
Round sharp elevator
Square sharp elevator
Angled sharp elevator
Bailey approximator, 2
Finochietto retractor (medium)
Finochietto retractor (large)
Bethune rongeur
Bone cutter
Box rongeur
Leksell rongeur

GU MICRO INSTRUMENTS

Bishop-Harmon forceps, 2
Weck tying forceps, 2
Pierce forceps, 2
Micro bipolar forceps
Vessel dilator
Jeweler's forceps, 2
Micro curved forceps
Tenotomy scissors
Micro needle holders, 2
Bipolar cord
Small towel clips, 4
Vas approximators
Heifitz clips, 2
Vas irrigating cannula
Lacrimal duct probes, 5
Straight micro scissors
Curved micro scissors
Plastic needle holder
Vannas micro scissors, curved
Vannas micro scissors, straight

VASOVASOSTOMY CART

Sterile Instruments

GU micro instruments
Mosquito clamps, curved, 4
Towel clips, small, 4
Skin hooks, fine doubles, 2
Jeweler's forceps
Vascular forceps, medium
Brown-Adson forceps
Lahey scissors
Plastic needle holder
Vascular needle holder, medium
Baby Deaver retractor
Thyroid Richardson retractor
Lateral retractors, 2
Sterile slides
Weck spears
Micro knife
Hand-controlled Bovie
Bovie cleaner
20-gauge 1¼″ Angiocath for irrigation
Unsterile coverslips for slides
Sperm collection supplies
    Pipettes
    Sterile test tubes
Control syringes

Vail-jet dispensers
Butterfly IV set (19, 21, 23, and 25 gauge)
Retract-o-Tapes
TB syringe
Visibility background material
Micro wipe
Needle Bovie tip
Tongue blades
Labels
Microscope drapes
Various balloon catheters
    Latex (8 to 24 F)
    Silastic (8 to 18 F)
Catheter stilet (adult, pediatric)

Sutures

9-0 Ethilon VAS 100-4
9-0 Dermalon LE 100
7-0 Dermalon PRE 20
10-0 Ethilon VAS 100-3
10-0 Dermalon TE 100
2-0 chromic T5
3-0 chromic T5
4-0 chromic C4
4-0 chromic RB1
5-0 chromic RB1
3-0 plain gut SH
4-0 plain gut SH
2-0 plain gut ties
3-0 plain gut ties
4-0 Dexon T31
5-0 Dexon PRE2
3-0 Dermalon CE4
4-0 Dermalon CE4
2-0 Surgilene

Medications

Lidocaine (Xylocaine, 1%)
Bupivacaine (Marcaine, 0.25%)
Collodion
Papaverine
Methylene blue
Cefazolin (Kefzol)
Tobramycin
Gentamicin

SPE MICRO SET

Bipolar cord
Calipers
Micro curved scissors
Micro straight scissors
Castroviejo needle holder, locking and nonlocking (8″),
    1 each
Jeweler's forceps, 2
Bipolar forceps
Fine long forceps, 2

GI SPECIALS

Curved mosquito clamps, 4
Curved Kelly clamps, 4
Mayo clamps, 6

Kocher bowel clamps, 4
Babcock clamps (8″), 2
Doyen straight clamps, 2
Doyen curved clamps, 2
Glassman straight clamps, 2
Glassman angled clamps, 2
GI needle holder (7″)
Metzenbaum scissors (9″)
Jones clamps, 2
Thumb forceps (10″)
Tissue forceps (8″), 2
Cushing forceps with teeth, 2
Abdominal Poole suction
Tonsil suction
Ruler

Additions

Allen clamps
Bonney forceps
Babcock clamps
Deep pelvic retractor
D-tach Balfour retractor
Fine-tipped instruments
Foss clamps
Gelpi retractors
Harvey stone clamps
Jones straight clamps
Russian forceps
Pennington clamps
Weck clip appliers
Wertheim clamps

RETROPUBIC PROSTATECTOMY INSTRUMENTS

Curette
Bladder neck spreader
Mastoid retractor
T clamp
Lobe forceps (large), 2
Lobe forceps (medium), 2
Lobe forceps (small), 2
Curved stick sponge, 2
Mayo straight scissors (9″)
Mayo curved scissors (9″)
Jones clamps, 2

PERINEAL PROSTATECTOMY INSTRUMENTS

Anterior retractors, 4
Posterior retractors, 4 assorted

Lateral retractors, 4 assorted
Posterior retractor with fiberoptic carrier
Long Lowsley or Young tractor
Short Lowsley or Young tractor

CYSTOSCOPY SET (ADULT AND PEDIATRIC)

Cystoscope with bridge and lenses
Fiberoptic light source and light cord
Cysto pack
Cysto tubing
Prep tray
Lubricant in syringe
Curved and straight sounds
Sterile water in 1-L bags
Stirrups and booties
Pouch drape with suction
Barrier sheet for buttocks
Adjustable stool

KIDNEY TRANSPLANT RECOVERY SET

Basic Pack

Kocher clamps with teeth, 4
Perforating towel clips (small or large), 12
Curved mosquito clamps, 6
Medium and large hemoclips and appliers
10-ml syringe (with 8 ml water/saline)
Suction set-up
Laparotomy tapes (used dry), 3 pkgs

Sutures

2-0 silk ties (18″)
4-0 silk ties (18″)
3-0 silk GI with round needle
Heavy retention suture on a cutting needle (for closure)
Umbilical tapes (used dry), 4

Other

Bucket of ice
Specimen labels with patient's name stamped on each

References*

SURGICAL BASICS

Adamson RJ, Musco F, Enquist IF: The clinical dimensions of a healing incision. Surg Gynecol Obstet 123:515, 1966.

Adzick NS: Comparison of fetal, newborn and adult wound healing by histologic enzyme-histochemical, and hydroxyproline determination. J Pediatr Surg 20:315, 1985.

Adzick NS, Lonaker MT: The biology of fetal wound healing: A review. Plast Reconstr Surg 87:788, 1991.

Allen L: Lymphatics and lymphoid tissues. Annu Rev Physiol 29:197, 1967.

Anson BJ, McVay CB: Surgical Anatomy, 6th ed. Philadelphia, WB Saunders, 1984.

Arey LB: Developmental Anatomy. Philadelphia, WB Saunders, 1974.

Baker BH, Borchardt KA: Sump drains and airborne bacteria as a cause of wound infections. J Surg Res 17:407, 1974.

Bardenleben K von: Handbuch der Anatomie des Menschen. Jena, Germany, Fischer, 1911.

Bazeed MA: A new use of ureteroscopy. J Urol 150:922, 1993.

Bell PRF, Jamieson CW, Packley CV (eds): Surgical Management of Vascular Disease. London, Bailliere Tindall, 1992, chap 68.

Bloch EC: Anesthetic considerations in the neonate. In King LR (ed): Urologic Surgery in Neonates and Young Infants. Philadelphia, WB Saunders, 1988, p 119.

Bo WJ, Meschan I, Krueger WA: Basic Atlas of Cross-Sectional Anatomy. Philadelphia, WB Saunders, 1980.

Borges AF: Electrical Incisions and Scar Revision. Boston, Little, Brown & Co, 1973.

Britt BA: Malignant hyperthermia. Can Anaesth Soc J 32:666, 1985.

Byrne JJ (ed): General Surgery. Goldsmith HS (ed-in-chief): Practice of Surgery. Hagerstown, MD, Harper & Row, 1984.

Cassady JF Jr: Regional anesthesia for urologic procedures. Urol Clin North Am 14:43, 1987.

Clark P: Operations in Urology. Edinburgh, Churchill Livingstone, 1985.

Cockett ATK, Koshiba K: Manual of Urologic Surgery. Berlin, Springer-Verlag, 1979.

Crafts RC: Abdominopelvic cavity and perineum. In Crafts RC (ed): A Textbook of Human Anatomy, 2nd ed. New York, John Wiley & Sons, 1979, p 269.

Craig PH, Williams JA, Davis KW, et al: A biological comparison of polyglactin 910 and polyglycolic acid synthetic absorbable sutures. Surg Gynecol Obstet 141:1, 1975.

Crawford ED, Borden TA (eds): Genitourinary Cancer Surgery. Philadelphia, Lea & Febiger, 1982, p 126.

Culp DA, Fallon B, Loening SAH: Surgical Urology, 5th ed. Chicago, Year Book Medical Publishers, 1985.

Davis AT: Postoperative infection in surgical patients. In Raffensperger JG (ed): Swenson's Pediatric Surgery, 5th ed. Norwalk, CT, Appleton & Lange, 1990, p 29.

Davis MA, Das S: Psychosexual support for genitourinary cancer patients. In Crawford ED, Das S (eds): Current Genitourinary Cancer Surgery. Philadelphia, Lea & Febiger, 1990, p 669.

Dineen P: The Surgical Wound. Philadelphia, Lea & Febiger, 1981.

Ehrlich RM (guest ed): Symposium on Complications of Pediatric Urologic Surgery. Philadelphia, WB Saunders, 1983.

Flanigan RC: Pre- and postoperative nutritional and metabolic care of genitourinary cancer patients. In Crawford ED, Das S (eds): Current Genitourinary Cancer Surgery. Philadelphia, Lea & Febiger, 1990, p 660.

Flom LS, Maizels M: Evaluation of the urinary tract and principles of surgical care in the newborn and neonate. In Webster G, Kirby R, King L, Goldwasser B (eds): Reconstructive Urology. Boston, Blackwell Scientific Publications, 1993.

Fowler JE: Methods of Urologic Surgery. Chicago, Van Tec, 1987.

Frank JD, Johnston JH (eds): Operative Paediatric Urology. Edinburgh, Churchill Livingstone, 1990.

Giddins GE: Experience with a knot-free absorbable subcuticular suture. Ann R Coll Engl 76:405, 1994.

Gonzales ET Jr, Woodard JR (guest eds): Symposium on Pediatric Urology. Philadelphia, WB Saunders, 1980.

Gosling JA, Dixon JS, Humpherson JR: Functional Anatomy of the Urinary Tract. Baltimore, University Park Press, 1982.

Grabb WC, Smith JW: Plastic Surgery. Boston, Little, Brown & Co, 1979.

Gray SW, Skandalakis JE: Embryology for Surgeons. The Embryological Basis for the Treatment of Congenital Defects. Philadelphia, WB Saunders, 1972.

Hendren WH: In memoriam: Robert E. Gross MD, 1905–1988. J Pediatr Surg 24:623, 1989.

Hirsh RA: An approach to assessing perioperative risk. In Goldmann DR, Brown FH, Levy WK, et al (eds): Medical Care of the Surgical Patient. Philadelphia, JB Lippincott, 1982, p 31.

Hunt TK: Wound Healing and Wound Infection: Theory and Surgical Practice. New York, Appleton-Century-Crofts, 1980.

Hunt TK, Slavin JP, Goodson WH: Starch powder contamination of surgical wounds. Arch Surg 129:823, 1994.

Ingerman A, Stoller ML: Preoperative protection against occupationally acquired infectious agents. Contemp Urol 5(10):34, 1993.

King LR (guest ed): Symposium on Pediatric Urology. Philadelphia, WB Saunders, 1974.

Koritké JG, Sick H: Atlas of Sectional Human Anatomy. Baltimore, Urban & Schwarzenberg, 1988.

Langer CP: Zur Anatomie und Physiologie der Haut. Sitzungsb Acad Wissensch 45:223, 1861.

Larsen EH, Gasser TC, Madsen PO: Antimicrobial prophylaxis in urological surgery. Urol Clin North Am 13:591, 1986.

Libertino JA (ed): Pediatric and Adult Reconstructive Urologic Surgery, 2nd ed. Baltimore, Williams & Wilkins, 1987.

Liebert PS: Color Atlas of Pediatric Surgery. New York, Elsevier, 1989.

Livio M, Mannucci PM, Vigano G, et al: Conjugated estrogens for the management of bleeding associated with renal failure. N Engl J Med 315:731, 1986.

Londergan TA, Hochman HI, Goldberger N: Postoperative pain following outpatient pediatric urologic surgery: A comparison of anesthetic techniques. Urology 44:572, 1994.

Luck SR: Nutrition and metabolism. In Raffensperger JG (ed): Swenson's Pediatric Surgery, 5th ed. Norwalk, CT, Appleton & Lange, 1990, p 81.

Luck SR: Preoperative evaluation and preparation. In Raffensperger JG (ed): Swenson's Pediatric Surgery, 5th ed. Norwalk, CT, Appleton & Lange, 1990, p 7.

Mayor G, Zingg E: Urologic Surgery. Stuttgart, Georg Thieme, 1976.

McCarthy JG (ed): Plastic Surgery, vol 1, General Principles. Philadelphia, WB Saunders, 1990.

McDougal WS (ed): Rob & Smith's Operative Surgery: Urology, 4th ed. St. Louis, CV Mosby, 1983.

McMinn RMH, Hutchings RT: Color Atlas of Human Anatomy. Chicago, Year Book Medical Publishers, 1977.

Mellin P, Strohmenger P, Stocker L: Urologic surgery in infancy and childhood. English edition, arranged by H Lamm. Stuttgart, Georg Thieme, 1970.

Nguyen DH, Burns MW, Shapiro GG, et al: Intraoperative cardiovascular collapse secondary to latex allergy. J Urol 146:571, 1991.

Novick AC, Streem SB, Pontes EJ (eds): Stewart's Operative Urology. Baltimore, Williams & Wilkins, 1989.

Page CP, Bohnen JMA, Fletcher JR, et al: Antimicrobial prophylaxis for surgical wounds: Guidelines for clinical care. Arch Surg 128:79, 1993.

Paulson DF: Management of postoperative pain in the urologic patient. Probl Urol 3:219, 1989.

Pollack SV: Wound healing: A review. J Dermatol Surg Oncol 8:667, 1982.

Raffensperger JG: Fluid and electrolytes. In Raffensperger JG

---

*The numbers in the audiovisual references sections refer to the citations in the Ortho-McNeil/AUA Video Library Catalog: AUA 1996 Multi-Media Home Study Catalog.

(ed): Swenson's Pediatric Surgery, 5th ed. Norwalk, CT, Appleton & Lange, 1990, p 73.

Redman JF: An anatomic approach to the pelvis. *In* Crawford ED, Borden TA (eds): Genitourinary Cancer Surgery. Philadelphia, Lea & Febiger, 1982, p 126.

Resnick MI, Kursch E (eds): Current Therapy in Genitourinary Surgery. Toronto, BC Decker, 1987.

Rhodes RS: Hepatitis B virus, surgeons, and surgery. Bull Am Coll Surg 80:32, 1995.

Schecter WP, Gerberding JL: Human immunodeficiency virus and the surgeon. Probl Urol 8:237, 1994.

Schwartz BR, Gregg RV, Kessler DL, et al: Continuous postoperative epidural analgesia in the management of postoperative surgical pain. Urology 34:349, 1989.

See WA, Fuller JR, Toner ML: An outcome study of patient-controlled morphine analgesia, with or without ketorolac, following radical retropubic prostatectomy. J Urol 154:1429, 1995.

Smith RM, Fischer DC, Vester JW: Presurgical medical evaluation. *In* Crawford ED, Das S (eds): Current Genitourinary Cancer Surgery. Philadelphia, Lea & Febiger, 1990, p 654.

Staren ED, Cullen ML: Epidural catheter analgesia for the management of postoperative pain. Surg Gynecol Obstet 162:389, 1986.

Stephens FD: Congenital Malformations of the Urinary Tract. New York, Praeger, 1983.

Sundaresan R, Sheagren JN: Current understanding and treatment of sepsis. Infect Urol January-February, 1996.

Thomas R, Sharmen G: Urology cart. Urology 21:526, 1983.

Torda TA, Pybus DA: Extradural administration of morphine and bupivacaine. Br J Anaesth 56:141, 1984.

Walsh PC, Retik AB, Stamey TA, Vaughan ED (eds): Campbell's Urology, 6th ed. Philadelphia, WB Saunders, 1992.

Wheeless CR: Atlas of Pelvic Surgery. Philadelphia, Lea & Febiger, 1981.

Williams DI: Urology in Childhood. New York, Springer-Verlag, 1974.

Wind GG, Rich NM: Principles of Surgical Technique. Baltimore, Urban & Schwarzenberg, 1983.

Wishnow KI, Johnson DE, Babaian RJ, et al: Effective outpatient use of polyethylene glycol–electrolyte bowel preparation for radical cystectomy and ileal conduit urinary diversion. Urology 31:7, 1988.

Witman DH, Bergstein JM, Frantzides C: Calculated empiric therapy for mixed surgical infections. Infection 19 (Suppl 6):590, 1991.

Woo HH, Rosario DJ, Chapple CR: A simple technique for the intraoperative placement of a suprapubic catheter. Br J Urol 77:153, 1996.

Audiovisual

Hofsteller A: The Laser in Urology. Wilkes-Barre, PA, Karol Media, 1987 (30 minutes). AUA #919-0202.

THE UROLOGIST AT WORK

Adams JB, Schulam PG, Moore RG, et al: New laparoscopic suturing device: Initial clinical experience. Urology 46:242, 1995.

Adamson RJ, Musco F, Enquist IF: The clinical dimensions of a healing incision. Surg Gynecol Obstet 123:515, 1966.

Adzick NS, Lonaker MT (eds): Fetal Wound Healing. New York, Elsevier Scientific Publishing, 1992.

Alday ES, Goldsmith HS: Surgical technique for omental lengthening based on arterial anatomy. Surg Gynecol Obstet 135:103, 1972.

Andriole GL, Bettmann MA, Garnick MB, Richie JP: Indwelling double-J ureteral stents for temporary and permanent urinary drainage: Experience with 87 patients. J Urol 131:239, 1984.

Anson BJ, McVay CB: Surgical Anatomy, 6th ed. Philadelphia, WB Saunders, 1984.

Bagley DH, Huffman JL, Lyon ES (eds): Urologic Endoscopy: A Manual and Atlas. Boston, Little, Brown & Co, 1985.

Baker BH, Borchardt KA: Sump drains and airborne bacteria as a cause of wound infections. J Surg Res 17:407, 1974.

Banowsky LH: Basic microvascular techniques and principles. Urology 23:495, 1984.

Bardot SF, Montie JE, Jackson CL, Seiler JC: Laparoscopic surgical technique for the internal drainage of pelvic lymphocoele. J Urol 148:907, 1992.

Barham RE, Butz GW, Ansell JS: Comparison of wound strength in normal, radiated and infected tissue closed with polyglycolic and chromic catgut sutures. Surg Gynecol Obstet 146:901, 1978.

Barnes RW: Surgical handicraft: Teaching and learning surgical skills. Am J Surg 153:422, 1987.

Bartle EJ, Edwards ES: Vascular surgery for the urologic oncologist. *In* Crawford ED, Das S (eds): Current Genitourinary Cancer Surgery. Philadelphia, Lea & Febiger, 1990, p 646.

Bartone FF, Shires TK: The reaction of kidney and bladder tissue to catgut and reconstituted collagen sutures. Surg Gynecol Obstet 128:1221, 1969.

Bartone FF, Stinson W: Reaction of the urinary tract to polypropylene sutures. Invest Urol 14:44, 1976.

Baum NH, Brin E: Use of double J catheter in pyeloplasty. Urology 20:634, 1982.

Bell PRF, Jamieson CW, Packley CV (eds): Surgical Management of Vascular Disease. London, Bailliere Tindall, 1992, chap 68.

Berci G, Cuschieri A: Practical Laparoscopy. London, Bailliere Tindall, 1986.

Bevan PG: The craft of surgery: The anastomosis workshop. Ann R Coll Surg Engl 63:405, 1981.

Blandy J: Operative Urology, 2nd ed. Oxford, Blackwell Scientific Publications, 1986.

Bloom DA: Two-step orchidopexy with pelviscopic clip ligation of the spermatic vessels. J Urol 145:130, 1991.

Bloom DA, Ritchey ML, Jordan GH: Pediatric peritoneoscopy (laparoscopy). Clin Pediatr 32:100, 1993.

Bloom DA, Semm S: Advances in genitourinary laparoscopy. Adv Urol 4:167, 1991.

Borges AF: Electrical Incisions and Scar Revision. Boston, Little, Brown & Co, 1973.

Borges AF, Alexander SE: Relaxed skin tension lines, Z-plasties on scars and fusiform excision of lesions. Br J Plast Surg 15:242, 1962.

Borten M: Laparoscopic complications: Prevention and management. Toronto, BC Decker, 1986.

Brawer MK, Defalco AJ: New technique for repair of rectal injury. Urology 42:713, 1993.

Brigden RJ: Operating Theatre Technique. Edinburgh, Churchill Livingstone, 1980.

Briggs TP, Anson KM, Jones A, et al: Urological day case surgery in elderly and medically unfit patients using sedoanalgesia: What are the limits? Br J Urol 75:708, 1995.

Britt BA: Malignant hyperthermia. Can Anaesth Soc J 32:666, 1985.

Brown RP: Knotting technique and suture materials. Br J Surg 79:399, 1992.

Brunius ULF: Wound healing impairment from sutures. Acta Chir Scand Suppl 395:1, 1969.

Burow CA: Beschreibung eimer neuen Transplantations-methode (Methode der Seitlichen Dreiecke)-zum Wiedersatz Verlorengegangener. Theile des Gesichts. Berlin, Nauck, 1855.

Case GD, Glenn JE, Postlethwait RW: Comparison of absorbable sutures in urinary bladder. Urology 7:165, 1976.

Cassady JF Jr: Regional anesthesia for urologic procedures. Urol Clin North Am 14:43, 1987.

Chaffin RC: Drainage. Am J Surg 24:100, 1934.

Chassin JL, Rifkind KM, Turner JW: Errors and pitfalls in stapling gastrointestinal tract anastomoses. Surg Clin North Am 64:441, 1984.

Chu CC, Williams DF: Effects of physical configuration and chemical structure of suture material on bacterial absorption. Am J Surg 147:197, 1984.

Clark WR, Furlow W: Use of a balanced bowel preparation solution in urological surgery. J Urol 137:455, 1987.

Classen DC, Evans RS, Pestotnik SL, et al: The timing of prophylactic administration of antibiotics and the risk of surgical wound infection. N Engl J Med 326:281, 1992.

Clayman RV, Griffith DP, Kavoussi LR, et al: Laparoscopy: Tips on technique (symposium). Contemp Urol 3:28, 1991.

Clayman RV, Kavoussi LR, Firenshau RS, et al: Laparoscopic nephroureterectomy: Initial case report. J Laparoendosc Surg 1:343, 1991.

Clayman RV, Kavoussi LR, Soper NJ, et al: Laparoscopic nephrectomy: Initial case report. J Urol 146:278, 1991.

Clayman RV, McDougall EM (eds): Laparoscopic Urology. St. Louis, Quality Medical Publishing, 1993.

Cohn I Jr, Dennis C: Segmental resection of the small intestine and "aseptic" end-to-end anastomosis. In Madden JL (ed): Atlas of Technics in Surgery, 2nd ed. New York, Appleton-Century-Crofts, 1964.

Conlin MJ, Skoog SJ: Safe laparoscopic access in pediatric patients. Urology 44:579, 1994.

Cooperman AM, Zucker KA: Laparoscopic guided intestinal surgery. In Zucker KA (ed): Surgical Laparoscopy. St. Louis, Quality Medical Publishing, 1991, p 295.

Cormio L, Talja M, Koivusalo A, et al: Biocompatibility of various indwelling double-J stents. J Urol 153:494, 1995.

Craig PH, Williams JA, Davis KW, et al: A biological comparison of polyglactin 910 and polyglycolic acid synthetic absorbable sutures. Surg Gynecol Obstet 141:1, 1975.

Daniel RK, Taylor GI: Distant transfer of an island flap by microvascular anastomoses: A clinical technique. Plast Reconstr Surg 52:111, 1973.

Daniel RK, Williams HB: The free transfer of skin flaps by microvascular anastomosis: An experimental study and reappraisal. Plast Reconstr Surg 52:16, 1973.

Dauleh MI, Byrne DJ, Baxby K: Non-refluxing minimal irritation ureteric stent. Br J Urol 76:795, 1995.

Davis AT: Postoperative infection in surgical patients. In Raffensperger JG (ed): Swenson's Pediatric Surgery, 5th ed. Norwalk, CT, Appleton & Lange, 1990, p 29.

Davis DM: The process of ureteral repair: A recapitulation of the splinting question. Trans Am Assoc Genitourin Surg 49:71, 1959.

DeHoll D, Rodeheaver G, Edgerton MT, Edlich RF: Potentiation of infection by suture closure of dead space. Am J Surg 127:716, 1974.

Douglas DW: Tensile strength of sutures. Lancet 2:497, 1949.

Edlich RF, Panek PH, Rodeheaver GT, et al: Physical and chemical configuration of sutures in the development of surgical infection. Ann Surg 177:679, 1973.

El-Mahrouky A, McElhaney J, Bartone FF, King L: In vitro comparison of the properties of polydioxanone, polyglycolic acid and catgut sutures in sterile and infected urine. J Urol 138:913, 1987.

Eshghi M: Endoscopic surgery of the urinary tract: IV. Transitional cell carcinoma and laparoscopic surgery. Monogr Urol 13:57, 1992.

Finney RP: Double-J and diversion stents. Urol Clin North Am 9:89, 1982.

Finney RP: Experience with new double-J ureteral catheter stent. J Urol 120:678, 1978.

Gambee LP: A single-layer intestinal anastomosis applicable to the small as well as the large intestine. West J Surg Obstet Gynecol 59:1, 1951.

Gardner SM, Clayman RV, McDougall EM, et al: Laparoscopic pneumodissection: A unique means of tissue dissection. J Urol 154:591, 1995.

Gaur DD: Laparoscopic operative retroperitoneoscopy: Use of a new device. J Urol 148:1137, 1992.

Ger R, Duboys E: The prevention and repair of large abdominal-wall defects by muscle transposition: A preliminary communication. Plast Reconstr Surg 72:170, 1983.

Gilbert BR: Microsurgical equipment and instrumentation. In Goldstein M (ed): Surgery of Male Infertility. Philadelphia, WB Saunders, 1995, p 275.

Gillenwater JY, Grayhack JT, Howards SS, Duckett JW (eds): Adult and Pediatric Urology. Chicago, Year Book Medical Publishers, 1987.

Goldin AR: Percutaneous ureteral stenting. Urology 10:165, 1977.

Gomel V, James C: Intraoperative management of ureteral injury during operative laparoscopy. Fertil Steril 55:416, 1991.

Gomella LG, Kozminski M, Winfield HN (eds): Laparoscopic Urologic Surgery. New York, Raven Press, 1994.

Gomella LG, Lotfi MA, Ruckle HC: Management of laparoscopic complications. In Gomella LG, Kozminski M, Winfield HN (eds): Laparoscopic Urologic Surgery. New York, Raven Press, 1994.

Gomella LG, Strup S, Young C, et al: Combined laparoscopic lymphadenectomy and hernia repair. J Urol 147:44A, 1992.

Grainger DA, Soderstrom RM, Schiff SF, et al: Ureteral injuries at laparoscopy: Insights into diagnosis, management, and prevention. Obstet Gynecol 75:839, 1990.

Green LS, Loughlin KR, Kavoussi LR: Management of epigastric injury during laparoscopy. J Endourol 6:99, 1992.

Grossfeld JL (ed): Common Problems in Pediatric Surgery. St. Louis, Mosby-Year Book, 1991.

Hasson HM: Open laparoscopy: A report of 150 cases. J Reprod Med 12:234, 1974.

Hastings JC: The effect of suture materials on healing wounds of the bladder. Surg Gynecol Obstet 140:933, 1975.

Hastings JC, Van Winkle H Jr, Barker E, et al: Effect of suture materials on healing wounds of the stomach and colon. Surg Gynecol Obstet 140:701, 1975.

Herrmann JB: Tensile strength and knot security of surgical suture materials. Am J Surg 37:209, 1971.

Hinman F Jr: Accurate placement of the Penrose drain. Surg Gynecol Obstet 102:497, 1956.

Hinman F Jr: Bowel closure techniques: Large bowel: II. Houston, American Urological Association, AUA Update Series, vol IX, lesson 36, p 282, 1990.

Hinman F Jr: Bowel closure techniques: Small bowel: I. Houston, American Urological Association, AUA Update Series, vol IX, lesson 35, p 274, 1990.

Hinman F Jr: Differential diagnosis of flank pain. In Tanagho EA (guest ed): Pain of Genitourinary Origin. Probl Urol 3(2):182, 1989.

Hinman F Jr: Scalpel for operations on patients possibly infected with human immunodeficiency virus. Urology 32:350, 1988.

Hinman F Jr: Sources of pain. In Tanagho EA (guest ed): Pain of Genitourinary Origin. Probl Urol 3(2):179, 1989.

Hinman F Jr: Ureteral repair and the splint. J Urol 78:376, 1957.

Hirsch IH, Moreno JG, Lotfi MA, Gomella LG: Controlled balloon dilatation of the extraperitoneal space for laparoscopic urologic surgery. J Laparoendosc Surg 4:247, 1994.

Howes EL: Immediate strength of sutured wound. Surgery 7:24, 1940.

Howes EL: Strength studies of polyglycolic acid versus catgut sutures of the same size. Surg Gynecol Obstet 137:15, 1973.

Hulka JF: Textbook of Laparoscopy. Orlando, FL, Grune & Stratton, 1985.

Jackson FE, Fleming PM: Jackson Pratt brain drain. Int Surg 57:658, 1972.

Jacobson JH II, Suarez EL: Microsurgery in anastomosis of small vessels. Surg Forum 11:243, 1960.

Jarowenko MV, Bennett AH: Use of single J urinary diversion stents in intestinal urinary diversion. Urology 22:369, 1983.

Johnson DE, Fuerst DE: Use of auto suture for construction of ileal conduits. J Urol 109:821, 1973.

Jones PA, Moxon RA, Pittman MR, Edwards L: Double-ended pigtail polyethylene stents in the management of benign and malignant ureteral obstruction. J R Soc Med 76:458, 1983.

Jordan GH: The application of tissue transfer. In Webster G, Kirby R, King L, Goldwasser B (eds): Reconstructive Urology. Boston, Blackwell Scientific Publications, 1993.

Jordan GH, Bloom DA: Laparoendoscopic genitourinary surgery in children. In Gomella LG, Kozminski M, Winfield HN (eds): Laparoscopic Urologic Surgery. New York, Raven Press, 1994.

Jordan GH, McCraw JB: Tissue transfer techniques for genitourinary reconstructive surgery: IV. Houston, American Urological Association, AUA Update Series, vol VII, lesson 12, p 90, 1988.

Jordan J, Robey E, Winslow B: Laparoscopic management of the abdominal/trans-inguinal testis. J Endourol 6:157, 1992.

Kavoussi LR, Sosa RE, Capelouto C: Complications of laparoscopic surgery. J Endourol 6:95, 1992.

Kelalis PP, King LR, Belman AB (eds): Clinical Pediatric Urology, 2nd ed. Philadelphia, WB Saunders, 1985.

Kerbl K, Clayman RV: Acute hemostasis during laparoscopic procedures: Method for intraoperative application of hemostatic agent. J Urol 151:109, 1993.

Kiricuta I: Use of the Omentum in Plastic Surgery. Romania, Editura Medicala, 1980.

Koff SA, Brinkman J, Ulrich J, Deighton D: Extensive mobilization of the urethral plate and urethra for repair of hypospadias: The modified Barcat technique. J Urol 151:466, 1994.

Kozminski M, Richards WH III: Fly-casting method of intracorporeal laparoscopic knot tying. Urology 44:577, 1994.

Kronborg O, Tostergaard A, Steven KG, Toctrik JK: Polyglycolic acid versus chromic catgut in bladder surgery. Br J Urol 50:324, 1978.

Landes RR: An improved suction device for draining wounds. Arch Surg 104:707, 1972.

Lang EK: Antegrade ureteral stenting for dehiscence, strictures and fistulae. AJR 143:795, 1984.

Lange PH: Stirrups to minimize complications of prolonged dorsal lithotomy positioning. J Urol 139:326, 1988.

Langer CP: Zur Anatomie und Physiologie der Haut. Sitzungsb Acad Wissensch 45:223, 1861.

Larsen EH, Gasser TC, Madsen PO: Antimicrobial prophylaxis in urological surgery. Urol Clin North Am 13:591, 1986.

Larson DL: Musculocutaneous flaps. In Johnson DE, Boileau MA (eds): Genitourinary Tumors: Fundamental Principles and Surgical Techniques. New York, Grune & Stratton, 1982.

Laufman H, Rickel T: Synthetic absorbable sutures. Surg Gynecol Obstet 145:597, 1977.

Lerwick E: Studies on the efficacy and safety of polydioxanone monofilament absorbable sutures. Surg Gynecol Obstet 135:497, 1981.

Li PD, Goldstein M: Training in urologic microsurgery. In Goldstein M (ed): Surgery of Male Infertility. Philadelphia, WB Saunders, 1995, p 265.

Liebermann-Meffert D, White H (eds): The Greater Omentum. Berlin, Springer-Verlag, 1983.

Limberg AA: The planning of local plastic operations on the body surface. Lexington, MA, Collamore Press, 1984.

Loffer F, Pent D: Indications, contraindications and complications of laparoscopy. Obstet Gynecol Surg 30:4037, 1975.

Lowe BA, Novy MJ, Strang E: Laparoscopic segmental cystectomy. J Urol 147:408A, 1992.

Lumley JSP: The use of microsurgery in reconstruction. In Webster G, Kirby R, King L, Goldwasser B (eds): Reconstructive Urology. Boston, Blackwell Scientific Publications, 1993.

Magee WP, Gilbert DA, McInnis WD: Extended muscle and musculocutaneous flaps. Clin Plast Surg 7:57, 1980.

Mardis HK, Kroeger RM: Ureteral stents: Materials. Urol Clin North Am 15:471, 1988.

Mardis HK, Kroeger RM: Ureteral stents: Use and complications. Probl Urol 6:296, 1992.

Marrero MA, Corfman RS: Laparoscopic use of sutures. Clin Obstet Gynecol 34:387, 1991.

Marshall FF: Mini-laparotomy staging pelvic lymphadenectomy (minilap). Urology 41:201, 1993.

McAninch JW (guest ed): Urogenital Trauma. In Blaisdell FW, Trunkey DD (eds): Trauma Management, vol II. New York, Thieme-Stratton, 1985.

McCahy PJ, Ramsden PD: A computerized ureteric stent retrieval system. Br J Urol 77:147, 1996.

McCraw JB, Arnold PG (eds): McCraw and Arnold's Atlas of Muscle and Musculocutaneous Flaps. Norfolk, VA, Hampton Press, 1986.

McCraw JB, Dibbell DG, Carraway JH: Clinical definition of independent myocutaneous vascular territories. Plast Reconstr Surg 60:341, 1977.

McCullough CS, Soper NJ, Clayman RV, et al: Laparoscopic drainage of a posttransplant lymphocele. Transplantation 51:725, 1991.

McGregor IA: The theoretical basis of the Z-plasty. Br J Plast Surg 9:256, 1957.

McIntyre PB, Ritchie JK, Hawley PR, et al: Management of enterocutaneous fistulas: A review of 132 cases. Br J Surg 71:293, 1984.

Mitty HA, Train JS, Dan SJ: Antegrade ureteral stenting in the management of fistulae, strictures, and calculi. Radiology 149:433, 1983.

Monga M, Klein E, Castaneda-Zuniga WR, et al: The forgotten indwelling ureteral stent: A urologic dilemma. J Urol 153:1817, 1995.

Moore RG, Kavoussi LR, Bloom DA, et al: Postoperative adhesion formation after urological laparoscopy in the pediatric population. J Urol 153:792, 1995.

Morey AF, Deshon E Jr, Dresner ML: Adaptation of Foley catheter for hemostasis during urologic laparoscopy. Urology 42:583, 1993.

Morris AM: A controlled trial of closed wound suction. Br J Surg 60:357, 1973.

Morris MC, Baquero A, Redovan E, et al: Urolithiasis on absorbable and non-absorbable suture materials in the rabbit bladder. J Urol 135:602, 1986.

Morrow FA, Kogan SJ, Freed SZ, Laufman H: In vivo comparison of polyglycolic acid, chromic catgut and silk in tissue of the genitourinary tract: An experimental study of tissue retrieval and calculogenesis. J Urol 112:655, 1974.

Moss JP: Historical and current perspectives on surgical drainage. Surg Gynecol Obstet 152:517, 1981.

Murphy GF, Wood DP Jr: The use of mineral oil to manage nondeflating Foley catheter. J Urol 149:89, 1993.

Mykulak DJ, Herskowitz M, Glassberg KI: Use of magnetic internal ureteral stents in pediatric urology: Retrieval without routine requirement for cystoscopy and general anesthesia. J Urol 152:976, 1994.

Nadler RB, McDougall EM, Bullock AD, et al: Fascial closure of laparoscopic port sites: A new technique. Urology 45:1046, 1995.

Nash PA, Bruce JE, Indudhara H, Shinohara K: Transrectal ultrasound-guided prostatic nerve blockade eases systematic needle biopsy of the prostate. J Urol 155:607, 1996.

Nezhat C, Nezhat F, Green B, Gonzalez G: Laparoscopic ureteroureterostomy. J Endocrinol 6:143, 1992.

Nora PF, Vanecko RM, Brensfield JJ: Prophylactic abdominal drains. Arch Surg 105:173, 1972.

Nyhus LM, Baker RJ (eds): Masters of Surgery, 2nd ed. Boston, Little, Brown & Co, 1992.

Ochsner A: The relative merits of temporary gastrostomy and nasogastric suction of the stomach. Am J Surg 133:729, 1977.

Olivet RT, Nauss LA, Payne WS: A technique for continuous intercostal nerve block analgesia following thoracotomy. J Cardiovasc Surg 80:308, 1980.

Oneal RM, Dingman RO, Grabb WC: The teaching of plastic surgical techniques to medical students. Plast Reconstr Surg 40:494, 1967.

Page CP, Bohnen JMA, Fletcher JR, et al: Antimicrobial prophylaxis for surgical wounds: Guidelines for clinical care. Arch Surg 128:79, 1993.

Parra RO, Andrus CH, Jones JP, Boullier JA: Laparoscopic cystectomy: Initial report on a new treatment for the retained bladder. J Urol 148:1140, 1992.

Pearle MS, Nakada SY, McDougall EM, et al: Laparoscopic pneumodissection: Initial clinical experience. Urology 45:882, 1995.

Penrose CB: Drainage in abdominal surgery. JAMA 14:264, 1890.

Pocock RD, Stower MJ, Ferro MA, et al: Double-J stents: A review of 100 patients. Br J Urol 58:629, 1986.

Poole GV Jr: Mechanical factors in abdominal wound closure: The prevention of fascial dehiscence. Surgery 97:631, 1985.

Poppas DP, Gomella LG, Sosa RE: Basic laparoscopy: Pneumoperitoneum and trocar placement. In Gomella LG, Kozminski M, Winfield HN (eds): Laparoscopic Urologic Surgery. New York, Raven Press, 1994.

Powers JC, Fitzgerald JF, McAhranah MJ: The anatomic basis for the surgical detachment of the greater omentum from the transverse colon. Surg Gynecol Obstet 143:105, 1976.

Ramsay JWA, Payne SR, Gosling PT, et al: The effects of double-J stenting on unobstructed ureters: An experimental and clinical study. Br J Urol 57:630, 1985.

Read RA, Van Stiegemann G: Intestinal surgery for the urologic oncologist. In Crawford ED, Das S (eds): Current Genitourinary Cancer Surgery. Philadelphia, Lea & Febiger, 1990, p 631.

Redman JF: The anatomy of the genitourinary system. In Gillenwater JY, Grayhack JT, Howards SS, Duckett JW (eds): Adult and Pediatric Urology. Chicago, Year Book Medical Publishers, 1987, p 3.

Revington P, Bowyer RC: Sutures: The economics of knot tying techniques. Ann R Coll Surg Engl 76(Suppl):281, 1994.

Rodeheaver GF, Thacker JG, Edlich RF: Mechanical performance of polyglycolic acid and polyglactin 910 synthetic absorbable sutures. Surg Gynecol Obstet 153:835, 1981.

Ruckle H, Hadley R, Lui P, Stewart S: Laparoscopic pelvic lymph node dissection: Assessment of intraoperative and early postoperative complications. J Endourol 6:117, 1992.

Ruutu M, Talja M, Andersson LC, Alfthan OS: Biocompatibility of urinary catheters. Scand J Urol Nephrol 138:235, 1991.

Saleh JW: Laparoscopy. Philadelphia, WB Saunders, 1988, p 253.

Saltzman B: Ureteral stents: Indications, variations, and complications. Urol Clin North Am 15:481, 1988.

See WA: Overview of complications of urologic laparoscopy. In Gomella LG, Kozminski M, Winfield HN (eds): Laparoscopic Urologic Surgery. New York, Raven Press, 1994.

Seftel AD, Resnick MI, Boswell MV: Dorsal nerve block for management of intraoperative penile erection. J Urol 151:394, 1994.

Semjonow A, Roth S, Hertle L: Reducing trauma whilst removing long-term indwelling balloon catheters. Br J Urol 75:241, 1995.

Semm K: Operative pelviscopy. Br Med Bull 42:284, 1986.

Sharpe LA: Laparoscopic suturing techniques. In Gomella LG, Kozminski M, Winfield HN (eds): Laparoscopic Urologic Surgery. New York, Raven Press, 1994.

Singh B, Kim H, Wax SH: Stent versus nephrostomy: Is there a choice? J Urol 121:268, 1979.

Slaton JW, Kropp KA: Proximal ureteral stent migration: An avoidable complication? J Urol 155:58, 1996.

Smith AD: Retrieval of ureteral stents. Urol Clin North Am 9:109, 1982.

Smith MJV: Ureteral stents: Their use and misuse. Monogr Urol 14:1, 1993.

Stock JA, Packer MG, Kaplan GW: Pediatric urology facts and figures: Data useful in the management of pediatric urologic patients. Urol Clin North Am 22:205, 1995.

Thomas R: The evolving world of urological laparoscopy. J Urol 154:487, 1995. Editorial.

Topel HC (ed): Endoscopic Suturing and Knot Tying Manual. Somerville, NJ, Ethicon, 1991.

Trier WC: Considerations in the choice of surgical needles. Surg Gynecol Obstet 149:84, 1979.

Tuggle DW, Hoelzer DJ, Tunell WP, Smith EI: The safety and cost-effectiveness of polyethylene glycol electrolyte solution bowel preparation in infants and children. J Pediatr Surg 22:513, 1987.

Turner-Warwick R: The use of the omental pedicle graft in urinary tract reconstruction. J Urol 16:341, 1976.

Turner-Warwick R, Wynne EJ, Askhen MH: The use of the omental pedicle graft in the repair and reconstruction of the urinary tract. Br J Surg 54:849, 1967.

Van Arsdalen KN, Pollack HH, Wein AJ: Ureteral stenting. Semin Urol 2:180, 1984.

Van Winkle W Jr, Hastings J: Considerations in the choice of suture materials for various tissues. Surg Gynecol Obstet 135:113, 1972.

Van Winkle W Jr, Hastings J, Barker E, et al: Effect of suture materials on healing skin wounds. Surg Gynecol Obstet 140:7, 1975.

Van Winkle W Jr, Salthouse TN: Biological Response to Sutures and Principles of Suture Selection. Somerville, NJ, Ethicon, 1976.

Wein AJ, Malloy TR, Greenberg SH, et al: Omental transposition as an aid in genitourinary reconstructive procedures. J Trauma 10:473, 1980.

Wickham JEA, Miller RA: Percutaneous renal access. In Wickham JEA, Miller RA (eds): Percutaneous Renal Surgery. New York, Churchill Livingstone, 1983, p 33.

Winfield HN, Donovan JF, See WA, et al: Laparoscopic pelvic lymph node dissection for genitourinary malignancies: Indications, techniques and results. J Endourol 6:103, 1992.

Winfield HN, Donovan JF, See WA, et al: Urological laparoscopic surgery. J Urol 146:941, 1991.

Winfield HN, Ryan KJ: Experimental laparoscopic surgery: Potential clinical applications in urology. J Endourol 4:37, 1990.

Wishnow KI, Johnson DE, Babaian RJ, et al: Effective outpatient use of polyethylene glycol-electrolyte bowel preparation for radical cystectomy and ileal conduit urinary diversion. Urology 31:7, 1988.

Wolf JS Jr, Stoller ML: The physiology of laparoscopy: Basic principles, complications and other considerations. J Urol 152:294, 1994.

Woltering EA, Flye MW, Huntley S, et al: Evaluation of bupivacaine nerve blocks in modification of pain and pulmonary function changes after thoracotomy. Ann Thorac Surg 30:122, 1980.

Young GPH, Li PS, Gardner TA, Goldstein M: Animal models for microsurgical training and research. In Goldstein M (ed): Surgery of Male Infertility. Philadelphia, WB Saunders, 1995, p 297.

Yu D-S, Yang T-H, Ma C-P: Snail-headed catheter retriever: A simple way to remove catheters from female patients. J Urol 154:167, 1995.

Yuzpe AA: Pneumoperitoneum needle and trocar injuries in laparoscopy: A survey on possible contributing factors and prevention. J Reprod Med 25:485, 1990.

Audiovisuals

Griffith DR (moderator): Laparoscopy. Wilkes-Barre, PA, Karol Media, 1991 (51 minutes). AUA #919-2070.

Guerriero WG (moderator): Laparoscopic Surgery. Wilkes-Barre, PA, Karol Media, 1993 (77 minutes). AUA #919-2068.

Ryan K, Winfield HN: Urologic Applications of Laparoscopic Surgery. Wilkes-Barre, PA, Karol Media, 1990 (13 minutes). AUA #919-1162.

PENIS: PLASTIC OPERATIONS

Allen TD, Spence HM: The surgical treatment of coronal hypospadias and related problems. J Urol 100:504, 1968.

Altemus AR, Hutchins GM: Development of the human anterior urethra. J Urol 146:1084, 1991.

Arap S, Mitre AI, de Goes GM: Modified meatal advancement and glanuloplasty for distal hypospadias. J Urol 131:1140, 1984.

Arneri V: Reconstruction of the male genitalia. In Converse JM (ed): Reconstructive and Plastic Surgery, 2nd ed, vol 7. Philadelphia, WB Saunders, 1977, p 3902.

Asopa R, Asopa HS: One-stage repair of hypospadias using double island preputial skin tube. Indian J Urol 1:41, 1984.

Asopa HS, Elhence IP, Atri SP, Bansal NK: One stage correction of penile hypospadias using a foreskin tube: A preliminary report. Int Surg 55:435, 1971.

Ballesteros JJ: Personal technique for surgical repair of balanic hypospadias. J Urol 118:983, 1977.

Barcat J: Current concepts of treatment. In Horton CE (ed): Plastic and Reconstructive Surgery of the Genital Area. Boston, Little, Brown & Co, 1973, p 249.

Barcat J: Les hypospadias: III. Les urethroplasties, les resultats, les complications. Ann Chir Infect 10:310, 1969.

Bartone F, Shore N, Newland J, et al: The best suture for hypospadias? Urology 29:517, 1987.

Baskin L, Duckett JW: Buccal mucosa grafts in hypospadias surgery. Br J Urol 76:23, 1995.

Baskin L, Duckett JW: Dorsal tunica albuginea plication for hypospadias curvature. J Urol 151:1668, 1994.

Baskin L, Duckett JW: The versatility of the onlay island flap procedure for urethral replacement in hypospadias. In McAninch JW (ed): New Techniques in Reconstructive Urology. New York, Igaku-Shoin, 1996, p 24.

Baskin L, Duckett JW, Ueoka K, et al: Changing concepts of hypospadias curvature lead to more onlay island flap procedures. J Urol 151:191, 1994.

Beck C: Hypospadias and its treatment. Surg Gynecol Obstet 24:511, 1917.

Bellinger MF: Embryology of the male external genitalia. Urol Clin North Am 8:375, 1981.

Belman AB: De-epithelialized skin flap coverage in hypospadias repair. J Urol 140:1273, 1988.

Belman AB: The de-epithelialized flap and its influence on hypospadias repair. J Urol 152:2332, 1994.

Belman AB: The modified Mustardé hypospadias repair. J Urol 127:88, 1982.

Belt E: Diseases of the urinary system (surgical): Diagnostic and operative techniques for the urinary system. Annu Rev Med 6:377, 1955.

Bergman R, Howard AH, Barnes RW: Plastic reconstruction of the penis. J Urol 59:1174, 1948.

Bevan AD: A new operation for hypospadias. JAMA 68:1032, 1917.

Bhandari M, Kumar S: Modified single-stage hypospadias repair using double island preputial skin tube. Br J Urol 62:189, 1988.

Blandy JP, Singh M: The technique and results of one-stage island patch urethroplasty. Br J Urol 47:83, 1975.

Boxer JB: Reconstruction of the male genitalia. Surg Gynecol Obstet 141:939, 1975.

Bracka A: Hypospadias repair: The two-stage alternative. Br J Urol 76:31, 1995.

Broadbent TR, Woolf RM, Toksu E: Hypospadias: One-stage repair. Plast Reconstr Surg 27:154, 1961.

Brock JW III: Autologous buccal mucosal graft for urethral reconstruction. Urology 44:753, 1994.

Browne D: An operation for hypospadias. Lancet 1:141, 1936.

Bürger RA, Müller SC, El-Damanhoury H, et al: The buccal mucosal graft for urethral reconstruction: A preliminary report. J Urol 147:662, 1992.

Byars LT: Functional restoration of hypospadias deformities. Surg Gynecol Obstet 92:149, 1951.

Byars LT: A technique for consistently satisfactory repair of hypospadias. Surg Gynecol Obstet 100:184, 1955.

Cabral BHP, Gonzales R: Use of urethral drainage tube and dressing in hypospadias repair. Urology 33:327, 1989.

Cecil AB: Repair of hypospadias and urethral fistula. J Urol 56:237, 1946.

Cecil AB: Surgery of hypospadias and epispadias in the male. J Urol 67:1006, 1932.

Chen S, Wang G, Wang M: Modified longitudinal preputial island flap urethroplasty for repair of hypospadias: Results in 60 patients. J Urol 149:814, 1993.

Churchill BW, Van Savage J, Khoury AE, et al: The dartos flap as an adjunct in preventing urethrocutaneous fistulas in repeat hypospadias surgery. J Urol 156:2047, 1996.

Coleman JW: The bladder mucosal graft technique for hypospadias repair. J Urol 125:708, 1981.

Coleman JW, McGovern JH, Marshall VF: The bladder mucosal graft technique for hypospadias repair. Urol Clin North Am 8:457, 1981.

Cromie WJ, Bellinger MF: Hypospadias dressing and diversions. Urol Clin North Am 8:545, 1981.

Das S, Brosman SA: Duplication of male urethra. J Urol 117:452, 1977.

Daskalopous EL, Baskin L, Duckett JW, Snyder HM III: Congenital penile curvature (chordee without hypospadias). Urology 42:708, 1993.

Davits RJAM, Van Den Aker ESS, Scholtmeijer RJ, et al: Effect of parenteral testosterone therapy on penile development in boys with hypospadias. Br J Urol 71:593, 1993.

Decter RM: Inverted V glansplasty: A procedure for distal hypospadias. J Urol 146:641, 1991.

DeJong TPVM, Boemers TM: Improved Mathieu repair for coronal and distal shaft hypospadias with moderate chordee. Br J Urol 72:972, 1993.

Dessanti A, Rigamonti W, Merulla V, et al: Autologous buccal mucosa graft for hypospadias repair: An initial report. J Urol 147:1081, 1992.

De Sy WA: Aesthetic repair of meatal stricture. J Urol 132:678, 1984.

Devine CJ Jr: Editorial comment. J Urol 144:283, 1990.

Devine CJ Jr: Embryology of the male external genitalia. Clin Plast Surg 7:141, 1980.

Devine CJ Jr, Blackley SK, Horton CE, Gilbert DA: The surgical treatment of chordee without hypospadias in men. J Urol 146:325, 1991.

Devine CJ Jr, Gonzalez-Serva L, Stecker JF Jr, et al: Utricular configuration in hypospadias and intersex. Trans Am Assoc Genitourin Surg 71:154, 1979.

Devine CJ Jr, Horton CE: Chordee without hypospadias. J Urol 110:264, 1973.

Devine CJ Jr, Horton CE: A one-stage hypospadias repair. J Urol 85:166, 1961.

Devine CJ, Horton CE, Snyder HM III, et al: Chordee without hypospadias. Dialogues Pediatr Urol 9(2), 1986.

Dresner ML: Surgical revision of scrotal engulfment. Urol Clin North Am 9:305, 1982.

Duckett JW: Advances in hypospadias repair. Festschrift honoring Sir David I. Williams. Postgrad Med J 66:62, 1990.

Duckett JW: The current hype in hypospadiology. Br J Urol 76:1, 1995.

Duckett JW: Hypospadias. In Gillenwater JY, Grayhack JT, Howards SS, Duckett JW (eds): Adult and Pediatric Urology, 2nd ed. St. Louis, Mosby–Year Book, 1991, p 2103.

Duckett JW: Hypospadias. In Walsh PC, Gittes RF, Perlmutter AD, Stamey TA (eds): Campbell's Urology, 5th ed. Philadelphia, WB Saunders, 1986, p 1969.

Duckett JW: Hypospadias. In Webster G, Kirby R, King L, Goldwasser B (eds): Reconstructive Urology. Boston, Blackwell Scientific Publications, 1993.

Duckett JW: Hypospadias repair. In Frank SJ, Johnston JH (eds): Operative Paediatric Urology. London, Churchill Livingstone, 1990, p 197.

Duckett JW: The island flap technique for hypospadias repair. Urol Clin North Am 8:503, 1981.

Duckett JW: MAGPI (meatoplasty and glanuloplasty): A procedure for subcoronal hypospadias. Urol Clin North Am 8:513, 1981.

Duckett JW, Coplen D, Ewalt D, Baskin LS: Buccal mucosal urethral replacement. J Urol 153:1660, 1995.

Duckett JW, Keating MA: Technical challenge of the megameatus intact prepuce hypospadias (MIP) variant: The pyramid procedure. J Urol 141:1407, 1989.

Duckett JW, Snyder HM: Meatal advancement and glanuloplasty hypospadias repair after 1,000 cases: Avoidance of meatal stenosis and regression. J Urol 147:665, 1992.

Duplay S: Sur le traitement chirurgical de l'hypospadias et l'epispadias. Arch Gen Med 145:257, 1980.

Eardley I, Whitaker RH: Surgery for hypospadias fistula. Br J Urol 69:306, 1992.

Eberle J, Überreiter S, Radmayr C, et al: Posterior hypospadias: Long-term follow-up after reconstructive surgery in the male direction. J Urol 150:1474, 1993.

Ehrlich RM, Alter G: Split-thickness skin graft urethroplasty and tunica vaginalis flaps for failed hypospadias repairs. J Urol 155:131, 1996.

Ehrlich RM, Reda EF, Koyle MA, et al: Complications of bladder mucosal graft. J Urol 142:626, 1989.

Elder JS: Influence of glans morphology on choice of island flap technique in children with proximal hypospadias. J Urol 147:317, 1992.

Elder JS, Duckett JW, Snyder HM: Onlay island flap in the repair of mid and distal penile hypospadias without chordee. J Urol 138:376, 1987.

Feldman KW, Smith DW: Fetal phallic growth and penile standards for newborn male infants. J Pediatr 86:395, 1975.

Fichtner J, Filipas D, Mottrie AM, et al: Analysis of meatal location in 500 men: Wide variation questions need for meatal advancement in all pediatric anterior hypospadias cases. J Urol 154:833, 1995.

Firlit CF: The mucosal collar in hypospadias surgery. J Urol 137:80, 1987.

Firlit CF: Stents, splints. Dial Pediatr Urol 13:4, 1990.

Flack CE, Walker RD III: Onlay-tube-onlay urethroplasty technique in primary perineal hypospadias surgery. J Urol 154:837, 1995.

Fuqua F: Renaissance of urethroplasty: The Belt technique of hypospadias repair. J Urol 106:782, 1971.

Gaylis FD, Zaontz MR, Dalton D, et al: Silicone foam dressing for penis after reconstructive pediatric surgery. Urology 33:296, 1989.

Gearhart JP, Borland RN: Onlay island flap urethroplasty: Variation on a theme. J Urol 148:1507, 1992.

Gearhart JP, Rock JA: Total ablation of the penis after circumcision with electrocautery: A method of management and long-term follow-up. J Urol 142:799, 1989.

Germiyanoglu G, Ozkardes H, Altug U, et al: Reconstruction of penoscrotal transposition. Br J Urol 73:200, 1993.

Gibbons MD: Nuances of distal hypospadias. Urol Clin North Am 12:169, 1985.

Gilpin D, Clements WDB, Boston VE: GRAP repair: Single-stage reconstruction of hypospadias as an outpatient procedure. Br J Urol 71:226, 1993.

Glenister TW: The origin and fate of the urethral plate in man. J Anat 288:413, 1954.

Gonzales ET: Hypospadias repair. In Glenn JF (ed): Urologic Surgery, 4th ed. Philadelphia, JB Lippincott, 1990, p 817.

Greenfield SP, Sadler BT, Wan J: Two-stage repair for severe hypospadias. J Urol 152:498, 1994.

Hendren WH: The Belt-Fuqua technique for repair of hypospadias. Urol Clin North Am 8:431, 1981.

Hendren WH, Caesar RE: Chordee without hypospadias: Experience with 33 cases. J Urol 147:107, 1992.

Hendren WH, Crawford JD: The child with ambiguous genitalia. Curr Probl Surg 1:64, 1972.

Hendren WH, Horton CE Jr: Experience with 1-stage repair of hypospadias and chordee using free graft of prepuce. J Urol 140:1259, 1988.

Hendren WH, Keating MA: Use of dermal grafts and free urethral grafts in penile reconstruction. J Urol 140:1265, 1988.

Hensle RW, Mollitt DL: Experience with the Belt-Fuqua hypospadias repair. J Urol 125:703, 1981.

Hill GA, Wacksman J, Lewis AG, et al: The modified pyramid hypospadias procedure: Repair of megameatus and deep glanular groove variants. J Urol 150:1208, 1993.

Hinman F Jr: The blood supply to preputial island flaps. J Urol 145:1232, 1991.

Hinman F Jr, Spence HF, Culp OS, et al: Panel discussion: Anomalies of external genitalia in infancy and childhood. J Urol 93:1, 1965.

Hodgson NB: Editorial comment. J Urol 149:816, 1993.

Hodgson NB: Hypospadias and urethral duplications. In Harrison JH, Gittes RF, Perlmutter A, et al (eds): Campbell's Urology, 4th ed. Philadelphia, WB Saunders, 1979, p 1566.

Hollowell JG, Keating MA, Snyder HM III, Duckett JW: Preservation of the urethral plate in hypospadias repair: Extended applications and further experience with the onlay island flap urethroplasty. J Urol 143:98, 1990.

Horton CE, Devine CJ Jr: A one-stage repair for hypospadias cripples. Plast Reconstr Surg 66:407, 1970.

Howard FS: Hypospadias with enlargement of the prostatic utricle. Surg Gynecol Obstet 86:307, 1948.

Issa MM, Gearhart JP: The failed MAGPI: Management and prevention. Br J Urol 64:169, 1989.

Jayanthi VR, McLorie GA, Khoury AE, Churchill BM: Can previously relocated penile skin be successfully used for salvage hypospadias repair? J Urol 152:740, 1994.

Jones FW: The development and malformations of the glans and prepuce. BMJ 1:137, 1910.

Joseph VT: Concepts in the surgical technique of one-stage hypospadias correction. Br J Urol 76:504, 1995.

Juskiewenski S, Vaysse PH, Moscovici J, et al: A study of the arterial blood supply to the penis. Anat Clin 4:101, 1982.

Kaplan GW: Repair of proximal hypospadias using a preputial free graft for neourethral construction and a preputial pedicle flap for ventral skin coverage. J Urol 140:1270, 1988.

Kass EJ: Dorsal corporeal rotation: An alternative technique for the management of severe chordee. J Urol 150:635, 1993.

Kass EJ, Bolong D: Single-stage hypospadias reconstruction without fistula. J Urol 144:520, 1990.

Keating MA, Duckett JW Jr: Failed hypospadias repair. In Cohen MS, Resnick MI (eds): Reoperative Urology. Boston, Little, Brown & Co, 1995, p 187.

Keating MA, Duckett JW Jr: Recent advances in the repair of hypospadias. In Nyhus L (ed): Surgery Annual, vol 22. New York, Appleton-Century-Crofts, 1991.

Klimberg I, Walker RD: Comparison of Mustardé and Horton-Devine flip-flap techniques of hypospadias repair. J Urol 134:103, 1985.

Koff SA, Brinkman J, Ulrich J, et al: Extensive mobilization of the urethral plate and urethra for repair of hypospadias: The modified Barcat technique. J Urol 151:466, 1994.

Koff SA, Eakins M: The treatment of penile chordee using corporal rotation. J Urol 131:931, 1984.

Kropfl D, Schardt M, Fey S: Modified meatal advancement and glanuloplasty with complete foreskin reconstruction. Eur Urol 22:57, 1992.

Lau JTK, Ong GB: Subglandular urethral fistula following circumcision: Repair by the advancement method. J Urol 126:702, 1981.

Li ZC, Zheng ZH, Sheh YX, et al: One-stage urethroplasty for hypospadias using a tube constructed with bladder mucosa: A new procedure. Urol Clin North Am 8:463, 1981.

Livne PM, Gibbons MD, Gonzales ET Jr: Correction of disproportion of corpora cavernosa as cause of chordee in hypospadias. Urology 22:608, 1983.

Malament M: Repair of the recurrent fistula of the penile urethra. J Urol 106:704, 1971.

Marberger H, Pauer W: Experience in hypospadias repair. Urol Clin North Am 8:403, 1981.

Marshall VF, Spellman RM: Construction of urethra in hypospadias using vesical mucosal grafts. J Urol 73:335, 1955.

Mathieu P: Traitement en un temps de l'hypospadias balanique et juxtabalanique. J Chir 39:481, 1932.

McCormack RM: Simultaneous chordee repair and urethral reconstruction for hypospadias. Plast Reconstr Surg 13:257, 1954.

McMillan RDH, Churchill BM, Gilmore RF: Assessment of urinary stream after repair of anterior hypospadias by meatoplasty and glanuloplasty. J Urol 134:100, 1985.

Mettauer JP: Practical observations on those malformations of the male urethra and penis, termed hypospadias and epispadias, with an anomalous case. Am J Med Sci 4:43, 1842.

Mitchell ME: Dressing for hypospadias repair. Dial Pediatr Urol 13:6, 1990.

Mitchell ME, Kalb TB: Hypospadias repair without a bladder drainage catheter. J Urol 135:321, 1986.

Mollard P, Castagnola C: Hypospadias: The release of chordee without dividing the urethral plate and onlay island flap (92 cases). J Urol 152:1238, 1994.

Mollard P, Mouriquand P, Bringeon G, et al: Repair of hypospadias using bladder mucosal graft in 76 cases. J Urol 142:1548, 1989.

Mollard P, Mouriquand P, Felfela T: Application of the onlay island flap urethroplasty to penile hypospadias with severe chordee. Br J Urol 68:317, 1991.

Moscona AR, Govrin-Yehudain J, Hirshowitz B: Closure of urethral fistulae by transverse Y-V advancement flap. Br J Urol 56:313, 1984.

Mouriquand PDE, Persad A, Sharma S: Hypospadias repair: Current principles and procedures. Br J Urol 76:9, 1995.

Mureau MAM, Slijper FME, Nijman RJM, et al: Psychosexual adjustment of children and adolescents after different types of hypospadias surgery: A norm-related study. J Urol 154:1902, 1995.

Mustardé JC: One-stage correction of distal hypospadias and other people's fistulae. Br J Plast Surg 18:413, 1965.

Nesbit RM: Operation for correction of distal penile ventral curvature with or without hypospadias. J Urol 97:470, 1967.

Nesbit RM: Plastic procedure for correction of hypospadias. J Urol 45:699, 1941.

Nesbit RM, MacKinney CC, Dingman R: Z-plasty for correction of meatal ureteral stricture after hypospadias repair. J Urol 72:681, 1954.

Nonomura K, Koyanagi T, Imanaka K, et al: One-stage total repair of severe hypospadias with scrotal transposition: Experience in 18 cases. J Pediatr Surg 23:177, 1988.

Oesterling JE, Gearhart JP, Jeffs RD: Urinary diversion after hypospadias surgery. Urology 29:513, 1987.

Passerini G, Maio G, Cisternino A, et al: One-stage repair of severe hypospadias. Presented before the International Congress of Pediatric Urology, Florence, Italy, 1986. Abstract. Cited in Gillenwater JY, Grayhack JT, Howards SS, Duckett JW (eds): Adult and Pediatric Urology. Chicago, Year Book Medical Publishers, 1986, p 1902.

Perovic S: Hypospadias sine hypospadias. World J Urol 10:85, 1992.

Perovic S, Vukadinovic V: Onlay island flap urethroplasty for severe hypospadias: A variant of the technique. J Urol 151:711, 1994.

Perovic S, Vukadinovic V: Penoscrotal transposition with hypospadias: 1-stage repair. J Urol 148:1510, 1992.

Ransley PG, Duffy PG, Oesch IL, et al: The use of bladder mucosa and combined bladder mucosa/preputial skin grafts for urethral reconstruction. J Urol 138:1096, 1987.

Redman JF: The Barcat balanic groove technique for the repair of distal hypospadias. J Urol 137:83, 1987.

Retik AB, Bauer SB, Mandell J, et al: Management of severe hypospadias with 2-stage repair. J Urol 152:749, 1994.

Rickwood AMK, Anderson PAM: One-stage hypospadias repair: Experience with 367 cases. Br J Urol 67:424, 1991.

Ritchey ML, Benson RC Jr, Kramer SA, et al: Management of müllerian duct remnants in the male patient. J Urol 140:795, 1988.

Rober PE, Perlmutter AD, Reitelman C: Experience with 81 one-stage hypospadias/chordee repairs using free graft urethroplasties. J Urol 144:526, 1990.

Roberts AHN: A new operation for the repair of hypospadias fistulae. Br J Plast Surg 35:386, 1982.

Saad MN, Khoo CTK, Lochaitis AS: A simple technique for repair of urethral fistula by Y-V advancement. Br J Plast Surg 33:410, 1980.

Scherz HC, Kaplan GW, Packer MG: Modified meatal advancement and glanuloplasty (ARAP hypospadias repair): Experience in 31 patients. J Urol 142:620, 1989.

Schultz JB, Klykylo WM, Wacksman J: Timing of elective hypospadias repair in children. Pediatrics 71:342, 1983.

Secrest CL, Jordan GH, Winslow BH, et al: Repair of complications of hypospadias surgery. J Urol 150:1415, 1993.

Smith ED: Commentary: Multiple stage repair of hypospadias. In Whitehead ED, Leiter E (eds): Current Operative Urology, 2nd ed. Philadelphia, Harper & Row, 1984, p 1251.

Smith ED: A de-epithelialized overlap technique in the repair of hypospadias. Br J Plast Surg 26:106, 1973.

Smith ED: Durham-Smith repair of hypospadias. Urol Clin North Am 8:451, 1981.

Smith ED: Malformations of the bladder, urethra and hypospadias. In Holder TM, Ashcraft KW (eds): Pediatric Surgery. Philadelphia, WB Saunders, 1990, p 752.

Smith ED: Timing of surgery in hypospadias repair. Aust NZ J Surg 53:396, 1983.

Snodgrass W: Tubularized, incised plate urethroplasty for distal hypospadias. J Urol 151:464, 1994.

Snodgrass W, Decter RM, Roth DR, et al: Management of the penile shaft skin in hypospadias repair: Alternative to Byars flaps. J Pediatr Surg 23:181, 1988.

Snow BW: Transverse corporeal plication for persistent chordee. Urology 34:360, 1989.

Snow BW: Use of tunica vaginalis to prevent fistulas in hypospadias surgery. J Urol 136:861, 1986.

Snow BW, Cartwright PC, Unger K: Tunica vaginalis blanket wrap to prevent urethrocutaneous fistula: An 8-year experience. J Urol 153:472, 1995.

Snow BW, Georges LS, Tarry WF: Techniques for outpatient hypospadias surgery. Urology 35:327, 1990.

Snyder HM: Does glans configuration indicate the type of chordee present in hypospadias? Soc Pediatr Urol Newsl 5/24:38, 1991.

Spaulding MH: The development of external genitalia in the human embryo. Contr Embryol Carnegie Inst, publication 276, p 67, 1921.

Speakman MJ, Azmy AF: Skin chordee without hypospadias: An unrecognized entity. Br J Urol 69:428, 1992.

Spencer JR, Perlmutter AD: Sleeve advancement hypospadias repair. J Urol 144:523, 1990.

Standoli L: One-stage repair of hypospadias: Preputial island flap technique. Ann Plast Surg 9:81, 1982.

Stock JA, Cortez J, Scherz HC, Kaplan GW: The management of proximal hypospadias using a 1-stage hypospadias repair with a preputial free graft for neourethral construction and a preputial pedicle flap for ventral skin coverage. J Urol 152:2335, 1994.

Teague JL, Roth DR, Gonzales ET: Repair of hypospadias complications using the meatal based flap urethroplasty. J Urol 151:470, 1994.

Thiersch C: On the origin and operative treatment of epispadias (in German). Arch Heilkd 10:20, 1869.

Turner-Warwick R: Hypospadiac and epispadiac retrievoplasty. In Webster G, Kirby R, King L, Goldwasser B (eds): Reconstructive Urology. Boston, Blackwell Scientific Publications, 1993.

Turner-Warwick R: Observations upon techniques for reconstruction of the urethral meatus, the hypospadiac glans deformity and the penile urethra. Urol Clin North Am 6:643, 1979.

Van Horn AC, Kass EJ: Glanuloplasty and in situ tubularization of the urethral plate: A simple reliable technique for the majority of boys with hypospadias. J Urol 154:1505, 1995.

Wacksman J: Modification of the one stage flip-flap procedure to repair distal penile hypospadias. Urol Clin North Am 8:527, 1981.

Wacksman J: Results of early hypospadias surgery using optical magnification. J Urol 131:516, 1984.

Wacksman J: Use of the Hodgson XX (modified Asopa) procedure to correct hypospadias with chordee: Surgical technique and results. J Urol 136:1264, 1986.

Wacksman J, Sheldon C, King L: Distal hypospadias repair. In Webster G, Kirby R, King L, Goldwasser B (eds): Reconstructive Urology. Boston, Blackwell Scientific Publications, 1993.

Walker RD: Outpatient repair of urethral fistulae. Urol Clin North Am 8:582, 1981.

Wehrbein HL: Hypospadias. J Urol 50:335, 1943.

Williams DI: The development and abnormalities of the penile urethra. Acta Anat 15:176, 1952.

Winslow BH, Vorstman B, Devine CJ Jr: Complications of hypospadias surgery. In Marshall F (ed): Urologic Complications. Chicago, Year Book Medical Publishers, 1986.

Wise HA II, Berggren RB: Another method of repair for urethrocutaneous fistulae. J Urol 118:1054, 1977.

Yachia D: Pedicled scrotal skin advancement for one-stage anterior urethral reconstruction in circumcised patients. J Urol 139:1007, 1988.

Young F, Benjamin JA: Preschool age repair of hypospadias with free inlay skin graft. Surgery 26:384, 1949.

Young F, Benjamin JA: Repair of hypospadias with free inlay skin graft. Surg Gynecol Obstet 5:86, 1948.

Zagula EM, Braren V: Management of urethrocutaneous fistulas following hypospadias repair. J Urol 130:743, 1983.

Zaontz MR: The GAP (glans approximation procedure) for glanular/coronal hypospadias. J Urol 141:359, 1989.

Zhong-Chu L, Yu-Hen Z, Ya-Xiong S, Yu-Feng C: One-stage urethroplasty for hypospadias using a tube constructed with bladder mucosa: A new procedure. Urol Clin North Am 8:463, 1981.

Audiovisual

Nonomura K, Koyanagi T, Kakizaki H, et al: One-Stage Urethroplasty. Wilkes-Barre, PA, Karol Media, 1992 (14 minutes). AUA #919-2000.

PENIS: EXCISION

Abraham V, Ravi R, Shrivastava BR: Primary reconstruction to avoid wound breakdown following groin block dissection. Br J Plast Surg 45:211, 1992.

Bandieramonte G, Santoro O, Boracchi P, et al: Total resection of the glans penis surface by CO_2 laser microsurgery. Acta Oncol 27:575, 1988.

Bare RL, Assimos DG, McCullough DL, et al: Inguinal lymphadenectomy and primary groin reconstruction using rectus abdominis muscle flaps in patients with penile cancer. Urology 44:557, 1994.

Brown MD, Zachary CB, Grekin RC, et al: Penile tumors: Their management by Mohs micrographic surgery. J Dermatol Surg Oncol 13:1163, 1987.

Cabanas RM: Anatomy and biopsy of sentinel lymph nodes. Urol Clin North Am 2:267, 1992.

Cabanas RM, Whitmore WF Jr: The use of testicular lymphatics to bypass obstructed lymphatics in the dog. Invest Urol 18:262, 1981.

Carroll PR: Surgical management of urethral carcinoma. In Crawford ED, Das S (eds): Current Genitourinary Cancer Surgery. Philadelphia, Lea & Febiger, 1990, p 380.

Catalona WJ: Modified inguinal lymphadenectomy for carcinoma of the penis with preservation of the saphenous veins: Technique and preliminary results. J Urol 140:306, 1988.

Crawford ED: Technique of ilioinguinal lymph node dissection. In Skinner DG, Lieskovsky G (eds): Diagnosis and Management of Genitourinary Cancer. Philadelphia, WB Saunders, 1988, p 817.

Das S, Crawford ED: Carcinoma of the penis: Management of the primary. In Crawford ED, Das S (eds): Current Genitourinary Cancer Surgery. Philadelphia, Lea & Febiger, 1990, p 367.

Das S, Crawford ED: Carcinoma of the penis: Management of the regional lymphatic drainage. In Crawford ED, Das S (eds): Current Genitourinary Cancer Surgery. Philadelphia, Lea & Febiger, 1990, p 363.

Fowler JE Jr: Sentinel lymph node biopsy for staging penile cancer. Urology 23:352, 1984.

Fraley EE, Hutchens HD: Radical ilio-inguinal node dissection: The skin bridge technique: A new procedure. J Urol 108:279, 1972.

Fraley EE, Zhang G, Sazama R, Lange PH: Cancer of the penis: Prognosis and treatment plans. Cancer 55:1618, 1985.

Goldman HB, Dmochowski RR, Cox CE: Penetrating trauma to the penis: Functional results. J Urol 155:551, 1996.

Horenblas S, van Tinteren H, Delemarre JFM, et al: Squamous cell carcinoma of the penis: II. Treatment of the primary tumor. J Urol 147:1533, 1992.

Johnson DE, Ames FC: Surgical anatomy and lymphatic drainage of the ilioinguinal region. In Johnson DE, Ames FC (eds): Groin Dissection. Chicago, Year Book Medical Publishers, 1985.

Klein FA: Inferior pubic rami resection with en bloc radical excision for invasive proximal urethral carcinoma. Cancer 52:1238, 1983.

McLoughlin KR: The rosebud technique for creation of a neomeatus after partial or total penectomy. Br J Urol 76:123, 1995.

Mohs FE, Snow SN, Messing EM, Kuglitsch ME: Microscopically controlled surgery in the treatment of carcinoma of the penis. J Urol 133:961, 1985.

Ornellas AA, Seixas ALC, De Moraes JR: Analyses of 200 lymphadenectomies in patients with penile carcinoma. J Urol 146:330, 1991.

Parkash S, Ananthrakrishnan N, Roy P: Refashioning of phallus stumps and phalloplasty in the treatment of carcinoma of the penis. Br J Surg 73:902, 1986.

Parra RO: Accurate staging of carcinoma of the penis in men with nonpalpable inguinal lymph nodes by modified inguinal lymphadenectomy. J Urol 155:560, 1996.

Ravi R: Morbidity following groin dissection for penile carcinoma. Br J Urol 72:941, 1993.

Santucci RA, Berger RE: "Finger trap" penile lengthening after partial penectomy by multiple incisions in the tunica albuginea. J Urol 154:530, 1995.

See WA: Overview of complications of urologic laparoscopy. In Gomella LG, Kozminski M, Winfield HN (eds): Laparoscopic Urologic Surgery. New York, Raven Press, 1994.

Spaulding JT, Grabstald H: Surgery of penile carcinoma. In Harrison JH, Gittes RF, Perlmutter A, et al (eds): Campbell's Urology, 4th ed. Philadelphia, WB Saunders, 1979, p 2965.

Thomas JA, Matanhelia SS, Dickson WA, et al: Use of the abdominis myocutaneous flap in treating advanced carcinomas of the penis. Br J Urol 75:214, 1995.

Wespes E, Simon J, Schulman CC: Cabanas approach: Is sentinel node biopsy reliable for staging penile carcinoma? Urology 28:278, 1986.

Whitmore WF Jr, Vagaiwala MR: A technique of ilioinguinal lymph node dissection for carcinoma of the penis. Surg Gynecol Obstet 159:573, 1984.

Zabro A, Montie JE: Management of the urethra in men undergoing radical cystectomy for bladder cancer. J Urol 131:267, 1984.

Audiovisuals

Catalona WJ, Andriole GL: Modified Groin Dissection for Carcinoma of the Penis with Preservation of the Saphenous Veins. Wilkes-Barre, PA, Karol Media, 1988 (13 minutes). AUA #919-1151.

DeSouza A, Seizas A, De Campos ES, et al: Inguinal Lymphadectomy of Penile Carcinoma. Wilkes-Barre, PA, Karol Media, 1992 (11 minutes). AUA #919-2004.

Donohue JR, Foster RS, Rowland RG, Bihrle R: Nerve-sparing Retroperitoneal Lymph Node Dissection. Wilkes-Barre, PA, Karol Media, 1992 (18 minutes). AUA #919-2003.

Guerriero WG (moderator): Retroperitoneal Node Dissection in the 90's. Wilkes-Barre, PA, Karol Media, 1993 (73 minutes). AUA #919-2067.

Russo P, Winter H, Fair WR, et al: Radical Groin Dissection with Tensor Lata Myocutaneous Island Flap. Wilkes-Barre, PA, Karol Media, 1990 (20 minutes). AUA #919-1195.

Wacksman J: Repair of Distal Hypospadias Using the Flip-Flap Technique with the Operating Room Microscope. Wilkes-Barre, PA, Karol Media, 1985 (12 minutes). AUA #919-1136.

PENIS: CORRECTION

Allen TD: Microphallus: Clinical and endocrinological characteristics. J Urol 119:750, 1978.

Arnett RM, Jones JS, Horger EO III: Effectiveness of 1% lidocaine dorsal penile nerve block in infant circumcision. Am J Obstet Gynecol 163:1074, 1990.

Azmy A, Eckstein HB: Surgical correction of torsion of the penis. Br J Urol 53:378, 1981.

Badlani GH: Management of complications of penile prostheses. Mediguide Urol 5:1, 1992.

Blandy JP: Circumcision. In Chamberlain GVP (ed): Contemporary Obstetrics and Gynaecology. London, Northwood, 1977, p 240.

Blandy JP, Tresidder GC: Meatoplasty. Br J Urol 39:633, 1967.

Boemers TML, De Jong TPVM: The surgical correction of buried penis: A new technique. J Urol 154:550, 1995.

1094 REFERENCES

Brown TC, Weidner NJ, Bouwmeester J: Dorsal nerve of penis block: Anatomical and radiological studies. Anaesth Intens Care 17:34, 1989.

Burkholder GV, Newell ME: New surgical treatment for micropenis. J Urol 129:832, 1983.

Caldamone AA: Micropenis. In Resnick MI, Caldamone AA, Spirnak JP (eds): Decision Making in Urology, 2nd ed. Philadelphia, BC Decker, 1991, p 196.

Coran AG, Polley TZ Jr: Surgical management of ambiguous genitalia in the infant and child. J Pediatr Surg 26:812, 1991.

Crawford BS: Buried penis. Br J Plast Surg 30:96, 1977.

Cuckow PM, Rix G, Mouriquand PDE: Preputial plasty: A good alternative to circumcision. J Pediatr Surg 29:561, 1994.

Dalens B, Vanneuville G, Dechelotte P: Penile block via the subpubic space in 100 children. Anesth Analg 69:41, 1989.

Das S, Brosman SA: Duplication of male urethra. J Urol 117:452, 1977.

De Sy WA: Aesthetic repair of meatal strictures. J Urol 132:678, 1984.

Diamond DA, Ransley PG: Improved glanuloplasty in epispadias repair: Technical aspects. J Urol 152:1243, 1994.

Donahoe PK, Keating MA: Preputial unfurling to correct the buried penis. J Pediatr Surg 21:1055, 1986.

Ebbehoj J, Metz P: New operation for "Krummerik" (penile curvature). Urology 26:76, 1985.

Ehrlich RM, Scardino PT: Surgical correction of scrotal transposition and perineal hypospadias. J Pediatr Surg 17:175, 1982.

Feldman KW, Smith DW: Fetal phallic growth and penile standards for newborn male infants. J Pediatr 86:395, 1975.

Frank JD, Johnston JH: Operative Paediatric Urology. New York, Churchill Livingstone, 1990.

Gearhart JP, Leonard MP, Burgers JK, Jeffs RD: The Cantwell-Ransley technique for repair of epispadias. J Urol 148:851, 1992.

Gearhart JP, Peppas DS, Jeffs RD: Complete genitourinary reconstruction in female epispadias. J Urol 149:1110, 1993.

Glenn JF, Anderson E: Surgical correction of incomplete penoscrotal transposition. J Urol 110:603, 1973.

Heaton BW, Snow BW, Cartwright PC: Repair of urethral diverticulum by plication. Urology 44:749, 1944.

Hendren WH: Surgical management of urogenital sinus abnormalities. J Pediatr Surg 12:339, 1977.

Hendren WH, Keating MA: Use of dermal grafts and free urethral grafts in penile reconstruction. J Urol 140:1265, 1988.

Herschorn S, Ordorica RC: Penile prosthesis insertion with corporeal reconstruction with synthetic vascular graft material. J Urol 154:80, 1995.

Hester TR, Hill HL, Jurkewicz MJ: One-stage reconstruction of the penis. Br J Plast Surg 31:279, 1978.

Hinman F Jr, Spence HF, Culp OS, et al: Panel discussion: Anomalies of external genitalia in infancy and childhood. J Urol 93:1, 1965.

Horton CE, Devine CJ Jr: Plication of the tunica albuginea to straighten the curved penis. Plast Reconstr Surg 52:32, 1973.

Horton CE, McCraw JB, Devine CJ Jr, Devine PC: Secondary reconstruction of the genital area. Urol Clin North Am 4:133, 1977.

Horton CE, Vorstman B, Teasley D, Winslow B: Hidden penis release: Adjunctive suprapubic lipectomy. Ann Plast Surg 19:131, 1987.

Huffman WC, Culp DA, Flocks RH: Injuries of the external male genitalia. In Converse JM (ed): Reconstructive Plastic Surgery. Philadelphia, WB Saunders, 1964, chap 70.

Huffman WC, Culp DA, Greenleaf JS, et al: Injuries to the male genitalia. Plast Reconstr Surg 18:344, 1956.

Jordan GH: Reconstruction of the fossa navicularis. J Urol 138:102, 1987.

Jordan GH: Reconstruction of the meatus/fossa navicularis using flap techniques. In Schreiter F (ed): Plastic Reconstructive Surgery in Urology. Stuttgart, Theime Verlag (in press).

Kaplan I, Wesser D: A rapid method for constructing a functional sensitive penis. Br J Plast Surg 24:342, 1971.

Kelami A: Congenital penile deviation and its treatment with the Nesbit-Kelami technique. Br J Urol 60:261, 1987.

Koff SA, Eakins M: The treatment of penile chordee using corporal rotation. J Urol 131:931, 1984.

Kramer SA: Intersex states and ambiguous genitalia. In Webster G, Kirby R, King L, Goldwasser B (eds): Reconstructive Urology. Boston, Blackwell Scientific Publications, 1993.

Kroovand RL: Complications of neonatal circumcision. In Cohen MS, Resnick MI (eds): Reoperative Urology. Boston, Little, Brown & Co, 1995, p 205.

Kubota Y, Ishii N, Watanabe H, et al: Buried penis: A surgical repair. Urol Int 46:61, 1991.

Larson DL: Musculocutaneous flaps. In Johnson DE, Boileau MA (eds): Genitourinary Tumors: Fundamental Principles and Surgical Techniques. New York, Grune & Stratton, 1982.

Lau JTK, Ong GB: Subglandular urethral fistula following circumcision: Repair by the advancement method. J Urol 126:702, 1981.

Maizels M, Zaontz M, Donovan J, et al: Surgical correction of the buried penis: Description of a classification system and a technique to correct the disorder. J Urol 136:268, 1986.

Malament M: Repair of the recurrent fistula of the penile urethra. J Urol 106:704, 1971.

Maxwell LG, Yaster M, Wetzel RC, Niebyl JR: Penile nerve block for newborn circumcision. Obstet Gynecol 70:415, 1987.

McAninch JW (guest ed): Urogenital trauma. In Blaisdell FW, Trunkey DD (eds): Trauma Management, vol 2. New York, Thieme-Stratton, 1985.

McAninch JW, Kahn RI, Jeffrey RB, et al: Major traumatic and septic genital injuries. J Trauma 24:291, 1984.

McCraw JB, Myers B, Shanklin KD: The value of fluorescein in predicting the viability of arterialized flaps. Plast Reconstr Surg 60:710, 1977.

McFarlane RM: The use of continuous suction under skin flaps. Br J Plast Surg 17:77, 1959.

McGowan AJ, Waterhouse K: Mobilization of the anterior urethra. Bull NY Acad Med 40:776, 1964.

Mitchell ME, Bagli DJ: Complete penile disassembly for epispadias repair: The Mitchell technique. J Urol 155:300, 1996.

Money J, Mazur T: Microphallus: The successful use of a prosthetic phallus in a 9-year-old boy. J Sex Marital Ther 3:187, 1977.

Monfort G: Transvesical approach to utricular cysts. J Pediatr Surg 17:406, 1982.

Monfort G, Morrisson-Lacombe G, Guys JM, Coquet M: Transverse island flap and a double flap procedure in the treatment of congenital epispadias in 32 patients. J Urol 138:1069, 1987.

Moriel EZ, Grinwald A, Rajfer J: Vein grafting of tunical incisions combined with contralateral plication in the treatment of penile curvature. Urology 43:697, 1994.

Mufti GR, Aitchison M, Bramwell SP, et al: Corporeal plication for surgical correction of Peyronie's disease. J Urol 144:281, 1990.

Nesbit RM: Congenital curvature of the phallus: Report of 3 cases with description of corrective operation. J Urol 93:230, 1965.

Nesbit RM: Operation for correction of distal penile ventral curvature with or without hypospadias. J Urol 97:470, 1967.

Oesch IL, Pinter A, Ransley PG: Penile agenesis: Report of six cases. J Pediatr Surg 22:172, 1987.

Oesterling JE, Gearhart JP, Jeffs RD: A unified approach to early reconstructive surgery of the child with ambiguous genitalia. J Urol 138:1079, 1987.

Ohjimi H, Ogata K, Ohjimi T: A new method for the relief of adult phimosis. J Urol 153:1607, 1995.

Orticochea M: A new method of total reconstruction of the penis. Br J Plast Surg 25:347, 1972.

Peña A: Atlas of Surgical Management of Anorectal Malformations. New York, Springer-Verlag, 1990.

Perovic S, Vukadinovic V: Penoscrotal transposition with hypospadias: 1-stage repair. J Urol 148:1510, 1992.

Persad R, Sharma S, Mctavish J, et al: Clinical presentation and pathophysiology of meatal stenosis following circumcision. Br J Urol 75:91, 1995.

Persky L, Resnick M, Desprez J: Penile reconstruction with gracilis pedicle grafts. J Urol 129:603, 1983.

Peters CA, Hendren WH: Splitting the pubis for exposure in difficult reconstructions for incontinence. J Urol 142:527, 1989. Discussion 542.

Peters PC: Complications of penile surgery. *In* Smith RB, Skinner DG (eds): Complications of Urologic Surgery: Prevention and Management. Philadelphia, WB Saunders, 1976, p 420.

Pond HS, Brannan W: Correction of congenital curvature of the penis: Experiences with the Nesbit operation at Ochsner Clinic. J Urol 112:491, 1974.

Ransley PH: Epispadias repair. *In* Spitz L, Homewood NH (eds): Operative Surgery: Paediatric Surgery, 4th ed. London, Butterworths, 1988, p 624.

Redman JF: Circumcision revision in prepubertal boys: Analysis of a 2-year experience and description of a technique. J Urol 153:180, 1995.

Redman JF: Extended application of Nesbit ellipses in the correction of childhood penile curvature. J Urol 119:122, 1978.

Redman JF: Technique for phalloplasty. Urology 27:360, 1986.

Redman JF: A technique for repair of penoscrotal fusion. J Urol 133:432, 1985.

Redman JF, Bissada NK: One-stage correction of chordee and 180-degree penile rotation. Urology 7:632, 1976.

Reilly JM, Woodhouse CRJ: Small penis and the male sexual role. J Urol 142:569, 1989.

Reilly JM, Woodhouse CRJ: Surgical and hormonal approaches to the small penis. *In* Webster G, Kirby R, King L, Goldwasser B (eds): Reconstructive Urology. Boston, Blackwell Scientific Publications, 1993.

Sadove RC, Jordan GH, Sagher U, et al: Use of the rectus abdominis muscle flap in secondary reconstruction of exstrophy-epispadias. Plast Reconstr Surg 91:511, 1993.

Schuhrke TD, Kaplan GW: Prostatic utricle cysts (Müllerian duct cysts). J Urol 119:765, 1978.

Serour F, Reuben S, Ezra S: Circumcision in children with penile block alone. J Urol 153:474, 1995.

Shapiro SR: Surgical treatment of the "buried" penis. Urology 30:554, 1987.

Sharp RJ, Holder TM, Howard CD, Grunt JA: Neonatal genital reconstruction. J Pediatr Surg 22:168, 1987.

Shepard GH, Wilson CS, Sallade RL: Webbed penis. Plast Reconstr Surg 66:453, 1980.

Sislow JG, Ireton RC, Ansell JS: Treatment of congenital penile curvature due to disparate corpora cavernosa by the Nesbit technique: A rule of thumb for the number of wedges required to achieve correction. J Urol 141:92, 1989.

Slawin KM, Nagler HM: Treatment of congenital penile curvature with penile torsion: A new twist. J Urol 147:152, 1992.

Smith ED: Malformations of the bladder, urethra and hypospadias. *In* Holder TM, Ashcraft KW (eds): Pediatric Surgery. Philadelphia, WB Saunders, 1990, p 752.

Snow BW: Transverse corporeal plication for persistent chordee. Urology 34:360, 1989.

Snow BW, Cartwright PC: Cosmetic epispadias skin coverage. Urology 43:232, 1994.

Snyder HMcC III: Management of ambiguous genitalia in the neonate. *In* King LR (ed): Urologic Surgery in Neonates and Young Infants. Philadelphia, WB Saunders, 1988, p 346.

Soderdahl DW, Brosman SA, Goodwin WE: Penile agenesis. J Urol 108:496, 1972.

Soliman MG, Tremblay NA: Nerve block of the penis for postoperative pain relief in children. Anesth Analg 57:495, 1978.

Spaulding MH: The development of external genitalia in the human embryo. Contr Embryol Carnegie Inst, publication 276, p 67, 1921.

Staerman F, Nouri M, Coeurdacier P, et al: Treatment of the intraoperative penile erection with intracavernous phenylephrine. J Urol 153:1478, 1995.

Stephens FD: Congenital imperforate rectum, rectourethral and rectovaginal fistulae. Aust NZ J Surg 22:161, 1953.

Thomalla JV, Mitchell ME: Ventral preputial island flap technique for the repair of epispadias with or without exstrophy. J Urol 132:985, 1984.

Turner-Warwick R: The use of pedicle grafts in repair of urinary fistulae. Br J Urol 44:644, 1972.

Walker RD: Outpatient repair of urethral fistulae. Urol Clin North Am 8:582, 1981.

Walsh PC, Wilson JD, Allen TD, et al: Clinical and endocrinological evaluation of patients with congenital microphallus. J Urol 120:90, 1978.

Webster GD, Robertson CN: The vascularized skin island urethroplasty: Its role and results in urethral stricture management. J Urol 133:31, 1985.

Wegner HEH, Anderson R, Knispel HH, et al: Evaluation of penile arteries with color-coded duplex sonography: Prevalence and possible therapeutic implications of connections between dorsal and cavernous arteries in impotent men. J Urol 153:1469, 1995.

Williams DI: The development and abnormalities of the penile urethra. Acta Anat 15:176, 1952.

Wilson MC, Wilson CL, Thickstein JN: Transposition of the external genitalia. J Urol 94:600, 1965.

Wise HA II, Berggren RB: Another method of repair for urethrocutaneous fistulae. J Urol 118:1054, 1977.

Wollin M, Duffy G, Malone PS, Ransley PG: Buried penis: A novel approach. Br J Urol 65:97, 1990.

Yachia D: Modified corporoplasty for the treatment of penile curvature. J Urol 143:80, 1990.

Yeoman PM, Cooke R, Hain WR: Penile block for circumcision? A comparison with caudal block. Anesthesia 38:862, 1983.

Young HH: Genital Abnormalities. Baltimore, Williams & Wilkins, 1937.

Audiovisuals

Aboseif SR, Breza J, Kuala N, et al: Surgical Anatomy of the Penis. Wilkes-Barre, PA, Karol Media, 1988 (15 minutes). AUA #919-1156.

Hirsch IH, Moreno JG, Gomella LG: The Concept of Controlled Distention for Inflatable Penile Prosthesis Implantation. Wilkes-Barre, PA, Karol Media, 1995 (10 minutes). AUA #919-2051.

PENIS: RECONSTRUCTION

Abercrombie GF, Branicki F, Smart CJ: Partial amputation of the penis. Proc R Soc Med 68:783, 1975.

Anson BF, Morgan EH, McVay CB: Surgical anatomy of the inguinal region based upon a study of 500 body halves. Surg Gynecol Obstet 3:707, 1960.

Asgari MA, Hosseini SY, Safarinejad MR, et al: Penile fractures: Evaluation, therapeutic approaches and long-term results. J Urol 155:148, 1996.

Bailey MJ, Yande S, Walmsley B, et al: Surgery for Peyronie's disease: A review of 200 patients. Br J Urol 57:746, 1985.

Ball TP: Surgical repair of penile SST deformity. Urology 15:603, 1980.

Baronofsky ID: Technique of inguinal node dissection. Surgery 24:555, 1948.

Barry JM, Seifort A: Penoscrotal approach for placement of paired penile implants for impotence. J Urol 122:325, 1979.

Bennett AH: Venous arterialization for erectile impotence. Urol Clin North Am 15:111, 1988.

Bennett AH, Rivard DJ, Blanc RP, et al: Reconstructive surgery for vasculogenic impotence. J Urol 136:599, 1986.

Benson RC Jr, Patterson DE: The Nesbit procedure for Peyronie's disease. J Urol 130:692, 1983.

Bertram RA, Carson CC, Altaffer LF: Severe penile curvature after implantation of an inflatable penile prosthesis. J Urol 139:743, 1988.

Biemer E: Penile construction by the radial arm flap. Clin Plast Surg 15:425, 1988.

Block NL, Rosen P, Whitmore WF Jr: Hemipelvectomy for advanced penile cancer. J Urol 110:703, 1973.

Boxer RJ: Reconstruction of the male external genitalia. Surg Gynecol Obstet 141:939, 1975.

Brant MD, Ludlow JK, Mulcahy JJ: The prosthesis salvage operation: Immediate replacement of the infected penile prosthesis. J Urol 155:155, 1996.

Brock G, Breza J, Lue TF, Tanagho EA: High flow priapism: A spectrum of disease. J Urol 150:968, 1993.

Brock G, Kadioglu A, Lue TF: Peyronie's disease: A modified treatment. Urology 42:300, 1993.

Brock G, Nunes L, von Heyden B, et al: Can a venous patch graft be a substitute for the tunica albuginea of the penis? J Urol 150:1306, 1993.

Burkholder GV, Newell MF: Amelioration of problems of partial penile amputation. J Urol 122:562, 1979.

Buvat J, Lemaire A, Dehaene JL: Critical study of the organic basis of the venous "leakages" detected by the artificial erection test. In Virag R, Virag-Lappas H (eds): Proceedings of the 1st World Meeting on Impotence. Paris, Les Editions du CERI, 1984, p 179.

Bux R, Carroll P, Berger M, Yarbrough W: Primary penile reanastomosis. Urology 11:500, 1978.

Bystrom J, Alfthan O, Johansson B, Korlof B: Induratio penis plastica (Peyronie's disease): Results after excision and dermo-fat grafting. Scand J Plast Reconstr Surg 7:137, 1973.

Cabanas RM: An approach for the treatment of penile carcinoma. Cancer 39:456, 1977.

Carroll PR, Lue TF, Schmidt RA, et al: Penile reimplantation: Current concepts. J Urol 133:282, 1985.

Carson CC: Infections in genitourinary prosthesis. Urol Clin North Am 16:139, 1989.

Carson CC: Inflatable penile prosthesis: Experience with 100 patients. South Med J 76:1139, 1983.

Carson CC: Penile prostheses. In Webster G, Kirby R, King L, Goldwasser B (eds): Reconstructive Urology. Boston, Blackwell Scientific Publications, 1993.

Carson CC, Hodge GB, Anderson EE: Penile prosthesis in Peyronie's disease. Br J Urol 35:417, 1983.

Carter RG, Thomas CE, Tomskey GC: Cavernospongiosum shunts in the treatment of priapism. Urology 7:292, 1976.

Cartwright PC, Snow BW, Reid BS, Shultz PK: Color Doppler ultrasound in newborn testis torsion. Urology 45:667, 1995.

Cass AS: Testicular trauma. J Urol 129:299, 1983.

Catalona WJ: Role of lymphadenectomy in carcinoma of the penis. Urol Clin North Am 7:785, 1980.

Chang T-S, Hwang W-Y: Forearm flap in one-stage reconstruction of the penis. Plast Reconstr Surg 74:251, 1984.

Cherup LL, Gottlieb LJ, Zachary LS, Levine LA: The sensate functional total phallic reconstruction. Plast Surg Forum 12:25, 1989.

Cohen BE, May JW, Daly JE, Young HH II: Successful clinical replantation of an amputated penis by microneurovascular repair. Plast Reconstr Surg 59:276, 1977.

Cormack GC, Lamberty BGH: Fasciocutaneous vessels in the upper arm: Application to the design of new fasciocutaneous flaps. Plast Reconstr Surg 74:244, 1984.

Culp DA: Genital injuries: Etiology and initial management in genitourinary trauma. Urol Clin North Am 4:143, 1977.

Daseler EH, Anson BJ, Feimans AF: Radical excision of the inguinal and iliac lymph glands: A study based on 450 anatomical dissections and upon supportive clinical observations. Surg Gynecol Obstet 87:679, 1943.

DasGupta TK: Radical groin dissection. Surgery 129:1275, 1969.

de Souza LJ: Subtotal amputation for carcinoma of the penis with reconstruction of penile stump. Ann R Coll Surg Engl 58:398, 1976.

De Stefani S, Simonato A, Capone M, et al: The benefit of glans fixation in prosthetic penile surgery. J Urol 152:1533, 1994.

Dean AL: Conservative amputation of the penis for carcinoma. J Urol 68:374, 1952.

Dekernion JB, Persky L: Neoplastic lesions of the penis. In Skinner DG, Dekernion JB (eds): Genitourinary Cancer. Philadelphia, WB Saunders, 1978.

Devine CJ Jr, Horton CE: Peyronie's disease. Clin Plast Surg 15:405, 1988.

Devine CJ Jr, Horton CE: Surgical treatment of Peyronie's disease with a dermal graft. J Urol 111:44, 1974.

Devine CJ Jr, Jordan GH, Schlossberg SM: Peyronie's disease. In

Cohen MS, Resnick MI (eds): Reoperative Urology. Boston, Little, Brown & Co, 1995, p 221.

Devine CJ Jr, Jordan GH, Schlossberg SM, Horton CE: Surgical treatment of patients with Peyronie's disease. Progr Clin Biol Res 370:359, 1991.

Devine PC: Peyronie's disease and penile curvature. In Glenn JF (ed): Urologic Surgery, 3rd ed. Philadelphia, JB Lippincott, 1983, p 89.

Devine PC, Winslow BH, Jordan GH, et al: Reconstructive phallic surgery. In Libertino JA (ed): Pediatric and Adult Reconstructive Urologic Surgery, 2nd ed. Baltimore, Williams & Wilkins, 1987.

DeVries PA, Peña A: Posterior sagittal anorectoplasty. J Pediatr Surg 17:638, 1982.

Eadie DGA, Brock TP: Corpus-saphenous bypass in the treatment of priapism. Br J Surg 57:172, 1970.

Edgerton MT, Knorr NJ, Callison JR: The surgical treatment of transsexual patients: Limitations and indications. Plast Reconstr Surg 45:38, 1970.

Ehrlich RM, Scardino PT: Surgical correction of scrotal transposition and perineal hypospadias. J Pediatr Surg 17:175, 1982.

Eigner EB, Kabalin JN, Kessler R: Penile implants in the treatment of Peyronie's disease. J Urol 145:69, 1991.

Einarsson G, Goldstein M, Laungani G: Penile reimplantation. Urology 22:404, 1983.

Elder JS, Mostwin JL: Cyst of the ejaculatory duct/urogenital sinus. J Urol 132:768, 1994.

Essed E, Schroeder FH: New surgical treatment for Peyronie Disease. Urology 25:582, 1985.

Finney RP: Flexi-Flate penile prosthesis. Semin Urol 4:244, 1986.

Finney RP: Coring fibrotic corpora for penile implants. Urology 24:73, 1984.

Fishman IJ: Complicated implantations of inflatable penile prosthesis. Urol Clin North Am 14:217, 1987.

Fishman IJ: Corporeal reconstruction for complicated penile implants. Urol Clin North Am 16:73, 1989.

Fishman IJ: Experience with the Hydroflex penile prosthesis. Semin Urol 4:239, 1986.

Fishman IJ: Perforation and erosion of penile prosthesis. Contemp Urol 3:55, 1991.

Fishman MD, Scott FB, Light JK: Experience with inflatable penile prosthesis. Urology 123:86, 1984.

Fournier GR Jr, Lue TF, Tanagho EA: Peyronie's plaque: Surgical treatment with the carbon dioxide laser and a deep dorsal vein patch graft. J Urol 149:1321, 1993.

Fowler JE: Sentinel lymph node biopsy for staging penile cancer. Urology 23:352, 1984.

Fraley EE, Hutchens HC: Radical ilio-inguinal node dissection: The skin-bridge technique. J Urol 108:279, 1972.

Furlow WL: Surgery for male impotence. In Glenn JF (ed): Urologic Surgery, 3rd ed. Philadelphia, JB Lippincott, 1983, p 837.

Furlow WL, Barrett DM: Inflatable penile prosthesis: New device and patient-partner satisfaction. Urology 24:559, 1984.

Furlow WL, Fisher J, Knoll LD: Penile revascularization: Experience with deep dorsal vein arterialization—the Furlow-Fisher modification with 27 patients. In Proceedings of the Sixth Biennial International Symposium for Corpus Cavernosum Revascularization and Third Biennial World Meeting on Impotence. Boston, International Society for Impotence Research, 1988, p 139.

Furlow WL, Goldwasser B: Salvage of the eroded inflatable penile prosthesis: A new concept. J Urol 138:318, 1987.

Furlow WF, Motley RC: The inflatable penile prosthesis: Clinical experience with a new controlled expansion cylinder. J Urol 139:945, 1988.

Futral AA, Witt MA: A closed system for corporeal irrigation in the treatment of refractory priapism. Urology 46:403, 1995.

Ganabathi K, Dmochowski R, Zimmern PE, Leach GE: Peyronie's disease: Surgical treatment based on penile rigidity. J Urol 153:662, 1995.

Garrett RA, Rhamy DE: Priapism: Management with corpus saphenous shunt. J Urol 95:65, 1966.

Gelbard MK: Relaxing incisions in the correction of penile deformity due to Peyronie's disease. J Urol 154:1457, 1995.

Gelbard MK, Dorey F, James K: The natural history of Peyronie's disease. J Urol 144:1376, 1990.

Gelbard MK, Hayden B: Expanding contractures of the tunica albuginea due to Peyronie's disease with temporalis fascia free grafts. J Urol 145:772, 1991.

Gilbert DA, Horton CE, Terzis JK, et al: New concepts in phallic reconstruction. Ann Plast Surg 18:128, 1987.

Gilbert DA, Jordan GH, Devine CJ Jr, et al: Phallic construction in prepubertal and adolescent boys. J Urol 149:1521, 1993.

Gilbert DA, Jordan GH, Devine CJ Jr, Winslow BH: Microsurgical forearm "cricket bat–transformer" phalloplasty. Plast Reconstr Surg 90:711, 1992.

Gilbert DA, Williams MW, Horton CE, et al: Phallic innervation via the pudendal nerve. J Urol 140:295, 1988.

Goldstein I: Arterial revascularization procedures. Semin Urol 4:252, 1986.

Goldstein I: Penile revascularization. Urol Clin North Am 14:805, 1987.

Goldstein I: Penile revascularization. *In* Mundy AR (ed): Current Operative Surgery: Urology. East Sussex, Bailliere Tindall, 1986.

Goldstein I, Hatzichristou D, Seftel AD: Arterial reconstruction for erectile impotence. *In* Webster G, Kirby R, King L, Goldwasser B (eds): Reconstructive Urology. Boston, Blackwell Scientific Publications, 1993.

Goldstein M, Blumberg N: Correction of severe penile curves with tunica albuginea autografts. J Urol 139:1269, 1988.

Gottlieb LG, Levine LA: A new design for the radial forearm free-flap phallic construction. Plast Reconstr Surg 92:276, 1993.

Grace DA, Winter CC: Priapism: An appraisal of management of twenty-three patients. J Urol 99:301, 1968.

Grayhack JT, McCullough W, O'Connor VJ Jr, Trippel O: Venous bypass to control priapism. Invest Urol 1:509, 1964.

Gross M: Rupture of the testicle: The importance of early surgical treatment. J Urol 101:196, 1969.

Hakim LS, Kulaksizoglu H, Mulligan R, et al: Evolving concepts in the diagnosis and treatment of arterial high flow priapism. J Urol 155:541, 1996.

Hauri D: A new operative technique in vasculogenic erectile impotence. World J Urol 4:237, 1986.

Hawtrey CE, Culp DA, Hartford CE: The management of severe inflammation and traumatic injuries to the genital skin. J Urol 108:431, 1972.

Helal MA, Lockhart JL, Sanford E, Persky L: Tunica vaginalis flap for the management of disabling Peyronie's disease: Surgical technique, results and complications. Urology 46:390, 1995.

Herman PG, Benninghoff DL, Nelson JH Jr, Mellins HZ: Roentgen anatomy of the ilio-pelvic-aortic lymphatic system. Radiology 80:182, 1963.

Herschorn S, Barkin M, Comisarow R: New technique for difficult penile implants. Urology 27:463, 1986.

Heymann AD, Bell-Thomson J, Rathod DM, et al: Successful reimplantation of the penis using microvascular techniques. J Urol 118:879, 1977.

Hinman F Jr: Priapism. Reasons for failure of therapy. J Urol 83:420, 1960.

Horton CE, Devine CJ Jr: Peyronie's disease. Plast Reconstr Surg 52:503, 1973.

Hovnanian AP: Ilio-inguinal lymphatic excision. Surgery 54:592, 1963.

Huffman WC, Culp DA, Flocks RH: Injuries of the external male genitalia. *In* Converse JM (ed): Reconstructive and Plastic Surgery. Philadelphia, WB Saunders, 1964, chap 70.

Huffman WC, Culp DA, Greenleaf JS, et al: Injuries to the male genitalia. Plast Reconstr Surg 18:344, 1956.

Hutson JM, Donohoe PK, Budzil GP: Müllerian inhibiting substance: A fetal hormone with surgical implications. Aust NZ J Surg 55:599, 1985.

Johnson DE, Schoenwald MB, Bracken B, et al: Rotational skin flaps to cover wound defect in groin. Urology 6:461, 1975.

Jonas U, Jacobi GH: Silicone-silver-penile prosthesis: Description, operative approach, and results. J Urol 123:865, 1980.

Jordan GH, Alter GJ, Gilbert DA, et al: Penile prosthesis implantation in total phalloplasty. J Urol 152:410, 1994.

Jordan GH, Gilbert DA: Male genital trauma. Clin Plast Surg 15:431, 1988.

Jordan GH, Gilbert DA: Management of amputation injuries of the male genitalia. Urol Clin North Am 16:359, 1989.

Juskiewenski S, Vaysse P, Moscovici J, et al: A study of the arterial blood supply to the penis. Anat Clin 4:101, 1982.

Kabalin JN, Kessler R: Experience with the Hydroflex penile prosthesis. J Urol 141:58, 1989.

Kalash SS, Young JD: Fracture of the penis: controversy of surgical versus conservative treatment. Urology 24:21, 1984.

Kaplan GW, Piconi JR, Schuhrke TD: Posterior approach to müllerian duct and seminal vesicle cysts. Birth Defects 13:241, 1977.

Kaplan I, Wesser D: A rapid method for constructing a functional sensitive penis. Br J Plast Surg 24:342, 1971.

Kaufman JJ, Lindner A, Raz S: Complications of penile prosthesis surgery for impotence. J Urol 128:1192, 1982.

Kelami A: Congenital penile deviation and its treatment with the Nesbit-Kelami technique. Br J Urol 60:261, 1987.

Kelami A: Infrapubic approach for Small-Carrion prosthesis in erectile impotence. Urology 8:164, 1976.

Kessler R: Complications of inflatable penile prostheses. Urology 18:470, 1981.

Keuhn CA, Roberts RR: Amputation and radical lymph gland dissection in carcinoma of the penis: An operative approach. J Urol 69:173, 1953.

Kim ED, McVary KT: Long-term follow-up of treatment of Peyronie's disease with plaque incision, carbon dioxide laser plaque ablation and placement of a deep dorsal vein patch graft. J Urol 153:1843, 1995.

Klevmark B, Andersen M, Schultz A, Talseth T: Congenital and acquired curvature of the penis treated surgically by plication of the tunica albuginea. Br J Urol 74:501, 1994.

Knoll LD, Furlow WL, Benson RC: Management of Peyronie's disease by implantation of inflatable penile prosthesis. Urology 36:406, 1990.

Koga S, Shiraishi K, Saito Y: Post-traumatic priapism. J Trauma 30:1591, 1990.

Konnak JW, Ohl DA: Microsurgical penile revascularization using central corporeal penile artery. J Urol 142:305, 1989.

Koshima I, Tai T, Yamasaki M: One-stage reconstruction of the penis using an innervated radial forearm osteocutaneous flap. J Reconstr Microsurg 3:19, 1986.

Krane RJ: Omniphase penile prosthesis. Semin Urol 4:247, 1986.

Krane RJ, Goldstein I: Surgery for impotency: Prosthesis implantation and penile revascularization. *In* Libertino JA, Zinman L (eds): Pediatric and Adult Reconstructive Urologic Surgery. Baltimore, Williams & Wilkins, 1986.

Lamont GL, Gough DCS: Transtrigonal approach for excision of müllerian duct structures. Br J Urol 72:834, 1993.

Larson DL: Musculocutaneous flaps. *In* Johnson DE, Boileau MA (eds): Genitourinary Tumors: Fundamental Principles and Surgical Techniques. New York, Grune & Stratton, 1982.

Lee ES: Ilio-inguinal block dissection with primary healing. Lancet 2:520, 1955.

Lee GW, Khouri RK: Reconstruction of a near total male urethral defect with a microvascular free flap. J Urol 149:1548, 1993.

Leiter E, Futterweit W, Brown GR: Gender reassignment: Psychiatric, endocrinologic, and surgical management. *In* Webster G, Kirby R, King L, Goldwasser B (eds): Reconstructive Urology. Boston, Blackwell Scientific Publications, 1993.

Levine FJ, Goldstein I: Reconstructive vascular surgery for impotence. *In* Jonas U, Thon WF, Stief CG (eds): Erectile Dysfunction. Berlin, Springer-Verlag, 1991, p 240.

Levine LA, Gottlieb LJ: Penile construction. *In* Whitfield HN (ed): Genitourinary Surgery. Oxford, Butterworth-Heinemann, 1993.

Levine LA, Gottlieb LJ: Phallic reconstruction for trauma. *In* Webster G, Kirby R, King L, Goldwasser B (eds): Reconstructive Urology. Boston, Blackwell Scientific Publications, 1993.

Levine LA, Zachary LS, Gottlieb LJ: Prosthesis placement after total phallic reconstruction. J Urol 149:593, 1993.

Lewis RW: Venous surgery for impotence. Urol Clin North Am 15:115, 1988.

Lewis RW, McLaren R: Reoperation for penile prosthesis implantation. *In* Carson C (ed): Problems in Urology—Prosthetics in Urology. Philadelphia, JB Lippincott, 1993, p 382.

Lewis RW, Morgan WR: Failure of the penile prosthesis. *In* Cohen MS, Resnick MI (eds): Reoperative Urology. Boston, Little, Brown & Co, 1995, p 235.

Lowsley OS, Rueda A: Further experience with an operation for the cure of certain types of impotence. J Int Coll Surg 19:69, 1953.

Lue TF: Penile venous surgery. Urol Clin North Am 16:607, 1989.

Lue TF, Hricak H, Schmidt RA, Tanagho EA: Functional evaluation of penile veins by cavernosography in papaverine-induced erection. J Urol 135:479, 1986.

Lue T, Zeineh SJ, Schmidt RA, Tanagho EA: Neuroanatomy of penile erection: Its relevance to iatrogenic impotency. J Urol 131:273, 1984.

Lund GO, Winfield HN, Donovan JF: Laparoscopically assisted penile revascularization for vasculogenic impotence. J Urol 153:1923, 1995.

MacDonald I, Smith GK, Guiss LW, et al: Exposure and suction drainage in the management of major dissective wounds. Surg Gynecol Obstet 107:532, 1958.

Mark SD, Webster GD: Reconstruction of penile curvature and Peyronie's disease. *In* Webster G, Kirby R, King L, Goldwasser B (eds): Reconstructive Urology. Boston, Blackwell Scientific Publications, 1993.

Marshall VF: Excision of locally extensive carcinoma of the urethra in male patients. J Urol 788:252, 1957.

McAninch JW: Management of genital skin loss. Urol Clin North Am 16:387, 1989.

McAninch JW (guest ed): Urogenital trauma. *In* Blaisdell FW, Trunkey DD (eds): Trauma Management, vol 2. New York, Thieme-Stratton, 1985.

McAninch JW, Kahn RI, Jeffrey RB, et al: Major traumatic and septic genital injuries. J Trauma 24:291, 1984.

McConnell JD, Peters PC, Lewis SE: Testicular rupture in blunt scrotal trauma: A review of 15 cases with recent application of testicular scanning. J Urol 128:309, 1982.

McDougal WS: Scrotal reconstruction using thigh pedicle flaps. J Urol 129:757, 1983.

McDougal WS, Jeffery RF: Microscopic penile revascularization. J Urol 129:517, 1983.

McDougal WS, Persky LI (eds): Traumatic Injuries of the Genitourinary System. Baltimore, Williams & Wilkins, 1981.

McFarlane RM: The use of continuous suction under skin flaps. Br J Plast Surg 17:77, 1959.

Merrill D: Mentor inflatable penile prosthesis. Urology 22:504, 1983.

Merrill D: Mentor inflatable penile prostheses. Urol Clin North Am 16:51, 1989.

Meyer R, Daverio PJ, Dequesne J: One-stage phalloplasty in transsexuals. Ann Plast Surg 16:472, 1986.

Michal V, Kramar R, Hejhal L: Revascularization procedures of the cavernous bodies. *In* Zorgniotti AW, Rossi G (eds): Proceedings of the First International Conference on Corpus Cavernosum Revascularization. Springfield, IL, Charles C Thomas, 1980, p 239.

Michal V, Kramar R, Pospichal J: Femoropudendal bypass, internal iliac thromboendarterectomy and direct arterial anastomosis to the cavernous body in the treatment of erectile impotence. Bull Soc Int Chir 33:343, 1974.

Michal V, Kramar R, Pospichal J, et al: Vascular surgery in the treatment of impotence: Its present possibilities and prospects. Czech Med 3:213, 1980.

Michal V, Kramar R, Pospichal J, Hejhal L: Arterial epigastrico-cavernous anastomosis for the treatment of sexual impotence. World J Surg 1:515, 1977.

Michal V, Kramar R, Pospichal J, Hejhal L: Direct arterial anastomosis to the cavernous body in the treatment of erectile impotence. Rozhl Chir 52:587, 1973.

Montague DK: Penile prosthesis implantation. *In* Marshall FF (ed): Operative Urology. Philadelphia, WB Saunders, 1991.

Montague DK: Periprosthetic infections. J Urol 138:68, 1987.

Moul JW, McCleod DG: Experience with the AMS 600 malleable penile prosthesis. J Urol 135:929, 1986.

Mufti GR, Aitchison M, Bramwell SP, et al: Corporeal plication for surgical correction of Peyronie's disease. J Urol 144:281, 1990.

Mulcahy JJ: A technique of maintaining penile prosthesis position to prevent proximal migration. J Urol 137:294, 1987.

Mulcahy JJ: Update: Penile prosthesis. Contemp Urol, October 1994, p 15.

Nesbit RM: Congenital curvature of the phallus: Report of three cases with description of corrective operation. J Urol 93:230, 1965.

Nicolaisen G, Melamud A, Williams RD, et al: Rupture of the corpus cavernosum: Surgical management. J Urol 130:917, 1983.

Nooter RI, Bosch JLHR, Schröder FH: Peyronie's disease and congenital penile curvature: Long-term results of operative treatment with the plication procedure. Br J Urol 74:497, 1994.

O'Donnell PD: Operative approach for secondary placement of penile prosthesis. Urology 28:108, 1986.

Oesch IL, Pinter A, Ransley PG: Penile agenesis: Report of six cases. J Pediatr Surg 22:172, 1987.

Olsson CA: Metastatic squamous cell carcinoma. *In* Resnick MI, Kursh E (eds): Current Therapy in Genitourinary Surgery. Toronto, BC Decker, 1987, p 120.

Orticochea M: A new method of total reconstruction of the penis. Br J Plast Surg 25:347, 1972.

Orvis BR, McAninch JW: Penile rupture. Urol Clin North Am 16:369, 1989.

Ovrum E: Rupture of the penis. Scand J Urol Nephrol 12:83, 1978.

Perinetti E, Crane DB, Catalona WJ: Unreliability of sentinel lymph node biopsy for staging penile carcinoma. J Urol 124:734, 1980.

Perovic S: Phalloplasty in children and adolescents using the extended pedicle island groin flap. J Urol 154:848, 1995.

Persky L, Resnick M, Desprez J: Penile reconstruction with gracilis pedicle grafts. J Urol 129:603, 1983.

Pryor JP, Fitzpatrick JM: A new approach to the correction of the penile deformity in Peyronie's disease. J Urol 122:622, 1979.

Puech-Leao P, Reis JM, Glina S, Reichelt AC: Leakage through the crural edge of corpus cavernosum. Eur Urol 13:163, 1987.

Quackles R: Cure d'un cas de priapisme par anastomose cavernospongieuse. Acta Urol Belg 32:5, 1964.

Rabinovitch HH: Urethral duplication. *In* Webster G, Kirby G, King L, Goldwasser B (eds): Reconstructive Urology. Boston, Blackwell Scientific Publications, 1993.

Raz S, Dekernion JB, Kaufman JK: Surgical treatment of Peyronie's disease: A new approach. J Urol 117:598, 1977.

Redman JF: Extended application of Nesbit ellipses in the correction of childhood penile curvature. J Urol 119:122, 1978.

Redman JF: Technique for phalloplasty. Urology 27:360, 1986.

Redman JF, Bissada NK: One-stage correction of chordee and 180-degree penile rotation. Urology 7:632, 1976.

Rigaud G, Berger RE: Corrective procedures for penile shortening due to Peyronie's disease. J Urol 153:368, 1995.

Sadove RC, Sengezer M, McRoberts JW, et al: One-stage total penile reconstruction with a free sensate osteocutaneous fibula flap. Plast Reconstr Surg 92:1314, 1993.

Santucci RA, Berger RE: "Finger Trap" penile lengthening after partial penectomy by multiple incisions in the tunica albuginea. J Urol 154:530, 1995.

Sarranon JP, Janssen T, Rischman P, et al: Deep dorsal vein arterialization for vascular impotence. Eur Urol 25:29, 1994.

Sassine AM, Wespes E, Schulman CC: Modified corporoplasty for penile curvature: 10 years' experience. Urology 44:419, 1994.

Sawhney CP: Management of the urethra following total amputation of the penis. Br J Urol 39:405, 1967.

Schellhammer PF, Grabstald H: Tumors of the penis. *In* Walsh PC, Perlmutter AD, Gittes RF, Stamey TA (eds): Campbell's Urology, 5th ed. Philadelphia, WB Saunders, 1986, p 1595.

Schellhammer PF, Spaulding JT: Carcinoma of the penis. *In* Paulson DF (ed): Genitourinary Surgery. New York, Churchill Livingstone, 1984.

Schulman ML: Re-anastomosis of the amputated penis. J Urol 109:432, 1973.

Scott FB, Bradley WE, Timm GW: Management of erectile impotence: Use of implantable inflatable prosthesis. Urology 2:80, 1973.

Seftel AD, Oates RD, Goldstein I: Use of polytetrafluoroethylene tube graft as a circumferential neotunica during placement of a penile prosthesis. J Urol 148:1531, 1992.

Shapiro SR: Surgical treatment of the "buried" penis. Urology 30:554, 1987.

Sharlip ID: The role of vascular surgery in arteriogenic and combined arteriogenic and venogenic impotence. Semin Urol 8:129, 1990.

Sharlip ID: Vasculogenic impotence secondary to atherosclerosis/dysplasia. *In* Bennett AH (ed): Impotence: Diagnosis and Management of Erectile Dysfunction. Philadelphia, WB Saunders, 1994.

Siegel JF, Brock WA, Peña A: Transrectal posterior sagittal approach to prostatic utricle (müllerian duct cyst). J Urol 153:785, 1995.

Silvis RS, Potter LE, Robinson DW, et al: The use of continuous suction negative pressure instead of pressure dressing. Ann Surg 142:252, 1955.

Skinner DG, Leadbetter WF, Kelley SB: The surgical management of squamous cell carcinoma of the penis. J Urol 107:273, 1972.

Small MP, Carrion HM, Gordon JA: Small-Carrion penile prosthesis: A new implant for management of impotence. Urology 5:479, 1975.

Song R, Gao Y, Song Y, et al: The forearm flap. Clin Plast Surg 9:21, 1982.

Sonn DJ, Smith AD, Moldwin RM: Other urologic laparoscopic applications. *In* Gomella LG, Kozminski M, Winfield HN (eds): Laparoscopic Urologic Surgery. New York, Raven Press, 1994.

Spaulding JT: Tumors of the penis. *In* Javadpour N (ed): Principles and Management of Urologic Cancer. Baltimore, Williams & Wilkins, 1979, p 475.

Spaulding JT, Grabstald H: Surgery of penile and urethral carcinoma. *In* Walsh PC, Perlmutter AD, Gittes RF, Stamey TA (eds): Campbell's Urology, 5th ed. Philadelphia, WB Saunders, 1986, p 2916.

Spratt JS, Shieber W, Dillard BM: Anatomy and Surgical Technique of Groin Dissection. St. Louis, CV Mosby, 1965.

Still EF II, Goodman RC: Total reconstruction of a two-compartment scrotum by tissue expansion. Plast Reconstr Surg 85:805, 1990.

Tamai S, Nakamura Y, Motomiya Y: Microsurgical replantation of a completely amputated penis and scrotum: Case report. Plast Reconstr Surg 60:287, 1977.

Tank ES, Hatch DA: Müllerian remnant causing bladder outlet obstruction. J Pediatr Surg 21:77, 1986.

Thon LA, Levine FJ, Gasior BL, Goldstein I: Reconstructive arterial surgery for impotence. Semin Int Radiol 6:220, 1989.

Tiwari IN, Seth HP, Mehdiratta KS: Reconstruction of the scrotum by thigh flaps. Plast Reconstr Surg 66:605, 1980.

Tuerk M, Weir WH Jr: Successful replantation of a traumatically amputated glans penis. Plast Reconstr Surg 48:499, 1971.

Vale JA, Feneley MR, Lees WR, Kirby RS: Venous leak surgery: Long-term follow-up of patients undergoing excision and ligation of the deep dorsal vein of the penis. Br J Urol 76:192, 1995.

Vincent MP, Horton CE, Devine CJ: An evaluation of skin grafts for reconstruction of penis and scrotum. Clin Plast Surg 15:411, 1988.

Virag R: Revascularization of the penis. *In* Bennett AH (ed): Management of Male Impotence. Baltimore, Williams & Wilkins, 1982, p 219.

Virag R, Zwang G, Demange H, et al: Vasculogenic impotence: A review of 92 cases with 54 surgical operations. Vasc Surg 15:9, 1981.

Wagner G: Surgical treatment of erectile failure. *In* Wagner G, Green R (eds): Impotence: Physiological, Psychological, Surgical Diagnosis and Treatment. New York, Plenum Press, 1981, p 155.

Wahle GR, Mulcahy JJ: Ventral penile approach in unitary component penile prosthesis placement. J Urol 149:537, 1993.

Wear JB Jr, Crummy AB, Munsen BO: A new approach to the treatment of priapism. J Urol 117:252, 1977.

Webster GD, Khoury JM: Management of acute urethral trauma. *In* Webster G, Kirby R, King L, Goldwasser B (eds): Reconstructive Urology. Boston, Blackwell Scientific Publications, 1993.

Wespes E: Pathogenesis, diagnosis, and treatment of cavernovenous leak as a cause of erectile impotence. *In* Webster G, Kirby R, King L, Goldwasser B (eds): Reconstructive Urology. Boston, Blackwell Scientific Publications, 1993.

Wespes E, Corbusier A, Delcour C, et al: Deep dorsal vein arterialization in vascular impotence. Br J Urol 64:535, 1989.

Wespes E, Libert M, Simon J, Schulman CC: Fracture of the penis: Conservative versus surgical treatment. Eur Urol 13:166, 1987.

Wespes E, Moreira de Goes P, Sattar AA, et al: Objective criteria in the long-term evaluation of penile venous surgery. J Urol 152:888, 1994.

Wespes E, Schulman CC: Venous leakage: Surgical treatment of a curable cause for impotence. J Urol 133:796, 1985.

Whitmore WF Jr, Vagaiwala MR: A technique of ilioinguinal lymph node dissection for carcinoma of the penis. Surg Gynecol Obstet 159:573, 1984.

Wild RM, Devine CJ Jr, Horton CE: Dermal graft repair of Peyronie's disease: Survey of 50 patients. J Urol 121:47, 1979.

Williams JL: Surgical treatment of carcinoma of the penis. Proc R Soc Med 68:781, 1975.

Wilson SK, Cleves MA, Delk JR II: Ultrex cylinders: Problems with uncontrolled lengthening (the S-shaped deformity). J Urol 155:135, 1996.

Wilson SK, Delk JR II: Inflatable penile implant infection: Predisposing factors and treatment suggestions. J Urol 153:659, 1995.

Winter CC: Cure of idiopathic priapism: A new procedure for creating fistula between glans penis and corpora cavernosa. Urology 8:389, 1976.

Winter CC: Priapism. *In* Cohen MS, Resnick MI (eds): Reoperative Urology. Boston, Little, Brown & Co, 1995, p 215.

Yachia D: Modified corporoplasty for the treatment of penile curvature. J Urol 143:80, 1990.

Audiovisuals

Carmingnani G, Simonato A: Microsurgical Neuroprotective Dissection of the Neurovascular Bundle and Vascularized Preputial Skin Flap for Albuginea Replacement in Peyronie's Disease. Wilkes-Barre, PA, Karol Media, 1993 (10 minutes). AUA #919-2021.

Lue TF, Tanagho EA, Kenny S: Modified Surgical Approach to Peyronie's Disease: Plaque Incision and Venous Graft. Wilkes-Barre, PA, Karol Media, 1994 (11 minutes). AUA #919-2037.

Praun OH: Peyronie's Disease: Surgical Treatment with Free Patch of Fascia Lata. Wilkes-Barre, PA, Karol Media, 1995 (9 minutes). AUA #919-2049.

Scott FB: Implantation of the Inflatable Penile Prosthesis. Wilkes-Barre, PA, Karol Media, 1983 (24 minutes). AUA #919-1110.

FEMALE GENITALIA: RECONSTRUCTION

Abbé R: New method of creating a vagina in a case of congenital absence. Med Rec, December 10, 1898.

Allen LE, Hardy BE, Churchill BM: The surgical management of the enlarged clitoris. J Urol 128:351, 1982.

Allen TD: Microphallus: Clinical and endocrinological characteristics. J Urol 119:750, 1978.

Ansell JS, Rajfer J: A new and simplified method for concealing the hypertrophied clitoris. J Pediatr Surg 16:681, 1981.

Azmy A, Eckstein HB: Surgical correction of torsion of the penis. Br J Urol 53:378, 1981.

Bailez MM, Gearhart JP, Migeon C, Rock J: Vaginal reconstruction after initial construction of the external genitalia in girls with salt-wasting adrenal hyperplasia. J Urol 148:680, 1992.

Baldwin JF: Formation of an artificial vagina by intestinal transplantation. Am J Obstet Gynecol 56:636, 1907.

Barrett TM, Gonzales ET Jr: Reconstruction of the female external genitalia. Urol Clin North Am 7:455, 1980.

Beck RP, McCormick S, Nordstrom L: The fascia lata sling procedure for the treatment of recurrent genuine stress incontinence of urine. Obstet Gynecol 72:699, 1988.

Beemer W, Hopkins MP, Morley GW: Vaginal reconstruction in gynecologic oncology. Obstet Gynecol 72:911, 1988.

Bellinger MF: Subtotal de-epithelialization and partial concealment of the glans clitoris: A modification to improve the cosmetic results of feminizing genitoplasty. J Urol 150:651, 1993.

Blaivas JG: Vaginal flap urethral reconstuction: An alternative to the bladder flap neourethra. J Urol 141:542, 1989.

Blandy JP: Circumcision. In Chamberlain GVP (ed): Contemporary Obstetrics and Gynaecology. London, Northwood, 1977, p 240.

Boyd SD, Raz S: Female urethral diverticula. In Raz S (ed): Female Urology. Philadelphia, WB Saunders, 1983, p 378.

Braren V: Vaginal amplification using a posterolateral Y-V plasty. J Urol 126:645, 1981.

Bürger RA, Riedmiller H, Knapstein PG, et al: Ileocecal vaginal construction. Am J Obstet Gynecol 161:162, 1989.

Cain JM, Diamond A, Tamimi HK, et al: The morbidity and benefits of concurrent gracilis myocutaneous graft with pelvic exenteration. Obstet Gynecol 74:185, 1989.

Chancellor MB, Liu J-B, Rivas DA, et al: Intraoperative endoluminal ultrasound evaluation of urethral diverticula. J Urol 153:72, 1995.

Christmas TJ, Kirby RS, Turner-Warwick R: Vaginal reconstruction using colon. In Webster G, Kirby R, King L, Goldwasser B (eds): Reconstructive Urology. Boston, Blackwell Scientific Publications, 1993, p 857.

Clarke-Pearson DL, Soper JT: Vaginal reconstruction with gracilis myocutaneous flaps. In Webster G, Kirby R, King L, Goldwasser B (eds): Reconstructive Urology. Boston, Blackwell Scientific Publications, 1993, p 837.

Conway H, Stark RB: Construction and reconstruction of the vagina. Surg Gynecol Obstet 97:573, 1953.

Coran AG, Polley TZ Jr: Surgical management of ambiguous genitalia in the infant and child. J Pediatr Surg 26:812, 1991.

Crawford BS: Buried penis. Br J Plast Surg 30:96, 1977.

Culp DA: Genital injuries: Etiology and initial management in genitourinary trauma. Urol Clin North Am 4:143, 1977.

Davis RS, Linke CA, Kraemer GK: Use of labial tissue in repair of urethrovaginal fistula and injury. Arch Surg 115:628, 1980.

Dean GE, Hensle TW: Intestinal vaginoplasty. In Olsson CA (ed): Current Surgical Techniques in Urology, vol 7, issue 2, 1994.

De Jong TPVM, Boemers TML: Neonatal management of female intersex by clitorovaginoplasty. J Urol 154:830, 1995.

Devine CJ Jr, Jordan GH: Strictures of the anterior urethra. Houston, American Urological Association, AUA Update Series, vol II, lesson 26, p 202, 1990.

Donahoe PK, Hendren WH III: Perineal reconstruction in ambiguous genitalia in infants raised as females. Ann Surg 200:363, 1984.

Downs RA: Urethral diverticula in females: Alternative surgical treatment. Urology 29:201, 1987.

Elkins TE, Drescher C, Martey JO, Fort D: Vesicovaginal fistula revisited. Obstet Gynecol 72:307, 1988.

Flack CE, Barraza MA, Stevens PS: Vaginoplasty: Combination therapy using labia minora flaps and Lucite dilators: Preliminary report. J Urol 150:654, 1993.

Frank RT: The formation of an artificial vagina without operation. Am J Obstet Gynecol 35:1053, 1938.

Ganabathi K, Leach GE, Zimmern PE, Dmochowski R: Experi-ence with the management of urethral diverticulum in 63 women. J Urol 152:1445, 1994.

Glassberg KI, Laungani G: Reduction clitoroplasty. Urology 17:604, 1981.

Gonzales R, Fernandes ET: Single-stage feminization genitoplasty. J Urol 143:776, 1990.

Goodwin WE: Partial (segmental) amputation of the clitoris for female pseudohermaphroditism. Soc Pediatr Urol Newsl, 1981.

Gunst MA, Ackerman D, Zingg EJ: Urethral reconstruction in females. Eur Urol 13:62, 1987.

Hagerty RC, Vaughn TR, Lutz MH: The perineal artery axial flap in reconstruction of the vagina. Plast Reconstr Surg 82:344, 1988.

Hanna MK: Vaginal construction. Urology 29:272, 1987.

Heckler FR: Gracilis myocutaneous and muscle flaps. Clin Plast Surg 7:27, 1980.

Hedden RJ, Husseinzadeh N, Bracken RB: Bladder sparing surgery for locally advanced female urethral cancer. J Urol 150:1135, 1993.

Hendren WH: Construction of a female urethra from vaginal wall and perineal flap. J Urol 123:657, 1980.

Hendren WH: Reconstructive problems of the vagina and female urethra. Clin Plast Surg 7:207, 1980.

Hendren WH: Surgical management of urogenital sinus abnormalities. J Pediatr Surg 12:339, 1977.

Hendren WH, Atala A: Use of bowel for vaginal reconstruction. J Urol 152:752, 1994.

Hendren WH, Caesar RE: Chordee without hypospadias: Experience with 33 cases. J Urol 147:107, 1992.

Hendren WH, Crawford JD: Adrenogenital syndrome: The anatomy of the anomaly and its repair: Some new concepts. J Pediatr Surg 4:49, 1969.

Hendren WH, Crawford JD: The child with ambiguous genitalia. Curr Probl Surg 1:64, 1972.

Hendren WH, Donahoe PK: Correction of congenital abnormalities of the vagina and perineum. J Pediatr Surg 15:751, 1980.

Hensle TW, Dean GE: Vaginal replacement in children. J Urol 148:677, 1992.

Hester TR, Hill HL, Jurkewicz MJ: One-stage reconstruction of the penis. Br J Plast Surg 31:279, 1978.

Hinman F Jr: Surgical reversal of the female adrenal intersex. Urol Int 19:211, 1965.

Hitchcock RJI, Malone PS: Colovaginoplasty in infants and children. Br J Urol 73:196, 1994.

Horton CE, Devine CJ Jr: Plication of the tunica albuginea to straighten the curved penis. Plast Reconstr Surg 52:32, 1973.

Horton CE, McCraw JB, Devine CJ Jr, Devine PC: Secondary reconstruction of the genital area. Urol Clin North Am 4:133, 1977.

Hudson CN, Setchell ME: Vaginal reconstruction using flaps and grafts. In Webster G, Kirby R, King L, Goldwasser B (eds): Reconstructive Urology. Boston, Blackwell Scientific Publications, 1993.

Huffman WC, Culp DA, Flocks RH: Injuries of the external male genitalia. In Converse JM (ed): Reconstructive and Plastic Surgery. Philadelphia, WB Saunders, 1964, chap 70.

Huffman WC, Culp DA, Greenleaf JS, et al: Injuries to the male genitalia. Plast Reconstr Surg 18:344, 1956.

Ingram JM: The bicycle seat stool in the treatment of vaginal agenesis and stenosis: A preliminary report. Am J Obstet Gynecol 140:867, 1981.

Johnson N, Lilford RJ, Batchelor A: The free flap vaginoplasty: A new surgical procedure for the treatment of vaginal agenesis. Br J Obstet Gynaecol 98:184, 1991.

Jones HW Jr, Garcia SC, Klingensmith GJ: Secondary surgical treatment of the masculinized external genitalia of patients with virilizing adrenal hyperplasia. Obstet Gynecol 48:73, 1976.

Jordan GH, McCraw JB: Tissue transfer techniques for genitourinary reconstruction: IV. Houston, American Urological Association, AUA Update Series, vol VII, lesson 12, p 90, 1988.

Juma S, Little NA, Raz S: Vaginal wall sling: Four years later. Urology 39:424, 1992.

Kogan SJ, Smey P, Leavitt S: Subtunical total reduction clitoroplasty: A safe modification of existing techniques. J Urol 130:746, 1983.

Kramer SA, Mesrobian HG, Kelalis PP: Long-term follow-up of cosmetic appearance and genital function in male epispadias: Review of 70 cases. J Urol 135:543, 1986.

Kreder KJ: Female urethral diverticulum and fistula. *In* Webster G, Kirby R, King L, Goldwasser B (eds): Reconstructive Urology. Boston, Blackwell Scientific Publications, 1993, p 861.

Lacey CG, Stern JL, Feigenbaum S, et al: Vaginal reconstruction after exenteration with use of gracilis myocutaneous flaps: The University of California San Francisco experience. Am J Obstet Gynecol 158:1278, 1988.

Larson DL: Musculocutaneous flaps. *In* Johnson DE, Boileau MA (eds): Genitourinary Tumors: Fundamental Principles and Surgical Techniques. New York, Grune & Stratton, 1982.

Lattimer JK: Relocation and recession of the enlarged clitoris with preservation of the glans: An alternative to amputation. J Urol 86:113, 1961.

Lattimer JK, MacFarlane MT: A urethral lengthening procedure for epispadias and exstrophy. J Urol 123:544, 1980.

Leach GE, Bavendan TG: Female urethral diverticulum. Urology 30:407, 1987.

Leach GE, Schmidbauer CP, Hadley HR, et al: Surgical treatment of female urethral diverticulum. Semin Urol 4:33, 1986.

Lesavoy MA: Vaginal reconstruction. Urol Clin North Am 12:369, 1985.

Livne PM, Gibbons MD, Gonzales ET Jr: Correction of disproportion of corpora cavernosa as cause of chordee in hypospadias. Urology 22:608, 1983.

Lockhart JL, Nazir CA: Proximal vaginal flap and needle suspension procedure in management of large urethral fistulas in females. Urology 27:24, 1986.

Maizels M, Zaontz M, Donovan J, et al: Surgical correction of the buried penis. J Urol 136:268, 1986.

McCraw J, Massey F, Shanklin K, Horton C: Vaginal reconstruction using gracilis myocutaneous flaps. Plast Reconstr Surg 58:176, 1970.

McCraw J, Myers B, Shanklin K: The value of fluorescein in predicting the viability of arterialized flaps. Plast Reconstr Surg 60:710, 1977.

McFarlane RM: The use of continuous suction under skin flaps. Br J Plast Surg 17:77, 1959.

McIndoe A: The treatment of congenital absence and obliterative conditions of the vagina. Br J Plast Surg 2:254, 1950.

Meyer R, Kesselring UK: One-stage reconstruction of the vagina with penile skin as an island flap in male transsexuals. Plast Reconstr Surg 66:401, 1980.

Michalowski E, Modelski W: The surgical treatment of epispadias. Surg Gynecol Obstet 117:465, 1963.

Mininberg DT: Phalloplasty in congenital adrenal hyperplasia. J Urol 128:355, 1982.

Mitchell ME, Hensle TW, Crooks KK: Urethral reconstruction in the young female using a perineal pedicle flap. J Pediatr Surg 17:687, 1982.

Moir JC: The Gauze-Hammock operation. J Obstet Gynaecol Br Commonw 75:1, 1968.

Mollard P, Juskiewenski S, Sarkissian J: Clitoroplasty in intersex: A new technique. Br J Urol 53:371, 1981.

Morley GW, de Lancey JOL: Full thickness skin graft vaginoplasty for treatment of the stenotic or foreshortened vagina. Obstet Gynecol 77:485, 1991.

O'Brien BM, Mellow CG, MacIsaac IA, et al: Treatment of vaginal agenesis with a new vulvovaginoplasty. Plast Reconstr Surg 85:942, 1990.

Oesterling JE, Gearhart JP, Jeffs RD: A unified approach to early reconstructive surgery of the child with ambiguous genitalia. J Urol 138:1079, 1987.

Parrott TS, Scheflan M, Hester TR: Reduction clitoroplasty and vaginal construction in a single operation. Urology 14:367, 1980.

Passerini-Glazel G: A new 1-stage procedure for clitorovaginoplasty in severely masculinized female pseudohermaphrodites. J Urol 142:565, 1989.

Pea A: Atlas of Surgical Management of Anorectal Malformations. New York, Springer-Verlag, 1990.

Pratt JH: Vaginal atresia corrected by use of small and large bowel. Clin Obstet Gynecol 15:639, 1972.

Radhakkrishnan J: Colon interposition vaginoplasty: A modification of the Wagner-Baldwin technique. J Pediatr Surg 22:1175, 1987.

Rajfer J, Ehrlich RM, Goodwin WE: Reduction clitoroplasty via ventral approach. J Urol 128:341, 1982.

Randolph JG, Hung W: Reduction clitoroplasty in females with hypertrophied clitoris. J Pediatr Surg 5:224, 1970.

Ransley PG: Epispadias repair. *In* Spitz L, Homewood NH (eds): Operative Surgery: Paediatric Surgery, 4th ed. London, Butterworths, 1988, p 624.

Sharp RJ, Holder TM, Howard CD, Grunt JA: Neonatal genital reconstruction. J Pediatr Surg 22:168, 1987.

Shaw A: Subcutaneous reduction clitoroplasty. J Pediatr Surg 112:331, 1977.

Sislow JG, Ireton RC, Ansell JS: Treatment of congenital penile curvature due to disparate corpora cavernosa by the Nesbit technique: A rule of thumb for the number of wedges required to achieve correction. J Urol 141:92, 1989.

Snyder HMcC III: Clitoroplasty: II. Dial Pediatr Urol 8:2, 1985.

Snyder HMcC III: Management of ambiguous genitalia in the neonate. *In* King LR (ed): Urologic Surgery in Neonates and Young Infants. Philadelphia, WB Saunders, 1988, p 346.

Snyder HMcC III, Retik AB, Bauer SB, Colodny AH: Feminizing genitoplasty: A synthesis. J Urol 129:1024, 1983.

Soderdahl DW, Brosman SA, Goodwin WE: Penile agenesis. J Urol 108:496, 1972.

Soper JT, Larson D, Hunter VJ, et al: Short gracilis myocutaneous flaps for vulvo-vaginal reconstruction after radical pelvic surgery. Obstet Gynecol 74:823, 1989.

Spence HM, Allen TD: Genital reconstruction in the female with the adrenogenital syndrome. Br J Urol 45:126, 1973.

Spence HM, Duckett JW Jr: Diverticulum of the female urethra: Clinical aspects and presentation of a simple operative technique for cure. J Urol 104:432, 1970.

Stefan H: Surgical reconstruction of the external genitalia in female pseudohermaphrodites. Br J Urol 39:347, 1967.

Symmonds RE, Hill M: Loss of the urethra: Report on 50 patients. Am J Obstet Gynecol 84:130, 1978.

Thomalla JV, Mitchell ME: Ventral preputial island flap technique for the repair of epispadias with or without exstrophy. J Urol 132:985, 1984.

Tobin GR, Day TG: Vaginal and pelvic reconstruction with distally based rectus abdominis myocutaneous flaps. Plast Reconstr Surg 81:62, 1988.

Turner UG, Edlich RF, Edgerton MT: Male transsexualism: A review of genital surgical reconstruction. Am J Obstet Gynecol 132:119, 1978.

Turner-Warwick R, Kirby RS: The construction and reconstruction of the vagina with the colocecum. Surg Gynecol Obstet 170:132, 1990.

Walsh PC, Wilson JD, Allen TD, et al: Clinical and endocrinological evaluation of patients with congenital microphallus. J Urol 120:90, 1978.

Wang Y, Hadley HR: The use of rotated vascularized pedicle flaps for complex transvaginal procedures. J Urol 149:590, 1993.

Webster GD, Shelnik SA, Stone AR: Urethrovaginal fistula: A review of the surgical management. J Urol 132:460, 1984.

Williams EA: Congenital absence of the vagina: A simple operation for its relief. J Obstet Gynaecol Br Commonw 71:511, 1964.

Wilson MC, Wilson CL, Thickstein JN: Transposition of the external genitalia. J Urol 94:600, 1965.

Woods JE, Alter G, Meland B, Podratz K: Experience with vaginal reconstruction utilizing the modified Singapore flap. Plast Reconstr Surg 90:270, 1992.

Young HH: Genital Abnormalities. Baltimore, Williams & Wilkins, 1937.

Audiovisuals

Kaplan GW, Strand WR: Posterior Sagittal Resection of Müllerian Duct Cysts. Wilkes-Barre, PA, Karol Media, 1995 (7 minutes). AUA #919-2060.

Leach GE (moderator): Management of Female Stress Incontinence. Wilkes-Barre, PA, Karol Media, 1992 (75 minutes). AUA #919-2065.

McCraw J, Nahai F, Mathes S, Arnold PG: Inferior Rectus Abdominis Flap. Norfolk, VA, Hampton Press, 1987 (44 minutes).

McCraw J, Nahai F, Mathes S, Arnold PG: Gracilis Muscle Flap. Norfolk, VA, Hampton Press, 1987 (31 minutes).

Peña A, Filmer RB: Transanorectal Repair of Urogenital Sinus. Wilkes-Barre, PA, Karol Media, 1991 (23 minutes). AUA #919-1171.

Raz S: Pelvic Reconstruction. Wilkes-Barre, PA, Karol Media, 1994 (37 minutes). AUA #919-2064.

URETHRA: RECONSTRUCTION

Angermeier KW, Jordan GH, Schlossberg SM: Complex urethral reconstruction. Urol Clin North Am 21:567, 1994.

Barbagli G, Selli C, Tosto A, Palminteri E: Dorsal free graft urethroplasty. J Urol 155:123, 1996.

Belman AB, King LR: Urinary tract abnormalities associated with imperforate anus. J Urol 108:823, 1972.

Blandy JP: Urethral stricture. Postgrad Med J 56:383, 1980.

Blandy JP, Singh M: The technique and results of one-stage island patch urethroplasty. Br J Urol 47:83, 1975.

Blandy JP, Tresidder GC: Meatoplasty. Br J Urol 39:633, 1967.

Brannan W, Ochsner M, Fuselier HA, Goodlet JS: Free full thickness skin graft urethroplasty for urethral stricture: Experience with 66 patients. J Urol 115:677, 1976.

Brannen GE: Meatal reconstruction. J Urol 116:319, 1976.

Breza J, Aboseif SR, Orvis BR, et al: Detailed anatomy of penile neurovascular structures: Surgical significance. J Urol 141:437, 1989.

Burbige KA: Transpubic-perineal urethral reconstruction in boys using a substitution graft. J Urol 148:1235, 1992.

Chilton CP: The urethra. In Webster G, Kirby R, King L, Goldwasser B (eds): Reconstructive Urology. Boston, Blackwell Scientific Publications, 1993.

Cohney BC: A penile flap procedure for the relief of meatal strictures. Br J Urol 35:182, 1963.

de la Rosette JJMCH, de Vries JDM, Lock MTWT, Debryne FMJ: Urethroplasty using the pedicled island flap technique in complicated urethral strictures. J Urol 146:40, 1991.

Dessanti A, Rigamonti W, Merulla V, et al: Autologous buccal mucosa graft for hypospadias repair: An initial report. J Urol 147:1081, 1992.

De Sy WA: Aesthetic repair of meatal stricture. J Urol 132:678, 1984.

De Sy WA, Oosterlinck W: Atlas of Reconstructive Urethral Surgery. Cadempino, Switzerland, Inpharzam Medical Publications, 1990.

De Sy WA, Oosterlinck W: Partial pubectomy: Technique and indications. Br J Urol 58:464, 1986.

De Sy WA, Verbaeys A, Roelandt R, Oosterlinck W: A simple approach to the entire urethra. Br J Urol 58:344, 1986.

Devine CJ Jr: Surgery of the urethra. In Walsh P, Gittes R, Perlmutter A, Stamey T (eds): Campbell's Urology, 5th ed. Philadelphia, WB Saunders, 1986, p 2853.

Devine PC, Devine CJ Jr, Horton CE: Anterior urethral injuries: Secondary reconstruction. Urol Clin North Am 4:157, 1977.

Devine PC, Horton CE, Devine CJ Jr, et al: Use of full thickness skin grafts in repair of urethral strictures. J Urol 90:67, 1963.

Devine PC, Sakati IA, Poutasse EF, Devine CJ Jr: One stage urethroplasty: Repair of urethral strictures with a free full thickness patch of skin. J Urol 99:191, 1968.

Devine PC, Wendelken JR, Devine CJ Jr: Free full thickness skin graft urethroplasty: Current technique. J Urol 121:282, 1979.

Dewan PA, Dinneen MD, Duffy PG, et al: Pedicle patch urethroplasty. Br J Urol 67:420, 1991.

Dhabuwala CB, Hamid S, Katsikas DM, Pierce JM: Impotence following delayed repair of prostatomembranous urethral disruption. J Urol 144:677, 1990.

Docimo SG, Gearhart JP, Jeffs RD: Ureteral graft in urological reconstruction: Clinical experience and review of the literature. J Urol 153:1648, 1995.

El-Kasaby AW, Fath-alla M, Noweir AM, et al: The use of buccal mucosa patch graft in the management of anterior urethral strictures. J Urol 149:276, 1993.

Finkelstein LH, Blatstein LM: Epilation of hair-bearing urethral grafts using the neodymium:YAG surgical laser. J Urol 146:840, 1991.

Gilbert DA, Jordan GH, Devine CJ Jr, Winslow BH: Microsurgical forearm "cricket bat–transformer" phalloplasty. Plast Reconstr Surg 90:711, 1992.

Johanson B: Reconstruction of the male urethra in strictures: Application of the buried intact epithelium technic. Acta Chir Scand 176(Suppl):3, 1953.

Jordan GH: Management of anterior urethral stricture disease. In Webster G, Kirby R, King L, Goldwasser B (eds): Reconstructive Urology. Boston, Blackwell Scientific Publications, 1993.

Jordan GH: Principles of plastic surgery. In Droller MJ (ed): Surgical Management of Urologic Disease: An Anatomic Approach. St. Louis, Mosby–Year Book, 1991, p 1218.

Jordan GH: Reconstruction for strictures of the fossa navicularis. In McAninch JW (ed): New Techniques in Reconstructive Urology. New York, Igaku-Shoin, 1996, p 3.

Jordan GH: Reconstruction of the fossa navicularis. J Urol 138:102, 1987.

Jordan GH: Reconstruction of the meatus/fossa navicularis using flap techniques. In Schreiter F (ed): Plastic Reconstructive Surgery in Urology. Stuttgart, Thieme (in preparation).

Jordan GH, Devine PC: Application of tissue transfer techniques to the management of urethral strictures. Semin Urol 5:228, 1987.

Jordan GH, Devine PC: Hairless scrotal island flap urethroplasty. J Urol 135:212A, 1986.

Jordan GH, McCraw JB: Tissue transfer techniques for genitourinary reconstructive surgery: I. Houston, American Urological Association. AUA Update Series, vol VII, lesson 9, p 66, 1988.

Jordan GH, Schelhammer PF: Urethral surgery and stricture disease. In Droller MJ (ed): Surgical Management of Urologic Disease: An Anatomic Approach. St. Louis, Mosby–Year Book, 1991, p 815.

Jordan GH, Secrest CL: Arteriography in select patients with posterior urethral distraction injuries. J Urol 147:289A, 1992.

Kirby RS: Reconstruction of the urethral meatus and fossa navicularis. In Webster G, Kirby R, King L, Goldwasser B (eds): Reconstructive Urology. Boston, Blackwell Scientific Publications, 1993.

Koyle MA, Ehrlich RM: The bladder mucosal graft for urethral reconstruction. J Urol 138:1093, 1987.

Leadbetter GW Jr, Leadbetter WF: Urethral strictures in male children. J Urol 87:409, 1962.

Lee YT, Lee JM: Delayed retropubic urethroplasty of completely transected female membranous urethra. Urology 22:499, 1988.

Lim PHC, Ching HC: Initial management of acute urethral injuries. Br J Urol 64:165, 1989.

MacDiarmid S, Rosario D, Chapple CR: The importance of accurate assessment and conservative management of the open bladder neck in patients with post-pelvic fracture membranous urethral distraction defects. Br J Urol 75:65, 1995.

Mark SD, Keane TE, Vandemark RM, Webster GD: Impotence following pelvic fracture urethral injury: Incidence, aetiology and management. Br J Urol 75:62, 1995.

McAninch JW: Management of genital skin loss. Urol Clin North Am 16:387, 1989.

McAninch JW: Pubectomy in repair of membranous urethral stricture. Urol Clin North Am 16:297, 1989.

McAninch JW: Reconstruction of extensive urethral strictures: Circular fasciocutaneous penile flap. J Urol 149:488, 1993.

McGowan AJ, Waterhouse K: Mobilization of the anterior urethra. Bull NY Acad Med 40:776, 1964.

McGuire EJ, Weiss RM: Scrotal flap urethroplasty for strictures of the deep urethra in infants and children. J Urol 110:599, 1973.

Moscona AR, Govrin-Yehudain J, Hirshowitz B: Closure of urethral fistulae by transverse Y-V advancement flap. Br J Urol 56:313, 1984.

Motiwala HG: Dartos flap: An aid to urethral construction. Br J Urol 72:260, 1993.

Mundy AR: The long-term results of skin inlay urethroplasty. Br J Urol 75:59, 1995.

Mundy AR: The role of delayed primary repair in the acute management of pelvic fracture injuries of the urethra. Br J Urol 68:273, 1991.

Mundy AR, Stephenson TP: Pedicled preputial patch urethroplasty. Br J Urol 61:48, 1988.

Netto NR Jr: Surgical repair of posterior urethral strictures by transpubic urethroplasty or pull-through technique. J Urol 133:411, 1985.

Orandi A: One-stage urethroplasty. Br J Urol 40:717, 1968.

Orandi A: One-stage urethroplasty: 4-year follow-up. J Urol 107:977, 1972.

Osegbe DN, Ntia I: One-stage urethroplasty for complicated urethral strictures using axial penile skin island flap. Eur Urol 17:79, 1990.

Patil UB, Ackerman NB, Waterhouse K: The transpubic approach in the management of problems of the lower genitourinary and intestinal tracts. Surg Gynecol Obstet 155:97, 1982.

Peirson EL: An easy method of removing large diverticula of the bladder. J Urol 43:686, 1940.

Peters CA, Hendren WH: Splitting the pubis for exposure in difficult reconstructions for incontinence. J Urol 142:527, 1989.

Pierce JM Jr: Exposure of the membranous and posterior urethra by total pubectomy. J Urol 88:256, 1962.

Presman D, Greenfield DL: Reconstruction of the perineal urethra with a free full-thickness skin graft from the prepuce. J Urol 69:677, 1953.

Pritchett TR, Shapiro RA, Hardy BE: Surgical management of traumatic posterior urethral strictures in children. Urology 42:59, 1993.

Quartey JKM: One-stage penile/preputial cutaneous island flap urethroplasty for urethral stricture: A preliminary report. J Urol 129:284, 1983.

Quartey JKM: One-stage penile/preputial island flap urethroplasty for urethral stricture. J Urol 134:474, 1985.

Rogers HS, McNicholas TA, Blandy JP: Long-term results of one-stage scrotal patch urethroplasty. Br J Urol 69:621, 1992.

Schreiter F: Mesh-graft-Urethroplastik. Aktuelle Urol 15:173, 1984.

Schreiter F, Noll F: Meshgraft urethroplasty using split thickness skin graft or foreskin. J Urol 142:1223, 1989.

Turner-Warwick R: The anatomical basis of functional reconstruction of the urethra. In Droller M (ed): Surgical Management of Urologic Disease: An Anatomic Approach. St. Louis, Mosby–Year Book, 1991, p 770.

Turner-Warwick R: Bulbar urethral reconstruction procedure. In Mundy AJ (ed): Operative Urology. London, Bailliere Tindall, 1988, p 160.

Turner-Warwick R: Complications of urethral surgery. In Smith RS, Ehrlich RM (eds): Complications of Urologic Surgery. London, WB Saunders, 1989, chap 34.

Turner-Warwick R: The functional anatomy of the urethra and its relation to the pelvic floor musculature. In Droller M (ed): Surgical Management of Urologic Disease: An Anatomic Approach. St. Louis, Mosby–Year Book, 1991, p 740.

Turner-Warwick R: Improving surgical access to retropubic space. Br J Urol 65:3078, 1990.

Turner-Warwick R: The management of traumatic urethral strictures and injuries. Br J Surg 60:775, 1973.

Turner-Warwick R: Observations upon techniques for reconstruction of the urethral meatus, the hypospadiac glans deformity and the penile urethra. Urol Clin North Am 6:643, 1979.

Turner-Warwick R: A personal view of the management of traumatic posterior urethral stricture. Urol Clin North Am 4:111, 1977.

Turner-Warwick R: Prevention of complications resulting from pelvic fracture urethral injuries and from their surgical management. Urol Clin North Am 16:335, 1989.

Turner-Warwick R: Principles of urethral reconstruction. In Webster G, Kirby R, King L, Goldwasser B (eds): Reconstructive Urology. Boston, Blackwell Scientific Publications, 1993.

Turner-Warwick R: Urethral stricture surgery. In Glenn JF (ed): Urologic Surgery, 4th ed. Philadelphia, JB Lippincott, 1991, chap 65.

Turner-Warwick R: Urethral stricture surgery. In Mundy AJ (ed): Current Operative Urology. London, Bailliere Tindall, 1988.

Turner-Warwick R: The use of pedicle grafts in repair of urinary fistulae. Br J Urol 44:644, 1972.

Turner-Warwick R, Kirby RS: Urodynamic studies and their effect upon management. In Chishold GD, Fair WR (eds): Scientific Foundations of Urology, 3rd ed. London, Heinemann, 1991.

Waterhouse K: The surgical repair of membranous urethral strictures in children. Trans Am Assoc Genitourin Surg 67:81, 1975.

Webster GD: Perineal repair of membranous urethral stricture. Urol Clin North Am 16:2, 1989.

Webster GD, Goldwasser B: Perineal transpubic repair: A technique for treating post-traumatic prostatomembranous urethral strictures. J Urol 135:278, 1986.

Webster GD, Koefoot RB, Sihelnik SA: Urethroplasty management in 100 cases of urethral stricture: A rationale for procedure selection. J Urol 134:892, 1985.

Webster GD, MacDiarmid SA: Posterior urethral reconstruction. In Webster G, Kirby R, King L, Goldwasser B (eds): Reconstructive Urology. Boston, Blackwell Scientific Publications, 1993.

Webster GD, Mathes G, Selli C: Prostatomembranous urethral injuries: A review of the literature and a rational approach to their management. J Urol 130:898, 1983.

Webster GD, Ramon J: Repair of pelvic fracture posterior urethral defects using an elaborated perineal approach: Experience with 74 cases. J Urol 145:535, 1991.

Webster GD, Ramon J, Kreder KJ: Salvage posterior urethroplasty after failed initial repair of pelvic fracture membranous urethral defects. J Urol 144:1370, 1990.

Webster GD, Robertson CN: The vascularized skin island urethroplasty: Its role and results in urethral stricture management. J Urol 133:31, 1985.

Webster GD, Sihelnik S: The management of strictures of the membranous urethra. J Urol 134:469, 1985.

Woodside JR: Urinary incontinence after urethral trauma in women. J Urol 138:527, 1987.

Yachia D: Pedicled scrotal skin advancement for one-stage anterior urethral reconstruction in circumcised patients. J Urol 139:1007, 1988.

Audiovisuals

Devine PC: Perineal Repair of Posterior Urethral Injury. Wilkes-Barre, PA, Karol Media, 1986 (25 minutes). AUA #919-1140.

Lee YT, Lee JM: Gracilis-myo-bladder-mucosa (Umbilical) Flap Neourethra: A New Technique of Urethral Reconstruction. Wilkes-Barre, PA, Karol Media, 1993 (23 minutes). AUA #919-2017.

Marshall FF, Chang R: Endoscopic Reconstruction of Traumatic Membranous Urethral Transection. Wilkes-Barre, PA, Karol Media, 1987 (8 minutes). AUA #919-1150.

Quartey JK: Modified Perineal Approach to Reconstruction of Membranous Urethra for Stricture. Wilkes-Barre, PA, Karol Media, 1986 (20 minutes). AUA #919-1138.

Quartey JK: One Stage Penile/Preputial Island Flap Urethroplasty for Urethral Strictures. Wilkes-Barre, PA, Karol Media, 1984 (21 minutes). AUA #919-1119.

Schlossberg SM, Jordan GH: Panurethral Reconstruction—Double Island Technique. Wilkes-Barre, PA, Karol Media, 1995 (15 minutes). AUA #919-2050.

Webster GD, Mark SD: Perineal Repair of Posterior Urethral

Distraction Defects Following Pelvic Fracture Urethral Injury. Wilkes-Barre, PA, Karol Media, 1993 (19 minutes). AUA #919-2014.

Winslow BH, McCraw JB, Burns CM, et al: Genitourinary Reconstructive Surgery. Wilkes-Barre, PA, Karol Media, 1982 (60 minutes). AUA #919-1122.

TESTIS: REPAIR AND RECONSTRUCTION

Aaberg RA, Vancaillie TG, Schuessler WW: Laparoscopic varicocele ligation: A new technique. Fertil Steril 56:776, 1991.

Abbassian A: A new surgical technique for testicular implantation. J Urol 107:618, 1972.

Aceland RD: Instrumentation for microsurgery. Orthop Clin North Am 8:281, 1977.

Action Committee on Surgery on the Genitalia of Male Children: The timing of elective surgery on the genitalia of male children with particular reference to undescended testes and hypospadias. Pediatrics 56:479, 1975.

Akgür FM, Kilin K, Aktug T, et al: The effect of allopurinol pretreatment before detorting testicular torsion. J Urol 151:1715, 1994.

Alfert HJ, Gillenwater JY: Ectopic vas deferens communicating with lower ureter: Embryological considerations. J Urol 108:172, 1972.

Backhouse KM: Embryology of the normal and cryptorchid testis. In Fonkelsrud EW, Mengel W (eds): The Undescended Testis. Chicago, Year Book Medical Publishers, 1981.

Backhouse KM: The gubernaculum testis Hunteri: Testicular descent and maldescent. Ann R Coll Surg 35:15, 1964.

Banwell PE, Hill ADK, Menzies-Gow N, et al: Laparoscopic management of cryptorchidism and associated inguinal hernia. Br J Urol 74:245, 1994.

Barbot DS, Gomella LG: Laparoscopic herniorrhaphy. In Gomella LG, Kozminski M, Winfield HN (eds): Laparoscopic Urologic Surgery. New York, Raven Press, 1994.

Beck EM, Schlegel PN, Goldstein M: Intraoperative varicocele anatomy: A macroscopic and microscopic study. J Urol 148:1190, 1992.

Bellinger MF, Abromowitz H, Brantley S, Marshall G: Orchiopexy: An experimental study of the effect of surgical technique on testicular histology. J Urol 142:553, 1989.

Belker AM: The failed vasovasostomy/vasoepididymostomy. In Cohen MS, Resnick MI (eds): Reoperative Urology. Boston, Little, Brown & Co, 1995, p 245.

Bianchi A: Microvascular orchidopexy for high undescended testes. Br J Urol 56:521, 1984.

Bloom DA: Two-step orchiopexy with pelviscopic clip ligation of the spermatic vessels. J Urol 145:1030, 1991.

Bloom DA, Guiney EJ, Ritchey ML: Normal and abnormal pelviscopic anatomy at the internal inguinal ring in boys and the vasal triangle. Urology 44:905, 1994.

Boddy S-AM, Gordon AC, Thomas DFM, et al: Experience with Fowler-Stephens and microvascular procedures in the management of the intraabdominal testis. J Urol 68:199, 1991.

Bogaert GA, Kogan BA, Mevorach RA: Therapeutic laparoscopy for intra-abdominal testes. Urology 42:182, 1993.

Borten M: Laparoscopic complications: Prevention and management. Philadelphia, BC Decker, 1986.

Bramwell RGB, Bullen C, Radford P: Caudal block for postoperative analgesia in children. Anaesthesia 37:1024, 1982.

Brock JW: Use of laparoscopy. In Cartwright PC (ed): Reoperative Orchiopexy. Dial Pediatr Urol 16(7):7, 1993.

Browne D: Diagnosis of undescended testicle. BMJ 2:168, 1938.

Browne D: Some anatomical points in the operation for undescended testicle. Lancet 1:460, 1933.

Bukowski TP, Wacksman J, Billmire DA, et al: Testicular autotransplantation: A 17-year review of an effective approach to the management of the intra-abdominal testis. J Urol 154:558, 1995.

Burton CC: A description of the boundaries of the inguinal rings and scrotal pouches. Surg Gynecol Obstet 104:142, 1957.

Burton CC: The embryologic development and descent of the testis in relation to congenital hernia. Surg Gynecol Obstet 107:294, 1958.

Cabot H, Nesbit RM: Undescended testis. Arch Surg 22:850, 1931.

Caldamone AA, Amaral JF: Laparoscopic stage 2 Fowler-Stephens orchiopexy. J Urol 152:1253, 1994.

Cartwright PC, Snow BW, Reid BS, et al: Color Doppler ultrasound in newborn testis torsion. Urology 45:667, 1995.

Cartwright PC, Velagapudi S, Snyder HM III, et al: A surgical approach to reoperative orchiopexy. J Urol 149:817, 1993.

Castanheira ACC, McAninch JW: Reconstruction for penile trauma. In Webster G, Kirby R, King L, Goldwasser B (eds): Reconstructive Urology. Boston, Blackwell Scientific Publications, 1993.

Cattolica EV, Karol JB, Rankin KN, Klein RS: High testicular salvage rate in torsion of the spermatic cord. J Urol 128:66, 1982.

Clatworthy HW Jr, Hollanbaugh RS, Grosfeld JL: The "long loop vas" orchiopexy for high undescended testis. Am Surg 38:69, 1972.

Coburn M, Wheeler T, Lipshultz LI: Testicular biopsy: Its use and limitations. Urol Clin North Am 14:551, 1987.

Cohen TD, Kay R, Knipper N: Reoperation for cryptorchid testis in prepubertal child. Urology 42:437, 1993.

Coolsaet BLRA: The varicocele syndrome: Venography determining the optimal level for surgical management. J Urol 124:833,1980.

Cooper BJ, Little TM: Orchidopexy: Theory and practice. BMJ 291:706, 1985.

Corbitt J: Laparoscopic herniorrhaphy. Surg Laparosc Endosc 1:23, 1991.

Corkery JJ: Staged orchiopexy: A new technique. J Pediatr Surg 10:515, 1975.

Cortes D, Thorup J, Frisch M, et al: Examination for intratubular germ cell neoplasia at operation for undescended testis in boys. J Urol 151:722, 1994.

Cortes D, Thorup J, Lenz K, et al: Laparoscopy in 100 consecutive patients with 128 impalpable testes. Br J Urol 75:281, 1995.

Cortesi N, Ferrari P, Zambarda E, et al: Diagnosis of bilateral abdominal cryptorchidism by laparoscopy. Endoscopy 8:33, 1976.

Cos LR, Valvo JR, Davis RS, Cockett ATK: Vasovasostomy: Current state of the art. Urology 22:56, 1983.

Dahl DS, Singh M, O'Conor VJ Jr, et al: Lord's operation for hydrocele compared with conventional techniques. Arch Surg 104:40, 1972.

Dajani AM: Transverse ectopia of the testis. Br J Urol 41:80, 1969.

Davenport M, Brain C, Vandenber C, et al: The use of the HCG stimulation test in the endocrine evaluation of cryptorchidism. Br J Urol 76:790, 1995.

Davits RJAM, Van Den Aker ESS, Scholtmeijer RJ, et al: Effect of parenteral testosterone therapy on penile development in boys with hypospadias. Br J Urol 71:593, 1993.

DeBoer A: Inguinal hernia in infants and children. Arch Surg 75:920, 1957.

Dewire DM, Thomas AJ Jr: Microsurgical end-to-side vasoepididymostomy. In Goldstein M (ed): Surgery of Male Infertility. Philadelphia, WB Saunders, 1995, p 128.

Diamond DA, Caldamone AA: The value of laparoscopy for 106 impalpable testes relative to clinical presentation. J Urol 148:632, 1992.

Docimo SG, Moore RG, Kavoussi LR: Laparoscopic orchidopexy in the prune belly syndrome: A case report and review of the literature. Urology 45:679, 1995.

Docimo SG, Moore RG, Adams J, Kavoussi LR: Laparoscopic orchiopexy for the high palpable undescended testis: Preliminary experience. J Urol 154:1513, 1995.

Donnell SC, Rickwood AMK, Lee LD, Jackson M: Congenital testicular maldescent: Significance of the complete hernial sac. Br J Urol 75:702, 1995.

Donovan JF Jr: Laparoscopic varix ligation. Urology 44:467, 1994.

Donovan JF Jr, Winfield HN: Laparoscopic varix ligation with the Nd:YAG laser. J Endourol 6:165, 1992.

Donovan JF Jr, Winfield HN: Laparoscopic varix ligation. *In* Gomella LG, Kozminski M, Winfield HN (eds): Laparoscopic Urologic Surgery. New York, Raven Press, 1994.

Dudai M, Sayfan J, Mesholam J, Sperber Y: Laparoscopic simultaneous ligation of internal and external spermatic veins for varicocele. J Urol 153:704, 1995.

Dwoskin JY, Kuhn JP: Herniograms in undescended testes and hydroceles. J Urol 109:520, 1973.

Editorial: Laparoscopic orchiopexy for the intra-abdominal testis. J Urol 152:1257, 1994.

Edmonds-Seal J, Paterson GM, Loach AB: Local nerve blocks for postoperative analgesia. J R Soc Med 73:111, 1980.

Elder JS: The failed orchiopexy. *In* Cohen MS, Resnick MI (eds): Reoperative Urology. Boston, Little, Brown & Co, 1995, p 251.

Elder JS: Laparoscopy and Fowler-Stephens orchiopexy in the management of the impalpable testis. Urol Clin North Am 16:399, 1989.

Elder JS: Laparoscopy for impalpable testes: Significance of the patent processus vaginalis. J Urol 152:776, 1994.

Elder JS: Two-stage Fowler-Stephens orchiopexy in the management of intra-abdominal testes. J Urol 148:1239, 1992.

Elder JS: The undescended testis: Hormonal and surgical management. Surg Clin North Am 68:983, 1988.

Elder JS, Keating MA, Duckett JW: Infant testicular prostheses. J Urol 141:1413, 1989.

Enquist E, Stein BS, Sigman M: Laparoscopic vs subinguinal varicocelectomy: A comparative study. Fertil Steril 61:1092, 1994.

Evans RM, Hulbert JC, Reddy PK: Complications in laparoscopy. Semin Urol 10:164, 1992.

Firor HV: Two-stage orchiopexy. Arch Surg 102:598, 1971.

Flinn RA, King LR: Experiences with the midline transabdominal approach in orchiopexy. Surg Gynecol Obstet 133:285, 1971.

Fogdestam I, Fall M, Nilsson S: Microsurgical epididymovasostomy in the treatment of occlusive azoospermia. Fertil Steril 46:925, 1986.

Fowler R, Stephens FD: The role of testicular vascular anatomy in the salvage of the high undescended testis. Aust NZ J Surg 29:92, 1959.

Fowler R, Stephens FD: The role of testicular vascular anatomy in the salvage of the high undescended testis. *In* Stephens FD (ed): Congenital Malformations of Rectum, Anus and Genitourinary Tract. Edinburgh, E & H Livingstone, 1963, p 306.

Fox M: Vasectomy reversal: Microsurgery for best results. Br J Urol 73:449, 1994.

Garibyan H, Hazebroek FWJ, Schulkes JAR, et al: Microvascular surgical orchiopexy in the treatment of high-lying undescended testes. Br J Urol 56:326, 1984.

Gaur DD, Agarwal DK, Purohit KC, Darshane AS: Laparoscopic orchiopexy for the intra-abdominal testis. J Urol 153:479, 1995.

Gearhart JB, Oesterman J, Jeffs RD: The use of parenteral testosterone therapy in genital reconstructive surgery. J Urol 138:1077, 1987.

Ger R: The laparoscopic management of groin hernias. Contemp Surg 39:15, 1991.

Ger R, Monroe K, Duvivier R, Mishrick A: Management of indirect inguinal hernias by laparoscopic closure of the neck of the sac. Am J Surg 159:370, 1990.

Goldberg LM, Skaist LB, Morrow JW: Congenital absence of testes: Anorchism and monorchism. J Urol 111:840, 1974.

Goldstein M: Hydrocelectomy. *In* Goldstein M (ed): Surgery of Male Infertility. Philadelphia, WB Saunders, 1995, p 199.

Goldstein M: Microsurgical vasoepididymostomy: End-to-end anastomosis. *In* Goldstein M (ed): Surgery of Male Infertility. Philadelphia, WB Saunders, 1995, p 120.

Goldstein M: Mini-incision microsurgical inguinal or subinguinal varicocelectomy with delivery of the testis. *In* Goldstein M (ed): Surgery of Male Infertility. Philadelphia, WB Saunders, 1995, p 173.

Goldstein M: Vasovasostomy: Surgical approach, decision making, and multilayer microdot technique. *In* Goldstein M (ed): Surgery of Male Infertility. Philadelphia, WB Saunders, 1995, p 46.

Goldstein M, Gilbert BR, Dicker AP, et al: Microsurgical inguinal varicocelectomy with delivery of the testis: An artery and lymphatic sparing technique. J Urol 148:1608, 1992.

Goluboff ET, Chang DT, Kirsch AJ, Fisch H: Incidence of external spermatic veins in patients undergoing inguinal varicocelectomy. Urology 44:893, 1994.

Gomella LG, Strup S, Young C, Barbot D: Laparoscopic pelvic lymphadenectomy combined with inguinal herniorrhaphy. Techn Urol 1:49, 1995.

Gomez RG, McAninch JW: Scrotal reconstruction using flaps and grafts. *In* Webster G, Kirby R, King L, Goldwasser B (eds): Reconstructive Urology. Boston, Blackwell Scientific Publications, 1993.

Gracia J, Gonzalez N, Gomez ME, et al: Clinical and anatomopathological study of 2000 cryptorchid testes. Br J Urol 75:697, 1995.

Grasso M, Lania C, Castelli M, Rigatti P: New technical expedient for epididymovasostomy. Br J Urol 73:207, 1994.

Gross RE: The Surgery of Infancy and Childhood: Its Principles and Techniques. Philadelphia, WB Saunders, 1953.

Gross RE, Jewett TC Jr: Surgical experiences from 1,222 operations for undescended testes. JAMA 160:634, 1956.

Guiney EJ, Corbally M, Malone PS: Laparoscopy and the management of the impalpable testis. Br J Urol 63:313, 1989.

Hadziselimovic F, Kogan SJ: Testicular development. *In* Gillenwater JY, Grayhack JT, Howards SS, Duckett JW (eds): Adult and Pediatric Urology. Chicago, Year Book Medical Publishers, 1987.

Hagood PG, Mehan DJ, Worischek JH, et al: Laparoscopic varicocelectomy: Preliminary report of a new technique. J Urol 147:73, 1992.

Harkins HN: Hernia. Philadelphia, JB Lippincott, 1964.

Harrison RG: The distribution of the vasal and cremasteric arteries to the testis and their functional importance. J Anat 83:267, 1949.

Harrison RG, McGregor GA: Anomalous origin and branching of the testicular arteries. Anat Rec 129:401, 1957.

Hart RR, Rushton HG, Belman AB: Intraoperative spermatic venography during varicocele surgery in adolescents. J Urol 148:1514, 1992.

Hass JA, Carrion HM, Sharkey J, Politano VA: Operative treatment of hydrocele: Another look at Lord's procedure. Urology 12:578, 1978.

Hazebroeck FWJ, Molenaar JC: The management of the impalpable testis by surgery alone. J Urol 148:629, 1993.

Hendry WF: Testicular obstruction: Causes, evaluation, and the results of surgery. *In* Webster G, Kirby R, King L, Goldwasser B (eds): Reconstructive Urology. Boston, Blackwell Scientific Publications, 1993.

Hill EC: The vascularisation of the human testis. Am J Anat 9:463, 1909.

Hinman F Jr: Alternatives to orchiopexy. J Urol 123:548, 1980.

Hinman F Jr: The case for primary orchiectomy for the unilateral abdominal testis. *In* Carlton CE Jr (ed): Controversies in Urology. Chicago, Year Book Medical Publishers, 1989, p 42.

Hinman F Jr: Indications and contraindications for orchiopexy and orchiectomy. *In* Fonkalsrud EW, Mengel W (eds): The Undescended Testis. Chicago, Year Book Medical Publishers, 1981.

Hinman F Jr: Indications and contraindications for orchiopexy. *In* Hadziselimovic F (ed): Cryptorchidism: Management and Implications. Berlin-Heidelberg, Springer-Verlag, 1983, p 99.

Hinman F Jr: Management of the intra-abdominal testis. Eur J Pediatr 146:549, 1987.

Hinman F Jr: Optimum time for orchiopexy in cryptorchidism. Fertil Steril 6:206, 1955.

Hinman F Jr: Survey: Localization and operation for non-palpable testes. Urology 30:193, 1987.

Hinman F Jr: Transmission of intra-abdominal pressure to the pampiniform plexus (in preparation).

Hinman F Jr: Unilateral abdominal cryptorchidism. J Urol 122:71, 1979.

Hunt JB, Witherington R, Smith AM: The midline preperitoneal approach to orchiopexy. Am Surg 47:184, 1981.

Hussman DA, Levy JB: Current concepts in the pathophysiology of testicular undescent. Urology 46:267, 1995.

Hutson JM, Beasley SW: Descent of the Testis. London, Edward Arnold, 1993.

Hutson JM, Williams MPL, Fallat ME, Attah A: Testicular descent: New insights into its hormonal control. Oxf Rev Reprod Biol 12:1, 1990.

Ivanissevich O: Left varicocele due to reflux: Experience with 4,470 operative cases in 42 years. J Int Coll Surg 34:742, 1918.

Ivanissevich O, Gregorini H: A new operation for the cure of varicocele. Semana Med 25:575, 1918.

Janecka IP, Romas NA: Microvascular free transfer of human testes. J Plast Reconstr Surg 63:42, 1979.

Jarow JP: Clinical significance of intratesticular arterial anatomy. J Urol 145:777, 1991.

Jarow JP: Intratesticular arterial anatomy. J Androl 11:255, 1990.

Jarow JP: Varicocele repair: Low ligation. Urology 44:470, 1994.

Jarow JP, Assimos DG, Pittaway DE: Effectiveness of laparoscopic varicocelectomy. Urology 42:544, 1993.

Jarow JP, Sigman M, Buch JP, Oates RD: Delayed appearance of sperm after end-to-side vasoepididymostomy. J Urol 153:1156, 1995.

Jasper WS: Combined open prostatectomy and herniorrhaphy. J Urol 111:370, 1974.

Jirásek JE: The relationship between differentiation of the testicle, genital ducts and external genitalia in fetal and postnatal life. In Rosenberg E, Paulsen AC (eds): The Human Testis. New York, Plenum Press, 1970.

Jones PF: Approaches to orchidopexy. Br J Urol 75:693, 1995.

Jordan GH, Winslow BH: Laparoscopic single stage and staged orchiopexy. J Urol 152:1249, 1994.

Jordan GH, Robey EL, Winslow BH: Laparoendoscopic surgical management of the abdominal/transinguinal undescended testicle. J Endourol 6:157, 1992.

Juskiewenski S, Vaysse PH: Arterial vascularisation of the testes and surgery for undescended testicles (testicular ectopia). Anat Clin 1:127, 1979.

Kass EJ, Belman AB: Reversal of testicular growth failure by varicocele ligation. J Urol 137:475, 1987.

Kass EJ, Chandra RS, Belman AB: Testicular histology in the adolescent with a varicocele. Pediatrics 79:996, 1987.

Kass EJ, Freitas JE, Bour JB: Pituitary-gonadal function in adolescents with a varicocele. J Urol 139:207, 1988.

Kaye KW, Lange PH, Fraley EE: Spermatic cord block in urologic surgery. J Urol 128:720, 1982.

Kelalis PP, King LR, Belman AB (eds): Clinical Pediatric Urology, 2nd ed. Philadelphia, WB Saunders, 1985.

Khamesra HL, Gupta AS, Malpani NK: Transverse testicular ectopia. Br J Urol 50:283, 1978.

Khan AB, Conn IG: Use of EMLA during local anaesthetic vasectomy. Br J Urol 75:761, 1995.

King LM, Sekaran SK, Sauer D, et al: Untwisting in delayed treatment of torsion of the spermatic cord. J Urol 112:217, 1974.

Kogan SJ, Houman BZ, Reda EF, Levitt SB: Orchiopexy of the high undescended testis by division of the spermatic vessels: A critical review of 38 selected transections. J Urol 141:1416, 1989.

Kursh ED, Persky L: Preperitoneal herniorrhaphy: Adjunct to prostatic surgery. Urology 5:322, 1975.

La Roque GP: The permanent cure of inguinal and femoral hernia. Surg Gynecol Obstet 29:507, 1919.

Lattimer JK, Vakili BF, Smith AM, et al: A natural-feeling testicular prosthesis. J Urol 110:81, 1973.

Lawson AL, Gornall P, Brick RG, et al: Impalpable testis: Testicular vessel division in treatment. Br J Surg 78:1111, 1991.

Lee PA, O'Leary LA, Songer NJ, et al: Paternity after cryptorchidism: Lack of correlation with age at orchiopexy. Br J Urol 75:704, 1995.

Lemoh CN: A study of the development and structural relationships of the testis and gubernaculum. Surg Gynecol Obstet 110:164, 1960.

Levitt SB, Kogan SJ, Engel RM, et al: The impalpable testis: A rational approach to management. J Urol 120:515, 1978.

Lewis EL: The Ivanissevich operation. J Urol 63:165, 1950.

Li SQ, Goldstein M, Zhu J, Huber D: The no-scalpel vasectomy. J Urol 145:341, 1991.

Livne PM, Savir A, Servadio C: Re-orchiopexy: Advantages and disadvantages. Eur Urol 18:137, 1990.

Lord PH: A bloodless operation for the radical cure of idiopathic hydrocele. Br J Surg 51:914, 1964.

Loughlin KR, Brooks DC: The use of a Doppler probe to facilitate laparoscopic varicocele ligation. Surg Gynecol Obstet 174:326, 1992.

Lynch WJ, Badenoch DF, McAnena OJ: Comparison of laparoscopic and open ligation of the testicular vein. Br J Urol 72:796, 1993.

Lyon RP: Torsion of the testicle in childhood: A painless emergency requiring contralateral orchiopexy. JAMA 178:702, 1961.

MacMahon RA, O'Brien BM, Cussen LJ: The use of microsurgery in the treatment of the undescended testis. J Pediatr Surg 11:52, 1976.

MacMillan EW: The blood supply of the epididymis in man. Br J Urol 26:60, 1954.

Maizels M, Gomez F, Firlit CF: Surgical correction of the failed orchiopexy. J Urol 130:955, 1983.

Markham SJ, Tomlinson J, Hain WR: Ilioinguinal nerve block in children: A comparison with caudal block for intra- and postoperative analgesia. Anaesthesia 41:1098, 1986.

Marmar JL, DeBenedictis TJ, Praiss D: The management of varicoceles by microdissection of the spermatic cord at the external inguinal ring. Fertil Steril 43:583, 1985.

Marmar JL, Kim Y: Subinguinal microsurgical varicocelectomy: A technical critique and statistical analysis of semen and pregnancy data. J Urol 152:1127, 1994.

Marmar JL, Kim Y: Varicocelectomy: Subinguinal approach. In Goldstein M (ed): Surgery of Male Infertility. Philadelphia, WB Saunders, 1995, p 178.

Marshall FF, Shermeta DW: Epididymal abnormalities associated with undescended testis. J Urol 121:341, 1979.

Martin DC, Menck HR: The undescended testis: Management after puberty. J Urol 114:77, 1975.

Matsuda T, Horii Y, Higashi S, et al: Laparoscopic varicocelectomy: A simple technique for clip ligation of the spermatic vessels. J Urol 147:636, 1992.

Matthews GJ, Schlegel PN, Goldstein M: Patency following microsurgical vasoepididymostomy and vasovasostomy: Temporal considerations. J Urol 154:2070, 1995.

McVay CB: The anatomic basis for inguinal and femoral hernioplasty. Surg Gynecol Obstet 139:931, 1974.

Middleton RG, Henderson D: Vas deferens reanastomosis without splints and without magnification. J Urol 119:763, 1978.

Moore RG, Peters CA, Bauer SB, et al: Laparoscopic evaluation of the nonpalpable testis: A prospective assessment of accuracy. J Urol 151:728, 1994.

Morse TS, Hollebaugh RS: The window orchiopexy for prevention of testicular torsion. J Pediatr Surg 12:237, 1977.

Moul JW, Belman AB: A review of surgical treatment of undescended testis with emphasis on anatomical position. J Urol 140:382, 1988.

Murnaghan GF: The appendages of the testis and epididymis: A short review with case reports. Br J Urol 31:190, 1959.

Nadelson EJ, Cohen M, Warner R, Leiter E: Update: Varicocelectomy—a safe outpatient procedure. Urology 14:259, 1984.

Neiderberger C, Ross LS: Microsurgical epididymovasostomy predictors of success. J Urol 149:1364, 1993.

Nguyen DH, Mitchell ME: Ureteral obstruction due to compression by the vas deferens following Fowler-Stephens orchiopexy. J Urol 149:94, 1993.

Nitapathpongporn A, Huber DH, Kreeger JN: No scalpel vasectomy at the King's birthday vasectomy celebration. Lancet 335:894, 1990.

Nunn LN, Stephens FD: The triad syndrome: A composite anomaly of the abdominal wall, urinary system, and testis. J Urol 86:782, 1961.

Nyhus LM: An anatomic reappraisal of the posterior inguinal wall. Surg Clin North Am 44:1305, 1964.

Nyhus LM: The preperitoneal approach and iliopubic tract repair on inguinal hernia. In Nyhus LM, Condon RE (eds): Hernia, 2nd ed. Philadelphia, JB Lippincott, 1978, p 212.

Nyhus LM, Condon RE, Harkins HN: Clinical experiences with preperitoneal hernial repair for all types of hernia of the groin. Am J Surg 100:234, 1960.

O'Brien BM, Rao VK, MacLeod AM, et al: Microvascular testicular transfer. Plast Reconstr Surg 71:87, 1983.

Odiase V, Whitaker RH: Analysis of cord length obtained during steps of orchiopexy. Br J Urol 54:308, 1982.

Ombredanne L: Sur l'orchiopexie. Bull Soc Pediatr 25:473, 1927.

Ottenheimer EJ: Testicular fixation in torsion of the spermatic cord. JAMA 101:116, 1933.

Palomo A: Radical cure of varicocele by a new technique: Preliminary report. J Urol 61:604, 1949.

Parkash S, Ramakrishnan K, Bagdi RK: Orchiopexy: Trans-septal ipsilateral positioning. Br J Urol 55:79, 1982.

Parker RM, Robison JR: Anatomy and diagnosis of torsion of the testicle. J Urol 106:243, 1971.

Parrott TS, Hewatt L: Ligation of the testicular artery and vein in adolescent varicocele. J Urol 152:791, 1994.

Pascual JA, Villanueva-Meyer J, Salido E, et al: Recovery of testicular blood flow following ligation of the testicular vessels. J Urol 142:549, 1989.

Perovic S, Janic N: Laparoscopy in the diagnosis of non-palpable testes. Br J Urol 73:310, 1994.

Persky L, Albert DJ: Staged orchiopexy. Surg Gynecol Obstet 132:43, 1971.

Petrivalsky J: Zur Behandlung des Leistenhodens. Zentralbl Chir 58:1001, 1931.

Pinsolle J, Drouillard J, Bruneton JN, Grenier FN: Anatomical bases of testicular vein catheterization and phlebography. Anat Clin 2:191, 1980.

Plottzker ED, Rushton HG, Belman AN, Skoog SJ: Laparoscopy for nonpalpable testes in childhood: Is inguinal exploration also necessary when the vas and vessels exit the external ring? J Urol 148:635, 1992.

Poenaru D, Homsy YL, Péloquin F, Andze GO: Laparoscopic management of the impalpable abdominal testis. Urology 42:574, 1993.

Popp L: Improvement on endoscopic hernioplasty: Transcutaneous aquadissection of the musculofascial defect and preperitoneal endoscopic patch repair. J Laparoendosc Surg 1:83, 1991.

Poppas DP, Schlegel PN, Sosa RE: Varicocelectomy: The laparoscopic approach. In Goldstein M (ed): Surgery of Male Infertility. Philadelphia, WB Saunders, 1995, p 185.

Prentiss RJ, Boatwright DC, Pennington RD, et al: Testicular prosthesis: Materials, methods and results. J Urol 90:208, 1963.

Prentiss RJ, Weickgenant CJ, Moses JJ, Frazier DB: Undescended testis: Surgical anatomy of spermatic vessels, spermatic surgical triangles and lateral spermatic ligament. J Urol 83:686, 1960.

Rajfer J, Binder S: Use of Biopty gun for transcutaneous testis needle biopsies. J Urol 142:1021, 1989.

Rajfer J, Pickett S, Klein SR: Laparoscopic occlusion of testicular veins for clinical varicocele. Urology 40:113, 1992.

Ralph DJ, Timoney AG, Parker C, Pryor JP: Laparoscopic varicocele ligation. Br J Urol 72:230, 1993.

Ransley PG, Vordermark JS, Caldamone AA, et al: Preliminary ligation of the gonadal vessels prior to orchiopexy for the intra-abdominal testicle: A staged Fowler-Stephens procedure. World J Urol 2:266, 1984.

Redman JF Barthold JS: A technique for atraumatic scrotal pouch orchiopexy in the management of testicular torsion. J Urol 154:1511, 1995.

Redman JF: Simplified technique for scrotal pouch orchiopexy. Urol Clin North Am 17:9, 1990.

Redman JF: The secondary internal ring: Applications to surgery of the inguinal canal. J Urol 155:170, 1996.

Ritchey ML, Bloom DA: Modified dartos pouch orchiopexy. Urology 45:136, 1995.

Rolnick D, Kawanoue S, Szanto P, et al: Anatomical incidence of testicular appendages. J Urol 100:755, 1968.

Salerno G, Fitzgibbons R Jr, Filipi C: Laparoscopic inguinal hernia repair. In Zucker K (ed): Surgical Laparoscopy. St. Louis, Quality Medical Publishing, 1991, p 281.

Schlegel PN, Goldstein M: Anatomical approach to varicocelectomy. Semin Urol 10:242, 1992.

Schlegel PN, Goldstein M: Microsurgical vasoepididymostomy: Refinements and results. J Urol 150:1165, 1993.

Schlegel PN, Goldstein M: Vasectomy. In Goldstein M (ed): Surgery of Male Infertility. Philadelphia, WB Saunders, 1995, p 35.

Schmidt SS: Prevention of failure in vasectomy. J Urol 109:296, 1973.

Schultz L, Graber J, Pietrafitta J, Hickok D: Laser laparoscopic herniorrhaphy: A clinical trial, preliminary results. J Laparosc Surg 1:41, 1990.

Scorer CG: The descent of the testis. Arch Dis Child 39:605, 1964.

Scorer CG, Farrington GH: Congenital Deformities of the Testis and Epididymis. London, Butterworth & Co, 1971.

Semm K: Operative Manual for Endoscopic Abdominal Surgery. Friedrich ER (trans). Chicago, Year Book Medical Publishers, 1987.

Shafik A: Obturator foramen approach: II. A new surgical approach for management of the short-pedicled undescended testis. Am J Surg 144:381, 1982.

Shafik A, Moftah A, Olfat S, et al: Testicular veins: Anatomy and role in varicocelogenesis and other pathologic conditions. Urology 35:175, 1990.

Sharlip ID: Microsurgical vasovasostomy: Modified one-layer technique. In Goldstein M (ed): Surgery of Male Infertility. Philadelphia, WB Saunders, 1995, p 67.

Sharlip ID: Surgery of scrotal contents. Urol Clin North Am 14:145, 1987.

Shenfeld O, Eldar I, Lotan G, et al: Intraoperative irrigation with bupivacaine for analgesia after orchiopexy and herniorrhaphy in children. J Urol 153:185, 1995.

Shokeir AA, Ghoneim MA: Further experience with the modified ileal ureter. J Urol 154:45, 1995.

Silber SJ: Microscopic vasectomy reversal. Fertil Steril 28:1191, 1977.

Silber SJ: Microsurgery for vasectomy reversal and vasoepididymostomy. Urology 5:505, 1984.

Silber SJ: Techniques for the resolution of testicular obstruction. In Webster G, Kirby R, King L, Goldwasser B (eds): Reconstructive Urology. Boston, Blackwell Scientific Publications, 1993.

Silber SJ, Kelly J: Successful autotransplantation of an intra-abdominal testis to the scrotum by microvascular technique. J Urol 115:452, 1976.

Skandalakis JE: Hernia: Surgical Anatomy and Technique. New York, McGraw-Hill, 1989.

Snyder WH Jr: Inguinal hernia complicated by descended testis. Am J Surg 94:325, 1955.

Solomon AA: The extrusion operation for hydrocele. NY State J Med 55:1885, 1955.

Solomon AA: Testicular prosthesis: A new insertion operation. J Urol 108:436, 1972.

Spaw AT, Ennis BN, Spaw LP: Laparoscopic hernia repair: The anatomic basis. J Laparoendosc Surg 1:269, 1991.

Steinhardt GF, Kroovand RL, Perlmutter AD: Orchiopexy: Planned 2-stage technique. J Urol 133:434, 1985.

Stephens FD (guest ed): Embryopathy of malformations. J Urol 127:13, 1982.

Stockton MD, Davis LE, Bolton KM: No-scalpel vasectomy: A technique for family physicians. Am Fam Physician 46:1153, 1992.

Stone KT, Kass EJ, Cacciarelli AA, Gibson DP: Management of suspected antenatal torsion: What is the best strategy? J Urol 153:782, 1995.

Tan SM, Ng FC, Ravintharan T, et al: Laparoscopic varicocelectomy: Technique and results. Br J Urol 75:523, 1995.

Tennenbaum SY, Lerner SE, McAleer IM, et al: Preoperative laparoscopic localization of the nonpalpable testis: A critical analysis of a 10-year experience. J Urol 151:732, 1994.

Toy F, Smoot R: Toy-Smoot laparoscopic hernioplasty. Surg Laparosc Endosc 1:151, 1991.

Turek PJ, Ewalt DH, Snyder HM III, et al: The absent cryptorchid testis: Surgical findings and their implications for diagnosis and etiology. J Urol 151:718, 1994.

Urquhart-Hay D: A low power magnification technique for re-anastomosis of the vas. Br J Urol 53:446, 1981.

Vergnes P, Midy D, Bondonny JM, Cabanie H: Anatomical basis of inguinal surgery in children. Anat Clin 7:257, 1985.

Viidik T, Marshall DG: Direct inguinal hernias in infancy and early childhood. J Pediatr Surg 15:646, 1980.

Wacksman J, Dinner M, Straffon R: Technique of testicular auto-transplantation using microvascular anastomosis. Surg Gynecol Obstet 150:399, 1980.

Waldron R, James M, Clain A: Technique and results of transscrotal operations for hydrocele and scrotal cysts. Br J Urol 58:303, 1986.

Weiss RM, Seashore JH: Laparoscopy in the management of the nonpalpable testis. J Urol 138:382, 1987.

Weissbach L: Alloplastic testicular prostheses. In Wagenknecht LV, Furlow WL, Auvert J (eds): Genitourinary Reconstruction with Prostheses. Stuttgart, Georg Thieme, 1981, p 173.

Winfield HN, Donovan JF, See WA, et al: Urological laparoscopic surgery. J Urol 146:941, 1991.

Woodard JR: Prune-belly syndrome. In Kelalis PP, King LR, Belman AB (eds): Clinical Pediatric Urology. Philadelphia, WB Saunders, 1985, p 805.

Woodard JR, Parrot TS: Orchiopexy in the prune-belly syndrome. Br J Surg 50:348, 1978.

Youngson GG, Jones PF: Management of the impalpable testis: Long-term results of the preperitoneal approach. J Pediatr Surg 26:618, 1991.

Zer M, Wolloch Y, Dintsman M: Staged orchiorrhaphy: Therapeutic procedure in cryptorchic testicle with a short spermatic cord. Arch Surg 110:387, 1975.

Audiovisuals

Donovan JE Jr, Winfield HN: Laparoscopic Varix Ligation. Wilkes-Barre, PA, Karol Media, 1991 (13 minutes). AUA #919-1135.

Schichman SJ, Sosa RE, Poppas D, Mininberg D: Laparoscopic Orchiopexy. Wilkes-Barre, PA, Karol Media, 1993 (9 minutes). AUA #919-2016.

Silber SJ: Microsurgery for Male Sterility. Wilkes-Barre, PA, Karol Media, 1985 (19 minutes). AUA #919-1135

Woodard JR (moderator): Pediatric Urology: Cryptorchidism. Wilkes-Barre, PA, Karol Media, 1990 (59 minutes). AUA #919-2071.

TESTIS: EXCISION

Bahnson RS, Slasky BS, Ernstoff MS, et al: Sonographic characteristics of epidermoid cysts of the testicle. Urology 35:508, 1990.

Baniel J, Foster RS, Donohue JP: Surgical anatomy of the lumbar vessels: Implications for retroperitoneal surgery. J Urol 153:1422, 1995.

Baniel J, Foster RS, Rowland RG, et al: Complications of post-chemotherapy retroperitoneal lymph node dissection. J Urol 153:976, 1995.

Baniel J, Foster RS, Rowland RG, et al: Complications of primary retroperitoneal lymph node dissection. J Urol 152:424, 1994.

Bihrle R, Donohue JP, Foster RS: Complications of retroperitoneal lymph node dissection. Urol Clin North Am 15:237, 1988.

Capelouto CC, Clark PE, Ransil BJ, Loughlin KR: A review of scrotal violation in testicular cancer: Is adjuvant local therapy necessary? J Urol 153:981, 1995.

Colleselli K, Poisel S, Schachtner W, et al: Nerve preserving bilateral retroperitoneal lymphadenectomy: An anatomical study and operative approach. J Urol 144:293, 1990.

Cooper JF, Leadbetter WF, Chute R: The thoracoabdominal approach for retroperitoneal gland dissection: Its application to testis tumors. Surg Gynecol Obstet 90:496, 1950.

Doerr A, Skinner EC, Skinner DG: Preservation of ejaculation through a modified retroperitoneal lymph node dissection in low stage testis cancer. J Urol 149:1472, 1993.

Donohue JP: Metastatic pathways of nonseminomatous germ cell tumors. Semin Urol 2:1, 1984.

Donohue JP: Nerve sparing retroperitoneal lymph node dissection for testis cancer: Evolution of surgical templates for low-stage disease. Eur Urol 23(Suppl 2):44, 1993.

Donohue JP: Retroperitoneal lymphadenectomy: The anterior approach including bilateral suprarenal-hilar dissection. Urol Clin North Am 4:509, 1977.

Donohue JP, Foster RS, Geirer G, et al: Preservation of ejaculation following nerve-sparing retroperitoneal lymphadenectomy. J Urol 139:206A, 1988.

Donohue JP, Foster RS, Rowland RG, et al: Nerve-sparing retroperitoneal lymphadenectomy with the preservation of ejaculation. J Urol 144:287, 1990.

Donohue JP, Rowland RG, Einhorn LH, et al: Cytoreductive surgery for metastatic testis cancer. J Urol 127:111, 1982.

Donohue JP, Thornhill JA, Foster RS, et al: Primary retroperitoneal lymph node dissection in clinical stage A non-seminomatous germ cell testis cancer: Review of the Indiana University experience 1965–1989. Br J Urol 71:326, 1993.

Donohue JP, Thornhill JA, Foster RS, et al: Retroperitoneal lymphadenectomy for clinical Stage A testis cancer (1965 to 1989): Modifications of technique and impact on ejaculation. J Urol 149:237, 1993.

Donohue JP, Zachary JM, Maynard BR: Distribution of nodal metastases in nonseminomatous testis cancer. J Urol 128:315, 1982.

Eisenmenger M, Lang S, Donner G, et al: Epidermoid cysts of the testis: Organ-preserving surgery following diagnosis by ultrasonography. Br J Urol 72:955, 1993.

Foster RS, Donohue JP: Nerve-sparing retroperitoneal lymphadenectomy. Urol Clin North Am 20:117, 1993.

Foster RS, Donohue JP, Bihrle R: Stage A nonseminomatous testis carcinoma: Rationale and results of nerve-sparing retroperitoneal lymphadenectomy. Urol Int 46:294, 1991.

Fraley EE, Lange PH: Technical nuances of extended retroperitoneal dissection for low stage nonseminomatous testicular germ cell cancer. World J Urol 2:43, 1984.

Fuse H, Shimazaki J, Katayama T: Ultrasonography of testicular tumors. Eur Urol 17:273, 1990.

Gaur DD: Laparoscopic operative retroperitoneoscopy: Use of a new device. J Urol 148:1137, 1992.

Gerber GS, Bissada NK, Hulbert JC, et al: Laparoscopic retroperitoneal lymphadenectomy: Multi-institutional analysis. J Urol 152:1188, 1994.

Giwercman A, von der Maase H, Berthelsen JG, et al: Localized irradiation of testes with carcinoma in situ: Effects on Leydig cell function and eradication of malignant germ cells in 20 patients. J Clin Endocrinol Metab 73:596, 1991.

Glenn JF: Subepididymal orchiectomy: The acceptable alternative. J Urol 144:942, 1990.

Gottesman JE: Radical inguinal orchiectomy. In Crawford ED, Das S (eds): Current Genitourinary Cancer Surgery. Philadelphia, Lea & Febiger, 1990, p 319.

Heidenreich A, Bonfig R, Derschum W, et al: A conservative approach to bilateral testicular germ cell tumors. J Urol 153:10, 1995.

Heidenreich A, Engelmann UH, Vietsch HV, Derschum W: Organ preserving surgery in testicular epidermoid cysts. J Urol 153:1147, 1995.

Hulbert JC, Fraley EE: Laparoscopic retroperitoneal lymphadenectomy: New approach to pathologic staging of clinical stage I germ cell tumors of the testis. J Endourol 6:123, 1992.

Janetschek G, Reissigl A, Peschel R, et al: Laparoscopic retroperitoneal lymph node dissection for clinical stage 1 nonseminomatous testicular tumor. Urology 44:382, 1994.

Lange PH, Brawer MK: Anterior transabdominal approach for radical retroperitoneal lymphadenectomy: Anatomy and nerve sparing technique. In Crawford ED, Das S (eds): Current Genitourinary Cancer Surgery. Philadelphia, Lea & Febiger, 1990, p 346.

Lange PH, Lightner DJ, Fraley EE: Surveillance vs. early lymphadenectomy for patients with stage 1 nonseminomatous germ cell testicular tumors. Adv Urol 2:41, 1989.

Leibovitch I, Rowland RG, Goldwasser B, Donohue JP: Incidental appendectomy during urological surgery. J Urol 154:1110, 1995.

Lerner SP: Testis cancer progress in risk assessment for occult retroperitoneal lymph node metastases. J Urol 155:593, 1996. Editorial.

McDougall EM, Clayman RV, Anderson K, et al: Laparoscopic gonadectomy in a case of testicular feminization. Urology 42:201, 1993.

Morey AF, Plymyer M, Rozanski TA, et al: Biopty gun testis needle biopsy: A preliminary clinical experience. Br J Urol 74:366, 1994.

Ray B, Hadju SI, Whitmore WF Jr: Distribution of retroperitoneal lymph node metastases in testicular germinal tumors. Cancer 33:340, 1974.

Recker F, Tscholl R: Monitoring of emission as direct intraoperative control for nerve sparing retroperitoneal lymphadenectomy. J Urol 150:1360, 1993.

Richie JP: Clinical stage 1 testicular cancer: The role of modified retroperitoneal lymphadenectomy. J Urol 144:1160, 1990.

Rozanski TA, Wojno KJ, Bloom DA: The remnant orchiectomy. J Urol 155:712, 1996.

Rukstalis DB, Chodak GW: Laparoscopic retroperitoneal lymph node dissection in a patient with stage 1 testicular carcinoma. J Urol 148:1907, 1992.

Saxman SB, Nichols CR, Foster RS, et al: The management of patients with clinical stage 1 nonseminomatous testicular tumors and persistently elevated serologic markers. J Urol 155:587, 1996.

Scardino PT: Thoracoabdominal retroperitoneal lymphadenectomy for testicular carcinoma. In Crawford ED, Borden TA (eds): Genitourinary Cancer Surgery. Philadelphia, Lea & Febiger, 1982, p 27.

Schlecker BA, Siegel A, Weiss J, Wein A: Epidermoid cyst of the testes: A surgical approach for testicular preservation. J Urol 133:610, 1985.

Shapeero LG, Vordermark JS: Epidermoid cysts of testes and role of sonography. Urology 41:75, 1993.

Skinner DG: Considerations for management of large retroperitoneal tumors: Use of the modified thoracoabdominal approach. Urology 117:605, 1977.

Skinner DG: Non-seminomatous testis tumors: A plan of management based on 96 patients. J Urol 115:65, 1976.

Stone NN: Retroperitoneal laparoscopic surgery: Ureterolithotomy and retroperitoneal lymph node dissection. In Gomella LG, Kozminski M, Winfield HN (eds): Laparoscopic Urologic Surgery. New York, Raven Press, 1994.

Stone NN, Schluessel RN, Waterhouse RL, Unger P: Laparoscopic retroperitoneal lymph node dissection in stage A nonseminomatous testis cancer. Urology 42:610, 1993.

Wakefield SE, Elewa AA: Spermatic cord block: A safe technique for intrascrotal surgery. Ann R Coll Surg Engl 76:401, 1994.

Waterhouse RL, Stone NN, Schluessel RN: Laparoscopic retroperitoneal lymph node dissection for testicular cancer. J Urol 147:194A, 1992.

Wise PG, Scardino PT: Thoracoabdominal retroperitoneal lymphadenectomy. In Crawford ED, Das S (eds): Current Genitourinary Cancer Surgery. Philadelphia, Lea & Febiger, 1990, p 328.

Audiovisual

Skinner DG: The Thoracoabdominal Approach for Management of Nonseminomatous Germ Cell Tumors of the Testis. Wilkes-Barre, PA, Karol Media, 1986 (29 minutes). AUA #919-1144.

PROSTATE: EXCISION

Albert PS, Raboy A: Extraperitoneal endoscopic "gas-less" pelvic lymph node dissection. Curr Surg Techn Urol 7(5):1, 1994.

Angermeier KW, Jordan GH: Complications of the exaggerated lithotomy position: A review of 177 cases. J Urol 151:866, 1994.

Arai Y, Ishitoya S, Okuba K, et al: Mini-laparotomy staging pelvic lymph node dissection for localized prostate cancer. Int J Urol 2:121, 1995.

Bardot SF, Montie JE: Lymphocele drainage. In Gomella LG, Kozminski M, Winfield HN (eds): Laparoscopic Urologic Surgery. New York, Raven Press, 1994.

Bell DG: A simple technique to facilitate vesicourethral anastomosis following radical prostatectomy. Br J Urol 72:124, 1993.

Belt E: Radical perineal prostatectomy in early carcinoma of the prostate. J Urol 48:287, 1942.

Belt E, Ebert CE, Surber AC Jr: A new anatomic approach in perineal prostatectomy. J Urol 41:482, 1939.

Berger RE, Ireton R: Combined infrapubic and retropubic ligation of the dorsal vein of the penis during radical retropubic surgery. J Urol 130:1107, 1983.

Blandy JP: Surgery of the benign prostate. First Sir Peter Freyer memorial lecture. Irish Med J 70:517, 1977.

Bollman J, Zingg E: Retropubic prostatectomy. Prog Clin Biol Res 6:59, 1976.

Bonnin NJ: Plastic reconstruction of the bladder, neck, and prostatectomy: An operation suitable for all types of nonmalignant bladder neck obstruction. Aust NZ J Surg 27:161, 1957-1958.

Borland RN, Walsh PC: The management of rectal injury during radical retropubic prostatectomy. J Urol 147:905, 1992.

Bourque JP: The transvesico-capsular prostatic adenectomy. Urol Int 4:65, 1957.

Bourque JP: Transvesico-capsular prostatic adenomectomy (trans-commissural): Preliminary report on 80 cases. J Urol 72:918, 1954.

Breza J, Aboseif SR, Bradley RO, et al: Detailed anatomy of penile neurovascular structures: Surgical significance. J Urol 141:437, 1989.

Brock WA: Anorectal malformations: Urologic implications. Dial Pediatr Urol 10:1, 1987.

Bukowski TP, Chakrabarty A, Powell IJ, et al: Acquired rectourethral fistula: Methods of repair. J Urol 153:730, 1995.

Campbell EW: Total prostatectomy with preliminary ligation of the vascular pedicles. J Urol 81:464, 1959.

Chodak GW, Levine LA, Gerber GS, et al: Safety and efficacy of laparoscopic lymphadenectomy. J Urol 147:245, 1992.

Connolly JA, Presti JC Jr, Carroll PR: Anterior bladder neck tube reconstruction at radical prostatectomy preserves functional urethral length: A comparative urodynamic study. Br J Urol 75:766, 1995.

Councill WAH Jr: Retropubic prostatectomy: A modification of technique using a combined prostatovesical incision. J Urol 73:373, 1955.

Cox CE, Hinman F Jr: Retention catheterization and the bladder defense mechanism. JAMA 191:171, 1965.

Crawford ED: Radical retropubic prostatectomy: Antegrade approach. In Crawford ED, Das S (eds): Current Genitourinary Cancer Surgery. Philadelphia, Lea & Febiger, 1990, p 180.

Crawford ED, Kiker JD: Radical retropubic prostatectomy. J Urol 129:1145, 1983.

Culp OS: Radical perineal prostatectomy: Its past, present, and possible future. J Urol 98:618, 1967.

Culp OS, Calhoon HW: A variety of rectourethral fistulas: Experiences with 20 cases. J Urol 91:560, 1964.

Dahl DS, Howard PM, Middleton RG: The surgical management of rectourinary fistulas resulting from a prostatic operation: A report of 5 cases. J Urol 111:514, 1974.

Dalkin BL: Endoscopic evaluation and treatment of anastomotic strictures after radical retropubic prostatectomy. J Urol 155:206, 1996.

Danella JF, Dekernion JB, Smith RB, Steckel J: The contemporary incidence of lymph node metastases in prostate cancer: Implications for laparoscopic lymph node dissection. J Urol 149:1488, 1993.

Das S, Tashima M: Extraperitoneal laparoscopic staging pelvic lymph node dissection. J Urol 151:1321, 1994.

Evans JP, Smart JG, Bagshaw PF: Bacterial contents of enucleated prostate glands. Urology 17:328, 1981.

Firfer R, Berkson BM, Lipshitz S, Hsieh WHH: The combined prostatectomy. J Urol 132:687, 1984.

Fisher RE, Koch MO: Recognition and management of delayed disruption vesicourethral anastomosis in radical prostatectomy. J Urol 147:1579, 1992.

Flanagan WF, Webster GD, Brown MW, Massey EW: Lumbosacral plexus stretch injury following the use of the modified lithotomy position. J Urol 134:567, 1985.

Flocks RH: The arterial distribution within the prostate gland: Its role in transurethral prostatic resection. J Urol 37:524, 1937.

Flocks RH, Culp DA: A modification of technique for anastomosing membranous urethra and bladder neck following total prostatectomy. J Urol 69:411, 1953.

Fourcade RO: Urethrovesical anastomosis: Urethral suturing under direct vision. J Urol 151:943, 1994.

Frazier HA, Robertson JE, Paulson DF: Radical prostatectomy: The pros and cons of the perineal versus retropubic approach. J Urol 147:888, 1992.

Freyer PJ: A new method of performing prostatectomy. Lancet 1:774, 1900.

Fuller E: Six successful and successive cases of prostatectomy. J Cutan Genitourin Dis 13:229, 1895.

Gadhvi NP: Sushruta's lateral perineal approach for prostatectomy and repair of the ruptured posterior urethra. Br J Urol 61:333, 1988.

Gaur DD: Laparoscopic operative retroperitoneoscopy: Use of a new device. J Urol 148:1137, 1992.

Gecelter L: Transanorectal approach to the posterior urethra and bladder neck. J Urol 109:1011, 1973.

Gibbons RP, Correa RJ, Branner GE, et al: Total prostatectomy for localized prostatic cancer. J Urol 131:73, 1984.

Gill IS, Hodge EE, Munch LC, et al: Transperitoneal marsupialization of lymphoceles: A comparison of laparoscopic and open techniques. J Urol 153:706, 1995.

Godec CJ, Plawker M, Rudberg A, Sharma N: Radical retropubic prostatectomy with minimal blood loss. *In* Olsson CA (ed): Current Surgical Techniques in Urology, vol 8, issue 4. Wilmington, DE, Medical Publications, 1995.

Goldberg MG, Surya BV, Catanese A, et al: Effect of patient positioning on urethral mobility: Implications for radical pelvic surgery. J Urol 146:1252, 1991.

Golimbu M, Morales P, Al-Askari S, Brown J: Extended pelvic lymphadenectomy for prostatic cancer. J Urol 121:617, 1979.

Goodfellow GE: Median perineal prostatectomy. JAMA 43:194, 1904.

Goodwin WE: Complications of perineal prostatectomy. *In* Smith RB, Skinner DG (eds): Complications of Urologic Surgery: Prevention and Management. Philadelphia, WB Saunders, 1976, p 252.

Goodwin WE: Radical prostatectomy after previous prostatic surgery. JAMA 148:799, 1952.

Goodwin WE, Turner RD, Winter CC: Rectourinary fistula: Principles of management and a technique of surgical closure. J Urol 80:246, 1958.

Goodwin WE, Winter CC, Turner RD: Fistula between bowel and urinary tract. J Urol 84:95, 1960.

Grass JA, Sakima NT, Valley M, et al: Assessment of ketorolac as an adjuvant to fentanyl patient-controlled epidural analgesia after radical retropubic prostatectomy. Anesthesiology 78:642, 1993.

Gregoir W: Haemostatic prostatic adenomectomy. Eur Urol 4:1, 1978.

Griffith DP, Schuessler WW, Nickell KG, Meaney JT: Laparoscopic pelvic lymphadenectomy for prostatic adenocarcinoma. Urol Clin North Am 19:407, 1992.

Gupta NP, Mohanty NK, Reddy PS, et al: A high risk factor score in the management of benign prostatic hyperplasia. Br J Urol 58:296, 1986.

Harpster LE, Rommel FM, Sieber PR, et al: The incidence and management of rectal injury associated with radical prostatectomy in a community based urology practice. J Urol 154:1435, 1995.

Harris SH: Suprapubic prostatectomy with closure. Br J Urol 1:285, 1929.

Hayashi T, Taki Y, Hiura M, et al: Simplified technique for management of Santorini plexus and puboprostatic ligaments during radical retropubic prostatectomy. Urology 28:322, 1986.

Hedican SP, Walsh PC: Postoperative bleeding following radical retropubic prostatectomy. J Urol 152:1181, 1994.

Henderson DJ, Middleton RG, Dahl DS: Single stage repair of rectourinary fistula. J Urol 125:592, 1981.

Hinman F: Perineal prostatectomy. Surg Gynecol Obstet 49:669, 1929.

Hinman F: Surgery in cancer of the prostate. JAMA 119:669, 1942.

Hinman F Jr: Capsular influence on benign prostatic hyperplasia. Urology 28:347, 1986.

Hinman F Jr: The early diagnosis and radical treatment of prostatic carcinoma. Calif Med 68:336, 1948.

Hinman F Jr: Perineal prostatectomy. *In* Encyclopedia of Medicine, Surgery and Specialties. Philadelphia, FA Davis, 1965, part 1, p 355.

Hodges CV: Vesicourethral anastomosis after radical perineal prostatectomy: Experience with the Jewett modification. J Urol 118:209, 1977.

Hohenfellner R: Suprapubic prostatectomy. *In* Marberger H (ed): Prostatic Disease, vol 6. New York, Alan R. Liss, 1976, p 49.

Hohenfellner R: Suprapubic prostatectomy. Prog Clin Biol Res 6:49, 1976.

Hrebinko RL, O'Donnel WF: Control of the deep dorsal venous complex in radical retropubic prostatectomy. J Urol 149:799, 1993.

Hryntschak T: Suprapubic transvesical prostatectomy with primary closure of the bladder. J Int Coll Surg 15:366, 1951.

Huber A, von Hochstetter A, Allgower M: Anatomy of the pelvic floor for translevatoric-transsphincteric operations. Am Surg 53:247, 1987.

Hudson PB: Perineal prostatectomy. Urol Clin North Am 2:69, 1975.

Hudson PB, Stout AP: An Atlas of Prostatic Surgery. Philadelphia, WB Saunders, 1962.

Igel TC, Barrett DM, Rife CC: Comparison of techniques for vesicourethral anastomosis: Simple direct versus modified Vest traction sutures. Urology 31:474, 1988.

Igel TC, Barrett DM, Segura JW, et al: Perioperative and postoperative complications from bilateral pelvic lymphadenectomy and radical retropubic prostatectomy. J Urol 137:1189, 1987.

Jasper WS Sr: Combined open prostatectomy and herniorrhaphy. J Urol 111:370, 1974.

Johnson CM: Perineal prostatectomy. J Urol 44:821, 1940.

Jønler M, Messing EM, Rhodes PR, Bruskewitz RC: Sequelae of radical prostatectomy. Br J Urol 74:352, 1994.

Kaufman JJ, Katske FA: Simple technique to control venous bleeding during radical retropubic prostatectomy and cystectomy. Urology 20:309, 1982.

Kavoussi LR, Schuessler WW, Vancaillie TG, Clayman RV: Laparoscopic approach to the seminal vesicles. J Urol 150:417, 1993.

Kavoussi LR, Sosa E, Chandhoke P, et al: Complications of laparoscopic pelvic lymph node dissection. J Urol 149:322, 1993.

Kerbl K, Clayman RV, Petros JA, et al: Staging pelvic lymphadenectomy: A comparison of laparoscopic and open techniques. J Urol 150:396, 1993.

Kilpatrick FR, Thompson HR: Post-operative rectoprostatic fistula and closure by Kraske's approach. Br J Urol 34:470, 1962.

Kilpatrick FR, Mason AY: Post-operative recto-prostatic fistula. Br J Urol 41:649, 1969.

Kischeff S: Combined transvesicoretropubic approach in bladder neck obstruction. Urol Int 6:92, 1963.

Klein EA: Early continence after radical prostatectomy. J Urol 148:92, 1992.

Koch MO, Brandell RA, Lin D, Smith JA Jr: The effect of sequential compression devices on intraoperative blood loss during radical prostatectomy. J Urol 152:1178, 1994.

Kursh ED, Resnick MI: Radical transpubic prostatectomy. J Urol 132:1131, 1984.

Laird DR: Procedures used in treatment of complicated fistulas. Am J Surg 76:701, 1948.

Lang GS, Ruckle HC, Hadley HR, et al: One hundred consecutive laparoscopic pelvic lymph node dissections: Comparing complications of the first 50 cases to the second 50 cases. Urology 44:221, 1994.

Lange PH, Reddy PK: Technical nuances and surgical results of radical retropubic prostatectomy in 150 patients. J Urol 138:348, 1987.

Lassen PM, Kearse WF Jr: Rectal injuries during radical perineal prostatectomy. Urology 45:266, 1995.

Lawson RK: Prostatectomy for benign disease. In Cohen MS, Resnick MI (eds): Reoperative Urology. Boston, Little, Brown & Co, 1995, p 267.

Leadbetter GW Jr, Duxbury JH, Leadbetter WF: Can prostatectomy be improved? J Urol 82:600, 1959.

Leff RG, Shapiro SR: Lower extremity complications of the lithotomy position: Prevention and management. J Urol 122:138, 1979.

Leibovitch I, Foster RS, Wass JL, et al: Color Doppler flow imaging for deep venous thrombosis screening in patients undergoing pelvic lymphadenectomy and radical retropubic prostatectomy for prostatic carcinoma. J Urol 153:1866, 1995.

Leiskovsky G, Skinner DG, Weisenburger T: Pelvic lymphadenectomy in the management of carcinoma of the prostate. J Urol 124:635, 1980.

Lepor H, Gregerman M, Crosby R, et al: Precise localization of the autonomic nerves from the pelvic plexus to the corpora cavernosa: A detailed anatomic study of the adult male pelvis. J Urol 133:207, 1985.

Levy JB, Ramchandani P, Berlin JW, et al: Vesicourethral healing following radical prostatectomy: Is it related to surgical approach? Urology 44:889, 1994.

Levy DA, Resnick MI: Laparoscopic pelvic lymphadenectomy and radical perineal prostatectomy: A viable alternative to radical retropubic prostatectomy. J Urol 151:905, 1994.

Loffer F, Pent D: Indications, contraindications and complications of laparoscopy. Obstet Gynecol Surg 30:4037, 1975.

Malament M: Maximal hemostasis in suprapubic prostatectomy. Surg Gynecol Obstet 120:1307, 1965.

Malizia AA, Banks DW, Newton NE, et al: Modified radical retropubic prostatectomy: Double continence technique. J Urol 141:316A, 585, 1989.

Mark S, Perez LM, Webster GD: Synchronous management of anatomic contracture and stress urinary incontinence following radical prostatectomy. J Urol 151:1202, 1994.

Mason AY: Trans-sphincteric exposure of the rectum. Ann R Coll Surg Engl 51:320, 1972.

Masters JE, Fraundorfer MR, Gilling PJ: Extraperitoneal laparoscopic pelvic lymph node dissection using the Gaur balloon technique. Br J Urol 74:128, 1994.

McCullough CS, Soper NJ, Clayman RV, et al: Laparoscopic drainage of a posttransplant lymphocele. Transplantation 51:725, 1991.

McLaren RH, Barrett DM, Zincke H: Rectal injuries occurring at radical retropubic prostatectomy for prostate cancer: Etiology and treatment. Urology 42:401, 1993.

McLin PH, Fisher R, Hinman F Jr: Rapid sensitivity testing in the prevention of sepsis from genitourinary instrumentation. J Urol 100:787, 1968.

Merritt WA: Bacterial endocarditis as a complication of transurethral prostatic resection. J Urol 65:100, 1951.

Miles WE: Rectal Surgery. London, Cassel & Co, 1939.

Miller JI, Larson TR: Simplified technique for improving exposure of the apical prostate during radical prostatectomy. Urology 44:117, 1994.

Millin T: Retropubic prostatectomy: New extravesical technique: Report on 20 cases. Lancet 2:693, 1945.

Millin T: Retropubic Urinary Surgery. Baltimore, Williams & Wilkins, 1947.

Mohler JL: Outpatient pelvic lymph node dissection. J Urol 154:1439, 1995.

Monfort G: Transvesical approach to utricular cysts. J Pediatr Surg 17:406, 1982.

Myers RP: Improving the exposure of the prostate in radical retropubic prostatectomy: Longitudinal bunching of the deep venous plexus. J Urol 142:1282, 1989.

Narayan P: Nerve sparing radical prostatectomy. In Crawford ED, Das S (eds): Current Genitourinary Cancer Surgery. Philadelphia, Lea & Febiger, 1990, p 171.

Narayan P: Nerve sparing and continence preservation during radical prostatectomy. Urol Int 46:266, 1991.

Nicoll GA, Riffle GN, Anderson FO: Suprapubic prostatectomy: The removable purse string: A continuing comparative analysis of 300 consecutive cases. J Urol 120:702, 1978.

Nishijima Y, Koiso K: The role of the vertebral veins in the dissemination of prostatic carcinoma. Jpn J Urol 86:927, 1995.

Noldus J, Huland H: Dyeing: A simple method for detecting positive or negative surgical margins. Urology 45:133, 1995.

Norgan WR, Lieber MM: Pelvic lymphadenectomy. In Crawford ED, Das S (eds): Current Genitourinary Cancer Surgery. Philadelphia, Lea & Febiger, 1990, p 162.

Novicki DE, Larson TR, Ferrigni RG, et al: A comparison of the modified Vest and direct anastomosis for radical retropubic prostatectomy. Urology (in press).

O'Conor VJ Jr: An aid for hemostasis in open prostatectomy: Capsular plication. J Urol 127:448, 1982.

O'Conor VJ Jr: Suprapubic prostatectomy. In Landes RR, Bush RB, Zorgniotti AW (eds): Perspectives in Urology, vol 1. Nutley, NJ, Roche Laboratories 1976, p 135.

O'Conor VJ, Bulkley GJ, Sokol JK: Low suprapubic prostatectomy: Comparison of results with standard operation in two comparable groups of 142 patients. J Urol 90:301, 1963.

O'Conor VJ Jr, Nanninga JB: Low suprapubic prostatectomy: A continuing report. J Urol 108:453, 1972.

O'Donnell PD, Finan BF: Continence following nerve-sparing radical prostatectomy. J Urol 142:1227, 1989.

Page BH: The pathological anatomy of digital enucleation for benign prostatic hyperplasia and its application to endoscopic resection. Br J Urol 52:111, 1980.

Parra RO, Hagood PG, Boullier JA, et al: Complications of laparoscopic urological surgery: Experience at St. Louis University. J Urol 151:681, 1994.

Partin AW, Yoo J, Carter HB, et al: The use of prostate specific antigen clinical stage and Gleason score to predict pathological stage in men with localized prostate cancer. J Urol 150:110, 1993.

Paulson DF: Radical perineal prostatectomy. Urol Clin North Am 7:847, 1980.

Paulson DF: The surgical technique of radical perineal prostatectomy. Houston, American Urological Association, AUA Update Series, vol V, lesson 38, 1986.

Peña A: Anatomical considerations relevant to fecal incontinence. Semin Surg Oncol 3:1141, 1987.

Peña A: Posterior sagittal anorectoplasty as a secondary operation for the treatment of fecal incontinence. J Pediatr Surg 18:762, 1983.

Peters PC: Radical retropubic prostatectomy. In Glenn JF (ed): Urologic Surgery, 3rd ed. Philadelphia, JB Lippincott, 1983, p 949.

Peterson NE: Management of operative prostatic hemorrhage. Monogr Urol 5:66, 1984.

Petros JA, Catalona WJ: Lower incidence of unsuspected lymph node metastases in 521 consecutive patients with clinically localized prostate cancer. J Urol 147:1574, 1992.

Plorde JJ, Kennedy RP, Bourne HH, et al: Course and prognosis of prostatectomy: With a note on the incidence of bacteremia and effectiveness of chemoprophylaxis. N Engl J Med 272:269, 1965.

Polascik TJ, Walsh PC: Radical retropubic prostatectomy: The influence of accessory pudendal arteries on the recovery of sexual function. J Urol 153:150, 1995.

Pontes JE: Radical prostatectomy. *In* Cohen MS, Resnick MI (eds): Reoperative Urology. Boston, Little, Brown & Co, 1995, p 271.

Prasas ML, Nelson R, Hambrick E, et al: York-Mason procedure for repair of postoperative rectoprostatic urethral fistula. Dis Colon Rectum 26:716, 1983.

Pressman D, Rolnick D: Retropubic prostatectomy: Mortality complications and functional end results. J Urol 88:814, 1962.

Presti JC Jr, Schmidt RA, Narayan PA, et al: Pathophysiology of urinary incontinence after radical prostatectomy. J Urol 143:975, 1990.

Rainwater LM, Segura JW: Technical considerations in radical prostatectomy: Blood loss after ligation of dorsal vein complex. J Urol 143:1163, 1990.

Ramchandani P, Banner MP, Berlin JW, et al: Vesicourethral anastomotic strictures after radical prostatectomy: Efficacy of transurethral balloon dilation. Radiology 193:345, 1994.

Randall A: The Surgical Pathology of Prostatic Obstructions. Baltimore, Williams & Wilkins, 1931.

Randall A, Hinman F Jr: Surgical anatomy of the prostatic lobes. *In* Hinman F Jr (ed): Benign Prostatic Hypertrophy. New York, Springer-Verlag, 1983, p 672.

Reddy PK, Kaye KW: Deep posterior compartmental syndrome: A serious complication of the lithotomy position. J Urol 132:144, 1984.

Redman JF: Anatomic approach to the pelvis. *In* Crawford ED, Borden TA (eds): Genitourinary Cancer Surgery. Philadelphia, Lea & Febiger, 1982, p 126.

Reiner WG, Walsh PC: An anatomical approach to the surgical management of the dorsal vein and Santorini's plexus during radical retropubic surgery. J Urol 121:198, 1979.

Resnick MI: Complications of laparoscopic pelvic lymphadenectomy. Urologists' Correspondence Club Letter, June 25, 1992.

Resnick MI: Editorial comment to Lassen PM, Kearse WF Jr: Rectal injuries during radical perineal prostatectomy. Urology 45:266, 1995.

Rinker R Jr: Retropubic seminal vesiculectomy for chronic seminal vesiculitis with preservation of potency. J Urol 104:463, 1970.

Ruckle H, Hadley R, Lui P, Stewart S: Laparoscopic pelvic lymph node dissection: Assessment of intraoperative and early postoperative complications. J Endourol 6:117, 1992.

Ruckle HC, Zincke H: Potency-sparing radical retropubic prostatectomy simplified anatomical approach. J Urol 153:1875, 1995.

Rukstalis DB, Gerber GS, Vogelzang NJ, et al: Laparoscopic pelvic lymph node dissection: A review of 103 consecutive cases. J Urol 151:670, 1994.

Sattar AA, Noel JC, Vanderhaeghen JJ, et al: Prostate capsule: Computerized morphometric analysis of its components. Urology 46:178, 1995.

Schellhammer PF, Jordan GH, Schlossberg SM: Transurethral balloon dilation of anastomotic stricture after radical prostatectomy. Contemp Urol 6:16, 1994.

Schlegel PN, Walsh PC: Neuroanatomical approach to radical cystoprostatectomy with preservation of sexual function. J Urol 138:1402, 1987.

Schlossberg S, Jordan G, Schellhammer P: Repair of obliterative vesicourethral stricture after radical prostatectomy: A technique for preservation of continence. Urology 45:510, 1995.

Schmidt JD: Indications for perineal prostatectomy. Prog Clin Biol Res 303:315, 1989.

Schmidt JD: Nerve sparing radical prostatectomy. West J Med 151:450, 1989.

Schmidt JD: Total perineal prostatectomy. *In* Crawford ED, Das S (eds): Current Genitourinary Cancer Surgery. Philadelphia, Lea & Febiger, 1990, p 194.

Schoenberg HW, Gregory JG: Anterior bladder tube in radical retropubic prostatectomy. Urology 7:495, 1976.

Schuessler WW, Vancaillie TG, Reich H, Griffith DP: Transperitoneal endosurgical lymphadenectomy in patients with localized prostate cancer. J Urol 145:988, 1991.

Schuhrke TD, Kaplan GW: Prostate utricle cysts. J Urol 119:765, 1978.

Selikowitz SM, Albala DM: A method of exposing the vesicourethral anastomotic site during radical retropubic prostatectomy. J Urol 154:1461, 1995.

Shah PJ, Abrams PH, Feneley RC, Green NA: The influence of prostatic anatomy on the differing results of prostatectomy according to the surgical approach. Br J Urol 51:549, 1979.

Shah PJR, Williams G, Chaudary M, et al: Short term antibiotic prophylaxis and prostatectomy. Br J Urol 53:339, 1981.

Smith AM, Veenema RJ: Management of rectal injury and rectourethral fistulas following radical retropubic prostatectomy. J Urol 108:778, 1972.

Stanley BK, Noble MJ, Gilliland C, et al: Comparison of patient-controlled analgesia versus intramuscular narcotics in resolution of post-operative ileus after radical retropubic prostatectomy. J Urol 150:1434, 1993.

Steiner MS: The puboprostatic ligament and the male urethral suspensory mechanism: An anatomic study. Urology 44:530, 1994.

Steiner MS, Burnett AL, Brooks JD, et al: Tubularized neourethra following radical retropubic prostatectomy. J Urol 150:407, 1993

Steiner MS, Marshall FF: Mini-laparotomy staging pelvic lymphadenectomy (minilap): Alternative to standard and laparoscopic pelvic lymphadenectomy. Urology 41:201, 1993.

Stone NN, Stock RG, Unger P: Indications for seminal vesicle biopsy and laparoscopic pelvic lymph node dissection in men with localized carcinoma of the prostate. J Urol 154:1392, 1995.

Stone NN, Wesson MF: Laparoscopic pelvic lymph node dissection with biplanar transperitoneal prostate implantation. *In* Gomella LG, Kozminski M, Winfield HN (eds): Laparoscopic Urologic Surgery. New York, Raven Press, 1994.

Surya BV, Provet J, Johanson K-E, Brown J: Anastomotic strictures following radical prostatectomy: Risk factors and management. J Urol 143:755, 1990.

Teichman JMH, Reddy PK, Hulbert JC: Laparoscopic pelvic lymph node dissection, laparoscopically assisted seminal vesicle mobilization, and total perineal prostatectomy versus radical retropubic prostatectomy for prostatic cancer. Urology 45:823, 1995.

Terris MK, McNeal JE, Freiha FS, Stamey TA: Efficacy of transrectal ultrasound-guided seminal vesicle biopsies in the detection of seminal vesicle invasion by prostate cancer. J Urol 149:1035, 1993.

Thomas DD, Levison MA, Dykstra BJ, Bender JS: Management of rectal injuries: Dogma versus practice. Am Surg 56:507, 1990.

Thomas GG, Molenaar JC: The management of a fistula between the rectum and lower urinary tract. J Pediatr Surg 14:65, 1979.

Thomas R, Steele R, Smith R, Brannan W: One-stage laparoscopic pelvic lymphadenectomy and radical perineal prostatectomy. J Urol 152:1174, 1994.

Tobin CE, Benjamin JA: Anatomical and surgical restudy of Denonvilliers' fascia. Surg Gynecol Obstet 80:373, 1945.

Turner-Warwick R: The sphincter mechanisms: Their relation to prostatic enlargement and its treatment. *In* Hinman F Jr (ed): Benign Prostatic Hypertrophy. New York, Springer-Verlag, 1983, p 809.

Turner-Warwick R, Whiteside CG, Worth PHC, et al: A urodynamic view of clinical problems associated with bladder neck dysfunction and its treatment by endoscopic incision and transtrigonal posterior prostatectomy. Br J Urol 45:44, 1973.

Uhlenhuth E, Wolfe WM, Smith EM, Middleton EB: The rectogenital septum. Surg Gynecol Obstet 86:148, 1948.

Van den Beviere H, Vossaert R, DeRoose J, Derom F: Our experience in the treatment of imperforate anus: Anterior Mollard's technique versus posterior approach (Stephen's technique). Acta Chir Belg 82:205, 1983.

Vest SA: Radical perineal prostatectomy: Modification of closure. Surg Gynecol Obstet 70:935, 1940.

Villers A, McNeal JE, Freiha FS, et al: Invasion of Denonvilliers' fascia in radical prostatectomy specimens. J Urol 149:793, 1993.

Villers A, Vannier JL, Abecassis R, et al: Extraperitoneal endosurgical lymphadenectomy with insufflation in the staging of bladder and prostate cancer. J Endourol 7:229, 1993.

Walker G: Symphysiotomy as an aid to the removal of cancer of the prostate. Ann Surg 73:609, 1921.

Walker WC, Bowles WT: Transvesical seminal vesiculostomy in treatment of congenital obstruction of seminal vesicles: Case report. J Urol 99:324, 1968.

Walsh PC, Donker PJ: Impotence following radical prostatectomy: Insight into etiology and prevention. J Urol 128:492, 1982.

Walsh PC, Lepor H, Eggleston JC: Radical prostatectomy with preservation of sexual function: Anatomical and pathological considerations. Prostate 4:473, 1983.

Walsh PC, Mostwin JL: Radical prostatectomy and cystoprostatectomy with preservation of potency: Results utilizing a new nerve-sparing technique. Br J Urol 56:694, 1984.

Walsh PC, Oesterling JE: Improved hemostasis during simple retropubic prostatectomy. J Urol 143:1202, 1990.

Walsh PC, Quinlan DU, Morton RA, et al: Radical retropubic prostatectomy: Improved anastomosis and urinary continence. Urol Clin North Am 17:679, 1990.

Waples MJ, Wegenke JD, Vega RJ: Laparoscopic management of lymphocoele after pelvic lymphadenectomy and radical retropubic prostatectomy. Urology 39:82, 1992.

Ward RO: Vesicocapsular prostatectomy. Lancet 1:472, 1948.

Weiss JP, Schlecker BA, Wein AJ, Hanno PL: Preservation of periprostatic autonomic nerves during total perineal prostatectomy by intrafascial dissection. Urology 26:160, 1985.

Weldon VE, Tavel FR: Potency-sparing radical perineal prostatectomy: Anatomy, surgical technique and initial results. J Urol 140:559, 1988.

Weyrauch HM: A critical study of surgical principles used in repair of urethrorectal fistula. Stanford Med Bull 9:2, 1951.

Weyrauch HM: Surgery of the Prostate. Philadelphia, WB Saunders, 1959.

Wheeler JS Jr, Krane RJ: Blood vessels and lymphatics of the prostate gland. *In* Abramson DI, Dobrin PB (eds): Blood Vessels and Lymphatics in Organ Systems. New York, Academic Press, 1984, p 548.

Wilbert DM, Buess G, Bichler KH: Combined endoscopic closure of rectourethral fistula. J Urol 155:256, 1996.

Wilson CS, Dahl DS, Middleton RG: Pelvic lymphadenectomy for the staging of apparently localized prostatic cancer. J Urol 117:197, 1977.

Winfield HN: Laparoscopic pelvic lymph node dissection: Application to genitourinary malignancies. *In* Gomella LG, Kozminski M, Winfield HN (eds): Laparoscopic Urologic Surgery. New York, Raven Press, 1994, p 111.

Winfield HN, Donovan JF, See WA, et al: Laparoscopic pelvic lymph node dissection for genitourinary malignancies: Indications, techniques and results. J Endourol 6:103, 1992.

Winfield HN, Ryan KJ: Experimental laparoscopic surgery: Potential clinical applications in urology. J Endourol 4:37, 1990.

Witherington R, Rinker JR: Retropubic seminal vesiculectomy for chronic seminal vesiculitis with preservation of potency. J Urol 104:463, 1970.

Witherington R, Shelor WC Jr: Suprapubic prostatectomy: Modified Hryntschak technique. Urology 4:550, 1974.

Wolf JS Jr, Shinohara K, Kerlikowske KM, et al: Selection of patients for laparoscopic pelvic lymphadenectomy prior to radical prostatectomy: A decision analysis. Urology 42:680, 1993.

Wood DP, Peretsman SJ, Seay TM: Incidence of benign and malignant prostate tissue in biopsies of the bladder neck after a radical prostatectomy. J Urol 154:1443, 1995.

Wood TW, Middleton RG: Single-stage transrectal transsphincteric (modified York-Mason) repair of rectourinary fistulas. Urology 35:27, 1990.

Young HH: Conservative perineal prostatectomy: Presentation of new instruments and technique. JAMA 41:999, 1903.

Young HH: Cure of cancer of prostate by radical perineal prostatectomy (prostatoseminal vesiculectomy): History, literature and statistics of Young's operation. J Urol 53:188, 1945.

Young HH: The early diagnosis and radical cure of carcinoma of the prostate. Bull Johns Hopkins Hosp 16:315, 1903.

Young HH, Stone HB: The operative treatment of urethrorectal fistula. Presentation of a method of radical cure. J Urol 1:289, 1917.

Zvara P, Carrier S, Kour N-W, Tanagho EA: The detailed neuro-anatomy of the human striated urethral sphincter. Br J Urol 74:182, 1994.

Audiovisuals

Camey M: Radical Cystoprostatectomy with Ileocystoplasty. Wilkes-Barre, PA, Karol Media, 1985 (23 minutes). AUA #919-1137.

Carlton E Jr, Chin JL, Denstedt JD, et al: Radical Perineal Prostatectomy: A Detailed Anatomic Depiction. Wilkes-Barre, PA, Karol Media, 1995 (28 minutes). AUA #919-2053.

Catalona WJ: Nerve-sparing Radical Retropubic Prostatectomy: 1995 Technique. Wilkes-Barre, PA, Karol Media, 1995 (25 minutes). AUA #919-2052.

Catalona WJ: Technique of Nerve-Sparing Radical Retropubic Prostatectomy. Wilkes-Barre, PA, Karol Media, 1990 (34 minutes). AUA #919-1163.

D'Ancona CAL, Netto NR Jr, Ferreira U, et al: Radical Perineal Prostatectomy. Wilkes-Barre, PA, Karol Media, 1994 (8 minutes). AUA #919-2024.

Griffith DP, Schuessler WW, Vancaillie TG: Laparoscopic Pelvic Lymphadenectomy: An Endoscopic Technique for Staging Pelvic Malignancies. Wilkes-Barre, PA, Karol Media, 1991 (12 minutes). AUA #919-1177.

Harris MJ, Thompson IM Jr: The Anatomical Radical Perineal Prostatectomy. Wilkes-Barre, PA, Karol Media, 1994 (16 minutes). AUA #919-2026.

McNeal JE (moderator): Clinical Anatomy of the Prostate: Normal, BPH and Cancer. Wilkes-Barre, PA, Karol Media, 1992 (51 minutes). AUA #919-2006.

Mueller EJ, Zeidman EJ, Thompson IM, et al: Anatomic Approach to Radical Prostatectomy. Wilkes-Barre, PA, Karol Media, 1992 (10 minutes). AUA #919-2005.

Parra RO, Mavrich V, Laguna P: Nerve-Sparing Radical Perineal Prostatectomy. Wilkes-Barre, PA, Karol Media, 1994 (11 minutes). AUA #919-2028.

Rigatti P, DaPozzo L, Francesca F, et al: Radical Transcoccygeal Prostatectomy. Wilkes-Barre, PA, Karol Media, 1994 (10 minutes). AUA #919-2029.

Stamey TA: The Stanford Radical Retropubic Prostatectomy. Wilkes-Barre, PA, Karol Media, 1991 (23 minutes). AUA #919-1178.

Zimmern PE, Himsl K, Kaswick J: Radical Perineal Prostatectomy. Wilkes-Barre, PA, Karol Media, 1995 (11 minutes). AUA #919-2054.

Zincke H, Cheng WS: Modifications to the Radical Prostatectomy. Wilkes-Barre, PA, Karol Media, 1992 (20 minutes). AUA #919-2002.

BLADDER: APPROACHES

Albert DJ, Persky L: Conjoined end-to-end uretero-intestinal anastomosis. J Urol 105:201, 1971.

Basmajian JV: The main arteries of the large intestine. Surg Gynecol Obstet 101:585, 1959.

Bennett RC, Duthie HL: The functional importance of the internal anal sphincter. Br J Surg 51:355, 1964.

Boucher BJ: Sex differences in the fetal pelvis. Am J Phys Anthropol 15:581, 1957.

Browning GG, Parks AG: A method and the results of loop colostomy. Dis Colon Rectum 26:223, 1983.

Cauldwell EW, Anson BJ: The visceral branches of the abdominal aorta: Topographical relationships. Am J Anat 73:27, 1943.

Cherney LS: A modified transverse incision for low abdominal operations. Surg Gynecol Obstet 72:92, 1941.

Chevrel JP, Gueraud JP: Arteries of the terminal ileum. Diaphanization study and surgical applications. Anat Clin 1:95, 1979.

Clark SS: Electrolyte disturbance associated with jejunal conduit. J Urol 112:42, 1974.

Connar RG, Sealy WC: Gastrostomy and its complications. Am Surg 138:732, 1979.

Coppa GF, Eng K, Gouge TH, et al: Parenteral and oral antibiotics in elective colon and rectal surgery: A prospective, randomized trial. Am J Surg 145:62, 1983.

Courtney H: Anatomy of the pelvic diaphragm and anorectal musculature as related to sphincter preservation in anorectal surgery. Am J Surg 79:155, 1950.

Couvelaire R: "La petite vessie" des tuberculeaux genito-urinaires: Essae de classification place et varidentes des cysto-intestino-plasties. J Urol (Paris) 56:381, 1950.

Droes JTPM: Observations on the musculature of the urinary bladder and the urethra in the human foetus. Br J Urol 46:179, 1974.

Fasth S, Hulten L: Loop ileostomy: A superior diverting stoma in colorectal surgery. World J Surg 8:401, 1984.

Gecelter L: Transanorectal approach to the posterior urethra and bladder neck. J Urol 109:1011, 1973.

Goligher JC, Leacock AG, Brossy JJ: The surgical anatomy of the anal canal. Br J Surg 43:51, 1955.

Goligher JC, Morris C, McAdam WAF, et al: A controlled trial of inverting versus everting suture in clinical large bowel surgery. Br J Surg 57:817, 1970.

Golimbu M, Al-Askari S, Morales P: Transpubic approach for lower urinary tract surgery: A 15-year experience. J Urol 143:72, 1990.

Gorsch RV: Perineopelvic Anatomy. New York, Tilghman, 1941.

Gosling JA: Structure of the bladder and urethra in relation to function. Urol Clin North Am 6:31, 1979.

Gosling JA, Dixon JS, Humpherson JR: Functional Anatomy of the Urinary Tract. Baltimore, University Park Press, 1982.

Griffiths DA: A reappraisal of the Pfannenstiel incision. Br J Urol 48:469, 1976.

Hodges CV: Surgical anatomy of the urinary bladder and pelvic ureter. Surg Clin North Am 44:1327, 1964.

Keisling VJ, Tank ES: Postoperative intussusception in children. Urology 33:387, 1989.

Lierse W: Applied Anatomy of the Pelvis. Berlin, Springer-Verlag, 1987.

MacKenzie AR, Whitmore WF Jr: Resection of pubic rami for urologic cancer. J Urol 100:546, 1968.

Montie J: Bladder injuries. Urol Clin North Am 4:59, 1977.

Mostwin JL: Current concepts of female pelvic anatomy and physiology. Urol Clin North Am 18:175, 1991.

O'Connor VJ Jr: Transperitoneal transvesical repair of vesicovaginal fistula with omental interposition. Houston, American Urological Association, AUA Update Series, vol X, lesson 13, 1991.

Pfannenstiel J: Über die Vorheile des suprasymphasaren Faschenquerschnitts für die gynkologischen Koliolomien, zugleich ein Beitrag zu der Indikatior stellung der Operationswege. Sanmburg Klin Vortr 268:1736, 1900.

Redman JF: An anatomic approach to the pelvis. In Crawford ED, Das S (eds): Current Genitourinary Cancer Surgery. Philadelphia, Lea & Febiger, 1990, p 140.

Reynolds EL: The bony pelvis in prepuberal childhood. Am J Phys Anthropol 5:165, 1947.

Silver PHS: The role of the peritoneum in the formation of the septum recto-vesical. J Anat 90:538, 1956.

Smith DR: The Cherney incision as applied to the surgery of the lower ureter and bladder. Surg Gynecol Obstet 83:364, 1946.

Uhlenhuth E, Wolfe WM, Smith EM: The rectogenital septum. Surg Gynecol Obstet 86:148, 1948.

BLADDER: EXCISION

Ahlering TE, Lieskovsky G: Surgical treatment of urethral cancer in the male patient. In Skinner DG, Lieskovsky G (eds): Diagnosis and Management of Genitourinary Cancer. Philadelphia, WB Saunders, 1988, p 622.

Babaian RJ: Radical cystectomy: Female. In Johnson DE, Boileau MA (eds): Genitourinary Tumors: Fundamental Principles and Surgical Techniques. New York, Grune & Stratton, 1982, p 477.

Barnes RW: Surgical treatment of large vesical diverticula: Presentation of a new technique. J Urol 42:794, 1939.

Bauer SB, Retik AB: Urachal anomalies and related umbilical disorders. Urol Clin North Am 5:195, 1978.

Beck AD, Gaudin HJ, Bonham DG: Carcinoma of the urachus. Br J Urol 42:555, 1970.

Begg RC: The urachus and umbilical fistulae. Surg Gynecol Obstet 45:165, 1927.

Begg RC: The urachus: Its anatomy, histology and development. J Anat 64:170, 1930.

Belman AB, King LR: Urinary tract abnormalities associated with imperforate anus. J Urol 108:823, 1972.

Berman SM, Tolia BM, Laor E, et al: Urachal remnants in adults. Urology 31:17, 1988.

Blichert-Toft M, Nielson OV: Congenital patent urachus and acquired variants. Acta Chir Scand 137:807, 1971.

Bowles WT, Cordonnier JJ: Total cystectomy for carcinoma of the bladder. J Urol 90:731, 1963.

Bracken RB, McDonald M, Johnson DE: Complications of single-stage radical cystectomy and ileal conduit. Urology 17:141, 1981.

Brand E: Pelvic exenteration in the female. In Crawford ED, Das S (eds): Current Genitourinary Cancer Surgery. Philadelphia, Lea & Febiger, 1990, p 616.

Brannan W, Ochsner MC, Fuselier HA Jr, Landry GR: Partial cystectomy in the treatment of transitional cell carcinoma of the bladder. J Urol 119:213, 1978.

Brendler CB, Schlegel PN, Walsh PC: Urethrectomy with preservation of potency. J Urol 144:270, 1990.

Bricker EM, Modlin J: The role of pelvic evisceration in surgery. Surgery 30:76, 1951.

Brunschwig A: Complete excision of pelvic viscera for advanced carcinoma: A one-stage abdominoperineal operation with end colostomy and bilateral ureteral implantation into the colon above the colostomy. Cancer 1:177, 1948.

Buchsbaum HJ, Christopherson W, Lifshitz S, et al: Vicryl mesh in pelvic floor reconstruction. Arch Surg 120:1389, 1985.

Burnett AL, Brendler CB: Femoral neuropathy following major pelvic surgery: Etiology and prevention. J Urol 151:163, 1994.

Cancrini A, De Carli P, Fattahi H, et al: Orthotopic ileal neobladder in female patients after radical cystectomy: 2-year experience. J Urol 153:956, 1995.

Clarke-Pearson DL, Soper JT, Creasman WT: Absorbable synthetic mesh (polyglactin 910) for the formation of a pelvic "lid" after radical pelvic resection. Am J Obstet Gynecol 158:158, 1988.

Clayman RV, Shahin S, Reddy P, et al: Transurethral treatment of bladder diverticula. Urology 13:573, 1984.

Colodny AJ: An improved surgical technique for intravesical resection of bladder diverticulum. Br J Urol 47:399, 1975.

Couvelaire R, Magder E: Total female cystectomy by vagino-perineal approach. J Urol Nephrol 72:661, 1966.

Crawford ED, Skinner DG: Salvage cystectomy after irradiation failure. J Urol 123:32, 1980.

Cummings KB, Mason JT, Correa RJ Jr, Gibbons RP: Segmental resection in the management of bladder carcinoma. J Urol 119:56, 1978.

Dalkin BL: Endoscopic evaluation and treatment of anastomotic strictures after radical retropubic prostatectomy. J Urol 155:206, 1996.

Das S: Laparoscopic bladder diverticulectomy. J Urol 147:407A, 1992.

Droller MJ: Bladder cancer. In Cohen MS, Resnick MI (eds): Reoperative Urology. Boston, Little, Brown & Co, 1995, p 99.

Flanigan RC, Rapp RP, McRoberts JW: Nutritional assessment and therapy in advanced urothelial cancer. Urol Clin North Am 11:671, 1984.

Flechner SM, Spaulding JT: Management of rectal injury during cystectomy. Urology 19:143, 1982.

Fox M, Power RF, Bruce AW: Diverticulum of the bladder: Presentation and evaluation of treatment of 115 cases. Br J Urol 34:286, 1962.

Freeman JA, Tarter TA, Esrig D, et al: Urethral recurrence in patients with orthotopic ileal neobladders. J Urol 156:1615, 1996.

Freiha FS: Complications of cystectomy. J Urol 123:168, 1980.

Freiha FS, Faysal MH: Salvage cystectomy. Urology 22:496, 1983.

Gerridzen RG, Futter NG: Ten year review of vesical diverticula. Urology 20:33, 1982.

Goldman HJ: A rapid, safe technique for removal of a large vesical diverticulum. J Urol 106:380, 1971.

Hammond G, Iglesias L, Davis JE: The urachus, its anatomy and associated fascias. Anat Rec 80:271, 1941.

Hautmann RE, Paiss T, de Petriconi R: The ileal neobladder in women: 9 years of experience with 18 patients. J Urol 155:76, 1996.

Hendry WF, Gowing NFC, Wallace DM: Surgical treatment of urethral tumors associated with bladder cancer. Proc R Soc Med 67:304, 1974.

Hinman F Jr: Patent urachus and urachal cysts. In Gellis SS, Kagan BM (eds): Current Pediatric Therapy, 12th ed. Philadelphia, WB Saunders, 1986, p 391.

Hinman F Jr: Surgical disorders of the bladder and umbilicus of urachal origin. Surg Gynecol Obstet 113:605, 1961.

Hinman F Jr: Urologic aspects of alternating urachal sinus. Am J Surg 102:339, 1961.

Jarow JP, Brendler CB: Urinary retention caused by a large bladder diverticulum: A simple method of diverticulectomy. J Urol 139:1260, 1988.

Johnson DE, Guinn GA: Surgical management of urethral carcinoma occurring after cystectomy. J Urol 103:314, 1970.

Johnson DE, Lamy S, Bracken RB: Salvage cystectomy after radiation failure in patients with bladder carcinoma. South Med J 70:11, 1977.

Johnson DE, Wishnow KI, Tenney D: Are frozen-section examinations of ureteral margins required for all patients undergoing radical cystectomy for bladder cancer? Urology 33:451, 1989.

Kenworthy P, Tanguay S, Dinney CPN: The risk of upper tract recurrence following cystectomy in patients with transitional cell carcinoma involving the distal ureter. J Urol 155:501, 1996.

Klein FA, Whitmore WF, Herr HW, et al: Inferior pubic rami resection with en bloc radical excision for invasive proximal urethral carcinoma. Cancer 51:1238, 1983.

Kozminski M, Konnak JW, Grossman H: Management of rectal injuries during radical cystectomy. J Urol 142:1204, 1989.

Kraybill WG, Lopez MJ, Bricker EM: Total pelvic evisceration as a therapeutic option in advanced malignant disease of the pelvis. Surg Gynecol Obstet 166:259, 1988.

Linker DG, Whitmore WF: Ureteral carcinoma in situ. J Urol 113:777, 1975.

Loughlin KR, Retik AB, Weinstein HJ, et al: Genitourinary rhabdomyosarcoma in children. Cancer 63:1600, 1989.

Mackenzie AR, Whitmore WF: Resection of pubic rami for urologic cancer. J Urol 100:546, 1968.

Marshall FF, Trieger BFG: Radical cystectomy (anterior exenteration) in the female patient. Urol Clin North Am 18:765, 1991.

Masina F: Segmental resection for tumours of the urinary bladder. Br J Surg 41:494, 1954.

Mayor F, Crawford ED: Partial cystectomy. In Crawford ED, Das S (eds): Current Genitourinary Cancer Surgery. Philadelphia, Lea & Febiger, 1990, p 247.

Mazeman E, Wurtz A, Gilliot P, Biserte J: Extraperitoneal pelvioscopy in lymph node staging of bladder and prostatic cancer. J Urol 147:366, 1992.

McDougal WS, Koch MO: Phallic reconstruction during exenterative surgery for invasive urethral carcinoma. J Urol 141:1201, 1989.

McLaren RH, Barrett DM, Zincke H: Rectal injury occurring at radical retropubic prostatectomy for prostate cancer: Etiology and treatment. Urology 42:401, 1993.

Miller A: The aetiology and treatment of diverticulum of the bladder. Br J Urol 30:43, 1958.

Minevich E, Wacksman J, Lewis AG, et al: The infected urachal cyst: Primary excision versus a staged approach. J Urol 155:824A, 1996.

Mohler JL, Flanigan RC: The effect of nutritional status and support on morbidity and mortality of bladder cancer patient treated by radical cystectomy. J Urol 137:404, 1987.

Montie FE, Pavone-Macaluso M, Tazaki H, et al: What are the risks of cystectomy and the advances in perioperative care? Int J Urol 2(Suppl 2):89, 1995.

Morley GW, Lindenauer SM, Youngs D: Vaginal reconstruction following pelvic exenteration: Surgical and psychological considerations. Am J Obstet Gynecol 116:996, 1973.

Nabors W, Crawford ED: Salvage cystectomy after radiation failure. In Crawford ED, Das S (eds): Current Genitourinary Cancer Surgery. Philadelphia, Lea & Febiger, 1990, p 253.

Nargund VH, Hamilton-Stewart PA: Endoscopic localization prior to partial cystectomy. Br J Urol 73:455, 1994.

Nelson JH Jr, Huston JW: Lymphocyst formation following pelvic lymphadenectomy. Am J Obstet Gynecol 78:1298, 1959.

Netto NR Jr, Lemos GC, deAlmeida Claro JF, Hering FLO: Congenital diverticulum of male urethra. Urology 24:239, 1984.

Nix JT, Menville JG, Albert M, Wendt DL: Congenital patent urachus. J Urol 79:264, 1958.

Novick AC, Stewart BH: Partial cystectomy in the treatment of primary and secondary carcinoma of the bladder. J Urol 116:570, 1976.

Olsson CA: Management of invasive carcinoma of the bladder. In deKernion JB, Paulson DF (eds): Genitourinary Cancer Management. Philadelphia, Lea & Febiger, 1987, p 59.

Parra RO, Jones JP, Andrus CH, Hagood PG: Laparoscopic diverticulectomy: Preliminary report of a new approach for the treatment of bladder diverticulum. J Urol 148:869, 1992.

Peirson EL: An easy method of removing large diverticula of the bladder. J Urol 43:686, 1940.

Pisters LL, Wajsman Z: A simple test for the detection of intraoperative rectal injury in major urological pelvic surgery. J Urol 148:354, 1992.

Prout GR Jr: The surgical management of bladder carcinoma. Urol Clin North Am 3:149, 1976.

Pyrah LN, Keates PG: The transperitoneal removal of certain vesical diverticula and a radiological technique for diagnosis. Br J Urol 30:168, 1958.

Raz S, McLorie G, Johnson S, Skinner DG: Management of the urethra in patients undergoing radical cystectomy for bladder carcinoma. J Urol 120:298, 1978.

Redman JF: An anatomic approach to the pelvis. In Crawford ED, Borden TA (eds): Genitourinary Cancer Surgery. Philadelphia, Lea & Febiger, 1982, p 126.

Rich RH, Hardy BE, Filler RM: Surgery for anomalies of the urachus. J Pediatr Surg 18:4, 1983.

Richie JP, Skinner DG: Carcinoma in-situ of the urethra associated with bladder carcinoma: The role of urethrectomy. J Urol 119:80, 1978.

Richie JP, Skinner DG, Kaufman JJ: Radical cystectomy for carcinoma of the bladder: 16 years of experience. J Urol 113:186, 1975.

Rutledge FN, Burns BS: Pelvic exenteration. Am J Obstet Gynecol 91:692, 1965.

Schlegel PN, Walsh PC: Neuroanatomical approach to radical cystoprostatectomy with preservation of sexual function. J Urol 138:1402, 1987.

Schmidt G, Ortiz J: Perineal procto-cystectomy. Rev Argent Urol Nefrol 37:42, 1968.

Schmitz BL, Schmitz HE, Smith CJ, Molitar JJ: Details of pelvic exenteration evolved during an experience with 75 cases. Am J Obstet Gynecol 80:43, 1960.

Schoenberg MP, Walsh PC, Breazeale DR, et al: Local recurrence and survival following nerve sparing radical cystoprostatectomy for bladder cancer: 10-year followup. J Urol 155:490, 1996.

Schreck WR, Campbell WA: The relationship of bladder outlet obstruction to urinary umbilical fistula. J Urol 108:641, 1972.

Schuessler WW, Pharand D, Vancaillie TG: Laparoscopic standard pelvic node dissection for carcinoma of the prostate: Is it accurate? J Urol 150:898, 1993.

Schuessler WW, Vancaillie TG, Reich H, Griffith DP: Transperitoneal endosurgical lymphadenectomy in patients with localized prostate cancer. J Urol 145:988, 1991.

Sheldon CA, Clayman RV, Gonzalez R, et al: Malignant urachal lesions. J Urol 131:1, 1984.

Shuttleworth KED, Lloyd-Davies RW: Radical resection for tumours involving the posterior urethra. Br J Urol 41:739, 1969.

Sims JM: On the treatment of vesicovaginal fistula. Am J Med Sci 23:59, 1952.

Skinner DG: Cystectomy for bladder cancer. *In* Crawford ED, Das S (eds): Current Genitourinary Cancer Surgery. Philadelphia, Lea & Febiger, 1990, p 235.

Skinner DG: Management of invasive bladder cancer: A meticulous node dissection can make a difference. J Urol 128:34, 1982.

Skinner DG: Technique of radical cystectomy. Urol Clin North Am 8:353, 1981.

Skinner DG, Crawford ED, Kaufman JJ: Complications of radical cystectomy for carcinoma of the bladder. J Urol 123:640, 1980.

Skinner DG, Lieskovsky G: Contemporary cystectomy with pelvic node dissection compared to preoperative radiation therapy plus cystectomy in management of invasive bladder cancer. J Urol 131:1336, 1984.

Skinner DG, Sherrod A: Total pelvic exenteration with simultaneous bowel and urinary reconstruction. J Urol 144:1443, 1990.

Skinner EC, Skinner DG: Management of carcinoma of the female urethra. *In* Skinner DG, Lieskovsky G (eds): Genitourinary Cancer. Philadelphia, WB Saunders, 1988, p 490.

Smith JA, Whitmore WF: Salvage cystectomy for bladder cancer after failure of definitive irradiation. J Urol 125:643, 1981.

Sonn DJ, Smith AD, Moldwin RM: Other urologic laparoscopic applications. *In* Gomella LG, Kozminski LG, Winfield HN (eds): Laparoscopic Urologic Surgery. New York, Raven Press, 1994, chap 24.

Soper JT, Berchuck A, Creasman WT, Clarke-Pearson DL: Pelvic exenteration: Factors associated with major surgical morbidity. Gynecol Oncol 35:93, 1989.

Stein JP, Cote RJ, Freeman JA, et al: Indications for lower tract reconstruction in women after cystectomy for bladder cancer: A pathological review of female cystectomy specimens. J Urol 154:1329, 1995.

Stenzl A, Colleselli K, Poisel S, et al: Rationale and technique of nerve sparing radical cystectomy before an orthotopic neobladder procedure in women. J Urol 154:2044, 1995.

Stenzl A, Draxl H, Posch B, et al: The risk of urethral tumors in female bladder cancer: Can the urethra be used for orthotopic reconstruction of the lower urinary tract? J Urol 153:950, 1995.

Symmonds RE, Pratt JH, Webb MJ: Exenteration operations: Experience with 198 patients. Am J Obstet Gynecol 191:907, 1975.

Wesselhoeft CWJ, Perlmutter AD, Berg S, et al: Pathogenesis and surgical treatment of diverticulum of the bladder. Surg Gynecol Obstet 116:719, 1963.

Wheeless CR Jr: Atlas of Pelvic Surgery. Philadelphia, Lea & Febiger, 1981.

Whitmore WF Jr, Batata MA, Ghoneim MA, et al: Radical cystectomy with or without prior irradiation in the treatment of bladder cancer. J Urol 18:184, 1977.

Whitmore WF Jr, Mount BM: A technique of urethrectomy in the male. Surg Gynecol Obstet 131:303, 1970.

Young HH: A new radical operation for carcinoma of the bulbous urethra: New use for penis. Surg Gynecol Obstet 68:77, 1939.

Young HH: The operative treatment of vesical diverticulum with report of four cases. Johns Hopkins Hosp Rep 13:411, 1906.

Zimmern PE, Cukier J: Prostatic and membranous urethrorectal fistulas: A new technique of surgical closure. J Urol 134:355, 1985.

Zinman L, Libertino JA: Techniques in the management of recurrent vesicovaginal fistula. Surg Clin North Am 53:479, 1973.

Audiovisuals

Austoni E, Trinchieri A, Zanetti G, et al: Radical Cystectomy with Total Urethrectomy in Bladder Carcinoma Surgery.

Wilkes-Barre, PA, Karol Media, 1994 (10 minutes). AUA #919-2023.

Fischer CG, Weidner W, Hummel G, Ringert R: Radical Cystoprostatovesiculectomy with Automatic Stapling Devices. Wilkes-Barre, PA, Karol Media, 1994 (11 minutes). AUA #919-2025.

Marshall FF, Steinberg G: Radical Cystectomy in the Female. Wilkes-Barre, PA, Karol Media, 1993 (22 minutes). AUA #919-2019.

BLADDER: RECONSTRUCTION

Adams MC, Mitchell ME, Rink RC: Gastrocystoplasty: An alternative solution to the problem of urological reconstruction in the severely compromised patient. J Urol 140:1152, 1988.

Albala DM, Schuessler WW, Vancaillie TG: Laparoscopic bladder neck suspension. J Endourol 6:137, 1992.

Albala DM, Vancaillie TG, Schuessler WW: Laparoscopic suspension of the bladder neck. *In* Gomella LG, Kozminski M, Winfield HN (eds): Laparoscopic Urologic Surgery. New York, Raven Press, 1994.

Aldridge AH: Transplantation of fascia for the relief of urinary stress incontinence. Am J Obstet Gynecol 44:398, 1942.

Alexander J, Karl RC, Skinner DB: Results of changing trends in the surgical management of complications of diverticular disease. Surgery 94:683, 1983.

Allen TD: The surgical management of total urinary incontinence in the female patient. J Urol 138:521, 1987.

Appell RA: Retropubic procedures for female stress incontinence. *In* Webster G, Kirby R, King L, Goldwasser B (eds): Reconstructive Urology. Boston, Blackwell Scientific Publications, 1993.

Appell RA: Techniques and results in the implantation of the artificial urinary sphincter in women with type III stress urinary incontinence by a vaginal approach. Neurourol Urodyn 7:613, 1988.

Avni EF, Matos C, et al: Midline omphalocele anomalies in children: Contribution of ultrasound imaging. Urol Radiol 10:189, 1988.

Badenoch DF, Tiptaft RC, Thakar DR, et al: Early repair of accidental injury to the ureter or bladder following gynaecological surgery. Br J Urol 59:516, 1987.

Baker KR, Drutz HP: Retropubic colpourethropexy: Clinical and urodynamic evaluation of 289 cases. Int Urogynecol J 12:196, 1991.

Barrett DM, Furlow WL: The management of severe urinary incontinence in patients with myelodysplasia by implantation of the AS 791/792 urinary sphincter device. J Urol 128:484, 1982.

Barrett DM, Malek RS, Kelalis P: Observations on vesical diverticulum in childhood. J Urol 116:234, 1976.

Barrett DM, Parulkar BG, Kramer SA: Experience with AS800 artificial sphincter in pediatric and young adult patients. Urology 42:431, 1993.

Barrington JW, Roberts A: Burch colposuspension facilitated by means of the Ferguson speculum. Br J Urol 75:242, 1995.

Bauer SB, Retik AB: Urachal anomalies and related umbilical disorders. Urol Clin North Am 5:195, 1978.

Beck RP, McCormick S, Nordstrom L: The fascia lata sling procedure for the treatment of recurrent genuine stress incontinence of urine. Obstet Gynecol 72:699, 1988.

Belman AB, King LR: Urinary tract abnormalities associated with imperforate anus. J Urol 108:823, 1972.

Birkhoff JD, Weschler M, Romas NA: Urinary fistulas: Vaginal repair using a labial fat pad. J Urol 117:595, 1977.

Blaivas JG: Female urethral reconstruction. *In* Webster G, Kirby R, King L, Goldwasser B (eds): Reconstructive Urology. Boston, Blackwell Scientific Publications, 1993.

Blaivas JG: The use of slings for female stress incontinence. *In* Webster G, Kirby R, King L, Goldwasser B (eds): Reconstructive Urology. Boston, Blackwell Scientific Publications, 1993.

Blaivas JG: Vaginal flap neourethra: An alternative to bladder flap urethral reconstruction. J Urol 141:542, 1989.

Blaivas JG, Heritz DM, Romanzi LJ: Early versus late repair of vesicovaginal fistulas: Vaginal and abdominal approaches. J Urol 153:1110, 1995.

Blaivas JG, Jacobs BZ: Pubovaginal sling in the treatment of complicated stress incontinence. J Urol 145:1214, 1994.

Blaivas JG, Olsson CA: Stress incontinence: Classification and surgical approach. J Urol 139:727, 1988.

Blandy JP, Badenoch DF, Fowler CG, et al: Early repair of iatrogenic injury to the ureter of bladder after gynecological surgery. J Urol 146:761, 1991.

Blichert-Toft M, Nielson OV: Congenital patent urachus and acquired variants. Acta Chir Scand 137:807, 1971.

Borzyskowski M, Mundy E (eds): Neuropathic Bladder in Childhood. New York, Cambridge University Press, 1991.

Boyce WH, Kroovand RL: The Boyce-Vest operation for exstrophy of the bladder: 35 years later. Urol Clin North Am 13:307, 1986.

Boyce WH, Vest SA: A new concept concerning treatment of exstrophy of the bladder. J Urol 67:503, 1952.

Boyd SD, Raz S: Needle bladder neck suspension for female stress incontinence. Urol Clin North Am 11:357, 1984.

Brito CG, Mulcahy JJ, Mitchell ME, Adams MC: Use of a double cuff AMS800 urinary sphincter in severe stress incontinence. J Urol 149:283, 1993.

Brock WA: Anorectal malformations: Urologic implications. Dial Pediatr Urol 10:1, 1987.

Browne D: Congenital deformities of the anus and the rectum. Arch Dis Child 30:42, 1955.

Burbige KA, Hensle TW: The complications of urinary tract reconstruction. J Urol 136:292, 1986.

Burch JC: Urethrovaginal fixation to Cooper's ligament for correction of stress incontinence, cystocele, and prolapse. Am J Obstet Gynecol 81:281, 1961.

Burgio KL, Robinson JC, Engel BT: The role of biofeedback in Kegel exercise training from stress urinary incontinence. Am J Obstet Gynecol 154:58, 1986.

Canning DA, Gearhart JP, Peppas DS, Jeffs RD: The cephalotrigonal reimplant in bladder neck reconstruction for patients with exstrophy or epispadias. J Urol 150:156, 1993.

Cantwell FV: Operative technique of epispadias by transplantation of the urethra. Ann Surg 22:689, 1895.

Carr LK: An alternative to manage a nondeflating Foley catheter in women. J Urol 153:716, 1995.

Carson CC, Malek RS, Remine WH: Urologic aspects of vesicoenteric fistulas. J Urol 119:744, 1978.

Chancellor MB, Erhard MJ, Kiilholma PJ, et al: Functional urethral closure with pubovaginal sling for destroyed female urethra after long-term catheterization. Urology 43:499, 1995.

Chapple CR, Osborne JL: Laparoscopic colposuspension—a new procedure. J Urol 147:280A, 1992.

Chapple CR: Lower urinary tract fistulae. In Webster G, Kirby R, King L, Goldwasser B (eds): Reconstructive Urology. Boston, Blackwell Scientific Publications, 1993.

Cobb OE, Ragde H: Correction of female stress incontinence. J Urol 20:418, 1978.

Colodny AJ: An improved surgical technique for intravesical resection of bladder diverticulum. Br J Urol 47:399, 1975.

Couillard DR, Deckard-Janatpour KA, Stone AR: The vaginal wall sling: A compressive suspension procedure for recurrent incontinence in elderly patients. Urology 43:203, 1994.

Couillard DR, Vapnek JM, Stone AR: Proximal artificial sphincter cuff repositioning for urethral atrophy incontinence. Urology 45:653, 1995.

Courtney H: Anatomy of the pelvic diaphragm and anorectal musculature as related to sphincter preservation in anorectal surgery. Am J Surg 79:155, 1950.

Cruikshank SH: Early closure of posthysterectomy vesicovaginal fistulas. South Med J 81:152, 1988.

Curtis AH, Anson BJ, McVay CB: The anatomy and urogenital diaphragms in relation to urethrocele and cystocele. Surg Gynecol Obstet 68:161, 1939.

Das S, Palmer JK: Laparoscopic colposuspension. J Urol 154:1119, 1995.

Decter RM: Use of the fascial sling for neurogenic incontinence: Lesson learned. J Urol 150:683, 1994.

Dees J: Congenital epispadias with incontinence. J Urol 62:513, 1949.

Deshmukh AS, Bansal NK, Kropp KA: Use of methylene blue in suspected colovesical fistula. J Urol 118:819, 1977.

deVries PA, Peña A: Posterior sagittal anorectoplasty. J Pediatr Surg 17:638, 1982.

Drutz HP, Baker KR, Lemieux MC: Retropubic colpourethropexy with transabdominal anterior and/or posterior repair for the treatment of genuine stress urinary incontinence and genital prolapse. Int Urogynecol J 2:201, 1991.

Eid JF, Rosenberg P, Rothaus K, et al: Use of tissue expanders in final reconstruction of infrapubic midline scar, mons pubis, and vulva after bladder exstrophy repair. Urology 41:426, 1993.

Eisen M, Jurkovick K, Altwein JE, et al: Management of vesicovaginal fistulas with peritoneal flap interposition. J Urol 112:195, 1974.

Elkins TE, DeLancey JOL, McGuire EJ: The use of modified Martius graft as an adjunctive technique in vesicovaginal and rectovaginal fistula repair. Obstet Gynecol 75:727, 1990.

Elkins TE, Ghosh TS, Tagoe GA, et al: Transvaginal mobilization and utilization of the anterior bladder wall to repair vesicovaginal fistulas involving the urethra. Obstet Gynecol 79:455, 1992.

Englemann UH, Light JK, Scott FB: Use of artificial urinary sphincter with lower urinary tract reconstruction and continent urinary diversion: Clinical and experimental studies. In King LR (ed): Bladder Reconstruction and Continent Urinary Diversion. Chicago, Year Book Medical Publishers, 1986.

Enhörning G, Miller ER, Hinman F Jr: Urethral closure studied with cine-roentgenography and simultaneous bladder urethra pressure recording. Surg Gynecol Obstet 118:507, 1964.

Eshgi AM, Roth JS, Smith AD: Percutaneous transperitoneal approach to a pelvic kidney for endourological removal of staghorn calculus. J Urol 134:525, 1985.

Falk H, Orkin L: Nonsurgical closure of vesicovaginal fistulas. J Obstet Gynecol 9:538, 1957.

Feneley RCL: The management of female incontinence by suprapubic catheterisation, with or without urethral closure. Br J Urol 55:203, 1983.

Ferzli G, Trapasso J, Raboy A, et al: Extraperitoneal endoscopic pelvic lymph node dissection. J Laparoendosc Surg 2:39, 1992.

Fishman IJ, Shabsigh R, Scott FB: Experience with the artificial urinary sphincter model AS800 in 148 patients. J Urol 141:307, 1989.

Fitzpatrick C, Elkins TE: Plastic surgical techniques in the repair of vesicovaginal fistulas: A review. Int Urogynecol J 4:287, 1993.

Flah LM, Alpuche JO, Castro RS: Repair of posttraumatic stenosis of the urethra through a posterior sagittal approach. J Pediatr Surg 127:1465, 1992.

Fleischmann J, Picha G: Abdominal approach for gracilis muscle interposition and repair of recurrent vesicovaginal fistulas. J Urol 140:552, 1987.

Flocks RH, Boldus R: The surgical treatment and prevention of urinary incontinence associated with disturbance of the internal sphincter mechanism. J Urol 109:279, 1973.

Flocks RH, Culp DA: A modification of technique for anastomosing membranous urethra and bladder neck following prostatectomy. J Urol 69:411, 1953.

Foote JE, Zimmern PE, Leach GE: Vaginal reconstruction for pelvic floor laxity. In Webster G, Kirby R, King L, Goldwasser B (eds): Reconstructive Urology. Boston, Blackwell Scientific Publications, 1993, p 819.

Foster HE, McGuire EJ: Management of urethral obstruction with transvaginal urethrolysis. J Urol 150:1448, 1993.

Fox M, Power RF, Bruce AW: Diverticulum of the bladder: Presentation and evaluation of treatment of 115 cases. Br J Urol 34:286, 1962.

Furlow WL: Implantation of a new semiautomatic artificial genitourinary sphincter: Experience with primary activation and deactivation in 47 patients. J Urol 126:741, 1981.

Gallagher PV, Mellon JK, Ramsden PD, Neal DE: Tanagho bladder neck reconstruction in the treatment of adult incontinence. J Urol 153:1451, 1995.

Galloway NTM, Davies N, Stephenson TP: The complications of colposuspension. Br J Urol 60:122, 1987.

Garcia VF, Bloom DA: Inversion appendectomy. Urology 2:142, 1986.

Gecelter L: Transanorectal approach to the posterior urethra and bladder neck. J Urol 109:1011, 1973.

Gerber GS, Schoenberg HW: Female urinary tract fistulas. J Urol 149:229, 1993.

Ghoniem GM: Bladder neck wrap: A modified fascial sling in treatment of incontinence in meningomyelocele patients. Eur Urol 25:340, 1994.

Ghoniem GM, Elgamasy A-N: Simplified surgical approach to bladder outlet obstruction following pubovaginal sling. J Urol 154:181, 1995.

Gil-Vernet JM, Gil-Vernet A, Campos JA: New surgical approach for treatment of complex vesicovaginal fistula. J Urol 141:513, 1989.

Gilja I, Sarac S, Radej M: A modified Raz bladder neck suspension operation (Transvaginal Burch). J Urol 153:1455, 1995.

Gittes RF, Loughlin KR: No-incision pubovaginal suspension for stress incontinence. J Urol 138:568, 1987.

Glenn JF, Stevens PS: Simplified vesicovaginal fistulectomy. J Urol 110:521, 1973.

Goebell R: Zur Operativen Beseitigung der Angeborenen Incontinentia Vesical. Ztschr Urol Gynäkol 2:187, 1910.

Goldenberg SL, Fenster H, McLoughlin MG: Female bladder neck reconstruction: Anatomic and physiologic approach. Urology 25:139, 1985.

Goldwasser B, Ramon J: Prosthetics for urinary incontinence. In Webster G, Kirby R, King L, Goldwasser B (eds): Reconstructive Urology. Boston, Blackwell Scientific Publications, 1993.

Goligher JC, Leacock AG, Brossy JJ: The surgical anatomy of the anal canal. Br J Surg 43:51, 1955.

Gonzalez R: Reconstruction of the female urethra to allow intermittent catheterization for neurogenic bladders and urogenital sinus anomalies. J Urol 133:478, 1985.

Gonzalez R, Fraley EE: Surgical repair of post-hysterectomy vesico-vaginal fistulas. J Urol 115:660, 1976.

Gonzalez R, Koleilat N, Austin C, et al: The artificial sphincter AS800 in congenital urinary incontinence. J Urol 142:512, 1989.

Gonzalez R, Sheldon CA: Artificial sphincters in children with neurogenic bladders: Long-term results. J Urol 128:1270, 1982.

Goodwin WE, Scardino PT: Vesicovaginal and ureterovaginal fistulas: A summary of 25 years of experience. J Urol 123:370, 1980.

Goodwin WE, Turner RD, Winter CC: Rectourinary fistula: Principles of management and a technique of surgical closure. J Urol 80:246, 1958.

Gundian JC, Barrett DM, Parulkar BG: Mayo Clinic experience with the use of the AMS 800 artificial urinary sphincter for urinary incontinence following radical prostatectomy. J Urol 142:1459, 1989.

Hadley HR, Staskin DR, Schmidbauer CP: Operative correction for female urethral incompetence. Semin Urol 4:13, 1986.

Hanna MK: Results of Millin's pedicled fascial sling for urinary incontinence, due to sphincter incompetence. Annual Meeting, American Academy of Pediatrics, 1995. Abstract.

Harewood LM: Laparoscopic needle colposuspension for genuine stress incontinence. J Endourol 6:S145, 1992.

Harrison MR, Glick PL, Nakayama DL, et al: Loop colon rectovaginoplasty for high cloacal anomaly. J Pediatr Surg 18:885, 1983.

Hayes SN: Operative technique of complicated vesicovaginal fistulas. Surg Gynecol Obstet 81:346, 1945.

Heckler FR, Aldridge JE Jr, Songcharden S, Jabaley ME: Muscle flaps and musculocutaneous flaps in the repair of urinary fistulas. Plast Reconstr Surg 66:94, 1980.

Helmbrecht LJ, Goldstein AMB, Morrow JW: The use of pedicled omentum in the repair of large vesicovaginal fistulas. Invest Urol 13:104, 1975.

Hernandez RD, Himsl K, Zimmern PE: Transvaginal repair of bladder injury during vaginal hysterectomy. J Urol 152:2061, 1994.

Herr HW: Urachal carcinoma: The case for extended partial cystectomy. J Urol 151:365, 1994.

Hinman F Jr: Male incontinence: Relationship of physiology to surgery. J Urol 115:274, 1976.

Hinman F Jr: The non-neurogenic neurogenic bladder (Hinman syndrome): Fifteen years later. J Urol 136:769, 1986.

Hinman F Jr: Obstruction to voiding. In Resnick MI (ed): Current Therapy in Genitourinary Surgery. Toronto, BC Decker, 1987.

Hinman F Jr, Boyarsky S, Pierce JM Jr, Zinner NR (eds): Hydrodynamics of Micturition. Springfield, IL, Charles C Thomas, 1971.

Hinman F Jr, Schmaelzle JF, Cass AS: Autogenous perineal bone graft for post-prostatectomy incontinence: II. Technique and results of prosthetic fixation of urogenital diaphragm in man. J Urol 104:888, 1970.

Jones JA, Mitchell ME, Rink RC: Improved results using a modification of the Young-Dees-Leadbetter bladder neck repair. Br J Urol 71:555, 1993.

Karamchandani MC, West CF Jr: Vesicoenteric fistulas. Am J Surg 147:681, 1984.

Kelemen Z, Lehoczky G: Closure of severe vesico-vagino-rectal fistulas using Lehoczky's island flap. Br J Urol 59:153, 1987.

Kelly HA: Incontinence of urine in women. Urol Cutan Rev 17:291, 1913.

King RM, Beart RW Jr, McIlrath DC: Colovesical and rectovesical fistulas. Arch Surg 117:680, 1982.

Klauber GT: Posterior bladder tube for CIC. Soc Pediatr Urol Newsl, May 20, 1992, p 9.

Kroovland RL, Boyce WH: Isolated vesicorectal internal urinary diversion: A 37-year review of the Boyce-Vest procedure. J Urol 140:572, 1988.

Kropp KA, Angwafo FF: Urethral lengthening and reimplantation for neurogenic incontinence in children. J Urol 135:534, 1986.

Kursh ED: Vesicovaginal fistulas. In Cohen MS, Resnick MI (eds): Reoperative Urology. Boston, Little, Brown & Co, 1995, p 123.

Kurzrock EA, Lowe P, Hardy BE: Bladder wall pedicle wraparound sling for neurogenic urinary incontinence in children. J Urol 155:305, 1996.

Latzko W: Postoperative vesicovaginal fistulas. Am J Surg 58:211, 1942.

Leach GE: Bone fixation technique for transvaginal needle suspension. Urology 31:388, 1988.

Leach GE: Incontinence after artificial urinary sphincter placement: The role of perfusion sphincterometry. J Urol 138:529, 1987.

Leach GE, O'Donnel P, Raz S: Needle urethral-vesical suspension procedures. In Raz S (ed): Female Urology. Philadelphia, WB Saunders, 1983, p 276.

Leach GE, Raz S: Vaginal flap technique: A method of transvaginal vesicovaginal fistula repair. In Raz S (ed): Female Urology. Philadelphia, WB Saunders, 1983, p 372.

Leadbetter GW Jr: Surgical correction of total urinary incontinence. J Urol 91:261, 1964.

Leadbetter GW Jr, Fraley EE: Surgical correction for total urinary incontinence: 5 years later. J Urol 97:869, 1967.

Leadbetter GW Jr, Leadbetter WF: Ureteral reimplantation and bladder neck reconstruction. JAMA 175:676, 1976.

Lee RA, Symmonds RE, Williams TJ: Current status of genitourinary fistula. Obstet Gynecol 72:313, 1988.

Leonard MP, Gearhart JP, Jeffs RD: Continent urinary diversion in childhood. J Urol 144:330, 1990.

Light JK: Abdominal approach for implantation of the A.S. 800 artificial urinary sphincter in females. Neurourol Urodyn 7:603, 1988.

Light JK: The artificial urinary sphincter in children: Experience with the A.S. 800 series and bowel reconstruction. Urol Clin North Am 12:103, 1985.

Light JK: Long-term clinical results using the artificial urinary sphincter around bowel. J Urol 64:56, 1989.

Light JK, Flores FN, Scott FB: Use of the AS792 artificial sphincter following urinary undiversion. J Urol 129:548, 1983.

Light JK, Lapin S, Vohra S: Combined use of bowel and the artificial urinary sphincter in reconstruction of the lower urinary tract: Infectious complications. J Urol 153:331, 1995.

Light JK, Scott FB: Complications of the artificial urinary sphincter in pediatric patients. Urol Clin North Am 10:551, 1983.

Light JK, Scott FB: Management of urinary incontinence in women with the artificial urinary sphincter. J Urol 134:476, 1985.

Liu CY, Paek W: Laparoscopic retropubic colposuspension (Burch procedure). J Am Assoc Gynecol Laparosc 1:31, 1993.

Lockhart-Mummery HE: Vesico-intestinal fistula. Proc R Soc Med 51:1032, 1958.

Lowe DH, Scherz HC, Parsons CL: Urethral pressure profilometry in Scott artificial urinary sphincter. Urology 31:82, 1988.

Maileski WJ, Joehl RJ, Rege RV, Nahrwold DL: One-stage resection and anastomosis in the management of colovesical fistula. Am J Surg 153:75, 1987.

Marchetti AA, Marshall VF, Shultis LD: Simple vesicourethral suspension: A survey. Am J Obstet Gynecol 74:57, 1957.

Marconi F, Messina P, Pavanello P, Castro RD: Cosmetic reconstruction of the mons veneris and lower abdominal wall by skin expansion as the last stage of the surgical treatment of bladder exstrophy: A report of three cases. Plast Reconstr Surg 91:551, 1993.

Marshall VF, Marchetti AA, Krantz KE: The correction of stress urinary incontinence by simple vesico-urethral suspension. Surg Gynecol Obstet 88:590, 1949.

Martius H: Gynecologic Operations: With Emphasis on Topographic Anatomy. Boston, Little, Brown & Co, 1957.

Martius H: Die operative Wiedeherstellung der volkommen fehlenden Harnrohre und des Schiessmuskels derselben (The repair of vesicovaginal fistulae with interposition pedicle graft of labial tissue). Zentralbl Gynakol 52:480, 1928.

Mathes SJ, Nahai F: Clinical Applications for Muscle and Musculocutaneous Flaps. St. Louis, CV Mosby, 1982.

McBeath RB, Schiff M Jr, Allen V, et al: A 12-year experience with enterovesical fistulas. Urology 44:661, 1994.

McCraw JB, Dibbell DG, Carraway JH: Clinical definition of independent myocutaneous vascular territories. Plast Reconstr Surg 60:341, 1977.

McDougall EM, Klutke CG, Cornell T: Comparison of transvaginal versus laparoscopic bladder neck suspension for stress urinary incontinence. Urology 45:641, 1995.

McGuire EJ: Abdominal procedures for stress incontinence. Urol Clin North Am 12:285, 1985.

McGuire EJ: Stress incontinence in females. In Resnick MI, Kursch E (eds): Therapy in Genitourinary Surgery. Toronto, BC Decker, 1987, p 464.

McGuire EJ, Bennett CJ, Konnak JA, et al: Experience with pubovaginal slings for urinary incontinence at University of Michigan. J Urol 138:525, 1987.

McGuire EJ, Lytton B: The pubovaginal sling in stress urinary incontinence. J Urol 119:82, 1978.

McGuire EJ, Wang C-C, Usitalo H, Savastano J: Modified pubovaginal sling in girls with myelodysplasia. J Urol 135:94, 1985.

Mendez-Fernandez MA, Hollan C, Frank DH, Fisher JC: The scrotal myocutaneous flap. Plast Reconstr Surg 78:676, 1986.

Middleton RG: Further experience with the Young-Dees procedure for urinary incontinence in selected cases. J Urol 115:159, 1976.

Miller A: The aetiology and treatment of diverticulum of the bladder. Br J Urol 30:43, 1958.

Mitchell ME, Adams MC, Rink RC: Urethral replacement with ureter. J Urol 139:1282, 1988.

Mitchell ME, Hensle TW, Crooks KK: Urethral reconstruction in the young female using a perineal pedicle flap. J Pediatr Surg 17:687, 1982.

Mollard P, Mouriquand PDE, Joubert P: Urethral lengthening for neurogenic urinary incontinence (Kropps procedure): Results of 16 cases. J Urol 143:95, 1990.

Monfort G: Transvesical approach to utricular cysts. J Pediatr Surg 17:406, 1982.

Monga M, Ghoniem GM: Ilioinguinal nerve entrapment following needle bladder suspension procedures. Urology 44:447, 1994.

Morgan JE: A sling operation using Marlex polypropylene mesh for treatment of recurrent stress incontinence. Am J Obstet Gynecol 106:369, 1970.

Morgan JE, Heritz DM, Stewart FE, et al: The polypropylene pubovaginal sling for the treatment of recurrent stress urinary incontinence. J Urol 154:1013, 1995.

Morley GW, Delancey JO: Sacrospinous ligament fixation for eversion of the vagina. Am J Obstet Gynecol 158:872, 1988.

Mraz JP, Sutory M: An alternative in surgical treatment of postirradiation vesicovaginal and rectovaginal fistulas: The seromuscular intestinal graft (patch). J Urol 151:357, 1994.

Mundy AR: An anatomical explanation of bladder dysfunction following rectal and uterine surgery. Br J Urol 54:501, 1982.

Narik G, Palmrich AH: A simplified sling operation suitable for routine use. Am J Obstet Gynecol 84:400, 1962.

Netto NR Jr, Lemos GC, deAlmeida Claro JF, Hering FLO: Congenital diverticulum of male urethra. Urology 24:239, 1984.

Nichols DH: Vaginal prolapse affecting bladder function. Urol Clin North Am 12:222, 1985.

Nitti VW, Raz S: Obstruction following anti-incontinence procedures: Diagnosis and treatment with transvaginal urethrolysis. J Urol 152:93, 1994.

Norton P, Baker J, Sharp H, Warenski J: Genitourinary prolapse: Relationship with joint mobility. Neurourol Urodyn 9:2, 1990.

Nurse DE, Mundy AR: Metabolic complications of cystoplasty. Br J Urol 63:165, 1988.

O'Conor VJ Jr: Female urinary incontinence and vesico-vaginal fistula. In Glenn JF (ed): Urologic Surgery. Hagerstown, MD, Harper & Row, 1975, p 767.

O'Conor VJ Jr: Review of experience with vesicovaginal fistula repair. J Urol 123:367, 1980.

O'Conor VJ Jr: Transperitoneal transvesical repair of vesicovaginal fistula with omental interposition. Houston, American Urological Association, AUA Update Series, vol X, lesson 13, 1991.

O'Conor VJ Jr, Sokol JK, Bulkley GJ, et al: Suprapubic closure of vesico-vaginal fistulas. J Urol 109:51, 1973.

O'Sullivan DC, Chilton CP, Munson KW: Should Stamey colposuspension be our primary surgery for stress incontinence? Br J Urol 75:457, 1995.

Parry JRW, Nurse DE, Baucat HAP, et al: Surgical management of the congenital neurogenic bladder. Br J Urol 65:164, 1990.

Parulkar BG, Barrett DM: Intractable urinary incontinence in females: Application of the AS-800 artificial sphincter. Surg Gynecol Obstet 171:131, 1990.

Patil U, Waterhouse K, Laungani G: Management of 18 difficult vesico-vaginal and urethro-vaginal fistulas with modified Ingelmann-Sundberg and Martius operations. J Urol 123:653, 1980.

Peña A: Anatomical considerations relevant to fecal incontinence. Semin Surg Oncol 3:1141, 1987.

Peña A: Posterior sagittal anorectoplasty as a secondary operation for the treatment of fecal incontinence. J Pediatr Surg 18:762, 1983.

Peña A: Posterior sagittal approach for the correction of anorectal malformations. Adv Surg 19:69, 1986.

Peña A: Surgical treatment of high imperforate anus. World J Surg 9:236, 1985.

Peña A, DeVries P: Posterior sagittal anorectoplasty: Important technical considerations and new applications. J Pediatr Surg 17:796, 1982.

Pereyra AJ: A simplified surgical procedure for the correction of stress incontinence in women. West J Surg Obstet Gynecol 67:223, 1959.

Perez JJ: Laparoscopic presacral neurectomy. J Reprod Med 34:625, 1990.

Perez LM, Webster GD: Successful outcome of artificial urinary sphincters in men with post-prostatectomy urinary incontinence despite adverse implantation features. J Urol 148:1166, 1992.

Persky L, Herman G, Guerrier K: Non-delay in vesicovaginal fistula repair. J Urol 13:273, 1979.

Petrou SP, Barrett DM: The use of artificial genitourinary sphincter (AGUS) in female urinary incontinence. *In* Webster G, Kirby R, King L, Goldwasser B (eds): Reconstructive Urology. Boston, Blackwell Scientific Publications, 1993, p 915.

Pidutti RW, George SW, Morales A: Correction of recurrent stress urinary incontinence by needle urethropexy with a vaginal wall sling. Br J Urol 73:418, 1994.

Polascik TJ, Moore RG, Rosenberg MT, Kavoussi LR: Comparison of laparoscopic and open retropubic urethropexy for treatment of stress urinary incontinence. Urology 45:647, 1995.

Pow-Sang JM, Lockhart JL, Saurez A, et al: Female urinary incontinence: Preoperative selection, surgical complications and results. J Urol 136:831, 1986.

Radomski SB, Herschorn S: Laparoscopic Burch bladder neck suspension: Early results. J Urol 155:515, 1996.

Raboy A, Albert P: Extraperitoneal endoscopic vesicourethral suspension (EEVUS). J Laparoendosc Surg 3:505, 1993.

Ral PN, Knox R, Barnar RJ, Schofield PF: Management of colovesical fistula. Br J Surg 74:362, 1987.

Ray JE, Hughes JP, Gathright JB Jr: Surgical treatment of colovesical fistula: The value of a one-stage procedure. South Med J 69:40, 1976.

Raz S: Atlas of Transvaginal Surgery. Philadelphia, WB Saunders, 1992.

Raz S: Modified bladder neck suspension for female stress incontinence. Urology 18:82, 1981.

Raz S, Bregg KJ, Nitti VW, Sussman E: Transvaginal repair of vesicovaginal fistula using a peritoneal flap. J Urol 150:56, 1993.

Raz S, Erickson DR, Sussman EM: Vaginal procedures for female stress incontinence. *In* Webster G, Kirby R, King L, Goldwasser B (eds): Reconstructive Urology. Boston, Blackwell Scientific Publications, 1993, p 885.

Raz S, Klutke CG, Golomb J: Four-corner bladder and urethral suspension for moderate cystocele. J Urol 142:712, 1989.

Raz S, Little NA, Juma S, Sussman EM: Repair of severe anterior vaginal wall prolapse (grade IV cystourethrocele). J Urol 146:98, 1991.

Raz S, McGuire EJ, Ehrlich RM, et al: Fascial sling to correct male neurogenic sphincter incompetence: The McGuire/Raz approach. J Urol 139:528, 1988.

Raz S, Siegel AL, Short JL, Snyder JA: Vaginal wall sling. J Urol 141:43, 1989.

Raz S, Sussman EM, Erickson DB, et al: The Raz bladder neck suspension: Results in 206 patients. J Urol 148:845, 1992.

Reich HA: Laparoscopic treatment of extensive pelvic adhesions, including hydrosalpinx. J Reprod Med 32:735, 1987.

Reich HA, McGlynn F: Laparoscopic repair of bladder injury. Obstet Gynecol 76:909, 1990.

Reid K, Schneider K, Fruchtman B: Closure of the bladder neck in patients undergoing continent vesicostomy for urinary incontinence. J Urol 120:40, 1978.

Rich RH, Hardy BE, Filler RM: Surgery for anomalies of the urachus. J Pediatr Surg 18:4, 1983.

Rink RC, Adams MC, Keating MA: The flip-flap technique to lengthen the urethra (Salle procedure) for treatment of neurogenic urinary incontinence. J Urol 152:799, 1994.

Rink RC, Retik AB: Ureteroileocecal sigmoidostomy and avoidance of carcinoma of the colon. *In* King LR, Stone AR, Webster GD (eds): Bladder Reconstruction and Continent Urinary Diversion. St. Louis, Mosby–Year Book, 1991, p 221.

Robertson JR: Vesicovaginal fistula: Vaginal repair. *In* Ostergard DR, Bent AE (eds): Urogynecology and Urodynamics: Theory and Practice, 3rd ed. Baltimore, Williams & Wilkins, 1991, p 189.

Rosen M: A simple artificial implantable sphincter. Br J Urol 48:676, 1976.

Salle JLP, De Fraga JCS, Amarante A, et al: Urethral lengthening with anterior bladder wall flap for urinary incontinence: A new approach. J Urol 152:803, 1994.

Sasaki H, Yoshida T, Noda K, et al: Urethral pressure profiles following radical hysterectomy. Obstet Gynecol 59:101, 1982.

Sauer HA, Klutke CG: Transvaginal sacrospinous ligament fixation for treatment of vaginal prolapse. J Urol 154:1008, 1995.

Schneider KM, Reid RE, Fruchtman B: Closure of the bladder neck in patients undergoing continent vesicostomy. J Urol 120:40, 1978.

Schreck WR, Campbell WA: The relationship of bladder outlet obstruction to urinary umbilical fistula. J Urol 108:641, 1972.

Schuessler WW, Vancaillie TG: Laparoscopic bladder neck suspension. J Laparoendosc Surg 3:169, 1991.

Scott FB, Bradley WE, Timm GW: Treatment of urinary incontinence by an implantable prosthetic sphincter. Urology 1:252, 1973.

Scott FB, Light JK, Fishman I, et al: Implantation of an artificial sphincter for urinary incontinence. Contemp Surg 18:11, 1981.

Shatila AH, Ackerman NB: Diagnosis and management of colovesical fistulas. Surg Gynecol Obstet 143:71, 1976.

Shaw PJR: Supravesical bladder neck closure. *In* Whitfield HH (ed): Genitourinary Surgery. Oxford, Butterworth-Heinemann, 1993, p 283.

Sidi AA, Reinberg Y, Gonzalez R: Comparison of the artificial sphincter implantation and bladder neck reconstruction in patients with neurogenic urinary incontinence. J Urol 138:1120, 1987.

Siegel AL, Raz S: Surgical treatment of anatomical stress incontinence. Neurourol Urodyn 7:569, 1988.

Spence HM, Allen TD: Vaginal vesicostomy for empyema of the defunctionalized bladder. J Urol 106:862, 1971.

Stamey TA: Cystoscopic suspension of the vesical neck for urinary incontinence. Surg Gynecol Obstet 136:547, 1973.

Stephens FD: Form of stress incontinence in children: Another method for bladder neck repair. Aust NZ J Surg 40:124, 1970.

Stone AR: Male incontinence. *In* Krane RJ, Siroky M, Fitzpatrick J (eds): Clinical Urology. Philadelphia, JB Lippincott, 1994, p 580.

Stovsky MD, Ignatoff JM, Blum MD, et al: Use of electrocoagulation in the treatment of vesicovaginal fistulas. J Urol 152:1443, 1994.

Stower MJ, Massey JA, Feneley RCL: Urethral closure in management of urinary incontinence. Urology 34:246, 1989.

Strawbridge LR, Kramer SA, Castillo OA, Barrett DM: Augmentation cystoplasty and the artificial genitourinary sphincter. J Urol 142:297, 1989.

Sussman EM, Erickson DR, Raz S: Stress incontinence. *In* Cohen MS, Resnick MI (eds): Reoperative Urology. Boston, Little, Brown & Co, 1995, p 173.

Tanagho EA: Bladder neck reconstruction for total urinary incontinence: 10 years of experience. J Urol 125:321, 1981.

Tanagho EA: Urethrosphincteric reconstruction for congenitally absent urethra. J Urol 116:237, 1976.

Tanagho EA, Smith DR: Clinical evaluation of a surgical technique for the correction of complete urinary incontinence. J Urol 107:402, 1972.

Tanagho EA, Smith DR, Meyers FH, Fisher R: Mechanism of urinary continence: II. Technique for surgical correction of incontinence. J Urol 101:305, 1969.

Trendelenburg F: Operations for vesico-vaginal fistula and the elevated pelvic position for operations within the abdominal cavity. Med Classics 4:964, 1940.

Turner-Warwick R: The use of the omental pedicle graft in urinary tract reconstruction. J Urol 16:341, 1976.

Turner-Warwick R: The use of pedicle grafts in the repair of urinary tract fistulae. Br J Urol 44:644, 1972.

Turner-Warwick R, Kirby RS: Principles of sphincteroplasty. *In* Webster G, Kirby R, King L, Goldwasser B (eds): Reconstructive Urology. Boston, Blackwell Scientific Publications, 1993, p. 657.

Turner-Warwick R, Wynne EJ, Askhen MH: The use of the omental pedicle graft in the repair and reconstruction of the urinary tract. Br J Surg 54:849, 1967.

Twombly GH, Marshall VF: Repair of vesicovaginal fistula caused by radiation. Surg Gynecol Obstet 83:348, 1946.

Ueda T, Iwatsubo E, Osada Y, et al: Closure of vesicovaginal fistula using a vaginal flap. J Urol 119:742, 1978.

Van den Beviere H, Vossaert R, DeRoose J, Derom F: Our experience in the treatment of imperforate anus: Anterior

Mollard's technique versus posterior approach (Stephen's technique). Acta Chir Belg 82:205, 1983.

Vancaillie TG, Schuessler W: Laparoscopic bladder neck suspension. J Laparoendosc Surg 1:169, 1991.

Walker RD III, Flack CE, Hawkins-Lee B, et al: Rectus fascial wrap: Early results of a modification of the rectus fascial sling. J Urol 154:771, 1995.

Walters W: Omental flap in the transperitoneal repair of recurring vesicovaginal fistulas. Surg Gynecol Obstet 64:74, 1937.

Wang Y, Hadley HR: Nondelayed transvaginal repair of high lying vesicovaginal fistula. J Urol 144:34, 1990.

Ward JN, Lavengood RW Jr, Nay HR, Draper JW: Diagnosis and treatment of colovesical fistula. Surg Gynecol Obstet 130:1082, 1970.

Webster GD, Kreder KJ: Voiding dysfunction following cystourethropexy: Its evaluation and management. J Urol 144:670, 1990.

Wein AJ, Malloy TR, Capiniello VL, et al: Repair of vesicovaginal fistula by a suprapubic transvesical approach. Surg Gynecol Obstet 150:57, 1980.

Wein AJ, Malloy TR, Greenberg SH, et al: Omental transposition as an aid in genitourinary reconstructive procedures. J Trauma 10:473, 1980.

Wesselhoeft CWJ, Perlmutter AD, Berg S, et al: Pathogenesis and surgical treatment of diverticulum of the bladder. Surg Gynecol Obstet 116:719, 1963.

Williams DI, Snyder HW: Anterior detrusor tube repair for urinary incontinence in children. Br J Urol 48:671, 1976.

Woodard JR, Marshall VF: Reconstruction of the female urethra to reduce post-traumatic incontinence. Surg Gynecol Obstet 113:687, 1961.

Woodside JR, Borden TA: Pubovaginal sling procedure for the management of urinary incontinence in myelodysplastic girls. J Urol 127:744, 1982.

Zeidman EJ, Chiang H, Alarcon A, Raz S: Suprapubic cystostomy using Lowsley retractor. Urology 32:54, 1988.

Zimmern PE, Hadley HR, Leach GE, et al: Trans-vaginal closure of bladder neck and placement of a suprapubic catheter for destroyed urethra after long-term indwelling catheter. J Urol 134:554, 1985.

Audiovisuals

Dickson JC, Boone T, Preminger GM: Laparoscopic Urethral Sling. Wilkes-Barre, PA, Karol Media, 1994 (6 minutes). AUA #919-2033.

Ghoniem GM: Modified Pubovaginal Sling with Pubocervical Fixation for Treatment of Complicated Stress Urinary Incontinence in Females. Wilkes-Barre, PA, Karol Media, 1991 (9 minutes). AUA #919-1174.

Goldenberg SL: Technical Aspects of Periurethral Collagen Implant in Females with Stress Urinary Incontinence. Wilkes-Barre, PA, Karol Media, 1993 (19 minutes). AUA #919-2018.

Klutke CG, Petros J: Sacrospinalis Ligament Vaginal Fixation: Operative Technique. Wilkes-Barre, PA, Karol Media, 1994 (5 minutes). AUA #919-2035.

Kreder KJ, Nygaard IE: Fascia Lata Sling Cystourethropexy. Wilkes-Barre, PA, Karol Media, 1995 (9 minutes). AUA #919-2053.

Kropp KA, Filmer RB, Spencer JR, Figeroa TE: Bladder Tube Urethral Lengthening/Reimplantation Procedure for Urinary Incontinence. Wilkes-Barre, PA, Karol Media, 1990 (22 minutes). AUA #919-1199.

Loughlin KR: The Endoscopic Fascial Sling for Treatment of Female Stress Urinary Incontinence. Wilkes-Barre, PA, Karol Media, 1995 (7 minutes). AUA #919-2047.

McDougall EM, Clayman RV: Retropubic Laparoscopic Bladder Neck Suspension. Wilkes-Barre, PA, Karol Media, 1994 (26 minutes). AUA #919-2034.

Royce P, Reisner G: Laparoscopic Extraperitoneal Bladder Neck Suspension. Wilkes-Barre, PA, Karol Media, 1995 (6 minutes). AUA #919-2044.

Winfield HN, Kreder KJ, Narepalem N: Laparoscopically-Assisted Fascia Lata Sling for Type-III Stress Urinary Incontinence. Wilkes-Barre, PA, Karol Media, 1995 (6 minutes). AUA #919-2041.

Zimmern PE, Leach GE, Dmochowski R: Transvaginal Rectocele Repair and Perineorrhaphy. Wilkes-Barre, PA, Karol Media, 1995 (9 minutes). AUA #919-2039.

Zimmern PE, Leach GE, Ganabathiand K, Sirls LT: Transvaginal Repair of Stress Urinary Incontinence Associated with a Moderate Cystocele Using the 4 Corner Suspension Procedure. Wilkes-Barre, PA, Karol Media, 1994 (11 minutes). AUA #919-2036.

NONCONTINENT URINARY DIVERSION

Abrams JS: Abdominal Stomas: Indications, Operative Techniques and Patient Care. Boston, Wright, 1984.

Adams JT: Z-stitch suture for inversion of appendiceal stump. Surg Gynecol Obstet 127:1320, 1968.

Ahlering TE, Weinberg AC, Razor B: A comparative study of the ileal conduit, Kock pouch and modified Indiana pouch. J Urol 142:1193, 1989.

Albert DJ, Persky L: Conjoined end-to-end uretero-intestinal anastomosis. J Urol 105:201, 1971.

Allen TD: Vesicostomy for the temporary diversion of the urine in small children. J Urol 123:929, 1980.

Althausen AF, Hagen-Cook K, Hendren WH III: Non-refluxing colon conduit: Experience with 70 cases. J Urol 120:35, 1978.

Arango O, Llado C, Nohales G, et al: Incidental "aseptic appendectomy" in urologic surgery. Br J Urol 73:707, 1994.

Ariyoshi A, et al: Catheterless cutaneous ureterostomy. J Urol 114:533, 1975.

Arnarson O, Straffon RA: Clinical experience with the ileal conduit in children. J Urol 102:768, 1969.

Ashken MH: Stomas continent and incontinent. Br J Urol 59:203, 1987.

Ashken MH: Urinary Diversion. Berlin, Springer-Verlag, 1982.

Atta MA: A new technique for ileal nipple fixation: Preliminary report. J Urol 144:1192, 1990.

Bagley DH, Glazier W, Osias M, et al: Retroperitoneal drainage of uretero-intestinal conduits. J Urol 121:271, 1979.

Barry JM, Pitre TM, Hodges CV: Ureteroileourethrostomy: 16-year follow-up. J Urol 115:29, 1976.

Basmajian JV: The main arteries of the large intestine. Surg Gynecol Obstet 101:585, 1959.

Bauer SB, Hendren WH, Kozakewich H, et al: Perforation of the augmented bladder. J Urol 148:699, 1992.

Beckley S, Wajsman W, Pontes JE, Murphy G: Transverse colon conduit: A method of urinary diversion after pelvic irradiation. J Urol 128:464, 1982.

Beland G, Laberge I: Cutaneous transureterostomy in children. J Urol 114:588, 1975.

Blocksom BH Jr: Bladder pouch for prolonged tubeless cystostomy. J Urol 78:398, 1957.

Bloom DA, Lieskovsky G, Rainwater G, et al: The Turnbull loop stoma. J Urol 129:715, 1983.

Bloom DA, McGuire EJ: Complications of urinary stomas. In Smith RB, Ehrlich RM (eds): Complications of Urologic Surgery. Philadelphia, WB Saunders, 1990, p 319.

Bloom DA, Turner WRJ, Skinner DG: Urological Stomas. In Ehrlich RM (ed): Modern Techniques in Surgery: Urologic Surgery. Mt. Kisco, NY, Futura Publishing Co, 1981, p 19-1.

Bricker EM: Bladder substitution after pelvic evisceration. Surg Clin North Am 30:1511, 1950.

Bricker EM: The evolution of the ileal segment bladder substitution operation. Am J Surg 135:834, 1978.

Browning GG, Parks AG: A method and the results of loop colostomy. Dis Colon Rectum 26:223, 1983.

Bruce RB, Gonzales ET: Cutaneous vesicostomy: A useful form of temporary diversion in children. J Urol 123:927, 1980.

Bryniak SR, Bruce AW, Awad SA: Skin flap technique in formation of urinary conduit stoma. Urology 15:275, 1980.

Burbige KA, Hensle TW: The complications of urinary tract reconstruction. J Urol 136(pt 2):292, 1986.

Burgers JK, Quinlan DM, Brendler CB: Improved technique for creation of ileal conduit stoma. J Urol 144:1188, 1990.

Bystrom J: Early and later complications of ileal conduit urinary diversion. Scand J Urol Nephrol 12:233, 1978.

Chancellor M, Grossman HB, Konnak J, et al: Biocarbon ureterostomy device for urinary diversion. Urology 34:18, 1989.

Clark SS: Electrolyte disturbance associated with jejunal conduit. J Urol 112:42, 1974.

Cohen JS, Harbach LB, Kaplan GW: Cutaneous vesicostomy for temporary diversion in infants with neurogenic bladder dysfunction. J Urol 119:120, 1978.

Coleman TW, Libertino JA: Complications associated with ileal and colon conduits. In Cohen MS, Resnick MI (eds): Reoperative Urology. Boston, Little, Brown & Co, 1995, p 275.

Connar RG, Sealy WC: Gastrostomy and its complications. Am Surg 138:732, 1979.

Cukier J, Charbit L, Terdjman S, Nahas W: Direct cutaneous ureterostomy: A new technique. J Urol 90:345, 1984.

Dager JE, Sanford EJ, Rohner TJ Jr: Complications of the nonrefluxing colon conduit. J Urol 123:585, 1980.

Daniel O, Shackman R: The blood supply of the human ureter in relation to ureterocolic anastomosis. Br J Urol 24:334, 1952.

David FDR: A new surgical procedure for revision of the ileal conduit stoma in children. J Urol 115:188, 1976.

Donovan JF, Winfield HN, Williams RD: Construction of the intestinal stoma with an intraluminal stapling device. J Urol 142:1279, 1989.

Dretler SP: The pathogenesis of urinary tract calculi occurring after ileal conduit diversion: I. Clinical study. II. Conduit study. III. Prevention. J Urol 109:204, 1973.

Duckett JW Jr: Cutaneous vesicostomy in childhood: The Blocksom technique. Urol Clin North Am 1:485, 1974.

Dwoskin JY: Management of the massively dilated urinary tract in infants by temporary diversion and single-stage reconstruction. Urol Clin North Am 1:515, 1974.

Dyber R, Jeter K, Lattimer JK: Comparison of intraluminal pressures in ileal and colon conduits in children. J Urol 108:477, 1972.

Eckstein HB: Cutaneous ureterostomy. Proc R Soc Med 56:749, 1963.

Eigner EB, Freiha FS: The fate of the remaining bladder following supravesical diversion. J Urol 144:31, 1990.

Eiseman B, Bricker EM: Electrolyte absorption following bilateral ureteroenterostomy into an isolated intestinal segment. Ann Surg 136:761, 1952.

Ekman H, Jacobsson B, Kock N, Sundin T: The functional behavior of different types of intestinal urinary bladder substitutes. Cong Soc Int Urol 11:213, 1964.

Elder JS, Snyder HM, Hulbert WC, Duckett JW: Perforation of the augmented bladder in patients undergoing clean intermittent catheterization. J Urol 140:1159, 1988.

Emmett D, Noble MJ, Mebust WK: A comparison of end versus loop stomas for ileal conduit urinary diversion. J Urol 133:588, 1985.

Esho J, Cass AS: Management of stomal encrustations in children. J Urol 108:797, 1972.

Fasth S, Hulten L: Loop ileostomy: A superior diverting stoma in colorectal surgery. World J Surg 8:401, 1984.

Faxén A, Kock NG, Sundin T: Long-term functional results after ileocystoplasty. Scand J Urol Nephrol 7:127, 1973.

Feneley RCL: The management of female incontinence by suprapubic catheterisation, with or without urethral closure. Br J Urol 55:203, 1983.

Flinn RA, King LR, McDonald JH, et al: Cutaneous ureterostomy: An alternative urinary diversion. J Urol 105:358, 1971.

Garcia VF, Bloom DA: Inversion appendectomy. Urology 2:142, 1986.

Gil-Vernet JM Jr: The ileocolic segment in urologic surgery. J Urol 94:418, 1965.

Gonzales ET Jr: Vesicostomy, ureterostomy, and pyelostomy. In Cohen MS, Resnick MI (eds): Reoperative Urology. Boston, Little, Brown & Co, 1995, p 303.

Goodwin WE: Ileocystoplasty. In Cooper P (ed): Craft of Surgery. Boston, Little, Brown & Co, 1964, p 1139.

Goodwin WE, Turner RD, Winter CC: Results of ileocystoplasty. J Urol 80:461, 1958.

Goodwin WE, Winter CC: Technique of sigmoidocystoplasty. Surg Gynecol Obstet 108:370, 1959.

Green D, Mitcheson HD, McGuire EJ: Management of the bladder by augmentation ileocecocystoplasty. J Urol 130:133, 1981.

Hendren WH, Radopoulous D: Complications of ileal loop and colon conduit urinary diversion. Urol Clin North Am 10:451, 1983.

Hendren WH: Complications of ureterostomy. J Urol 120:269, 1978.

Hendren WH: Non-refluxing colon conduit for temporary or permanent urinary diversion in children. J Pediatr Surg 10:381, 1975.

Hinman F, Weyrauch HM: A critical study of the different principles of surgery which have been used in uretero-intestinal implantation. Int Abstracts Med 64:313, 1937.

Hinman F Jr: Leakage and reflux in uretero-intestinal anastomosis: I. The free peritoneal graft. J Urol 70:419, 1953.

Hinman F Jr: Ureteral implantation: II. Clinical results from a method of open submucosal anastomosis. J Urol 64:567, 1950.

Hinman F Jr: Urinary conduction versus storage by isolated ileal segment. In Proceedings of the 11th Congress of the International Society of Urology, Stockholm, June 25–30, 1958, p 37.

Hinman F Jr, Hinman F Sr: Ureteral implantation: I. Experiments on the surgical principles involved in an open submucosal method of ureterointestinal anastomosis. J Urol 64:457, 1950.

Hinman F Jr, Oppenheimer R: Functional characteristics of the ileal segment as a valve. J Urol 80:448, 1958.

Jaffe BM, Bricker EM, Butcher HR Jr: Surgical complications of ileal segment urinary diversion. Ann Surg 167:367, 1968.

Jeter KF: The flush versus the protruding urinary stoma. J Urol 116:424, 1976.

Jeter KF, Lattimer JK: Common stomal problems following ileal conduit urinary diversion. Urology 3:399, 1974.

Johnston JH: Temporary cutaneous ureterostomy in the management of advanced congenital urinary obstruction. Arch Dis Child 38:161, 1963.

Kalble T, Tricker AR, Friedl P, et al: Ureterosigmoidostomy: Long-term results, risk of carcinoma and aetiological factors for carcinogenesis. J Urol 145:1110, 1990.

Kass EJ, Koff SA: Bladder augmentation in the pediatric neuropathic bladder. J Urol 129:552, 1983.

Kaufman JJ: Repair of parastomal hernia by translocation of the stoma without laparotomy. J Urol 129:278, 1983.

Kelalis PP: Urinary diversion in children by the sigmoid conduit: Its advantages and limitations. J Urol 112:666, 1974.

Kennedy HA, Adams MC, Mitchell ME, et al: Chronic renal failure and bladder augmentation: Stomach versus sigmoid colon in the canine model. J Urol 140:1138, 1988.

King LR: Technique of ileal conduit: Evolution of the Brady method. Papers presented in honor of WW Scott. New York, Plenum Publications, 1972.

King LR, Scott WW: Pyeloileocutaneous anastomosis. Surg Gynecol Obstet 119:281, 1964.

King LR, Stone AR, Webster GD (eds): Bladder Reconstruction and Continent Urinary Diversion. Chicago, Year Book Medical Publishers, 1987.

Koch ME, McDougal WS, Reddy PK, Lange PH: Metabolic alterations following continent urinary diversion through colonic segments. J Urol 145:270, 1991.

Kock NG, Hultén L, Leandoer L: A study of the motility in different parts of the human colon: Resting activity, response to feeding and to prostigmine. Scand J Gastroenterol 3:163, 1968.

Kozminski M, Partamian KO: Case report of laparoscopic ileal loop conduit. J Endourol 6:147, 1992.

Kramolowsky EV, Clayman RV, Weyman PJ: Management of ureterointestinal anastomotic strictures: Comparison of open surgical and endourological repair. J Urol 139:1195, 1988.

Kretschner KP: The intestinal stoma. Major Probl Clin Surg 24:98, 1978.

Kristjánsson A, Bajc M, Wallin L, et al: Renal function up to 16 years after conduit (refluxing or anti-reflux anastomosis) or continent urinary diversion. 2. Renal scarring and location of bacteriuria. Br J Urol 76:546, 1995.

Lapides J: The abdominal neourethra. J Urol 95:350, 1966.

Lapides J: Butterfly cutaneous ureterostomy. J Urol 88:735, 1962.

Lapides J, Ajemian EP, Lichtwardt JR: Cutaneous vesicostomy. J Urol 84:609, 1960.

Lapides J, Diokno AC, Gould FR, et al: Clean intermittent self-catheterization in the treatment of urinary tract disease. J Urol 107:458, 1972.

Leibovitch I, Rowland RG, Goldwasser B, Donohue JP: Incidental appendectomy during urological surgery. J Urol 154:1110, 1995.

Libertino JA, Zinman L: Ileocecal antirefluxing conduit. Surg Clin North Am 62:999, 1982.

Lieskovsky G, Bloom DA: Creation of a Turnbull loop stoma. In Skinner DG (ed): Genitourinary Cancer. Philadelphia, WB Saunders, 1987, p 649.

Light JK: Enteroplasty to ablate bowel contractions in the reconstructed bladder: A case report. J Urol 134:958, 1985.

Linder A, Leach GE, Raz S: Augmentation cystoplasty in the treatment of neurogenic bladder dysfunction. J Urol 129:491, 1983.

Lingam K, Paterson PJ, Lingam MK, et al: Subcutaneous urinary diversion: An alternative to percutaneous nephrostomy. J Urol 152:70, 1994.

Lrimpi HD, Khubchandovic IT, Sheets JA, Stasik JJ: Advances in intestinal anastomoses. Dis Colon Rectum 20:107, 1977.

Lytton B, Weiss RM: Cutaneous vesicostomy for temporary urinary diversion in infants. J Urol 105:888, 1971.

Marshall FF, Leadbetter WF, Dretler SP: Ileal conduit parastomal hernias. J Urol 144:40, 1975.

Martin EC, Fankuchen EI, Casarella WJ: Percutaneous dilation of ureteroenteric strictures or occlusions in ileal conduit. Urol Radiol 4:19, 1982.

Mathisen W: A new method of ureterointestinal anastomosis: Preliminary report. Surg Gynecol Obstet 96:255, 1953.

Mathisen W: Open-loop sigmoido-cystoplasty. Acta Chir Scand 110:227, 1955.

Matsuura T, Tsujihashi H, Park YC, et al: Assessment of the long-term results of ileocaecal conduit urinary diversion. Urol Int 46:154, 1991.

Mayo ME, Chapman WH: Management of ileal conduit obstruction: A urodynamic study. J Urol 125:828, 1981.

Michie AJ, Borns P, Ames MD: Improvement following tubeless suprapubic cystostomy of myelomeningocele patients with hydronephrosis and recurrent acute pyelonephritis. J Pediatr Surg 1:347, 1966.

Mingledorff WE, Rinker JR, Owen G: Experimental study of the blood supply of the distal ureter with reference to cutaneous ureterostomy. J Urol 92:424, 1964.

Mininberg DT, Genvert HP: Posterior urethral valves: Role of temporary and permanent urinary diversion. Urology 33:205, 1989.

Mitchell ME: The role of bladder augmentation in undiversion. J Pediatr Surg 16:790, 1981.

Mitchell ME, Rink RC: Urinary diversion and undiversion. Urol Clin North Am 12:111, 1985.

Mitchell ME, Yoder IC, Pfister RC, et al: Ileal loop stenosis: A late complication of urinary diversion. J Urol 118:957, 1977.

Mogg RA: The result of urinary diversion using the colonic conduit. Br J Urol 97:684, 1967.

Mogg RA: The treatment of urinary incontinence using the colonic conduit. J Urol 97:684, 1967.

Monfort G, Guy JM, Morrisson-Lacombe G: Appendicovesicostomy: An alternative urinary diversion in the child. Eur Urol 10:361, 1984.

Moorcraft J, DuBoulay CEH, Isaacson P, Atwell JD: Changes in the mucosa of colon conduits with particular reference to the risk of malignant change. Br J Urol 55:185, 1983.

Mor Y, Ramon J, Raviv G, et al: Low loop cutaneous ureterostomy and subsequent reconstruction: 20 years of experience. J Urol 147:1595, 1992.

Namiki T, Yanagi S: A new technique for bilateral single stoma loop cutaneous ureterostomy. J Urol 154:361, 1995.

Naude JH: The hidden vesicostomy. Br J Urol 541:686, 1982.

Nesbit RM: Ureterosigmoid anastomosis by direct elliptical connection: A preliminary report. J Urol 61:728, 1949.

Netto NR Jr, et al: Ileocecal cystoplasty: Videotape poster. J Urol 131:141, 1984.

Ochsner A: The relative merits of temporary gastrostomy and nasogastric suction of the stomach. Am J Surg 133:729, 1977.

Parra RO, Cummings JM, Boullier JA: Simple detubularization technique for construction of continent colonic urinary reservoirs. Urology 44:35, 1994.

Perlmutter AD: Spiral advancement skin flap for stomal revision. J Urol 114:131, 1975.

Perlmutter AD, Tank ES: Ileal conduit stasis in children: Recognition and treatment. J Urol 101:688, 1969.

Perlmutter AD, Tank ES: Loop cutaneous ureterostomy. J Urol 99:559, 1968.

Persky L: Relocation of ileal stomas. J Urol 96:702, 1966.

Pitts WR, Muecke EC: A 20-year experience with ileal conduit: The fate of the kidneys. J Urol 122:154, 1979.

Pokorny M, Pontes JE, Pierce JM Jr: Ureterostomy in-situ. Urology 8:447, 1976.

Rabinowitz R, Barkin M, Schillinger JF, et al: Surgical treatment of the massively dilated ureter in children: I. Management by cutaneous ureterostomy. J Urol 117:658, 1977.

Rabinowitz R, Barkin M, Schillinger JF, et al: Upper tract management when posterior urethral valve ablation is insufficient. J Urol 122:370, 1979.

Ravitch MM: Observations on the healing of wounds of the intestines. Surgery 77:665, 1975.

Redman JF: Extensive shortening of ileal conduit through peristomal incision. Urology 9:45, 1977.

Redman JF: Techniques to enhance the ileal conduit. Urol Clin North Am 17:125, 1990.

Resnick MJ, Caldamone AA (eds): Use of large and small bowel in urologic surgery. Urol Clin North Am 13:177, 1986.

Richardson JR Jr, Linton PC, Leadbetter GW Jr: A new concept in the treatment of stomal stenosis. J Urol 108:159, 1972.

Richie JP: Nonrefluxing sigmoid conduit for urinary diversion. Urol Clin North Am 6:469, 1979.

Rickwood AMK: Urinary diversion in children. In Ashken MH (ed): Urinary Diversion. Berlin, Springer-Verlag, 1982, p 22.

Rosen MA, Roth DR, Gonzales ET Jr: Current indications for cutaneous ureterostomy. Urology 43:92, 1994.

Rovner E, Turek P, Duckett J: Ureterostomy in-situ: Rediscovering an old technique. Soc Pediatr Urol Newsl, December 5, 1991.

Rowland RG: Continent cutaneous diversion using ileocecal segment. In Crawford ED, Das S (eds): Current Genitourinary Cancer Surgery. Philadelphia, Lea & Febiger, 1990, p 284.

Sagalowsky AI: Further experience with the ileocecal conduit urinary diversion. J Urol 135:39, 1986.

Salley R, Bucher RM, Rodring CB: Colostomy closure: Morbidity reduction employing a semi-standardized protocol. Dis Colon Rectum 26:319, 1983.

Scardino PT, Bagley DH, Javadpour N, Ketchom AS: Sigmoid conduit urinary diversion. Urology 6:167, 1975.

Scherster T: Studies of the motorial function in the ileal segment in cutaneous uretero-ileostomy. Acta Clin Scand 124:149, 1962.

Schlesinger RE, Berman ML, Ballon SC, et al: The choice of an intestinal segment for a urinary conduit. Surg Gynecol Obstet 148:45, 1979.

Schmidt JD, Buchsbaum HJ, Jacobo EC: Transverse colon conduit for supravesical urinary tract diversion. Urology 8:542, 1976.

Schmidt JD, Buchsbaum HJ, Nachtsheim DA: Long-term follow-up, further experience with and modifications of the transverse colon conduit in urinary tract diversion. Br J Urol 57:284, 1985.

Schultz LS, Petrafitta JJ, Graber JN, et al: Retrograde laparoscopic appendectomy: Report of a case. J Laparoendosc Surg 1:111, 1991.

Schrock TR, Deveney CW, Dunphy JE: Factors contributing to leakage of colonic anastomoses. Ann Surg 177:513, 1973.

Schwartz SL, Kennelly MJ, McGuire EJ, et al: Incontinent ileovesicostomy urinary diversion in the treatment of lower urinary tract dysfunction. J Urol 152:99, 1994.

Senn E, Thüroff JW, Barandhauer K: Urodynamics of ileal conduits in adults. Eur Urol 10:401, 1984.

Shafik A: Stomal stenosis after cutaneous ureterostomy: Etiology and management. J Urol 105:65, 1971.

Shaw PJR: Supravesical urinary diversion. In Webster G, Kirby R, King L, Goldwasser B (eds): Reconstructive Urology. Boston, Blackwell Scientific Publications, 1993, p 283.

Sidi AA, Reinberg Y, Gonzalez R: Influence of intestinal segment and configuration on the outcome of augmentation enterocystoplasty. J Urol 136:1201, 1986.

Skinner DG, Gottesman JE, Richie JP: The isolated sigmoid segment: Its value in temporary urinary diversion and reconstruction. J Urol 113:614, 1975.

Smith ED: Follow-up study on 150 ileal conduits in children. J Pediatr Surg 7:1, 1972.

Smith GI, Hinman F Jr: The intussuscepted ileal cystostomy. J Urol 73:261, 1955.

Smith RB, Van Cangh P, Skinner DG, et al: Augmentation enterocystoplasty: A critical review. J Urol 118:35, 1977.

Spence HM, Allen TD: Vaginal vesicostomy for empyema of the defunctionalized bladder. J Urol 106:862, 1971.

Stevens PS, Eckstein HB: Ileal conduit diversion in children. Br J Urol 49:379, 1977.

Stone AR: Ileocystoplasty. In King LR, Stone AR, Webster GD (eds): Bladder Reconstruction and Continent Urinary Diversion. Chicago, Mosby–Year Book, 1991, p 58.

Straffon RA, Kyle K, Corvalan J: Techniques of cutaneous ureterostomy and results in 51 patients. J Urol 103:138, 1970.

Tasker JH: Ileo-cystoplasty: A new technique (an experimental study with report of a case). Br J Urol 25:349, 1953.

Turner-Warwick R: Cystoplasty. In Blandy JP (ed): Urology. Oxford, Blackwell Scientific Publications, 1976, p 840.

Turner-Warwick R, Ashken MH: The functional results of partial, subtotal and total cystoplasty with special reference to ureterocaecocystoplasty, selective sphincterotomy and cystocystoplasty. Br J Urol 39:3, 1967.

Van Poppel H, Baert L: The percutaneous operative gastrostomy for gastric decompression in major urological surgery. J Urol 145:100, 1991.

Vose SN, Dixey GM: Ureterostomy in-situ. J Urol 69:503, 1953.

Wallace DM: Ureteric diversion using a conduit: Simplified technique. Br J Urol 38:522, 1966.

Walsh A: Ureterostomy in-situ. Br J Urol 39:744, 1967.

Weakley FL, Turnbull RB Jr: Special intestinal procedures. In Stewart BH (ed): Operative Urology. Baltimore, Williams & Wilkins, 1975, p 322.

Weiss JP: Sigmoidocystoplasty to augment bladder capacity. Surg Gynecol Obstet 159:377, 1984.

Wells CA: The use of the intestine in urology. Br J Urol 28:335, 1956.

Wespes E, Stone AR, King LR: Ileocaecocystoplasty in urinary tract reconstruction in children. J Urol 58:266, 1986.

Wilbert DM, Hohenfellner R: Colonic conduit: Preoperative requirements, operative techniques, postoperative management. World J Urol 2:159, 1984.

Williams DI, Cromie WJ: Ring ureterostomy. Br J Urol 47:789, 1976.

Williams DI, Rabinovitch HH: Cutaneous ureterostomy for the grossly dilated ureter of childhood. Br J Urol 39:696, 1967.

Williams DI, Snyder H: Anterior detrusor tube repair for urinary incontinence in children. Br J Urol 48:671, 1976.

Zinman L, Libertino JA: The ileocecal conduit for temporary and permanent urinary diversion. J Urol 113:317, 1975.

Zinman L, Libertino JA: The ileocecal segment: An antirefluxing colonic conduit form of urinary diversion. Surg Clin North Am 56:733, 1976.

Audiovisual

Marberger M: Transverse Colon Conduit. Wilkes-Barre, PA, Karol Media, 1981 (25 minutes). AUA #919-1126.

CONTINENT DIVERSION

Adams MC, Bihrle R, Foster RS, et al: Conversion of ileal conduit to continent catheterizable stoma. J Urol 147:751, 1991.

Adams MC, Retik AB: Complications of ureterosigmoidostomy. In Cohen MS, Resnick MI (eds): Reoperative Urology. Boston, Little, Brown & Co, 1995, p 297.

Ahlering TE, Weinberg AC, Razor B: A comparative study of the ileal conduit, Kock pouch and modified Indiana pouch. J Urol 142:1193, 1989.

Ahlering TE, Weinberg AC, Razor B: Modified Indiana Pouch. J Urol 145:1156, 1991.

Akerlund S, Delin K, Kock N, et al: Renal function and upper urinary tract configuration following urinary diversion to a continent ileal reservoir (Kock pouch): A prospective 5 to 11 year followup after reservoir construction. J Urol 142:964, 1989.

Arai Y, Kawakita M, Terachi T, et al: Long-term follow-up of Kock and Indiana pouch procedures. (Editorial Comment by R. G. Rowland.) J Urol 150:51, 1993.

Arai Y, Okada Y, Matsuda T, et al: Afferent nipple valve malfunction caused by anchoring collar: An unexpected late complication of the Kock continent ileal reservoir. J Urol 145:29, 1991.

Ashken MH: An appliance-free ileocaecal urinary diversion: Preliminary communication. Br J Urol 46:631, 1974.

Ashken MH: Stomas continent and incontinent. Br J Urol 59:203, 1987.

Bejany DE, Politano VA: Stapled and nonstapled tapered distal ileum for construction of a continent colonic urinary reservoir. J Urol 140:491, 1988.

Bejany DE, Suarez G, Penalver M, Politano V: Nontunneled ureterocolonic anastomosis: An alternate to the tunneled implantation. J Urol 142:961, 1989.

Benchekroun A: Continent caecal bladder. Br J Urol 54:505, 1982.

Benchekroun A: The ileocecal continent bladder. In King LR, Stone AR, Webster GD (eds): Bladder Reconstruction and Continent Urinary Diversion. Chicago, Mosby–Year Book, 1991, p 324.

Benchekroun A, Essakalli N, Falk M, et al: Continent urostomy with hydraulic ileal valve in 136 patients: 13 years of experience. J Urol 142:46, 1989.

Bennett RC, Duthie HL: The functional importance of the internal anal sphincter. Br J Surg 51:355, 1964.

Berglund B, Kock NG, Norlen L, Philipson BM: Volume capacity and pressure characteristics of the continent ileal reservoir used for urinary diversion. J Urol 137:29, 1987.

Bissada NK: Characteristics and use of in situ appendix as continent catheterization stoma for continent urinary diversion in adults. J Urol 150:151, 1993.

Bissada NK: New continent ileocolonic urinary reservoir: Charleston pouch with minimally altered in situ appendix stoma. Urology 41:524, 1993.

Bissada NK, Morcos RR, Morgan WM, Hanash KA: Ureterosigmoidostomy: Is it a viable procedure in the age of continent urinary diversion and bladder substitution? J Urol 153:1429, 1995.

Bloom DA, Grossman HB, Konnak JW: Stomal construction and reconstruction. Urol Clin North Am 13:275, 1986.

Boyd SD: Continent urinary diversion: Koch pouch. In Webster G, Kirby R, King L, Goldwasser B (eds): Reconstructive Urology. Boston, Blackwell Scientific Publications, 1993, p 517.

Camey M: Bladder replacement by ileocystoplasty following radical cystectomy. World J Urol 3:161, 1985.

Canning DA, Perman JA, Gearhart JP: Nutritional consequences of bowel segments in the lower urinary tract. J Urol 142:509, 1989.

Carini M, Serni S, Lapini A, et al: Second stage reconfiguration of Camey 1 ileal bladder improves its urodynamic and clinical characteristics. Urology 44:425, 1994.

Cartwright PC, Snow BW, Reid BS, Shultz PK: Color Doppler ultrasound in newborn testis torsion. Urology 45:667, 1995.

Cendron M, Gearhart JP: The Mitrofanoff principle: Technique and application in urinary diversion. Urol Clin North Am 18:615, 1991.

Coffey RC: Transplantation of the ureters into the large intestine in the absence of the functioning urinary bladder. Surg Gynecol Obstet 32:383, 1921.

Cordonnier JJ: Ureterosigmoid anastomosis. J Urol 63:275, 1950.

Cordonnier JJ: Urinary diversion. Arch Surg 71:818, 1955.

Crane JM, Scherz HS, Billman GF, Kaplan GW: Ischemic necrosis: A hypothesis to explain the pathogenesis of spontaneously ruptured enterocystoplasty. J Urol 146:141, 1991.

Creevy CD: Facts about ureterosigmoidostomy. JAMA 151:120, 1953.

Davidsson T, Barker SB, Mansson W: Tapering of intussuscepted ileal nipple valve or ileocecal valve to correct secondary incontinence in patients with urinary reservoir. J Urol 147:144, 1992.

Decter RM: Use of the fascial sling for neurogenic incontinence: Lessons learned. J Urol 150:683, 1993.

DeKernion JB, DenBesten L, Kaufman JJ, Ehrlich R: The Kock pouch as a urinary reservoir: Pitfalls and perspectives. Am J Surg 150:83, 1985.

Diamond DA, Ransley PG: Bladder neck reconstruction with omentum, silicone and augmentation cystoplasty—a preliminary report. J Urol 136:252, 1986.

Dounis A, Abel BJ, Gow JG: Cecocystoplasty for bladder augmentation. J Urol 123:164, 1980.

Dretler SP, Hendren WH, Leadbetter WF: Urinary tract reconstruction following ileal conduit diversion. J Urol 109:217, 1973.

Duckett JW: Ureterosigmoidostomy: The pros and cons. Dial Pediatr Urol 5:4, 1982.

Duckett JW, Gazak JM: Complications of ureterosigmoidostomy. Urol Clin North Am 10:473, 1983.

Duckett JW, Lotfi A-H: Appendicovesicostomy (and variations) in bladder reconstruction. J Urol 149:567, 1993.

Duckett JW, Snyder HMc III: Use of the Mitrofanoff principle in urinary reconstruction. World J Urol 3:191, 1985.

Eiseman B, Bricker EM: Electrolyte absorption following bilateral ureteroenterostomy into an isolated intestinal segment. Ann Surg 136:761, 1952.

Engelmann UH, Light JK, Scott FB: Use of artificial urinary sphincter with lower urinary tract reconstruction and continent urinary diversion: Clinical and experimental studies. In King LR (ed): Bladder Reconstruction and Continent Urinary Diversion. Chicago, Year Book Medical Publishers, 1986.

Fekety R, Shah AB: Diagnosis and treatment of Clostridium difficile colitis. JAMA 269:71, 1993.

Ferris DO, Odel HM: Electrolyte pattern of the blood after bilateral ureterosigmoidostomy. JAMA 142:634, 1950.

Figueroa TE, Sabogal L, Helal M, Lockhart JL: The tapered and reimplanted small bowel as a variation of the Mitrofanoff procedure: Preliminary results. J Urol 152:73, 1994.

Filmer RB: Malignant tumors arising in bladder augmentations, and ileal and colon conduits. Soc Pediatr Urol Newsl, December 9, 1986.

Firlit CF, Sommer JT, Kaplan WE: Pediatric urinary undiversion. J Urol 123:748, 1980.

Fisch M, Wammack RE, Hohenfellner R: The Mainz Pouch procedure (mixed augmentation, ileum and cecum). In Webster G, Kirby R, King L, Goldwasser B (eds): Reconstructive Urology. Boston, Blackwell Scientific Publications, 1993, p. 459.

Fisch M, Wammack R, Müller SC, Hohenfellner R: The Mainz Pouch II (sigma rectum pouch). J Urol 149:258, 1993.

Fisch M, Wammack R, Spies, F et al: Ileocecal valve reconstruction during continent urinary diversion. J Urol 151:861, 1994.

Freiha FS: Continent diversion to the urethra (bladder substitution). In Crawford ED, Das S (eds): Current Genitourinary Cancer Surgery. Philadelphia, Lea & Febiger, 1990, p 294.

Gadacz TR, Kelly KA, Phillips SF: The continent ileal pouch: Absorptive and motor features. Gastroenterology 72:1287, 1977.

Gardiner RA: The invaginated sleeve technique for a continent cystostomy—five years' clinical experience. Br J Urol 74:35, 1994.

Gasparini ME, Hinman F Jr, Presti JC, et al: Continence after radical cystoprostatectomy and total bladder replacement: Urodynamic analysis. J Urol 148:1861, 1992.

Gersuny R, cited by Foges: Officielles protokoll der k.k. gesellshaft der Aerzte in Wien. Wien Klin Wochenschr 11:990, 1898.

Ghoneim MA: Urinary diversion to the modified rectal bladder: An anal sphincter controlled bladder substitute. In Webster G, Kirby R, King L, Goldwasser B (eds): Reconstructive Urology. Boston, Blackwell Scientific Publications, 1993, p 549.

Ghoneim MA, Ashamallah AK, Mahran MR, Kock NG: Further experience with the modified rectal bladder (the augmented and valved rectum) for urine diversion. J Urol 147:1252, 1992.

Ghoneim MA, Kock NG, Lycke G, el-Din AB: An appliance-free sphincter-controlled bladder substitute: The urethral Kock pouch. J Urol 138:1150, 1987.

Ghoneim MA, Shehab-El-Din AB, Ashamallah AK, Gaballah MA: Evolution of the rectal bladder as a method for urinary diversion. J Urol 126:737, 1981.

Ginsberg D, Huffman JL, Lieskovsky G, et al: Urinary tract stones: A complication of the Kock pouch continent urinary diversion. J Urol 145:956, 1991.

Gittes RF: Carcinogenesis in ureterosigmoidostomy. Urol Clin North Am 13:201, 1986.

Golimbu M, Farcon E, Provet J, et al: Bellevue pouch: Ileocolonic continent urinary reservoir. Urology 41:511, 1993.

Golomb J, Klutke CG, Raz S: Complications of bladder substitution and continent urinary diversion. Urology 34:329, 1989.

Gonzalez R: Reconstruction of the female urethra to allow intermittent catheterization for neurogenic bladders and urogenital sinus anomalies. J Urol 133:478, 1985.

Gonzalez R, LaPointe S, Sheldon CA, Mauer SM: Undiversion in children with renal failure. J Pediatr Surg 19:632, 1984.

Gonzalez R, Sheldon CA: Artificial sphincters in children with neurogenic bladders: Long-term results. J Urol 128:1270, 1982.

Gonzalez R, Sidi AA: Preoperative prediction of continence after enterocystoplasty or undiversion in children with neurogenic bladder. J Urol 134:705, 1985.

Goodwin WE, Harris AP, Kaufman JJ, Beal JM: Open, transcolonic ureterointestinal anastomosis: A new approach. Surg Gynecol Obstet 97:295, 1953.

Goodwin WE, Scardino PT: Ureterosigmoidostomy. J Urol 118:169, 1977.

Goodwin WE, Smith RB, Skinner DG (eds): Complications of ureterosigmoidostomy. In Smith RB, Skinner GD (eds): Complications of Urologic Surgery: Prevention and Management. Philadelphia, WB Saunders, 1976, p 229.

Gosalbez R, Padron OF, Singla AK, et al: The gastric augment single pedicle tube catheterizable stoma: A useful adjunct to reconstruction of the urinary tract. J Urol 152:2005, 1994.

Gosalbez R Jr, Woodard JR, Broecker BH, et al: The use of stomach in pediatric urinary reconstruction. J Urol 150:438, 1993.

Griffiths DM, Malone PS: The Malone antegrade continence enema. J Pediatr Surg 30:68, 1995.

Harrison MR, Glick PL, Nakayama DL, et al: Loop colon rectovaginoplasty for high cloacal anomaly. J Pediatr Surg 18:885, 1983.

Hasan ST, Marshall C, Neal DE: Continent urinary diversion using the Mitrofanoff principle. Br J Urol 74:454, 1994.

Hautmann RE, Egghart G, Frohneberg D, Miller K: The ileal neobladder. J Urol 139:39, 1988.

Hawley PR, Hunt TK, Dunphy JE: Etiology of colonic anastomotic leaks. Proc R Soc Med 63:28, 1970.

Heitz-Boyer M, Hovelacque A: Creation a une nouvelle vessie et un nouvel uretre. J Urol (Paris) 1:237, 1912.

Helal MA, Figueroa TE, Pow-Sang J, et al: A trans-reservoir technique for correction of ureterointestinal obstruction in continent urinary diversion. J Urol 153:1108, 1995.

Helal MA, Pow-Sang J, Sanford E, et al: Direct (nontunneled) ureterocolonic reimplantation in association with continent reservoirs. J Urol 150:835, 1993.

Hendren WH: Further experience in reconstructive surgery for cloacal anomalies. J Pediatr Surg 17:695, 1982.

Hendren WH: Ileal nipple for continence in cloacal exstrophy. J Urol 148:372, 1992.

Hendren WH: Non-refluxing colon conduit for temporary or permanent urinary diversion in children. J Pediatr Surg 10:381, 1975.

Hendren WH: Reconstruction of previously diverted urinary tracts in children. J Pediatr Surg 8:135, 1973.

Hendren WH: Some alternatives to urinary diversion in children. J Urol 119:652, 1978.

Hendren WH: Techniques for urinary undiversion. In King LR, Stone AR, Webster GD (eds): Bladder Reconstruction and Continent Urinary Diversion. Chicago, Year Book Medical Publishers, 1987, p 147.

Hendren WH: Ureterocolic diversion of urine: Management of some difficult problems. J Urol 129:719, 1983.

Hendren WH: Urinary diversion and undiversion in children. Surg Clin North Am 56:425, 1976.

Hendren WH: Urinary tract re-functionalization after long-term diversion: A 20-year experience with 177 patients. Ann Surg 212:478, 1990.

Hendren WH: Urinary tract refunctionalization after prior diversion in children. Ann Surg 180:494, 1974.

Hendren WH: Urinary undiversion and augmentation cystoplasty. In Kelalis PP, King LR, Belman AB (eds): Clinical Pediatric Urology, 2nd ed, vol 1. Philadelphia, WB Saunders, 1985, p 620.

Henriet MP, Neyra P, Elman B: Kock pouch procedures: Continuing experience and evolution in 135 cases. J Urol 145:16, 1991.

Hensle TW, Connor JP, Burbidge KA: Continent urinary diversion in childhood. J Urol 143:981, 1990.

Hensle TW, Dean GE: Complications of urinary tract reconstruction. Urol Clin North Am 18:755, 1991.

Hill DE, Kramer SA: Management of pregnancy after augmentation cystoplasty. J Urol 144:457, 1990.

Hinman F, Weyrauch HM: A critical study of the different principles of surgery which have been used in uretero-intestinal implantation. Int Abstracts Med 64:313, 1937.

Hinman F Jr: Functional classification of conduits for continent diversion. J Urol 144:27, 1990.

Hinman F Jr: Leakage and reflux in uretero-intestinal anastomosis: I. The free peritoneal graft. J Urol 70:419, 1953.

Hinman F Jr: Overview: The choice between ureterosigmoidostomy with perineal (Gersuny, Heitz-Boyer) or abdominal (Mauclaire) colostomy. In Whitehead ED, Leiter E (eds): Current Operative Urology, 2nd ed. Philadelphia, Harper & Row, 1984, p 783.

Hinman F Jr: Pascal, Laplace and a length of bowel. J Urol (Paris) 95:11, 1989.

Hinman F Jr: Reservoirs and continent conduits. Int Urogynecol 3:208, 1992.

Hinman F Jr: Selection of intestinal segments for bladder substitution: Physical and physiological characteristics. J Urol 139:519, 1988.

Hinman F Jr: The technique of the Gersuny operation (ureterosigmoidostomy with perineal colostomy) in vesical exstrophy. J Urol 80:126, 1959.

Hinman F Jr: Ureteral implantation: II. Clinical results from a method of open submucosal anastomosis. J Urol 64:567, 1950.

Hinman F Jr, Hinman F Sr: Ureteral implantation: I. Experiments on the surgical principles involved in an open submucosal method of ureterointestinal anastomosis. J Urol 64:457, 1950.

Hinman F Jr, Oppenheimer R: Functional characteristics of the ileal segment as a valve. J Urol 80:448, 1958.

Husman DA, Spence HM: Current status of tumour of the bowel

following ureterosigmoidostomy: A review. J Urol 144:607, 1990.

Issa MM, Oesterling JE, Canning DA, Jeffs RD: A new technique of using the in situ appendix as a catheterizable stoma for continent urinary reservoirs. J Urol 141:1385, 1989.

Jacobs A, Stirling WB: The late results of ureterocolic anastomoses. Br J Urol 24:259, 1952.

Jordan GH, Winslow BH: Laparoscopically assisted continent catheterizable cutaneous appendicovesicostomy. J Endourol 7:517, 1993.

Juma S, Nickel JC: Appendix interposition of the ureter. J Urol 144:130, 1990.

Kalble T, Tricker AR, Friedl P, et al: Ureterosigmoidostomy: Long-term results, risks of carcinoma and etiological factors for carcinogenesis. J Urol 144:1110, 1990.

Katz AE, Benson MC, Olsson CA: Complications of continent diversion. In Cohen MS, Resnick MI (eds): Reoperative Urology. Boston, Little, Brown & Co, 1995, p 287.

Keating MA, Bradley PK, Adams M, et al: Seromuscular trough modification in construction of continent urinary stomas. J Urol 150:734, 1993.

Keetch DW, Basler JW, Kavoussi LR, et al: Modification of Mitrofanoff principle for continent urinary diversion. Urology 41:507, 1993.

Kim KS, Susskind MR, King LR: Ileocecal ureterosigmoidostomy: An alternative to conventional ureterosigmoidostomy. J Urol 140:1494, 1988.

King LR, Robertson CN, Bertram RA: A new technique for the prevention of reflux in those undergoing bladder substitution or undiversion using bowel segments. World J Urol 3:194, 1985.

Kirsch AJ, Hensle TW, Olsson CA: Rapid construction of right colon pouch: Initial clinical experience. Urology 43:228, 1993.

Koch MO, McDougal WS: Nicotinic acid: Treatment for the hyperchloremic acidosis following urinary diversion through intestinal segments. J Urol 134:162, 1985.

Kock NG: Ileostomy without external appliance: A survey of 25 patients provided with intestinal reservoir. Ann Surg 173:545, 1971.

Kock NG, Ghoneim MA, Lycke KG, et al: Urinary diversion to the augmented and valved rectum: Preliminary results with a novel surgical procedure. J Urol 140:1375, 1988.

Kock NG, Nilson AE, Nilson LO, et al: Urinary diversion via a continent ileal reservoir: Clinical results in 12 patients. J Urol 128:469, 1982.

Kock NG, Norlen L, Philipson BM, et al: Current status of the ileal reservoir for continent urinary diversion. Surg Rounds, January 1985, p 32.

Koff SA: Abdominal neourethra in children: Technique and long-term results. J Urol 133:244, 1985.

Kosko JW, Kursh ED, Resnick MI: Metabolic complications of urologic intestinal substitutes. Urol Clin North Am 13:193, 1986.

Kozminski M: Laparoscopic ileal loop conduit and other urologic bowel surgery. In Gomella LG, Kozminski M, Winfield HN (eds): Laparoscopic Urologic Surgery. New York, Raven Press, 1994, p 211.

Kozminski M, Partamian KO: Case report of laparoscopic ileal loop conduit. J Endourol 6:147, 1992.

Kramolowsky EV, Clayman RV, Weyman PJ: Management of ureterointestinal anastomotic strictures: Comparison of open surgical and endourological repair. J Urol 139:1195, 1988.

Kroovand RL: Personal communication, 1995.

Kurzrock EA, Tomasic NA, Razi S, et al: Fluorourodynamic and clinical evaluation in males following construction of a Kock ileal-urethral reservoir. Urology 46:801, 1995.

Lampel A, Hohenfellner M, Schultz-Lampel D, Thüroff JW: In situ tunnelled bowel flap tubes: 2 new techniques of a continent outlet for Mainz pouch cutaneous diversion. J Urol 153:308, 1995.

Leadbetter GW Jr, Zickermin P, Pierce E: Ureterosigmoidostomy and carcinoma of the colon. J Urol 121:732, 1979.

Leadbetter WF: Considerations of problems incident to performance of uretero-enterostomy: Report of a technique. J Urol 68:818, 1951.

Leadbetter WF, Clarke BG: Five years experience with ureteroenterostomy by the "combined" technique. J Urol 73:67, 1954.

Le Duc A, Camey M: Un procédé d'implantation uréteroiléale anti-reflux dans l'entéro-cystoplastie. J Urol Nephrol 85:449, 1979.

Le Duc A, Camey M, Teillac P: An original anti-reflux ureteral ileal implantation technique: Long-term follow-up. J Urol 137:1156, 1987.

Leibovitch I, Kaefer M, Bihrle R: An alternative surgical technique for the management of afferent limb stricture in Kock pouch continent urinary diversion. Urology 46:867, 1995.

Leisinger HJ: Continent urinary diversion: Review of the intussuscepted ileal valve. World J Urol 4:231, 1986.

Leonard MP, Gearhart JP, Jeffs RD: 50 Continent urinary reservoirs in pediatric urological practice. J Urol 144:330, 1990.

Leonard MP, Quinlan DM: The Benchekroun ileal valve. Urol Clin North Am 18:717, 1991.

Leong CH: Use of the stomach for bladder replacement and urinary diversion. Ann R Coll Surg Engl 60:283, 1978.

Levinson AK, Johnson DE, Wishnow KI: Indication for urethrectomy in an era of continent urinary diversion. J Urol 144:73, 1990.

Lieskovsky G, Boyd SD, Skinner DG: Cutaneous Kock pouch urinary diversion. Probl Urol 5:256, 1991.

Lieskovsky G, Boyd SD, Skinner DG: Management of late complications of the Kock pouch form of urinary diversion. J Urol 137:1146, 1987.

Lieskovsky G, Skinner DG, Boyd SD: Complications of the Kock pouch. Urol Clin North Am 15:195, 1988.

Light JK, Engelmann UH: Le Bag: Total replacement of the bladder using an ileocolonic pouch. J Urol 136:27, 1986.

Light JK, Flores FN, Scott FB: Use of the AS792 artificial sphincter following urinary undiversion. J Urol 129:548, 1983.

Lobe TE: Conversion of an ileal conduit into a neourethral entero-plication for urinary continence: Tips in its proper construction. J Pediatr Surg 21:1040, 1986.

Lockhart JL: Remodeled right colon: An alternative urinary reservoir. J Urol 138:730, 1987.

Lockhart JL, Bejany DW: The antireflux uretero-ileal reimplantation. J Urol 137:867, 1987.

Lockhart JL, Davies R, Cox C, et al: The gastroileoileal pouch: An alternative continent urinary reservoir for patients with short bowel, acidosis and/or extensive pelvic radiation. J Urol 150:46, 1993.

Lockhart JL, Pow-Sang JM, Persky L, et al: A continent colonic urinary reservoir: The Florida pouch. J Urol 144:864, 1990.

Lockhart JL, Pow-Sang JM, Persky L, et al: Detubularized right colon for continent urinary diversion. In Webster G, Kirby R, King L, Goldwasser B (eds): Reconstructive Urology. Boston, Blackwell Scientific Publications, 1993, p 527.

Lrimpi HD, Khubchandovic IT, Sheets JA, Stasik JJ: Advances in intestinal anastomoses. Dis Colon Rectum 20:107, 1977.

Mahran MR, Ghaly AM, Sheir KZ, et al: The modified rectal bladder (the augmented and valved rectum) for urine diversion in children. Urology 44:737, 1994.

Malkowicz SB, Avon MR, Thangathurai D, et al: Intravenous papaverine in constructing continent urinary reservoir. Urology 33:431, 1989.

Malone PS, Ransley PG, Kiely EM: Preliminary report: The antegrade continence enema. Lancet 335:1217, 1990.

Mansson W: The continent cecal reservoir for urine (review). Scand J Urol S85:1, 1984.

Mansson W, Mattiasson A, White T: Acute effects of full urinary bladder and full caecal urinary reservoir on regional renal function: A study with scintillation camera renography. Scand J Urol Nephrol 18:299, 1984.

Marberger M, Walz P, Hohenfellner R: Urétérosigmoidostomie et urétérostomie cutanée transcolique: Indications, techniques et resultats. J Urol (Paris) 88:591, 1982.

Marshall FF: Creation of an ileocolic bladder after cystectomy. J Urol 139:1264, 1988.

Mathisen W: A new method of ureterointestinal anastomosis: Preliminary report. Surg Gynecol Obstet 96:255, 1953.

McDougal WS: The continent urinary diversion. J Urol 137:1214, 1987. Editorial.

McDougal WS: Mechanics and neurophysiology of intestinal segments as bowel substitutes. J Urol 138:1438, 1987.

McDougal WS: Metabolic complications of urinary intestinal diversion. J Urol 147:1199, 1992.

McLeod RS, Fazio VW: Quality of life with the continent ileostomy. World J Surg 8:90, 1984.

McLoughlin MG: Koch pouch: External and internal diversion. In Marshall FF (ed): Operative Urology. Philadelphia, WB Saunders, 1991, p 214.

Melchior H, Spehr C, Knop-Wagemann I, et al: The continent ileal bladder for urinary tract reconstruction after cystectomy: Survey of 44 patients. J Urol 139:714, 1988.

Mikami O, Osawa O, Matsuda T, et al: The augmented rectal bladder for urinary diversion: Experience with the original valved rectum and a valve-less modification. Int J Urol 1:57, 1994.

Mitchell ME: Urinary tract diversion and undiversion in the pediatric age group. Surg Clin North Am 61:1147, 1981.

Mitchell ME: Use of bowel in undiversion. Urol Clin North Am 13:349, 1986.

Mitchell ME, Rink RC: Urinary diversion and undiversion. Urol Clin North Am 12:111, 1985.

Mitrofanoff P: Cystostomie continente trans-appendiculaire dans le traitement des vessies neurologiques. Chir Pediatr 21:297, 1980.

Mitrofanoff P, Bonnet O, Annoot M, et al: Continent urinary diversion using an artificial urinary sphincter. Br J Urol 70:26, 1992.

Monfort G, Guy JM, Morrisson-Lacombe G: Apendicovesicostomy: An alternative urinary diversion in the child. Eur Urol 10:361, 1984.

Moorcraft J, DuBoulay CEH, Isaacson P, Atwell JD: Changes in the mucosa of colon conduits with particular reference to the risk of malignant change. Br J Urol 55:185, 1983.

Mor Y, Ramon J, Raviv G, et al: Low loop cutaneous ureterostomy and subsequent reconstruction: 20 years of experience. J Urol 147:1595, 1992.

Mraz JP, Sutory M, Zerhau P: Simple flap valve for continent urinary diversion. Br J Urol 74:328, 1994.

Mundy AR: A technique for total substitution of the lower urinary tract without the use of a prosthesis. Br J Urol 42:334, 1988.

Nesbit RM: Ureterosigmoid anastomosis by direct elliptical connection: A preliminary report. J Urol 61:728, 1949.

Nguyen DH, Ganesan GS, Sumfest JM, et al: The use of the AMS 800 artificial urinary sphincter in combination with the gastric tube for continence in the canine model. J Urol 150:737, 1994.

Noble JR, Mata JA, Humble RL, Culkin DJ: Maxi-pouch: A new technique for ileal conduit conversion to continent urinary reservoir. J Urol 143:116, 1990.

Norlén L, Trasti H: Functional behavior of the continent ileum reservoir for urinary diversion: Experimental and clinical study. Scand J Urol Nephrol (Suppl) 49:33, 1978.

Oesterling JE, Gearhart JP: Utilization of an ileal conduit in construction of a continent urinary reservoir. Urology 36:15, 1990.

Parra RO: A simplified technique for continent urinary diversion: An all-stapled colonic reservoir. J Urol 146:1496, 1991.

Pow-Sang J, Helal M, Figueroa TE, et al: Conversion from external appliance wearing or internal urinary diversion to a continent urinary reservoir (Florida pouch I or II): Surgical technique, indications and complications. J Urol 147:356, 1992.

Quinlan DM, Leonard MP, Brendler CB, et al: Use of the Benchekroun hydraulic valve as a catheterizable continence mechanism. J Urol 145:1151, 1991.

Reid K, Schneider K, Fruchtman B: Closure of the bladder neck in patients undergoing continent vesicostomy for urinary incontinence. J Urol 120:40, 1978.

Resnick MJ, Caldamone AA (eds): Use of large and small bowel in urologic surgery. Urol Clin North Am 13:177, 1986.

Richie JP: Ileal conduit urinary diversion. *In* Crawford ED, Das S (eds): Current Genitourinary Cancer Surgery. Philadelphia, Lea & Febiger, 1990, p 262.

Reidmiller H, Bürger R, Müller S, et al: Continent appendix stoma: A modification of the Mainz pouch technique. J Urol 143:1115, 1990.

Rink RC, Retik AB: Ureteroileocecal sigmoidostomy and avoidance of carcinoma of the colon. *In* King LR, Stone AR, Webster GD (eds): Bladder Reconstruction and Continent Urinary Diversion. Chicago, Mosby–Year Book, 1991, p 221.

Rosenberg ML: The physiology of hyperchloremic acidosis following ureterosigmoidostomy: A study of urinary reabsorption with radioactive isotopes. J Urol 70:569, 1953.

Rowland RG: Continent urinary diversion. J Urol 136:76, 1986.

Rowland RG, Bihrle R, Mitchell ME: The Indiana continent urinary reservoir. J Urol 137:1136, 1987.

Rowland RG, Bihrle R, Scheidler D, et al: Update on the Indiana continent reservoir. Probl Urol 5:269, 1991.

Rowland RG, Mitchell ME, Bihrle R: The cecoileal continent urinary reservoir. World J Urol 3:185, 1985.

Rudick J, Schonholz S, Weber HN: The gastric bladder: A continent reservoir for urinary diversion. Surgery 82:1, 1977.

Sagalowsky A: Mechanisms of continence in urinary reconstructions. Houston, American Urological Association, AUA Update Series, vol XI, lesson 4, 1991.

Scheidler DM, Klee LW, Rowland RG, et al: Update on the Indiana continent urinary reservoir. J Urol 141(pt 2):302A, 1989.

Schmidbauer CP, Chiang H, Raz S: Compliance of tubular and detubularized ileal reservoirs. J Urol 137:171A, 1987.

Schneider KM, Reid RE, Fruchtman B: Closure of the bladder neck in patients undergoing continent vesicostomy. J Urol 120:40, 1978.

Schrock TR, Deveney CW, Dunphy JE: Factors contributing to leakage of colonic anastomoses. Ann Surg 177:513, 1973.

Scott FB, Light JK, Fishman I, et al: Implantation of an artificial sphincter for urinary incontinence. Contemp Surg 18:11, 1981.

Sinaiko E: Artificial bladder from segment of stomach and study of urine on gastric secretion. Surg Gynecol Obstet 102:433, 1956.

Skinner DG: Further experience with the ileocecal segment in urinary reconstruction. J Urol 128:252, 1982.

Skinner DG: Secondary urinary reconstruction: Use of the ileocecal segment. J Urol 112:48, 1974.

Skinner DG, Boyd SD, Lieskovsky G, et al: Lower urinary tract reconstruction following cystectomy: Experience and results in 126 patients using the Kock ileal reservoir with bilateral uretero-ileo-urethrostomy. J Urol 146:756, 1991.

Skinner DG, Lieskovsky G, Boyd S: Continent urinary diversion. J Urol 141:1323, 1989.

Smith GI, Hinman F Jr: The intussuscepted ileal cystostomy. J Urol 73:261, 1955.

Smith GI, Hinman F Jr: The rectal bladder (colostomy with ureterosigmoidostomy): Experimental and clinical aspects. J Urol 74:354, 1955.

Spence HM: Ureterosigmoidostomy for exstrophy of the bladder: Results in a personal series of 31 cases. Br J Urol 38:36, 1966.

Spence HM, Hoffman WW, Fosmire GP: Tumour of the colon as a late complication of ureterosigmoidostomy for exstrophy of the bladder. Br J Urol 51:466, 1978.

Stamey TA: Pathogenesis and implications of electrolyte imbalance in ureterosigmoidostomy. Surg Gynecol Obstet 103:736, 1956.

Stein JP, Huffman JL, Freeman JA, et al: Stenosis of the afferent antireflux valve in the Kock pouch continent urinary diversion: Diagnosis and management. J Urol 151:338, 1994.

Stenzl A, Klutke CG, Golomb J, Raz S: Tapered intraluminal versus imbricated extraluminal valve: Comparison of two continence mechanisms for urinary diversion. J Urol 143:607, 1990.

Stockle M, Becht E, Voges G, et al: Ureterosigmoidostomy: An outdated approach to bladder exstrophy? J Urol 143:770, 1990.

Stower MJ, Massey JA, Feneley RCL: Urethral closure in management of urinary incontinence. Urology 34:246, 1989.

Straffon RA, Kyle K, Corvalan J: Techniques of cutaneous ureterostomy and results in 51 patients. J Urol 103:138, 1970.

Sundin T, Mansi MK: The valved S-shaped rectosigmoid pouch for continent urinary diversion. J Urol 150:838, 1993.

Sweitzer SJ, Kelalis PP: Cutaneous transureteroureterostomy as a form of diversion in children with a compromised urinary tract. J Urol 120:589, 1978.

Terai A, Ueda T, Kakehi Y, et al: Urinary calculi as late complication of the Indiana continent urinary diversion: Comparison with the Kock pouch procedure. J Urol 155:66, 1996.

Thüroff JW, Alken P, Riedmiller H, et al: The Mainz-pouch (mixed augmentation ileum and cecum) for bladder augmentation and continent diversion. J Urol 11:152, 1985.

Wagstaff KE, Woodhouse CRJ, Rose GA, et al: Biochemical and bacteriological consequences of enterocystoplasty. Br J Urol 68, 1991.

Wan J, McGuire EJ, Bloom DA, Ritchey ML: Stress leak point pressure: A diagnostic tool for incontinent children. J Urol 150:700, 1993.

Wear JB Jr, Barquin OP: Ureterosigmoidostomy: Long-term results. Urology 1:192, 1973.

Webster GD (guest ed): Problems in reconstructive urology. Probl Urol 1(2):1, 1987.

Weingarten JL, Cromie JW: The Mitrofanoff principle: An alternative form of urinary diversion in the child. J Urol 140:1529, 1988.

Wells CA: The use of the intestine in urology. Br J Urol 28:335, 1956.

Weyrauch HM, Young BW: Evaluation of common methods of uretero-intestinal anastomosis: An experimental study. J Urol 67:880, 1952.

Wolf JS, Stoller MC: Management of upper tract calculi in patients with tubularized urinary diversions. J Urol 145:266, 1991.

Woodhouse CRJ: The Mitrofanoff principle for continent urinary diversion. *In* Webster G, Kirby R, King L, Goldwasser B (eds): Reconstructive Urology. Boston, Blackwell Scientific Publications, 1993, p 539.

Woodhouse CRJ, Macneily AE: The Mitrofanoff principle: Expanding upon a versatile technique. Br J Urol 74:447, 1994.

Woodhouse CRJ, Malone PR, Cumming J, et al: The Mitrofanoff principle for continent urinary diversion. Br J Urol 63:53, 1989.

Zimmern PE, Hadley HR, Leach GE, Raz S: Transvaginal closure of the bladder neck and placement of a suprapubic catheter for destroyed urethra after long-term indwelling catheterization. J Urol 134:554, 1985.

Zincke H, Malek RS: Experience with cutaneous and transureteroureterostomy. J Urol 111:760, 1974.

Zingg E, Tscholl R: Continent cecoileal conduit: Preliminary report. J Urol 118:724, 1977.

Zinman L: Continent urinary reservoirs. J Urol 150:843, 1993. Editorial.

Zinman L, Libertino JA: Right colocystoplasty for bladder replacement. Urol Clin North Am 13:321, 1986.

Audiovisuals

Bihrle R: Profiles in Urology: The Indiana Pouch: A Continent Urinary Reservoir. Wilkes-Barre, PA, Karol Media, 1990 (15 minutes). AUA #919-2063.

Guille E, Coeurdacier P, Cipolla B, et al: Continent Urinary Diversion: The Florida Pouch, a Good Solution. Wilkes-Barre, PA, Karol Media, 1995 (10 minutes). AUA #919-2058.

Hohenfellner R: The Mainz Pouch—One Solution to Variety of Problems. Wilkes-Barre, PA, Karol Media, 1987 (14 minutes). AUA #919-1149.

Marshall FF: Ileocolic Urinary Bladder Post Cystectomy: Continent Micturition. Wilkes-Barre, PA, Karol Media, 1988 (13 minutes). AUA #919-1153.

BLADDER AUGMENTATION

Adams MC, Mitchell ME, Rink RC: Gastrocystoplasty: An alternative solution to the problem of urological reconstruction in the severely compromised patient. J Urol 140:1152, 1988.

Anderson PAM, Rickwood AMK: Detrusor hyper-reflexia as a factor in spontaneous perforation of augmentation cystoplasty for neuropathic bladder. Br J Urol 67:210, 1991.

Atala A, Bauer SB, Hendren WH, Retik AB: The effect of gastric augmentation on bladder function. J Urol 149:1099, 1993.

Atala A, Lailis NG, Cilento BG, et al: Progressive ureteral dilation for subsequent ureterocystoplasty. J Urol 156:1996.

Barrington JW, Fern-Davies H, Adams RJ, et al: Bile acid dysfunction after clam enterocystoplasty. Br J Urol 76:169, 1995.

Bauer SB, Hendren WH, Kozakewich H, et al: Perforation of the augmented bladder. J Urol 148:699, 1992.

Bellinger MF: Ureterocystoplasty: A unique method for vesical augmentation in children. J Urol 149:811, 1993.

Ben-Chaim J, Shenfeld O, Goldwasser B, et al: Does the use of the ileocecal region in reconstructive urology cause persistent diarrhea? Eur Urol 27:315, 1995.

Benchekroun A: Continent caecal bladder. Eur Urol 3:248, 1977.

Bissada SA, Bissada NK: Choice of gastroepiploic vessels for gastrocystoplasty. J Urol 148:101, 1992.

Bogaert GA, Mevorach RA, Kogan BA: Urodynamic and clinical follow-up of 28 children after gastrocystoplasty. Br J Urol 74:469, 1994.

Braren V: Laparoscopic bladder autoaugmentation. Soc Pediatr Urol Newsl, February 25, 1994.

Cartwright PC, Snow BW: Bladder augmentation: Early clinical experience. J Urol 142:505, 1989.

Cartwright PC, Snow BW: Bladder augmentation: Partial detrusor excision to augment the bladder without the use of bowel. J Urol 142:1050, 1989.

Chan SL, Ankenman GJ, Wright JE, McLoughlin MG: Cecocystoplasty in the surgical management of the small contracted bladder. J Urol 124:338, 1980.

Cheng C, Whitfield HN: Cystoplasty: Tubularisation or detubularisation? Br J Urol 66:30, 1990.

Churchill BM, Aliabadi H, Landau EH, et al: Ureteral bladder augmentation. J Urol 150:716, 1993.

Couvelaire R: "La petite vessie" des tuberculeaux genito-urinaires: Essae de classification place et varidentes des cysto-intestino-plasties. J Urol (Paris) 56:381, 1950.

Dewan PA, Stefanek W: Autoaugmentation gastrocystoplasty: Early clinical results. Br J Urol 74:460, 1994.

Dounis A, Abel BJ, Gow JG: Cecocystoplasty for bladder augmentation. J Urol 123:164, 1980.

Ehrlich RM, Gershman A: Laparoscopic seromyotomy (autoaugmentation) for non-neurogenic neurogenic bladder in a child: Initial case report. Urology 42:175, 1993.

Elder JS, Snyder HM, Hulbert WC, Duckett JW: Perforation of the augmented bladder in patients undergoing clean intermittent catheterization. J Urol 140:1159, 1988.

Faxén A, Kock NG, Sundin T: Long-term functional results after ileocystoplasty. Scand J Urol Nephrol 7:127, 1973.

Fenn N, Conn IG, German KA, et al: Complications of clam enterocystoplasty with particular reference to urinary tract infection. Br J Urol 69:366, 1992.

Filmer RB, Spencer JR: Malignancies in bladder augmentations and intestinal conduits. J Urol 143:671, 1990.

Gearhart JP, Peppas DS, Jeffs RD: The application of continent urinary stomas to bladder augmentation or replacement in the failed exstrophy reconstruction. Br J Urol 75:87, 1995.

Gil-Vernet JM Jr: The ileocolic segment in urologic surgery. J Urol 94:418, 1965.

Goldwasser B, Webster GD: Augmentation and substitution enterocystoplasty. J Urol 135:214, 1986.

Gonzalez R: Sigmoid cystoplasty. In King LR, Stone AR, Webster GD (eds): Bladder Reconstruction and Continent Urinary Diversion. Chicago, Mosby–Year Book, 1991, p 88.

Gonzalez R: Bladder augmentation with sigmoid or descending colon. In Webster G, Kirby R, King L, Goldwasser B (eds): Reconstructive Urology. Boston, Blackwell Scientific Publications, 1993, p 433.

Gonzalez R: Undiversion. In Glenn JF (ed): Urologic Surgery. Philadelphia, JB Lippincott, 1991, p 1068.

Gonzalez R, Buson H, Reid C, Reinberg Y: Seromuscular colocystoplasty lined with urothelium: Experience with 16 patients. Urology 45:124, 1995.

Gonzalez R, LaPointe S, Sheldon CA, Mauer SM: Undiversion in children with renal failure. J Pediatr Surg 19:632, 1984.

Gonzalez R, Ruiz E, de Badiola FIP, et al: Results and complications of sigmoid cystoplasty. J Urol 145:300A, 1991.

Gonzalez R, Sidi AA: Preoperative prediction of continence after enterocystoplasty or undiversion in children with neurogenic bladder. J Urol 134:705, 1985.

Goodwin WE: Ileocystoplasty. In Cooper P (ed): Craft of Surgery. Boston, Little, Brown & Co, 1964, p 1139.

Goodwin WE, Turner RD, Winter CC: Results of ileocystoplasty. J Urol 80:461, 1958.

Goodwin WE, Winter CC: Technique of sigmoidocystoplasty. Surg Gynecol Obstet 108:370, 1959.

Goodwin WE, Winter CC, Barker WF: "Cup-patch" technique of ileocystoplasty for bladder enlargement or partial substitution. Surg Gynecol Obstet 108:240, 1959.

Gosalbez R Jr, Woodard JR, Broecker BH, Warshaw B: Metabolic complications of the use of stomach for urinary reconstruction. J Urol 150:710, 1993.

Green D, Mitcheson HD, McGuire EJ: Management of the bladder by augmentation ileocecocystoplasty. J Urol 130:133, 1981.

Gudziak M, McGuire EJ, Rudy D: Detrusor myomectomy (bladder autoaugmentation): Report on 14 patients. J Urol 151:501, 1994.

Hautmann RE, Egghart G, Frohneberg D, Miller K: The ileal neobladder. J Urol 139:39, 1988.

Hendren WH: Urinary undiversion and augmentation cystoplasty. In Kelalis PP, King LR, Belman AB (eds): Clinical Pediatric Urology, 2nd ed. Philadelphia, WB Saunders, 1985, p 620.

Hendren WH, Hendren RB: Bladder augmentation: Experience with 129 children and young adults. J Urol 144:445, 1990.

Hitchcock RJI, Duffy PG, Malone PS: Ureterocystoplasty: The "bladder" augmentation of choice. Br J Urol 73:575, 1994.

Horowitz M, Mitchell ME, Nguyen DH: The DAWG procedure, gastrocystoplasty made better. J Urol 151:503, 1994.

Kass EJ, Koff SA: Bladder augmentation in the pediatric neuropathic bladder. J Urol 129:552, 1983.

Kennedy HA, Adams MC, Mitchell ME, et al: Chronic renal failure and bladder augmentation: Stomach versus sigmoid colon in the canine model. J Urol 140:1138, 1988.

Kennelly MJ, Gormley EA, McGuire EJ: Early clinical experience with adult bladder auto-augmentation. J Urol 152:303, 1994.

Khoury JM, Webster GD: Augmentation cystoplasty. World J Urol 8:203, 1990.

Koch MO, McDougal WS: The pathophysiology of hyperchloraemic metabolic acidosis after urinary diversion through intestinal segments. Surgery 93:561, 1985.

Kock NG, Ghoneim MA, Lycke KG, et al: Urinary diversion to an augmented and valved rectum: Preliminary results with a novel surgical procedure. J Urol 140:1375, 1988.

Kockelbergh RC, Tan JBL, Bates CP, et al: Clam enterocystoplasty in general urological practice. Br J Urol 68:38, 1991.

Kreder K, Das AK, Webster GD: The hemi-Kock ileocystoplasty: A versatile procedure in reconstructive urology. J Urol 147:1248, 1992.

Kreder KJ, Webster GD: Management of the bladder outlet in patients requiring enterocystoplasty. J Urol 147:38, 1992.

Landau EH, Jayanthi VR, Khoury AE, et al: Bladder augmentation: Ureterocystoplasty versus ileocystoplasty. J Urol 152:716, 1994.

Le Duc A, Camey M, Teillac P: An original antireflux ureteroileal implantation technique: Long-term follow-up. J Urol 137:1156, 1987.

Leong CH: Use of the stomach for bladder replacement and urinary diversion. Ann R Coll Surg Engl 60:283, 1978.

Lima SV, Aranjo LA, Vilar FO, et al: Nonsecretory sigmoid cystoplasty: Experimental and clinical results. J Urol 153:1651, 1995.

Linder A, Leach GE, Raz S: Augmentation cystoplasty in the treatment of neurogenic bladder dysfunction. J Urol 129:491, 1983.

Luangkhot R, Peng BCH, Blaivas JG: Ileocecocystoplasty for the management of refractory neurogenic bladder: Surgical technique and urodynamic findings. J Urol 146:1340, 1991.

Mathisen W: Open-loop sigmoido-cystoplasty. Acta Chir Scand 110:227, 1955.

McDougall EM, Clayman RV, Figenshay RS, Pearle MS: Laparoscopic retropubic auto-augmentation of the bladder. J Urol 153:123, 1995.

McKenna PH, Bauer MB: Bladder augmentation with ureter. Dial Pediatr Urol January:1, 1995.

Melchior HJ, Spehr C, Knop-Wagemann I, et al: The continent ileal bladder for urinary tract reconstruction after cystectomy: A survey of 44 patients. J Urol 139:714, 1988.

Menville JG, Nix JT, Pratt AM II: Cecocystoplasty. J Urol 79:78, 1958.

Miller K, Matsui U, Hautmann R: Functional, augmented rectal bladder: Early clinical experience. Eur Urol 19:269, 1991.

Mitchell ME: The role of bladder augmentation in undiversion. J Pediatr Surg 16:790, 1981.

Mitchell ME, Adams MC, Rink RC: Ureteral replacement with ureter. J Urol 139:1282, 1988.

Mitchell ME, Burns MW: Augmentation cystoplasty with stomach. In Webster G, Kirby R, King L, Goldwasser B (eds): Reconstructive Urology. Boston, Blackwell Scientific Publications, 1993, p 439.

Mundy AR: Cystoplasty. In Mundy AR (ed): Current Operative Surgery: Urology. Eastborne, England, Bailliere Tindall, 1986, p 140.

Mundy AR: A technique for total substitution of the lower urinary tract without the use of a prosthesis. Br J Urol 62:334, 1988.

Mundy AR, Stephenson TP: "Clam" ileocystoplasty for the treatment of refractory urge incontinence. Br J Urol 57:641, 1985.

Nguyen DH, Bain MA, Salmonson KL, et al: The syndrome of dysuria and hematuria in pediatric urinary construction with stomach. J Urol 150:707, 1993.

Nurse DE, Mundy AR: Assessment of the malignant potential of cystoplasty. Br J Urol 64:489, 1989.

Nurse DE, Mundy AR: Ileal augmentation cystoplasty. In Webster G, Kirby R, King L, Goldwasser B (eds): Reconstructive Urology. Boston, Blackwell Scientific Publications, 1993, p 421.

Nurse DE, Mundy AR: Metabolic complications of cystoplasty. Br J Urol 63:165, 1989.

Plawker MW, Rabinowitz SS, Etwaru DJ, Glassberg KI: Hypergastrinemia dysuria-hematuria and metabolic alkalosis: Complications associated with gastrocystoplasty. J Urol 154:546, 1995.

Raz S, Ehrlich JW, Babiarz JW, et al: Gastrocystoplasty without opening stomach. J Urol 150:713, 1993.

Reinberg Y, Allen RC Jr, Vaughn M, et al: Nephrectomy combined with lower abdominal extraperitoneal ureteral bladder augmentation in the treatment of children with vesicoureteral reflux dysplasia syndrome. J Urol 153:177, 1995.

Riedmiller H, Thüroff J, Stöckle M, et al: Continent urinary diversion and bladder augmentation in children: The Mainz pouch procedure. Pediatr Nephrol 3:68, 1989.

Roberts JP, Moon S, Malone PS: Treatment of neuropathic urinary and faecal incontinence with synchronous bladder reconstruction and the antegrade continence enema procedure. Br J Urol 75:386, 1995.

Rushton HR, Woodard JR, Parrott TS, et al: Delayed bladder rupture after augmentation enterocystoplasty. J Urol 140:344, 1988.

Sidi AA, Reinberg Y, Gonzalez R: Influence of intestinal segment and configuration on the outcome of augmentation enterocystoplasty. J Urol 136:1201, 1986.

Slaton JW, Kropp KA: Conservative management of suspected bladder rupture after augmentation enterocystoplasty. J Urol 152:713, 1994.

Smith RB, Van Cangh P, Skinner DG, et al: Augmentation enterocystoplasty: A critical review. J Urol 118:35, 1977.

Snow BW, Cartwright PC: Autoaugmentation of the bladder. Contemp Urol 4:41, 1992.

Stöhrer M, Kramer A, Goepel M, et al: Bladder auto-augmentation: An alternative for enterocystoplasty: Preliminary results. Neurourol Urodynam 14:11, 1995.

Stone AR: Ileocystoplasty. In King LR, Stone AR, Webster GD (eds): Bladder Reconstruction and Continent Urinary Diversion. Chicago, Mosby–Year Book, 1991, p 58.

Stothers L, Johnson H, Arnold W, et al: Bladder autoaugmentation by vesicomyotomy in the pediatric neurogenic bladder. Urology 44:110, 1994.

Tasker JH: Ileo-cystoplasty: A new technique (an experimental study with report of a case). Br J Urol 25:349, 1953.

Thüroff JW, Alken P, Riedmiller H, et al: The Mainz-pouch (mixed augmentation ileum and cecum) for bladder augmentation and continent diversion. J Urol 11:152, 1985.

Thüroff JW, Alken P, Riedmiller H, et al: 100 cases of Mainz pouch: Continuing experience and evolution. J Urol 140:283, 1988.

Turner-Warwick R: Cystoplasty. In Blandy JP (ed): Urology. Oxford, Blackwell Scientific Publications, 1976, p 840.

Turner-Warwick R, Ashken MH: The functional results of partial, subtotal and total cystoplasty with special reference to ureterocaecocystoplasty, selective sphincterotomy and cystocystoplasty. Br J Urol 39:3, 1967.

Walker RD III, Flack CE, Hawkins-Lee B, et al: Rectus fascial wrap: Early results of a modification of the rectus fascial sling. J Urol 154:771, 1995.

Weinberg AC, Boyd SD, Lieskovsky G, et al: Hemi-Kock augmentation ileocystoplasty: Low pressure antirefluxing system. J Urol 140:1380, 1988.

Weiss JP: Sigmoidocystoplasty to augment bladder capacity. Surg Gynecol Obstet 159:377, 1984.

Wespes E, Stone AR, King LR: Ileocaecocystoplasty in urinary tract reconstruction in children. J Urol 58:266, 1986.

Whitmore WF III, Gittes RF: Reconstruction of the urinary tract by cecal and ileocecal cystoplasty: Review of a 15-year experience. J Urol 130:494, 1983.

Wolf JS Jr, Turzan CW: Augmentation ureteroplasty. J Urol 149:1095, 1993.

Zingg E, Tscholl R: Continent cecoileal conduit: Preliminary report. J Urol 118:724, 1977.

Audiovisual

Mitchell ME: Gastrocystoplasty. Wilkes-Barre, PA, Karol Media, 1991 (23 minutes). AUA #919-1169.

BLADDER SUBSTITUTION

Atta MA: A new technique for continent urinary reservoir reconstruction. J Urol 145:960, 1991.

Bejany DE, Politano VA: Modified ileocolonic bladder: 5 years of experience. J Urol 149:1441, 1993.

Bogaert GA, Mevorach RA, Kim J, Kogan BA: The physiology of gastrocystoplasty: Once a stomach, always a stomach. J Urol 153:1977, 1995.

Burns MW, Watkins SL, Mitchell ME, et al: Treatment of bladder dysfunction in children with end-stage renal disease. J Pediatr Surg 27:170, 1992.

Camey M: Bladder replacement by ileocystoplasty following radical cystectomy. World J Urol 3:161, 1985.

Camey M, Richard F, Botto H: Bladder replacement by ileocystoplasty. In King LR, Stone AR, Webster GD (eds): Bladder Reconstruction and Continent Urinary Diversion. Chicago, Year Book Medical Publishers, 1987, p 336.

Carini M, Serni S, Lapini A, et al: Second stage reconfiguration of Camey I ileal bladder improves its urodynamic and clinical characteristics. Urology 44:425, 1994.

Casanova GA, Springer JP, Geriber E, et al: Urodynamic and

clinical aspects of ileal low pressure bladder substitutes. J Urol 72:728, 1993.

Chan SL, Ankenman GJ, Wright JE, McLoughlin MG: Cecocystoplasty in the surgical management of the small contracted bladder. J Urol 124:338, 1980.

Chen K-K, Chang LS, Chen M-T: Neobladder construction using completely detubularized sigmoid colon after radical cystoprostatectomy. J Urol 146:311, 1991.

Da Pozzo LF, Colombo R, Pompa P, et al: Detubularized sigmoid colon for bladder replacement after radical cystectomy. J Urol 152:1409, 1994.

De Geeter P, Melchior H: Orthotopic bladder replacement using detubularized ileum. *In* King LR, Stone AR, Webster GD (eds): Bladder Reconstruction and Continent Urinary Diversion, 2nd ed. Chicago, Mosby–Year Book, 1991, p 374.

Deklerk JN, Lambrechts W, Viljoen I: The bowel as substitute for the bladder. J Urol 121:22, 1979.

Ekman H, Jacobsson B, Kock N, Sundin T: The functional behavior of different types of intestinal urinary bladder substitutes. Cong Soc Int Urol 11:213, 1964.

Fisch M, Wammack R, Müller SC, Hohenfellner R: The Mainz Pouch II (sigma rectum pouch). J Urol 149:258, 1993.

Gadacz TR, Kelly KA, Phillips SF: The continent ileal pouch: Absorptive and motor features. Gastroenterology 72:1287, 1977.

Ganesan GS, Nguyen DH, Adams MC, et al: Lower urinary tract reconstruction using stomach and the artificial sphincter. J Urol 149:1107, 1993.

Gasparini ME, Hinman F Jr, Presti JC, et al: Continence after radical cystoprostatectomy and total bladder replacement: Urodynamic analysis. J Urol 148:1861, 1992.

Ghoneim MA, Kock NG, Lycke G, el-Din AB: An appliance-free sphincter-controlled bladder substitute: The urethral Kock pouch. J Urol 138:1150, 1987.

Ghoneim MA, Shehab-El-Din AB, Ashamallah AK, Gaballah MA: Evolution of the rectal bladder as a method for urinary diversion. J Urol 126:737, 1981.

Giertz G, Franksson C: Construction of a substitute bladder with preservation of urethral voiding after subtotal or total cystectomy. Acta Clin Scand 113:218, 1957.

Gil-Vernet JW, Escarpenter JM, Perez-Trujillo G, Bonet Vic J: A functioning artificial bladder: Results of 41 consecutive cases. J Urol 87:825, 1962.

Gilchrist RK, Merricks JW, Hamlin HH, et al: Construction of a substitute bladder and urethra. Surg Gynecol Obstet 90:752, 1950.

Goldwasser B: Bladder replacement. *In* Glenn JF, Graham SD (eds): Urologic Surgery, 4th ed. Philadelphia, JB Lippincott, 1991, p 1059.

Goldwasser B, Madgar I, Hanani Y: Urodynamic aspects of continent urinary diversion. Scand J Urol Nephrol 21:245, 1987.

Goldwasser B, Ramon J: Total bladder replacement using detubularized right colon. *In* Webster G, Kirby R, King L, Goldwasser B (eds): Reconstructive Urology. Boston, Blackwell Scientific Publications, 1993, p 477.

Golomb J, Klutke CG, Raz S: Complications of bladder substitution and continent urinary diversion. Urology 34:329, 1989.

Gonzalez R: Sigmoid cystoplasty. *In* King LR, Stone AR, Webster GD (eds): Bladder Reconstruction and Continent Urinary Diversion. Chicago, Mosby–Year Book, 1991, p 88.

Grunberger I, Catanese A, Hanna MK: Total replacement of bladder and urethra by cecum and appendix in bladder exstrophy. Urology 6:497, 1986.

Hautmann RE, Egghart G, Frohneberg D, Miller K: The ileal neobladder. J Urol 139:39, 1988.

Hautmann RE, Miller K, Steiner U, Wenderoth U: The ileal neobladder: 6 years of experience with more than 200 patients. J Urol 150:40, 1993.

Hautmann RE, Paiss T, de Petriconi R: The ileal neobladder in women: 9 years of experience with 18 patients. J Urol 155:76, 1996.

Hensle TW, Burbige KA: Bladder replacement in children and young adults. J Urol 133:1004, 1985.

Hensle TW, Dean GE: Complications of urinary tract reconstruction. Urol Clin North Am 18:755, 1991.

Hinman F Jr: Selection of intestinal segments for bladder substitution: Physical and physiological characteristics. J Urol 139:519, 1988.

Issa MM, Oesterling JE, Canning DA, Jeffs RD: A new technique of using the in situ appendix as a catheterizable stoma for continent urinary reservoirs. J Urol 141:1385, 1989.

Iwakiri J, Gill H, Anderson R, et al: Functional and urodynamic characteristics of an ileal neo-bladder. J Urol 149:1072, 1993.

Kakizaki H, Shibata T, Ameda K, et al: Continence mechanism of the orthotopic neobladder: Urodynamic analysis of ileocolic neobladder and external urethral functions. Int J Urol 2:267, 1995.

King LR, Stone AR, Webster GD (eds): Bladder Reconstruction and Continent Urinary Diversion. Chicago, Year Book Medical Publishers, 1987.

Klauber GT: Posterior bladder tube for CIC. Soc Pediatr Urol Newsl, May 20, 1992, p 9.

Koch MO, McDougal WS: Nicotinic acid: Treatment for the hyperchloremic acidosis following urinary diversion through intestinal segments. J Urol 134:162, 1985.

Koch MO, McDougal WS: The pathophysiology of hyperchloremic acidosis after urinary diversion through intestinal segments. Surgery 98:561, 1985.

Kock NG, Ghoneim MA, Lycke KG, Mahran MR: Replacement of the bladder by the urethral Kock pouch: Functional results, urodynamics and radiological features. J Urol 141:1111, 1989.

Koff SA: Abdominal neourethra in children: Technique and long-term results. J Urol 133:244, 1985.

Leisinger H, Säuberli H, Schauwecker H, et al: Continent ileal bladder: First clinical experience. Eur Urol 2:8, 1976.

Leonard MP, Gearhart JP, Jeffs RD: 50 continent urinary reservoirs in pediatric urological practice. J Urol 144:330, 1990.

Leong CH: Use of the stomach for bladder replacement and urinary diversion. Ann R Coll Surg Engl 60:283, 1978.

Lieskovsky G, Boyd SD, Skinner DG: Cutaneous Kock pouch urinary diversion. Probl Urol 5:256, 1991.

Light JK: Enteroplasty to ablate bowel contractions in the reconstructed bladder: A case report. J Urol 134:958, 1985.

Light JK: Long-term clinical results using the artificial urinary sphincter around bowel. Br J Urol 64:56, 1989.

Light JK: Total vesicourethral replacement in the female. *In* Webster G, Kirby R, King L, Goldwasser B (eds): Reconstructive Urology. Boston, Blackwell Scientific Publications, 1993, p 495.

Light JK, Engelmann UH: Le Bag: Total replacement of bladder using an ileocolonic pouch. J Urol 136:27, 1986.

Light JK, Marks JL: Total bladder replacement in the male and female using the ileocolonic segment (Le Bag). Br J Urol 65:467, 1990.

Lilien OM, Camey M: 25-year experience with replacement of the human bladder (Camey procedure). J Urol 132:886, 1984.

Lockhart JL, Davies R, Cox C, et al: Gastroileoileal pouch: Alternative continent urinary reservoir for patients with short bowel, acidosis and/or extensive pelvic radiation. J Urol 150:46, 1993.

Mansson W: The continent cecal reservoir for urine (review). Scand J Urol S85:1, 1984.

Mansson W, Mattiasson A, White T: Acute effects of full urinary bladder and full caecal urinary reservoir on regional renal function: A study with scintillation camera renography. Scand J Urol Nephrol 18:299, 1984.

Mark SD, Webster GD: Simplified urinary drainage following orthotopic or continent bladder replacement. J Urol 153:334, 1995.

Marshall FF: Creation of an ileocolic bladder after cystectomy. J Urol 139:1264, 1988.

Martins FE, Bennett CJ, Skinner DG: Options in replacement cystoplasty following radical cystectomy: High hopes or successful reality. J Urol 153:1363, 1995.

McDougal WS: Editorial comments. J Urol 148:810, 1992.

Melchior H, Spehr C, Knop-Wagemann I, et al: The continent ileal bladder for urinary tract reconstruction after cystectomy: A survey of 44 patients. J Urol 139:714, 1988.

Menville JG, Nix JT, Pratt AM II: Cecocystoplasty. J Urol 79:78, 1958.

Mitrofanoff P: Cystostomie continente trans-appendiculaire dans le traitement des vessies neurologiques. Chir Pediatr 21:297, 1980.

Nguyen DH, Mitchell ME: Gastric bladder reconstruction. Urol Clin North Am 18:649, 1991.

Norlén L, Trasti H: Functional behavior of the continent ileum reservoir for urinary diversion: Experimental and clinical study. Scand J Urol Nephrol (Suppl) 49:33, 1978.

Oesterling JE, Gearhart JP: Utilization of an ileal conduit in construction of a continent urinary reservoir. Urology 36:15, 1990.

Parra RO: A simplified technique for continent urinary diversion: An all-stapled colonic reservoir. J Urol 146:1496, 1991.

Quinlan DM, Leonard MP, Brendler CB, et al: Use of the Benchekroun hydraulic valve as a catheterizable continence mechanism. J Urol 145:1151, 1991.

Ramon J, Leandri P, Rossignol G, Botto H: Orthotopic bladder replacement using ileum: Techniques and results. In Webster G, Kirby R, King L, Goldwasser B (eds): Reconstructive Urology. Boston, Blackwell Scientific Publications, 1993, p 445.

Reddy PK: The colonic neobladder. Urol Clin North Am 18:4, 1991.

Reddy PK: Detubularized sigmoid reservoir for bladder replacement after cystoprostatectomy: Preliminary report of new configuration. Urology 29:625, 1987.

Reddy PK: Total bladder replacement using left colon. In Webster G, Kirby R, King L, Goldwasser B (eds): Reconstructive Urology. Boston, Blackwell Scientific Publications, 1993, p 487.

Reddy PK, Lange PH: Bladder replacement with sigmoid colon after radical cystoprostatectomy. Urology 29:268, 1987.

Reddy PK, Lange PH, Fraley EE: Total bladder replacement using detubularized sigmoid colon: Technique and results. J Urol 145:51, 1991.

Reddy PK, Sidi AA: Use of artificial urinary sphincter in patients with neobladder. J Urol 143:335A, 1990. Abstract.

Reidmiller H, Bürger R, Müller S, et al: Continent appendix stoma: A modification of the Mainz pouch technique. J Urol 143:1115, 1990.

Robertson CN, King LR: Bladder substitution in children. Urol Clin North Am 13:333, 1986.

Rogers E, Scardino PT: A simple ileal substitute bladder after radical cystectomy: Experience with a modification of the Studer pouch. J Urol 153:1432, 1995.

Rowland RG: Continent urinary diversion. J Urol 136:76, 1986.

Rowland RG, Mitchell ME, Bihrle R, et al: The Indiana continent urinary reservoir. J Urol 137:1136, 1987.

Schmidbauer CP, Chiang H, Raz S: Compliance of tubular and detubularized ileal reservoirs. J Urol 137:171A, 1987.

Shimizu TS, Fimbo H, Satoh F, et al: The colonic neobladder: A stoma-free bladder substitute after radical cystectomy: Preliminary results in six patients. Int J Urol 1:237, 1994.

Siegel AL, Snyder JA, Raz S: Total bladder substitution in the female. J Urol 139:312A, 1988.

Sinaiko ES: Artificial bladder from gastric pouch. Surg Gynecol Obstet 111:155, 1960.

Skinner DG: Further experience with the ileocecal segment in urinary reconstruction. J Urol 128:252, 1982.

Skinner DG: Secondary urinary reconstruction: Use of the ileocecal segment. J Urol 112:48, 1974.

Skinner DG, Boyd SD, Lieskovsky G, et al: Lower urinary tract reconstruction following cystectomy: Experience and results in 126 patients using the Kock ileal reservoir with bilateral uretero-ileo-urethrostomy. J Urol 146:756, 1991.

Skinner DG, Lieskovsky G, Boyd S: Continent urinary diversion. J Urol 141:1323, 1989.

Smith GI, Hinman F Jr: The intussuscepted ileal cystostomy. J Urol 73:261, 1955.

Snyder HMcC III: Foreword. In King LR, Stone AR, Webster GD (eds): Bladder Reconstruction and Continent Urinary Diversion. Chicago, Year Book Medical Publishers, 1986, p xi.

Steiner MS, Morton RA, Marshall FF: Vitamin B_{12} deficiency in patients with ileocolic neobladders. J Urol 149:255, 1993.

Stone AR, MacDermott JPA: The split-cuff ureteral nipple reimplantation technique: Reliable reflux prevention from bowel segments. J Urol 142:707, 1989.

Studer UE, Casanova GA, Mottaz AE, Zingg EJ: Results with a bladder substitute made from cross-folded ileal segments. (Goodwin's cup-patch technique). Prog Urol 1:13, 1991.

Studer UE, Turner WH: The ileal orthotopic bladder. Urology 45:185, 1995.

Webster GD, Goldwasser B: Management of incontinence after cystoplasty. In King LR, Stone AR, Webster GD (eds): Bladder Reconstruction and Continent Urinary Diversion. Chicago, Year Book Medical Publishers, 1986, p 75.

Webster GD, Ramon J: Bladder reconstruction by augmentation and substitution. In Droller MJ (ed): Genitourinary Surgery. Chicago, Mosby–Year Book, 1992, p 601.

Whitmore WF III, Gittes RF: Reconstruction of the urinary tract by cecal and ileocecal cystoplasty: Review of a 15-year experience. J Urol 130:494, 1983.

Zingg E, Tscholl R: Continent caecoileal reservoir in urinary diversion. Br J Urol 56:359, 1984.

Audiovisuals

Hautmann RE, Egghart G, Frohneberg DH, Miller K: The Ileal Neobladder. Wilkes-Barre, PA, Karol Media, 1987 (16 minutes). AUA #919-1148.

Mitchell ME, Lang PH: Gastric Neobladder. Wilkes-Barre, PA, Karol Media, 1991 (19 minutes). AUA #919-1169.

Raz S: UCLA Pouch in the Female: Total Bladder and Urethral Substitution with Enterovaginoplasty. Wilkes-Barre, PA, Karol Media, 1988 (18 minutes). AUA #919-1154.

Seemann O, Rassweiler J, Junemann K, Aiken P: The Sigmoid Neobladder—Technique and First Experience. Wilkes-Barre, PA, Karol Media, 1994 (10 minutes). AUA #919-2030.

Stenzl A, Colleselli K, Bartsch G: Continent Reservoir to the Urethra in the Female. Wilkes-Barre, PA, Karol Media, 1994 (10 minutes). AUA #919-2031.

Studer UE: Ileal Bladder Substitute. Wilkes-Barre, PA, Karol Media, 1988 (17 minutes). AUA #919-1155.

URETERAL RECONSTRUCTION AND EXCISION

Aaronson IA: Current status of the "Sting": An American perspective. Br J Urol 75:121, 1995.

Agran MA, Kratzman EA: Inferior vena cava on the left side: Its relationship to the right ureter. J Urol 101:149, 1969.

Allen TD: Congenital ureteral strictures. J Urol 104:196, 1970.

Amar AD: Reimplantation of completely duplicated ureters. J Urol 107:230, 1972.

Amar AD, Egan RM, Das S: Ipsilateral ureteroureterostomy combined with ureteral reimplantation for treatment of disease in both ureters in a child with complete ureteral duplication. J Urol 125:581, 1981.

Amin H: Experience with the ileal ureter. Br J Urol 48:19, 1976.

Anderson JC, Hynes W: Retrocaval ureter: A case diagnosed preoperatively and treated successfully by plastic operation. Br J Urol 21:209, 1949.

Ao T, Endo T, Suyama I, et al: Four cases of laparoscopic nephrectomy. Jpn J Clin Urol 47:833, 1993.

Arrivé L, Hricak H, Tavares NJ, et al: Malignant versus nonmalignant retroperitoneal fibrosis: Differentiation with MR imaging. Radiology 172:139, 1989.

Atala A, Kavoussi LR, Goldstein DS, et al: Laparoscopic correction of vesicoureteral reflux. J Urol 150:748, 1993.

Baker LRI, Mallinson WJW, Gregory MC, et al: Idiopathic retroperitoneal fibrosis: A retrospective analysis of 60 cases. Br J Urol 60:497, 1988.

Barone JG, Vates TS, Vasseli AJ: A simple technique for intraoperatively stenting a transected ureter. J Urol 149:535, 1994.

Barrett DM, Malek RS, Kelalis PP: Problems and solutions in surgical treatment of 100 consecutive ureteral duplications in children. J Urol 114:126, 1975.

Barry JM: Unstented extravesical ureteroneocystostomy in kidney transplantation. J Urol 129:918, 1983.

Barry JM, Hefty TR, Sasaki T: Clam-shell technique for right renal vein extension in cadaver kidney transplantation. J Urol 140:1479, 1988.

Baum WC: The clinical use of terminal ileum as a substitute ureter. J Urol 72:16, 1954.

Belman AB, Filmer RB, King LR: Surgical management of duplication of the collecting system. J Urol 112:316, 1974.

Bischoff P: Operative treatment of megaureter. J Urol 85:268, 1961.

Bishop MC, Askew AR, Smith JC: Reimplantation of the wide ureter. Br J Urol 50:383, 1978.

Blandy JP, Badenoch DF, Fowler CG, et al: Early repair of iatrogenic injury to the ureter or bladder after gynecological surgery. J Urol 146:761, 1991.

Blok C, Van Venroolj EPM, Mokhless I, Coolsaet BLRA: Dynamics of the ureterovesical junction: Its fluid transport mechanism in the pig. J Urol 134:175, 1985.

Blyth B, Passerini-Glazel G, Camuffo C, et al: Endoscopic incision of ureteroceles: Intravesical versus ectopic. J Urol 149:556, 1993.

Boari A: Chirurgia dell'uretere. Rome, Societa Editrice Dante Alighieri, 1900, p 176.

Bogaert GA, Mevorach RA, Kim J, Kogan BA: The physiology of gastrocystoplasty: Once a stomach, always a stomach. J Urol 153:1977, 1995.

Bogaert GA, Mevorach RA, Kogan BA: Urodynamic and clinical follow-up of 28 children after gastrocystoplasty. Br J Urol 74:469, 1994.

Boxer RJ, Fritzsche P, Skinner DG, et al: Replacement of the ureter by small intestine: Clinical applications and results of ileo-ureter in 89 patients. J Urol 121:128, 1979.

Brown S: Open versus endoscopic surgery in the treatment of vesicoureteral reflux. J Urol 142(pt 2): 499, 1989.

Bullock N: Retroperitoneal fibrosis. *In* Webster G, Kirby R, King L, Goldwasser B (eds): Reconstructive Urology. Boston, Blackwell Scientific Publications, 1993, p 389.

Caldamone AA, Snyder HM, Duckett JW: Ureteroceles in children: Follow-up of management with upper tract approach. J Urol 131:1130, 1984.

Carini M, Selli C, Lenzi R, et al: Surgical treatment of vesicoureteral reflux with bilateral medialization of the ureteral orifices. Eur Urol 11:181, 1985.

Carini M, Selli C, Rizzo M, et al: Surgical treatment of retroperitoneal fibrosis with omentoplasty. Surgery 91:137, 1982.

Carrion H, Safewood J, Politano V, et al: Retrocaval ureter: Report of 8 cases and the surgical management. J Urol 121:514, 1979.

Casati E, Boari A: Contributo sperimentale alla plastica dell' uretere: Communicazione preventia. Ferrara, Italy, Atti della Academia delle Scierze Mediche e Naturali, anno 68, fasc 3. 1894.

Cass AS, Schmaelzle JF, Hinman F Jr: Ureteral anastomosis in the dog: Comparing continuous with interrupted sutures. Invest Urol 6:94, 1968.

Caulk JR: Megaloureter—the importance of the ureterovesical valve. J Urol 9:315, 1923.

Cendron J, Melin Y, Valayer J: Simplified treatment of ureterocele with pyelo-ureteric duplication. Eur Urol 7:321, 1981.

Chan SL, Johnson HW, McLoughlin MG: Idiopathic retroperitoneal fibrosis in children. J Urol 122:103, 1979.

Chilton CP, Vordermark JS, Ransley PG: Transuretero-ureterostomy: A review of its use in modern pediatric urology. Br J Urol 56:604, 1984.

Cohen SJ: The Cohen reimplantation technique. *In* Bergsma D, Duckett JW, Paul NW, Dickman F (eds): Urinary System Malformations in Children. New York, Alan R. Liss, 1977, p 391.

Coplen DE, Duckett JW: The modern approach to ureteroceles. J Urol 153:166, 1995.

Cormio L, Crovace A, Lacalandra G, et al: Bladder Z-plasty for the repair of ureteric injuries: Experimental study in sheep. Br J Urol 71:66, 1993.

Couvelaire R, Auvert J, Moulonguet A, et al: Implantations et anastomoses urétéro-calicielles: Techniques et indications. J Urol Nephrol 70:437, 1964.

Creevy CD: The atonic distal ureteral segment (ureteral achalasia). J Urol 97:457, 1969.

Creevy CD: Misadventures following replacement of ureters with ileum. Surgery 58:497, 1965.

Dauler MI, Byrne DJ, Baxby K: Non-refluxing minimal irritation ureteric stent. Br J Urol 76:795, 1995.

Decter RM, Roth DR, Gonzales ET: Individualized treatment of ureteroceles. J Urol 142:535, 1989.

Dolff C: Verbesserung der Ergebnisse der Ureterimplantation in die Blase mit Hilfe einer elastischen Fixation der Blase. Zentralbl Gynaekol 74:1777, 1952.

Donohue JP, Hostetter M, Glover J, Madura J: Ureteroneocystostomy versus ureteropyelostomy: A comparison in the same renal allograft series. J Urol 114:202, 1975.

Dowd JB, Chen F: Ileal replacement of the ureter in the solitary kidney. Surg Clin North Am 51:739, 1971.

Duckett JW, Pfister RR: Ureterocalicostomy for renal salvage. J Urol 128:98, 1982.

Ehrlich RM: The ureteral folding technique for megaureter surgery. J Urol 134:668, 1986.

Ehrlich RM, Gershman A, Fuchs G: Laparoscopic vesicoureteroplasty in children: Initial case reports. Urology 43:255, 1993.

Ehrlich RM, Skinner DG: Complications of transuretero-ureterostomy. J Urol 113:467, 1975.

Esrig D, Huffman JL: Ureteral strictures. *In* Cohen MS, Resnick MI (eds): Reoperative Urology. Boston, Little, Brown & Co, 1995, p 63.

Foley FEB: Management of ureteral stones: Operation versus expectancy and manipulation. JAMA 104:1314, 1935.

Fort KF, Selman SH, Kropp KA: A retrospective analysis of the use of ureteral stents in children undergoing ureteroneocystostomy. J Urol 129:545, 1983.

Fowler JW: Peritoneal flap ureteropexy for idiopathic retroperitoneal fibrosis. Br J Urol 60:18, 1987.

Gaur DD: Retroperitoneal laparoscopic ureterolithotomy. J Urol 11:175, 1993.

Gearhart JP, Woolfenden KA: The vesico-psoas hitch as an adjunct to megaureter repair in childhood. J Urol 127:505, 1982.

Gibbons WS, Barry JM, Hefty TR: Complications following unstented parallel incision extravesical ureteroneocystostomy in 1,000 kidney transplants. J Urol 148:38, 1992.

Gil-Vernet JM: Lowering of the left renal artery. J Urol 128:686, 1982.

Gil-Vernet JM: A new technique for surgical correction of vesicoureteral reflux. J Urol 131:456, 1984.

Glassberg KI, Laungani G, Wasnick RJ, Waterhouse K: Transverse ureteral advancement technique of ureteroneocystostomy (Cohen reimplant) and modification for difficult cases (experience with 121 ureters). J Urol 134:304, 1985.

Glenn JF, Anderson EE: Distal tunnel ureteral reimplantation. J Urol 97:623, 1967.

Gomez-Avraham I, Nguyen T, Drach GW: Ileal patch ureteroplasty for repair of ureteral strictures: Clinical application and results in 4 patients. J Urol 152:2000, 1994.

Gonzales ET Jr: Reconstruction of anomalies of the distal ureter and ureterovesical junction. *In* Webster G, Kirby R, King L, Goldwasser B (eds): Reconstructive Urology. Boston, Blackwell Scientific Publications, 1993, p 361.

Gonzales ET Jr, Decter RM: Management of ureteroceles in the newborn. *In* King LR (ed): Urologic Surgery in Neonates and Young Infants. Philadelphia, WB Saunders, 1988, p 204.

Goodwin WE, Burke DE, Muller WH: Retrocaval ureter. Surg Gynecol Obstet 104:337, 1957.

Goodwin WE, Winter CC, Turner RD: Replacement of the ureter by small intestine: Clinical application and results of the ileal ureter. J Urol 81:406, 1959.

Gregoir W: Lich-Gregoir operation. *In* Epstein HB, Hohenfellner R, Williams DI (eds): Surgical Pediatric Urology. Stuttgart, Thieme, 1977, p 265.

Gregoir W, Schulman CC: Die extravesikale Antirefluxplastik. Urologe A 16:124, 1977.

Gregoir W, Van Regemorter GV: Le reflux vésico-urétéral congenital. Urol Int 18:122, 1964.

Gross M, Peng B, Waterhouse L: Use of the mobilized bladder to replace the pelvic ureter. J Urol 101:40, 1969.

Guerriero WG, Devine CJ Jr (eds): Urologic Injuries. East Norwalk, CT, Appleton-Century-Crofts, 1984.

Gutierrez J, Chang CY, Nesbit RM: Ipsilateral ureteroureterostomy for vesicoureteral reflux in duplicated ureter. J Urol 101:36, 1969.

Halpern GN, King LR, Belman AB: Transureteroureterostomy in children. J Urol 109:504, 1973.

Hanany Y, Nativ O, Madgar I, et al: The transvesical approach for the removal of distal ureteral calculi. J Urol 139:1177, 1988.

Hanna MK: Megaureter. In King LR (ed): Urologic Surgery in Neonates and Young Infants. Philadelphia, WB Saunders, 1988, p 160.

Hanna MK: New surgical method for one-stage total remodeling of massively dilated and tortuous ureter: Tapering in situ technique. Urology 14:453, 1979.

Harewood LM, Webb DR, Pope AJ: Laparoscopic ureterolithotomy: The results of an initial series and an evaluation of its role in the management of ureteric calculi. Br J Urol 74:170, 1994.

Harney J, Rodgers E, Campbell E, Hickey DP: Loin pain-hematuria syndrome: How effective is renal autotransplantation in its treatment? [See comments.] Urology 44:493, 1994.

Harrill HC: Retrocaval ureter: Report of a case with operative correction of the defect. J Urol 44:450, 1940.

Hawthorne NJ, Zincke H, Kelalis PP: Ureterocalycostomy: An alternative to nephrectomy. J Urol 115:583, 1976.

Hendren WH: Complications of megaureter repair in children. J Urol 113:238, 1975.

Hendren WH: Complications of ureteral reimplantation and megaureter repair. In Smith RB, Skinner DG (eds): Complications of Urologic Surgery: Prevention and Management. Philadelphia, WB Saunders, 1976, p 151.

Hendren WH: Functional restoration of decompensated ureters in children. Am J Surg 119:477, 1970.

Hendren WH: A new approach to infants with severe obstructive uropathy: Early complete reconstruction. J Pediatr Surg 5:184, 1970.

Hendren WH: Operative repair of megaureter in children. J Urol 101:49, 1969.

Hendren WH: Reoperation for the failed ureteral reimplantation. J Urol 111:403, 1974.

Hendren WH: Reoperative ureteral implantation: Management of the difficult case. J Pediatr Surg 15:770, 1980.

Hendren WH: Technical aspects of megaureter repair. Birth Defects 13:21, 1977.

Hendren WH, Hensle TW: Transureteroureterostomy: Experience with 75 cases. J Urol 123:826, 1980.

Hendren WH, McLorie GA: Late stricture of intestinal ureters. J Urol 129:584, 1983.

Hendren WH, Mitchell ME: Surgical correction of ureteroceles. J Urol 121:590, 1979.

Hendren WH, Monfort GJ: Surgical correction of ureteroceles in childhood. J Pediatr Surg 6:235, 1971.

Hensle TW, Burbige KA, Levin RK: Management of the short ureter in urinary tract reconstruction. J Urol 137:707, 1987.

Higgins CC: Transuretero-ureteral anastomosis. J Urol 34:349, 1935.

Hinman F Jr: Ureteral repair and the splint. J Urol 78:376, 1957.

Hinman F Jr, Baumann FW: Complications of vesicoureteral operations from incoordination of micturition. J Urol 116:638, 1976.

Hinman F Jr, Miller ER: Mural tension in vesical disorders and ureteral reflux. J Urol 91:33, 1964.

Hirschorn RC: The ileal sleeve: II. Surgical technique in clinical application. J Urol 92:120, 1964.

Hodges CV, Barry JM, Fuchs EF, et al: Transureteroureterostomy: 25 years experience with 100 patients. J Urol 123:834, 1980.

Hodges CV, Moore RJ, Lehman TH, Benham AM: Clinical experiences with transureteroureterostomy. J Urol 90:552, 1963.

Hodgson NB: Urinary tract infections in childhood. In Kendall AR, Karafin L (eds): Urology, vol 1. Philadelphia, Harper & Row, 1982, p 22.

Hodgson NB, Thompson LW: Technique of reductive ureteroplasty in the management of megaureter. J Urol 113:118, 1975.

Homsy YL, Nsouli I, Hamburger B, et al: Effects of oxybutynin on vesicoureteral reflux in children. J Urol 134:1168, 1985.

Houle AM, McLorie GA, Heritz DM, et al: Extravesical nondismembered ureteropyeloplasty with detrusorrhaphy: A renewed technique to correct vesicoureteral reflux in children. J Urol 148:704, 1992.

Hutch JA: The Uretero-vesical Junction. Berkeley, University of California Press, 1958.

Irby PB III, Wolfe JS Jr, Schaeffer CS, et al: Long-term follow-up of ventriculoureteral shunts for treatment of hydrocephalus. Urology 42:193, 1993.

Jameson SG, McKinney JS, Rushton JF: Ureterocalycostomy: A new surgical procedure for correction of ureteropelvic stricture associated with an intrarenal pelvis. J Urol 77:135, 1957.

Jayanthi VR, McLorie GA, Khoury AE, Churchill BM: Extravesical detrusorrhaphy for refluxing ureters associated with paraureteral diverticula. Urology 45:664, 1995.

Johnston JH: Reconstructive surgery of mega-ureter in childhood. Br J Urol 39:17, 1967.

Johnston JH, Farkas A: The congenital refluxing megaureter: Experiences with surgical reconstruction. Br J Urol 47:153, 1975.

Johnston JH, Heal MR: Reflux in complete duplicated ureters in children: Management and techniques. J Urol 105:881, 1971.

Johnston JH, Johnson LM: Experiences with ectopic ureteroceles. Br J Urol 41:61, 1971.

Juskiewenski S, Vaysse P, Moscovici J, et al: The ureterovesical junction. Anat Clin 5:251, 1984.

Kalicinski ZH, Kansy J, Kotarbínska B, Joszt W: Surgery of megaureters: Modification of Hendren's operation. J Pediatr Surg 12:183, 1977.

Kass EJ: Recurrent vesicoureteral reflux. In Cohen MS, Resnick MI (eds): Reoperative Urology. Boston, Little, Brown & Co, 1995, p 87.

Kavoussi LR, Clayman RV, Brunt LM, et al: Laparoscopic ureterolysis. J Urol 147:426, 1992.

Keating MA, Escala J, Snyder HM, et al: Changing concepts in management of primary obstructive megaureter. J Urol 142:636, 1989.

Kennelly MJ, Bloom DA, Ritchey ML, Panzl A: Outcome analysis of bilateral Cohen cross-trigonal ureteroneocystostomy. Urology 46:393, 1995.

Keramidas DC: Reimplantation of the ureter in a transtrigonal mucosal groove. Br J Urol 72:962, 1993.

King LR: Megaloureter: Definition, diagnosis and management. J Urol 123:222, 1980.

King LR, Koglowski JM, Schacht MJ: Ureteroceles in children: A simplified and successful approach to management. JAMA 249:1461, 1983.

Landes RR, Gavican JR, Fehrenbaker LG: Transvesical meatal-sparing ureterolithotomy. J Urol 109:587, 1972.

Lapides J: The physiology of the intact human ureter. J Urol 59:501, 1948.

Levitt SB, Nabizadek I, Javaid M, et al: Primary calycoureterostomy for pelvicoureteral junction obstructions. J Urol 126:382, 1981.

Lich R Jr, Howerton LW, Davis LA: Recurrent urosepsis in children. J Urol 86:554, 1961.

Lindell OI, Lehtonen TA: Surgical treatment of ureteric obstruction in idiopathic retroperitoneal fibrosis. Scand J Urol Nephrol 110(Suppl):299, 1988.

Lyon RP, Marshall S, Tanagho EA: The ureteral orifice: Its configuration and competency. J Urol 102:504, 1969.

Malek RS, Kelalis PP, Burke EC, et al: Simple and ectopic ureterocele in infancy and childhood. Surg Gynecol Obstet 134:611, 1972.

Mathisen W: Vesicoureteral reflux and its surgical correction. Surg Gynecol Obstet 118:965, 1964.

McCoy GB, Barry JM: Transplant techniques applied to general urology. Urology 33:110, 1989.

McDougall EM, Urban DA, Kerbl K, et al: Laparoscopic repair of vesicoureteral reflux utilizing the Lich-Gregoir technique in the pig model. J Urol 153:497, 1995.

Mering JM, Steel JF, Gittes RF: Congenital ureteral valves. J Urol 107:737, 1972.

Mesrobian H-GJ, Kramer SA, Kelalis PP: Reoperative ureteroneocystostomy: Review of 69 patients. J Urol 133:388, 1985.

Michalowski VE, Modelski W, Kmak A: Die End-zu-End Anastomose zwischen dem unteren Nierenkelch und Harnleiter (Ureterocalicostomie). Z Urol Nephrol 63:1, 1970.

Mikkelsen D, Lepor H: Innovative surgical management of idiopathic retroperitoneal fibrosis. J Urol 141:1192, 1989.

Mollard P, Braun P: Primary ureterocalycostomy for severe hydronephrosis in children. J Pediatr Surg 15:87, 1980.

Monga M, Klein E, Wilfrido R, et al: The forgotten indwelling ureteral stent: A urology dilemma. J Urol 153:1817, 1995.

Moore EV, Weber R, Woodward ER, et al: Isolated ileal loops for ureteral repair. Surg Gynecol Obstet 102:87, 1956.

Mulligan SA, Holley HC, Koehler RE, et al: CT and MR imaging in the evaluation of retroperitoneal fibrosis. J Comput Assist Tomogr 13:277, 1989.

Nesbit RM: Elliptical anastomosis and urologic surgery. Ann Surg 130:796, 1949.

Nezhat C, Nezhat F, Green B: Laparoscopic treatment of obstructed ureter due to endometriosis by resection and ureteroureterostomy: A case report. J Urol 148:865, 1992.

Novick AC, Jackson CL, Straffon RA: The role of renal autotransplantation in complex urological reconstruction. J Urol 143:452, 1990.

Ockerblad N: Reimplantation of the ureter into the bladder by a flap method. J Urol 57:845, 1947.

Okamura K, Ono Y, Yamada Y, et al: Endoscopic trigonoplasty for primary vesico-ureteric reflux. Br J Urol 75:390, 1995.

Ormond JK: Bilateral ureteral obstruction due to envelopment and compression by an inflammatory retroperitoneal process. J Urol 59:1072, 1948.

Osborn DE, Rao PN, Barnard RJ, et al: Surgical management of idiopathic retroperitoneal fibrosis. Br J Urol 53:292, 1981.

O'Sullivan DC, Lemberger RJ, Bishop MC, et al: Ureteric stricture formation following ureteric instrumentation in patients with a nephrostomy drain in place. Br J Urol 74:165, 1994.

Palleschi J, McAninch JW: Renal autotransplantation for retroperitoneal fibrosis. J Urol 125:408, 1981.

Paquin AJ Jr: Ureterovesical anastomosis: The description and evaluation of a technique. J Urol 82:573, 1959.

Perovic S: Surgical treatment of megaureters using detrusor tunneling extravesical ureteroneocystostomy. J Urol 152:622, 1994.

Perovic S, Vukadinovic V: Onlay island flap urethroplasty for severe hypospadias: A variant of the technique. J Urol 151:711, 1994.

Peters CA, Mandell J, Lebowitz RL, et al: Congenital obstructed megaureter in early infancy: Diagnosis and treatment. J Urol 142:641, 1989.

Pisters LL, Cohen MC: Extrinsic ureteral obstruction (including retroperitoneal fibrosis). In Cohen MS, Resnick MI (eds): Reoperative Urology. Boston, Little, Brown & Co, 1995, p 75.

Politano VA, Leadbetter WF: An operative technique for the correction of ureteric reflux. J Urol 79:932, 1958.

Prout GR Jr, Stuart WT, Witus WS: Utilization of ileal segments to substitute for extensive ureteral loss. J Urol 90:541, 1963.

Rainwater LM, Leary FJ, Rife CC: Transureteroureterostomy with cutaneous ureterostomy: A 25-year experience. J Urol 146:13, 1991.

Reddy PK, Evans RM: Laparoscopic ureteroneocystostomy. J Urol 152:2057, 1994.

Reha WC, Gibbons MD: Neonatal ascites and ureteral valves. Urology 33:468, 1989.

Reid R, Schneider K, Fruchtman B: Closure of the bladder neck in patients undergoing continent vesicostomy for urinary incontinence. J Urol 120:40, 1978.

Reinberg Y, Aliabadi H, Johnson P, et al: Congenital ureteral valves in children: Case report and review of the literature. J Pediatr Surg 22:379, 1987.

Retik AB, McEvoy JP, Bauer SB: Megaureters in children. Urology 11:231, 1978.

Rickwood AMK, Reiner I, Jones M, Pournaras C: Current management of duplex-system ureteroceles: Experience with 41 patients. Br J Urol 70:196, 1992.

Riedmiller H, Becht E, Hertle L, et al: Psoas hitch ureteroneocystostomy: Experience with 181 cases. Eur Urol 10:145, 1984.

Rose MC, Novick AC, Rybka SJ: Renal autotransplantation in patients with retroperitoneal fibrosis. Cleve Clin Q 51:357, 1984.

Ruano-Gil D, Coca-Payeras A, Tejedo-Mateu A: Obstruction and normal recanalization of the ureter in the human embryo: Its relation to congenital ureteric obstruction. Eur Urol 1:287, 1975.

Sant GR, Barbalias GA, Klauber GT: Congenital ureteral valves: An abnormality of ureteral embryogenesis? J Urol 133:427, 1985.

Scherz HC, Kaplan GW, Packer MG, Brock WA: Ectopic ureteroceles: Surgical management with preservation of continence: Review of 60 cases. J Urol 142:538, 1989.

Schulman CC, Gregoir W: Ureteric duplication. In Eckstein HB, Hohenfellner R, Williams DI (eds): Surgical Pediatric Urology. Stuttgart, Georg Thieme, 1977, p 244.

Selzman AA, Spirnak JP, Kursh ED: The changing management of ureterovaginal fistulas. J Urol 153:626, 1995.

Shapiro SR, Peckler MS, Johnston JH: Transureteroureterostomy for urinary diversion in children. Urology 8:35, 1976.

Sharp NW: Transureteroureteral anastomosis. Ann Surg 44:687, 1906.

Shehata R: A comparative study of the urinary bladder and the intramural portion of the ureter. Acta Anat 98:380, 1977.

Shokeir AA, Ghoneim MA: Further experience with the modified ileal ureter. J Urol 154:45, 1995.

Smith C, Gosalbez R, Parrott TS, et al: Transurethral puncture of ectopic ureteroceles in neonates and infants. J Urol 152:2110, 1994.

Smith FL, Ritchie EL, Maizels M, et al: Surgery for duplex kidneys with ectopic ureters: Ipsilateral ureterostomy vs. polar nephrectomy. J Urol 142:532, 1989.

Smith IB, Smith JC: Transureteroureterostomy: British experience. Br J Urol 47:519, 1975.

Smith JA Jr, Lee RE, Middleton RG: Ventriculoureteral shunt for hydrocephalus without nephrectomy. J Urol 123:224, 1980.

Sober J: Pelviureterostomy-en-Y. Urology 107:473, 1972.

Sole GM, Randall J, Arkell DG: Ureteropyelostomy: A simple and effective treatment for symptomatic ureteroureteric reflux. Br J Urol 60:325, 1987.

Starr A: Ureteral plication: A new concept in ureteral tailoring for megaureter. Invest Urol 17:153, 1979.

Stephanovic KB, Bukurov NS, Marinkovic JM: Non-antireflux versus antireflux ureteroneocystostomy in adults. Br J Urol 67:263, 1991.

Stephens FD: Treatment of megaureters by multiple micturition. Aust NZ J Surg 27:130, 1957.

Stephens FD: The vesicoureteral hiatus and paraureteral diverticula. J Urol 121:786, 1979.

Stephens FD, Lenaghan D: The anatomical basis and dynamics of vesicoureteral reflux. J Urol 87:669, 1962.

Stone AR, Moran ME: Management of the ureteral defect. In Webster G, Kirby R, King L, Goldwasser B (eds): Reconstructive Urology. Boston, Blackwell Scientific Publications, 1993, p 343.

Sumfest JM, Burns MW, Mitchell ME: The Mitrofanoff principle in urinary reconstruction. J Urol 150:1875, 1993.

Tanagho EA: Anatomy and management of ureteroceles. J Urol 107:729, 1972.

Tanagho EA: A case against incorporation of bowel segments into the closed urinary system. J Urol 113:796, 1975.

Tanagho EA: Embryologic basis for lower ureteral anomalies: A hypothesis. Urology 7:451, 1976.

Tanagho EA: Ureteral tailoring. J Urol 106:194, 1971.

Tanagho EA, Meyers FH, Smith DR: The trigone: Anatomical and physiological considerations: In relation to the ureterovesical junction. J Urol 100:623, 1968.

Tanagho EA, Pugh RCB: The anatomy and function of the ureterovesical junction. Br J Urol 35:151, 1963.

Tresidder CG, Blandy JP, Singh M: Omental sleeve to prevent recurrent retroperitoneal fibrosis under the ureter. Urol Int 27:144, 1972.

Turner-Warwick R: Lower pole pyelocalycostomy, retrograde partial nephrectomy and ureterocalycostomy. Br J Urol 37:673, 1965.

Wacksman J: Initial results with the Cohen cross-trigonal ureteroneocystotomy. J Urol 129:1198, 1983.

Wacksman J, Gilbert A, Sheldon CA: Results of the renewed extravesical reimplant for surgical correction of vesicoureteral reflux. J Urol 148:359, 1992.

Waldeyer W: Ureter-scheide. Verh Anat Ges 6:259, 1892.

Weinstein AJ, Bauer SB, Retik AB, et al: The surgical management of megaureters in duplex systems: The efficacy of ureteral tapering and common sheath reimplantation. J Urol 139:328, 1988.

Wesolowski S: Corrective operative procedure after unsuccessful pelvi-ureteric plastic surgery. Br J Urol 43:679, 1971.

Wesolowski S: Ureterocalycostomy. Eur Urol 1:18, 1975.

Wickramasinghe SF, Stephens FD: Paraureteral diverticula. Associated renal morphology and embryogenesis. Invest Urol 14:381, 1977.

Williams DI, Eckstein HB: Surgical treatment of reflux in children. Br J Urol 37:13, 1965.

Williams DI, Hulme-Moir I: Primary obstructive megaureter. Br J Urol 42:140, 1970.

Williams DI, Woodard JR: Problems in the management of ectopic ureteroceles. J Urol 92:635, 1964.

Zaontz MR, Maizels M, Sugar EC, Firlit CF: Detrusorrhaphy: Extravesical ureteral advancement to correct vesicoureteral reflux in children. J Urol 138:947, 1987.

SURGICAL APPROACHES TO THE KIDNEY

Anderson JC: Hydronephrosis: A fourteen years' survey of results. Proc R Soc Med 55:93, 1962.

Barbaric Z: Renal fascia in urinary tract disease. Radiology 117:17, 1976.

Barelare B: The Foley lumbar ureterolithotomy. J Urol 65:980, 1951.

Barry JM, Hodges CV: The supracostal approach to the kidney and adrenal. J Urol 114:666, 1975.

Bartone FF, Shires TK: The reaction of kidney and bladder tissue to catgut and reconstituted collagen sutures. Surg Gynecol Obstet 128:1221, 1969.

Bazy L: La nephrectomie sous-péritonéale par incision antérieure transversale. Presse Méd 22:186, 1914.

Benjamin JA, Tobin CE: Abnormalities of the kidneys, ureters, and perinephric fascia: Anatomic and clinical study. J Urol 65:715, 1951.

Bensimon H: Muscle protective incisions in renal surgery. Urology 4:476, 1974.

Bolkier M, Mosokovitz B, Ginesin Y, Levin DR: An operation for incisional lumbar hernia. Eur Urol 20:52, 1991.

Browse NL, Hurst P: Repair of long, large midline incisional hernias using reflected flaps of anterior rectus sheath reinforced with Marlex mesh. Am J Surg 138:738, 1979.

Buntain WL, Lynn HB: Splenorrhaphy: Changing concepts for traumatized spleen. Surgery 86:748, 1979.

Chute R, Baron JA, Olsson CA: The transverse upper abdominal "chevron" incision in urological surgery. Trans Am Assoc Genitourin Surg 29:14, 1967.

Chute R: The thoracoabdominal incision in urological surgery. J Urol 65:784, 1951.

Cieslik R, Cerkownik L: Management of the posterior peritoneum after transperitoneal renal surgery. Br J Urol 57:279, 1985.

Cole AT, Fried FA: Experience with the thoraco-abdominal incision for nephroblastoma in children less than 3 years old. J Urol 114:114, 1975.

Congdon ED, Edson JN: The cone of renal fascia in the adult white male. Anat Rec 80:289, 1941.

Cooper MJ, Williams RC: Splenectomy: Indications, hazards and alternatives. Br J Surg 71:173, 1984.

Cox PJ, Ausobsky JR, Ellis H, Pollack AV: Towards no incisional hernias: Lateral paramedian versus midline incisions. J R Soc Med 79:711, 1986.

Crawford ED, Skinner DG, Capparell DB: Intercostal nerve block with thoracoabdominal incision. J Urol 121:290, 1978.

Culp OS: Anterior nephroureterectomy: Advantages and limitations of a single incision. J Urol 85:193, 1961.

Das S, Harris CJ, Amar AD, Egan RM: Dorso-vertical lumbotomy approach for surgery of upper urinary tract calculi. J Urol 129:266, 1983.

Delany HM, Porreca F, Mitsudo S, et al: Splenic capping: An experimental study of a new technique for splenorrhaphy using woven polyglycolic acid mesh. Ann Surg 196:187, 1982.

Delmas P, Ravasse PH, Mallet JF, Pheline Y: Anatomical basis of the surgical approach to the kidney in children. Anat Clin 7:267, 1985.

Dodds WJ, Darweesh RMA, Lawson TL, et al: The retroperitoneal spaces revisited. AJR 147:1155, 1986.

Feldman RA, Shearer JK, Shield DE, et al: Sensitive method for intraoperative roentgenograms. Urology 9:695, 1977.

Feller I, Woodburne RT: Surgical anatomy of the abdominal aorta. Ann Surg 154(Suppl):239, 1961.

Fey B: L'abord du rein par la voie thoraco-abdominale. Arch Urol Clin Necker 5:169, 1926.

Freiha F, Zeineh S: Dorsal approach to upper urinary tract. Urology 21:15, 1983.

Gillou CR, Hall TJ, Donaldson DR, et al: Vertical abdominal incisions: A choice? Br J Surg 67:395, 1980.

Gonzalez R: Extraperitoneal midline approach to retroperitoneum in children. Urology 20:13, 1982.

Greenall MJ, Evans M, Pollock AV: Midline or transverse laparotomy? A random controlled clinical trial: I. Influence on healing. Br J Surg 67:188, 1980.

Griffiths DA: A reappraisal of the Pfannenstiel incision. Br J Urol 48:469, 1976.

Hadar H, Gadoth N: Positional relationships of the colon and kidney determined by perirenal fat. AJR 143:773, 1984.

Hayes MA: Abdominopelvic fascias. Am J Anat 87:119, 1950.

Hess E: Resection of the rib in renal operations. J Urol 42:943, 1939.

Hudnall CH, Kirk JF, Radwin HM: The role of posterior lumbotomy in the management of surgical stone disease. J Urol 139:704, 1988.

Huu N, Person H, Hong R, et al: Anatomical approach to the vascular segmentation of the spleen (lien) based on controlled experimental partial splenectomies. Anat Clin 4:265, 1982.

Jenkins TPN: The burst abdominal wound: A mechanical approach. Br J Surg 63:873, 1976.

Kockelbergh RC, Chilton CP: The Vac-Pac in open renal surgery. Br J Urol 71:110, 1993.

Kreder KJ, Thrasher JB: Surgical approaches to the genitourinary tract. In Webster G, Kirby R, King L, Goldwasser B (eds): Reconstructive Urology. Boston, Blackwell Scientific Publications, 1993, p 203.

Love L, Meyers MA, Churchill RJ, et al: Computed tomography of the extraperitoneal spaces. AJR 136:781, 1981.

Lurz H: Ein muskelschonender lumbalschnitt zur Freilegung der Niere. Chirurg 27:125, 1956.

Lutzeyer W: Lumbodorsal exploration. In Glenn JF (ed): Urologic Surgery. New York, Harper & Row, 1975, p 127.

Lyon RP: An anterior extraperitoneal incision for kidney surgery. J Urol 79:383, 1958.

Lytton B: Surgery of the kidney. In Walsh PC, Gittes RF, Perlmutter AD, Stamey TA (eds): Campbell's Urology, 5th ed, vol 3. Philadelphia, WB Saunders, 1986, p 2406.

MacCallum DB: The arterial blood supply of the mammalian kidney. Am J Anat 38:153, 1926.

Marshall M Jr, Johnson SH III: A simple direct approach to the renal pedicle. J Urol 84:24, 1960.

Marx WJ, Patel SK: Renal fascia: Its radiographic importance. Urology 13:1, 1979.

Mayo WJ: The incision for lumbar exposure of the kidney. Ann Surg 55:63, 1912.

McVay CB, Anson BJ: Aponeurotic and fascial continuities in the abdomen, pelvis and thigh. Anat Rec 76:213, 1940.

McVay CB, Anson BJ: Composition of the rectus sheath. Anat Rec 77:213, 1940.

Merrill DC: Modified thoracoabdominal approach to the kidney and retroperitoneal tissue. J Urol 117:15, 1977.

Meyers MA: The extraperitoneal spaces. In Meyers MA (ed): Dynamic Radiology of the Abdomen: Normal and Pathologic Anatomy. New York, Springer-Verlag, 1976, p 113.

Milloy FJ, Anson BJ, Cauldwell EW: Variations in the inferior caval veins and in their renal and lumbar communications. Surg Gynecol Obstet 115:131, 1962.

Mitchell GAG: The innervation of the kidney, ureter, testicle and epididymis. J Anat 70:10, 1935.

Mitchell GAG: The intrinsic renal nerves. Acta Anat 13:1, 1951.

Mitchell GAG: The renal fascia. Br J Surg 37:257, 1950.

More RH, Duff GL: The renal arterial vasculature in man. Am J Pathol 27:95, 1950.

Morgenstern L, Shapiro SJ: Techniques of splenic conservation. Arch Surg 114:449, 1979.

Mosnier H, Frantz P, Calmat A, et al: A study of the anastomoses between the left renal vein and the intravertebral plexuses. Anat Clin 1:321, 1980.

Nagamatsu G: Dorsolumbar approach to the kidney and adrenal with osteoplastic flap. J Urol 63:569, 1959.

Novick A: Posterior surgical approach to the kidney and ureter. J Urol 124:192, 1980.

O'Donohoe MK, Flanagan F, Fitzpatrick JM, Smith JM: Surgical approach to inferior vena caval extension of renal carcinoma. Br J Urol 60:492, 1987.

Orda R, Rudberg Z: The adreno-renal-ureteral sheath. Surgical-anatomical study. Urol Int 31:179, 1976.

Orland SM, Snyder HM, Duckett JW: The dorsal lumbotomy incision in pediatric urological surgery. J Urol 138:963, 1987.

Pansadoro V: The posterior lumbotomy. Urol Clin North Am 10:573, 1983.

Papin E: Chirurgie du Rein. Paris, Ed. Doin, 1928.

Parienty RA, Pradel J: Radiological evaluation of the peri- and para-renal spaces by computed tomography. CRC Crit Rev Diagn Imaging 20:1, 1983.

Pick JW, Anson BJ: The renal vascular pedicle: An anatomical study of 430 body halves. J Urol 44:411, 1940.

Poutasse EF: Anterior approach to the upper urinary tract. J Urol 85:199, 1961.

Pressman D: Eleventh intercostal space incision for renal surgery. J Urol 74:578, 1955.

Prince CL: Lumbar ureterolithotomy. J Urol 54:368, 1945.

Ravitch MM: Ventral hernia. Surg Clin North Am 51:1341, 1971.

Redman JF: The anatomy of the genitourinary system. In Gillenwater JY, Grayhack JT, Howards SS, Duckett JW (eds): Adult and Pediatric Urology. Chicago, Year Book Medical Publishers, 1987, p 3.

Redman JF: An anatomic approach to the kidneys and retroperitoneum. In Crawford ED, Das S (eds): Current Genitourinary Cancer Surgery. Philadelphia, Lea & Febiger, 1990, p 1.

Redman JF: Anatomy of the retroperitoneal connective tissue. J Urol 130:45, 1983.

Reis RH, Esenther G: Variations in the pattern of renal vessels and their relation to the type of posterior vena cava in man. Am J Anat 104:295, 1959.

Riehle RA Jr, Lavengood R: The eleventh rib transcostal incision: Technique for an extrapleural approach. J Urol 132:1089, 1984.

Robin CE: The renal fascia and its relation to the transversalis fascia. Anat Rec 89:295, 1944.

Rodgers F, Baumgartner N, Nolan P, et al: Repair of traumatic splenic injuries by splenorrhaphy with polyglycolic acid mesh. Curr Surg 44:112, 1987.

Ross JA, Samuel E, Millar DR: Variations in the renal vascular pedicle (an anatomical and radiological study with particular reference to renal transplantation). Br J Urol 33:478, 1961.

Rouiller C: General anatomy and histology of the kidney. In Rouiller C, Miller AF (eds): The Kidney, vol 1. New York, Academic Press, 1969, p 61.

Rubenstein WA, Auh YH, Zirinsky K, et al: Posterior peritoneal recesses: Assessment using CT. Radiology 156:461, 1985.

Smith DR, Schulte JW, Smart WR: Surgery of the kidney. In Campbell M (ed): Urology, vol III. Philadelphia, WB Saunders, 1963, p 2324.

Spence HM: Some observations on the indications for and technique of transperitoneal renal surgery. Urol Corresp Club Lett, February 9, 1962.

Ssysganow AN: Über des Lymphsystem der Nieren und Nierenhilen beim Menschen. Z Gesamte Anat 91:771, 1930.

Sutherland RS, Gerow RR: Hernia after dorsal incision into lumbar region: A case report and review of pathogenesis and treatment. J Urol 153:382, 1995.

Swartz WT: Lumbar hernia. In Nyhus LM, Condon RE (eds): Hernia, 2nd ed. Philadelphia, JB Lippincott, 1978, p 409.

Tessler AN, Yuvienco F, Farcon E: Paramedian extraperitoneal incision for total nephroureterectomy. Urology 5:397, 1975.

Thornbury JR: Perirenal anatomy: Normal and abnormal. Radiol Clin North Am 17:321, 1979.

Tobin CE: The renal fascia and its relation to the transversalis fascia. Anat Rec 89:295, 1944.

Tuffier R, Lejars F: Les veines de la capsule adipeuse du rein. Arch Physiol 1:41, 1891.

Turner-Warwick RT: The supracostal approach to the renal area. Br J Urol 37:671, 1965.

Usher FC: New technique for repairing incisional hernias with Marlex mesh. Am J Surg 138:740, 1979.

Ward JP, Smart CJ, O'Donoghue EPN, et al: Synchronous bilateral lumbotomy. Eur Urol 2:102, 1976.

Witherington R: Improving the supracostal loin incisions. J Urol 124:73, 1980.

Zuckerkandl E: Beiträge zur Anatomie des menschlichen Körpers: I. Ueber den Fixationsapparat der Nieren. In Anatomie des Menschens, vol II. Tubingen, Germany, 1863, p 59.

Audiovisual

Das S, Amar AD: Dorsal Lumbotomy Revisited. Wilkes-Barre, PA, Karol Media, 1985 (20 minutes). AUA #919-1131.

KIDNEY: RECONSTRUCTION

Anderson JC: Hydronephrosis: A fourteen years' survey of results. Proc R Soc Med 55:93, 1962.

Anderson JC, Hynes W: Retrocaval ureter: A case diagnosed preoperatively and treated successfully by a plastic operation. Br J Urol 21:209, 1949.

Anson BJ, Cauldwell EW: Pararenal vascular system: Study of 425 anatomical specimens. Q Bull Northwest Univ Med Sch 21:320, 1947.

Anson BJ, Cauldwell EW, Pick JW, Beaton LE: The anatomy of the pararenal system of veins, with comments on the renal arteries. J Urol 60:714, 1948.

Anson BJ, Cauldwell EW, Pick JW, Beaton LE: The blood supply of the kidney, suprarenal gland, and associated structures. Surg Gynecol Obstet 84:313, 1947.

Anson BJ, Daseler EH: Common variations in renal anatomy, affecting blood supply, form, and topography. Surg Gynecol Obstet 112:439, 1961.

Anson BJ, Kurth LE: Common variations in the renal blood supply. Surg Gynecol Obstet 100:156, 1955.

Auvert J: La veine rénale gauche. Presse Méd 75:1405, 1967.

Banowsky LH: The role of adjuvant operations in renal transplantation. Urol Clin North Am 3:527, 1976.

Banowsky LH: Surgical complications of renal transplantation. In Glenn JF (ed): Urologic Surgery, 4th ed. Philadelphia, WB Saunders, 1991, p 252.

Banowsky LH: Vascular complications of renal transplantation. *In* Cohen MS, Resnick MI (eds): Reoperative Urology. Boston, Little, Brown & Co, 1995, p 11.

Banowsky LH, Stewart BH: Renal transplantation. *In* Stewart BH (ed): Operative Urology. Baltimore, Williams & Wilkins, 1975, chap 14, p 5.

Barnett M, Bruskewitz RC, Belzer FO, et al: Ileocecocystoplasty bladder augmentation and renal transplantation. J Urol 138:855, 1987.

Barnett M, Bruskewitz R, Glass N, et al: Long-term clean intermittent self-catheterization in renal transplant recipient. J Urol 134:654, 1985.

Barry JM: Spermatic cord preservation in kidney transplantation. J Urol 127:1076, 1982.

Barry JM, Fuchs EF: Right renal vein extension in cadaver kidney transplantation. Arch Surg 113:300, 1978.

Barry JM, Lawson RK, Strong B, Hodges CV: Urologic complications in 173 kidney transplants. J Urol 112:567, 1974.

Barry JM, Lemmers MJ: Patch and flap techniques to repair right renal vein defects caused by cadaver liver retrieval for transplantation. J Urol 153:1803, 1995.

Beaton LE: The anatomy of the pararenal system of veins, with comments on the renal arteries. J Urol 60:714, 1948.

Belzer FO, Kountz SL, Najarian JS, et al: Prevention of urological complications after renal allotransplantation. Arch Surg 101:449, 1970.

Belzer FO, Schweizer RT, Kountz S: Management of multiple vessels in renal transplantation. Transplant Proc 4:639, 1972.

Benoit G, Delmas V, Gillot C, Hureau J: Anatomical bases of kidney transplantation in man. Anat Clin 6:239, 1984.

Bérard P, Pouyet M: Les voies d'évacuation veineuse du rein après ligature de la veine rénale gauche. Lyon Chir 64:781, 1968.

Berger RE, Ansell JS, Tremann JA, et al: The use of self-retained ureteral stents in the management of urologic complications in renal transplant recipients. J Urol 124:781, 1980.

Binder C, Bonick P, Ciavarra V: Experience with Silastic U-tube nephrostomy. J Urol 106:499, 1977.

Blaivas JG, Pais VM, Spellman RM: Chemolysis of residual stone fragments after extensive surgery for staghorn calculi. Urology 6:680, 1975.

Blandy J: Surgery of renal cast calculi. *In* Libertino JA, Zinman L (eds): Reconstructive Urologic Surgery. Baltimore, Williams & Wilkins, 1977, p 17.

Blandy J, Tresidder GC: Extended pyelolithotomy for renal calculi. Br J Urol 39:1, 1967.

Boatman DL, Cornell SH, Kolin CP: The arterial supply of horseshoe kidneys. AJR 113:447, 1971.

Boyce WH, Elkins IB: Reconstructive renal surgery following anatrophic nephrolithotomy. J Urol 111:307, 1974.

Boyce WH, Harrison LH: Complications of renal stone surgery. *In* Smith RB, Skinner DG (eds): Complications of Urologic Surgery: Prevention and Management. Philadelphia, WB Saunders, 1976, p 87.

Boyd GL, Diethelm AG, Gelman S, et al: Correcting prolonged bleeding during renal transplantation with estrogen or plasma. Arch Surg 131:160, 1996.

Bredael JJ, Carson CC III, Weinerth JL: Bilateral nephrectomy by the posterior approach. Eur Urol 6:251, 1980.

Brooks JD, Kavoussi LR, Preminger GM, et al: Comparison of open and endourologic approach to the obstructed ureteropelvic junction. Urology 46:791, 1995.

Caldamone AA, Zabbo A: Failed pyeloplasty. *In* Cohen MS, Resnick MI (eds): Reoperative Urology. Boston, Little, Brown & Co, 1995, p 35.

Carini M, Selli C, Grechi G, Masini G: Pyelovesicostomy: An alternative to ureteropelvic junction-plasty in pelvic ectopic kidneys. Urology 26:125, 1983.

Carlton CE Jr, Scott R Jr, Goldman M: The management of penetrating injuries of the kidney. J Trauma 8:1071, 1968.

Carroll PR, Klosterman P, McAninch JW: Early vascular control for renal trauma: A critical review. J Urol 141:826, 1989.

Carroll PR, McAninch JW: Staging of renal trauma. Urol Clin North Am 16:193, 1989.

Carroll PR, McAninch JW, Klosterman P, Greenblatt M: Renovascular trauma: Risk assessment, surgical management and outcome. J Trauma 30:547, 1990.

Cass AS: Renovascular injuries from external trauma: diagnosis, treatment and outcome. Urol Clin North Am 16:3, 1989.

Cass AS, Bubrick M, Luxenberg M, et al: Renal pedicle injury in the patient with multiple injuries. J Trauma 25:892, 1985.

Cass AS, Ireland GW: Comparison of the conservative and surgical management of the more severe degrees of renal trauma in multiple injured patients. J Urol 109:8, 1973.

Cass AS, Luxenberg M: Conservative or immediate surgical management of blunt renal injuries. J Urol 130:11, 1983.

Chang R, Marshall FF, Mitchell S: Percutaneous management of benign ureteral strictures and fistulas. J Urol 137:1126, 1987.

Chin JL: Microvascular reconstructive "bench" surgery for donor kidneys before transplantation: Techniques and results. J Urol 142:23, 1989.

Chiverton SG, Murie JA, Allen RD, Morris PJ: Renal transplant nephrectomy. Surg Gynecol Obstet 164:324, 1987.

Clayman RV, Basler JW, Kavoussi L, et al: Ureteronephroscopic endopyelotomy. J Urol 144:246, 1990.

Cockrell SN, Hendren WH: The importance of visualizing the ureter before performing a pyeloplasty. J Urol 144:588, 1990.

Collins GM, Green RD, Boyer D, et al: Protection of kidneys from warm ischemic injury: Dosage and timing of mannitol administration. Transplantation 29:83, 1980.

Cook JH III, Lytton B: Intraoperative localization of renal calculi during nephrolithotomy by ultrasound scanning. J Urol 117:546, 1979.

Corriere JN, Perloff LJ, Barker CF, et al: The ureteropyelostomy in human renal transplantation. J Urol 110:24, 1973.

Cromie WJ: Complications of pyeloplasty. Urol Clin North Am 10:385, 1983.

Culp OS, DeWeerd JH: A pelvic flap operation for certain types of ureteropelvic obstruction: Preliminary report. Proc Staff Meet Mayo Clin 26:483, 1951.

Culp OS, Winterringer JR: Surgical treatment of horseshoe kidney: A comparison of results after various types of operations. J Urol 73:747, 1955.

Darner HL: Bilateral ectopic kidney. J Urol 12:193, 1924.

Daseler EH, Anson BJ: Anatomical relations of ectopic iliolumbar kidneys, bilateral in adult and unilateral in fetus. J Urol 49:789, 1943.

Davis DM: Intubated ureterotomy: A new operation for ureteral and ureteropelvic stricture. Surg Gynecol Obstet 76:513, 1943.

Dees JF: The use of an intraoperative coagulum in pyelolithotomy: A preliminary report. South Med J 49:497, 1943.

DeWeerd JH, Paulk SC, Tomera FM, et al: Renal autotransplantation for upper ureteral stenosis. J Urol 116:23, 1976.

Dixon JS, Gosling JA: The musculature of the human renal calices, pelvis and upper ureter. J Anat 135:129, 1982.

Dixon CM, McAninch JW: A practical approach for managing blunt renal trauma. Infect Urol, January/February, 1994.

Dixon CM, McAninch JW: Reconstruction of the traumatized kidney. *In* Webster G, Kirby R, King L, Goldwasser B (eds): Reconstructive Urology. Boston, Blackwell Scientific Publications, 1993, p 273.

Dixon CM, McAninch JW: Traumatic renal injuries: II. Operative management. Houston, American Urological Association, AUA Update Series, vol X, lesson 36, pp 282-288, 1991.

Djurhuus JC, Nerström B, Rask-Andersen H: Dynamics of upper urinary tract in man. Acta Chir Scand 472:49, 1976.

Doménech-Mateu JM, Gonzalez-Compta X: Horseshoe kidney: A new theory on its embryogenesis based on the study of a 16-mm human embryo. Anat Rec 222:408, 1988.

Donahoe PK, Hendren WH: Pelvic kidney in infants and children: Experience with 16 cases. J Pediatr Surg 15:486, 1980.

Donohue JP, Hostetter M, Glover J, Madura J: Ureteroneocystostomy versus ureteropyelostomy: A comparison in the same renal allograft series. J Urol 114:202, 1975.

Douville E, Hollingshead WH: The blood-supply of the normal renal pelvis. J Urol 73:906, 1955.

Dretler SP, Pfister RC, Newhouse JH: Renal stone dissolution via percutaneous nephrostomy. N Engl J Med 300:341, 1979.

Duckett JW Jr: When to operate on neonatal hydronephrosis. Urology 42:617, 1993.

Duckett JW, Pfister RR: Ureterocalicostomy for renal salvage. J Urol 128:98, 1982.

Eckstein HB, Kamal I: Hydronephrosis due to pelvi-ureteric obstruction in children: An assessment of the anterior transperitoneal approach. Br J Surg 58:663, 1971.

Edwards EA: Clinical anatomy of lesser variations of the inferior vena cava and a proposal for classifying the anomalies of this vessel. Angiology 2:85, 1951.

Erturk E, Novick AC, Vidt DG, et al: Secondary renorevascularization for recurrent renal artery stenosis. Cleve Clin J Med 56:427, 1989.

Escala JM, Keating MA, Boyd G, et al: Development of elastic fibers in the upper urinary tract. J Urol 141:969, 1989.

Facer MJ, Lynch RD, Evans HO, Chin FK: Inferior vena cava duplication: Demonstration by computed tomography. Radiology 130:707, 1979.

Faerber GJ, Ritchey ML, Bloom DA: Percutaneous endopyelotomy in infants and young children after failed open pyeloplasty. J Urol 154:1495, 1995.

Feldman RA, Shearer JK, Shield DE, et al: Sensitive method for intraoperative roentgenograms. Urology 9:695, 1977.

Fine H, Keen EN: The arteries of the human kidney. J Anat 100:881, 1966.

Flashner SC, Weinerth JL: Renal transplant and associated reconstructive procedures. *In* Webster G, Kirby R, King L, Goldwasser B (eds): Reconstructive Urology. Boston, Blackwell Scientific Publications, 1993, p 329.

Foley FEB: New plastic operation for stricture at ureteropelvic junction: Report of 20 operations. J Urol 38:643, 1937.

Foote JW, Blennerhasset JB, Eiglesworth FW, MacKinnon KJ: Observations on the ureteropelvic junction. J Urol 104:252, 1970.

Fourman J, Moffat DB: The Blood Vessels of the Kidney. Oxford, Blackwell Scientific Publications, 1971.

Fowler JE Jr: Bacteriology of branched renal calculi and accompanying urinary tract infection. J Urol 131:213, 1984.

Freed SZ: Bilateral nephrectomy in transplant recipients. Urology 10(Suppl):16, 1977.

Freed SZ, Veith FJ, Soberman R, Gliedman ML: Simultaneous bilateral posterior nephrectomy in transplant recipients. Surgery 68:468, 1970.

Freed SZ, Veith FJ, Tellis V, et al: Improved cadaveric nephrectomy for kidney transplantation. Surg Gynecol Obstet 137:101, 1973.

Friedland GW, DeVries P: Renal ectopia and fusion—embryologic basis. Urology 5:698, 1975.

Gelin LE, Claes G, Gustafsson A, Storm B: Total bloodlessness for extracorporeal organ repair. Rev Surg 28:305, 1971.

Gibbons RP, Correa RJ Jr, Cummings KB, Mason JT: Surgical management of renal lesions using in situ hypothermia and ischemia. J Urol 115:12, 1976.

Gil-Vernet JM: New surgical concepts in removing renal calculi. Urol Int 20:255, 1965.

Gil-Vernet JM, Caralps A, Revert I, et al: Extracorporeal renal surgery. Urology 5:444, 1975.

Golbus MS, Harrison MR, Filly RA, et al: In utero treatment of urinary tract obstruction. Am J Obstet Gynecol 142:383, 1982.

Goldstein I, Cho SI, Olsson CA: Nephrostomy drainage for renal transplant complications. J Urol 126:159, 1981.

Gordon MR, Carrion HM, Politano VA: Dissolution of uric acid calculi with THAM irrigation. Urology 12:393, 1978.

Gosling JA: The musculature of the upper urinary tract. Acta Anat 75:408, 1970.

Gosling JA, Constantinou CE: The origin and propagation of upper urinary tract contraction waves: A new in vitro methodology. Experientia 32:266, 1976.

Gosling JA, Dixon JS: The structure of the normal and hydronephrotic upper urinary tract. *In* O'Reilly PH, Gosling JA (eds): Idiopathic Hydronephrosis. London, Springer-Verlag, 1982.

Graves FT: The aberrant renal artery. J Anat 90:553, 1956.

Graves FT: The anatomy of the intra-renal arteries in health and disease. Br J Surg 43:605, 1956.

Graves FT: The arterial anatomy of the congenitally abnormal kidney. Br J Surg 56:533, 1969.

Greenberg SH, Wein AJ, Perloff LF, Barker CF: Ureteropyelostomy and ureteroneocystostomy in renal transplantation: Postoperative urological complications. J Urol 118:17, 1977.

Gruenwald P: The normal changes in the position of the embryonic kidney. Anat Rec 85:163, 1943.

Guar DD, Agarwal DK, Khochikar MV, Purohit KC: Laparoscopic renal biopsy via retroperitoneal approach. J Urol 151:925, 1994.

Guerriero WG: Ureteral injury. Urol Clin North Am 16:237, 1989.

Guerriero WG, Carlton CE Jr, Scott R Jr, Beall AC Jr: Renal pedicle injuries. J Trauma 11:53, 1971.

Hamm FC, Weinberg SR: Renal and ureteral surgery without intubation. J Urol 73:475, 1955.

Hanley HG: The pelvi-ureteric junction: A cine-pyelography study. Br J Urol 31:377, 1959.

Hanna MK, Jeffs RD, Sturgess JM, Barkin M: Ureteral structure and ultrastructure: I. The normal human ureter. II. Congenital ureteropelvic junction obstruction and primary obstructive megaureter. J Urol 116:718, 725, 1976.

Hardy JD: High ureteral injuries: Management by autotransplantation of the kidney. JAMA 184:97, 1963.

Harrison MR, Golbus MS, Filly RA, et al: Fetal hydronephrosis: Selection and surgical repair. J Pediatr Surg 22:556, 1987.

Harrison MR, Golbus MS, Filly RA, et al: Fetal surgery for congenital hydronephrosis. N Engl J Med 306:591, 1982.

Harrison MR, Golbus MS, Filly RA, et al: Management of the fetus with congenital hydronephrosis. J Pediatr Surg 17:728, 1982.

Hegedüs V: Arterial anatomy of the kidney. A three dimensional angiographic investigation. Acta Radiol Diagn 12:604, 1972.

Hellstrom J: Some observations on removal of kidney stones particularly by means of pyelolithotomy in situ. Acta Clin Scand 98:442, 1949.

Hellstrom J, Giertz G, Lindblom K: Pathogenesis and treatment of hydronephrosis. *In* Proceedings of the VIII Congress de Société Internationale d'Urologie, Paris, 1949.

Hendren WH, Radharkrishnan J, Middleton AW Jr: Pediatric pyeloplasty. J Pediatr Surg 15:133, 1980.

Henriksson C, Brynger H, Nilsson AE, et al: Reconstruction of urinary outflow obstructions by renal autotransplantation. Scand J Urol Nephrol 15(Suppl 59):1, 1980.

Herwig KR, Konnak JW: Vesicopyelostomy: A method for urinary drainage of the transplanted kidney. J Urol 109:955, 1973.

Heynes CF, van Gelderen WFC: 3-dimensional imaging of the pelviocaliceal system by computerized tomographic reconstruction. J Urol 144:1335, 1990.

Hinman F Jr: Ballottement of peripelvic cyst for operative diagnosis and localization. J Urol 97:7, 1967.

Hinman F Jr: Dismembered pyeloplasty without urinary diversion. *In* Scott R (ed): Current Controversies in Urologic Management. Philadelphia, WB Saunders Co, 1972, p 253.

Hinman F Jr: Hydronephrosis. *In* Goldman HS (ed): Practice of Surgery. Hagerstown, MD, Harper & Row, 1980, chap 2, p 1.

Hinman F Jr: Peripelvic extravasation during intravenous urography: Evidence for an additional route for backflow after ureteral obstruction. J Urol 85:385, 1961.

Hinman F Jr: Techniques for ureteropyeloplasty. Arch Surg 71:790, 1955.

Hinman F Jr, Belzer FO: Urinary tract infection and renal homotransplantation: I. Effect of antibacterial irrigations on defenses of the defunctionalized bladder. J Urol 101:477, 1969.

Hinman F Jr, Cattolica EV: Branched calculi: Shapes and operative approaches. J Urol 126:291, 1981.

Hinman F Jr, Oppenheimer R: Ureteral regeneration: VI. Delayed urinary flow in the healing of unsplinted ureteral defects. J Urol 78:138, 1957.

Hinman F Jr, Schmaelzle JF, Belzer FO: Urinary tract infection and renal homotransplantation: II. Posttransplantation bacterial invasion. J Urol 101:673, 1969.

Hjort EF: Partial resection of the renal pelvis and pole of the kidney for hydronephrosis. Br J Urol 43:406, 1971.

Hodge EE, Novick AC: Reconstructive surgery for renovascular disease. *In* Webster G, Kirby R, King L, Goldwasser B (eds): Reconstructive Urology. Boston, Blackwell Scientific Publications, 1993, p 299.

Hodges CV, Lawson RK, Pearse HD, Stranburg CO: Autotransplantation of the kidney. J Urol 110:20, 1973.

Hodson J: The lobar structure of the kidney. Br J Urol 44:246, 1972.

Hoeltl W, Hruby W, Aharinejad S: Renal vein anatomy and its implications for retroperitoneal surgery. J Urol 143:1108, 1990.

Hollowell JG, Altman HG, Snyder H III, et al: Co-existing ureteropelvic junction obstruction and vesicoureteral reflux: Diagnostic and therapeutic implications. J Urol 142:490, 1989.

Homsy Y, Simard J, Debs C, et al: Pyeloplasty: To divert or not to divert? Urology 16:577, 1980.

Hubner WA, Schramek P, Pfluger H: Laparoscopic nephropexy. J Urol 152:1184, 1994.

Immergut MA, Jacobson JJ, Culp DA: Cutaneous pyelostomy. J Urol 101:276, 1969.

Ivatury RR, Zubowski R, Stahl WM: Penetrating renovascular trauma. J Trauma 29:1620, 1989.

Jackson CL, Novick AC: Renovascular complications unrelated to renal transplantation. *In* Cohen MS, Resnick MI (eds): Reoperative Urology. Boston, Little, Brown & Co, 1995, p 27.

Janetschek G, Peschel R, Reissigl A, Bartsch G: Laparoscopic dismembered pyeloplasty. J Endourol 8:S83, 1994.

Johnston JH, Evans JP, Glassberg KI, et al: Pelvic hydronephrosis in children: A review of 9 personal cases. J Urol 117:97, 1977.

Kadir S, White RI Jr, Engel R: Balloon dilatation of a ureteropelvic junction obstruction. Radiology 143:263, 1982.

Kaneto H, Orikasa S, Chiba T, Takahashi T: Three-D muscular arrangement at the ureteropelvic junction and its changes in congenital hydronephrosis: A stereo-morphometric study. J Urol 146:909, 1991.

Kark RM: Renal biopsy. JAMA 105:220, 1968.

Karlin GS, Badlani GH, Smith AD: Endopyelotomy versus open pyeloplasty: Comparison in 88 patients. J Urol 140:476, 1988.

Karsburg W, Leary FJ: Nephrostomy tube replacement. Urology 13:301, 1979.

Kaylor WM, Novick AC, Ziegelbaum M, et al: Reversal of end stage renal failure with surgical revascularization in patients with atherosclerotic renal artery occlusion. J Urol 141:46, 1989.

Khauli R, Novick AC, Ziegelbaum M: Splenorenal bypass in the treatment of renal artery stenosis: Experience with 69 cases. J Vasc Surg 2:547, 1985.

Kiil F: The Function of the Ureter and Renal Pelvis. Oslo, Oslo University Press, 1957.

King LR: Management of multicystic kidney and ureteropelvic junction obstruction. *In* King LR (ed): Urologic Surgery in Neonates and Young Infants. Philadelphia, WB Saunders, 1988, p 140.

Koff SA, Hayden LJ, Cirulli C, Shore R: Pathophysiology of ureteropelvic obstruction: Experimental and clinical observations. J Urol 136:336, 1986.

Koff SA, Thrall JH, Keyes JW Jr: Diuretic radionuclide urography: A non-invasive method for evaluating nephroureteral dilatation. J Urol 1:153, 1979.

KooSee Lin LC, Bewick M, Koffman CG: Primary use of a double J silicone ureteral stent in renal transplantation. Br J Urol 72:697, 1993.

Kumar S, Bhandari M, Mohapatra TP: A simple ureteric function test: Intra-operative and post-operative uses in pyeloplasty. Br J Urol 71:625, 1993.

Landau R, Botha JR, Myburgh JA: Pyeloureterostomy or ureteroneocystostomy in renal transplantation? Br J Urol 58:6, 1986.

Lawson RK: Extracorporeal renal surgery. J Urol 123:301, 1980.

Lawson RK, Hodges CV: Extracorporeal renal artery repair and autotransplantation. Urology 4:532, 1974.

Leadbetter GW Jr, Monaco AP, Russell PS: A technique for reconstruction of the urinary tract in renal transplantation. Surg Gynecol Obstet 123:839, 1966.

Lee WJ, Badlani GH, Karlin GS, et al: Treatment of ureteropelvic

strictures with percutaneous pyelotomy: Experience in 62 patients. AJR 151:515, 1988.

Lerner SE, Griefer I, Taub HC, et al: A single center experience with renal transplantation in young children. J Urol 149:549, 1993.

Libertino JA, Zinman L: Surgery for renovascular hypertension. *In* Libertino JA (ed): Pediatric and Adult Reconstructive Urologic Surgery, 2nd ed. Baltimore, Williams & Wilkins, 1987, p 119.

Libertino JA, Zinman L, Breslin DJ, et al: Renal artery revascularization. Restoration of renal function. JAMA 244:1340, 1980.

Liebermann-Meffert D, White H (eds): The Greater Omentum. Berlin, Springer-Verlag, 1983.

Linke CA, Cockett ATK, Lai MK, Youseff AM: The use of pedicled grafts of omentum in the repair of transplant-related urinary tract problems. J Urol 120:532, 1978.

Linke CA, May AG: Autotransplantation in retroperitoneal fibrosis. J Urol 107:196, 1972.

Maatman TJ, Montie JE: Complications of renal surgery. *In* Marshall FF (ed): Urologic Complications. Chicago, Year Book Medical Publishers, 1986, p 103.

Madaio MP: Renal biopsy. Kidney Int 38:529, 1990.

Maizels M, Stephens FD: The induction of urologic malformations: Understanding the relationship of renal ectopia and congenital scoliosis. Invest Urol 17:209, 1979.

Margreit R, Steiner E, Aigner F, Hoyer J: A safe technique for renal transplantation in patients with severely infected bladders. Surg Gynecol Obstet 159:487, 1984.

Marshall FF: Intraoperative localization of renal calculi. Urol Clin North Am 10:629, 1983.

Marshall FF, Smolev JK, Spees EK, et al: The urological evaluation and management of patients with congenital lower urinary tract anomalies prior to renal transplantation. J Urol 127:1078, 1982.

Marshall VR, Singh M, Tresidder GC, Blandy JP: The place of partial nephrectomy in the management of renal calyceal calculi. Br J Urol 47:759, 1976.

Masaki Z, Iguchi A, Kinoshita N, et al: Intrasinusal pyelolithotomy with lower pole nephrotomy for removal of renal stones. Urology 26:461, 1985.

McAninch JW, Carroll PR: Renal trauma: Kidney preservation through improved vascular control—a refined approach. J Trauma 22:285, 1982.

McAninch JW, Carroll PR, Klosterman PW, et al: Renal reconstruction after injury. J Urol 145:932, 1991.

McClure CFW, Butler EG: The development of the vena cava inferior in man. Am J Anat 35:331, 1925.

McCowan RE: Bilateral renal ectopia. J Urol 22:653, 1929.

McCullough CS, Soper NJ, Clayman RV, et al: Laparoscopic drainage of a posttransplant lymphocele. Transplantation 51:725, 1991.

McDougal WS, Persky LI (eds): Traumatic Injuries of the Genitourinary System. Baltimore, Williams & Wilkins, 1981.

McDougall EM, Clayman RV, Fadden PT: Retroperitoneoscopy: The Washington University Medical School experience. Urology 43:446, 1994.

McLean PA, Gawley WF, Gorey TP: Technical modifications of Anderson-Hynes pyeloplasty for congenital pelviureteric junction obstruction. Br J Urol 57:114, 1985.

McLoughlin MG, Williams GM, Stonesifer GL: Ex vivo surgical dissection. JAMA 235:1705, 1976.

McQuitty DA, Boone TB, Preminger GM: Lower pole calicostomy for the management of iatrogenic ureteropelvic junction obstruction. J Urol 153:142, 1995.

Merkel FK, Straus AK, Andersen O, et al: Microvascular techniques for polar artery reconstruction in kidney transplants. Surgery 79:253, 1976.

Merklin RJ, Michels NA: The variant renal and suprarenal blood supply with data on the inferior phrenic, ureteral and gonadal arteries. J Int Coll Surg 29:41, 1958.

Milloy FJ, Anson BJ, Cauldwell EW: Variations in the inferior caval veins and in their renal and lumbar communications. Surg Gynecol Obstet 115:131, 1962.

Milsten R, Neifield J, Koontz WW: Extracorporeal renal surgery. J Urol 112:425, 1974.

Mitchell A, Morris PJ: Surgery for the spleen. Clin Haematol 12:565, 1983.

Morita T, Kondo S, Suzuki T, et al: Effect of calyceal resection on pelviureteral peristalsis in isolated pig kidney. J Urol 135:151, 1986.

Motola JA, Badlani GH, Smith AD: Results of 2 consecutive endopyelotomies: An 8-year followup. J Urol 149:453, 1993.

Murnaghan GF: The dynamics of the renal pelvis and ureter with reference to congenital hydronephrosis. Br J Urol 30:3, 1958.

Murnaghan GF: Mechanisms of congenital hydronephrosis with reference to factors influencing surgical treatment. Ann R Coll Surg Engl 23:25, 1958.

Murnaghan GF: Renal pelvis and ureter. *In* Wells C, Kyle J (eds): Scientific Foundations of Surgery. New York, Elsevier, 1967, p 280.

Nakada SY, McDougall EM, Clayman RV: Laparoscopic pyeloplasty for secondary ureteropelvic junction obstruction: Preliminary experience. Urology 46:257, 1995.

Namiki M, Shimoe S: Asymmetric fused kidney: A report of two cases and discussion on its classification. Acta Urol Jpn 24:1061, 1978.

Narath PA: The dynamics of the upper urinary tract. *In* Narath, PA: Renal Pelvis and Ureter. New York: Grune & Stratton, 1951, p 5.

Nesbit RM: Elliptical anastomosis in urologic surgery. Am Surg 130:796, 1949.

Nicol DL, P'ng K, Hardie DR, et al: Routine use of indwelling ureteral stents in renal transplantation. J Urol 150:1375, 1993.

Notley RG, Beaugle JM: The long-term follow-up of Anderson-Hynes pyeloplasty for hydronephrosis. Br J Urol 45:464, 1973.

Novick AC: Aortorenal bypass. *In* Novick AC, Streem SB, Pontes JE (eds): Stewart's Operative Urology, 2nd ed. Baltimore, Williams & Wilkins, 1989, p 250.

Novick AC: Extracorporeal renal surgery and autotransplantation. *In* Novick AC, Straffon RA (eds): Vascular Problems in Urologic Surgery. Philadelphia, WB Saunders, 1982, part 5, chap 20, p 305.

Novick AC: Partial nephrectomy for renal cell carcinoma. Urol Clin North Am 14:419, 1987.

Novick AC: Renal bench surgery. *In* Glenn J (ed): Urologic Surgery, 3rd ed. Philadelphia, JB Lippincott, 1983, p 137.

Novick AC: Renal hypothermia: In vivo and ex vivo. Urol Clin North Am 10:637, 1983.

Novick AC: Technique of renal transplantation. *In* Novick AC, Streem SB, Pontes JE (eds): Stewart's Operative Urology, 2nd ed. Baltimore, Williams & Wilkins, 1989, chap 32.

Novick AC, Cosgrove DM: Surgical approach for removal of renal cell carcinoma extending into the vena cava and the right atrium. J Urol 123:947, 1980.

Novick AC, Jackson CL, Straffon RA: The role of renal autotransplantation in complex urological reconstruction. J Urol 143:452, 1990.

Novick AC, Magnusson M, Braun WE: Multiple-artery renal transplantation: Emphasis on extracorporeal methods of donor arterial reconstruction. J Urol 122:731, 1979.

Novick AC, McElroy J: Renal revascularization by end-to-end anastomosis of the hepatic and renal arteries. J Urol 134:1089, 1985.

Novick AC, Stewart R: Use of the thoracic aorta for renal revascularization. J Urol 143:77, 1990.

Novick AC, Stewart BH, Straffon RA: Extracorporeal renal surgery and autotransplantation: Indications, techniques and results. J Urol 123:806, 1980.

Novick AC, Stewart BH, Straffon RA, Banowsky LH: Partial nephrectomy in the treatment of renal adenocarcinoma. J Urol 118:932, 1977.

Novick AC, Streem S, Montie JE, et al: Conservative surgery for renal cell carcinoma: A single-center experience with 100 patients. J Urol 141:835, 1989.

Novick AC, Ziegelbaum M, Vidt DG, et al: Trends in surgical revascularization for renal artery disease: Ten years' experience. JAMA 257:498, 1987.

Nylander WA Jr, Richie RE: Techniques of transplantation. *In*

Jacobson HR, Striker GE, Klahr S (eds): The Principles and Practice of Nephrology. Philadelphia, BC Decker, 1990.

Odiase V, Whitaker RH: Dynamic evaluation of the results of pyeloplasty using pressure-flow studies. Eur Urol 7:324, 1981.

Ohl DA, Konnak JW, Campbell DA, et al: Extravesical ureteroneocystostomy in renal transplantation. J Urol 139:499, 1988.

Olsson O, Wholey M: Vascular abnormalities in gross anomalies of kidneys. Acta Radiol (Diagn) 2:420, 1964.

O'Reilly PH: Open operation for ureteropelvic junction obstruction. *In* Webster G, Kirby R, King L, Goldwasser B (eds): Reconstructive Urology. Boston, Blackwell Scientific Publications, 1993, p 315.

Osathanondh V, Potter EL: Development of the human kidney as shown by microdissection (3 parts). Arch Pathol 76:271, 1963.

Ossandon F, Androulakakis P, Ransley PG: Surgical problems in pelviureteral junction obstruction of the lower moiety in incomplete duplex systems. J Urol 125:871, 1981.

Östling K: The genesis of hydronephrosis particularly with regard to the changes at the ureteropelvic junction. Acta Chir Scand 86(Suppl):72, 1942.

Özgök IY, Erduran D, Saglam R, et al: Intrarenal pressure following pyeloplasty or percutaneous surgery. Br J Urol 67:251, 1991.

Parker RM, Rudd RG, Wonderly RK, et al: Ureteropelvic junction obstruction in infants and children: Functional evaluation of the obstructed kidney preoperatively and postoperatively. J Urol 126:509, 1981.

Perlmutter AD, Kroovand RL, Lai Y-W: Management of ureteropelvic obstruction in the first year of life. J Urol 123:535, 1980.

Persky L, McDougal WS, Kedia K: Management of initial pyeloplasty failure. J Urol 125:695, 1981.

Peters CA, Schluessel RN, Retik AB: Pediatric laparoscopic dismembered pyeloplasty. J Urol 153:1962, 1995.

Peters PC, Bright TC III: Blunt renal injuries. Urol Clin North Am 4:17, 1977.

Pettersson S, Brynger H, Henriksson C, et al: Autologous renal transplantation with direct pyelocystostomy in the treatment of recurrent renal calculi. Br J Urol 55:154, 1983.

Pettersson S, Brynger H, Johansson S, Nilson AE: Extracorporeal surgery and autotransplantation for carcinoma of the pelvis and ureter. Scand J Urol Nephrol 13:89, 1979.

Pillet J, Cronier P: Observations on the development and migration of the human metanephros. Anat Clin 4:115, 1982.

Pitts WR Jr, Muecke EC: Horseshoe kidneys: A 40-year experience. J Urol 113:743, 1975.

Plaine LI, Hinman F Jr: Comparison of occlusion of the renal artery with occlusion of the entire pedicle on survival and serum creatinine levels of the rabbit. J Urol 93:117, 1965.

Pollak R, Veremis SA, Madux MS, Mozes MF: The natural history of and therapy for perirenal fluid collections following renal transplantation. J Urol 140:716, 1988.

Potter EL: Normal and Abnormal Development of the Kidney. Chicago, Year Book Medical Publishers, 1972.

Presti JC Jr, Carroll PR, McAninch JW: Ureteral and renal pelvic injuries from external trauma: Diagnosis and management. J Trauma 29:370, 1989.

Primack WA, Edelmann CM Jr: Technique of renal biopsy. *In* Edelmann CM Jr (ed): Pediatric Kidney Disease. Boston, Little, Brown & Co, 1978, p 262.

Provet JA, Hanna MK: Simultaneous repair of bilateral ureteropelvic junction obstruction. Urology 33:390, 1989.

Quinton W, Dillard D, Scribner BH: Cannulation of blood vessels for prolonged hemodialysis. Trans Am Soc Artif Intern Organs 6:104, 1960.

Rajfer J, Koyle MA, Ehrlich RM, Smith RB: Pyelovesicostomy as a form of urinary reconstruction in renal transplantation. J Urol 136:372, 1986.

Ramsay JWA, Miller RA, Kellett MJ, et al: Percutaneous pyelolysis: Indications, complications and results. Br J Urol 56:586, 1984.

Ranch T, Fall M, Henriksson C, et al: Urodynamic consequences of a direct pyelocystostomy at autotransplantation of the kidney. Urol Int 40:82, 1985.

Recker F, Subotic B, Goepel M, Tscholl R: Laparoscopic dismembered pyeloplasty: Preliminary report. J Urol 153:1601, 1995.

Reis RH, Esenther G: Variations in the pattern of renal vessels and their relation to the type of posterior vena cava in man. Am J Anat 104:295, 1959.

Rickwood AM, Phadke D: Pyeloplasty in infants and children with particular reference to the method of drainage postoperatively. Br J Urol 50:7, 1978.

Ritchie E, Reisman EM, Zaontz MR, et al: Use of kidney internal splint/stent (KISS) catheter in urinary diversion after pyeloplasty. Urology 42:55, 1993.

Roberts SD, Resnick MI: Complications of surgery for removal of renal and ureteral stones. In Marshall FF (ed): Urologic Complications. Chicago, Year Book Medical Publishers, 1986, p 143.

Robson WJ, Rudy SM, Johnston JH: Pelviureteric obstruction in infancy. J Pediatr Surg 11:57, 1976.

Rodman JS, Williams JJ, Peterson CM: Dissolution of uric acid calculi. J Urol 131:1039, 1984.

Rosenthal JT: Complications of renal transplantation and autotransplantation. In Smith RB, Ehrlich RM (eds): Complications of Urologic Surgery: Prevention and Management. Philadelphia, WB Saunders, 1990, p 231.

Rosenthal JT, Peaster ML, Laub D: The challenge of kidney transplant nephrectomy. J Urol 149:1395, 1993.

Ross G Jr: Fistula and obstruction following renal transplantation. In Resnick MI, Kursh E (eds): Current Therapy in Genitourinary Surgery. Toronto, BC Decker, 1987, p 419.

Roth RA: Residual stones. In Roth RA, Finlayson B (eds): Stones: Clinical Management of Urolithiasis. Baltimore, Williams & Wilkins, 1983, p 422.

Ruiz R, Novick AC, Braun WE, et al: Transperitoneal live donor nephrectomy. J Urol 123:819, 1980.

Sagalowsky AI, Hinnant CW Jr: Nonvascular complications of renal transplantation. In Cohen MS, Resnick MI (eds): Reoperative Urology. Boston, Little, Brown & Co, 1995, p 19.

Salvatierra O, Amend W, Vincenti F, et al: 1500 renal transplants at one center: The evolution of a strategy for optimum success. Am J Surg 142:14, 1981.

Salvatierra O, Belzer FO: Pediatric cadaver kidneys: Their use in renal transplantation. Arch Surg 110:181, 1975.

Salvatierra O, Kountz SL, Belzer FO: Prevention of ureteral fistula after renal transplantation. J Urol 112:445, 1974.

Salvatierra O, Olcott C, Amend WJ, et al: Urological complications of renal transplantation can be prevented or controlled. J Urol 117:4, 1977.

Sampaio FJB, Mandarim-De Lacerda CA: Anatomic classification of the kidney collecting system for endourologic procedures. J Endourol 2:247, 1988.

Sandler CM, Toombs BD: Computed tomographic evaluation of blunt renal injuries. Radiology 141:461, 1981.

Sant GR, Blaivas JG, Meares EM: Hemiacidrin irrigation in the management of struvite calculi: Long-term results. J Urol 130:1048, 1983.

Scardino PL, Prince CL: Vertical flap ureteropelvioplasty: Preliminary report. South Med J 46:325, 1953.

Schiff M Jr, McGuire EJ, Weiss RM, Lytton B: Management of urinary fistulas after renal transplantation. J Urol 115:251, 1976.

Schreiner GE: Renal biopsy. In Strauss MB, Welt LG (eds): Diseases of the Kidney, 2nd ed. Boston, Little, Brown & Co, 1971, p 197.

Schuessler WW, Grune MT, Tecuanhuey LV, et al: Laparoscopic dismembered pyeloplasty. J Urol 150:1795, 1993.

Scott HW Jr, Cantrell JR, Bunce PL: The principle of aortic compression in the management of massive hemorrhage from the renal pedicle after nephrectomy. J Urol 69:26, 1953.

Sherwood T, Ruutu M, Chisholm GD: Renal angiography problems in live kidney donors. Br J Radiol 51:99, 1978.

Siegfried MS, Rochester D, Bernstein JR, Miller JW: Diagnosis of inferior vena cava anomalies by computerized tomography. Comput Radiol 7:119, 1983.

Silverman DE, Stamey TA: Management of infection stones: The Stanford experience. Medicine 62:44, 1983.

Simmons RL, Kjellstrand CM, Najarian JS: Kidney: Technique, complications, and results. In Najarian JS, Simmons RL (eds): Transplantation. Philadelphia, Lea & Febiger, 1972, p 449.

Singh M, Marshall V, Blandy J: The residual renal stone. Br J Urol 47:125, 1975.

Smart WR: An evaluation of the intubation ureterotomy with a description of surgical technique. J Urol 85:512, 1961.

Smith AD, Lange PH, Fraley EE: Percutaneous nephrostomy: New challenges and opportunities in endo-urology. J Urol 1:382, 1979.

Smith JM, Butler MR: Splinting in pyeloplasty. Urology 8:8, 1976.

Smith MJV, Boyce WH: Anatrophic nephrotomy and plastic calyrhaphy. J Urol 99:5, 1968.

Smith P, Roberts M, Whitaker RH, et al: Primary pelvic hydronephrosis in children: A retrospective study. Br J Urol 48:549, 1976.

Smith RB, Ehrlich RM: Complications of renal transplant surgery (including autotransplantation). In Smith RB, Skinner DG, (eds): Complications of Urologic Surgery: Prevention and Management. Philadelphia, WB Saunders, 1976, p 459.

Snyder HM III, Lebowitz RL, Colodny AH, et al: Ureteropelvic junction obstruction in children. Urol Clin North Am 7:273, 1980.

Spanos PK, Simmons RL, Buselmeier TJ, et al: Kidney transplantation from living related donors with multiple vessels. Am J Surg 125:554, 1973.

Starzl TE, Miller C, Broznick B, et al: An improved technique for multiple organ harvesting. Surg Gynecol Obstet 165:343, 1987.

Stephenson TP, Bauer S, Hargreave TB, Turner-Warwick R: The technique and results of pyelocalycotomy for staghorn calculi. Br J Urol 47:751, 1976.

Stewart BH: Autotransplantation for extensive ureteral disease. In Bergman H (ed): The Ureter, 2nd ed. New York, Springer-Verlag, 1981, p 449.

Stewart BH, Hewitt CB, Banowsky LHW: Management of extensively destroyed ureter: Special reference to renal autotransplantation. J Urol 115:257, 1976.

Streem SB, Bretan PN: Considerations in donor nephrectomy. In Droller MJ (ed): Surgical Management of Urologic Disease—an Anatomical Approach. St. Louis, Mosby–Year Book, 1992, chap 87.

Streem SB, Novick AC, Steinmuller DR, et al: Flank donor nephrectomy: Efficacy in the donor and recipient. J Urol 141:1099, 1989.

Sutherland DER, Simmons RL, Howard RJ, Najarian JS: Intracapsular technique of transplant nephrectomy. Surg Gynecol Obstet 146:950, 1978.

Tandon SC, Stewart RJ, Boston VE: Watertight pyeloplasty: A novel approach. Br J Urol 72:986, 1993.

Taylor RJ: Cadaveric kidney recovery. In Resnick MI, Kursh E (eds): Current Therapy in Genitourinary Surgery. Toronto, BC Decker, 1987, p 485.

Tenckhoff H, Schechter H: A bacteriologically safe peritoneal access device. Trans Am Soc Artif Intern Organs 14:181, 1968.

Thompson IM, Latourette H, Montie JE, Ross G Jr: Results of nonoperative management of blunt renal trauma. J Urol 118:522, 1977.

Toguri AG, Emtage JB, Jarzylo SV: Management of total ureteral loss after kidney transplantation. Can J Surg 26:498, 1983.

Turner-Warwick R, Wynne EJ, Ashken MH: The use of the omental pedicle graft in the repair and reconstruction of the urinary tract. Br J Surg 54:849, 1967.

Underbjerg PE, Munch JT, Taagehøj-Jensen F, Djurhuus JC: The functional outcome of Anderson-Hynes pyeloplasty for hydronephrosis. Scand J Urol Nephrol 21:213, 1987.

Usher FC: New technique for repairing incisional hernias with Marlex mesh. Am J Surg 138:740, 1979.

Uson AC, Cox LA, Lattimer JK: Hydronephrosis in infants and children: II. Surgical management and results. JAMA 205:327, 1968.

Vaughan ED Jr, Sosa ER: Renovascular hypertension: Treatment options. Houston, American Urological Association, AUA Update Series, vol VIII, lesson 36, pp 282-287, 1989.

Voesten HG, Slooff MJ, Hooykaas JA, et al: Safe removal of failed transplanted kidneys. Br J Surg 69:480, 1982.

Wagner M, Dieckmann KP, Rudiger K, et al: Rescue of renal transplants with distal ureteral complications by pyelo-pyelostomy. J Urol 151:578, 1994.

Wein AJ, Murphy JJ, Mulholland SG, et al: A conservative approach to the management of blunt renal trauma. J Urol 117:425, 1977.

Williams DI, Cromie WJ: Ring ureterostomy. Br J Urol 47:789, 1975.

Williams DI, Karlaftis CM: Hydronephrosis due to pelviureteric obstruction in the newborn. Br J Urol 38:138, 1969.

Witters G, Baert L: Secondary pyelo-pyelic anastomosis in renal transplant patients. Urology 36:183, 1990.

Woodruff MFA, Doig A, Donald KW, Nolan B: Renal autotransplantation. Lancet 1:433, 1966.

Yang SC, Park DS, Lee DH, et al: Retroperitoneal endoscopic live donor nephrectomy: Report of 3 cases. J Urol 153:1884, 1995.

Zaontz MR, Hatch DA, Firlit CF: Urological complication in pediatric renal transplantation: Management and prevention. J Urol 140:1123, 1988.

Zincke H, Kelalis PP, Culp OS: Ureteropelvic obstruction in children. Surg Gynecol Obstet 139:873, 1974.

Zingg ES, Futterlieb A: Nephroscopy in stone surgery. Br J Urol 52:33, 1980.

Ziolkowski M, Kurlej W, Klak A: Typology of the renal pelvices in human fetuses. Fol Morphol 47:153, 1988.

Audiovisual

Smith A: Endourologic Management of Pelvic Kidneys. Wilkes-Barre, PA, Karol Media, 1986 (15 minutes). AUA #919-1145.

KIDNEY: EXCISION

Allen JE, Brecher MJ, Karp MP, et al: Wilms' tumor treatment and results: A five-decade experience. J Surg Oncol 30:235, 1985.

Anson BJ, Cauldwell EW: Pararenal vascular system: Study of 425 anatomical specimens. Q Bull Northwest Univ Med Sch 21:320, 1947.

Anson BJ, Cauldwell EW, Pick JW, Beaton LE: The anatomy of the pararenal system of veins, with comments on the renal arteries. J Urol 60:714, 1948.

Anson BJ, Kurth LE: Common variations in the renal blood supply. Surg Gynecol Obstet 100:156, 1955.

Assimos DG, Boyce WH, Harrison LH, et al: The role of open stone surgery since extracorporeal shock wave lithotripsy. J Urol 142:263, 1989.

Assimos DG, Wrenn JJ, Harrison LH, et al: A comparison of anatrophic nephrolithotomy and percutaneous nephrolithotomy with and without extracorporeal shock wave lithotripsy for management of patients with staghorn calculi. J Urol 145:710, 1991.

Attwood S, Lang DM, Goiti J, Grant J: Venous bypass for surgical resection of renal carcinoma invading the vena cava: A new approach. Br J Urol 61:402, 1988.

Auvert J: La veine rénale gauche. Presse Méd 75:1405, 1967.

Baniel J, Bihrle R, Wahle GR, Foster RS: Splenic rupture during occlusion of the porta hepatis in resection of tumors with vena caval extension. J Urol 151:992, 1994.

Barbaric Z: Renal fascia in urinary tract disease. Radiology 117:17, 1976.

Beaton LE: The anatomy of the pararenal system of veins, with comments on the renal arteries. J Urol 60:714, 1948.

Belzer FO, Salvatierra O, Palubinskas A, Stoney RJ: Ex vivo renal artery reconstruction. Ann Surg 182:456, 1975.

Bennett BC, Selby R, Bahnson RR: Surgical resection for management of renal cancer with hepatic involvement. J Urol 154:972, 1995.

Bérard P, Pouyet M: Les voies d'évacuation veineuse du rein après ligature de la veine rénale gauche. Lyon Chir 64:781, 1968.

Bernstein SM, Koyle MA, Gittes RF: Partial nephrectomy, extracorporeal surgery, and autotransplantation for renal cell carcinoma. In Crawford ED, Das S (eds): Current Genitourinary Cancer Surgery. Philadelphia, Lea & Febiger, 1990, p 50.

Blackley SK, Ladaga L, Woolfitt RA, et al: Ex situ study of the effectiveness of enucleation in patients with renal cell carcinoma. J Urol 140:6, 1988.

Blaivas JG, Pais VM, Spellman RM: Chemolysis of residual stone fragments after extensive surgery for staghorn calculi. Urology 6:680, 1975.

Blandy J: Surgery of renal cast calculi. In Libertino JA, Zinman L (eds): Reconstructive Urologic Surgery. Baltimore, Williams & Wilkins, 1977, p 17.

Blandy JP, Tresidder GC: Extended pyelolithotomy for renal calculi. Br J Urol 39:121, 1967.

Blute ML, Kelalis PP, Offord KP, et al: Bilateral Wilms' tumor. J Urol 138:968, 1987.

Boyce WH: Surgery of urinary calculi in perspective. Urol Clin North Am 10:585, 1983.

Boyce WH, Elkins IB: Reconstructive renal surgery following anatrophic nephrolithotomy. J Urol 111:307, 1974.

Boyce WH, Harrison LH: Complications of renal stone surgery. In Smith RB, Skinner DG (eds): Complications of Urologic Surgery: Prevention and Management. Philadelphia, WB Saunders, 1976, p 87.

Bredael JJ, Carson CC III, Weinerth JL: Bilateral nephrectomy by the posterior approach. Eur Urol 6:251, 1980.

Brödel M: The intrinsic blood vessels of the kidney and their significance in nephrotomy. Johns Hopkins Hosp Bull 12:10, 1901.

Broecker BH, Perlmutter AD: Management of unresectable Wilms' tumor. Urology 24:170, 1984.

Brynger H, Claes G, Gelin LE, et al: Extracorporeal resection for parenchymatous renal tumours. Scand J Urol Nephrol 15(Suppl 60):27, 1981.

Buntain WL, Lynn HB: Splenorrhaphy: Changing concepts for traumatized spleen. Surgery 86:748, 1979.

Butarazzi PJ, Devine PC, Devine CJ, et al: The indications, complications, and results of partial nephrectomy. J Urol 99:376, 1968.

Campbell SC, Novick AC, Streem SB, et al: Complications of nephron sparing surgery for renal tumors. J Urol 151:1177, 1994.

Capelouto CC, Moore RG, Silverman SG, Kavoussi LR: Retroperitoneoscopy: Anatomical rationale for direct retroperitoneal access. J Urol 152:2008, 1994.

Chopp RI, Shah BB, Addonaio JC: Use of ultrasonic aspirator in renal surgery. Urology 22:157, 1983.

Chute R, Soutter L, Kerr WS: The value of the thoracoabdominal incision in the removal of kidney tumors. N Engl J Med 241:951, 1949.

Clayman RV, Garske GL, Lange PH: Total nephroureterectomy with ureteral intussusception and transurethral ureteral detachment and pull-through. Urology 21:482, 1983.

Clayman RV, Gonzalez R, Fraley EE: Renal cell carcinoma invading the inferior vena cava: Clinical review and anatomical approach. J Urol 123:157, 1980.

Clayman RV, Kavoussi LR, McDougall EM, et al: Laparoscopic nephrectomy: A review of 16 cases. Surg Laparosc Endosc 2:29, 1992.

Clayman RV, Kavoussi LR, Soper NJ, et al: Laparoscopic nephrectomy. N Engl J Med 324:1370, 1991.

Clayman RV, Preminger GM, Frankline JR, et al: Percutaneous ureterolithotomy. J Urol 133:671, 1985.

Clayman RV, Sheldon CA, Gonzalez R: Wilms tumor: An approach to vena caval intrusion. Prog Pediatr Surg 15:285, 1982.

Cole AT, Fried FA: Experience with the thoraco-abdominal incision for nephroblastoma in children less than 3 years old. J Urol 114:114, 1975.

Cook JH III, Lytton B: Intraoperative localization of renal calculi during nephrolithotomy by ultrasound scanning. J Urol 117:546, 1979.

Cooper CS, Cohen MB, Donovan JF Jr: Splenectomy complicating left nephrectomy. J Urol 155:30, 1996.

Craven WM, Redmond PL, Kumpe DA, et al: Planned delayed nephrectomy after ethanol embolization of renal carcinoma. J Urol 146:704, 1991.

Crissey MM, Gittes RF: Dissolution of cystine ureteral calculus by irrigation with tromethamine. J Urol 121:811, 1979.

Culp OS: Anterior nephroureterectomy: Advantages and limitations of a single incision. J Urol 85:193, 1961.

Cummings KB: Nephroureterectomy: Rationale in the management of transitional cell carcinoma of the upper urinary tract. Urol Clin North Am 7:569, 1980.

Cummings KB: Surgical management of renal cell carcinoma with vena caval extension. *In* Crawford ED, Das S (eds): Current Genitourinary Cancer Surgery. Philadelphia, Lea & Febiger, 1990, p 69.

Cummings KB, Li W-I, Ryan JA, et al: Intraoperative management of renal cell carcinoma with supradiaphragmatic caval extension. J Urol 122:829, 1979.

D'Angio GJ, Evans A, Breslow N, et al: The treatment of Wilms' tumor: Results of the Second National Wilms' Tumor Study. Cancer 47:2302, 1981.

Das S: Radical nephrectomy: Thoracoabdominal intrapleural approach. *In* Crawford ED, Borden TA (eds): Genitourinary Cancer Surgery. Philadelphia, Lea & Febiger, 1982, p 30.

Daseler EH, Anson BJ: Anatomical relations of ectopic iliolumbar kidneys, bilateral in adult and unilateral in fetus. J Urol 49:789, 1943.

David IB, Diehl JT, Benak A, et al: Resection of retrohepatic inferior vena caval tumours: A new technique using the Biomedicus pump. Can J Surg 31:219, 1988.

Davis RA, Milloy FJ Jr, Anson BJ: Lumbar, renal and associated parietal and visceral veins based upon a study of 100 specimens. Surg Gynecol Obstet 107:122, 1958.

Dees JF: The use of an intraoperative coagulum in pyelolithotomy: A preliminary report. South Med J 49:497, 1943.

DeKernion JB: Lymphadenectomy for renal cell carcinoma: Therapeutic implications. Urol Clin North Am 7:697, 1980.

DeKernion JB: Radical nephrectomy. *In* Ehrlich RM (ed): Modern Techniques in Surgery (Urologic Surgery). Mt. Kisco, NY, Futura Publishing, 1980.

Donohue RE: Radical nephroureterectomy for carcinoma of the renal pelvis and ureter. *In* Crawford ED, Das S (eds): Current Genitourinary Cancer Surgery. Philadelphia, Lea & Febiger, 1990, p 88.

Dretler SP, Pfister RC, Newhouse JH: Renal stone dissolution via percutaneous nephrostomy. N Engl J Med 300:341, 1979.

Duckett JW: Neuroblastoma. *In* Glenn JF (ed): Urologic Surgery, 3rd ed. Philadelphia, JB Lippincott, 1983, p 55.

Duckett JW, Lifland JJ, Peters PC: Resection of the vena cava for adjacent malignant disease. Surg Gynecol Obstet 136:711, 1973.

Eden CG: Operative retroperitoneoscopy. Br J Urol 76:125, 1995.

Edwards EA: The anatomy of collateral circulation. Surg Gynecol Obstet 107:183, 1958.

Edwards EA: Clinical anatomy of lesser variations of the inferior vena cava and a proposal for classifying the anomalies of this vessel. Angiology 2:85, 1951.

Ehrlich RM, Gershman A, Fuchs G: Laparoscopic renal surgery in children. J Urol 151:735, 1994.

Ehrlich RM, Goodwin WE: The surgical treatment of nephroblastoma (Wilms' tumor). Cancer 32:1145, 1973.

Elder JS, Hladky D, Selzman AA: Outpatient nephrectomy for nonfunctioning kidneys. J Urol 154:712, 1995.

Erlich RM, Shanberg AM, Asch MJ, et al: Bilateral Wilms' tumor. J Urol 136:308, 1986.

Feldman RA, Shearer JK, Shield DE, et al: Sensitive method for intraoperative roentgenograms. Urology 9:695, 1977.

Feller I, Woodburne RT: Surgical anatomy of the abdominal aorta. Ann Surg 154 (Suppl):239, 1961.

Figenshau RS, Clayman RV, Kerbl K, et al: Laparoscopic nephroureterectomy in the child: Initial case report. J Urol 151:740, 1994.

Fine H, Keen EN: The arteries of the human kidney. J Anat 100:881, 1966.

Foster RS, Mahomed Y, Bihrle R, Strup S: Use of a caval-atrial shunt for resection of a caval tumor thrombus in renal cell carcinoma. J Urol 140:1370, 1988.

Fowler JE Jr: Bacteriology of branched renal calculi and accompanying urinary tract infection. J Urol 131:213, 1984.

Friedland GW, deVries PA, Nino-Murcia M, et al: Congenital anomalies of the inferior vena cava: Embryogenesis and MR features. Urol Radiol 13:237, 1992.

Gaur DD: Laparoscopic operative retroperitoneoscopy: Use of a new device. J Urol 148:1137, 1992.

Gaur DD: Retroperitoneal laparoscopy: A simple technique of balloon insertion and establishment of the primary port. Br J Urol 77:458, 1996.

Gaur DD, Agarwal DK, Khochikar MV, Purohit KC: Laparoscopic renal biopsy via retroperitoneal approach. J Urol 151:925, 1994.

Gaur DD, Agarwal DK, Purohit KC: Retroperitoneal laparoscopic nephrectomy: Initial case report. J Urol 149:103, 1993.

Gaur DD, Agarwal DK, Purohit KC: Retroperitoneal laparoscopic varicocelectomy. J Urol 151:825, 1994.

Gaur DD, Agarwal DK, Purohit KC, Darshane AS: Retroperitoneal laparoscopic pyelolithotomy. J Urol 151:927, 1994.

Gaur DD, Agarwal DK, Purohit KC, et al: Retroperitoneal laparoscopic ureterolithotomy for multiple upper mid ureteral calculi. J Urol 151:1001, 1994.

Gelin LE, Claes G, Gustafsson A, Storm B: Total bloodlessness for extracorporeal organ repair. Rev Surg 28:305, 1971.

Gibbons RP, Correa RJ Jr, Cummings KB, Mason JT: Surgical management of renal lesions using in situ hypothermia and ischemia. J Urol 115:12, 1976.

Gill IS, Kavoussi LR, Clayman RV, et al: Complications of laparoscopic nephrectomy in 185 patients: A multi-institutional review. J Urol 154:479, 1995.

Gill IS, McClennan BL, Kerbl K, et al: Adrenal involvement from renal carcinoma: Predictive value of computerized tomography. J Urol 152:1082, 1994.

Gill IS, Munch LC, Clayman RV, et al: A new renal tourniquet for open and laparoscopic partial nephrectomy. J Urol 154:1113, 1995.

Gil-Vernet JM: New surgical concepts in removing renal calculi. Urol Int 20:255, 1965.

Gil-Vernet JM, Caralps A, Revert I, et al: Extracorporeal renal surgery. Urology 5:444, 1975.

Giordano JM, Trout HH III: Anomalies of the inferior vena cava. J Vasc Surg 3:924, 1986.

Gittes RF: Management of transitional cell carcinoma of the upper tract: Case for conservative local excision. Urol Clin North Am 7:559, 1980.

Gittes RF: Partial nephrectomy and bench surgery: Techniques and applications. *In* Libertino R, Zinman L (eds): Reconstructive Urologic Surgery: Pediatric and Adult. Baltimore, Williams & Wilkins, 1977, p 45.

Gittes RF, McCullough DL: Bench surgery for tumor in a solitary kidney. J Urol 113:12, 1975.

Glazer AA, Novick AC: Long-term follow-up after surgical treatment for renal cell carcinoma extending into the right atrium. J Urol 155:448, 1996.

Gohji K, Kamidono S, Yamanaka N: Renal carcinoma in a solitary kidney. Br J Urol 66:248, 1990.

Goldfarb DA, Novick AC, Lorig R, et al: Magnetic resonance imaging for assessment of vena caval tumor thrombi: A comparative study with venacavography and computerized tomography scanning. J Urol 144:1100, 1990.

Goldwasser B, Carson CC, Shalaby NF, et al: Kidney tourniquet: A new instrument for regional blood control in partial nephrectomy. Urology 30:162, 1987.

Gordon MR, Carrion HM, Politano VA: Dissolution of uric acid calculi with THAM irrigation. Urology 12:393, 1978.

Graham SD Jr, Glenn JF: Enucleative surgery for renal malignancy. J Urol 122:546, 1979.

Graves FT: The anatomy of the intra-renal arteries in health and disease. Br J Surg 43:605, 1956.

Graves FT: The aberrant renal artery. J Anat 90:553, 1956.

Graves FT: The anatomy of the intrarenal arteries and its application to segmental resection of the kidney. Br J Surg 43:132, 1954.

Graves FT: Renal hypothermia: An aid to partial nephrectomy. Br J Surg 50:362, 1963.

Gschwend JE, Vogel U, Bader C, et al: Predictive value of magnetic resonance imaging and computerized tomography for conservative renal surgery in an ex vivo tumor enucleation study followed by step-sectioning. J Urol 155:451, 1996.

Harris DD, Ruckle HC, Gaskill DM, et al: Intraoperative ultrasound: Determination of the presence and extent of vena caval tumor thrombus. Urology 44:189, 1994.

Hegedüs V: Arterial anatomy of the kidney: A three dimensional angiographic investigation. Acta Radiol Diagn 12:604, 1972.

Hellstrom J: Some observations on removal of kidney stones particularly by means of pyelolithotomy in situ. Acta Clin Scand 98:442, 1949.

Heppe RK, Crawford ED: Radical nephrectomy: Thoracoabdominal intrapleural approach. In Crawford ED, Das S (eds): Current Genitourinary Cancer Surgery. Philadelphia, Lea & Febiger, 1990, p 39.

Heynes CF, van Gelderen WFC: 3-dimensional imaging of the pelviocaliceal system by computerized tomographic reconstruction. J Urol 144:1335, 1990.

Hinman F Jr: Ballottement of peripelvic cyst for operative diagnosis and localization. J Urol 97:7, 1967.

Hinman F Jr, Cattolica EV: Branched calculi: Shapes and operative approaches. J Urol 126:291, 1981.

Hodges CV, Lawson RK, Pearse HD, Stranburg CO: Autotransplantation of the kidney. J Urol 110:20, 1973.

Hoeltl W, Hruby W, Aharinejad S: Renal vein anatomy and its implications for retroperitoneal surgery. J Urol 143:1108, 1990.

Howard FS, Hinman F Jr: The ureteral splint in the repair of ureteropelvic avulsion. J Urol 68:916, 1952.

Hurwitz RS: Easy method of upper-pole heminephrectomy in duplex systems in children. Urol Clin North Am 17:115, 1990.

Hussmann DA, Ewalt DH, Glenski WJ, Bernier PA: Ureterocele associated with ureteral duplication of a nonfunctioning upper pole segment: Management by partial nephroureterectomy alone. J Urol 154:723, 1995.

Jacobs SC: Role of conservative surgery for patients with bilateral kidney tumors. In Catalona WJ, Ratliff TL (eds): Urologic Oncology. Boston, Martinus Nijhoff, 1984, p 139.

Janetschek G, Reissigl A, Peschel R, et al: Laparoscopic nephroureterectomy. Br J Urol 72:987, 1993.

Janosko EO, Powell CS, Spence PA, et al: Surgical management of renal cell carcinoma with extensive intracaval involvement using a venous bypass system suitable for rapid conversion to total cardiopulmonary bypass. J Urol 145:555, 1991.

Jordan GH, Winslow BH: Laparoendoscopic upper pole partial nephrectomy with ureterectomy. J Urol 150:940, 1993.

Kane CJ, Bolton DM, Stoller ML: Current indications for open stone surgery in an endourology center. Urology 45:218, 1995.

Kark RM: Renal biopsy. JAMA 105:220, 1968.

Kavoussi LR, Clayman RV: Laparoscopic renal surgery: Nephrectomy, nephroureterectomy and ureterolysis. In Gomella LG, Kozminski M, Winfield HN (eds): Laparoscopic Urologic Surgery. New York, Raven Press, 1994, p 151.

Kavoussi LR, Kerbl K, Capelouto CC, et al: Laparoscopic nephrectomy for renal neoplasms. Urology 42:603, 1993.

Kearney GP, Waters WB, Klein LA, et al: Results of inferior vena cava resection for renal cell carcinoma. J Urol 125:769, 1981.

Kelalis PP: Wilms' tumor. J Urol 135:989, 1986.

Kerbl K, Clayman RV, McDougall EM, Kavoussi LR: Laparoscopic nephrectomy: The Washington University experience. Br J Urol 73:231, 1994.

Klimberg I, Sirois R, Wajsman Z, Baker J: Intraoperative autotransfusion in urologic oncology. Arch Surg 121:1326, 1986.

Kolln CP, Boldus RA, Brandon NK, Flocks RH: Bilateral partial nephrectomy for bilateral renal cell carcinoma. J Urol 105:45, 1971.

Koo AS, Koyle MA, Hurwitz RS, et al: Necessity of contralateral exploration in Wilms tumor with modern noninvasive imaging technique: Reassessment. J Urol 144:416, 1990.

Koontz WW: The difficult nephrectomy. J Urol 110:16, 1973.

Koontz WW: Nephrectomy and the difficult nephrectomy. In Ehrlich RM (ed): Modern Techniques in Surgery (Urologic Surgery). Mt. Kisco, NY, Futura Publishing, 1981.

Koop CE, Schnaufer L: The management of abdominal neuroblastoma. Cancer 35:905, 1975.

Koyle MA, Ehrlich RM: Wilms tumor in neonates and young infants: Current considerations and controversies. In King LR (ed): Urologic Surgery in Neonates and Young Infants. Philadelphia, WB Saunders, 1988, p 429.

Krane RJ, deVere White R, Davis Z, et al: Removal of renal cell carcinoma extending into the right atrium using cardiopulmonary bypass, profound hypothermia and circulatory arrest. J Urol 131:945, 1984.

Kusunoki T: Partial nephrectomy. Urol Int 1:243, 1955.

Lawson RK: Extracorporeal renal surgery. J Urol 123:301, 1980.

Lawson RK, Hodges CV: Extracorporeal renal artery repair and autotransplantation. Urology 4:532, 1974.

Lawson RK, Hodges CV, Pitre TM: Nephrectomy, microvascular repair and autotransplantation. Surg Forum 23:539, 1972.

Leape LL, Breslow NE, Bishop HC: The surgical management of Wilms' tumor. Am Surg 187:351, 1978.

Leibovitch I, Raviv G, Mor Y, et al: Reconsidering the necessity of ipsilateral adrenalectomy during radical nephrectomy for renal cell carcinoma. Urology 46:316, 1995.

Leinonen A, Suramo I, Paivansalo M, Kontturi M: Ultrasonography, computed tomography and arteriography in the evaluation of the local spreading of malignant renal neoplasm. Ann Clin Res 16(Suppl 40):27, 1984.

Lytton B: Surgery of the kidney. In Harrison JH, Gittes RF, Perlmutter AD, et al (eds): Campbell's Urology, 4th ed, vol 3. Philadelphia, WB Saunders, 1979, p 1993.

Maatman TJ, Montie JE: Complications of renal surgery. In Marshall FF (ed): Urologic Complications. Chicago, Year Book Medical Publishers, 1986, p 103.

MacCallum DB: The arterial blood supply of the mammalian kidney. Am J Anat 38:153, 1926.

Malloy TR, Schultz RE, Wein AJ, et al: Renal preservation using neodymium:YAG laser. Urology 27:99, 1986.

Marsh CL, Lange PH: Application of liver transplant and organ procurement techniques to difficult upper abdominal urological cases. J Urol 151:1652, 1994.

Marshall FF: Intraoperative localization of renal calculi. Urol Clin North Am 10:629, 1983.

Marshall FF, Dietrick DD, Baumgartner WA, Reitz BA: Surgical management of renal cell carcinoma with intracaval neoplastic extension above the hepatic veins. J Urol 139:1166, 1988.

Marshall FF, Reitz BA: Technique for removal of renal cell carcinoma with suprahepatic vena caval tumor thrombus. Urol Clin North Am 13:551, 1986.

Marshall FF, Reitz BA, Diamond DA: A new technique for management of renal cell carcinoma involving the right atrium: Hypothermia and cardiac arrest. J Urol 131:103, 1984.

Marshall FF, Walsh PC: In situ management of renal tumors: Renal cell carcinoma and transitional cell carcinoma. J Urol 131:1045, 1984.

Marshall M Jr, Johnson SH III: A simple direct approach to the renal pedicle. J Urol 84:24, 1960.

Marshall VR, Singh M, Tresidder GC, Blandy JP: The place of partial nephrectomy in the management of renal calyceal calculi. Br J Urol 47:759, 1976.

Martin LW, Reyes PM Jr: An evaluation of 10 years experience with retroperitoneal lymph node dissection for Wilms' tumor. J Pediatr Surg 4:683, 1969.

Martin LW, Schaffner DP, Cox JA, et al: Retroperitoneal lymph node dissection for Wilms' tumor. J Pediatr Surg 14:704, 1979.

Masaki Z, Iguchi A, Kinoshita N, et al: Intrasinusal pyelolithotomy with lower pole nephrotomy for removal of renal stones. Urology 26:461, 1985.

McCullough DL, Gittes RF: Vena cava resection for renal cell carcinoma. J Urol 112:162, 1974.

McDougall EM, Clayman RV, Chandhoke PS, et al: Laparoscopic partial nephrectomy in the pig model. J Urol 149:1663, 1993.

McDougall EM, Clayman RV, Elashry O: Laparoscopic nephroureterectomy for upper tract transitional cell cancer: The Washington University experience. J Urol 154:975, 1995.

McLoughlin MG, Williams GM, Stonesifer GL: Ex vivo surgical dissection. JAMA 235:1705, 1976.

Merklin RJ, Michels NA: The variant renal and suprarenal blood supply with data on the inferior phrenic, ureteral and gonadal arteries. J Int Coll Surg 29:41, 1958.

Mesrobian H-GJ: Experience with a novel approach to upper-pole nephrectomy and partial ureterectomy. Pediatr Surg Int 9:150, 1994.

Mesrobian H-GJ: Wilms' tumor: Past, present and future. J Urol 140:231, 1988.

Middleton RG, Presto AJ III: Radical thoracoabdominal nephrectomy for renal cell carcinoma. J Urol 110:36, 1973.

Milsten R, Neifield J, Koontz WW: Extracorporeal renal surgery. J Urol 112:425, 1974.

Montie JE, Jackson CL, Cosgrove DM, et al: Resection of large inferior vena caval thrombi from renal cell carcinoma with the use of circulatory arrest. J Urol 139:25, 1987.

Mor Y, Goldwasser B, Ben-Chaim J, et al: Upper pole hemi-nephrectomy for duplex systems in children: A modified technical approach. Br J Urol 73:584, 1994.

Morita T, Kondo S, Suzuki T, et al: Effect of calyceal resection on pelviureteral peristalsis in isolated pig kidney. J Urol 135:151, 1986.

Mosnier H, Frantz P, Calmat A, et al: A study of the anastomoses between the left renal vein and the intravertebral plexuses. Anat Clin 1:321, 1980.

Mulvaney WP: The clinical use of Renacidin in urinary calcifications. J Urol 84:206, 1960.

Murnaghan GF: Surgical exposure of the kidney. *In* McDougal WS (ed): Rob and Smith's Operative Surgery: Urology, 4th ed. St. Louis, CV Mosby, 1983, p 21.

Murphy JJ, Glantz W, Schoenberg HW: The healing of renal wounds: III. A comparison of electrocoagulation and suture ligation for hemostasis in partial nephrectomy. J Urol 85:882, 1961.

Nativ O, Goldwasser B: Preservation of renal function in malignant disease of the kidney. *In* Webster G, Kirby R, King L, Goldwasser B (eds): Reconstructive Urology. Boston, Blackwell Scientific Publications, 1993, p 283.

Nemoy WJ: Renacidin in the treatment of infection stones. *In* Kaufman JJ (ed): Current Urologic Therapy. Philadelphia, WB Saunders, 1980, p 145.

Nicol DL, Winkle DC, Nathanson LK, Smithers BM: Laparoscopic nephrectomy for benign renal disease. Br J Urol 73:237, 1994.

Nishiyama T, Terunuma M: Laparoscopy-assisted radical nephrectomy in combination with minilaparotomy: Report of initial 7 cases. Int J Urol 2:124, 1995.

Novick AC: Extracorporeal renal surgery and autotransplantation. *In* Novick AC, Straffon RA (eds): Vascular Problems in Urologic Surgery. Philadelphia, WB Saunders, 1982, part 5, chap 20, p 305.

Novick AC: Partial nephrectomy for renal cell carcinoma. Urol Clin North Am 14:419, 1987.

Novick AC: Renal bench surgery. *In* Glenn J (ed): Urologic Surgery, 3rd ed. Philadelphia, JB Lippincott, 1983, p 137.

Novick AC: Renal hypothermia: In vivo and ex vivo. Urol Clin North Am 10:637, 1983.

Novick AC, Cosgrove DM: Surgical approach for removal of renal cell carcinoma extending into the vena cava and the right atrium. J Urol 123:947, 1980.

Novick AC, Jackson CL, Straffon RA: The role of renal autotransplantation in complex urological reconstruction. J Urol 143:452, 1990.

Novick AC, Stewart BH, Straffon RA: Extracorporeal renal surgery and autotransplantation: Indications, techniques and results. J Urol 123:806, 1980.

Novick AC, Stewart BH, Straffon RA, Banowsky LH: Partial nephrectomy in the treatment of renal adenocarcinoma. J Urol 118:932, 1977.

Novick AC, Straffon RA: Management of locally recurrent renal cell carcinoma after partial nephrectomy. J Urol 138:607, 1987.

Novick AC, Straffon RA, Stewart BH: Experience with extracorporeal renal operations and autotransplantation in the management of complicated urologic disorders. Surg Gynecol Obstet 153:10, 1981.

Novick AC, Streem S, Montie JE, et al: Conservative surgery for renal cell carcinoma: A single-center experience with 100 patients. J Urol 141:835, 1989.

Novick AC, Zincke H, Neves RJ, Topley MH: Surgical enucleation for renal cell carcinoma. J Urol 135:235, 1986.

O'Brien W, Lynch J: Adrenal metastases by renal cell carcinoma. Urology 19:605, 1987.

O'Conor VJ, Logan DJ: Nephroureterectomy. Surg Gynecol Obstet 122:601, 1966.

O'Donohoe MK, Flanagan F, Fitzpatrick JM, Smith JM: Surgical approach to inferior vena caval extension of renal carcinoma. Br J Urol 60:492, 1987.

Ono Y, Katoh N, Kinukawa T, et al: Laparoscopic nephrectomy, radical nephrectomy and adrenalectomy: Nagoya experience. J Urol 152:1962, 1994.

Ono Y, Ohshima S, Hirabayashi S, et al: Laparoscopic nephrectomy using a retroperitoneal approach: Comparison with a transabdominal approach. Int J Urol 2:12, 1995.

Oravisto KJ: Transverse partial nephrectomy. Acta Chir Scand 130:331, 1965.

Palou J, Caparros J, Orsola A, et al: Transurethral resection of the intramural ureter as the first step of nephroureterectomy. J Urol 154:43, 1995.

Parry WL, Finelli JF: Some considerations in the technique of partial nephrectomy. J Urol 82:562, 1959.

Patil U, Mathews R: Minimal surgery with renal preservation in anomalous complete duplicated systems: Is it feasible? J Urol 154:727, 1995.

Perez CA, Kaiman HA, Keith J, et al: Treatment of Wilms' tumor and factors affecting prognosis. Cancer 32:609, 1973.

Peters PC: Radical nephrectomy: Anterior transabdominal approach. *In* Crawford ED, Das S (eds): Current Genitourinary Cancer Surgery. Philadelphia, Lea & Febiger, 1990, p 45.

Pettersson S, Aamot P, Brynger H, et al: Extracorporeal renal surgery, autotransplantation and calicovesicostomy for renal pelvic and ureteric tumours. Scand J Urol Nephrol 15(Suppl 60):33, 1980.

Pettersson S, Brynger H, Henriksson C, et al: Treatment of urothelial tumors of the upper urinary tract by nephroureterectomy, renal autotransplantation and pyelocystostomy. Cancer 54:379, 1984.

Plaine LI, Hinman F Jr: Comparison of occlusion of the renal artery with occlusion of the entire pedicle on survival and serum creatinine levels of the rabbit. J Urol 93:117, 1965.

Plaine LI, Hinman F Jr: Malignancy in asymptomatic renal masses. J Urol 94:342, 1965.

Poutasse EF: Partial nephrectomy: New techniques, approach, operative indications, and review of 51 cases. J Urol 88:153, 1962.

Primack WA, Edelmann CM Jr: Technique of renal biopsy. *In* Edelmann CM Jr (ed): Pediatric Kidney Disease. Boston, Little, Brown & Co, 1978, p 262.

Pritchett TR, Raval JK, Benson RC, et al: Preoperative magnetic resonance imaging of vena caval tumor thrombi: Experience with 5 cases. J Urol 138:1220, 1987.

Rassweiler JJ, Henkel TO, Potempa DM, et al: The technique of transperitoneal laparoscopic nephrectomy, adrenalectomy, and nephroureterectomy. Eur Urol 23:425, 1993.

Reservitz GB: A historic review of nephroureterectomy. Surg Gynecol Obstet 125:853, 1967.

Retik AB, Peters CA: Ectopic ureter and ureterocele. *In* Walsh PC, Retik AB, Stamey TA, Vaughan ED (eds): Campbell's Urology, 6th ed, vol 2. Philadelphia, WB Saunders, 1992, p 1743.

Ritchey ML, Kelalis PP, Breslow N: Intracaval and atrial involvement with nephroblastoma: Review of National Wilms' Tumor Study-III. J Urol 140:1113, 1988.

Roberts SD, Resnick MI: Complications of surgery for removal of renal and ureteral stones. *In* Marshall FF (ed): Urologic Complications. Chicago, Year Book Medical Publishers, 1986, p 143.

Robey EL, Schellhammer PF: The adrenal gland and renal carcinoma: Is ipsilateral adrenalectomy a necessary component of radical nephrectomy? J Urol 135:453, 1986.

Robson CJ: Radical nephrectomy for renal cell carcinoma. J Urol 89:37, 1963.

Robson CJ, Churchill BM, Anderson W: The results of radical nephrectomy for renal cell carcinoma. Trans Am Assoc Genitourin Surg 60:122, 1968.

Rodman JS, Williams JJ, Peterson CM: Dissolution of uric acid calculi. J Urol 131:1039, 1984.

Ross JA, Samuel E, Millar DR: Variations in the renal vascular pedicle (an anatomical and radiological study with particular reference to renal transplantation). Br J Urol 33:478, 1961.

Roth RA: Residual stones. In Roth RA, Finlayson B (eds): Stones: Clinical Management of Urolithiasis. Baltimore, Williams & Wilkins, 1983, p 422.

Rubenstein SC, Hulbert JC, Pharand D, et al: Laparoscopic ablation of symptomatic renal cysts. J Urol 150:1103, 1993.

Sagalowsky AI: Indications and techniques for nephron sparing surgery. J Urol 154:1319, 1995. Editorial.

Sampaio FJB, Aragao AHM: Anatomical relationship between the intrarenal arteries and the kidney collecting system. J Urol 143:679, 1990.

Sampaio FJB, Mandarim-De Lacerda CA: Anatomic classification of the kidney collecting system for endourologic procedures. J Endourol 2:247, 1988.

Sant GR, Blaivas JG, Meares EM: Hemiacidrin irrigation in the management of struvite calculi: Long-term results. J Urol 130:1048, 1983.

Sawczuk I: Renal cell carcinoma: Local recurrence/splenic injury. J Urol 155:37, 1996. Editorial.

Schefft P, Novick AC, Straffon RA, Stewart BH: Surgery for renal cell carcinoma extending into the inferior vena cava. J Urol 120:28, 1977.

Schmeller NT, Hofstetter AG: Laser treatment of ureteral tumors. J Urol 141:840, 1989.

Scott HW Jr, Cantrell JR, Bunce PL: The principle of aortic compression in the management of massive hemorrhage from the renal pedicle after nephrectomy. J Urol 69:26, 1953.

Scott RF Jr, Selzman HM: Complications of nephrectomy: Review of 450 patients and a description of a modification of the transperitoneal approach. J Urol 95:307, 1966.

Semb C: Conservative renal surgery. J R Coll Surg Edinb 10:9, 1964.

Shalev M, Cipolla B, Guille F, et al: Is ipsilateral adrenalectomy a necessary component of radical nephrectomy? J Urol 153:1415, 1995.

Silverman DE, Stamey TA: Management of infection stones: The Stanford experience. Medicine 62:44, 1983.

Singh M, Marshall V, Blandy J: The residual renal stone. Br J Urol 47:125, 1975.

Skinner DG: Considerations for management of large retroperitoneal tumors: Use of the modified thoracoabdominal approach. J Urol 117:605, 1977.

Skinner DG, Colvin R, Vermillion CD: The surgical management of renal cell carcinoma. J Urol 107:705, 1972.

Skinner DG, Gloege GM: Technique of nephroureterectomy with regional node dissection. Urol Clin North Am 5:253, 1978.

Smith AD, Orihuela E, Crowley AR: Percutaneous management of renal pelvic tumors: A treatment option in selected cases. J Urol 137:852, 1987.

Smith MJV, Boyce WH: Anatrophic nephrotomy and plastic calyrhaphy. J Urol 99:521, 1968.

Smith RB: Surgical management of retroperitoneal tumors. In Crawford ED, Das S (eds): Current Genitourinary Cancer Surgery. Philadelphia, Lea & Febiger, 1990, p 140.

Snyder JA, Smith AD: Endourologic diagnosis and management of upper tract urothelial carcinoma. In Crawford ED, Das S (eds): Current Genitourinary Cancer Surgery. Philadelphia, Lea & Febiger, 1990, p 29.

Spencer WF, Novick AC, Montie JE, et al: Surgical treatment of localized renal cell carcinoma in von Hippel-Lindau disease. J Urol 140:129, 1988.

Squadrito JF Jr, Ellis DJ: Renal biopsy. In Gomella LG, Kozminski M, Winfield HN (eds): Laparoscopic Urologic Surgery. New York, Raven Press, 1994, p 175.

Stanley KE, Winfield HN, Donovan JF, Fallon B: Laparoscopic nephrectomy in crossed fused renal ectopia. Urology 42:375, 1993.

Stephenson TP, Bauer S, Hargreave TB, Turner-Warwick R: The technique and results of pyelocalycotomy for staghorn calculi. Br J Urol 47:751, 1976.

Stewart BH: Radical nephrectomy. In Stewart BH (ed): Operative Urology. Baltimore, Williams & Wilkins, 1975, p 114.

Stoller ML, Irby PB, Osman M, et al: Laparoscopic marsupialization of a simple renal cyst. J Urol 150:1486, 1993.

Storm FK, Kaufman JJ, Longmire WP: Kidney resection clamp: New instrument. Urology 6:494, 1975.

Straffon RA, Siegel DF: Saphenous vein bypass graft in the treatment of renovascular hypertension. Urol Clin North Am 2:337, 1975.

Streem SB, Pontes EJ: Percutaneous management of upper tract transitional cell carcinoma. J Urol 135:773, 1986.

Strong DW, Pearse HD, Tank ES Jr, Hodges CV: The ureteral stump after nephroureterectomy. J Urol 115:654, 1976.

Sullivan MJ, Joseph E, Taylor JC: Extracorporeal renal parenchymal surgery with continuous perfusion. JAMA 229:1780, 1974.

Sykes D: The arterial supply of the human kidney with special reference to accessory renal arteries. Br J Surg 50:368, 1963.

Sykes D: The morphology of renal lobulations and calices, and their relationship to partial nephrectomy. Br J Surg 51:294, 1964.

Tanguay S, Pisters LL, Lawrence DD, Dinney CPN: Therapy of locally recurrent renal cell carcinoma after nephrectomy. J Urol 155:26, 1996.

Thompson SD, Resnick MI: Stone surgery. In Cohen MS, Resnick MI (eds): Reoperative Urology. Boston, Little, Brown & Co, 1995, p 43.

Thüroff JW, Frohneberg D, Riedmiller R, et al: Localisation of segmental arteries in renal surgery by Doppler sonography. J Urol 127:863, 1982.

Treiger BFG, Humphrey LS, Peterson CV Jr, et al: Transesophageal echocardiography in renal cell carcinoma: An accurate diagnostic technique for intracaval neoplastic extension. J Urol 145:1138, 1991.

Vandeput JJ, Tanner JC, Eberhart C: Partial nephrectomy: Experimental closure with a free peritoneal graft. J Urol 93:364, 1967.

Vermootin V: Indications for conservative surgery in certain renal tumors: A study based on the growth pattern of the clear cell carcinoma. J Urol 64:200, 1950.

Wagget J, Koop CE: Wilms' tumor: Preoperative radiotherapy and chemotherapy in the management of massive tumors. Cancer 26:338, 1970.

Wald U, Caine M, Solomon H: Partial nephrectomy in surgical treatment of calculous disease. Urology 11:343, 1978.

Walther MM, Choyke PL, Hayes W, et al: Evaluation of color Doppler intraoperative ultrasound in parenchymal sparing renal surgery. J Urol 152:1984, 1994.

Ward JP, Smart CJ, O'Donoghue EPN, et al: Synchronous bilateral lumbotomy. Eur Urol 2:102, 1976.

Watts HG: Heminephrectomy: A simplified technique. Aust NZ J Surg 37:256, 1968.

Wein AJ, Carpiniello VL, Murphy JJ: A simple technique for partial nephrectomy. Surg Gynecol Obstet 146:620, 1978.

Wickham JEA: Conservative renal surgery for adenocarcinoma: Natural history and results of treatment. J Urol 119:722, 1978.

Wickham JEA: Conservative renal surgery for adenocarcinoma: The place of bench surgery. Br J Urol 47:25, 1975.

Williams DF, Schapiro AE, Arconti JS, et al: A new technique of partial nephrectomy. J Urol 97:955, 1967.

Winfield HN, Donovan JF, Lund GO, et al: Laparoscopic partial nephrectomy: Initial experience and comparison to the open surgical approach. J Urol 153:1409, 1995.

Winfield HN, Donovan JF Jr: Marsupialization of simple renal cysts. In Gomella LG, Kozminski M, Winfield HN (eds): Laparoscopic Urologic Surgery. New York, Raven Press, 1994, p 169.

Winfield HN, Donovan JF, Lund GO, et al: Laparoscopic partial nephrectomy: Initial experience and comparison to the open surgical approach. J Urol 153:1409, 1995.

Yang SC, Park DS, Lee DH, et al: Retroperitoneal live donor nephrectomy: Report of 3 cases. J Urol 153:1884, 1995.

Zingg ES, Futterlieb A: Nephroscopy in stone surgery. Br J Urol 52:333, 1980.

Audiovisuals

Clayman RV: Laparoscopic Nephrectomy. Wilkes-Barre, PA, Karol Media, 1991 (14 minutes). AUA #919-2062.

Kavoussi LR, Clayman RV, Figenshau RS, et al: Clinical Experience with Laparoscopic Nephrectomy. Wilkes-Barre, PA, Karol Media, 1992 (11 minutes). AUA #919-2007.

Marshall FF: Suprahepatic Renal Cell Carcinoma Tumor Thrombus: Surgical Management Utilizing Cardiopulmonary Bypass, Hypothermia, Temporary Cardiac Arrest. Wilkes-Barre, PA, Karol Media, 1985 (11 minutes). AUA #919-1134.

Marshall FF, Brooks JD, Schoenberg MP: Partial Nephrectomy: New Techniques. Wilkes-Barre, PA, Karol Media, 1994 (17 minutes). AUA #919-2027.

Marshall FF, Reitz B: The Management of Renal Cell Carcinoma with Suprahepatic Intracaval Neoplastic Extension. Wilkes-Barre, PA, Karol Media, 1990 (12 minutes). AUA #919-1161.

Menezes de Goes G: Anatrophic Nephrolithotomy with In Situ Renal Hypothermia. Wilkes-Barre, PA, Karol Media, 1981 (25 minutes). AUA #919-1102.

Niles BS, Smith AD: Techniques of Percutaneous Access to the Upper Tract. Wilkes-Barre, PA, Karol Media, 1995 (10 minutes). AUA #919-1150.

Novick AC: Partial Nephrectomy for Renal Cell Carcinoma. Wilkes-Barre, PA, Karol Media, 1995 (21 minutes). AUA #919-1146.

Rassweiler J, Henkel T, Stock C, et al: Retroperitoneoscopy—Technique and Indications. Wilkes-Barre, PA, Karol Media, 1995 (15 minutes). AUA #919-2059.

Rosenberg MT, Tutrone RF, Macleod S, et al: Laparoscopic Radical Nephrectomy. Wilkes-Barre, PA, Karol Media, 1993 (13 minutes). AUA #919-2015.

ADRENAL EXCISION

Aird I: Bilateral anterior transabdominal adrenalectomy. BMJ 2:708, 1955.

Angermeier KW, Montie JE: Perioperative complications of adrenal surgery. Urol Clin North Am 16:597, 1989.

Caty MG, Coran AG, Geagan M, Thompson NW: Current diagnosis and treatment of pheochromocytoma in children: Experience with 22 consecutive tumors in 14 patients. Arch Surg 125:978, 1990.

Chino ES, Thomas CG: An extended Kocher incision for bilateral adrenalectomy. Am J Surg 149:292, 1985.

Deoreo GA Jr, Stewart BH, Tarazi RC, Gifford RW: Preoperative blood transfusion in the safe surgical management of pheochromocytoma: A review of 46 cases. J Urol 111:715, 1974.

Donohue JP: Surgery of the adrenal gland. In Crawford ED, Das S (eds): Current Genitourinary Cancer Surgery. Philadelphia, Lea & Febiger, 1990, p 8.

Fonkalsrud EW: Adrenal pheochromocytoma in childhood. Progr Pediatr Surg 26:103, 1991.

Gil-Vernet J: New surgical concepts in removing renal calculi. Urol Int 20:255, 1965.

Gittes RF, Mahoney EM: Pheochromocytoma. Urol Clin North Am 4:239, 1977.

Gleason PE, Weinberger MH, Pratt JH, et al: Evaluation of diagnostic tests in the differential diagnosis of primary hyperaldosteronism: Unilateral adenoma versus bilateral micronodular hyperplasia. J Urol 150:1365, 1993.

Goldfein A: Pheochromocytoma: Diagnosis and anesthetic and surgical management. Anesthesiology 24:462, 1963.

Guazzoni G, Montorsi F, Bocciardi A, et al: Transperitoneal laparoscopic versus open adrenalectomy for benign hyperfunctioning adrenal tumors: A comparative study. J Urol 153:1597, 1995.

Hume DM: Pheochromocytoma in the adult and in the child. Am J Surg 99:458, 1960.

Hureau J, Hidden G, Thanh Minh TA: The vascularisation of the suprarenal glands. Anat Clin 2:127, 1980.

Jovenich JJ: Anesthesia in adrenal surgery. Urol Clin North Am 16:583, 1989.

Kaufman BH, Telander RL, van Heerden JA, et al: Pheochromocytoma in the pediatric age group: Current status. J Pediatr Surg 18:879, 1983.

Koyle MA: Neuroblastoma. In Vaughan ED Jr, Carey RM (eds): Adrenal Disorders. New York, Thieme Medical Publishers, 1989, p 275.

Libertino JA, Novick AC (eds): Adrenal surgery. Urol Clin North Am 16:417, 1989.

Mahoney EM, Crocker DW, Friend DG, et al: Adrenal and extraadrenal pheochromocytomas: Localization by vena cava: A sampling and observations on renal juxtaglomerular apparatus. J Urol 108:4, 1972.

Malone MJ, Libertino JA, Tsapatasaris NP, et al: Preoperative and surgical management of pheochromocytoma. Urol Clin North Am 16:567, 1989.

Nakada T, Kubota Y, Sasagawa I, et al: Therapeutic outcome of primary aldosteronism: Adrenalectomy versus enucleation of aldosterone-producing adenoma. J Urol 153:1775, 1995.

Novick AC, Straffon RA, Kaylor W: Posterior transthoracic approach for adrenal surgery. J Urol 141:254, 1989.

O'Neal LW: Surgery of the Adrenal Glands. St. Louis, CV Mosby, 1968.

Reckler JM, Vaughan ED Jr, Tjeuw M, Carey RM: Pheochromocytoma. In Vaughan ED Jr, Carey RM (eds): Adrenal Disorders. New York, Thieme Medical Publishers, 1989, p 259.

Revillon Y, Daher P, Jan D, et al: Pheochromocytoma in children: 15 cases. J Pediatr Surg 27:910, 1992.

Schlund JF, Kenney PJ, Brown ED, et al: Adrenocortical carcinoma: MR imaging appearance with current techniques. J MR Imaging 5:171, 1995.

Scott HW Jr: The pituitary and adrenals. In Sabiston DC Jr (ed): Textbook of Surgery: The Biological Basis of Modern Surgical Practice, 11th ed. Philadelphia, WB Saunders, 1977, p 776.

Scott HW Jr, Dean RH, Oates JA, et al: Surgical management of pheochromocytoma. Am Surg 47:6, 1981.

Shandling B, Wesson D, Filler RM: Recurrent pheochromocytoma in children. J Pediatr Surg 25:1063, 1990.

Shulkin BL, Wieland DM, Schwaiger M, et al: PET scanning with hydroxyephedrine: An approach to the localization of pheochromocytoma. J Nucl Med 33:1125, 1992.

Siragy HM, Vaughan ED Jr, Carey RM: Cushing's syndrome. In Vaughan ED Jr, Carey RM (eds): Adrenal Disorders. New York, Thieme Medical Publishers, 1989, p 147.

Suzuki K, Kageyama S, Ueda D, et al: Laparoscopic adrenalectomy: Clinical experience with 12 cases. J Urol 150:1099, 1993.

Vaughan ED Jr, Phillips H: Modified posterior approach for right adrenalectomy. Surg Gynecol Obstet 165:453, 1987.

Vaughan ED Jr, Carey RM: Adrenal carcinoma. In Vaughan ED Jr, Carey RM (eds): Adrenal Disorders. New York, Thieme Medical Publishers, 1989, p 231.

Whalen RK, Althausen AF, Daniels GH: Extra-adrenal pheochromocytoma. J Urol 147:1, 1992.

Young HH: A technique for simultaneous exposure and operation on the adrenals. Surg Gynecol Obstet 54:179, 1936.

Audiovisual

Cerny JC: Adrenalectomy via the Transabdominal Approach: A Differential Diagnosis of Cushing's Syndrome. Wilkes-Barre, PA, Karol Media, 1983 (15 minutes). AUA #919-1111.

Index

Note: Page numbers in *italics* refer to illustrations;
page numbers followed by t refer to tables.

ISBN 0-7216-6404-0